CONTENTS

Fourth Edition

COMMUNITY HEALTH NURSING
Caring for Populations

Fourth Edition

COMMUNITY HEALTH NURSING
Caring for Populations

MARY JO CLARK, PhD, RN

Associate Dean and Professor
Hahn School of Nursing and Health Science
University of San Diego
San Diego, California

Prentice
Hall

Upper Saddle River, New Jersey 07458

Library of Congress Cataloging-in-Publication Data

Clark, Mary Jo Dummer.
   Community health nursing : caring for populations / Mary Jo Clark.—4th ed.
     p. ; cm.
   Rev. ed. of: Nursing in the community. Stamford, Conn. : Appleton & Lange, c1999.
   Includes bibliographical references and index.
   ISBN 0-13-094149-2
   1. Community health nursing. I. Nursing in the community. II. Title.
   [DNLM: 1. Community Health Nursing. 2. Nursing Process. WY 106 C594ca 2003]
  RT98 .N88 2003
  610.73'43—dc21

2001058837

Publisher: Julie Levin Alexander
Executive Assistant: Regina Bruno
Executive Editor: Maura Connor
Acquisitions Editor: Nancy Anselment
Marketing Manager: Nicole Benson
Development Editor: Elisabeth Garofalo
Editorial Assistant: Sarah Caffrey
**Director of Manufacturing
  and Production:** Bruce Johnson
Managing Editor: Patrick Walsh
Production Editor: Linda Begley, Rainbow Graphics
Production Liaison: Cathy O'Connell
Manufacturing Buyer: Pat Brown
Design Director: Cheryl Asherman
Senior Design Coordinator: Maria Guglielmo
Cover/Interior Design: Donna Wickes
Cover/Interior Art: Don Bishop/Artville
Photographer: Al Dodge
Illustration Studio: ElectraGraphics
Media Editor: Sarah Hayday
Media Production Manager: Amy Peltier
Media Project Manager: Stephen Hartner
Composition: Rainbow Graphics
Printing and Binding: Von Hoffmann

Pearson Education LTD.
Pearson Education Australia PTY, Limited
Pearson Education Singapore, Pte. Ltd
Pearson Education North Asia Ltd
Pearson Education, Canada, Ltd
Pearson Educación de Mexico, S.A. de C.V.
Pearson Education—Japan
Pearson Education Malaysia, Pte. Ltd

Notice: Care has been taken to confirm the accuracy of information presented in this book. The authors, editors, and the publisher, however, cannot accept any responsibility for errors or omissions or for consequences from application of the information in this book and make no warranty, express or implied, with respect to its contents.

The authors and publisher have exerted every effort to ensure that drug selections and dosages set forth in this text are in accord with current recommendations and practice at time of publication. However, in view of ongoing research, changes in government regulations, and the constant flow of information relating to drug therapy and drug reactions, the reader is urged to check the package inserts of all drugs for any change in indications of dosage and for added warnings and precautions. This is particularly important when the recommended agent is a new and/or infrequently employed drug.

10 9 8 7 6 5 4 3 2

ISBN 0-13-094149-2

This book is lovingly dedicated to Phil the elder and Phil the younger, who motivate me to do the best I can, and to Elisabeth, who knows how to fight the important battles.
Thank you.

CONTENTS

viii   Contents

Unit II

Unit III

PROCESSES USED IN COMMUNITY HEALTH NURSING   207

Unit V

Unit VI

COMMON HEALTH PROBLEMS OF POPULATIONS   655

CHAPTER 28 ■ Communicable Diseases   657

CHAPTER 29 ■ Chronic Physical Health Problems   683

CHAPTER 30 ■ Community Mental Health Problems   711

CHAPTER 31 ■ Substance Abuse   729

PREFACE

This book represents the lessons learned and the progress made in more than 100 years of community health nursing in the United States. The year 1993 marked the 100th anniversary of the founding of the Henry Street Settlement, the acknowledged beginning of modern American community health nursing. Since then, the work of community health nurses has led to better health for individuals, families, and population groups. In this book, I have tried to distill the wisdom of early pioneers and present-day practitioners to guide and direct future generations of community health nurses.

Locally, nationally, and globally, society is in greater need of community health nursing services than at any time since our beginning. Although expected longevity has increased significantly in the last century, quality of life has not kept pace for large segments of the world's population. Previously controlled communicable diseases are resurfacing and new diseases are emerging to threaten the public's health. Malnutrition is a fact of life for many people. Chronic physical and emotional diseases are taking their toll on the lives of large numbers of people. Substance abuse and societal violence are rampant, and more and more frequently environmental conditions do not support health. All of these are problems that community health nurses can and do help to solve.

Community health nurses must have the depth and breadth of knowledge that allows them to work independently and in conjunction with others to improve the health of the world's populations. In part, this improvement occurs through care provided to individuals and families, but it must occur on a larger scale through care provided to communities and population groups. *Community Health Nursing: Caring for Populations* provides community health nurses with the knowledge needed to provide care at all these levels. This knowledge is theoretically and scientifically sound, yet practical and applicable to society's changing demands. This book has been written to give students a strong, balanced foundation for community health nursing.

Community Health Nursing: Caring for Populations is written for all students in community health nursing courses and provides a thorough introduction to all aspects of the specialty. The book is designed to prepare nurse generalists who can function in any setting, providing care to individuals, families, communities, and population groups.

Each unit in this fourth edition is introduced by the work of Veneta Masson. Her writing reflects some of the realities of day-to-day community health nursing practice. The following dialogue between nurse and client is excerpted from one of Ms. Masson's poems, "Christmas Eve at Maggie's," and portrays the sometimes differing perspectives of nurse and client. Throughout the text the poetry presents other intimate glimpses of individual clients and the profession for students to ponder.

Guess what today is Maggie.
  What is today? I prod
  tense with expectation
  as her fingers tighten
  round her empty wallet

Why, I reckon . . . Well, praise the Lord!
  It must be the first of the month
  and my check come!
  No, Maggie, it's Christmas Eve.
  I came to wish you Merry Christmas.
  Sorry.

She fumbles with the stale debris
  of yesterday's carry-out sandwich.
  That so? she says, wiping the wreath
  of crumbs from her mouth.
  And here I thought it was the first of the month.

The overall approach of this book is to convey to nursing students at the beginning of the twenty-first century the excitement and challenge of providing nursing care in the community. As we begin a new era of community health nursing, I believe that well-educated community health nurses can provide a focal point for resolution of the global health problems presented above. Early community health nurses changed the face of society, and we can be a strong force in molding the society of the future.

I am convinced that when the bicentennial anniversary of American community health nursing occurs in 2093, community health nurses will be able to look back on the accomplishments of our second century with as much pride as the first.

Organization

This textbook is designed to present general principles of community health nursing and to assist students to apply those principles in practice. It is organized in six units. The first three units address general concepts of community health nursing practice and the last three examine the application of those concepts to specific populations, settings, and community health problems.

Unit I sets the stage for practice by describing the context in which community health nursing occurs. Readers are introduced to the concept of populations as recipients of nursing care and to the historical underpinnings and development of community health nursing as an area of specialty practice. Other chapters in this unit address the influences of the health care, political, economic, sociocultural, and environmental contexts that influence the health of populations and the practice of community health nursing.

Unit II examines community health nursing as a specialized area of practice, exploring its population focus and the attributes and features that make it unique. Standards for practice and typical roles and functions of community health nurses are also addressed. The second chapter in this unit provides several theoretical perspectives on community health nursing and discusses theoretical models applicable to population groups, as well as individuals and families, as recipients of care.

A unique feature of this textbook is the consistent use of the Dimensions Model of Community Health Nursing to structure the discussion of principles of practice. In Units III through VI, elements of the model are used to examine the processes used in community health nursing practice and the provision of care to selected populations, in specialized settings, and with specific community health problems. A change from the previous edition is the elimination of some redundancy in the use of the model across chapters; however, the model remains as an organizing framework for the chapters in these units, systematizing assessment in terms of the six dimensions of health (addressing relevant biophysical, psychological, physical environmental, sociocultural, behavioral, and health systems considerations) and framing nursing interventions in terms of primary, secondary, and tertiary prevention activities. This consistent approach permits students to readily identify commonalities and differences among processes, populations, settings, and problems.

Unit III presents common processes used in community health nursing. In each chapter, the elements of the Dimensions Model are applied to a specific process used by community health nurses. For example, in Chapter 10, students are acquainted with general principles of epidemiol-ogy and then apply those principles in the context of the model to the process of health promotion for individuals, families, and groups of clients. Considerations in each of the six dimensions of health are examined in light of their influence on health promotion. Other processes examined in this unit include the health education, case management, and change, leadership, and group processes.

Unit IV examines community health nursing care provided to special population groups. In each chapter, students are assisted to apply principles of care to individuals and families, as well as to these populations as aggregates. For example, in Chapter 16, emphasis is placed on community health nursing care for individual children and their families as well as on strategies for improving the health of children as a population group. Similar approaches are taken to the other population groups addressed in the unit: families, communities, women, men, the elderly, and the homeless.

Unit V presents community health nursing practice in specialized settings such as the home, school, work, correctional, and disaster settings. Chapter 22, a new chapter in this edition examines the role of the community health nurse in official and voluntary agencies as specialized settings. The local health department is used as an exemplar of official agencies and parish or faith community nursing is the exemplar for community health nursing practice in a voluntary agency. In each of the chapters in the unit, students are guided in the use of the nursing process in the special practice setting. Consideration is given to factors influencing health in each of the six dimensions of health, and nursing interventions at the primary, secondary, and tertiary levels of prevention are discussed.

Unit VI focuses on community health nursing practice related to common population health problems such as communicable diseases, chronic physical and mental health conditions, substance abuse, and societal violence. Again, students are assisted to apply the nursing process to identify factors contributing to problems in each of these areas and in designing relevant nursing interventions at primary, secondary, and tertiary levels of prevention. Consideration is given to care of individuals and families with these problems as well as to resolving common community health problems at the population level.

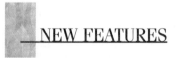

NEW FEATURES

- **New Chapter,** *"Care of Clients in Official and Voluntary Agencies,"* includes detailed discussion of parish nursing and its roles and functions as an exemplar of a voluntary health agency. Standards, functions, and services of community/public health nursing serve as a starting point for exploring an official health agency.
- **Cultural Considerations** highlight cultural factors that influence health, health care delivery, and community

health nursing practice. Readers are encouraged to examine the effects of their own cultural traditions, as well as those of clients, on health, illness, and nurse–client interactions.

- **Ethical Awareness** introduces readers to ethical dilemmas faced by community health nurses and assists them to apply principles of ethical decision making.
- **Healthy People 2010: Goals for the Population** provides a focus for health-related initiatives as well as a snapshot of the current state of health of the U.S. population.
- **Focus on Public Health Aspects of Terrorism** incorporates information related to the public health aspects of terrorism. For example, the concept of terrorism and types of terrorist activities and their health effects are introduced in the discussion of global health issues in Chapter 3. Chapter 10 incorporates information on the epidemiology of selected biological weapons. This information is expanded in Chapter 28 and Appendix B, both of which address control of communicable diseases. Finally, terrorist attacks as a form of disaster are addressed in Chapter 27.

HALLMARK FEATURES

Chapter Structure

Each chapter of *Community Health Nursing: Caring for Populations* includes:

- **Chapter objectives** that summarize important points and assist the reader in identifying key issues addressed in the chapter.
- **Key terms** that direct the reader's attention to critical issues addressed in the chapter.
- **Numerous tables and figures** that highlight important concepts and assist readers in their understanding.
- **Highlights** that summarize content and assist students to identify major points presented in the text.
- **Assessment Tips** that provide a series of questions to assist readers in tailoring their nursing assessment to the specific needs of the client population, setting, or health problem addressed in the chapter.
- **Critical Thinking in Research** boxes that stimulate readers to consider research related to chapter topics and to broaden their understanding of research principles and methods.
- **Case Studies** that assist the reader to apply the principles addressed in the chapter to community health nursing practice situations. Each case study is followed by questions designed to promote critical thinking in nursing practice.
- **Testing Your Understanding** is a feature that assists readers to evaluate their comprehension of concepts and principles presented in the chapter. These challenging review questions stimulate thought and discussion of important chapter concepts. Each question is followed by page references for a quick review of content addressed.
- **Think About It** poses thought-provoking questions to stimulate individual thought or class discussion on issues addressed in the chapter. These questions encourage the reader to go beyond the content presented and to examine related issues and application to their own areas of practice.
- **References** contained in each chapter present an up-to-date picture of principles and concepts related to the topic addressed. References provide a balanced view of community health nursing, exploring a variety of issues from several perspectives, and provide a wide range of supplemental material for the interested reader.
- **Full-color photographs** serve to bring home to readers the concepts discussed in the chapters while presenting a realistic picture of community health nursing practice.

Appendices

Several of the assessment tools contained in the Appendices of previous editions of the textbook, as well as additional tools previously contained in the *Community Health Nursing Handbook,* have been moved to the companion Web site for the fourth edition. This move was made to permit readers to download immediately usable assessment tools as desired. The remaining appendices present the reader with detailed information that supplements content in the chapters in the book.

COMPREHENSIVE TEACHING AND LEARNING PACKAGE

Companion Web Site

The companion Web site for the fourth edition of the textbook contains a variety of supplemental information and assessment tools that will be of immediate use to readers. The Web site includes the following new features:

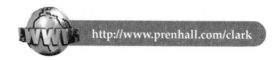

http://www.prenhall.com/clark

- **Chapter outlines:** Detailed chapter outlines assist readers to organize their learning of chapter content and to easily refer back to important portions of the chapter.
- **Chapter objectives:** Chapter objectives assist readers in identifying key concepts contained in each chapter.
- **Key terms:** A list of key terms and audio glossary from the text are included to assist students to grasp basic concepts of community health nursing.

- **Multiple-choice questions:** Multiple-choice review questions are provided for each chapter to assist readers to evaluate their comprehension of chapter content. Answers and rationale are provided for questions posed.

- **Challenge Your Knowledge:** The *Challenge Your Knowledge* feature presents readers with thought-provoking short essay questions that test and expand comprehension of important concepts presented in each chapter. These questions assist students in the application of principles of community health nursing in practice.

- **Expanding Your Perspective:** This feature presents summaries of full-text articles that assist readers to examine a topic in more depth or additional case studies that promote the application of theoretical principles to practice. Links to several full-text research articles are provided related to selected chapters in the text. These articles present research studies related to the content in relevant chapters. Each article summary is followed by questions that assist the reader to evaluate the study and the applicability of findings to community health nursing practice in their own locations.

  Case studies assist readers in applying principles presented in the chapter to actual community health nursing practice. Each case study is followed by questions to stimulate thought on the part of the reader; potential answers to these questions are provided.

- **Assessment tools:** Assessment tools provided on the Web site include those previously included in the appendices to the text as well as several additional tools from the *Community Health Nursing Handbook.* Some new assessment tools are included as well. Tools are based on a consistent assessment format and address considerations in each of the six dimensions of health (biophysical, psychological, physical environmental, sociocultural, behavioral, and health system) as they affect the health status of specific population groups or in specific settings.

- **Web links:** Web links are provided to additional sources of information related to chapter topics.

- **Information updates:** This feature provides periodic updates on information that changes more frequently than a textbook can be revised (for example, immunization schedules, new epidemiologic information for selected conditions). Updated incidence and prevalence maps for selected conditions are also included.

INSTRUCTOR'S RESOURCE CD-ROM

The *Instructor's Resource CD-ROM* includes the following features:

- **Detailed chapter outlines** that pinpoint the main issues discussed in each chapter.

- **Learning objectives** that provide instructors with student goals for each chapter.

- **Key terms** and definitions provided in the core text.

- **PowerPoint slides** for each chapter that can be used to structure class presentations.

- **Suggested teaching strategies** that actively involve students and help bring community health nursing practice to life.

- **Discussion topics** that will evoke active student participation in the classroom. The topics presented can also be used for out-of-class activities by students.

- **Answers to case study questions** presented in the text that allow for their use as examinations or for class discussion.

- **Test questions** in multiple-choice format that test students' grasp of content provided in each chapter. Answers and rationale are also provided.

- **Discussion guides** for the *Critical Thinking in Research, Cultural Considerations,* and *Ethical Awareness* features that allow faculty members to make the most effective use of these features to expand students' knowledge and understanding.

ACKNOWLEDGMENTS

I wish to extend a sincere thank you to the talented team involved in the fourth edition of this book:

- All of the **reviewers** who provided so many helpful comments. They are listed on page xix.

- **Nancy Anselment,** Acquisitions Editor, and **Elisabeth Garofalo,** Developmental Editor. Their dedication and commitment to excellence made this revision possible.

- **Sarah Caffrey,** Editorial Assistant, who always provided help when needed.

- **Patrick Walsh,** Managing Production Editor, **Marilyn Meserve,** Senior Managing Development Editor, and **Cathy O'Connell,** Senior Production Editor. Their guidance and expertise is revealed in the final product.

- **Yesenia Kopperman,** Assistant Editor, coordinated the Instructor's CD-ROM, and **Sarah Hayday,** Media Editor, led the way to bring the Companion Web site "live."

- **Cheryl Asherman,** Art and Design Manager, has created a visually appealing book.

- **Linda Begley** of Rainbow Graphics, who has carefully monitored this project throughout composition.

- **Bobby Starnes,** Art Director of Electragraphics, Inc. rendered the line drawings.

- **Al Dodge,** who provided most of the striking photographs for the book.

• **Sara Kolb** and her colleagues, who expended multiple roles of film to get the perfect parish nursing center picture.

Thank you for a highly educational experience!

Mary Jo Clark, RN, PhD

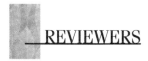

REVIEWERS

Jackie Birmingham, RN, BSN, MS
Adjunct Faculty
St. Joseph College
West Hartford, Connecticut

Mary Bittle, MA, RNC
Associate Clinical Professor
Texas Women's University College of Nursing
Dallas, Texas

Janet S. Brookman, DSN, RN
Clinical Assistant Professor
The University of Alabama in Huntsville
College of Nursing
Huntsville, Alabama

Dianne Jackson, MSN, RN
Clinical Instructor
University of Arizona College of Nursing
Tucson, Arizona

Dawna Martich, RN, BSN, MSN
Clinical Trainer
American Healthways
Pittsburgh, Pennsylvania

Dr. Victoria Rizzo Nikou, PhD, RN, CS
Assistant Professor
Pace University Lienhard School of Nursing
New York, New York

Janine Saulpaugh, RN, MS, WHNP
Lecturer, Assistant Professor
University of Arizona College of Nursing
Tucson, Arizona

Ann Tamule, RNC, MS, ANP
Assistant Professor of Nursing
Simmons College
Boston, Massachusetts

Elizabeth Johnston Taylor, PhD, RN
Associate Professor
Loma Linda University School of Nursing
Loma Linda, California

Donna Zazworsky, MS, RN, CCM
Adjunct Clinical Assistant Professor
University of Arizona
Tucson, Arizona

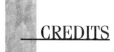

CREDITS

The poetry that introduces each unit in this textbook is from *Rehab at the Florida Avenue Grill* by Veneta Masson. Veneta is a community health nurse and nurse practitioner who brings the insights of compassion to her work with underserved populations in Washington, D.C. *Rehab at the Florida Avenue Grill* was published by Sage Femme Press in 1999, and is available from Window on Nursing, P.O. Box 1253, Olney, MD 20830-1253. Mary Jo Clark and Prentice Hall express our appreciation to the poet for her heartfelt expressions of nursing in the community and for her generosity in permitting us to reprint her work.

Historical photographs used in Chapter 2 were provided courtesy of the Visiting Nurse Association of Boston. Mt. Auburn Hospital provided great assistance with sites and locations for specific photographs. Other photographs are the work of Al Dodge of Boston, Sara Kolb of the St. Philip of Jesus Ministeria de Salud, San Antonio, Texas, and the author.

The ANA Standards for Public Health Nursing listed on pages 174–175 are reprinted with permission from the American Nurses Association, *Scope and Standards of Public Health Nursing Practice,* copyright 1999 American Nurses Association, 600 Maryland Avenue, SW, Suite 100 West, Washington, DC 20024-2571.

The standards for parish nursing practice presented on pages 529–530 are reprinted with permission from the Health Ministries Association and American Nurses Association, *Scope and Standards of Parish Nursing Practice,* copyright 1998 American Nurses Association, 600 Maryland Avenue, SW, Suite 100 West, Washington, DC 20024-2571.

Standards for school nursing practice are reprinted on page 540 with permission of the National Association of School Nurses from *Standards of Professional School Nursing Practice,* copyright 1998 National Association of School Nurses, Inc., P.O. Box 1300 Scarborough, ME 04070-1300.

The occupational health nursing standards presented on pages 563–564 are reprinted with permission of the American Association of Occupational Health Nurses from *Standards of Occupational and Environmental Health Nursing,* copyright 1999 American Association of

Occupational Health Nurses, Inc., Suite 100 2920 Brandywine Road, Atlanta, Georgia 30341.

Standards for nursing practice in correctional settings included on page 607 are reprinted with permission from the American Nurses Association, *Scope and Standards of Nursing Practice in Correctional Facilities*, copyright 1995 American Nurses Association, 600 Maryland Avenue, SW, Suite 100 West, Washington, DC 20024-2571.

Standards for nursing practice in home health settings included on pages 507–508 are reprinted with permission from the American Nurses Association, *Scope and Standards of Home Health Nursing Practice*, copyright 1999 American Nurses Association, 600 Maryland Avenue, SW, Suite 100 West, Washington, DC 20024-2571.

Tenets of public health nursing included on page 174 and page 524 are reprinted with permission from the American Nurses Association, *Scope and Standards of Public Health Nursing Practice*, copyright 1999 American Nurses Association, 600 Maryland Avenue, SW, Suite 100 West, Washington, DC 20024-2571.

Guide to Key Features

CHAPTER OBJECTIVES

Chapter objectives identify essential learning concepts, stimulate thought, and assist readers in reviewing chapter content.

KEY TERMS

Key terms list the important vocabulary covered in each chapter. At the point of definition within the chapter, each term is set in boldface type.

MEDIA LINK

Icon integrated throughout the book which directs students to additional online content.

CULTURAL CONSIDERATIONS

This special feature points out cultural considerations relevant to chapter content, presenting cultural information or posing questions related to cultural influences on health and health care delivery that assist readers to apply cultural concepts in clinical practice.

THE POLITICAL CONTEXT

4

Chapter Objectives

After reading this chapter, you should be able to:

- Describe potential nursing contributions to policy development.
- Identify four competencies required for effective policy development.
- Identify at least three levels at which health policy development occurs.
- Outline the legislative process.
- Describe the regulatory process at the state and federal levels.
- Describe at least four aspects of the policy development process.
- Identify four criteria for evaluating health policy development.

KEY TERMS

allocative policies 64
bill 65
campaigning 74
coalitions 72
community organizing 72
electioneering 74
executive orders 69
health care policy 63
judicial decisions 69
laws 64
legislative proposals 65
lobbying 73
macropolicy 64
pocket veto 68
policy 63
political process 62
politics 64
public policy 64
public health policy 64
regulation 68
regulatory policies 64
social policy 63
stakeholders 70

Media Links

http://www.prenhall.com/clark

Additional interactive resources for this chapter can be found on the companion Web site. Click on Chapter 4 and "Begin" to select the activities for this chapter.

---

102 Unit I ■ The Context for Community Health Nursing

When the provider prescribes a single drug, credibility may be lost and compliance will suffer.

THINK ABOUT IT

What are some aspects of the culture of professional nursing? How might nursing's professional culture interfere with effective interaction with clients?

NURSING AND CULTURE

The interface between community health nursing and culture occurs in one of three arenas: one's personal culture, the professional culture of nursing, and care of clients from a culture different from one's own. All of us are the products of our own cultural heritage. Many nurses adhere to the major tenets of the dominant American culture, but maintain many beliefs, values, and practices derived from familial culture and our cultures of origin. We have attitudes toward time, cleanliness, the value of religious affiliation, "proper behavior" and so on that may enhance or impede our interactions with others. Community health nurses should become aware of these cultural influences in their own lives and their impact on interactions with others.

Nursing, as a profession, also has a distinct culture as do other health care professionals and people with whom community health nurses collaborate in their practice. Differences between these cultures may give rise to as much misunderstanding or conflict as differences between nurse and client. For example, a cultural emphasis on cure among physicians may hamper their ability to understand the motivations of a nurse who advocates for termination of life support in keeping with a client's or family's wishes. In this instance, the cultural values of cure and advocacy, arising out of the medical and nursing cultures, respectively, are in conflict. Similarly, nursing has its own language, which may or may not be understood by persons from another culture (ethnic or professional). In addition to the general professional culture, subcultures exist in specific health care settings that may make it difficult even for two nurses to understand each other (Andershed & Ternestedt, 1999).

The final aspect of the interface between nursing and culture lies in our interactions with clients. In this interaction, we may need not only to address the differences between the client's ethnic culture and our cultural heritage, but we must examine the effects of differences on effective professional and lay cultures on effective health care.

Community health nurses should cultivate an awareness of their own cultural beliefs, values, and attitudes

CULTURAL CONSIDERATIONS

Many large health care organizations employ a culturally diverse staff and serve several different cultural population groups. In some such organizations, staff whose first language is other than English are prohibited from speaking to each other in their native language in front of clients.

- In what ways does this prohibition demonstrate or not demonstrate culturally competent organizations?
- What interventions might these organizations employ to demonstrate respect and acceptance of the cultural values and behaviors of both clients and staff?

and their potential interactions with the cultures of clients and other health care providers. To do this, nurses may explore their own cultures using the cultural assessment tips presented on page 135. Introspection, interviews with family members, and discussions of changes from "my day" to now with older family members may uncover previously unrecognized cultural influences on the nurse's behavior.

Attention to cultural issues related to clients can be traced to Florence Nightingale, who was interested in the health of indigenous groups in Australia. Early public health nurses in the United States and Canada devoted their efforts to improving the health status of immigrant groups. More formalized attention to cultural issues in nursing is seen in nursing's documents. Although cultural sensitivity is implicit in *Nursing's Social Policy Statement*, it is explicitly noted as a required feature of nursing practice in the American Nurses Association's *Position Statement on Cultural Diversity in Nursing Practice* (Poss, 1999). As noted earlier, it is increasingly important for community health nurses to be prepared to care for a highly culturally diverse population.

Community health nurses employ knowledge of culture and culturally sensitive health care with populations as well as with individual clients. At the level of the individual, the nurse devises health care interventions congruent with the client's culture, being sensitive to cultural influences affecting health and incorporating cultural health beliefs and practices whenever possible. At the population level, community health nurses must be involved in the development of culturally sensitive health care delivery systems and programs.

CULTURAL COMPETENCE

In order to interact effectively with clients, health professionals, or other people from cultures different from their own cultures of origin, community health nurses must develop cultural competence. The United States Health

---

xxiii

ETHICAL AWARENESS

Legislation aimed at preventing exposure to second-hand smoke in public places has been criticized because it infringes on the rights of individuals to decide for themselves whether, when, and where they will smoke. What approaches to ethical decision making would support the rights of smokers to self-determination? Which position would you support? Why?

An example of tertiary control measures at this level might include political activity to mandate standards that prevent the recurrence of a leak at a nuclear power plant or to pass a bond issue to renovate a water treatment plant and prevent recontamination of drinking water with sewage. Other possible tertiary preventive interventions by community health nurses are presented in Table 7–4 ■.

In addition to political activity and community health that help to protect the environment, community health nurses can also model environmentally conscious behaviors in their personal and professional lives. Some of these measures are summarized below.

EVALUATING ENVIRONMENTAL MEASURES

Community health nurses are also involved in evaluating the effectiveness of environmental control measures.

Evaluation would focus on the effectiveness of primary, secondary, and tertiary preventive measures related to individuals, families, and population groups. For example, the nurse might monitor blood lead levels of children in housing with lead-based paint to determine whether primary preventive measures have prevented initial elevation. For those children who already have elevated blood lead levels, evaluation would focus on the effects of chelating agents in reducing blood levels and the prevention of symptoms of lead poisoning. Evaluation of tertiary measures would be aimed at the effectiveness of abatement procedures in preventing

HIGHLIGHTS

Personal and Professional Environmental Protection Strategies

Personal Strategies

- Avoid unnecessary driving or gasoline consumption by combining trips or carpooling.
- Install water-conserving bathroom and kitchen fixtures.
- Reduce power use to minimum requirements by turning off appliances, computers, and so on when not in use; engage in family activities in one room to decrease use of lights; run major appliances during off-peak use hours; replace worn-out appliances with energy-conserving models; use cold water to wash clothes; wash full loads of clothing and hang them to dry; wash dishes by hand or run the dishwasher only when full.
- Use grass clippings and fallen leaves as mulch rather than burning them or taking them to a landfill.
- Dispose of hazardous wastes appropriately.
- Recycle materials whenever possible.
- Use environmentally safe household cleaning products.
- Limit use of aerosol sprays.
- Buy recycled goods.
- Refrain from smoking.

Professional Strategies

- Encourage health care institutions and agencies to use recyclable materials where possible.
- Promote recycling in the work setting.
- Promote appropriate disposal of hazardous medical wastes.
- Promote use of nontoxic, environmentally safe cleaning products in health care settings.
- Promote carpool programs among fellow employees.
- Promote a smoke-free workplace.

ETHICAL AWARENESS

This new feature presents an ethical dilemma or issue related to the chapter that stimulates student thought on the course or courses of action they might take in a similar practice situation.

■ **TABLE 7–5**   Sample Questions for Evaluating Primary, Secondary, and Tertiary Prevention of Environmental Hazards *(continued)*

ENVIRONMENTAL HAZARD	PRIMARY PREVENTION	SECONDARY PREVENTION	TERTIARY PREVENTION
Air pollution	Has the level of pollutants in ambient or indoor air been reduced? Has the incidence of diseases due to air pollution declined?	Have individuals with diseases due to air pollution received adequate diagnostic and treatment services?	Has further contamination of ambient or indoor air been prevented?
Water pollution	Has the number of exposures to polluted water been reduced? Has the incidence of diseases due to polluted water declined?	Have individuals with diseases due to water pollution been adequately treated?	Have recurrent episodes of diseases due to water pollution been prevented? Has recontamination of water by pollutants been prevented?

HEALTHY PEOPLE 2010

GOALS FOR THE POPULATION

Status of Selected National Objectives Related to Environmental Health

Objective	Target	Status
■ 8-1. Reduce the proportion of people exposed to harmful air pollutants (1997)		
Ozone	0%	43%
Particulate matter	0%	12%
Carbon monoxide	0%	18%
Nitrogen dioxide	0%	5%
Sulfur dioxide	0%	2%
Lead	0%	<1%
■ 8-5. Increase the proportion of people receiving safe drinking water from community water systems (1995)	95%	73%
■ 8-6. Reduce waterborne disease outbreaks (1987–1996 average)	2	6
■ 8-7. Reduce daily per capita water withdrawals (1995)	90.9 gal	101 gal
■ 8-11. Eliminate elevated BLLs in children (1991–1994)	0	4.4%
■ 8-13. Reduce pesticide exposures resulting in visits to health care facilities (1997)	13,500	27,156
■ 8-15. Increase recycling of municipal solid waste (1996)	38%	27%
■ 8-18. Increase the proportion of homes tested for radon (1998)	20%	17%
■ 8-22. Increase the proportion of pre-1950s homes tested for lead-based paint (1998)	50%	16%
■ 8-23. Reduce the proportion of substandard homes (1995)	3%	6.2%
■ 8-29. Reduce the global burden of disease deaths due to poor water quality, sanitation, and personal/domestic hygiene (1990)	2.1 mil	2.6 mil

Source: U.S. Department of Health and Human Services. (2000). Healthy people 2010. (Conference edition, in two volumes). Washington, DC: Author.

tions are not met, screening is unlikely to be effective in improving the health of communities. Disease, test, and target group considerations in planning large-scale screening programs are summarized below.

HIGHLIGHTS

Diseases, Test, and Target Group Considerations in Screening

Disease Considerations

- The disease affects a sufficient number of people to make screening cost-effective.
- The disease is relatively serious.
- An effective treatment is available for the disease.
- The preclinical period is sufficient to allow treatment before symptoms occur.
- Early diagnosis and treatment make a difference in terms of outcome.

Test Considerations

- The screening test is sensitive enough to detect most cases of the disease.
- The screening test is specific enough to exclude most other causes of positive results.
- The screening test costs little, is easy to administer, and has minimal side effects.

Target Group Considerations

- The target group is identifiable.
- The target group is accessible.

HEALTHY PEOPLE 2010: GOALS FOR THE POPULATION

Tables present relevant Healthy People 2010 objectives as well as information on the current status of related objectives for 2000.

Control Programs

Some of the same programs described as primary preventive measures may also be employed in secondary prevention designed to alleviate existing health problems. When a community or target group is already experiencing a high rate of sexually transmitted diseases (STDs), education on the transmission and prevention of STDs would be a secondary preventive measure. The intent of the program is to control an existing problem (high rate of STDs), rather than prevent a problem from occurring.

The kind of secondary prevention programs planned in a given community or target group varies with the types of problems identified in the assessment. For example, if child abuse is prevalent in the community, parenting classes for abusive parents would be an appropriate secondary preventive measure. Similarly, if there is a high rate of hypertension among group members, clinics would be established to screen for, diagnose, and treat this problem. In another community, a program to enforce seat belt legislation could be used as a secondary preventive measure for a high rate of motor vehicle accident fatalities.

Tertiary prevention programs for communities or target groups are designed to prevent complications of identified problems or prevent the recurrence of a problem. For example, if a community is experiencing an epidemic of measles, mass immunization programs to control the epidemic would be used as a secondary preventive measure. When the epidemic is under control, a program designed to maintain immunity levels among commu-

CRITICAL THINKING IN RESEARCH

Healey (1998) conducted a study to determine the prevalence and characteristics of tobacco use in three counties in Pennsylvania. He examined the extent of cigarette use in children under 18 years of age and the age of onset of cigarette use as well as gender differences in cigarette use. He also noted the extent of continued cigarette use among children. Study findings were used to provide the impetus for two community initiatives to reduce the prevalence of tobacco use among children in the area.

- What other kinds of prevalence data might be used as a catalyst for community action?
- How might you go about obtaining similar data related to another health behavior (e.g., bicycle helmet or seat belt use)?
- Who would you involve in participatory community-based research related to your topic? Why would you include these people in your research team?
- To whom should your findings be disseminated? Why? How would you go about disseminating your findings to these individuals or groups?

CRITICAL THINKING IN RESEARCH

This feature presents a potential research question or findings of a study related to chapter content to assist readers to incorporate research findings and methodology into everyday practice in community health nursing.

CASE STUDIES

Case studies allow students to apply concepts and principles addressed in the chapter to realistic practice situations.

TESTING YOUR UNDERSTANDING

Review questions test the reader's understanding of concepts and principles addressed in each chapter. Page references are provided to direct readers to related content in the chapter.

ASSESSMENT TIPS

Assessment tips direct the reader in health assessment with particular clients and specific population groups.

THINK ABOUT IT

Think About It questions stimulate thought and discussion beyond the content of the chapter to permit more in-depth exploration of selected concepts and issues.

The effects of intervention at the aggregate level can be assessed in terms of the accomplishment of national health objectives. The current status of selected objectives related to men's health is presented on page 434. Information about objectives related to men's health is available on the Healthy People 2010 Web site, which may be accessed through links provided on the companion Web site for this book.

Men have a variety of health care needs that they may or may not acknowledge. Community health nurses can be actively involved in encouraging men to seek health care as needed. They may also provide direct services to male clients, particularly with respect to education for primary prevention.

APPLYING YOUR KNOWLEDGE IN PRACTICE

CASE STUDY
Caring for the Adolescent Male

You are a community health nurse working with a hypertensive, diabetic, middle-aged single mother for the past year. Her 17-year-old son has had hand surgery and has been added to your caseload for wound and cast care. On your next meeting with the mother, you discover that she is very upset about her son's behavior. He broke his hand when he punched a wall in a fit of anger, and the necessary care he has hurt the family's very limited finances. The mother reports that she believes her son is drinking, and she is especially angry and upset about this because her ex-husband had deserted the family largely because of his own alcohol abuse. While the mother answers a phone call, you attempt to speak to the son. He seems wary but does concede he punches walls when angry. His view at present is that "It's no big deal—the cast will handle it." When asked about alcohol, he replies, "It's what we do . . . a little doesn't hurt anyone." When you begin to address the risks involved in this behav-

ior, he cuts you off by angrily retorting, "It's none of your damn business! Get lost and leave me alone!"

- What psychological and sociocultural dimension factors may be influencing the son's behavior? Are these typical or atypical of men in general? Of adolescent boys?
- What actual and potential health issues are raised by the lifestyle of the son and his past and present family situation?
- What primary interventions are indicated for the health risks present in the son?
- What secondary interventions are indicated for the health concerns affecting the son?
- How should the nurse respond to the client's denial and anger?
- How might the nurse's interventions be evaluated?

TESTING YOUR UNDERSTANDING

- What are the major considerations in assessing the biophysical, psychological, physical environmental, sociocultural, behavioral, and health system factors influencing men's health? (pp. 414–423)
- What are some of the factors that contribute to adverse health effects for gay, bisexual, and transgender men? (pp. 423–429)
- Identify at least four areas for primary prevention with male clients. How might the community health nurse be involved in each? (pp. 430–432)

- What are the major secondary prevention considerations for male clients. Give an example of at least one community health nursing intervention related to each consideration. (pp. 432–433)
- Identify areas of emphasis in tertiary prevention for male clients. How might the community health nurse be involved in each? In what kinds of situations might tertiary prevention be required? (pp. 433–434)

THINK ABOUT IT

How might health [...] meet the needs of gay men [...]

assessment tips ASSESSING MEN'S HEALTH

Biophysical Considerations

- What is the man's age? Has he accomplished the developmental tasks relevant to his current and previous developmental stages? Has the man achieved sexual maturity?
- Does the man have any existing physical health problems? Is the man experiencing impotence or other sexual problems?

Psychological Considerations

- What is the extent of stress in the client's life? How has he been socialized to deal with stress? How effective are his coping strategies?
- Is the man depressed? Is he suicidal? Does the man have a history of mental illness? Signs of PTSD?

Physical Environmental Considerations

- Where does the man live? Is he exposed to safety or environmental health hazards?

Sociocultural Considerations

- How does the man deal with conflict? What is the quality of interpersonal interactions?
- Is the man a victim or perpetrator of family violence?
- What is the extent of the man's social support network?

- What effect do the [...] occupation, and income have on his health [...]

Behavioral Considerations

- What are the man's typical behavior patterns? How do they affect health?
- Is the man sexually active? What is his sexual orientation? Is he comfortable with his sexual identity? Does he engage in unsafe sexual practices? Does he practice regular testicular self-examination?
- To what extent has the gay, bisexual, or transgender client disclosed his sexual identity? Is confidentiality a particularly important issue for him?

Health System Considerations

- How does the man define health? What is his attitude to health and health care? What is his usual source of health care? To what extent does he utilize health care services? Does he engage in preventive health care practices?
- How does the man finance health care?
- What is the reaction of health care providers to the gay, bisexual, or transgender client? How does this reaction influence attitudes toward and use of health care services?

[...] masculine [...] to inform that [...] man may view the [...] frailties to a community [...] who believe that taking [...] to their masculinity may [...] frequent health impairment may [...] from these examples, when societal [...] roles are internalized by men, they [...] psychological factors influencing health-related behaviors.

THINK ABOUT IT

In what ways were you socialized into gender roles? How closely do your internalized gender roles conform to those expected of society? What problems, if any, has gender created in your life?

[...] te [...] ph [...]

T [...] ered [...] tion lev [...] nized aga [...] pneumococc [...] receive varic [...] are more likel [...] in the last 10 ye [...] 64 years of age) [...] influenza vaccine [...] pneumococcal vaccine [...] & Strikas 2000).

Community health nurses should assess individual male clients for risk factors for physiologic dysfunction as well as signs and symptoms of existing disorders. In addition, when existing conditions are noted, the nurse should assess the degree of limitation posed by the problem. As men are often reluctant to seek care for health problems, conditions tend to be more severe when help is sought. At the population level, community health nurses obtain information on the incidence and prevalence of acute and chronic conditions among men as well as the prevalence of risk factors for these conditions (e.g., smoking or overweight as risk factors for cardiovascular disease). In addition, they would assess immunization levels among the male population.

Psychological Considerations

Two related elements of the psychological dimension are of concern to community health nurses caring for men. These elements include socialization, stress, and coping abilities, as well as suicide as an outcome of ineffective coping.

Socialization, Stress, and Coping

Men, like women, have several basic psychological needs. These include the needs to know and be known to others,

Although men [...] received Td vaccines [...]% among persons 50 to [...] past year or to ever have received [...] (Singleton, Greby, Wooten, Walker, [...]) should also [...] less likely to have received [...]

Men may also have a stronger psychological need than women to see themselves as healthy and even invulnerable. Because men tend to value strength and endurance more than women, they are more likely to conceal or suppress pain and other perceived indicators of frailty. An example of this state of mind can be seen in the male post–myocardial infarction client who resumes shoveling snow against the recommendations of health care professionals and his family, and who continues it despite the return of the now-familiar angina. As a result of this need for strength in his self-image, the male client minimizes the importance of the problem. Consequently, when shoveling snow causes further angina, he may seek shoveling snow less readily and use it less effectively than would a female client in a similar situation.

Conversely, it should be noted that male values of strength and endurance do not always adversely affect a male client's health. Some men who value strength actually may be more motivated to exercise and maintain a higher level of general fitness and to seek preventive

tice guidelines, agency procedures and protocols, or elements of clinical pathways. The federal Agency for Healthcare Research and Quality (AHRQ) (formerly the Agency for Health Care Policy and Research [AHCPR]) has developed practice guidelines for several problems relevant to home health nursing. Current guidelines include those related to pressure ulcer prevention and treatment and cardiac rehabilitation. Prior guidelines include those for acute pain management, urinary incontinence, cataracts, depression, sickle cell disease, early HIV infection, unstable angina, heart failure, otitis media with effusion, benign prostatic hypertrophy, acute low back pain, poststroke rehabilitation, smoking cessation, and early Alzheimer's disease (Agency for Healthcare Research and Quality, 2001). Because of recent developments in treatment, these prior guidelines are no longer considered current, but may be of interest to home health nurses anyway. Current and prior guidelines may be accessed through the AHRQ Web page for this book.

Agency procedures and protocols and clinical pathways may also be used as guides for planning nursing interventions during a home visit. Clinical pathways were addressed in detail in Chapter 12. Clinical pathways may differ from agency to agency and should be tailored to the goals and resources of the particular agency (Peters & McKeon, 1998). Components of clinical pathways are summarized below.

The activities planned reflect the nurse's assessment of health care needs and the factors influencing them. In the previous example, referral to a Head Start program may provide assistance with child care, but only if the children involved are of the right ages. If the youngsters are of school age, the appropriate nursing intervention might be to help the father explore the possibility of an after-school program, if one is available, or have the children go home with the parents of a friend until the father can pick them up after work.

Nursing activities can focus on both health promotion and resolution of health-related problems. For example, the community health nurse might provide the parents of a toddler with anticipatory guidance regarding toilet training or assist parents to discuss sexuality with their preteen daughter. Other positive interventions might focus on providing adequate nutrition for a young child or promoting a healthy pregnancy for the pregnant female.

Specific interventions employed by the nurse include referral, education, and technical procedures. For example, the nurse might refer a family to social services for financial assistance, teach a mother about appropriate nutrition for the family, or check a hypertensive client's blood pressure. The actions selected should be geared to achieving the goals and objectives established while taking into account the constraints and supports in the individual client situation.

Obtaining Necessary Materials

One aspect of planning the home visit that does not apply to many of the other processes discussed in this unit is obtaining materials and supplies that may be needed to implement planned interventions. Because the nurse is going to be in the client's home, one cannot assume that necessary supplies will be available there. If the nurse plans to engage in nutrition education, he or she might want to leave a selection of pamphlets with the client to reinforce teaching. If planned activities involve weighing a premature infant, the nurse will want to take along a scale.

Equipment and supplies may also be needed for other procedures such as dressing changes, catheterizations, injections, and blood pressure checks. Because the nurse frequently does a physical assessment of one or more clients, additional equipment such as a stethoscope, percussion hammer, tongue blade, flashlight, and otophthalmoscope will need to be obtained prior to setting out for the visit.

Planning Evaluation

As with every other process employed by community health nurses, the planning phase of the home visit process concludes with plans for evaluation. The nurse determines criteria to be used to evaluate the effectiveness of the home visit. Criteria for evaluating client outcomes are derived from the outcome objectives developed for the visit. Because the outcome of nursing interventions undertaken during a home visit may not be immediately apparent, the nurse needs to develop both long-term and short-term evaluative criteria. Short-term

HIGHLIGHTS

Characteristic Elements of Clinical Pathways

Scope: The extent of the client episode to which the pathway is applicable (e.g., only home care services, or a continuum of care from hospital to home care)

Condition: The health problem or condition to which the pathway applies (e.g., pregnancy or congestive heart failure)

Activity categories: Activities required in the care of typical clients with the specific condition, may be more or less detailed, but ideally reflects activities for which reimbursement is sought

Outcomes: Expected outcomes of care for the client and family

Format: The way in which activities are organized and presented in the pathway (e.g., in a linear form, by treatment day or visit, by discipline)

Documentation: Use of the pathway itself to document interventions, in which case the pathway becomes part of the client's permanent record.

Adapted with permission from Peters, D. A., & McKeon, T. (1998). *Transforming home care: Quality, cost, and data management*. Gaithersburg, MD: Aspen.

HIGHLIGHTS BOXES

Highlights boxes summarize important concepts presented in the chapter and assist the reader in identifying key principles.

ADDITIONAL ONLINE RESOURCES

RESOURCE LINKS

Special icons refer the reader to the companion Web site where links to other sources of information are provided.

ASSESSMENT GUIDE LINKS

Special icons refer the reader to the companion Web site to obtain printable assessment guides specific to a given population, setting, or health problem.

SUMMARIES OF FULL-TEXT ARTICLES

Icons refer the reader to the companion Web site to review summaries of selected full-text articles that provide more detailed information or another perspective on chapter content.

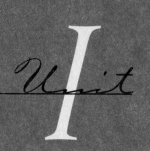

Unit I

THE CONTEXT FOR COMMUNITY HEALTH NURSING

ANOTHER CASE OF CHRONIC PELVIC PAIN

Like the others, she is not from here
and when she came she left
all of what matters behind—
four children, a village
a father (not well), the lingering
scent of her man (who had fled)
Sunday walks in the plaza after mass
on days when the soldiers were gone
on days when no bodies were found.

The journey from home was perilous—
sometimes on foot, or crowded
into the back of a truck, over hills
through dense forests, arroyos
dark rivers, toward menacing lights,
the eyes of hostile cities.

The trip cost her more than
she wanted to pay—
all the crumpled bills
from the earthenware jar
in the wall of the house,
the silver bracelets and earrings
passed down from her mother.
Her body they took along the way
again and again as if for a debt
that can never be paid.
What drove her on was a woman's
fixed and singular faith that
she is the giver of life
the mother of God.

By bus from the border
by phone from the station
by foot to the room of the friend
of a cousin who knew of a place
and jobs cleaning offices at night
where no questions were asked
and dollars were paid
unless you missed work

or were caught by the migra—
all this distance she came
numb to the pain in her feet and back
and the ache in her lower heart.

She spent her days trying to sleep.
Nights she roamed large empty halls
as wide as the streets
that gave onto the plaza
pushing a cart full of cleaning supplies
bagging the trash, sweeping the floors
washing away the stains of another
day in the upper world.
Paydays she sent her money home
by the man at Urgente Express.
Sunday she sometimes walked
down the street at the edge
of the park, watching
with shaded eyes among the men
for one she might know.

Months passed this way
and with each one she wept
the tears of blood that women weep
and felt the ache in her belly
grow stronger until at last
there was no relief,
come new moon or full,
and no poultice, tea or prayer
that helped her bear
what she must bear.

She sits in the clinic—
"a 32-year-old Hispanic female
complaining of chronic pelvic pain."

The results of all the tests
are negative they say.
That means there's nothing we can find
to blame for all the pain.

his poem highlights the complex interaction of the many contexts that influence health and community health nursing practice.

There is a cause, of course—
perhaps a scar deep inside.
Surgery might tell us more—or not,
but then there's the matter of money.

I see, *she says simply*.
Well, if you can't find
anything wrong—and you know
there is no money. . .

There are some pills
you could take, they say,
for the pain, when it
bothers you most.

You are kind, *she says*
and stands up to go,
like the others,
from here to her job,
her room, and perhaps twice a year
to a telephone that spans the miles

of dense forest, dark river
to the house of a friend
of an aunt of her father
to ask if the children
are well and in school
on days when the soldiers are gone
on days when no bodies are found.

I will send for them
one day soon, *she says*.
For now there is only the ache in her belly,
come new moon or full,
and no poultice, pill, or prayer
to help her bear
what she must bear.

What drives her on is a woman's
fixed and singular faith that
she is the giver of life
the mother of God.

Reprinted with permission from V. Masson (1999),
Rehab at the Florida Avenue Grill. *Washington,*
DC: Sage Femme Press.

THE POPULATION CONTEXT

1

Media Link

http://www.prenhall.com/clark

Additional interactive resources for this chapter can be found on the companion Web site. Click on Chapter 1 and "Begin" to select the activities for this chapter.

The hallmark of community health nursing is that the primary client or recipient of care is a group of people, or population, rather than an individual or a particular family. Although nurses who engage in community health nursing practice may also provide services to individuals and families, they do so with the express purpose of improving the health of the overall population. The focus of their care is the population group, not the individuals and families who are its members (Kuss, Proulx-Girouard, Lovitt, Katz, & Kennelly, 1997).

DEFINING POPULATIONS AS A FOCUS FOR CARE

The population groups that form the focus for community health nursing can be many and varied. *Population* refers to the general public or society or a collection of communities. Populations generally do not display social action among all members, but among selected subgroups within the population (Kuss et al., 1997). Three other commonly used, similar but different terms for these smaller subgroups are *aggregate, neighborhood,* and *community.*

Aggregates are populations with some common characteristics who frequently have common concerns, but, like populations, may not interact with each other to address those concerns (Kuss et al., 1997). School-aged children, persons with human immunodeficiency virus (HIV) infection, and the elderly are all examples of aggregates. The term aggregate is often used to refer to populations at high risk for certain health conditions (Helvie, 1998).

A *neighborhood* is a smaller, more homogeneous group than a community (Matteson, 2000) and involves an inter-face with others living nearby and a level of identification with those others. Neighborhoods are self-defined, and although they may be constrained by natural or man-made factors, they often do not have specifically demarcated boundaries (Matteson, 1999). For example, a major highway may limit interactions between residents on either side, thus creating separate neighborhoods. Or a neighborhood may be defined by a common language or cultural heritage. Thus, non-Hispanic residents of a "Hispanic neighborhood" are not usually considered, nor do they consider themselves, part of the neighborhood.

A community may be composed of several neighborhoods (Matteson, 2000). Some authors define communities as geographic entities (Stackhouse, 1998), but the majority of writers have moved away from locale as a primary defining characteristic of communities (Baldwin, Conger, Abegglen, & Hill, 1998). In addition to location, other potential defining aspects of communities include a social system or social institutions designed to carry out specific functions (Cassells, 1997; Matteson, 2000); identity, commitment, or emotional connection (Israel, Shulz, Parker, & Becker, 1998; Kuss et al., 1997); common norms and values (Matteson, 2000; Schulz, et al., 1998); common history or interests (Kone et al., 2000); common symbols; social interaction (Kuss et al., 1997); and intentional action to meet common needs (Kulbok, Gates, Vicenzi, & Schultz, 1999). Although most of these characteristics are also true of neighborhoods, the critical distinction between neighborhoods and communities would appear to be a defined social structure containing institutions designed to accomplish designated community functions such as education, social support, and so on. For our purposes, then, a *community* is defined as a group of people who share common interests, who interact with each other, and who function

Communities may consist of several types of neighborhoods.

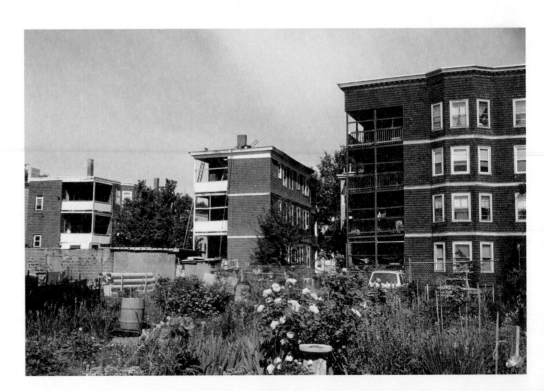

CULTURAL CONSIDERATIONS

Some cultural groups traditionally think of people in the aggregate rather than as individuals. What cultural groups in your area have a community orientation? How might a community health nurse capitalize on this orientation? What aspects of traditional American culture make it more difficult to adopt aggregate thinking? What strategies by community health nurses might help people adopt a community orientation?

collectively within a defined social structure to address common concerns. By this definition, geopolitical entities, such as the city of San Diego, a school of nursing, and a religious congregation can be considered communities. A *geopolitical community* is one characterized by geographic and jursidictional boundaries.

All three communities (city, nursing program, and religious group), however, can be considered *communities of identity*—communities with a common identity and interests (Israel et al., 1998).

Community health nurses may work with any or all of these population groups—aggregates, neighborhoods, and communities—in their efforts to enhance the health status of the general public or overall population.

DEFINING THE HEALTH OF POPULATIONS

The health of a population group goes beyond the health status of the individuals or groups who comprise it

(Frankish, Veenstra, & Moulton, 1999). *Population health,* or community health, can be defined as the attainment of the greatest possible biologic, psychological, and social well-being of the population as an entity and of its individual members. Population health results when knowledge of determinants of individual and group health is used to develop programs and policies that support conditions conducive to health (Butler-Jones, 1999). Health is derived from opportunities and choices provided to the public as well as the population's response to those choices (Wilcox & Knapp, 2000). Healthy populations provide their members with the knowledge and opportunities to make choices that improve health.

In large part, the health of a population is defined and determined by the perceptions, norms, and values of its members (Kuss et al., 1997). Despite the resulting variability in definitions of *health,* there are certain characteristics that healthy populations have in common. The Health Cities initiative, begun in 1983 and followed by the Healthy Communities movement a decade later (Duhl, 2000), has generated several characteristics of healthy communities that can be applied to populations at large. Chief among these are the 11 parameters of a healthy city identified by the World Health Organization (WHO). These parameters include:

- A healthful physical environment (including housing)
- A stable, sustainable ecosystem
- A strong, supportive, and nonexploitive population
- Extensive public participation in decisions affecting health
- Provisions for meeting members' basic needs
- Wide access to resources and opportunities for interaction among members

Children created a mural incorporating personal perceptions of their community.

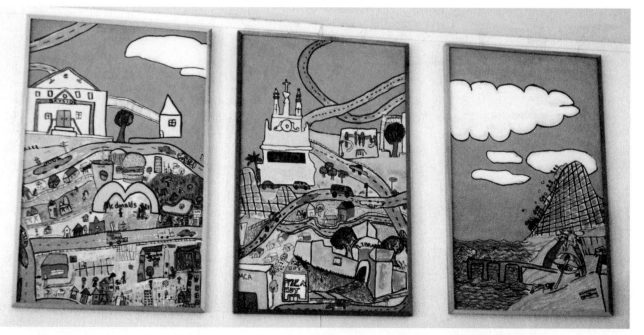

- A vital economy
- Connectedness with cultural and biological heritage
- Governance structures that promote health
- Appropriate and accessible services for all
- A high health status, including strong positive health indicators as well as low incidence of disease (cited in Lipschutz, 1995).

Other characteristics of healthy cities include abilities to change and adapt to changing circumstances, create a shared vision, embrace the diversity of members, assess assets and needs, create a sense of responsibility and belonging, and manage conflict effectively (Duhl, 2000; Kuss et al., 1997; Norris & Pitman, 2000). These characteristics of healthy populations are summarized below.

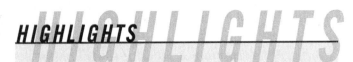

HIGHLIGHTS

Characteristics of Healthy Populations

- Provide a healthful physical environment
- Maintain a stable ecosystem
- Comprise a strong, supportive, nonexploitive membership
- Provide for extensive participation in decision making
- Provide for members' basic needs
- Provide access to resources and opportunities for interaction
- Sustain a vital economy
- Maintain connectedness with their cultural and biological heritages
- Provide governance structures that promote health
- Provide appropriate and accessible services for all members
- Display strong positive health indicators and low incidence of health problems
- Adapt to changing conditions and circumstances
- Create a shared vision for future development
- Celebrate diversity among members
- Periodically assess needs and assets
- Create a sense of group responsibility and belonging in members
- Deal effectively with conflict among members

ⓖTHINK ABOUT IT

What changes in perspective are required when you think of a group of people rather than an individual as your client?

PUBLIC HEALTH PRACTICE

The principle avenue for creating healthy populations is public health practice. According to the Institute of Medicine (IOM) (1988), in its report *The Future of Public Health*, **public health practice** "is what we, as a society, do to assure the conditions in which people can be healthy." In community health nursing, public health practice is combined with nursing practice to create a unique field focused on the health of population groups. For this reason, it is important for community health nurses to be conversant with some of the basic concepts of public health practice. Three of these concepts—the goals of public health, its core functions, and its outcomes—are addressed here. Others, such as the science of epidemiology and principles of disease causation, are presented later in this book.

Goals of Public Health Practice

Public health practice differs from the practice of medicine in a number of ways, particularly in its goals. Public health practice focuses on the health of population groups while medicine addresses the health of individuals. In medical practice, emphasis is placed on healing; in public health, the emphasis is on health promotion and prevention of illness. Achievement of the goals of public health and medicine also require different strategies. In medical practice, care requires individual decisions on the part of the practitioner and client. In public health practice, on the other hand, action to improve the public's health often requires political decisions and legislative activity (Brandt, 1999; Lasker, 1997; Schneider, 2000). Additional goals of medical practice include relief of suffering and enhanced capacity to function, while public health assumes responsibility for informing health care providers and the public regarding health issues (Keck, 1999).

Core Public Health Functions

Public health and medical practice also differ in terms of their core functions. Those of medicine include diagnosis and treatment of existing illness. The *core functions of public health* are its primary responsibilities, identified by the IOM as assessment, policy development, and assurance (Fahrenwald, Fischer, Boysen, & Maurer, 1999). These core functions form the foundation for public health and community health nursing activities (Baldwin et al., 1998; Keller, Strohschein, Lia-Hoagberg, & Schaffer, 1998).

In its *assessment* function, public health practice is responsible for assessing and monitoring the occurrence of health-related problems within the population, as well as identifying factors that contribute to, or prevent, those problems. The *policy development* function of public health involves advocacy and political action to develop local, state, and national policies conducive to population health. This may also include planning for health care delivery at the population level and assuring core funding for public health activities (Milio, 1998). The third core function, *assurance,* reflects the responsibility of the public health sector to assure availability of and access to health care services essential to sustain and improve the health of the population. This may involve the actual provision of services, but more often involves developing mechanisms whereby essential services are available within the community. For example, public health agencies may arrange for indigent members of the population to receive medical services from local providers rather than provide them directly to the public.

Outcomes of Public Health Practice

Public health practice is directed toward achieving four major outcomes: promotion of health, protection of the public, prevention of health problems, and access to services (Kuss et al., 1997). These outcomes reflect provision of services at three levels of prevention: primary, secondary, and tertiary.

Health promotion involves activities designed to promote the overall health of the population and has been defined by the World Health Organization (1984) as "a process of enabling individuals and communities to increase control over the determinants of health partly through political actions, to create a healthier environment." Interventions designed to provide healthy diets and exercise are examples of health promotion. *Health protection* is minimization of health risks arising from the environment. Control of water pollution is an example of a health protection activity. *Illness prevention* involves activities designed to prevent the occurrence of specific health problems. For example, diphtheria immunization is directed toward preventing cases of diphtheria in individuals and preventing diphtheria outbreaks in the population at large.

Health promotion, health protection, and illness prevention all reflect primary prevention. *Primary prevention* was defined by the originators of the term as "measures designed to promote general optimum health or . . . the specific protection of man against disease agents" (Leavell & Clark, 1965, p. 20). Primary prevention is action taken prior to the occurrence of health problems and is directed toward avoiding their occurrence (Hunt, 1998). Primary prevention may include increasing people's resistance to illness (as in the case of immunization), decreasing or eliminating the causes of health problems, or creating an environment conducive to health rather than health problems (Helvie, 1998).

Access to health care, as an outcome of public health practice, is related to the core function of assurance as well as to all three levels of prevention. With respect to primary prevention, access involves the ability of the population to obtain goods and services necessary to promote health and prevent illness. For example, at this level access would include the availability of immunization services.

Secondary prevention is the early identification and treatment of existing health problems (Hunt, 1998) and takes place after the health problem has occurred. Emphasis is on resolving health problems and preventing serious consequences. Secondary prevention activities include screening and early diagnosis, as well as treatment for existing health problems. Screening for hypertension is an example of secondary prevention. Secondary prevention would also include the actual diagnosis and treatment of a person with hypertension.

Tertiary prevention is activity aimed at returning the client to the highest level of function and preventing further deterioration in health (Scutchfield & Keck, 1997). Tertiary prevention also focuses on preventing recurrences of the problem. Placing a client on a maintenance diet after the loss of a desired number of pounds constitutes tertiary prevention.

A particular intervention may be viewed as a primary, secondary, or tertiary preventive measure depending on its relationship to the occurrence of a problem. Take, for example, nutrition education as an intervention. Nutrition education is a primary preventive measure when the nurse is teaching concepts of good nutrition in an effort to promote health and prevent overweight; the intervention is employed prior to the occurrence of a problem. Nutrition education for the client who is already overweight is a secondary preventive measure; the problem has already occurred and the education program is designed to help the client lose weight. Nutrition education may also be a tertiary preventive measure when the client goes on a "maintenance diet" after weight loss has occurred.

The Interface Between Public Health and Medicine

In spite of considerable mutual interdependence in their early history, the practice of medicine and public health have become increasingly divergent. Recently, the Committee on Medicine and Public Health, a joint initiative of the American Medical Association (AMA) and the American Public Health Association (APHA), identified the need for closer collaboration and interface between the two disciplines. The committee identified six areas for synergy in public health practice and medicine. These include:

1. Improving health care by coordinating services to individuals. This may involve combining clinical services with "wraparound" services that address barriers to health care, education regarding risk factor reduction, outreach services such as home visits, case management services, and social services that address socioeconomic factors that influence health.

2. Improving access to care by creating frameworks for providing care to uninsured and underinsured individuals. Synergy in this area is necessary as public health *safety net providers* (those who provide health care services to persons who cannot access mainstream medical care in the private sector) lose revenue derived from serving Medicaid and Medicare populations when these clients are absorbed by managed care organizations. There is a need to move the uninsured and underinsured into mainstream health care provision to allow public health agencies to focus on the core functions of public health rather than use limited resources in the provision of direct care services to these populations.

3. Improving the quality and cost-effectiveness of care by applying a population perspective to medical practice. It is becoming apparent that viable health care systems must be designed to address health problems common to the populations served and that those problems will vary from one population group to another. Therefore, it is essential for medical practice to identify and focus on population-based problems and to become involved in population-based strategies to resolve them.

4. Using clinical medical practice to identify and address community health problems. Because of their frequent interaction with members of the public, medical practitioners have opportunities to gather data for community-wide data bases as well as to educate clients to reduce or eliminate lifestyle risk factors.

5. Strengthening health promotion and health protection by mobilizing community campaigns. Synergy in this area would include collaborative efforts between medicine and public health to mount community education or advocacy campaigns. For example, the AMA might use its considerable lobbying influence to promote health-related legislation.

6. Shaping the future direction of health care delivery through collaboration in policy making, education of practitioners, and research (Lasker, 1997).

Medical authors have suggested means by which primary practice physicians can incorporate a community perspective into their medical practice. These include participating in health-related activities in their communities, becoming conversant with the cultural and social factors that influence their clientele, making appropriate use of existing community resources, and becoming involved in health-related and non–health-related organizations within the community (Pathman, Steiner, Williams, & Riggins, 1998). Additional activities include incorporating more of a health promotion and prevention focus into practice, advocating public policies that promote health, and mitigating the health effects of population problems until means to prevent them are developed (Butler-Jones, 1999).

CRITICAL THINKING IN RESEARCH

How might population-focused and person/family-focused nurses collaborate in research that would improve the health of population groups? What specific research questions might be addressed? What roles might each group of nurses play in conducting the research?

The interface between medical and public health practice described here has parallels in the interaction between population-focused and person/family-focused nursing. Nursing authors have noted that "the best population-focused practice emerges when the practitioner is well grounded in expert individual/family practice" (Diekemper, SmithBattle, & Drake, 1999). Although health promotion is not a primary focus of nursing in acute care settings that parallel medical practice, nurses practicing in these settings need to bring these aspects of primary prevention into their practice to minimize rehospitalizations. Similarly, nurses who care for individuals and families need to be aware of population trends in the health problems encountered. A population focus in the acute care setting serves to improve services to the individuals seen in that setting (Baldwin et al., 1998). Like the medical practitioner, the nurse caring for individuals and families can use client encounters as opportunities to gather population-based data and to educate clients regarding risk factors for health problems present in their population or community.

OBJECTIVES FOR POPULATION HEALTH

The goals and desired outcomes of public health practice have been operationalized more specifically in several sets of national objectives for improving the health of the U.S. population. The first set of objectives was established in 1980 in the publication *Promoting Health/ Preventing Disease: Objectives for the Nation* (U.S. Department of Health and Human Services, 1980) and targeted 15 priority intervention areas in three strategic action categories: preventive health, health protection, and health promotion. The primary goal of this initiative was to reduce mortality (Friedrich, 2000). Approximately one third of the 226 objectives were met by the target date of 1990 (National Center for Health Statistics, 1992).

A subsequent set of National Health Objectives, *Healthy People 2000: National Health Promotion and Disease Prevention Objectives*, was established for the year 2000 (U.S. Department of Health and Human Services, 1990). The broad goals for this second set of objectives were to (a) increase the span of healthy life (not just longevity), (b) reduce health disparities among subpopulations, and (c) achieve access to preventive health services for all (U.S. Department of Health and Human Services, 1995). The year 2000 objectives differed from those for 1990 in several ways. First, priority intervention areas were increased from 15 to 22 to include cancer screening, HIV infection, and preventive services. Second, the focus of the objectives was moved beyond reduction of mortality to improving the quality of life. A third difference was the special attention given to the needs of high-risk populations such as the elderly and minority groups. Fourth, the year 2000 objectives reflected concern for access to basic health services for all (Jamison & Mosley, 1991). Finally, responsibility for overseeing and monitoring achievement in each priority area was delegated to a specific agency of the U.S. Public Health Service (U.S. Department of Health and Human Services, 1996). A report in June of 1999 indicated that 15% of the year 2000 objectives had been met and another 44% were moving toward the established targets. Unfortunately, another 18% of objectives were moving away from the targets. Others had not been evaluated due to the lack of baseline and follow-up data (Friedrich, 2000).

⑥THINK ABOUT IT

Is longer life an objective to be achieved in and of itself? Would it be appropriate to use public health funds to prolong life? Why or why not?

The most recent set of objectives were published in January of 2000 in *Healthy People 2010* (U.S. Department of Health and Human Services, 2000a). This latest document was produced with input from the Healthy People Consortium, a coalition of more than 600 national and state health agencies, organizations, and experts (Davis, Okuboye, & Ferguson, 2000). The Surgeon General has identified four major strategies that will lead to the two overall goals of the new objectives. The four strategies are (a) promoting healthy behaviors, (b) promoting healthy and safe communities, (c) improving personal and public health systems, and (d) preventing and reducing diseases and disorders (Richmond, 1999).

The development of the objectives was based on a systematic approach consisting of four elements: goals, objectives, determinants of health, and health status (U.S. Department of Health and Human Services, 2000b). The goals provide direction for the development of more specific objectives. The two overarching goals are to increase quality and length of healthy life and to eliminate health disparities (Vinicor, Burton, Forster, & Eastman, 2000). The first goal continues the emphasis of *Healthy People 2000* on improved quality of life versus reduced mortality emphasized in the objectives for 1990. The second

expands the year 2000 goal of reducing disparities to eliminating them altogether.

The objectives specify the amount of progress expected in improving the health status of the population in the next 10 years. The 2010 objectives have been expanded to cover 28 focus areas and 467 objectives. Some of the focus areas from the year 2000 objectives have been separated and others added. Table 1–1 ■ provides a summary of focus areas included in the *Healthy People 2010* document with the agencies responsible for monitoring progress toward the objectives in each area. *Healthy People 2010* incorporates a common structure for each focus area that includes:

- Identification of the lead agency responsible for monitoring progress toward achievement of objectives.

- A concise goal statement for the focus area that delineates the overall purpose of the focus area.

- An overview of context and background for the objectives related to the focus area. This overview includes related issues, trends, disparities among population subgroups, and opportunities for prevention or intervention.

- Data on progress toward meeting related objectives for 2000.

- Objectives related to the focus area. These objectives are of two types: measurable outcome objectives and developmental objectives. Measurable objectives include baseline data, the target for 2010, and potential data sources for monitoring progress toward the target. Unlike the year 2000 objectives, which set separate targets for subpopulations, a single target is set for the entire population. The targets for each objective have been set at a level that is "better than the best" resulting in improved health status for all segments of the population (U.S. Department of Health and Human Services, 2000c). Developmental objectives relate to areas for which data systems do not exist and will direct the development of data systems related to emerging health issues.

- A standard data table including a set of population variables by which progress will be monitored. The minimum set of variables includes race and ethnicity, gender, family income, and education level. Additional categories of variables will be included where relevant and include geographic location, health insurance status, disability status, and other selected populations (e.g., school grade levels, etc.) (U.S. Department of Health and Human Services, 2000a).

The third element in the systematic approach to health improvement exemplified by the document is related to the determinants of health. These determinants are the "combined effects of individual and community physical and social environments and the policies and interventions used to promote health, prevent disease, and ensure access to quality health care" (U.S. Department of Health and Human Services, 2000b, p. 7).

■ **TABLE 1–1   Healthy People 2010: Focus Areas and Responsible Agencies**

FOCUS AREA	RESPONSIBLE AGENCIES
Access to quality health services	Agency for Health Care Research and Quality Health Resources and Services Administration
Arthritis, osteoporosis, and chronic back pain	Centers for Disease Control and Prevention National Institutes of Health
Cancer	Centers for Disease Control and Prevention National Institutes of Health
Chronic kidney disease	National Institutes of Health
Diabetes	Centers for Disease Control and Prevention National Institutes of Health
Disability and secondary conditions	Centers for Disease Control and Prevention National Institute on Disability and Rehabilitation Research U.S. Department of Education
Educational and community-based programs	Centers for Disease Control and Prevention Health Resources and Services Administration
Environmental health	Agency for Toxic Substances and Disease Registry Centers for Disease Control and Prevention National Institutes of Health
Family planning	Office of Population Affairs
Food safety	Food and Drug Administration Food Safety and Inspection Service U.S. Department of Agriculture
Health communication	Office of Disease Prevention and Health Promotion
Heart disease and stroke	Centers for Disease Control and Prevention National Institutes of Health
HIV	Centers for Disease Control and Prevention Health Resources and Services Administration
Immunization and infectious diseases	Centers for Disease Control and Prevention
Injury and violence prevention	Centers for Disease Control and Prevention
Maternal, infant, and child health	Centers for Disease Control and Prevention Health Resources and Services Administration
Medical product safety	Food and Drug Administration
Mental health and mental disorders	National Institutes of Health Substance Abuse and Mental Health Services Administration
Nutrition and overweight	Food and Drug Administration National Institutes of Health
Occupational safety and health	Centers for Disease Control and Prevention
Oral health	Centers for Disease Control and Prevention Health Resources and Services Administration National Institutes of Health
Physical fitness and activity	Centers for Disease Control and Prevention President's Council on Physical Fitness and Sports
Public health infrastructure	Centers for Disease Control and Prevention Health Resources and Services Administration

FOCUS AREA	RESPONSIBLE AGENCIES
Respiratory diseases	Centers for Disease Control and Prevention National Institutes of Health
Sexually transmitted diseases	Centers for Disease Control and Prevention
Substance abuse	National Institutes of Health Substance Abuse and Mental Health Services Administration
Tobacco use	Centers for Disease Control and Prevention
Vision and hearing	National Institutes of Health

Source: U.S. Department of Health and Human Services. (2000). *Healthy people 2010* (Conference edition, in two volumes). Washington, DC: Author.
Note: The Web address for Healthy People 2010 is *http://www.health.gov/healthypeople.*

Health status of the overall population, the fourth element of the approach, is the expected outcome and measure of success of the approach. Health status is reflected in the extent to which each of the 467 objectives is met, but is also reflected at a more general level in 10 leading health indicators. These indicators are presented in Table 1–2 ■ and are designed to reflect the major public health issues in the nation. A small set of two to three objectives is identified for each health indicator and will be used to track and report trends in the indicator. Information related to health indicators includes health impacts, trends, populations particularly affected, and related issues (U.S. Department of Health and Human Services, 2000a). Figure 1–1 ■ depicts the interrelationships among the four elements of the systematic approach taken to improving the health of the nation.

Table 1–3 ■ presents an overview of trends in the national objectives for population health from 1990 to 2010.

As we have seen in this chapter, the community or population group is the primary focus of care in community health nursing. Care is provided to individuals and families with an eye toward improving the health care of

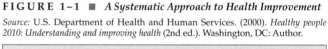

ETHICAL AWARENESS

One of the major changes in the *Healthy People 2010* objectives is the shift from minimizing health disparities among various groups within the population to eliminating them altogether. What are the ethical implications of achieving this goal if it means reducing the level of service provided to groups with better health status in order to to provide additional services to those with poorer health status? What models of ethical decision making would justify such an approach? What ethical arguments could be made against such reductions?

the total population. National health objectives guide the provision of care and serve as a means of evaluating the effectiveness of population health care.

FIGURE 1–1 ■ *A Systematic Approach to Health Improvement*
Source: U.S. Department of Health and Human Services. (2000). *Healthy people 2010: Understanding and improving health* (2nd ed.). Washington, DC: Author.

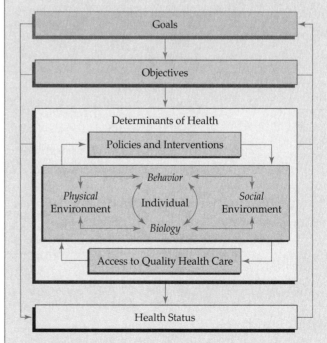

■ **TABLE 1–2   Leading Health Indicators**

Physical activity

Overweight and obesity

Tobacco use

Substance abuse

Responsible sexual behavior

Mental health

Injury and violence

Environmental quality

Immunization

Access to care

■ TABLE 1–3   Trends in National Health Objectives: 1990, 2000, and 2010

Overall Goal

1990:   Reduce mortality

2000:   Increase the span of healthy life
        Reduce disparities in health status among subpopulations
        Achieve access to preventive health services for all

2010:   Increase quality and years of healthy life
        Eliminate disparities in health status among subpopulations

Objective Categories

1990:   Preventive health objectives
        Health protection objectives
        Health promotion objectives

2000:   Health status objectives
        Risk reduction objectives
        Services and protection objectives

2010:   Objectives promoting healthy behaviors
        Objectives promoting healthy and safe communities
        Objectives to improve systems for personal and public health
        Objectives to prevent and reduce diseases and disorders

Focus Areas

1990:   15 priority areas designated

2000:   22 priority areas designated

2010:   28 focus areas designated

Objectives

1990:   226 objectives identified

2000:   319 objectives identified

2010:   467 objectives identified

Progress Toward Achievement

1990:   One third of objectives achieved by target date

2000:   15% of objectives achieved by target date
        44% making progress toward achievement
        18% moving away from the target
        23% untracked

2010:   Not applicable

Other Changes

1990:   Not applicable

2000:   Lead agencies responsible for monitoring progress identified
        Emphasis placed on quality of life as well as longevity
        Special attention given to high-risk groups
        Emphasis given to access to health services
        Baseline data provided where available

2010:   Widespread input into the development of the objectives
        Designation of leading health indicators
        Included a single target for each measurable objective, identified as "better than the best"
        Included developmental objectives
        Development of a common structure for each focus area
        Development of a standard data table for reporting
        progress toward achievement of objectives

APPLYING YOUR KNOWLEDGE IN PRACTICE

❧ CASE STUDY
Caring for Populations

Identify some of the neighborhoods in the area where your nursing program is located.

- What defines these neighborhoods—geographic boundaries, culture, or some other defining feature?
- What kinds of neighborhoods make up the communities in the area? What similarities and differences are there among neighborhoods in a given community? What effects do differences among neighborhoods have on planning health care services? Have these differences been taken into consideration in planning community health services?
- What are some of the subpopulations or aggregates in your community? Select one of these aggregates and determine whether or not the health needs of that group are met within the community. If not, what health needs remain unmet? What could be done to meet the health needs of this aggregate?

❧ TESTING YOUR UNDERSTANDING

- What is the difference between a neighborhood, a community, and an aggregate? (pp. 4–5)
- What are some of the differences between public health and medical practice? What are some ways in which they interface? In what ways could that interface be strengthened? (pp. 6–8)
- What are some of the interactions that might occur between population-focused and person/family-focused nursing? (p. 8)
- Describe trends in national health objectives for 1990, 2000, and 2010. What are the overall goals of each document? What additional features have been added over time? (pp. 8–12)

REFERENCES

Baldwin, J. H., Conger, C. O., Abegglen, J. C., & Hill, E. M. (1998). Population-focused and community-based nursing—Moving toward clarification of concepts. *Public Health Nursing, 15*, 12–18.

Brandt, A. (1999). The challenge: An analysis of past and current practices to identify problems and opportunities of synergistic practice in order to derive educational objectives. In M. Hager (Ed.), *Education for more synergistic practice of medicine and public health* (pp. 23–34). New York: Josiah Macy, Jr. Foundation.

Butler-Jones, D. (1999). Applying a population health approach. *Canadian Journal of Public Health, 90*(Suppl. 1), S62–S64.

Cassells, H. (1997). Community assessment and epidemiology. In J. M. Swanson and M. A. Nies (Eds.), *Community health nursing: Promoting the health of aggregates* (2nd ed.) (pp. 83–116). Philadelphia: Saunders.

Davis, L. J., Okuboye, S., & Ferguson, S. L. (2000). Healthy people 2010: Examining a decade of maternal & infant health. *AWHONN Lifelines, 4*(3), 26–33.

Diekemper, M., SmithBattle, L., & Drake, M. A. (1999). Sharpening the focus on populations: An intentional community health nursing approach. Part II. *Public Health Nursing, 16*(1), 11–16.

Duhl, L. J. (2000). A short history and some acknowledgments. (Healthy communities.) *Public Health Reports, 115*, 116–117.

Fahrenwald, N. L., Fischer, C., Boysen, R., & Maurer, R. (1999). Population-based clinical projects: Bridging community-based and public health concepts. *Nurse Educator, 24*(6), 28–32.

Frankish, J., Veenstra, G., & Moulton, G. (1999). Population health in Canada: Issues and challenges for policy, practice, and research. *Canadian Journal of Public Health, 90*(Suppl. 1), S71–S75.

Friedrich, M. J. (2000). More healthy people in the 21st century? *JAMA, 283*, 37–38.

Helvie, C. O. (1998). *Advanced practice nursing in the community*. Thousand Oaks, CA: Sage.

Hunt, R. (1998). Community-based nursing: Philosophy or setting? *American Journal of Nursing, 98*, 44–47.

Institute of Medicine. (1988). *The future of public health*. Washington, DC: National Academy Press.

Israel, B. A., Schulz, A. J., Parker, E. A., & Becker, A. B. (1998). Review of community-based research: Assessing partnership approaches to improve public health. *Annual Reviews Public Health, 19*, 173–202.

Jamison, D. T., & Mosley, W. H. (1991). Disease control priorities in developing countries: Health policy responses to epidemiological change. *American Journal of Public Health, 81*, 15–22.

Keck, C. W. (1999). Core competencies for the synergistic practice of medicine and public health. In M. Hager (Ed.), *Education for more synergistic practice of medicine and public health* (pp. 238–261). New York: Josiah Macy, Jr. Foundation.

Keller, L. O., Strohschein, S., Lia-Hoagberg, B., & Schaffer, M. (1998). Population-based public health nursing interventions: A model from practice. *Public Health Nursing, 15,* 207–215.

Kone, A., Sullivan, M., Senturia, K., Chrisman, N., Ciske, S. J., & Krieger, J. W. (2000). Improving collaboration between researchers and communities. *Public Health Reports, 115,* 243–250.

Kulbok, P. A., Gates, M. F., Vicenzi, A. E., & Schultz, P. R. (1999). Focus on community: Directions for nursing knowledge development. *Journal of Advanced Nursing, 29,* 1188–1196.

Kuss, T., Proulx-Girouard, L., Lovitt, S., Katz, C. B., & Kennelly, P. (1997). A public health nursing model. *Public Health Nursing, 14,* 81–91.

Lasker, R. D., & the Committee on Medicine and Public Health. (1997). *Public health and medicine: The power of collaboration.* New York: New York Academy of Medicine.

Leavell, H. R., & Clark, E. G. (1965). *Preventive medicine for the doctor in his community: An epidemiologic approach* (3rd ed.). New York: McGraw-Hill.

Lipschutz, R. D. (1995). Healthy environment, healthy community: Promoting community health in California through effective environmental protection, regulation, and education. In California Wellness Foundation/ University of California, *1995 wellness lectures* (pp. 126–157). San Francisco: Author.

Matteson, P. S. (1999). Environmental survey. In *Implementing community based education in the undergraduate nursing curriculum.* Proceedings of the American Association of Colleges of Nursing and Helene Fuld Trust 1999 Faculty Development Workshops on Community-based Education (pp. 31–37). Washington, DC: American Association of Colleges of Nursing.

Matteson, P. S. (2000). Preparing nurses for the future. In P. S. Matteson (Ed.), *Community-based nursing education* (pp. 1–7). New York: Springer.

Milio, N. (1998). Priorities and strategies for promoting community-based prevention policies. *Public Health Management Practice, 4*(3), 14–28.

National Center for Health Statistics. (1992). *Health United States, 1991.* Washington, DC: Government Printing Office.

Norris, T., & Pittman, M. (2000). The healthy communities movement and the coalition for healthier cities and communities. *Public Health Reports, 115,* 118–124.

Pathman, D. E., Steiner, B. D., Williams, E., & Riggins, T. (1998). The four community dimensions of primary care practice. *The Journal of Family Practice, 46,* 293–303.

Richmond, J. B. (1999). Building the next generation of healthy people. *Public Health Reports, 114,* 213–217.

Schneider, M. J. (2000). *Introduction to public health.* Gaithersburg, MD: Aspen.

Schulz, A. J., Parker, E. A., Israel, B. A., Becker, A. B., Maciak, B. J., & Hollis, R. (1998). Conducting a participatory community-based survey for a community health intervention on Detroit's east side. *Journal of Public Health Management Practice, 4*(2), 10–24.

Scutchfield, F. D., & Keck, C. W. (1997). Concepts and definitions of public health practice. In D. F. Scutchfield & C. W. Keck (Eds.), *Principles of public health practice* (pp. 3–9). Albany, NY: Delmar.

Stackhouse, J. C. (1998). *Into the community: Nursing in ambulatory and health care.* Philadelphia: Lippincott.

U.S. Department of Health and Human Services. (1980). *Promoting health/preventing disease: Objectives for the nation.* Washington, DC: Government Printing Office.

U.S. Department of Health and Human Services. (1990). *Healthy people 2000: National health promotion and disease prevention objectives.* Washington, DC: Government Printing Office.

U.S. Department of Health and Human Services. (1995, fall). Healthy people 2000—A mid-decade review. *Prevention Report,* 1–6.

U.S. Department of Health and Human Services. (1996). *Healthy people 2000: Fact sheet.* Washington, DC: Author.

U.S. Department of Health and Human Services. (2000a). *Healthy people 2010* (Conference edition, in two volumes). Washington, DC: Author.

U.S. Department of Health and Human Services. (2000b). *Healthy people 2010: Understanding and improving health* (2nd ed.). Washington, DC: Author.

U.S. Department of Health and Human Services. (2000c). Healthy people 2010: Understanding and improving health. *Prevention Report, 14*(4), 1–2, 4.

Vinicor, F., Burton, B., Forster, B., & Eastman, R. (2000). Healthy people 2010: Diabetes. *Diabetes Care, 23,* 853–855.

Wilcox, R., & Knapp, A. (2000). Building communities that create health. *Public Health Reports, 115,* 139–143.

World Health Organization Regional Office for Europe. (1984). A discussion document on the concept and principles of health promotion. *Health Promotion, 1*(1), 73–76.

THE HISTORICAL CONTEXT

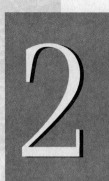

Chapter Objectives

After reading this chapter, you should be able to:

- Identify the contributions of Florence Nightingale and Lillian Wald to the development of community health nursing.
- Discuss the contributions of community health nurses to social and health care reform.
- Discuss the report that prompted creation of the forerunner of the modern board of health.
- List significant historical events in the development of community health nursing in the United States.
- Describe the influence of diagnosis-related groups (DRGs) on community health nursing.
- Describe evidence for a shift in public health policy toward a greater emphasis on health promotion.

KEY TERMS

Media Link

http://www.prenhall.com/clark

Additional interactive resources for this chapter can be found on the companion Web site. Click on Chapter 2 and "Begin" to select the activities for this chapter.

One work on the history of community health nursing stated the "task of the true historian is to relate the past with the present that our future work is more clearly outlined in the light of former mistakes or seemingly feeble beginnings" (Foley, 1985). Knowledge of past social and political events that have shaped the present allows us to identify factors that promote or undermine the health of the public. Such historical awareness also gives us a sense of the direction that community health nursing should take to achieve its goal—improved health for all people. Historical events that gave rise to a concern for the health of population groups influenced the development of both public health science and community health nursing. As noted by Rear Admiral Julia Plotnick (1994), Chief Nurse of the U.S. Public Health Service:

> The profession of public health nursing was created in response to the social, political, and environmental forces that threatened the health of Americans a century ago. Previous generations of public health nurses saw the need for community-based programs that connected the work of health departments and the people at risk. They led many of the policy revolutions that helped bring family planning, workplace safety, and maternal child health services to people in need.

This chapter examines some of the forces that shaped community health nursing practice, with an eye toward understanding how it is practiced today and how it should be practiced in the future.

HISTORICAL ROOTS

The roots of modern public health and community health nursing practice go far back in history. Early historical records provide evidence of concern for health and prevention of disease in several ancient civilizations. As early as 3000 to 1000 B.C., Minoans and Cretans had established drainage systems and flush sewage disposal (Harper & Lambert, 1994). Around 2000 B.C., Hammurabi, king of Babylonia, codified the laws of that land. Portions of the *Code of Hammurabi* specified health practices and regulated the conduct of physicians (Anderson, Morton, & Green, 1978).

In ancient Egypt there was a well-developed system of sewage disposal and personal hygiene measures were encouraged, while Hebrew Mosaic law addressed many aspects of health. Hebrew segregation of lepers and proscriptions against eating pork are examples of early population health measures. Other aspects of Mosaic law specified personal and community responsibilities for maternal health, communicable disease control, fumigation, decontamination of buildings, protection of food and water supplies, waste disposal, and sanitation of campsites (Benson, 1993).

The early Greeks were more concerned with personal than population health, but they practiced many health-promoting behaviors that are encouraged today. These included emphasis on a healthy diet, exercise, and hygiene. Ancient Rome, on the other hand, emphasized the welfare of the total population and developed a number of regulations related to population health. Roman concern for public sanitation was evident in systematic efforts at street cleaning and rubbish removal and in the construction of elaborate water and sewage systems. The Romans also regulated building construction, ventilation, and heating, and mandated nuisance prevention and destruction of decaying goods. In 494 B.C., the Roman Office of Aedile was created to supervise health concerns (Winslow, 1923). This official was the forerunner of today's state or county health officer.

Nursing of the sick at this period in history was the function of the women of the family (Bullough & Bullough, 1993). In the case of large and wealthy households, the matron of the family cared for the health needs of both family members and servants or slaves. The care provided, however, was primarily palliative and was only slightly related to today's concept of nursing.

THE INFLUENCE OF CHRISTIANITY

The Early Church

The advent of Christianity brought an emphasis on personal responsibility for the corporal and spiritual welfare of others. Care of the sick was seen as one means of fulfilling this responsibility, and early Christians employed their time and monetary wealth ministering to the sick. Such efforts were intended to provide comfort and material goods to the sick and suffering (Brainerd, 1985) and bore little resemblance to modern community health nursing. Such services, although lacking an emphasis on prevention and health promotion or cure, did serve to bring about an awareness of illness within the population.

With the growth of Christianity and charitable giving by Christians, the wealth of the early Christian Church began to accumulate. A large portion of this wealth was used for organized care of the sick and needy through almshouses, asylums, and hospitals rather than through personal visitation of the sick. Hospitals or hospices of this time were not designed exclusively for care of the sick but ministered to all in need, including the sick, the poor, and travelers or pilgrims. The first hospital exclusively for the care of the sick was the Nosocomia or "house for the sick," established by the Roman matron Fabiola in the fourth century (Bullough & Bullough, 1993).

The Middle Ages

The mystical tradition of Christianity during the Middle Ages (500–1500 A.D.) led to a decline in population and personal health status. Castigation and neglect of the body to purify the soul resulted in a number of health problems. Many health-promotive activities of antiquity were abandoned in favor of fasting and the wearing of sackcloth and ashes. The need for healthy warriors to fight in the Crusades sparked a slight renewal of interest in health and led to the development of military nursing orders such as the Ancient Order of the Knights of Malta. The function of this order and similar groups was not only military service but also care of the sick and wounded (Kelly, 1981). The creation of these orders was justified in the light of evidence that the majority of casualties suffered in the Crusades were the result of illness rather than battle wounds.

Although the European Crusaders took home with them the Byzantine model of hospital care for the sick with the growth of the military nursing orders, they failed to import the concept of paid professionals to care for the sick. Institutional care for the sick had evolved into a paid occupation in the Byzantine Empire as early as the sixth century, but remained a charitable or family function until the nineteenth century in the West. Eastern nurses, both men and women, received a basic education and passed a qualifying examination making them forerunners of today's registered nurse (Bullough & Bullough, 1993).

Following the Crusades, other religious orders were formed to look after the sick. Groups of monks and nuns established hospitals to care for the ill. In many instances, particular orders would focus on the care of specific groups or illnesses. For instance, the Knights Templar cared for pilgrims, travelers, and soldiers, whereas the Lazarists emphasized care of those with leprosy, smallpox, and pustular fevers (Brainerd, 1985). The concept of specialization among health care providers is not as recent as one might believe.

In addition to the religious orders, groups of laypeople also cared for the sick. One such group was the Beguines, an order of laywomen who tended the sick in both the hospital and the home. The Beguines was a forerunner of modern visiting nurse associations and is an early example of political influence by nurses. Because they refused to accept rules for cloistered orders, they were often at odds with the Church hierarchy and were periodically excommunicated. Their exemplary service to their communities, however, allowed them to enlist the aid of wealthy and influential patrons who prevented the Church from disbanding the order (Brainerd, 1985). The focus of nursing care remained the easing of distress rather than therapeutic or preventive activity.

The concept of quarantine, developed in response to repeated epidemics of bubonic plague, was one of the few advances in public health science during the Middle Ages. Venice banned the entry of infected ships in 1348, and quarantine was officially legislated in Marseilles in 1383 (Anderson, Morton, & Green, 1978).

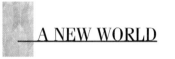

THE EUROPEAN RENAISSANCE

From 1500 to 1700, the European Renaissance gave rise to the beginnings of scientific thought. Also evident were the development of a social conscience and early recognition of social responsibility for the health and welfare of the population. England enacted the first Poor Law in 1601, making families financially responsible for the care of their aged and disabled members and creating publicly funded almshouses for those with no families.

For most of the population, nursing was performed by family members. In 1610, however, St. Francis DeSales and Madame de Chantal established a Parisian voluntary organization of well-to-do women to care for the sick in their homes, and in 1617 St. Vincent De Paul founded the order of the Sisters of Charity to care for the needs of the sick poor (Byrd, 1995). The activities of this order approximated those of a modern visiting nurse service and incorporated the use of field supervisors for sisters making home visits (Brainerd, 1985).

A NEW WORLD

The Colonial Period

While new avenues of scientific thought were being opened in Europe, some of the ideas generated were being translated into a new way of life on a new continent. In the early colonial period in America, the health status of those living in the colonies was good compared with that of their European counterparts, and longevity at that time approached today's figures for life expectancy. The relative good health of the population was due primarily to low population density and, interestingly, poor transportation. Communities remained relatively isolated, and the spread of communicable diseases, the major health problem of the era, was curtailed by lack of movement between population groups (Fee, 1997).

Because doctors were few, health care was primarily a function of the family. Nursing care in the United States was provided by the women of the family, with assistance from neighbors where this was possible. In Canada, early public health practice was carried out by Christian religious orders as early as the seventeenth century. One of the early Canadian public health activitists was nurse Jeanne Mance, who arrived in "New France" in 1659. Mance co-founded the Hotel Dieu in Montreal and provided leadership for a variety of other community health efforts (Duncan, Leipart, & Mill, 1999).

Early Public Health Efforts

The growth of population centers led to concern for sanitation and vital statistics, the foci of early public health efforts in the colonies. In 1639, both Massachusetts and Plymouth colonies mandated the reporting of all births and deaths, instituting the official reporting of vital statistics in what would later become the United States. Environmental health and sanitation were also of concern in the early colonies. Evidence of such concern is found in legislation passed in 1647 prohibiting pollution of Boston Harbor (Anderson, Morton, & Green, 1978).

Control of communicable disease was another concern as populations increased in size. In 1701, Massachusetts passed legislation regarding isolation of smallpox victims and quarantine of ships in Boston Harbor. For the most part, health was seen as a personal responsibility with little governmental involvement. Temporary boards of health were established in response to specific health problems, usually epidemics of communicable disease, and were disbanded after the crisis had passed. The first such board of health in the United States was established in Petersburg, Virginia, in 1780. Similar temporary state boards of health were established in New York and Massachusetts in 1797 (Smolensky, 1982). Early public health efforts in Canada were also crisis oriented, and centralized action on public health issues was strongly resisted (Duncan et al., 1999).

Recognition of the need for a consistent and organized approach to health problems was growing, however, and in 1797, the state of Massachusetts granted local jurisdictions legal authority to establish health services and regulations. The following year, Congress passed the Act for Relief of Sick and Disabled Seamen to create hospitals for the care of members of the merchant marine. The group of hospitals created under this act was renamed the Marine Hospital Service in 1871 (Fee, 1997). The act also provided for a systematic approach to quarantine of seaports as one of the first efforts to deal with health problems at a national, rather than a state or local, level.

Nursing during this period remained a function of the family. Although the care given was primarily palliative, the women of the house might also engage in some health-promotive practices, such as regular purging with castor oil. Treatment tended to rely on home remedies, and the literature of the era is replete with housewives' recipes for a variety of ailments.

In 1813, the Ladies' Benevolent Society of Charleston, South Carolina, was established. This was the first organized approach to home nursing of the sick in the United States. This organization was initiated in response to a yellow fever epidemic and was completely nondenominational and nondiscriminatory in an era characterized by widespread racial discrimination. Care was provided to the sick in their homes by upper-class women. Because these women had no background in nursing, care focused on relieving suffering and providing material aid (Brainerd, 1985). With the exception of a 20-year period during and after the Civil War, the Ladies' Benevolent Society provided services until the 1950s.

A similar service was instituted in 1819 in Philadelphia's Jewish community by the Hebrew Female Benevolent Society of Philadelphia. This service was organized by Rebecca Gratz, a Jewish society woman believed to be the model for Sir Walter Scott's Rebecca (Benson, 1993).

Another early attempt at home care nursing also saw upper-class women visiting the homes of indigent women during childbirth. The Lying-in Charity for Attending Indigent Women in Their Homes was established in 1832. The purpose of this organization was to assist poor women during and after delivery. Because of their lack of training, the services provided by these women emphasized social and emotional support for the woman in labor and assistance to her after delivery.

THE INDUSTRIAL REVOLUTION

The *Industrial Revolution* profoundly influenced health in both Europe and the United States. Movement on both continents from agricultural to industrial economies led to the development of large industrial centers and the need for a large work force to labor under unhealthy conditions in mines, mills, and factories. The demand for manufactured goods and the necessity to get goods to market prompted advancements in transportation that increased mobility and the potential for spreading communicable diseases. In the United States, rural–urban migration and the presence of large contingents of poor immigrants, who came to escape the poverty of their homelands, created crowded living conditions that further enhanced the potential for disease (Estabrooks, 1995).

The poor were overworked and underpaid. Poor nutrition contributed to increased incidence of a variety of diseases, particularly tuberculosis. Recognition of tuberculosis as a growing problem led to the creation of the first tuberculosis hospital in England in 1840 (Zilm & Warbinek, 1995). The use of children in the workforce, coupled with low wages, inadequate food, and hazardous living and working conditions, led to many preventable illnesses and deaths among the children of the poor (Estabrooks, 1995).

The nineteenth century saw a beginning recognition of the effects of these social and economic conditions on health, and the concept of social responsibility for public health began to take root. The growth of this concept was fostered by the publication in the mid-1800s of several landmark reports. The first of these publications was C. Turner Thackrah's treatise on occupational health, *The Effects of Arts, Trades, and Professions . . . on Health and Longevity*. In this document, Thackrah described the effects of working conditions on health. In 1842, Edwin Chadwick's *Inquiry into the Sanitary Conditions of the Labouring Population of Great Britain* provided additional fuel for reformers' efforts to change the working and social conditions that contributed to disease.

While Thackrah and Chadwick addressed the effects of working conditions on health and instigated reforms to prevent disease, Henry W. Rumsey focused on health promotion. Rumsey's *Essays on State Medicine* emphasized health promotion and illness prevention as social obligations of government. His description of the functions of a proposed district medical officer embodied most aspects of modern community health programs (Rosen, 1974).

Similar documents were published in the United States. The Massachusetts Sanitary Commission was established in response to concern over the effects of crowded living conditions, poverty, and poor sanitation on health. In 1850, Lemuel Shattuck drafted the commission's findings, aptly titled the ***Report of the Massachusetts Sanitary Commission.*** This report included recommendations for establishing state and local health departments, systematic collection of vital statistics, and sanitation inspections and instituting programs for school health and control of mental illness, alcohol abuse, and tuberculosis. Other recommendations included public education regarding sanitation, control of nuisances, periodic physical examinations, supervision of the health of immigrants, and construction of model tenements. In addition, the report recommended improved education for nurses and the inclusion of content on preventive medicine and sanitation in medical school curricula.

Publication of the *Report of the Massachusetts Sanitary Commission* marks the beginning of community health practice as we know it today (Epidemiology Program Office, 1999). Recommendations of the report form the basis for much of the present work of official state and local public health agencies. The eventual effect of the commission's report was the establishment of state boards of health. The first state board was established in Louisiana in 1855, but has been described as a "paper organization." In 1869, nearly 90 years after the advent of the first temporary boards of health and 19 years after publication of Shattuck's report, Massachusetts established the first working board of health, followed by California in 1870 (Fee, 1997). These first permanent boards, similar to modern boards of health, emphasized six aspects of community health practice: inspection of housing, public education in hygiene, investigation of disease, regulation of slaughterhouses, regulation of the sale of poisons, and health care for the poor (Anderson, Morton, & Green, 1978).

Collection of vital statistics at the national level was another activity undertaken in the later half of the nineteenth century. The first national mortality statistics, for example, were published by the U.S. federal government in 1950 (Epidemiology Program Office, 1999).

Community health nurses visited clients in many different settings. (Photo courtesy of the Visiting Nurse Association of Boston)

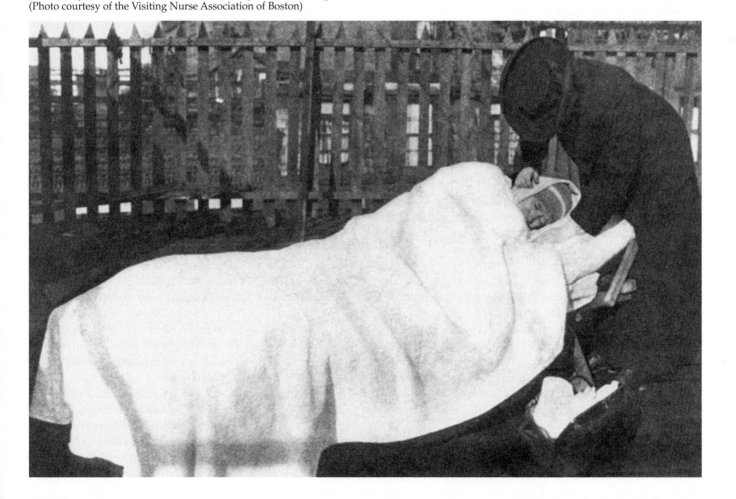

HIGHLIGHTS

Reports Influencing Early Public Health Efforts

- *The Effects of Arts, Trades and Professions . . . on Health and Longevity* (C. Turner Thackrah)
  Addressed the effects of working conditions on health.
- *Inquiry into the Sanitary Conditions of the Labouring Population of Great Britain* (Edwin Chadwick, 1842)
  Exposed the health effects of occupational and social conditions in Great Britain.
- *Essays on State Medicine* (Henry W. Rumsey)
  Proposed that public health promotion and illness prevention were social responsibilities of government.
- *Report of the Massachusetts Sanitary Commission* (Lemuel Shattuck, 1850)
  Reported on health-related conditions in Massachusetts and recommended several approaches for dealing with them including establishing permanent boards of health, collection of vital statistics, sanitation inspections, school health programs, nuisance control, and public education.

During this period, great strides were being made in the fledgling science of epidemiology. In 1856, without knowledge of the nature of the causative organism, John Snow determined the source of a London epidemic of cholera to be something in the water of the Broad Street pump. It was not, however, until 1877 that Louis Pasteur and Robert Koch, working independently, identified specific bacteria. These and other epidemiologic findings allowed more scientific measures to be applied to the control of communicable disease and contributed greatly to the armamentarium used by later community health nurses in preventing disease.

DISTRICT NURSING IN ENGLAND

The "three great revolutions" of the late eighteenth and early nineteenth centuries—the intellectual revolution, the French and American political revolutions, and the Industrial Revolution—set the stage for the development of community health nursing. In England, the same spirit that motivated industrial and prison reform led to concern for the health of large urban populations and development of nursing practices to address these concerns.

In addition to being the acknowledged founder of modern hospital nursing, *Florence Nightingale* was instrumental in the development of community health or

district nursing. Nightingale received her training in nursing at the school for deaconesses established by Theodor Fliedner. Fliedner's second wife, Caroline Bertheau, conceived the idea of extending the nursing services offered in the hospital to the sick in their homes. This concept influenced Nightingale, who endorsed the idea of health promotion as well as home care for illness (Falk Rafael, 1999).

In 1859, Nightingale assisted William Rathbone to form the first district public health nursing association in England. The organization was funded by philanthropic citizens and hired trained nurses who were assigned to specific districts in London. Each nurse was responsible for the health needs of the people in her district. The nurses were viewed as social reformers as well as providers of care for the sick, evidence of the early development of the advocacy role of the community health nurse (Falk Rafael, 1999).

The need to standardize community health nursing services was recognized early in the development of the district nursing associations. The East London Nursing Society was established for this purpose but proved ineffective. Subsequently, investigation of the district nursing system revealed a need for a national association. As a result, the Metropolitan and National Nursing Association for Providing Trained Nurses for the Sick Poor was established in 1875. This group fostered employment of educated women in public health nursing as a step toward the professionalization of nursing.

One of the first activities of the association, which was headed by Florence Lees, a protege of Nightingale, was a study of the need for public health nursing, the personnel available, and the training required and work done by district nurses. Results of the study of 115 district nurses employed by various organizations throughout London indicated that the work done by those nurses who were trained was effective. Unfortunately, more than half of those studied had no training in public health and were found to be insufficiently prepared for their role in the unsupervised care of the sick. Hospital training was found to be inadequate for district nursing, and a recommendation was made that district nurses receive three months of training in public health in addition to their year of hospital training (Brainerd, 1985).

The district nursing associations embodied three of the principles of modern community health nursing. The first of these, as noted above, was the need for special training for nurses working in the community. By 1889, this need had been widely recognized. At that time, monies donated to Queen Victoria's Jubilee fund were allocated to Queen Victoria's Jubilee Institute for Nursing (Cohen, 1997). The Institute was established to prepare nurses for community health practice and to extend community health nursing throughout the British Empire. A program was instituted to provide an additional six-month educational experience for community health

HIGHLIGHTS

Contributions of Florence Nightingale to Public Health Nursing

- Endorsed the concept of health promotion as well as care of the sick
- Established, with William Rathbone, the first district public health nursing association
- Promoted advanced education for public health nursing practice
- Divorced nursing care from provision of material assistance
- Divorced care of the sick in their homes from religious proselytizing

nurses following the initial three years of training in the hospital (Gardner, 1952).

The second principle of modern community health nursing embodied in the district nursing associations was the separation of nursing care from the provision of material goods. As noted earlier, many early efforts at visiting the sick focused on dealing with material needs through the distribution of money, food, or clothing. The district nursing concept eliminated such charitable activities from the role of the nurse and focused on the provision of nursing care per se. This principle was strongly supported by Florence Nightingale as a primary difference between district nurses and "philanthropic visitors" (Montiero, 1987).

The third principle was the prohibition of religious proselytizing by the nurses. Again, because much prior visiting of the sick had been done in the name of Christian charity, visits had been used as an opportunity to encourage supposed sinners to mend their evil ways. Much of this type of activity derived from convictions that poverty, illness, and suffering were punishment for sins and that repentance was needed.

CULTURAL CONSIDERATIONS

Early community health nursing leaders were products of the culture and society of their times, yet many of them put aside cultural expectations of marriage and family to devote their energies to improving the health of the public. Explore the life and times of one of these leaders. What factors in her development led her to move outside of cultural prescriptions for women? In what ways did they continue to display their cultural heritage? Would these women face similar challenges today? Why or why not?

VISITING NURSES IN AMERICA

In the United States, proselytizing was also part of the role of nurses who provided early home care to the sick poor; however, efforts had been made to incorporate the provision of *nursing care* in addition to proselytizing and providing for material needs. In 1877, the Women's Branch of the New York City Mission employed Frances Root as the first salaried American nurse to visit the sick poor. Her role, and that of many *missionary nurses* to follow her, was to provide nursing care and religious instruction for the sick poor (Brainerd, 1985).

In 1878, the Ethical Culture Society of New York employed four nurses in dispensaries, inaugurating the ambulatory care role of the community health nurse. These nurses worked under the supervision of a physician and emphasized health teaching as well as illness care (Brainerd, 1985). In the next few years, *visiting nurse associations* were established in Buffalo (1885), and in Boston and Philadelphia (1886). The Philadelphia agency was the first to institute a nurse's uniform, a fee for services, and the community nursing supervisor. The Boston Instructive Visiting Nurse Association emphasized the community health nurse's educative function as well as her role in the care of the sick, signaling the beginning of the health promotion emphasis that now characterizes community health nursing. Similar events were taking place in Canada with the establishment of the *Victorian Order of Nurses (VON)* in 1897 and the hiring of the first community health nurse in British Columbia in 1901 (Zilm & Warbinek, 1995). Although initiated to provide midwifery services on the Northwest frontier, medical opposition to nurse midwifery led to a shift in focus to home visiting services in urban areas (Richardson, 1998). By 1890, visiting nurse services were available in 21 U.S. cities (Novak, 1988), and 22 years later, when the National Organization for Public Health Nursing (NOPHN) was founded, there were 3,000 visiting nurses in the United States (Winslow, 1993). Similarly, Alberta's District Nursing Service, founded in 1919 with three nurses, grew to encompass 13 nurses by 1935 and 35 by 1950 (Richardson, 1998).

NURSING AND THE SETTLEMENT HOUSES

The settlement movement was based on the belief espoused by Arnold Toynbee that educated persons could promote learning, morality, and civic responsibility in the poor by living among them and sharing certain aspects of their poverty. Groups of students from Oxford and Cambridge, acting on this belief, "settled" in homes in the London slums with the idea that their poor neighbors would learn through watching their behavior (Erickson, 1987).

⑤THINK ABOUT IT

Would the settlement house concept be an effective approach to meeting the health care needs of the U.S. public today? Why or why not?

___

In the United States, the settlement idea was adapted by nurses such as **Lillian Wald,** who believed that the most effective way to bring health care to the poor immigrant population was for nurses to live and work among them. Accordingly, Wald and her associate Mary Brewster established the forerunner of the **Henry Street Settlement** in New York City in 1893. The actual Henry Street establishment was purchased in 1895 and incorporated in 1901. The house on Henry Street differed from many other settlement houses of the era in its incorporation of visiting nurse services (Estabrooks, 1995).

The Henry Street Settlement is usually considered the first American community health agency because of its incorporation of modern concepts of community health nursing. The nurses of the Henry Street Settlement did more than visit the sick in their homes. Health promotion and disease prevention were heavily emphasized, as was political activism. Wald herself was a prime example of the political activist, supporting many changes in social conditions that would benefit the health of the public (Coss, 1989). Lillian Wald is said to have coined the term *public health nurse* (Kuss, Proulx-Girouard, Lovitt, Katz, & Kennelly, 1997) and, as noted by one historian, "has been credited with being the first person to view nursing as a relationship between the nurse and the public rather than the nurse and the individual or hospital ward" (Fritz, 1995, p. 214).

⑤THINK ABOUT IT

What would the modern equivalent of a settlement house be like?

___

Many families who received community health nurses lived in a single room.
(Photo courtesy of the Visiting Nurse Association of Boston)

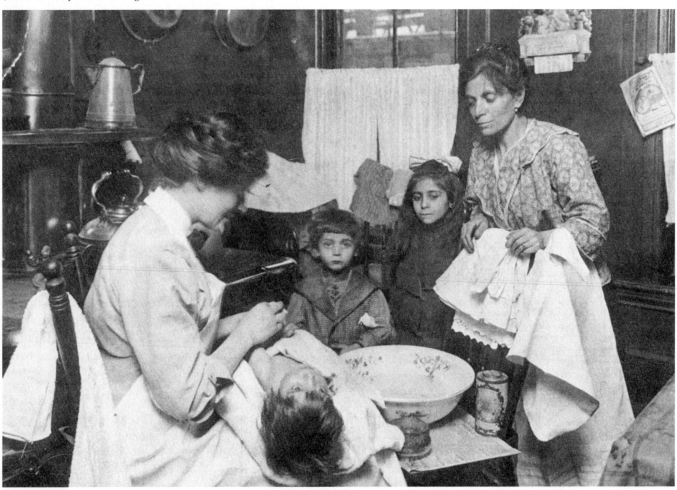

CRITICAL THINKING IN RESEARCH

It is important for community health nurses to understand the forces that shaped their practice in the past and continue to influence community health nursing today. Historical research can provide us with this understanding.

- When did community health nursing originate in your area? What was the impetus for its development? Who were the nurses who were influential in its development? How has local community health nursing changed with time? What factors prompted those changes?
- Where would you begin to look for answers to the questions posed above? What documents might provide information? Where might you find them?
- Are there people still living who might be able to shed light on those events? How would you go about finding them? What would you want to ask them? Why?

Other Henry Street nurses like *Lavinia Dock* and *Margaret Sanger* were also actively involved in promoting social change (Estabrooks, 1995). In fact, the Henry Street nurses have been described as "virtually independent practitioners in sick and preventive care, health, education, and school nursing" in an era when other nurses were experiencing medical domination (Roberts & Group, 1995, p. 82).

Other nursing settlement houses patterned on the Henry Street model were established. One particularly inspiring example was the Nurse's Settlement established in 1900 in Richmond, Virginia, by the graduating class of Old Dominion Hospital. These nurses had been exposed to the needs of Richmond's poor during student experiences with the Instructive Visiting Nurse Association of Richmond. The settlement they founded differed from the Henry Street Settlement in that it did not have any wealthy patrons to provide support and was initiated with the limited resources of the graduates themselves. Like Henry Street, the Richmond settlement focused on health promotion and education as well as care of the sick (Erickson, 1987).

EXPANDING THE FOCUS ON PREVENTION

The effectiveness of community health nurses in preventing sickness and death among the poor was recognized and became the basis for visiting nurse services offered by the Metropolitan Life Insurance Company (Hamilton, 1988). This program was begun at the instigation of Lee Frankel and Lillian Wald. Wald convinced the Metropolitan board that providing nursing services to its policyholders would improve the public image of an industry tarnished by economic scandal. The telling argument, though, was evidence that community health nursing reduced mortality and would limit the benefits paid by the company. Services were begun on an experimental basis in 1909 with one of the Henry Street nurses.

The three-month experiment was such a success that the program was extended and continued to provide services until 1953. This association with the business world was an education for community health nurses who had no conception of marketing or economic bases for programs. The program was finally discontinued because of nursing's failure to grasp economic realities and the realization of diminishing returns by the insurance company (Hamilton, 1989).

The emphasis of community health nursing on health promotion began with health in the home during visits to the poor in large cities. Gradually, however, the concepts of health promotion and illness prevention were expanded to other population groups to include services to mothers and young children, school-age youngsters, employees, and the rural population.

Concern for the health of mothers and children was growing, and the nurses of the Henry Street Settlement and other similar programs spent a large portion of their time in health promotion for this group of clients. Because they recognized that services to individual families would not overcome the effects of poverty, they worked actively to improve social conditions affecting health (SmithBattle, Diekemper, & Drake, 1999). Because of the efforts of Lillian Wald and other social activists, the first White House Conference on Children was held in 1909. As a result of the conference, the U.S. Children's Bureau was established in 1912 to address the issue of child labor. Its efforts were later expanded to encompass a variety of initiatives related to child health (Hefland, Lazarus, & Theerman, 2000).

School nursing, another arena for health promotion, actually began in London in 1892 and was introduced in the United States by Lillian Wald of the Henry Street Settlement (Igoe, 1994). The initial impetus for school health nursing was the high level of school absenteeism due to illness. In New York City in 1902, 15 to 20 children per school were being sent home daily. In response, Wald assigned Lina Struthers from the Henry Street Settlement to a pilot project in school nursing. Because of the overwhelming success of the project, the New York Board of Health absorbed the program and hired additional nurses to continue the work (Jossens & Ferjancsik, 1996).

The concept of school nursing spread to other parts of the country and to Canada. In 1904, Los Angeles became the first of many municipalities to employ nurses in schools (Gardner, 1952). In 1906, the Montreal Board of Health initiated medical inspections of school children, later appointing a VON nurse to a school nursing position. School nurses were also appointed in Hamilton in 1909 and Toronto in 1910 (Duncan et al., 1999).

Early school nursing focused on preventing the spread of communicable diseases and treating ailments related

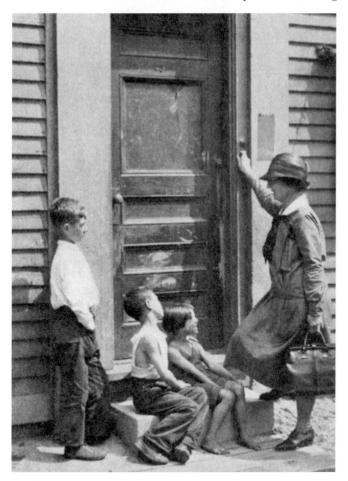

In addition to school inspections, community health nurses made home visits to children excluded from school for communicable diseases.
(Photo courtesy of the Visiting Nurse Association of Boston)

to compulsory school life. By the 1930s, however, the focus had shifted to preventive and promotive activities including case finding, integrating health concepts into school curricula, and maintaining a healthful school environment (Igoe, 1980).

The first rural nursing service was established in 1896 in Westchester County, New York, by Ellen Morris Wood and was followed in 1906 with the initiation of a nursing service for both the poor and the well-to-do of Salisbury, Connecticut. Despite her usual sphere of activity in the city, Lillian Wald was also involved in the growth of rural community health nursing. She convinced the **American Red Cross,** founded in 1881, to direct its peacetime attention to expanding community health services in rural America. In 1912, the Red Cross established the **Rural Nursing Service** (later the Town and Country Nursing Service) to extend community health nursing services to rural areas (Brainerd, 1985). In Canada, rural nursing services were provided to large immigrant populations by such organizations as the Victorian Order of Nurses for Canada, the Canadian Red Cross Society, and the Women's Missionary Society (Bramadat & Saydak, 1993).

Other largely rural populations experiencing significant health problems were the Native American population on federal reservations and the African Americans in the South. Community health nursing services on the reservations arose out of a 1922 study of health conditions by the American Red Cross commissioned by the Bureau of Indian Affairs (Ruffing-Rahal, 1995). Nurses in this setting often found themselves breaking official rules in order to provide effectively for the needs of their clients (Abel, 1996). To meet the needs of black women in the South, some states co-opted local black midwives to work closely with public health nurses. As on the reservations, the rules imposed frequently violated accepted cultural health practices. For example, the nurses "forbade midwives to use any folk medicine or herbal remedies in their childbirth work" (Smith, 1994). In spite of the cultural insensitivity displayed, the partnership between public health nurses and midwives helped to create a modern public health system in the rural South.

Occupational health nursing provided another avenue for health promotion by community health nurses. This specialty area began in 1895 when Vermont's Governor Proctor employed nurses to see to the health needs of villages where employees of his Vermont Marble Company lived (Novak, 1988). In 1897, the Employees' Benefit Association of John Wanamaker's department store in New York City hired nurses to visit employee's homes. These nurses soon expanded their role to include first aid and prevention of illness and injury in the work setting. The number of firms employing nurses increased rapidly from 66 in 1910 to 871 by 1919 (Brainerd, 1985). About this same time, Simmons College offered a certificate program in industrial nursing, acknowledging the need for advanced educational preparation for this specialty area (Golden & Moore, 1986). Based on the demonstrated efficacy of nurses in occupational settings, a 1943 study by the U.S. Public Health Service recommended one nurse

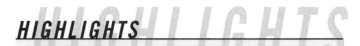

HIGHLIGHTS

Contributions of Lillian Wald to Public Health Nursing

• Establishment of the Henry Street Settlement
• Establishment of the Metropolitan Life Insurance home visiting program
• Promotion of social and political activism by public health nurses
• Initiation of school nursing practice
• Emphasis on health promotion and health education
• Establishment of the U.S. Children's Bureau
• Establishment of the Red Cross Nursing Service

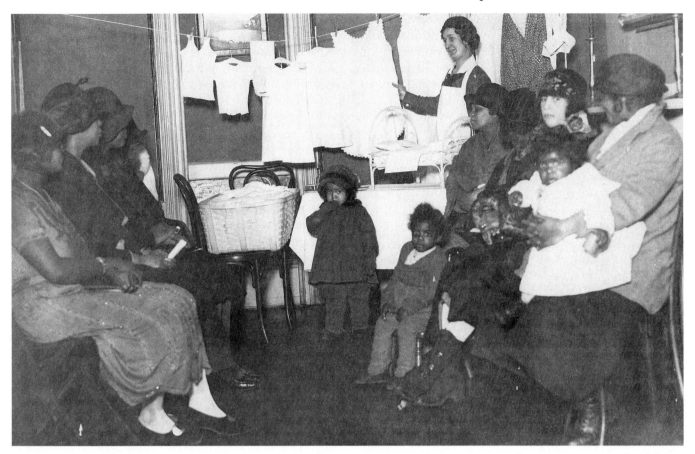

Health education has always been an important role for community health nurses.
(Photo courtesy of the Visiting Nurse Association of Boston)

for every 300 factory workers to provide health services and engage in advocacy (Anglin, 1990).

Health promotion activities by community health nurses were often combined with advocacy efforts. The work of Margaret Sanger is a striking example. Sanger was instrumental in initiating the National Birth Control League in 1913, and in 1916 opened the first birth control clinic in the United States. Despite serious opposition and her arrest, Sanger persisted. She eventually succeeded in her efforts to make contraceptive information and services available to American women and after World War II founded the International Planned Parenthood Federation to carry on her work (Fritz, 1995; Roberts & Group, 1995).

ETHICAL AWARENESS

> Part of the impetus for the Children's Bureau was the use of child labor. This practice occurs today in underdeveloped countries and on U.S. farms. What are the ethical implications of child labor that allows families to meet basic survival needs? Are the implications similar or different for underdeveloped countries and U.S. farm families? Why?

STANDARDIZING PRACTICE

The need to standardize community nursing practice was recognized in both the United States and England. Early American attempts to standardize visiting nursing services included publications related to public health nursing and development of a national logo by the Cleveland Visiting Nurse Association (VNA). This logo, or seal, was made available to any visiting nurse organization that met established standards. Both the Chicago (1906) and Cleveland (1909) VNAs published newsletters titled *Visiting Nurse Quarterly* to aid attempts to standardize care (Brainerd, 1985).

In 1911, a joint committee of the American Nurses Association and the Society for Superintendents of Training Schools for Nurses met to consider the need for standardization. The result was a second meeting held in 1912. Letters inviting representation were sent to 1,092 organizations employing visiting nurses at that time. These organizations included VNAs, city and state boards of health and education, private clubs and societies, tuberculosis leagues, hospitals and dispensaries, businesses, settlements and day nurseries, churches, and charitable organizations. A total of 69 agencies responded with their intent to send a representative to the meeting.

The result of this second meeting was the formation of the *National Organization for Public Health Nursing (NOPHN)* (Brainerd, 1985). The objective of this organization was to provide for stimulation and standardization of public health nursing. This was the first professional body in the United States to include lay membership. In Canada, similar activity was undertaken, leading to the creation in 1920 of the public health section of the Canadian Association of Trained Nurses (Duncan et al., 1999).

The NOPHN was influential in maintaining public health nursing services at home during World War I and in the organization of the Division of Public Health Nursing within the U.S. Public Health Service in 1944. The NOPHN also provided advisory services regarding postgraduate education for public health nursing in colleges and universities. The NOPHN was incorporated into the *National League for Nursing (NLN)* in the 1952 restructuring of professional nursing organizations.

EDUCATING COMMUNITY HEALTH NURSES

During the 1920s, nursing education was under study. The *Goldmark Report, Nursing and Nursing Education in the United States,* published in 1923, dealt with nursing education in general and pointed out the need for advanced preparation for community health nursing. The report recommended that nursing education take place in institutions of higher learning. At the same time, the American Medical Association's Committee on Trained Nursing recommended university education for management or teaching functions in specialty areas (Krampitz, 1987). As a result, the Yale University School of Nursing and the Frances Payne Bolton School of Nursing at Western Reserve University opened in 1923. Canada's first baccalaureate program in nursing (also the first in the British Empire) was established in 1919 at the University of British Columbia (Duncan et al., 1999). The curricula of both U.S. and Canadian programs included community health nursing content.

Prior to the education of nurses in university settings, special postgraduate courses in public health nursing had been established by various agencies. The first of these in the United States was undertaken by the Instructive District Nursing Association of Boston in 1906. In 1910, Teachers' College of Columbia University offered the first course in public health nursing in an institution of higher learning (Brainerd, 1985). In 1949, NOPHN developed criteria for evaluating courses in public health nursing (Golden & Moore, 1986). In Canada, the Canadian Red Cross Society instituted a 14-week certificate course for public health nurses in 1920 (Zilm & Warbinek, 1995). The

first such course was offered by the University of Alberta in 1918 (Duncan et al., 1999).

In addition to witnessing the movement of community health nursing education to institutions of higher learning, the 1920s saw a shift in employment of public health nurses. Before this time, most public health nursing services were provided by voluntary agencies such as the Red Cross and similar organizations. During the 1920s, however, public health nursing services began to be taken over by official governmental agencies such as local and state health departments (Bigbee & Crowder, 1985). In 1937, 67% of all community health nurses were employed by official public health agencies (Winslow, 1993). This same incorporation of public health nurses into governmental agencies began in Canada in the early 1900s (Matuk & Horsburgh, 1989).

The *Brown Report* of 1948, *Nursing for the Future,* reemphasized the need for nurses to be educated in institutions of higher learning so as to prepare them to meet community health needs (Benson & McDevitt, 1976). A similar, but earlier, report in Canada, *Survey of Nursing Education in Canada* (Weir, 1932), also known as the *Weir Report,* had recommended advanced educational preparation for community health nurses, particularly those practicing in rural areas. In 1964, the American Nurses Association (ANA) formally defined the public health nurse as a graduate of a baccalaureate program in nursing. In 1995, the Pew Health Professions Commission report, *Critical Challenges: Revitalizing the Health Professions,* reinforced baccalaureate education as the entry level for community-based practice. Today, in some states, such as California, only graduates from baccalaureate programs in nursing can be certified as public health nurses. Moreover, there are now master's and doctoral programs with a community health nursing focus.

FEDERAL INVOLVEMENT IN HEALTH CARE

For most of its history the federal government has left health matters to the states. It was not until 1879 that the United States established a National Board of Health in response to a yellow fever epidemic. This board continued to function until 1883 when it was dissolved. In 1912, the need for a permanent national agency responsible for the country's health was recognized, and the *U.S. Public Health Service (USPHS)* was created out of the reorganization of the Marine Hospital Service (Fee, 1997). In that same year, federal legislation was passed creating the office of the Surgeon General and mandating federal involvement in health promotion. It was not until 1953, however, that the need for advisement on health matters at the cabinet level was recognized with the creation of the Department of Health, Education, and Welfare. This department was reorganized in 1980 to create the present Department of Health and Human Services (DHHS).

Since the beginning of the twentieth century, the federal government has become progressively more involved in health care delivery. Unfortunately, this involvement has been rather haphazard, dependent on the interests and concerns of differing administrations. In the early years of the twentieth century, the health needs of specific segments of the population began to be recognized, resulting in federal programs designed to enhance the health of mothers and children, the poor, those with sexually transmitted diseases, the mentally ill, and others. For example, in 1921, Congress passed the Sheppard–Towner Act to help state and local agencies meet the health needs of mothers and children (Pollit, 1991). In addition to providing funds for maternity centers, prenatal care, and child health clinics, the legislation provided monies to enhance visiting nurse services (Krampitz, 1987). These funds allowed local agencies, for example, the San Diego County Health Department, to hire additional community health nurses known as "Sheppard–Towner nurses" (Interview). Later, recognition of the need for federal support of health care research to address the health needs of mothers and children and other special groups led to the development of the National Institutes of Health in 1930.

As a result of the Great Depression of the 1930s, the federal government became even more active in health and social welfare programs. Jobs were created to employ thousands of the unemployed. Nurses were also employed at this time to meet the health needs of the population. The first public health nurse was employed by USPHS in 1934.

Recognition of the economic plight of the elderly led to passage of the *Social Security Act* in 1935, 60 years after the efforts of Lavinia Dock and others to provide health care to the elderly poor. This act established the Old Age Survivors Insurance Program (OASI, better known as Social Security) to improve the financial status of the elderly. In 1966, the Social Security Act was amended to create the Medicare program funding health care for older Americans. Medicaid, a program that funds health care for the indigent, was instituted in 1967. These two programs contributed to increased demands for health care services and resulted in rapid increases in the cost of health care.

World War II also influenced health care delivery. Wage and price freezes and a dearth of skilled labor led industries to offer health insurance benefits in an attempt to compete for competent workers (McGuire & Anderson, 1999). During the war, some 15 million U.S. service members were exposed to quality health care, some for the first time in their lives. Afterward, these veterans began to demand the same quality of care for themselves and their families in the civilian sector. This increased demand for care led to new arrangements for

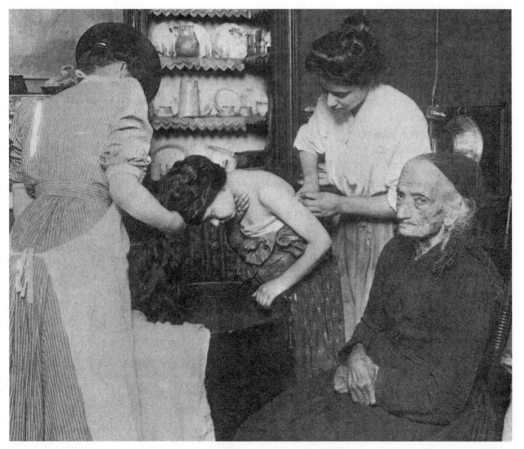

Community health nurses often demonstrated appropriate hygiene practices as well as teaching about them.
(Photo courtesy of the Visiting Nurse Association of Boston)

financing health care and a subsequent burgeoning of the health insurance industry. The growth in health insurance was further influenced by the 1954 inclusion of premiums as legitimate tax deductions (Ginzberg, 1985). This development led to the use of insurance benefits as a tax-deductible substitute for higher wages in business and industry. Because such benefits were tax exempt for employees, they were readily accepted in lieu of salary increases by unions and other bargaining agents.

Increased demands for services also led to a lack of adequate facilities, especially in nonurban areas. In 1946, pressured by USPHS officials, Congress responded with passage of the Hill–Burton Act to finance hospital construction in underserved areas (Lasker, 1997). Hospital construction and insurance coverage for care provided in the hospital further strengthened the national emphasis on curative rather than preventive care and widened the gap between bedside nursing and health promotion and prevention. In fact, a 1928 Bureau of Indian Affairs (BIA) circular directed BIA public health field nurses that it was "unwise to make bedside care the greatest factor, as the hospital should be used to a larger extent than is customary at present" (Abel, 1996). Hospitals became a major focus for health and illness care. Ironically, during this same period, the first hospital-based home care program was established at Montefiore Hospital (Jonas & Rosenberg, 1986), setting a precedent for the burgeoning home care industry of today. The present emphasis on cost containment has led to a shift away from institutional care and more home and community-based care. This development has also resulted in a growing need for community health nurses to provide home health services.

Acknowledging the growing demand for health care and recognizing the differing abilities of certain areas of the country to meet those needs, the U.S. federal government responded with the Comprehensive Health Planning Act of 1966 and the National Health Planning and Resources Development Act of 1974. Both pieces of legislation were attempts to organize the planning of health care delivery to meet differing needs throughout the country (Sofaer, 1988). Unfortunately, both efforts failed. One positive effect of the 1974 act was recognition of the contribution of nurse practitioners to the health status of the public, nine years after the establishment of the first nurse practitioner program in 1965 (Jenkins & Sullivan-Marx, 1994).

The Child Health Act of 1967 and the Health Maintenance Organization Act of 1973 also recommended use of nurses in extended roles. The 1971 publication of a report entitled *Extending the Scope of Nursing Practice* provided additional support for the use of nurses in expanded capacities. Subsequent legislation has led to the increased use of nurse practitioners in a variety of settings. Over the last few years, there has been increased use of community health nurses with advanced educational preparation as nurse practitioners providing primary care to selected populations.

While the United States was attempting to decentralize health care policy making through health planning legislation, efforts were being made elsewhere to focus attention on risk factors for population health problems. The **Lalonde Report**, *New Perspectives for the Health of Canadians*, was published in Canada in 1974, identifying the importance of biological, environmental, and lifestyle risks as determinants of health and recommending greater attention to elimination of risks in each of these areas. The Lalonde Report marked the initial shift away from a treatment paradigm to a health promotion focus at the national level in Canada (Falk Rafael, 1999).

In 1978, at an international conference on primary health care, the Declaration of Alma Alta was developed calling for access to primary health care for all. This concept was further developed in the World Health Organization's *Global Strategies for Health for All by the Year 2000* published in 1981 and the *Ottawa Charter for Health Promotion* developed at the First International Conference on Health Promotion, both focusing on social, economic, and political reform and empowerment as strategies for improving the health of the world's populations (Harper & Lambert, 1994). The importance of health promotion at the global level has recently been reinforced in the *Jakarta Declaration on Health Promotion into the 21st Century* (Fourth International Conference on Health Promotion, 1998).

Reform efforts in the United States have focused more on health care financing and the organization of services than on changes in social conditions affecting health. The **Tax Equity and Fiscal Responsibility Act (TEFRA)** of 1982 had a profound effect on health care and community health nursing. This act, passed in an effort to reduce Medicare expenditures, led to the development of **diagnosis-related groups (DRGs)** as a mechanism for prospective payment for services provided under Medicare (Harris, 1988). Basically, prospective payment means that health care institutions are paid a flat fee set in advance under Medicare. The fee is based on the client's diagnosis. The effect of this legislation has been earlier discharge of sicker clients and greater demand for home health and community health nursing services. Diagnosis-related groups and their effects have changed the role of community health nurses, who may need to return to the earlier role of care of the sick in their homes, in addition to their roles in promoting health and preventing illness.

Another recent event that will probably have a significant impact on community health nursing is the development of the **Nursing Interventions Classification (NIC)** system to categorize nursing services and facilitate their direct reimbursement (McCloskey & Bulechek, 1996). The NIC system should lend itself to direct reimbursement for nursing services under managed care, the new focus of the U.S. federal government. Both Medicare and Medicaid clients have been encouraged to enroll in managed care programs in pilot projects throughout the country. Unfortunately, several managed care organizations are discontinuing services to Medicare enrollees because of the reduced profit margin in providing care to the elderly. Continued growth of managed care could lead to a resurgence of the case management role traditionally played by the community health nurse. Community health nurses, however, will need to seize this opportunity with alacrity to prevent encroachment on this area of practice already underway from other professional groups.

THINK ABOUT IT

Does public health history reveal any repeated patterns or trends that might be of assistance in dealing with today's health problems? If so, what are they? What messages do they have for community health nurses today?

THE PRESENT AND THE FUTURE

Community health nursing, as practiced today, differs somewhat from the practice arena envisioned by Lillian Wald and her associates. Over the past 100 years, community health nursing practice has changed to meet the changing needs and demands of society. The Henry Street nurses and their contemporaries combined personal care and health promotion services as two aspects of community health nursing practice. When official health agencies began to provide population-based screening and education services, community health nurses employed by these agencies began to emphasize the health-promotive and disease-preventive aspects of their practice, leaving the provision of personal health services for the sick in their homes to visiting nurse associations (Jenkins & Sullivan-Marx, 1994). More recently, community health nurses have assumed a more clinical, illness-oriented role, downplaying their previous home- and community-based preventive role, as official agencies have begun to provide more direct clinical care. This shift has occurred, in part, in response to societal need, but also in large part to the reimbursability of these services as opposed to traditional public health services.

This situation has led to what a 1988 report on the status of the nation's public health system, *The Future of Public Health,* described as a system in disarray. The report concluded that major reforms will be required to promote and protect the health of the public. Unfortunately, the report did not address the contribution of community health nursing to public health. This, in itself, may be ominous. Community health nursing may not survive as an area of specialty practice if it is not seen as contributing to public health. To forestall this possibility, community health nurses in several areas are engaged in efforts to reframe and reorganize community health nursing in terms of the core functions of public health (Gebbie, 1996; Josten, Aroskar, Reckinger, & Shannon, 1996; Virginia Department of Health, 1996). Some groups, like the Washington State Department of Health, have identified core competencies for health professionals related to the core functions of public health and have instituted specific training to develop those competencies in community health nurses and other public health professionals (Joint Council of Governmental Public Health Agencies, 1996).

There are, however, some indications of greater concern for community health. Growing evidence indicates a shift to greater emphasis on health promotion and illness prevention in national health policy. The national health objectives, published first in 1980 and again in 1990 and discussed in Chapter 1, are one sign of this shift. A second bit of evidence is the 1988 creation of the Center for Nursing Research (now the **National Institute for Nursing Research**) within the National Institutes of Health. One reason given in Senate testimony favoring the center was the health promotion and illness prevention focus in much of nursing research. Another somewhat encouraging sign is the passage of the **Public Health Improvement Act** of 2000, which provides funds for the development of public health activities at state and local levels (*The Nation's Health,* 2000). In addition, one of the new focus areas for *Healthy People 2010* is development of the public health infrastructure. The **public health infrastructure** includes the organizational structure of official government health agencies, the public health workforce, and the information systems employed in public health practice (U.S. Department of Health and Human Services, 2000).

In this chapter, we have seen how community health nursing grew to its present state. Some of the events influencing its development are summarized in Table 2–1 ■. The future direction of community health nursing will be determined by the community health nurses of today and tomorrow. As noted by one historian of the Henry Street nurses, "We live in times not unlike those of the early Henry Street days. Our inner cities—cities within cities—are frightening, bleak places of despair. I am struck by the similarity of issues—poverty, sanitation, prostitution, pornography, . . . violence, drugs, communicable diseases, hopelessness" (Estabrooks, 1995). It may be time to return to the dual nature of the initial community health nursing role: personal care in conjunction with population-based health promotion and illness prevention. Perhaps then we can achieve the goal, set in 1923 but never accomplished, of one community health nurse to every 2,000 Americans (Winslow, 1993).

■ **TABLE 2-1   Historical Events Influencing the Development of Community Health Nursing**

DATE	EVENT
1601	First Poor Law is enacted in Great Britain.
1639	Massachusetts and Plymouth colonies mandate reporting of births and deaths.
1647	Massachusetts enacts regulations regarding pollution of Boston harbor.
1701	Massachusetts enacts laws regarding quarantine of ships and isolation of persons with smallpox.
1780	First local board of health in the United States is established at Petersburg, Virginia.
1797	Temporary state boards of health are established in Massachusetts and New York. Massachusetts grants local jurisdictions the authority to establish local health services.
1798	National Quarantine Act provides a systematic national approach to quarantine of seaports.
1813	* Ladies' Benevolent Society is organized in South Carolina as the first home nursing service in the United States.
1819	* Visiting nursing services are organized through the Hebrew Female Benevolent Society of Philadelphia.
1831	**Thackrah's treatise on occupational health is published.**
1832	* Lying-in Charity for Attending Indigent Women in Their Homes is established.
1840	First tuberculosis hospital opened in England.
1842	**Chadwick's *Inquiry into the Sanitary Conditions of the Labouring Population of Great Britain* is published.**
1850	**Shattuck's *Report of the Massachusetts Sanitary Commission* is published.**
1856	Rumsey's *Essay on State Medicine* argues for government responsibility for public health. Snow's historic epidemiologic study of cholera is conducted.
1858	National board of health is established in the United States.
1869	**First modern state board of health is established in Massachusetts.**
1872	American Public Health Association is established.
1873	* Comstock Act made it illegal for anyone other than physicians to disseminate contraceptive information, spurring efforts by Margaret Sanger and others to educate women regarding contraception.
1875	* Metropolitan and National Nursing Association for Providing Trained Nurses for the Sick Poor is established in England.
1877	**Pasteur and Koch independently identify specific bacteria.** * Women's Branch of the New York City Mission is first to employ trained nurses for home visiting.
1878	* Ethical Culture Society of New York City places four nurses in dispensaries. Federal Quarantine Act is passed.
1881	* American Red Cross is founded.
1885–86	* **Visiting nurse associations are established in Buffalo, Boston, and Philadelphia.**
1892	* First school nurse is employed in London.
1893	* **Henry Street Settlement is founded by Lillian Wald.**
1895	* Vermont Marble Company employs first occupational health nurse.
1896	* First rural nursing service is established (Westchester County, New York).
1897	* Victorian Order of Nurses (VON) founded to pioneer community health nursing in Canada.
1899	* International Council of Nurses established by Lavinia Dock and others.
1900	* Richmond, Virginia, nurses' settlement house is founded.

DATE	EVENT
1902	* First school nursing program in the United States is established by Henry Street Settlement.
1903	* Henry Street Settlement school nursing program is absorbed by New York City Department of Health.
1904	* First school nurse is employed by a municipality (Los Angeles, California).
1906	* The *Visiting Nurse Quarterly* is first published (Chicago). * **First postgraduate course in public health nursing is established by Instructive District Nursing Association of Boston.** * Pure Food and Drug Act passed.
1909	White House Conference on Children has first meeting. * Metropolitan Life Insurance Company offers visiting nurse services to policyholders. * **Red Cross Nursing Service established.**
1910	* First postgraduate course in community health nursing in an institution of higher learning is established at Columbia University.
1912	Children's Bureau is set up to foster child health. First law empowering the Surgeon General to promote health is passed. Marine Hospital Services becomes U.S. Public Health Service (USPHS). * National Organization for Public Health Nursing (NOPHN) is established. * **Red Cross Town and Country Nursing Service is established.**
1918	* University of Alberta offered first Canadian course in public health nursing.
1919	* Alberta District Nursing Service established to meet the needs of frontier families.
1920	* Public health section of the Canadian National Association of Trained Nurses established.
1921	* Maternity and Infancy (Sheppard–Towner) Act passed to provide assistance to mothers and children.
1923	* Goldmark Report recommends education for nurses in institutions of higher learning and additional preparation for community health nursing.
1929	* NOPHN establishes criteria and procedures for grading courses in public health nursing, initiating the accreditation process. Blue Cross Insurance instituted.
1930	National Institutes of Health is set up to fund and conduct health research. Food and Drug Administration established.
1932	Weir report on nursing education in Canada recognized need for advanced education for public health nurses and recommended an increase in the public health nurse workforce.
1934	* First public health nurse is employed by USPHS.
1935	Social Security Act establishes Old Age Survivor's Insurance Program (OASI).
1938	Garfield/Kaiser Prepaid Group Practice established (forerunner of Kaiser Permanente).
1944	* Division of Nursing is established in USPHS.
1946	Hospital Survey and Construction (Hill–Burton) Act provides funds for hospital construction in underserved areas. Communicable Disease Center is established from Office of Malaria Control in War Areas.
1948	* **Brown Report reemphasizes the need to educate nurses in institutions of higher learning and to include community health nursing content in curricula.**
1952	* NOPHN is absorbed into National League for Nursing (NLN).
1953	U.S. Department of Health, Education, and Welfare is created.
1954	Health insurance premiums are first allowed as tax deductions.
1957	Nationalized Canadian health care begins with federal coverage of hospital and diagnostic services.

(continued)

■ **TABLE 2–1   Historical Events Influencing the Development of Community Health Nursing** *(continued)*

DATE	EVENT
1964	* **Public health nurse is defined by American Nurses Association as a graduate of a baccalaureate program in nursing.** Surgeon General's report on smoking is published.
1966	Comprehensive Health Planning and Public Health Services Act is passed. Medicare program is instituted to fund health care for the elderly.
1967	* Child Health Act recommends use of nurse practitioners in the care of children. Medicaid program is instituted to fund health care for the indigent.
1968	Medical insurance added to Canadian health care system to become current "Medicare" system.
1970	Occupational Safety and Health Administration is established. Environmental Protection Agency is instituted.
1974	National Health Planning and Resources Development Act is passed in an attempt at systematic health care planning. Lalonde Report, *New Perspectives for the Health of Canadians,* emphasizes the importance of health promotion and illness prevention.
1979	*Healthy People: Surgeon General's Report on Health Promotion and Disease Prevention* **is published.**
1980	U.S. Department of Health, Education, and Welfare is reorganized, creating the Department of Health and Human Services. *Promoting Health/Preventing Disease: Objectives for the Nation* is published, creating the first set of national health objectives for the United States.
1981	**World Health Organization report,** *Global Strategies for Health for All by the Year 2000,* **emphasizes the importance of primary health care.**
1982	Tax Equity and Fiscal Responsibility Act (TEFRA) is passed.
1983	**Prospective payment system based on diagnosis-related groups is instituted under Medicare.**
1986	*The Ottawa Charter for Health Promotion* **identifies prerequisites to, and five strategies for, achieving health for all.**
1988	Institute of Medicine report, *The Future of Public Health,* recommends changes in the U.S. health care system.
1989	*U.S. Public Health Services Task Force: Guide to Clinical Preventive Services* recommends standardized screening and prevention strategies for specific population groups.
1990	*Healthy People 2000: National Objectives for Health Promotion and Illness Prevention* is published.
1993–94	Clinton Health Security plan for U.S. health care reform fails.
1993	* **National Center for Nursing Research is established.** **Health Plan Employer Data and Information Set (HEDIS) is created.**
1995	* Pew Health Professions Commission reinforces baccalaureate as entry level for community health nursing practice.
1997	*Medicine and Public Health: The Power of Collaboration* is published, recommending closer integration of medicine and public health practice.
1998	*Jakarta Declaration on Health Promotion into the 21st Century* **reinforces the concepts of global health promotion.**
2000	*Healthy People 2010* is published. Public Health Improvement Act is passed to assist state and local agencies in enhancing public health services.

* Events affecting nursing directly.

APPLYING YOUR KNOWLEDGE IN PRACTICE

❧ CASE STUDY
Continuing the Focus on the Public's Health

Community health nursing in the United States arose in response to identified health needs among European immigrants. What recently arrived immigrant populations live in the area surrounding your nursing program? In what ways are these new immigrants similar to and different from those arriving in the United States at the end of the nineteenth century? How do their health needs compare to those encountered by the nurses on Henry Street?

❧ TESTING YOUR UNDERSTANDING

- Which of the many contributions made by Florence Nightingale are relevant to the development of community health nursing? To public health practice? (pp. 20–21)
- Describe the contributions of Lillian Wald to the development of community health nursing in the United States. What features of her Henry Street practice are relevant to today's community health nursing practice? (pp. 21–24)
- Describe some of the contributions made by early community health nurses to social and health care reform. (pp. 22–23)
- What report led to the creation of the forerunner of the modern board of health? List at least five recommendations from this report. (p. 19)

- List at least four major historical events in the development of community health nursing in the United States. (pp. 21–29)
- How have DRGs influenced community health nursing practice? Will a similar reimbursement system for ambulatory care services have the same kind of effect on community health nursing? (p. 28)
- What evidence is there for a shift to greater emphasis on health promotion and illness prevention in the United States? In Canada? (p. 29)

REFERENCES

Abel, E. K. (1996). "We are left so much alone to work out our own problems": Nurses on American Indian reservations during the 1930s. *Nursing History Review, 4,* 43–64.

Anderson, C. L., Morton, R. F., & Green, L. W. (1978). *Community health* (3rd ed.). St. Louis: C. V. Mosby.

Anglin, L. T. (1990). The roles of nurse: A history, 1900 to 1988. Unpublished doctoral dissertation, Illinois State University.

Benson, E. R. (1993). Public health nursing and the Jewish contribution. *Public Health Nursing, 10*(1), 55–57.

Benson, E. R., & McDevitt, J. Q. (1976). *Community health and nursing practice.* Englewood Cliffs, NJ: Prentice Hall.

Bigbee, J. L., & Crowder, E. L. M. (1985). The Red Cross Rural Nursing Service: An innovative model of public health nursing. *Public Health Nursing, 2,* 109–121.

Brainerd, A. M. (1985). *The evolution of public health nursing.* New York: Garland. Reprinted from A. M. Brainerd (1922), *The evolution of public health nursing.* Philadelphia: Saunders.

Bramadat, I. J., & Saydak, M. I. (1993). Nursing on the Canadian Prairies, 1900–1930: Effects of Immigration. *Nursing History Review, 1,* 105–117.

Bullough, V. L., & Bullough, B. (1993). Medieval nursing. *Nursing History Review, 1,* 89–104.

Byrd, M. E. (1995). A concept analysis of home visiting. *Public Health Nursing, 12*(2), 83–89.

Cohen, S. (1997). Miss Loane, Florence Nightingale, and district nursing in late Victorian Britain. *Nursing History Review, 5,* 83–103.

Coss, C. (1989). *Lillian Wald: A progressive activist.* New York: Feminist Press.

Duncan, S. M., Leipart, B. D., & Mill, J. E. (1999). "Nurses as health evangelists"?: The evolution of public health nursing in Canada, 1918–1939. *Advances in Nursing Science, 22*(1), 40–51.

Epidemiology Program Office, Centers for Disease Control and Prevention. (1999). Changes in the public health system. *Morbidity and Mortality Weekly Report, 48,* 1141–1147.

Erickson, G. (1987). Southern initiative in public health nursing. *Journal of Nursing History, 3*(1), 17–29.

Estabrooks, C. A. (1995). Lavinia Lloyd Dock: The Henry Street years. *Nursing History Review, 3,* 143–172.

Falk Rafael, A. R. (1999). The politics of health promotion: Influences on public health promotion nursing practice in Ontario, Canada from Nightingale to the nineties. *Advances in Nursing Science, 22*(1), 23–39.

Fee, E. (1997). History and development of public health. In F. D. Scutchfield & C. W.

Keck (Eds.), *Principles of public health practice* (pp. 10–30). Albany, NY: Delmar.

Foley, E. L. (1985). Introduction. In A. M. Brainerd (1922), *The evolution of public health nursing* (pp. i–vii). New York: Garland. Reprinted from A. M. Brainerd, *The evolution of public health nursing*. Philadelphia: Saunders.

Fourth International Conference on Health Promotion. (1998). The Jakarta Declaration on Health Promotion into the 21st Century. *Pan American Journal, 3*(1), 58–61.

Fritz, K. (1995). A history of the concept of creativity in western nursing: A cultural feminist perspective. Unpublished doctoral dissertation, University of San Diego.

Gardner, M. S. (1952). *Public health nursing* (3rd ed.). New York: Macmillan.

Gebbie, K. M. (1996). *Preparing currently employed public health nurses for changes in the health system: Meeting report and suggested action steps*. New York: Center for Health Policy and Health Sciences Research.

Ginzberg, E. (1985). *American medicine: The power shifts*. Totowa, NJ: Rowman & Allanheld.

Golden, J., & Moore, P. (1986). The Simmons Harvard graduate program in public health nursing. *Public Health Nursing, 4*, 123–127.

Hamilton, D. (1988). Clinical excellence, but too high a cost: The Metropolitan Life Insurance Company Visiting Nurse Service (1909–1952). *Public Health Nursing, 5*, 235–240.

Hamilton, D. (1989). The cost of caring: The Metropolitan Life Insurance Company's Visiting Nurse Service. *Bulletin of the History of Nursing, 63*, 414–434.

Harper, A. C., & Lambert, L. J. (1994). *The health of populations: An introduction* (2nd ed.). New York: Springer.

Harris, M. D. (1988). The changing scene in community health nursing. *Nursing Clinics of North America, 23*, 226–229.

Hefland, W. H., Lazarus, J., & Theerman, P. (2000). The Children's Bureau and public health at midcentury. *American Journal of Public Health, 90*, 1703.

Igoe, J. B. (1980). Changing patterns in school health and school health nursing. *Nursing Outlook, 28*, 486–492.

Igoe, J. B. (1994). School nursing. *Nursing Clinics of North America, 29*, 443–458.

Interview with Harney M. Cordua, son of Dr. Olive Cordua, San Diego County Medical Officer. San Diego: San Diego Historical Society.

Jenkins, M. L., & Sullivan–Marx, E. M. (1994). Nurse practitioners and community health nurses: Clinical partnerships and future visions. *Nursing Clinics of North America, 29*, 459–470.

Joint Council of Governmental Public Health Agencies Work Group on Human Resources Development. (1996). *Public health improvement plan: Education and training competency model*. Seattle, WA: Washington State Department of Health.

Jonas, S., & Rosenberg, S. (1986). Ambulatory care. In S. Jonas (Ed.), *Health care delivery in the United States* (3rd ed.) (pp. 125–165). New York: Springer.

Jossens, M. O. R., & Ferjancsik, P. (1996). Of Lillian Wald, community health nursing education, and health care reform. *Public Health Nursing, 13*(2), 97–103.

Josten, L., Aroskar, M., Reckinger, D., & Shannon, M. (1996). *Educating nurses for public health leadership*. Minneapolis, MN: University of Minnesota.

Kelly, L. Y. (1981). *Dimensions of professional nursing* (4th ed.). New York: Macmillan.

Krampitz, S. D. (1987). The Yale experiment: Innovation in nursing education. In C. Maggs (Ed.), *Nursing history: The state of the art* (pp. 60–73). London: Croom Helm.

Kuss, T., Proulx-Girouard, L., Lovitt, S., Katz, C., & Kennelly, P. (1997). A public health nursing model. *Public Health Nursing, 14*, 81–91.

Lasker, R. D., & the Committee on Medicine and Public Health. (1997). *Medicine & public health: The power of collaboration*. New York: New York Academy of Medicine.

Matuk, L. Y., & Horsburgh, M. C. (1989). Rebuilding public health nursing: A Canadian perspective. *Public Health Nursing, 6*, 169–173.

McCloskey, J. C., & Bulecheck, G. M. (Eds.). (1996). *Nursing interventions classification: Iowa Interventions Project* (2nd ed.). St. Louis: Mosby-Year Book.

McGuire, M. T., & Anderson, W. H. (1999). *The US healthcare dilemma: Mirrors and chains*. Westport, CT: Auburn House.

Montiero, L. A. (1987). Insights from the past. *Nursing Outlook, 35*, 65–69.

The Nation's Health. (December 2000/January 2001). Legislation to benefit key public health issues. 1.

Novak, J. C. (1988). The social mandate and historical basis for nursing's role in health promotion. *Journal of Professional Nursing, 4*(2), 80–87.

Pew Health Professions Commission. (1995). *Critical challenges: Revitalizing the health pro-

fessions for the twenty-first century*. San Francisco, UCSF Center for the Health Professions.

Plotnick, J. (1994, March). *Public health components of the Health Security Act*. Paper presented at the meeting of the Public Health Nursing Division, San Diego County Department of Health Services, San Diego, CA.

Pollit, P. (1991). Lydia Holman: Community health pioneer. *Nursing Outlook, 39*, 230–232.

Richardson, S. (1998). Political women, professional nurses, and the creation of Alberta's District Nursing Service, 1919–1925. *Nursing History Review, 6*, 25–50.

Roberts, J. I., & Group, T. M. (1995). Feminism and nursing: An historical perspective on power, status, and political activism in the nursing profession. Westport, CT: Praeger.

Rosen, G. (1974). *From medical police to social medicine: Essays on the history of health care*. New York: Science History Publications.

Ruffing-Rahal, M. A. (1995). The Navajo experience of Elizabeth Foster, public health nurse. *Nursing History Review, 3*, 173–188.

Smith, S. L. (1994). White nurses, black midwives, and public health in Mississippi, 1920–1950. *Nursing History Review, 2*, 29–49.

SmithBattle, L., Diekemper, M., & Drake, M. A. (1999). Articulating the culture and tradition of community health nursing. *Public Health Nursing, 16*, 215–222.

Smolensky, J. (1982). *Principles of community health* (3rd ed.). Philadelphia: Saunders.

Sofaer, S. (1988). Community health planning in the United States: A postmortem. *Family Community Health, 10*(4), 1–12.

U.S. Department of Health and Human Services. (2000). *Healthy people 2010* (Conference edition, in two volumes). Washington, DC: Author.

Virginia Department of Health. (1996). *The role of public health nursing in Virginia's changing health care environment*. Richmond, VA: Author.

Weir, G. M. (1932). *Survey of nursing education in Canada*. Toronto: University of Toronto Press.

Winslow, C. E. (1923). *The evolution and significance of the modern public health campaign*. New Haven, CT: Yale University Press.

Winslow, C. E. A. (1993). Nursing and the community. *Public Health Nursing, 10*, 58–63. (Reprinted from *The Public Health Nurse*, April 1938).

Zilm, G., & Warbinek, E. (1995). Early tuberculosis nursing in British Columbia. *Canadian Journal of Nursing Research, 27*(3), 65–81.

THE HEALTH SYSTEM CONTEXT

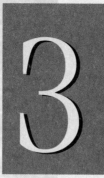

3

Chapter Objectives

After reading this chapter, you should be able to:

- Identify six core goals for effective health care systems.
- Describe the organizational structure of the U.S. health care delivery system.
- Compare and contrast official and voluntary health agencies.
- Describe at least five functions performed by voluntary health agencies.
- Identify 10 essential public health services.
- Discuss the involvement of local, state, and national governments in health care in the United States.
- Compare selected features of national health care systems.
- Describe two types of international health agencies.
- Discuss the role of the community health nurse with respect to international terrorism.
- Discuss the need for international collaboration on health issues.

Media Link

http://www.prenhall.com/clark

Additional interactive resources for this chapter can be found on the companion Web site. Click on Chapter 3 and "Begin" to select the activities for this chapter.

Community health nursing occurs in the context of a health care delivery system that creates constraints and provides opportunities for the practice of community health nursing. For example, lack of emphasis on health promotion in the health care delivery system increases the need for health promotion efforts by community health nurses, but simultaneously limits funds available for health promotion activities.

Health and health care are concerns throughout the world, and each jurisdiction (community, state, or nation) has developed a system to address these concerns. A system is defined as "a set of planned parts and their interrelationships" (Reagan, 1999, p. 19). A *health care system* is defined by the World Health Organization (WHO) (2000, p. 5) as "all the activities whose primary purpose is to promote, restore, or maintain health."

WHO (2000) has developed a list of core goals to be accomplished by health care systems. These include:

- Improving health status of the population
- Reducing health inequalities
- Promoting responsiveness to legitimate expectations of members of the populations
- Increasing efficiency of health care delivery
- Protecting individuals, families, and communities from health-related financial loss
- Promoting fairness in the financing and delivery of health care services

Accomplishment of these broad health system goals can be achieved through a variety of organizational structures. Although each jurisdiction has its own way of organizing and providing health care, some features are common to all systems.

Exploring the organization of health care delivery systems can help us to understand how these systems developed, how they work, and how and why they sometimes fail to work. Moreover, we can identify factors that positively or negatively influence community health nursing practice. Finally, we can identify areas where change is needed in the health care delivery system to best fulfill our goal as community health nurses, namely, promotion of the public's health. In this chapter, we will examine the organization of health care delivery in the United States, as well as in other countries, and make comparisons that permit us to see the advantages and disadvantages of various approaches to health care.

HEALTH CARE DELIVERY IN THE UNITED STATES

Health care delivery in the United States has been called a nonsystem or an "accidental system." It is accidental in that it has not been purposefully created and organized like the health care systems in other industrialized nations. Indeed, the health care system in the United

States is an amalgam of programs created to meet specific needs identified at different times within different political contexts with no thought to how the various parts of the system interact (Reagan, 1999). Despite the relative accuracy of this description, we can still examine U.S. health care delivery in terms of the structure depicted in Figure 3–1 ■.

The organizational structure for health care delivery in the United States consists of three major elements or subsystems depicted in Figure 3–1. These subsystems include the popular health care subsystem, the complementary or alternative health care subsystem, and the scientific health care subsystem.

The Popular Health Care Subsystem

Most health-related care is provided within the *popular health care subsystem.* In fact, it is estimated that 70% to 90% of illness care is provided within the home by family members and others (WHO, 2000). The popular subsystem component of the health care system includes health care that each of us provides for ourself and our family. When you have a headache, for example, you may take an over-the-counter analgesic. If you are constipated, you may either increase the bulk, fiber, and fluid in your diet or take a laxative. If your child has a mild fever, you might give him or her an antipyretic. All of these self-care or family care practices constitute popular subsystem health care.

Although health care in this subsystem is provided by oneself or by family members, community health nurses have an educational role in the popular subsystem. As we shall see in Chapter 11, one of the purposes of health

FIGURE 3–1 ■ *Organizational Structure of the U.S. Health Care Delivery System*

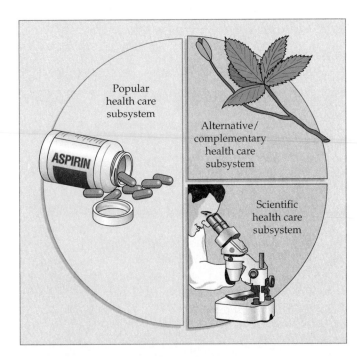

education is to prepare clients to make informed self-care decisions. For example, a community health nurse might caution a client against overuse of laxatives and suggest dietary approaches in dealing with constipation, or the nurse may inform parents about the hazards of giving aspirin to children and recommend a nonaspirin substitute.

The Complementary/Alternative Health Care Subsystem

When self-care fails or seems inappropriate, people often turn to other sources of health care. Some of these sources might be folk health practitioners found in the *complementary/alternative health care subsystem.* Alternative health care providers are individuals who are believed to have special health-related knowledge or training above that provided to the average member of the society. Examples of alternative health care providers are the *curandera* found among Latinos in the northeastern and southwestern regions of the United States and the herbalists found in these and other areas. The role of the community health nurse in the complementary/alternative health care subsystem is to assess the influence of this subsystem on health and to incorporate traditional health practices into the plan of care as appropriate. We discuss the complementary/alternative health care subsystem in more detail in Chapter 6.

The Scientific Health Care Subsystem

The professional or *scientific health care subsystem* is the system of care based on scientific research-derived evidence. Health care provided in the scientific subsystem is based on knowledge derived from the biological, physical, and behavioral sciences and includes the services of nurses, physicians, pharmacists, social workers, and other health care professionals.

The scientific health care subsystem consists of two sectors that differ primarily in their focus of care. These

Community health services are provided in a variety of settings.

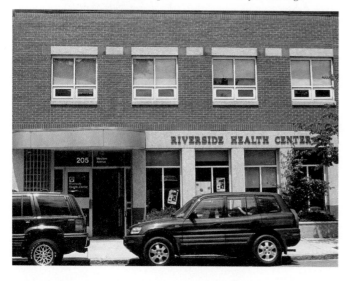

sectors are the personal health care sector and the public, or population, health care sector (Lasker, 1997).

THE PERSONAL HEALTH CARE SECTOR

The focus of care in the *personal health care sector* is the health of the individual. The primary emphasis in this sector is cure of disease and restoration of health, although individuals may also receive some health-promotive and illness-preventive services.

Personal health services are provided in office settings, clinics, hospitals, and other places where care is dispensed to individual clients. Institutions that provide personal health care, such as hospitals and clinics, may be either privately or publicly funded. For example, both private hospitals and publicly funded community hospitals are part of the personal health care sector.

THE POPULATION HEALTH CARE SECTOR

The *population health care sector* consists of both public and private organizations whose focus is the health of the total population (Mays, Halverson, & Miller, 1998). Care provided has traditionally centered on promoting health and preventing disease, although some curative care does occur in this sector. Emphasis is on designing health care programs that meet the needs of population groups.

In the last several years, there has been significant crossover in the activities of agencies and organizations in the personal and public health care sectors. For example, public health care sector organizations have begun to provide more personal health care services to people with no other source of health care. In this respect, the public health care sector has provided a "safety net" for those who would otherwise not receive care (Lasker, 1997). In many instances, public health agencies have become "providers of last resort" to assure access to services for underserved populations (Wall, 1998).

Provision of personal health services is seen by many as undermining the fundamental responsibility of the public health sector, and the burgeoning emphasis on a return to the core functions of public health has led many public health agencies to attempt to "privatize" personal health care services (Lasker, 1997). *Privatization* is the movement of personal health care services from public health agencies to private organizations in the personal health care sector.

At the same time, many organizations in the personal health care sector are absorbing functions, such as immunization and treatment of sexually transmitted diseases, which have traditionally been the purview of public health agencies. In fact, some studies indicate that personal sector organizations are also engaging in activities related to the core public health functions (Chapel, Stange, Gordon, & Miller, 1998). As noted in Chapter 1, there is a growing need for collaboration between the personal and public health care sectors. Collaborative efforts between the two sectors can accomplish more than either sector working in isolation.

Let us turn now, though, to a discussion of the organization of the public health care sector. Health care services in the public health sector may be provided by either official or voluntary agencies.

OFFICIAL HEALTH AGENCIES   *Official health agencies* are agencies of local, state, and national governments that are responsible for the health of the people in their jurisdiction. Official agencies are supported by tax revenues and other public funding. They are accountable to the citizens of their jurisdiction, usually through an elected or appointed governing body. Many of the activities conducted by official agencies are mandated by law. For example, local health departments are required by state law to report cases of certain diseases. We will discuss specific functions of official agencies at local, state, and national levels in more detail later in this chapter. Generally speaking, however, all official health agencies are responsible for carrying out the three core public health functions described in Chapter 1.

Under its assessment function, the public health sector is responsible for collecting and analyzing data to identify population health problems. The policy development function entails using a scientific knowledge base to provide direction for health program development. Finally, in its assurance function, the public health sector is responsible for assuring that the health care services needed by the population are available and accessible to those in need (Miller, Moore, Richards, & Monk, 1994).

VOLUNTARY HEALTH AGENCIES   *Voluntary health agencies* are private, nonprofit organizations that are formed by groups of people because of their interest in a particular health concern, such as diabetes, child abuse, or environmental pollution (Rovner, 2000). They may focus on a specific disease entity, an organ system, or a population group (Miller, 1995). Voluntary agencies are funded primarily by donations. They are accountable to their supporters, and their activities are determined by supported interest, rather than legal mandate. Their primary emphasis is on research, education, and policy development (primarily through legislative lobbying), although they may provide some direct health care services.

Voluntary agencies can be categorized on the basis of their source of funding. The first category consists of agencies supported by citizen contributions, such as the American Cancer Society. The first agency of this type in the United States was the Antituberculosis Society founded in Philadelphia in 1892. The focus of this type of agency frequently changes as health needs change. For example, the Antituberculosis Society is known today as the American Lung Association, indicating its broader focus on a variety of respiratory conditions. The second category consists of foundations established by private philanthropic contributions. An example of this type of voluntary organization would be the Kellogg Foundation, which provides funding for health care research. Today,

more than 3,000 philanthropic foundations support health efforts. The third category of voluntary agency is funded by member dues. The American Public Health Association and the American Nurses Association are examples of this type of agency.

Integrating agencies, such as the United Way, coordinate the fund-raising activities of several voluntary agencies. A fifth type of voluntary agency includes religious organizations that derive their funds from contributions by members of a congregation. These groups often focus on local needs and are particularly effective because of their ability to draw on volunteers (Miller, 1995). The final category of voluntary health agency is the commercial organization that engages in health care activities. For example, the American Dairy Association provides literature and visual aids for nutrition education. Similarly, health insurance companies often put out literature on health promotion and illness prevention.

Voluntary agencies perform eight basic functions within the scientific health care subsystem. The first of these is *pioneering* activities. Voluntary agencies explore areas that are underserved by the other components of the health care system. For example, research that culminated in the development of a vaccine for polio was the early focus of the March of Dimes. Now, polio immunization is largely a function of official agencies.

The second function of voluntary agencies is *demonstration* of pilot projects in health care delivery. For instance, the Planned Parenthood Association instituted clinics for contraceptive services long before most official health agencies became involved in this area of service. *Education* of the public and health professionals is the third function of voluntary agencies. For example, the American Cancer Society has spearheaded educational campaigns on the hazards of smoking. The fourth function of voluntary agencies is *supplementation* of services provided by official health agencies. For instance, some voluntary agencies provide transportation to clinics, respite care, special equipment, and other ancillary services.

⑥THINK ABOUT IT

What gaps do voluntary agencies fill in your community? What advantages do they have over official public health agencies in filling these gaps? What difficulties do they face?

Fifth, voluntary agencies *advocate* for the public's health. For example, a voluntary agency may campaign against reduction of health care services due to budget cuts. The sixth function, promoting *legislation* related to health, is a closely related function. In Tennessee, the Fraternal Order of Police and the Tennessee Nurses Association were instrumental in getting child car restraint legislation passed.

The seventh function of voluntary agencies relates to health *planning and organization.* Voluntary agencies often assist official agencies in determining health care needs in the population and in planning programs to address those needs. The final function of voluntary agencies is *assisting official agencies* in developing well-balanced community health programs. For example, in 1915, when the San Diego Common Council passed an ordinance creating the position of Municipal Tuberculosis Visiting Nurse, but could not afford to pay her salary, the State Tuberculosis Society agreed to fund the position for one year, allowing the city to hire its first community health nurse (Communication from the City Auditor, 1915). The functions of voluntary agencies are summarized below.

HIGHLIGHTS

Functions of Voluntary Health Agencies

- Pioneering: Exploring areas not addressed by other components of the health care system
- Demonstration: Initiating and testing innovative strategies for health care delivery
- Education: Educating both the public and health care professions regarding health issues
- Supplementation: Providing services that complement and strengthen those of official health agencies
- Advocacy: Speaking for the public's benefit in the development of health policy
- Legislation: Initiating and campaigning for health-related legislation
- Planning and organizing: Assisting official health agencies in determining health care needs, priorities, policies, and programs
- Assisting official agencies: Supporting the efforts of official health agencies in improving the health of the public

LEVELS OF HEALTH CARE DELIVERY

Health care delivery in the United States takes place on local, state, and national levels. Each level has certain responsibilities with respect to the health of the population. The Reforming States Group (1998), an alliance of officials and legislators from 40 states, has noted, however, that this distribution of responsibility is more often due to historical precedent than to reasoned decision making. Both official and voluntary agencies exist at each level, but official agencies are the focus of this discussion.

The core public health functions identified by the Institute of Medicine (1988) have been further operationalized by the Steering Committee and Working Group of the Public Health Functions Project convened under the auspices of the U.S. Assistant Secretary of Health (Health Resources and Services Administration, 1998) in 10 essential public health services. These services include:

- Monitoring health status to identify community health problems
- Diagnosing and investigating health problems and health hazards in the community
- Informing, educating, and empowering people regarding health issues
- Mobilizing community partnerships to identify and solve health problems
- Developing health policies and plans that support individual and community health efforts
- Enforcing laws and regulations that protect health and assure safety
- Linking people to needed personal health care services and assuring the provision of health care when otherwise unavailable
- Assuring a competent public health and personal health workforce
- Evaluating effectiveness, accessibility, and quality of personal and population-based health services
- Conducting research to develop new insights and innovative solutions to health problems (U.S. Department of Health and Human Services, 2000)

Public health agencies at each of the three levels—local, state, and national—perform these essential services, but the degree to which they are emphasized varies from level to level.

The Local Level

The official agency at the local level is usually the *local health department.* Local health agencies encompass the "resources (money, people, physical infrastructure, and technology) and the organizational configuration used to transform these resources into health care services" (Longest, cited in Aday, Begley, Lairson, & Slater, 1998, p. 49). Local health agencies in the United States include more than 3,000 city, county, and other municipal agencies (Wall, 1998). Several of these agencies are large health systems serving the populations of major jurisdictions such as New York City or Los Angeles County. Most, however, serve smaller populations that do not have the resources for performing all of the essential public health functions. In fact, half of these agencies serve populations of less than 25,000 people (Center for Studying Health System Change, 1997). The local health department's authority is derived, in part, from responsibilities delegated by the state. For example, the state delegates to the local level the responsibility for collecting statistics on births and deaths. Because this responsibility has been legally delegated, the local health department has the authority to ensure that a death certificate is filed for every death that occurs. The local agency also derives authority from local health ordinances. For instance, local government might pass an ordinance requiring all residential rental units to have functioning smoke detectors. Enforcement of this ordinance might then become the responsibility of the local health department.

Funding at the local level comes from both local taxes and state and federal subsidies. Approximately 40% of local public health agency funding comes from the state, including federal *passthrough funds,* money granted to the states by the federal government that is allocated to local government agencies. Another 34% of local operating funds, on average, derives from local revenues including local taxes. A small percentage of funding (6%) comes directly from federal monies (excluding Medicaid and Medicare funds). In recent years, local health departments have attempted to augment revenue sources by providing personal care services reimbursable under Medicare and Medicaid. These revenues account, on average, for about 10% of local health department budgets, but may be as high as 30% to 50% in some states (Wall, 1998). As many Medicare and Medicaid recipients are being enrolled in managed care organizations (MCOs) in the personal health care sector, these sources of revenue are being withdrawn from local health depart-

ments, in some cases jeopardizing their abilities to subsidize services for other indigent populations (Lasker, 1997). Another small percentage (about 10%) of local health department funding is derived from client fees, private health insurance, regulatory fees, and so on (Wall, 1998).

Figure 3–2 ■ depicts the typical organizational structure of a local health department. The staff and programs included will vary from place to place. In some areas, the district health officer might also fulfill the role of administrative officer. Small counties or districts may not be able to afford the full-time services of some types of personnel, and the services of nutritionists, social workers, dentists, and other personnel might be shared by several counties or provided at the state level. Nurses and clerical staff would be found in almost any health department. Other personnel who may be available include environmental specialists, physical therapists, psychologists, laboratory and X-ray technicians, and pharmacists.

Because delegation of specific responsibilities to local jurisdictions is the function of the state, the responsibilities assumed vary from state to state. Local responsibilities may also vary within regions of a particular state depending on the local jurisdiction's capabilities and resources. In general, local health agencies are responsible for several basic functions identified by the National Association of County and City Health Officials. These functions include conducting community assessments, controlling epidemics, providing a safe environment, evaluating health services, promoting healthy lifestyles and educating the public, assuring access to laboratory

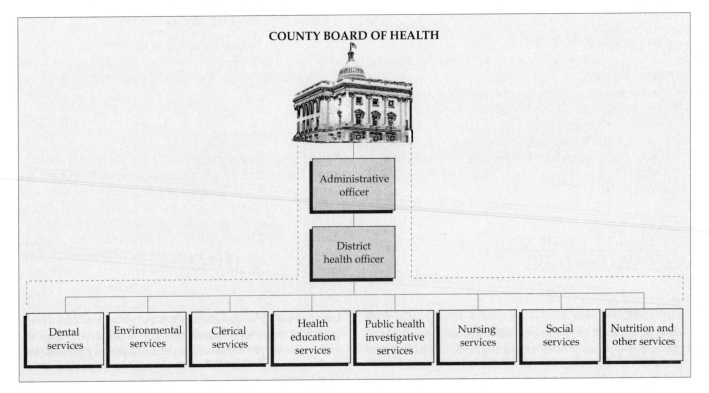

FIGURE 3–2 ■ *Typical Organizational Structure of a Local Health Department*

services, and engaging in outreach activities and partnership formation. Additional functions include providing some personal health services, research, and mobilizing communities for action (Rawding & Wasserman, 1997).

With increased emphasis on collaboration between the personal and public health care sectors, the specific functions performed by local health departments may vary even more widely (Reid & Mason, 1998). At one end of a continuum of potential roles envisioned for local health departments, depicted in Figure 3–3 ■, is performance of the core functions incorporating assessment of local health care needs and the development of health policies to meet those needs with assurance services monitoring the provision of services by elements of the personal health care sector (Wall, 1998). The next level would entail enactment of the core functions as well as performance of other traditional public health services. These services would include collection of vital statistics, control of communicable diseases, public sanitation, laboratory services, maternal and child health services, and health education, as well as community assessment and policy development. At the third position on the continuum, the health department would provide these traditional public health services as well as preventive services for specific populations. For example, the health department might contract with MCOs to provide childhood immunizations to Medicaid enrollees in the MCO or with local industry to provide influenza immunization for employees.

An intermediate level might include provision of *enabling services,* services, such as transportation, case management, and other services that enable clients to make effective use of personal health care sector resources (Wall, 1998). At the next level, local agency functions might include those of the previous levels in addition to the provision of primary care services to specific populations. For example, the local health department may contract with MCOs to provide ambulatory care for pediatric Medicaid enrollees or prenatal services for pregnant women covered by Medicaid. Similarly, at the next level, the agency may be involved in all of the preceding activities as well as provision of the full range of primary care to underserved areas within its jurisdiction. For example, the health department may provide primary care services in rural areas lacking in services by the personal health care sector. Finally, local health departments may decide to provide a full range of services to the entire population either under contract to or in competition with personal health care sector organizations (Reid & Mason, 1998). The position that any given local public health agency assumes on the continuum will be dictated by local needs, circumstances, resources, and capabilities.

The State Level

The official agency at the state level has traditionally been a state department of health. The state, not the federal government or the local jurisdiction, has primary authority in matters relating to health. This authority is derived from the sovereign powers reserved to the states under the U.S. Constitution. The state retains the ultimate responsibility for the health of the public and possesses essential power to make laws and regulations regarding health.

The state health department derives funding from state tax revenues and may also receive monies from the federal government. A general organizational schema for a state department of health is depicted in Figure 3–4 ■. The various divisions coordinate services at the state level and provide assistance to the local level.

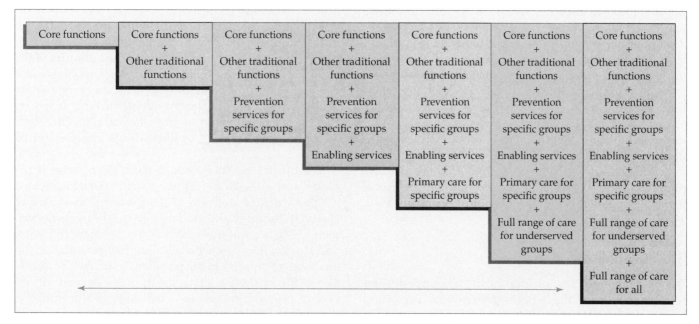

FIGURE 3–3 ■ *Continuum of Possible Roles for Local Health Departments*

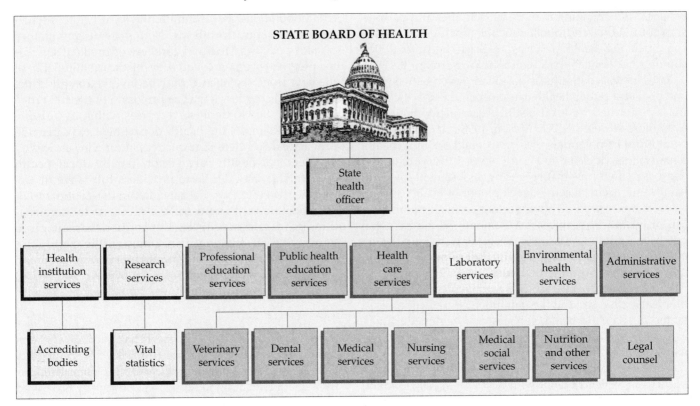

STATE BOARD OF HEALTH

FIGURE 3–4 ■ *Typical Organizational Structure of a State Health Department*

In general, the functions of state health agencies fall into five categories: health information, disease and disability prevention, health protection, health promotion, and improving the health care delivery system (Dandoy, 1997). Specific activities related to the information function include collecting and recording vital statistics and monitoring the incidence of specific health problems. Disease and disability prevention activities focus on screening and treatment services for specific conditions (e.g., tuberculosis) or special groups (e.g., children with disabilities), immunization, outbreak investigation, and laboratory services. Activities geared toward health protection include pollution control, inspections, and licensing of health care facilities and providers. Health promotion activities typically focus on providing specific services (e.g., family planning and prenatal care) and health education. Finally, activities under the health delivery system function include education of health professionals, policy development and priority setting, financing, and monitoring the performance of local health agencies (Mays, Halverson, & Miller, 1998; Wall, 1998).

The National Level

Because the Constitution makes no reference to any responsibilities of the federal government regarding health, the federal government has no direct authority to regulate health-related matters. The authority of the fed-eral government with respect to health is derived indirectly from three constitutional powers. The first of these is the *power to regulate foreign and interstate commerce.* For example, because most cosmetics are transported across state lines, the federal Food and Drug Administration has the authority to establish standards of purity for the manufacture of cosmetics.

The second constitutional source of authority over health matters is the *power to levy taxes and promote the general welfare.* For example, it can be argued that such programs as Medicaid and Medicare promote the general welfare and are therefore within the authority of the federal government. The *power to make treaties* is the third source of federal power in matters related to health. For example, a treaty with Mexico might specify that the Mexican government would take specific steps to control the shipment of illicit drugs into the United States.

The official health agency at the national level is the *Department of Health and Human Services* (DHHS), created in 1980 with the division of the former Department of Health, Education, and Welfare into two separate departments. The head of the agency is the Secretary of Health and Human Services, who fills a cabinet post and acts in an advisory capacity to the president in matters of health. The Office of the Secretary incorporates several offices. One of primary interest to community health nurses is the *Office of Public Health and Science,* which was only added to the division in 1996. The responsibilities of this

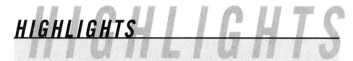

Constitutional Sources of Federal Authority for Health

- Power to regulate foreign and interstate commerce
- Power to levy taxes and promote the general welfare
- Power to make treaties

agency include national public health needs assessment and leadership in population-based health care and preventive services. Other agencies housed in the Secretary's Office include the Office of HIV/AIDS, the Office of Emergency Preparedness, and the Office of International and Refugee Health.

The major health-related agencies within DHHS are the Administration on Aging, the Administration for Children and Families, the Health Care Financing Administration, and the U.S. Public Health Service (Office of the Federal Register, 2000).

Figure 3–5 ■ depicts part of the organizational structure of DHHS. The public health component of the department is the *U.S. Public Health Service (USPHS)*. The USPHS consists of eight agencies. The *Food and Drug Administration (FDA)* is responsible for establishing and enforcing standards for the manufacture and processing of food, drugs, and cosmetics. It is also responsible for ascertaining the safety of new drugs and other health-related products such as food additives and medical devices. The *Centers for Disease Control and Prevention*

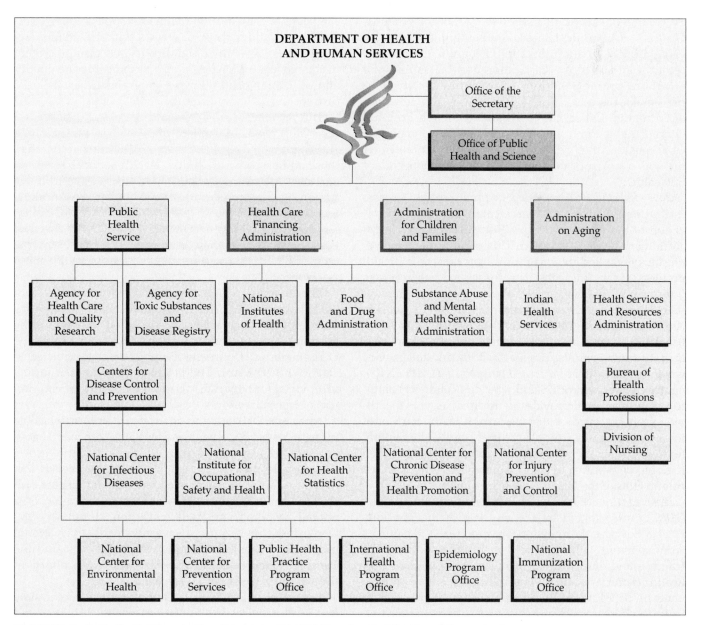

FIGURE 3–5 ■ *Partial Organizational Structure of the U.S. Department of Health and Human Services*

(CDC) investigates causes of disease and establishes policies and standards for the prevention, diagnosis, and treatment of a variety of health problems. The CDC consists of several component agencies depicted in Figure 3–5. The National Center for Infectious Diseases maintains the original focus of the CDC, investigating factors that contribute to communicable diseases, monitoring their occurrence, and developing policies and standards for their control. The National Center for Prevention Services focuses on health promotion and disease prevention activities and provides research and program support for these activities. The National Center for Environmental Health and the National Center for Injury Prevention and Control investigate factors underlying environmentally caused diseases and unintentional injuries and support policies and programs for their control. Control of occupational disease and injury is the focus of the National Institute for Occupational Safety and Health (NIOSH), and health promotion and prevention of chronic illness are the foci of the National Center for Chronic Disease Prevention and Health Promotion. The Immunization Program Office was recently added to the CDC and coordinates national efforts to promote immunization rates for vaccine-preventable diseases. The CDC also houses the Epidemiology Program Office, the International Health Program Office, and the Public Health Program Office. Finally, the CDC includes the National Center for Health Statistics, previously a part of the Office of the Assistant Secretary of Health.

The *Substance Abuse and Mental Health Services Administration (SAMHSA)* was created with the reorganization of the Alcohol, Drug Abuse, and Mental Health Administration (ADAMHA). This organization focuses on prevention and treatment programs for mental health problems, including substance abuse, and encompasses three centers: the Center for Substance Abuse Treatment (CSAT), the Center for Substance Abuse Prevention (CSAP), and the Center for Mental Health Services (CMHS). As part of the reorganization of ADAMHA, three research institutes previously housed in this agency were moved to the *National Institutes of Health (NIH)*, another component of USPHS. The NIH conducts health-related research and provides some direct services to individuals in the course of that research. With the transfer of the three institutes from ADAMHA, the NIH currently houses 25 research institutes, divisions, and centers, each focusing on research in a special interest area. The major components of the NIH are depicted in Figure 3–6 ■.

The *Health Resources and Services Administration (HRSA)* was created by the merging of the previous Health Services Administration and Health Resources Administration. This combined agency is responsible for training and employment of health professionals and health resources planning and utilization. Major components of the HRSA include the Bureau of Primary Health Care, the Bureau of Health Resources Development, and the Division of Immigration Health Services. One additional HRSA bureau of interest to community health nurses is the Bureau of Health Professionals, which houses the Division of Nursing.

Other agencies within the USPHS include the Agency for Toxic Substances and Disease Registry, the Indian Health Service, and the Agency for Health Care Research and Quality. The *Agency for Toxic Substances and Disease Registry* monitors exposures to toxic substances and the occurrence of disease related to toxic exposures. The *Indian Health Service*, previously housed under the Health Resources and Services Administration, is responsible for providing direct care services for large segments of the Native American population. The *Agency for Health Care Research and Quality* focuses on generating and disseminating information for use in policy formation, with emphasis on quality, effectiveness, and cost of health care.

The *Health Care Financing Administration (HCFA)* is responsible for federally funded programs under Medicare and Medicaid. HCFA is responsible for reimbursement under these programs and sets reimbursement rates under the diagnosis-related groups system discussed earlier. HCFA is also responsible for quality and utilization control for the programs under its jurisdiction.

The *Administration for Children and Families* addresses the health needs of children and families, persons with developmental disabilities, Native Americans (other than those addressed by the Indian Health Service), refugees, and legalized aliens. The agency consists of the Administration on Children, Youth, and Families; the Administration on Developmental Disabilities; the Administration for Native Americans; the Office of Child Support Enforcement; the Office of Community Services, the Office of Refugee Resettlement, and the Office of Family Assistance.

The *Administration on Aging* focuses on the needs of the elderly population in the United States, and develops policies, plans, and programs designed to enhance the health of this growing population. The components of the Department of Health and Human Services are listed in Table 3–1 ■. The World Wide Web address of each agency is provided for those who wish to obtain further information on specific services.

Although DHHS is the agency primarily responsible for national health, other agencies within the federal government are also involved in addressing health issues. For example, the Department of Defense provides health care for military personnel, dependents, and retirees, and the Department of the Interior addresses health concerns related to environmental pollution. Similarly, the Department of Labor is concerned with occupational health as well as other employment concerns, and the Treasury Department is actively involved in efforts to control drugs subject to abuse (Miller, 1995).

Agencies at the federal level provide assistance to state and local agencies in the form of health resources and professional education. Agencies also assist in improving

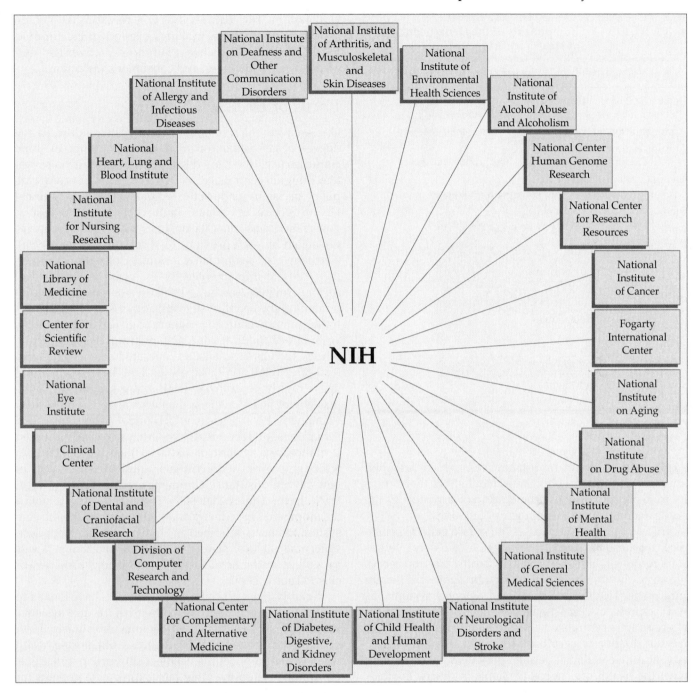

FIGURE 3–6   ■   *Major Components of the National Institutes of Health*

health care delivery and conduct, support, and disseminate findings of health-related research. Additional federal responsibilities related to health include protecting the public against unsafe food and drugs, controlling communicable diseases, and functioning as liaison between the United States and international health organizations or with other countries. Federal agencies also provide direct services to certain population groups such as Native Americans and military personnel, retirees, and dependents. Federal health-related agencies are included in the resource lists on the Web site for this book.

Although state public health agencies have primary responsibility for health matters and federal responsibility has been only indirectly derived from the Constitution, there is growing recognition of the need for a more explicit interface between federal and state public health efforts. This need arises out of the fact that many health problems cannot be solved within state jurisdictions and that broader efforts will be required for their resolution.

Members of the Reforming States Group (1998) have identified this need and have recommended a system of "balanced federalism" in which the federal government sets broad national standards in consultation with state

■ **TABLE 3–1**   **Components of the Department of Health and Human Services**

AGENCY	WORLD WIDE WEB ADDRESS
Department of Health and Human Services	*www.dhhs.gov*
Administration on Aging	*www.aoa.dhhs.gov*
Administration for Children and Families	*www.afc.gov*
Health Care Financing Administration	*www.hcfa.gov*
Agency for Toxic Substances and Disease Registry	*www.atsdr.gov*
Agency for Health Care Research and Quality	*www.ahrq.gov*
Centers for Disease Control and Prevention	*www.cdc.gov*
Food and Drug Administration	*www.fda.gov*
Health Services and Resources Administration	*www.hrsa.gov*
Indian Health Service	*www.ihs.gov*
National Institutes of Health	*www.nih.gov*
Substance Abuse and Mental Health Services Administration	*www.samhsa.gov*

and personal sector representatives, which are then implemented by the states. States would have the authority to expand upon these standards as warranted by the needs and circumstances of their populations.

This recommendation arises out of two general principles: the need for a clear delineation of federal versus state responsibilities in the area of health care and recognition of the capabilities that each brings to the health care arena. Health care plans and delivery systems, as well as problems, cross over state boundaries, and there is a need for a centralized effort to monitor and standardize the quality of services provided. In addition, the advent of telemedicine permits providers in one state to meet the health care needs of clients in others. Furthermore, there is a need to evaluate large for-profit health care endeavors in the light of antitrust laws. Finally, development of national standards will facilitate data collection and identification of population health problems (Reforming States Group, 1998).

INTERNATIONAL COMPARISONS

Other nations throughout the world have developed their own organizational structures for delivering health care services to their peoples. Examination of selected features of the health care systems in other countries can assist in identifying the strengths and weaknesses of the

U.S. system. The features that will be explored include the locus of decision making, expenditures, funding mechanisms, professional autonomy, coverage and access, health outcomes, and consumer satisfaction.

Locus of Decision Making

One area in which national health systems differ is the degree of centralization of decision making. In some countries (e.g., the United Kingdom), the health care system is highly centralized, with the majority of health care policy decisions made at the federal level by the National Health Service. In Canada, on the other hand, the federal government sets general principles which are then operationalized by each province as it sees fit (Reagan, 1999). Germany also has initiated a number of national principles that are implemented by the personal health care sector (Brown & Amelung, 1999). In Australia, some components of the health system are administered by the central Commonwealth government (e.g., care of the elderly, ambulatory medical care, and pharmaceuticals), while others, such as hospitals, are operated by the states and territories (Hall, 1999). Japan, like the United Kingdom, has a highly centralized health care system, with the majority of policy made at the national government level (Yamauchi, 1999). Russia, which under communism had the epitome of a centralized system, has recently adopted a mandatory system of national health insurance in which employers of individuals contract with a variety of new private insurance companies for coverage (Twigg, 1999). In the United States, the foci for health care policy development are so many and varied that the health care system has been described as "hyperpluralist" with decisions made at local, state, and national government levels as well as at the level of the organization, provider, or client (Tuohy, 1999).

Recently, many European governments have looked to decentralize some portions of their health care systems, promoting decision making at regional or municipal levels. Decentralization has the advantage of tailoring health care delivery to meet the needs of differing populations. Centralization, on the other hand, can create impetus for more rational planning and cost control (Reagan, 1999).

Successful decentralization requires several preexisting conditions. These include local administrative capacity to develop and implement health policy and readiness to accept several interpretations of problems and their solutions. When these conditions do not exist, decentralization can result in fragmentation, inequity, and weakening of public health regulatory functions (Saltman & Figueras, 1998). Fragmentation is certainly evident in the U.S. health care system, and inequities have been noted in the health services provided from one province to another in Canada (Gratzer, 1999).

There appear to be some areas of health decision making that are best centralized, even in a largely decentralized system. These include determination of basic policy directions, strategic planning for resource development,

CULTURAL CONSIDERATIONS

What traditional features of the dominant American culture would make it difficult for much of the U.S. public to accept a national health care system similar to that of the United Kingdom? Might such a system be more easily accepted by members of ethnic minority groups residing in the United States? Why or why not?

public safety regulation, and monitoring and assessing health status and the quality of health care (Saltman & Figueras, 1998).

To a large extent, decisions about the centralization or decentralization of health care policy making are based on national attitudes and values. The hyperpluralism and lack of centralization of the U.S. health care system, for example, is largely a result of strongly held values of individualism and limited government involvement in everyday life (Inglehart, 2000), and a centralized government-operated health care system is likely to be unacceptable to the U.S. population (Garson, 2000). Other nations (e.g., Canada and the United Kingdom) place higher priority on communal obligations and public primacy (Inglehart, 2000; Saltman & Figueras, 1998). German attitudes are characterized by a strong sense of mutual dependence and obligation between government and the private sector for creating a common good (Reagan, 1999). Health care systems, however they are designed, must support the values and beliefs of the populations served if they are to be effective in achieving established health goals.

Expenditures

Cost control has been a recent concern for health systems in all nations. Some countries, however, are more successful at controlling health care expenditures than others. For example, in 1998, Japan spent only 7.4% of its *gross domestic product (GDP)* (the total monetary value of all goods and services produced by a nation in a given period) on health care, whereas the United States expended 14.0% of its GDP, the highest percentage of any developed nation. To some extent, these higher expenditures are a result of greater incorporation of technology in health care practice, but also are due to limited control of health care costs. The economic aspects of the U.S. health care delivery system will be discussed in more detail in Chapter 5.

Most European countries and Canada lie between the United States and Japan in terms of their health care expenditures. Canada, for example, spent 9.3% of its GDP on health care in 1998, while Germany spent 10.6%. The United Kingdom, on the other hand, spent even less than Japan, at 6.9% of the GDP (Inglehart, 2000). Figures for Australia and Russia are from 1997 and include 7.8% and 5.4% of GDP, respectively. Despite greater expenditures,

health care outcomes are no better, and are sometimes worse, in the United States than elsewhere, as we will see later.

Another cost measure in which national health care systems differ is the percentage of health care expenditures paid out-of-pocket by consumers. Of the nations discussed here, the United Kingdom has the lowest out-of-pocket costs at just 3.1% and Russia the highest at 23.2%. Out-of-pocket expenditures in Australia (16.6%), Canada (17%), and the United States (16.6%) are roughly comparable, while those in Germany are somewhat lower (11.3%) and those in Japan higher (19.9%) based on 1997 figures (WHO, 2000).

Funding Mechanisms

Health care systems also vary widely in terms of the means by which services are funded and providers reimbursed. As we will see in Chapter 5, health care funding in the United States is derived from a number of sources, including out-of-pocket payment, private insurance, and federal and state tax dollars. Similarly, providers may be reimbursed on the basis of fee-for-service or flat rates per person or per service provided.

The majority of German health system funding is based on "sickness funds" provided by employers and employees. Employer and employee each pay half of the premium to a maximum of 13% of the employee's salary. All citizens with incomes less than $44,000 (in 1997 U.S. dollars) are required to enroll in this national insurance fund, and approximately 90% of the population are covered by this mechanism. Those with higher incomes can choose private insurance coverage, and many covered employees have supplemental private insurance plans (Reagan, 1999). Recent legislation has attempted to create competition among sickness funds in an effort to control rising health care costs (Brown & Amelung, 1999). German providers are paid on a fee-for-service basis by the sickness funds or insurance programs.

Initially, the Canadian national health care system "Medicare" was funded equally by federal and provincial revenues. Since 1977, however, the federal government has gradually reduced its contribution (Inglehart, 2000). For the most part, funds are derived from general tax revenues, although some provinces support the program by payroll taxes or insurance premiums (Gratzer, 1999). Approximately 30% of health care expenditures are funded by private sources (private insurance or out-of-pocket payment) (Naylor, 1999). Hospitals are paid an annual lump sum by provincial governments, but physicians are reimbursed on a fee-for-service basis at rates negotiated between the provincial government and regional medical associations.

In the United Kingdom, health care system funding is largely derived from federal tax revenues (Scully, Birchfield, & Munro, 1998). System reforms in 1991 created General Practitioner (GP) fundholders (general practices with a certain number of clients) that were given a budget to provide services and/or contract for them with secondary providers. Changes also made hospitals independent trusts that contract with local health authorities and GP fundholders to provide hospital services. These changes, initiated to promote internal competition, have had somewhat limited success (Le Grand, 1999). In more recent reforms, the GP fundholders will be replaced by primary care groups who will receive a lump sum payment, based on the number of clients served, to provide all necessary services to their client population (Davis, 1999). Specialists, in the British system, are salaried hospital employees (Tuohy, 1999).

Funding for the Japanese health care system arises out of three social insurance plans, each covering approximately a third of the population. The first covers employees and dependents in the public sector and in large private firms and consists of nearly 2,000 independent plans with premiums ranging from 6% to 9.5% of the employee's wages and shared by employer and employee. The second plan is administered by the Ministry of Health and Welfare and covers employees and dependents of small firms. Current premiums are 8.6% of wages up to a maximum amount, and half of the premium is paid by the employer. Those who are self-employed or pensioners are covered by Citizen's Health Insurance provided by local cities, villages, and towns. Premiums in this plan vary with family circumstances and are paid directly to the municipal government (Ikegami & Campbell, 1999).

In 2000, Japan initiated long-term care insurance for the elderly and disabled to cover institutional or community-based care. Every person 40 years of age and older must contribute to this program. Half of program funding will come from general revenues (50% at the national level and 25% each from the prefecture and municipality) and half from premiums. Persons aged 40 to 64 years will pay a supplement to their existing health insurance premium (about 0.9% of earnings). Those over 65 years of age will have graduated premiums deducted from their public pensions based on income (Campbell & Ikegami, 2000).

Hospitals and physicians in Japan are separate systems, with most physicians operating independently with no access to hospital care. Both are reimbursed on a fee-for-service basis by the insurance plans, but with differing rates of reimbursement (higher for physician care than hospital care for the same service).

The Australian "Medicare" system of universal health care insurance is funded through general tax revenues and a specific income tax. Hospital care is provided in public hospitals, and reimbursement rates are determined by the states and territories. Physician services are reimbursed on a fee-for-service basis in the personal health care sector (Hall, 1999).

Funding in the new Russian health care system is provided by a 3.6% payroll tax paid by employers to federal and regional health insurance funds. Municipal governments subsidize the funds for services to children, the elderly, and the unemployed. Reimbursement for specific

---

services provided may be on a fee-for-service or capitated basis or a combination of both, depending on the region (Twigg, 1999).

Autonomy

National health systems also vary in terms of the degree of autonomy exercised by clients and providers within the system. In the U.S. system, the degree of autonomy of both clients and providers varies greatly depending on the source of health care funding, as we will see in Chapter 5. For example, clients enrolled in some managed care organizations may be constrained in their choice of provider or in their ability to seek the services of a specialist. Similarly, providers may be limited in their choice of treatment options depending on the source of their funding. Some insurance plans, for instance, may cover certain procedures or medications and not others.

Expansion of consumer choice is one of the tenets of health care system reform in many European countries (Saltman & Figueras, 1998). In the Canadian, German, Japanese, Australian, and new Russian systems, clients have a choice in their primary providers. Choice of specialist care is constrained in Canada and the United Kingdom by limited availability and long waiting times in some areas (Donelan, Blendon, Schoen, Davis, & Binns, 1999; Inglehart, 2000). In other countries, such as Australia, primary care physicians constitute "gatekeepers" who make decisions on when specialist care is warranted (Hall, 1999). In fact, it has been noted that there is no general consensus on whether clients should have unlimited access to specialty care (Saltman & Figueras, 1998).

Providers may also be constrained in practice decisions either directly or by system factors. Providers in Japan and Germany are highly independent and there are few constraints on their practice. Health care professionals also have a high degree of autonomy in Canada and the United Kingdom, but are frequently constrained by the availability of special diagnostic or specialty care services. As noted by one disgruntled Canadian physician,

"In the past, we did the best we *could* for patients. Today we do the best we are *allowed* to do under the circumstances" (Gratzer, 1999, p. 19). In the United States, providers in some managed care organizations are hampered in providing what they consider to be optimal care by gag clauses that prevent them from discussing with clients treatment options not covered by the insurance plan (Rovner, 2000).

Finally, providers may be constrained in terms of their ability to access several revenue streams. In the United States, many providers are on the provider panels of several managed care organizations. Similarly, in Japan, most physicians belong to all three types of insurance plans (Yamauchi, 1999). Physicians in the United Kingdom have the ability to engage in private practice in addition to participation in the National Health System, and even public hospitals have a certain number of private-pay beds (Reagan, 1999). Similarly, in the United Kingdom, Australia, and Germany, citizens have the option to purchase supplemental private insurance, yet German physicians are prohibited by law from advertising (Brown & Amelung, 1999; Davis, 1999). In Canada, physicians can opt for private practice only if they choose not to participate in the national health care system, and private insurance companies are legally prohibited from offering coverage for any services covered under the national plan (Reagan, 1999; Inglehart, 2000).

Coverage and Access

The United States is the only health care system addressed here that does not provide universal access to health care for all citizens, and approximately 40 million people were uninsured in 1995 compared to none of the populations in other countries (Aday et al., 1998). The other systems discussed here provide nearly, if not perfect, universal coverage. For example, approximately 3% of Canadians are not covered by the "Medicare" system because they do not pay the payroll taxes levied by a few provinces (Gratzer, 1999). Similarly, the Russian system covers approximately 80% of the population (Twigg, 1999), and the German system provides service to 90% of its citizens (Brown & Amelung, 1999). The remaining percentages of these populations are covered by private forms of insurance.

Although the bulk of the population is covered under all of the national health systems discussed, except that of the United States, that does not mean that all conceivable services are provided. For example, the Japanese system covers prescription drugs (Ikegami & Campbell, 1999), as do many managed care plans in the United States. However, pharmaceuticals are covered only for the elderly in the Canadian system (Inglehart, 2000), although hospital and medical services are covered for all. The Australian system covers pharmaceuticals as well as medical and hospital care, but funding derives from different sources, with hospital funding from the states and territories and prescription drugs through the commonwealth government (Hall, 1999). In Japan, dental care and home care are also covered, although few other national systems provide such coverage (Ikegami & Campbell, 1999; Yamauchi, 1999).

Health Outcomes

Another way of comparing national health care delivery systems is in terms of the outcomes achieved. One of the principle outcomes is that of life expectancy. Despite the level of health expenditures in the United States, the nation ranked nineteenth among selected nations for female life expectancy in 1999 and twenty-fifth in male life expectancy. Life expectancies for both males and females in the United States lagged behind each of the other countries discussed here except the Russian Federation (WHO, 2000). These figures are displayed in Table 3–2 ■.

Life expectancy, however, measures longevity as an outcome of health care, but does not measure the burden of disease and disability. A more reflective measure of health care outcomes is *disability-adjusted life expectancy (DALE)*, or the number of years of healthy life that one can expect to attain. Again, the countries considered here vary considerably in terms of this outcome variable. According to 1999 estimates from WHO (2000), Japan again ranks highest, with 74.5 years of expected disability-free life, followed by Australia in second place (73.2), Canada at twelfth (72.0), the United Kingdom at fourteenth (71.7), and Germany at twenty-second (70.4). The United States ranks twenty-fourth at a disability-adjusted life expectancy of 70 years, and Russia is ninety-first, at only 61.3 years. Disability-adjusted life expectancy and longevity are compared for these nations in Table 3–2.

■ **TABLE 3–2   International Comparisons of Life Expectancy (LE) and Disability-Adjusted Life Expectancy (DALE) (1999)**

	LE				DALE	
	Female		Male		Total Population	
COUNTRY	Years	Rank	Years	Rank	Years	Rank
Australia	80.4	7	74.4	7	73.2	2
Canada	81.9	6	76.2	4	72.0	12
Germany	80.1	14	73.7	16	70.4	22
Japan	84.3	2	77.6	1	74.5	1
Russia	74.0	N/A	62.7	N/A	61.3	91
United Kingdom	79.7	16	74.7	11	71.7	14
United States	79.7	19	73.8	25	70.0	24

Sources: U.S. Department of Health and Human Services. (2000). *Healthy people 2010* (Conference edition, in two volumes). Washington, DC: Author; and World Health Organization. (2000). *The world health report 2000: Health systems: Improving performance.* Geneva, Switzerland: Author.

Goal attainment and overall system performance as measured by WHO are other ways of assessing health system outcomes. With respect to goal attainment for the national health sytems reviewed here, Japan is rated first of 191 member nations, followed by Canada, the United Kingdom, Australia, and Germany. The United States is rated fifteenth, and the Russian Federation at 100th. In terms of overall health system performance, defined as a ratio of achieved levels of health to levels achievable by the most efficient system, top ratings are held by France, followed by Australia, Japan, the United Kingdom, Germany, the United States (at thirty-seventh), and Russia.

The United States ranked first in terms of the level of responsiveness of its health care system, with a rating of 8.10 of a possible 10 points. Responsiveness was measured by several variables related to respect for persons (dignity, autonomy, and confidentiality) and client orientation (prompt attention, quality of basic amenities, access to social support as part of care, and provider choice). Other nations' health care systems were rated less favorably, with Germany ranked fifth, Japan at sixth, Canada tied for seventh position, Australia tied for twelfth, the United Kingdom tied at twenty-sixth, and Russia tied at sixty-ninth (WHO, 2000). National rankings on goal attainment, overall system performance, and responsiveness are summarized in Table 3–3 ■.

Child survival is another measure of the effectiveness of health care systems. According to 1997 data from WHO (2000), the United Kingdom and Japan rank second and third in the world in child survival (outranked only by Chile), followed by Australia, Canada, and Germany at positions 17, 18, and 20, respectively. The United States ranks thirty-second, and Russia lags behind at sixty-ninth of 191 nations.

Consumer Satisfaction

Consumer satisfaction is another way in which health care systems can be compared. Satisfaction studies have been conducted for some of the national health care sys-tems discussed here and not for others. Satisfaction ratings for several health care systems have declined in recent years, most noticeably Canada. For example, only 24% of Canadians rated their health care system as good or excellent in 1999 compared to 61% in 1991 (Inglehart, 2000). In 1998, a survey conducted by the Commonwealth Fund found that nearly one third of U.S. citizens and Australians and 23% of Canadians favored a complete restructuring of the health care system compared to only 14% of people in the United Kingdom. In the same study, roughly half of the respondents in each country indicated that some fundamental changes were needed in their national system. Sources of dissatisfaction varied somewhat, with people in countries with universal coverage more concerned about administrative issues, including long waiting periods for some services, and those in the United States concerned with financial access to services. Satisfaction with health care services declined from 1988 to 1998 for Australia, Canada, and the United Kingdom, but improved slightly in the United States (Donelan et al., 1999). Table 3–4 ■ summarizes information about the national systems discussed here related to locus of decision making, expenditures, funding mechanisms, autonomy, and coverage and access.

⑥THINK ABOUT IT

What are the advantages and disadvantages of a centralized, government-supported health care system for all citizens?

As we have seen, national health care systems vary in a number of ways, and each system has both positive and negative features. No nation has yet developed a perfect health care delivery system that meets what have

■ **TABLE 3–3** **National Rankings for Health System Goal Attainment, System Performance, and Responsiveness (1999)**

COUNTRY	GOAL ATTAINMENT	SYSTEM PERFORMANCE	RESPONSIVENESS
Australia	10	9	12
Canada	7	30	7
Germany	14	25	5
Japan	1	10	6
Russia	100	130	69
United Kingdom	9	18	26
United States	15	37	1

Source: World Health Organization. (2000). *The world health report 2000: Health systems: Improving performance.* Geneva, Switzerland: Author.

■ **TABLE 3–4   Comparison of Selected National Health System Features**

LOCUS OF DECISION MAKING

Australia: Decentralized
Canada: Decentralized
Germany: Centralized
Japan: Highly Centralized
Russian Federation: Decentralized
United Kingdom: Centralized, but becoming less so
United States: Hyperpluralistic

EXPENDITURES	PERCENT OF GDP	OUT-OF-POCKET
Australia	7.8%[a]	16.6%[a]
Canada	9.3%[b]	17.0%[a]
Germany	10.6%[b]	11.3%[a]
Japan	7.4%[b]	19.9%[a]
Russian Federation	5.4%[a]	23.2%[a]
United Kingdom	6.9%[b]	3.1%[a]
United States	14.0%[b]	16.6%[a]

[a] 1997 figures
[b] 1998 figures

FUNDING MECHANISMS

Australia: Tax revenues
Canada: Tax revenues (payroll tax in some provinces)
Germany: Payroll tax
Japan: Payroll tax, municipal revenues
Russian Federation: Payroll tax
United Kingdom: Tax revenues
United States: Variable

PROVIDER REIMBURSEMENT

Australia: Fee-for-service
Canada: Fee-for-service
Germany: Fee-for-service
Japan: Fee-for-service
Russian Federation: Fee-for-service
United Kingdom: Fee-for-service, moving toward per-person flat fee
United States: Variable

CONSUMER CHOICE

Australia: Open choice of primary provider, gatekeeper for specialty services, can obtain supplemental private insurance if desired
Canada: Open choice of provider or specialist, supplemental insurance only for uncovered services
Germany: Open choice of provider and insurance company, private insurance available for higher wage earners
Japan: Open choice of provider
Russian Federation: Open choice of provider and insurance company
United Kingdom: Open choice of primary provider within health authority
United States: Variable, often constrained in MCOs

(continued)

■ **TABLE 3–4   Comparison of Selected National Health System Features** *(continued)*

PROVIDER AUTONOMY

Australia: High

Canada: High in personal practice; specialty referrals often constrained by availability; MD cannot choose both private practice and participation in national program

Germany: High

Japan: High

Russian Federation: Unknown

United Kingdom: High in personal practice; specialty referrals often constrained by availability; MD able to engage in private practice as well

United States: Variable; often constrained in MCOs

COVERAGE

Australia: Universal

Canada: Universal; may have long waits for specialty or diagnostic services

Germany: Universal

Japan: Universal

Russian Federation: Universal, but resources not adequate to meet need

United Kingdom: Universal; may have long waits for specialty or elective services

United States: Approximately 40 million uninsured

CONSUMER SATISFACTION

Australia: Declining

Canada: Declining

Germany: Unknown

Japan: Unknown

Russian Federation: Unknown

United Kingdom: Relatively high

United States: Increasing slightly

---

been identified as five "basic pillars" of health care: quality, timeliness of diagnosis and treatment, cost-effectiveness, client orientation, and accessibility (Gratzer, 1999). Community health nurses in all countries need to be actively involved in the development of systems that meet these criteria. Even then, it is unlikely that all criteria can be met to the maximum, since some of them are mutually exclusive. For example, the highest quality of health care is incompatible with the lowest cost (Reagan, 1999), and balance will need to be achieved among criteria. Consumers and community health nurses must be involved in discussions that determine that balance.

GLOBAL HEALTH CARE

Thus far, we have been discussing systems of health care delivery within a single nation. Nations are interdependent, however, and people can travel to any place in the world in a matter of hours. International health is of increasing concern. Increased mobility means increased potential for the spread of disease from nation to nation. This remains true of communicable diseases traditionally spread by travelers from infected to noninfected areas. For example, wild polio virus was reintroduced into China by border crossers from northern India (Andrus et al., 2001), and several cases of malaria occurring near airports in developed countries are believed to have been spread by mosquitos imported on international flights (*The Nation's Health*, 2000).

In addition, increased global communication and mobility have led to changes in lifestyle that bring the attendant risks of many lifestyle-related chronic illnesses. For example, dietary changes that occur as many developing countries are exposed to Western culture have contributed to a rise in heart disease. Adoption of new lifestyles in many parts of the world has contributed to the development of stress-related disorders. Increased travel and import/export opportunities have increased the potential for trafficking in illegal substances and increased drug use around the world. Alcoholism is another growing concern worldwide. Finally, environmental concerns are now international, rather than local, in scope.

Since 1977, the major emphasis in international health care has been the achievement of *"health for all by the year 2000,"* the outcome of the World Health Assembly of that year. The following year, the International Conference on Primary Health Care held in Alma Alta, in what was then the USSR, produced a report entitled *Primary Health Care,* otherwise known as the **Declaration of Alma Alta.** The central goal of the "health for all" movement is the provision of basic health care to all peoples of the world by the year 2000. Its three main objectives are promotion of healthy lifestyles, prevention of preventable conditions, and therapy for existing conditions (Orr, 1992).

Primary health care is the major strategy to be employed in achieving these objectives. **Primary health care (PHC)** has been described as "both a philosophy of health care and an approach to providing health care resources. Its basic elements are essential health care, socially acceptable and affordable methods and technology, accessibility, public participation, and intersectoral collaboration" (Beddone, Clark, & Whyte, 1993).

International Health Agencies

On the global level, the organization of health services is somewhat less structured than in the national systems discussed earlier. A number of organizations and agencies are concerned with international health. Organizations addressing international health concerns can be divided into several groups: private voluntary agencies, philanthropic foundations, private industries, and official agencies. Private voluntary agencies include both religious and secular groups that provide health assistance at the international level. The efforts of many religious organizations are coordinated by the Evangelical Foreign Missions Association or the Church World Service, while coordination of secular groups is the function of the International Council of Voluntary Agencies. CARE and Project Hope are examples of secular voluntary agencies; Catholic Relief Services is an international religious organization providing health assistance to developing countries. Philanthropic foundations are similar to those discussed earlier, but with an international rather than a national focus for their efforts. One example is the Rockerfeller Foundation. Private industries such as pharmaceutical companies also provide overseas health assistance.

Official international health agencies include member countries participating via official governmental structures. These agencies can be described as either bilateral or multilateral. **Multilateral agencies** are those that involve several countries in joint activities related to health, whereas **bilateral agencies** usually involve only two countries in any single project.

MULTILATERAL AGENCIES

The primary agency dealing with health concerns at the international level is the **World Health Organization (WHO)**, a multilateral agency. A specialized agency attached to the United Nations by formal agreement, but not subordinate to the UN, WHO is funded through subscription by member nations and is responsible for monitoring the incidence of disease throughout the world. The organization also sets international standards for sanitation, biological products, laboratory techniques and procedures, and the manufacture of drugs. WHO supports graduate study and research efforts and assists member nations in controlling disease. A further responsibility is monitoring environmental pollution levels through a program called "Earthwatch" and providing assistance to underdeveloped countries to prevent or eliminate pollution. The World Health Assembly, held yearly in May, is the arena for policy formation within WHO.

The **Pan American Health Organization (PAHO)** is another multilateral organization of particular interest. This agency deals with health-related concerns in the Americas and provides an avenue for collective efforts to promote the health status of people in all nations in the Western Hemisphere.

One PAHO program provides profiles of the health assessment efforts of international agencies. The Health Situation and Trend Analysis Program develops health profiles of member nations as part of a continuing effort to identify factors influencing health. National profiles include information on the health status of citizens, the health system within the country, and the environmental context in which the society is evolving. This information provides direction for programs to enhance health status in member nations.

Other multilateral agencies include the health components of the North Atlantic Treaty Organization (NATO) and the Southeast Asia Treaty Organization (SEATO). The United Nations International Children's Emergency Fund (UNICEF) and the United Nations Educational, Scientific, and Cultural Organization (UNESCO) are two other agencies within the UN that provide assistance with matters of international health. The Food and Agricultural Organization (FAO) is a multilateral agency designed to enhance the world's food supply. Finally, the World Bank provides both funding and technical assistance in dealing with health problems around the world.

BILATERAL AGENCIES

A number of bilateral organizations with health concerns exist throughout the world. Virtually all developed countries provide some form of health-related aid to underdeveloped countries, with the contribution of some countries far in excess of that provided by the United States. This section will focus on the bilateral organizations involving the United States. Such organizations may be either governmental or nongovernmental. One of the federal agencies that is concerned with international health is the Agency for International Development (AID), which administers all federally financed projects for foreign development, including those that are health related. This agency is housed in the U.S. State Department.

The Department of Health and Human Services includes the International Health Program Office within the CDC. This agency is concerned with cooperative projects for improving international health. The Fogarty International Center is housed in the NIH and focuses on international health. Other branches of the NIH (e.g., the Geographic Medicine Branch of the Institute of Allergy and Infectious Diseases) are involved in activities that are international in focus, as is the CDC. ACTION, the volunteer organization of the federal government, houses both the domestic assistance programs of VISTA (Volunteers in Service to America) and the international programs of the Peace Corps, many of which have a health focus. Federally chartered institutions such as the Institute of Medicine and the National Science Foundation are also concerned with problems of international health, as well as with domestic problems.

Names and addresses of several international health organizations are included on the companion Web site for this book. Similar information on additional agencies is available in the *Encyclopedia of Associations* (published annually by the Gale Group, Farmington Hills, MI).

Global Health Issues

Global health concerns fall into several major categories: infectious disease, injury and chronic disease, mental health, poverty and malnutrition, women's health, care of the elderly, tobacco use, environmental health, disasters, and global terrorism (Brundtland, 1999; International Council of Nurses, 1999; Schieber & Maeda, 1999).

CRITICAL THINKING IN RESEARCH

Literature related to health economics and to medicine contains numerous articles comparing and contrasting various aspects of different health care delivery systems. As we have seen, there are research studies comparing relative costs, client satisfaction, and a variety of outcome measures. There are few, if any, studies, however, that examine the effects of health care delivery systems on nursing, yet nurses are the health professionals responsible for implementing a large segment of the care provided in any system.

- How would you design a study to examine the effects of different health care systems on nursing practice?
- What variables might you choose to examine? Why?
- Who would you select as subjects for your study? Would you choose certain categories of nurses? Why or why not?
- What kind of data collection strategies would be most appropriate to the study variables you have identified? Are there tools already available that you might use?

Infectious diseases continue to be a major area of concern throughout the world. Much of the infectious disease burden lies in vaccine-preventable childhood illnesses. According to 1999 estimates, measles accounted for 875,000 deaths, tetanus for 377,000, and pertussis for 295,000 (WHO, 2000). Each year 3 million children die from vaccine-preventable diseases and approximately 23% of the children born each year receive no immunizations. At current cost estimates, $226 million would be required each year to provide vaccine coverage with the six basic vaccines of the Global Alliance for Vaccines and Immunizations (GAVI) Expanded Program on Immunization (EPI). These are vaccines for poliomyelitis, diphtheria, pertussis, tetanus, measles, and tuberculosis. Coverage with additional newer vaccines used in developed countries would cost an additional $352 million (WHO, 2000). GAVI has instituted a world fund to provide children's vaccines worldwide, but additional efforts are needed.

Other infectious diseases also pose a considerable burden in international illness and death. For example, 1.6 million deaths due to tuberculosis, 2.6 million HIV/AIDS deaths, 2.2 million deaths due to diarrheal diseases, and more than 1 million malaria deaths were estimated for 1999. Mortality for respiratory infections was estimated at more than 4 million persons.

Some degree of global control has been achieved over certain infectious diseases. The last recorded case of smallpox in the world occurred in 1977, and smallpox was declared eradicated by WHO in 1980 (Centers for Disease Control and Prevention [CDC], 1993). The goal of eliminating poliomyelitis in the Americas appears to be within reach. *Eradication* is the "reduction of the worldwide incidence of a disease to zero as a result of deliberate efforts, obviating the need for further control measures" (CDC, 1993). *Elimination* is the same phenomenon on a smaller scale; that is, the disease in question no longer occurs in one area of the world (CDC, 1993). Diseases currently targeted for worldwide eradication include dracunculiasis (guinea worm disease), poliomyelitis, filariasis, mumps, rubella, and pork tapeworm. By 1994, cases of wild virus polio had been virtually eliminated from the entire Western Hemisphere (UNICEF, 1995).

Although infectious diseases continue to be the primary health concern in several countries, many nations are experiencing a shift in health problems to encompass more chronic disease, injury, mental illness, nutritional problems, and environmentally caused disease. The rising incidence of chronic diseases in developing countries is a result of rising incomes, dietary changes, changes in exercise and substance use behaviors, and an aging population due to lower death rates and greater life expectancy. A worldwide report predicts that by 2020 chronic diseases will account for 73% of all deaths. In some developing nations, such as India, noncommunicable disease mortality is expected to double by that time (WHO, 1999). Based on 1999 estimates, 7 million deaths occurred due to malignant neoplasms, 777,000 deaths from diabetes mellitus, and almost 17 million deaths due to cardiovascular disease (WHO, 2000).

Chronic disease mortality is only one measure of its effects on health. Another measure of the international burden of chronic disease is *disability-adjusted life years (DALYs)* or the number of years of disability-free healthy life lost due to disease. It is estimated that 43% of all DALYs lost globally in 1998 were the result of chronic disease (as much as 81% in high-income countries), with cardiovascular disease responsible for 10% of the loss in low- and middle-income countries and 18% in high-income countries and cancer accounting for 5% and 15%, respectively (WHO, 1999). Diabetes prevalence in developing nations is expected to increase almost 300% by 2025, rising from 84 million people affected to 228 million. Smaller increases are also anticipated in developed countries, with an expected rise in the number of cases from 51 million to 72 million (*The Nation's Health*, 1998a).

Economic growth brings about an increase in motor vehicle use with a concomitant increase in injury rates. Potential for injury from industrial accidents and toxic chemicals also increases with industrialization. Injury accounts for one in six years of life lived with disability worldwide and contributed to an estimated 5.1 million deaths in 1999. By far the greatest portion of these deaths (24%) were due to motor vehicle accidents, but 17% are self-inflicted, and 15% resulted from homicide, violence, and war (WHO, 1999, 2000).

A growing burden of mental illness is also being experienced worldwide. For example, in 1998, unipolar major depression ranked fourth among all causes of disease burden, and neuropsychiatric conditions including depression, alcohol and drug dependence, psychoses, and other disorders accounted for 10% of DALYs lost in low- and middle-income countries and 23% in high-income countries. With respect to mortality, neuropsychiatric disorders accounted for an estimated 911,000 deaths in 1999, and alcohol dependence alone resulted in more than 60,000 deaths (WHO, 1999, 2000).

Poverty and malnutrition are other areas of significant concern in international health. For example, poverty contributes to 70% of all deaths and 92% of communicable disease deaths in the poorest quartile of countries as well as 60% of all ill health. Although malaria incidence is high in many countries, persons living in the poorest countries are 250 times more likely to die from malaria that those in the richest nations. Poverty is particularly hazardous for the young, with half of all deaths occurring before age 15 years in the poorest countries compared to only 4% in the richest countries.

Malnutrition is closely associated with poverty and poses an increasing burden of disease throughout the world. Based on 1999 mortality estimates, nutritional deficiencies accounted for more than 493,000 deaths as well as untold illness (WHO, 1999, 2000).

Women's health is another area of concern in global health care. Violation of women's rights and violence against women have been the subject of several recent international conferences. Violence is particularly apparent in refugee situations that occur with regularity in the modern world (McGuire, 1998). Maternal mortality continues to be high in many parts of the world and may be as high as 1 in 16 births in developing countries (Brundtland, 1999).

Health care for a growing elderly population is also of concern throughout the world. It is estimated that by 2020 there will be more than 1 billion people aged 60 years and older in the world, with roughly 70% of this older population living in developing countries. Elderly populations in developing countries will increase by nearly 240% from 1980 to 2020, primarily due to fertility declines and increased life expectancy (International Council of Nurses, 1999). Increased population mobility, increased numbers of women in the workforce, and the decline of the extended family as a social institution have increased the social burden of care for these older adults, and many countries are experiencing serious difficulty in providing health care for this population (Campbell & Ikegami, 2000). Specific areas of concern include financial assistance, food, housing, assistive aids such as glasses and hearing aids, adult day care, safety hazards, and social isolation.

Economic growth, as well as international travel, promotes the importation of many poor health habits from one country to another. Perhaps the foremost of these bad habits is tobacco use, which, although declining in many industrialized nations, is increasing elsewhere in the world. It is estimated that close to 500 million people alive today will die as a result of tobacco-caused illnesses. During the first quarter of the new century, tobacco is expected to cause 150 million deaths, with another 300 million in the second quarter. Anti-tobacco campaigns in the United States have decreased the prevalence of smoking from 40% of the population in 1964 to 23% in 1997. Unfortunately, tobacco consumption in developing countries is increasing by approximately 3.4% per year. Overall prevalence of smoking among the global male population is 48%. WHO (1999) has developed a set of tobacco control principles that could significantly reduce worldwide tobacco consumption. These principles have been demonstrated to be effective in national campaigns and could be equally effective if adopted by more nations. They include:

- Banning tobacco advertising and expanding public health information

- Increasing taxes and regulations to reduce consumption (e.g., prohibiting smoking in public places)

- Encouraging cessation of tobacco use and deregulating nicotine-replacement products

- Building anti-tobacco coalitions to promote anti-tobacco policies

Environmental concerns are drawing greater concern in international health than ever before. Safe drinking water is an area of serious concern. Despite marked improvements in accessibility, half a billion people still do not have access to safe drinking water. By 2050 this number is expected to quintuple, with 35% of the world's population affected (*The Nation's Health*, 1998b). Air pollution, global climate change, and deforestation are other areas of concern. In addition to the depletion of global resources, land use changes contribute to the development of health problems in areas where they did not exist before. For example, construction of dams has created new breeding areas for snails that transmit schistosomiasis. Similarly, land use changes have led to rural–urban migrations with translation of a variety of parasites to new locations (McGuire, 1998).

Another concern in international health is that of human response to disasters. One can hardly pick up a newspaper without reading of natural or man-made disasters that affect large numbers of people. International efforts coordinated by WHO and the International Red Cross have led to the development of disaster planning groups throughout the world. These groups or collaborating centers provide information, services, research, and training in support of international disaster response. One group in the United States designated as a WHO collaborating center is the Center for Emergency Preparedness and Response at the CDC. The function of this group is to coordinate disaster response and to conduct field research related to disasters. Disaster preparedness and the community health nurse's role in disaster are addressed in some detail in Chapter 27.

Global terrorism poses many of the same health concerns that disasters do, with the primary difference being the intentional nature of the event. Although man-made disasters result from human action, they are often not intentional (e.g., a serious train wreck or airline disaster). Terrorist activity, on the other hand, creates intentional harm for individuals or for population groups.

Terrorism has been defined as "the deliberate creation and exploitation of fear through violence or the threat of violence in the pursuit of political change" (Hoffman, 1998, p. 43). Terrorist activity may be categorized as domestic or international. ***Domestic terrorism*** is perpetrated by individuals or groups within a given country without foreign direction or involvement. Domestic terrorism is directed against either the government or population segments of one's own country. White supremacist activities against African Americans, Jews, and other ethnic and religious groups are examples of domestic terrorism. ***International terrorism,*** on the other hand, is directed by foreign groups and may transcend national boundaries, affecting people in several countries (Federal Emergency Management Agency, 1997).

Although many of the effects of terrorism are similar to those experienced in war, they may be more far reaching and more devastating than warfare. The rules of war promulgated in the Geneva and Hague Conventions on Warfare in the late nineteenth and early to mid-twentieth centuries prohibited taking civilians hostage, maltreating prisoners of war, and engaging in reprisals against noncombatants and prisoners. Furthermore, the conventions recognized neutral territory and neutral parties. As is obvious from recent terrorist activities, these conventions are systematically violated by terrorists, which serves to enhance the fear their activities generate (Hoffman, 1998).

The terrorist attacks on the World Trade Center and the U.S. Pentagon on September 11, 2001, and the subsequent success in contaminating the U.S. mail suggest the increased sophistication of current world terrorist activities. The frequency of international terrorist activities is also increasing. In 2000, for example, there were 423 terrorist attacks throughout the world, an 8% increase from the previous year and a nearly 40% increase from the 304 attacks perpetrated in 1997. Attacks directed specifically against the United States increased from 169 in 1999 to 200 in 2000. The increased severity of attacks is also seen in the fact that all international attacks in 2000 resulted in 405 deaths (U.S. Department of State, 1998, 2001), compared to more than 4,000 deaths that occurred in the attack on the World Trade Center alone.

The devastation caused by terrorist attacks increases exponentially with the use of weapons of mass destruction (WMD). There are four categories of agents considered WMDs: nuclear, chemical, and biological weapons; and computers. While the potential effects of nuclear, chemical, and biological weapons seem rather obvious, it may seem strange to think of computers as a possible weapon of mass destruction. Potential computer-mediated effects may range from the availability of information on construction of homemade bombs to dissemination of hate propaganda to the ability to shut down information systems vital to national defense or to health operations in times of emergency (Laqueur, 1999). Although most computer interference would not directly cause disease and death, it may hamper response to other crises that result in these effects.

Nuclear weapons, although potentially devastating in their effects, are unlikely to be used by terrorist groups because of the advanced technology needed and the high cost of materials. In the World Trade Center attacks, however, terrorists demonstrated that similar, if more localized, effects could be achieved with aviation fuel. Probably of greater concern, though, is the fact that both biological and chemical weapons are relatively inexpensive to develop and readily available to most terrorist groups. In fact, they have been referred to as the "poor man's weapons of mass destruction" (Solomon, 1999, p. 81). It has been suggested, in fact, that if World War I was the chemist's war based on the use of chemical weapons, and World War II was the physicist's war due to the use of nuclear weapons, a third world war might very well be a "biologist's war" (Shubik, 1997/1999).

Biological weapons involve the use of microorganisms to cause serious or fatal diseases (Tucker, 2000). They are classified into three categories by the CDC (2001). Category A diseases are those that can be easily disseminated, cause high mortality with significant public health impact, may lead to public panic and social disruption, and require special response preparation. These diseases include anthrax, botulism, plague, smallpox, tularemia, and viral hemorrhagic fever. Category B diseases include Q fever, brucellosis, glanders, ricin toxin, epsilon toxin, and *Staphylococcus B,* each of which can be transmitted with moderate ease, cause moderate morbidity and relatively low mortality, and require special diagnostic and surveillance capabilities. Category C diseases include emerging organisms that could be developed for mass dissemination that would have significant public health impact in terms of morbidity and mortality. Diseases in this category include Nipah virus, hantaviruses, tickborne hemorrhagic fever and encephalitis viruses, yellow fever, and multidrug-resistant tuberculosis. More information about several of these diseases is presented in Chapter 28 and in Appendix B.

Chemical warfare agents are highly toxic chemicals that can be disseminated as vapors, gases, liquids, or aerosols or adsorbed to dust particles (Tucker, 2000). Chemical weapons are categorized by the major organ system affected. Categories include blister or vesicant agents, such as mustard, that affect the skin and lungs; chemicals that affect the blood such as arsine, hydrogen chloride, and hydrogen cyanide; and agents such as chlorine gas, nitrogen oxide, sulfur trioxide–chlorosulfonic acid, and zinc oxide that affect the respiratory system. Other categories of chemical agents include those that cause mental incapacitation, such as LSD and phenothiazines; those that affect the central and peripheral nervous systems like sarin and V-gas; those that are used for riot control such as tear gas; and those that induce vomiting such as adamsite and ciphenylcyanoarsine (CDC, 2001).

Community health nurses may be involved in public health responses to terrorist attacks or in educating the public regarding preventive measures or actions to be taken in the case of exposure. In addition, community health nurses may be actively involved in preventing panic in the general public or in dealing with the psychological effects of a terrorist attack. In the case of biological attacks, community health nurses may be among the first to note symptoms of unusual illness in the population and should be familiar with the signs and symptoms of infection with the most likely biological agents (e.g., anthrax, smallpox, plague). Signs and symptoms of these

diseases are included in Appendix B, and specific health education measures for the general public in the event of terrorist attacks are included on the companion Web site for this book.

Cooperating for Global Health

International cooperation and effort make a difference in the health status of the world population. The classic example of the benefits of such cooperation is the eradication of smallpox. It took just 13 years to wipe out a disease that was taken for granted by the populations of two millennia. Similar concerted international efforts in other areas can influence the health of population groups throughout the world.

Global collaboration will require cooperation across borders as well as international systems that can assist individual nations in addressing global health concerns (Andrus et al., 2001). Elements of global collaboration will include the following:

- Identification of global priorities
- Standardized surveillance systems that identify problems and target populations
- Global professional education for surveillance and intervention techniques
- Development and implementation of performance indicators
- Coordinated cross-national interventions targeted to specific problems
- An overall coordinating body to organize and oversee cooperative efforts
- An accredited laboratory network to support diagnosis and surveillance
- Global funding for collaborative efforts
- Global research related to interventions and delivery mechanisms
- Strong within-nation support to effectively lobby for international health policy

Community health nurses can be active, particularly in terms of the last of these requirements, but may also be involved in research and intervention at international levels.

Health care services are provided in the popular, complementary or alternative, and scientific health care subsystems. In the scientific health care subsystem, care is provided by agencies and organizations at local, state, national, and international levels. Community health nurses may be involved in activities at any of these levels, but the principle focus of care remains the same: improvement in the health status of populations.

APPLYING YOUR KNOWLEDGE IN PRACTICE

🦋 CASE STUDY
Health Care Delivery Systems

Design a health care delivery system that would meet the health needs of the American public. Diagram the organizational structure of the system, making sure that your system addresses the core functions of public health as well as the goals of medical care described in Chapter 1. Address the following questions:

- What features (if any) would you incorporate from the health care delivery systems described in the chapter?
- How would you fund your system? Would health care providers operate on a fee-for-service basis or be salaried employees of the system? Why?

- Would you offer comprehensive health care services? What would be included in the basic health services package? Would this basic coverage be available to all residents? Why or why not?
- How would your system address the three levels of prevention? Would one level receive priority over the others? If so, why?
- What political, economic, and social changes would need to occur before your proposed system could be implemented in the United States?

🦋 TESTING YOUR UNDERSTANDING

- What are the six core goals for effective health care systems? How well does the U.S. system achieve them? (p. 36)
- Diagram the organizational structure of the U.S. health care delivery system. Describe the interactions between the component parts. (pp. 37–46)
- Compare and contrast official and voluntary health agencies. What interactions occur between them? (pp. 38–39)
- Describe five functions performed by voluntary health agencies. Give an example of each. (pp. 38–39)
- What are the 10 essential public health services? How might they be carried out differently by local, state, and national public health agencies? (p. 39)
- How are local, state, and national governments involved in health care delivery? In what ways is

this involvement similar? How does it differ between levels? (pp. 39–46)
- Compare at least three different national health care systems on at least four criteria. In what ways are they similar? How do they differ? (pp. 46–52)
- Differentiate between multilateral and bilateral international health agencies. Give examples of each and discuss when each might be most appropriate for solving a particular kind of health problem. (pp. 53–54)
- Why is international collaboration needed to address global health problems? What requirements must be met for international collaboration to occur? (pp. 57)

REFERENCES

Aday, L. A., Begley, C. E., Lairson, D. R., & Slater, C. H. (1998). *Evaluating the health care system: Effectiveness, efficiency, and equity.* Chicago: Health Administration Press.

Andrus, J. K., Thapa, A. B., Withana, N., Fitzsimmons, J. W., Abeykoon, P., & Aylward, B. (2001). A new paradigm for international

disease control: Lessons learned from polio eradication in Southeast Asia. *American Journal of Public Health, 91,* 146–150.

Beddone, G., Clark, H. F., & Whyte, N. B. (1993). Vision for the future of public health nursing: A case for primary health care. *Public Health Nursing, 10,* 13–18.

Brown, L. D., & Amelung, V. E. (1999). "Manacled competition": Market reforms in German health care. *Health Affairs, 18,* 76–94.

Brundtland, G. H. (1999). WHO Director-General Dr. Gro Harlem Brundtland offers new vision for global health. Global Health Council E-mail broadcast, June 21, 1999.

Campbell, J. C., & Ikegami, N. (2000). Long-term care insurance comes to Japan. *Health Affairs, 19*, 26–39.

Center for Studying Health System Change. (1997). Tracking changes in the public health system. *Journal of Nursing Administration, 27*(2), 16–19.

Centers for Disease Control and Prevention. (1993). Recommendations of the International Task Force for Disease Eradication. *Morbidity and Mortality Weekly Report, 41*(RR-16), 1–38.

Centers for Disease Control and Prevention. (2001). Agents/Diseases. Retrieved October 25, 2001, from the World Wide Web, *http://www.bt.cdc.gov/agent/agentlist.asp.*

Chapel, T. J., Stange, P. V., Gordon, R. L., & Miller, A. (1998). Private sector health care organizations and essential public health services: Potential effects on the practice of local public health. *Journal of Public Health Management Practice, 4*(1), 36–44.

Communication from the City Auditor regarding tuberculosis nurse. (1915, August 20). San Diego, CA: City of San Diego Archives.

Dandoy, S. (1997). The state public health department. In F. D. Scutchfield & C. W. Keck (Eds.), *Principles of public health practice* (pp. 68–86). Albany, NY: Delmar.

Davis, K. (1999). International health policy: Common problems, alternative strategies. *Health Affairs, 18*, 135–143.

Donelan, K., Blendon, R. J., Schoen, C., Davis, K., & Binns, K. (1999). The cost of health system change: Public discontent in five nations. *Health Affairs, 18*, 206–216.

Federal Emergency Management Agency. (1997). Backgrounder: Terrorism. Retrieved October 25, 2001, from the World Wide Web, *http://www.fema.gov.*

Garson, A. (2000). The US healthcare system 2010: Problems, principles, and potential solutions. *Circulation, 101*, 2015–2016.

Gratzer, D. (1999). *Code blue: Reviving Canada's health care system.* Toronto, Ontario: ECW Press.

Hall, J. (1999). Incremental changes in the Australian health care system. *Health Affairs, 18*, 95–110.

Health Resources and Services Administration. (1998). The public health workforce in crisis. *Health Workforce Newslink, 4*(1), 1–2.

Hoffman, B. (1998). *Inside terrorism.* New York: Columbia University Press.

Ikegami, N., & Campbell, J. C. (1999). Health care reform in Japan: The virtues of muddling through. *Health Affairs, 18*, 56–75.

Inglehart, J. K. (2000). Revisiting the Canadian health care system. *Health Policy Report, 342*, 2007–2012.

Institute of Medicine. (1988). *The future of public health.* Washington, DC: National Academy Press.

International Council of Nurses. (1999). ICN on healthy aging: A public health and nursing challenge. *Journal of Advanced Nursing, 30*, 280–281.

Laqueur, W. (1999). *The new terrorism: Fanaticism and the arms of mass destruction.* New York: Oxford University Press.

Lasker, R. D., and the Committee on Medicine and Public Health. (1997). *Medicine & public health: The power of collaboration.* New York: New York Academy of Medicine.

Le Grand, J. (1999). Competition, cooperation, or control? Tales from the British National Health Service. *Health Affairs, 18*, 27–39.

Mays, G. P., Halverson, P. K., & Miller, C. A. (1998). Assessing the performance of local public health systems: A survey of state health agency efforts. *Journal of Public Health Management Practice, 4*(4), 63–78.

McGuire, S. (1998). Global migration and health: Ecofeminist perspectives. *Advanced Nursing Science, 21*(2), 1–16.

Miller, C. A., Moore, K. S., Richards, T. B., & Monk. J. D. (1994). A proposed method for assessing the performance of local public health functions and practices. *American Journal of Public Health, 84*, 1743–1749.

Miller, D. F. (1995). *Dimensions of community health* (5th ed.). Dubuque, IA: Brown.

The Nation's Health. (1998a, November). The global burden of diabetes. p. 10.

The Nation's Health. (1998b, November). Lack of water could cap development, report warns. p. 10.

The Nation's Health. (2000, October). World health leaders fear spread of "airport malaria." p. 14.

Naylor, C. D. (1999). Health care in Canada: Incrementalism under fiscal duress. *Health Affairs, 18*, 9–26.

Office of the Federal Register. (2000). *The United States Government Manual, 2000–2001.* Washington, DC: Government Printing Office.

Orr, J. (1992). The community dimension. In K. Luker & J. Orr (Eds.), *Health visiting: Towards community health nursing.* London: Blackwell Scientific.

Rawding, N., & Wasserman, M. (1997). The local health department. In F. D. Scutchfield & C. W. Keck (Eds.), *Principles of public health practice* (pp. 87–100). Albany, NY: Delmar.

Reagan, M. D. (1999). *The accidental system: Health care policy in America.* Boulder, CO: Westview Press.

Reforming States Group. (1998). Balanced federalism and health system reform. *Health Affairs, 17*, 181–191.

Reid, W. M., & Mason, K. P. (1998). Roles and opportunities for local health departments in managed care markets. *Journal of Public Health Management Practice, 4*(1), 21–28.

Rovner, J. (2000). *Health care policy and politics A to Z.* Washington, DC: CQ Press.

Saltman, R. B., & Figueras, J. (1998). Analyzing the evidence of European health care reforms. *Health Affairs, 17*, 85–108.

Schieber, G., & Maeda, A. (1999). Health care financing and delivery in developing countries. *Health Affairs, 18*, 193–205.

Scully, J., Birchfield, M., & Munro, L. (1998). An international nursing course: The health system, England. *Nursing and Health Care Perspectives, 19*, 208–213.

Shubik, M. (1999). Terrorism, technology, and the socioeconomics of death. In B. Solomon (Ed.), *Chemical and biological warfare* (pp. 96–115). New York: Wilson (reprinted from *Comparative Strategy, 16*, 399–414).

Solomon, B. (1999). Terrorism at home and abroad. In B. Solomon (Ed.), *Chemical and biological warfare* (pp. 81–82). New York: Wilson.

Tucker, J. B. (2000). Introduction. In J. B. Tucker (Ed.), *Toxic terror: Assessing terrorist use of chemical and biological weapons* (pp. 1–14). Cambridge, MA: MIT Press.

Tuohy, C. H. (1999). Dynamics of a changing health sphere: The United States, Britain, and Canada. *Health Affairs, 18*, 114–134.

Twigg, J. L. (1999). Obligatory medical insurance in Russia: The participants' perspective. *Social Science & Medicine, 49*, 371–382.

UNICEF. (1995). *The state of the world's children.* Oxford: Oxford University Press.

U.S. Department of Health and Human Services. (2000). *Healthy people 2010* (Conference edition, in two volumes). Washington, DC: Author.

U.S. Department of State. (1998). *Patterns of global terrorism 1997.* Washington, DC: Author.

U.S. Department of State. (2001). *Patterns of global terrorism 2000.* Washington, DC: Author.

Wall, S. (1998). Transformations in public health systems. *Health Affairs, 17*, 64–80.

World Health Organization. (1999). *The world health report 1999: Making a difference.* Geneva, Switzerland: Author.

World Health Organization. (2000). *The world health report 2000: Health systems: Improving performance.* Geneva, Switzerland: Author.

Yamauchi, T. (1999). Healthcare system in Japan. *Nursing and Health Sciences, 1*, 45–48.

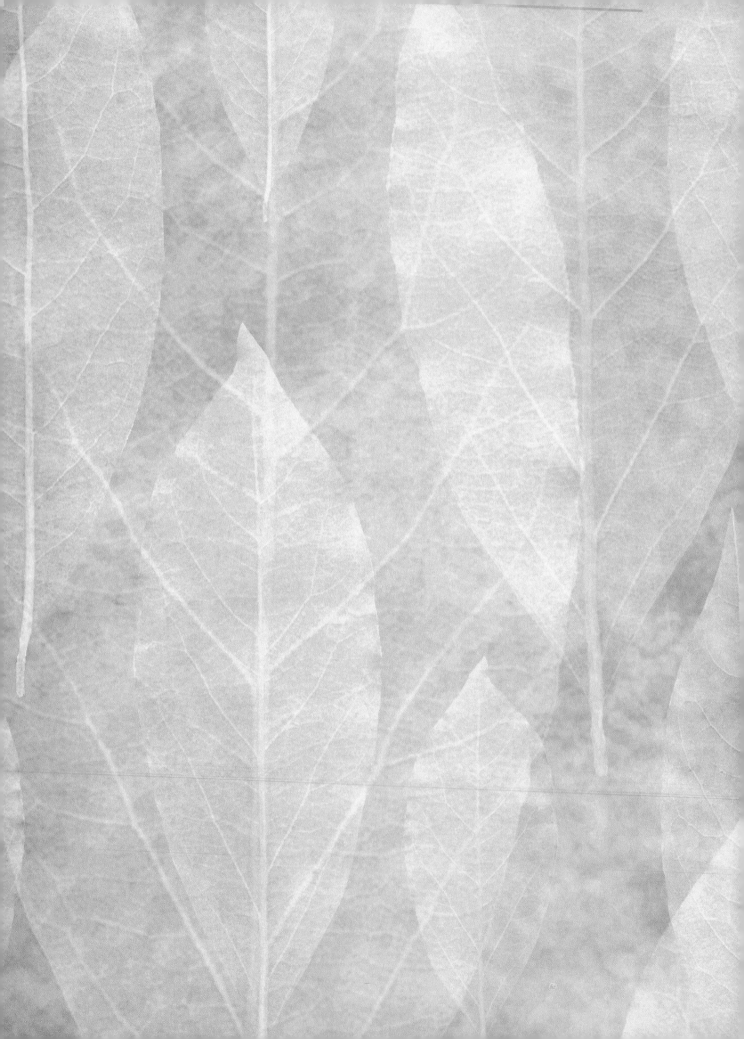

THE POLITICAL CONTEXT

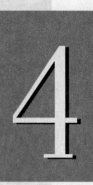

Chapter Objectives

After reading this chapter, you should be able to:

- Describe potential nursing contributions to policy development.
- Identify four competencies required for effective policy development.
- Identify at least three levels at which health policy development occurs.
- Outline the legislative process at the state and federal levels.
- Describe the regulatory process.
- Describe at least four aspects of the policy development process.
- Identify four criteria for evaluating health policy development.

Media Link

http://www.prenhall.com/clark

Additional interactive resources for this chapter can be found on the companion Web site. Click on Chapter 4 and "Begin" to select the activities for this chapter.

As we saw in Chapter 3, the effectiveness of community health nursing practice may be constrained by the features of the health care system context in which it occurs. The health care system context is shaped by political forces and health policy development at multiple levels in U.S. society. Community health nurses need an awareness of the political context in which their practice occurs and must possess the skills and abilities to influence health policy development to achieve their goals of improving the health of the public.

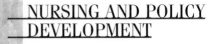

NURSING AND POLICY DEVELOPMENT

Florence Nightingale and other early community health nurses were adept at using the *political process* to promote the health of the population. We saw in Chapter 2 that Lillian Wald engaged in political activism to provide impetus for initiation of the Children's Bureau. She has been described as being alert to the political culture of her times and using that knowledge to gain important changes in societal conditions. Similar astuteness was displayed by Clara Barton and Florence Nightingale, who minimized their active support for women's suffrage issues in order to address what they considered more critical social issues. Others, such as Margaret Sanger and Lavinia Dock, were more confrontational in their political activism, but all achieved significant social changes (Fritz, 1995; Roberts & Group, 1995). These early leaders in community health nursing realized that the political process was a means of achieving their goal of improved health for all and that, because of its focus on the health of population groups, community health nursing is, by definition, political in nature.

Stages of Nursing Involvement in Policy Development

Over the years, many nurses became uncomfortable with the idea of political involvement, with the possible exception of exercising the right to vote. Politics had an unfavorable aura that was seen as incompatible with nursing's altruistic philosophy. More recently, nurses have begun to realize the need to influence health care policy decisions.

Some nursing authors (Cohen et al., 1996; Leavitt & Mason, 1998) describe a series of stages in nursing involvement in political activity after the era of Lillian Wald and her cohorts. The initial stage was one of marginal participation in political activity, primarily in terms of voting. Later, nurses began to engage in collective policy development efforts to benefit the profession. A third stage was one of participation in coalitions to address societal health issues. Nursing, as a profession, is just beginning to enter a fourth stage in which nurses provide leadership in mobilizing others to deal with health issues.

These stages of nursing involvement are akin to the levels of civil discourse often involved in policy making. At the first level, policies are made by individuals, institutions, and interest groups without much input from or consideration for the needs of those affected. In the second level of civil discourse, interested parties seek their own interests in the context of reciprocal endeavors. For example, nurses might agree to support a policy initiative of another group for an assurance of reciprocal support of nursing initiatives. At this level, people are focusing on their own rights with some consideration for the reciprocal rights of others. Level three involves the development of shared visions and consensus-oriented discourse. At level four, policy makers support principles of fairness and universal respect for others. Level five social discourse maintains this perspective on fairness and social justice but permits individuation to address the circumstances of each individual. At this level, policy making involves inclusive discourse among all involved in its development or affected by its outcomes (Kesler, 2000).

Nursing Contributions to Policy Development

There is a need for nursing input in health care policy that affects not only the health of the population but also nursing practice. This need is apparent at all levels of government, but particularly at the federal level. The need for nursing influence at the federal level is underscored by the recommendations of the Secretary's Commission on Nursing (1988) that policy making, regulatory, and accrediting bodies should foster nursing participation in decision activities and that employers of nurses should promote their participation in organizational governance.

Nurses bring professional skills to the policy arena not necessarily possessed by other players (Gebbie, Wakefield, & Kerfoot, 2000). For example, nurses possess interpersonal communication skills that allow them to work effectively with individuals with multiple perspectives and engage in consensus building. Similarly, nurses have a strong value for promoting self-efficacy among those served, which can foster public involvement in political action. In addition, nurses have abilities to rapidly process and act on both quantitative and qualitative information that may influence the policy context, as well as abilities to address multiple competing demands. Nurses also have a strong following both within the profession and among the population, due to nursing's credibility with respect to health issues.

Nurses, as a group, can have a tremendous impact on health care policy formation. There are over 2 million registered nurses in the United States, and one of every four women registered to vote is a registered nurse (RN). Nurses are politically active with respect to voting; 98% of nurses are "perennial voters" (Brydoff, 1996). Unfortunately, because we are less active in other spheres of political activity, we have less influence than we might otherwise have. As noted by Marla Salmon (1995), former director of the Division of Nursing, "Never before in the history of the United States has the relationship between public policy and the health of the American people been more apparent or more important." Community health nurses, who are responsible for the health of society at large, must become involved in the formation of health care policy.

Barriers to Nursing Participation in Policy Development

Despite the major contributions that nurses can make to policy development, there are some barriers that may inhibit their effectiveness in this arena. A major barrier is lack of education for participation in policy development activities at all levels. In addition, nursing in general has been fairly insular, and few nurses beyond those engaged in community health nursing have taken a "big picture view" of the societal conditions that affect health and health care delivery. Finally, because nurses are relatively new to higher education, they may be perceived as being "on a less intellectual plane" than others involved in health policy making, limiting their credibility with other policy makers. Such perceptions have led some nurse policy makers to divorce themselves from their nursing background to prevent devaluing of their input. This withdrawal from the profession furthers general perceptions that nurses have no interest in or capacity for policy development (Gebbie et al., 2000).

Effects of Nursing Involvement in Policy Development

Both society and the nursing profession can gain from nursing involvement in policy development. An assessment of the effects of nursing participation in the 1993–1994 efforts of the Clinton administration to initiate health system reform can highlight some of those benefits as well as some potential disadvantages of nursing involvement (Leavitt & Mason, 1998; Reagan, 1999).

Active nursing involvement in development of the Health Securities Act reinforced and expanded nursing awareness of the need for participation in policy development and provided salutary lessons in political strategizing. In addition, the proposal itself (although never successfully achieved) increased recognition of the need for health promotion and illness prevention, particularly among employers, but also in the general public. This recognition fosters achievement of the goal of community health nursing, improving the health of the population.

Even though the Health Security Act failed, it increased the familiarity of policy makers with advanced practice nursing (APN) roles and opened the way for Medicare reimbursement of APN services in 1997. The failure of a national health reform also led to a shift in the locus of control of health policy development from the federal to state and local levels. This will necessitate some

shift in nursing's political activity to the levels at which policy decisions are currently being made. Nurses' active participation in the development of the Health Security Act has also led to the appointment of nurses to high-level policy-making bodies.

Some of the negative effects of nursing participation included a growing rift between staff nurses and APNs, since the emphasis on APNs as a means of meeting societal health care needs seemed to devalue the contribution of other nurses. The failure of health system reform also left a vacuum filled by emphasis on market forces as a means of controlling health care costs. This has led to replacement of registered nurses by unlicensed personnel in some agencies as well as to the closure or absorption of many community hospitals in for-profit chains decreasing public access to health care services. The long-term effect of this consequence, however, may not be entirely negative, because it may serve to increase the public constituency for later comprehensive health system reforms (Leavitt & Mason, 1998).

Competencies Required for Effective Participation

As we noted earlier, one of the barriers to nursing participation in policy development is lack of education to foster skill in policy making. Some of the specific competencies that should be emphasized in such education include abilities to mobilize constituencies, abilities for organizational leadership, program planning capabilities, data collection skills, and understanding of health care financing (Milio, 1998). Nurses need the coalition-building and negotiation skills to mobilize effective constituencies to support policy initiatives. These skills necessitate interpersonal communication skills and skills in consensus building. Organizational leadership skills are also needed to promote priority setting and strategic planning for resource allocation. Nurses also need the ability to design programs to improve health at the population level rather than the level of the individual client. Data collection skills are needed to identify policy issues and the factors and constraints operating in the policy situation. Nurses also need the abilities to effectively disseminate information to policy makers. Finally, nurses involved in policy development require skills in fiscal management and in the development of creative funding strategies for health care programming.

HEALTH CARE POLICY

Policy is a set of principles directing activity toward a specific goal. Policy is typically concerned with complex issues, and its formation involves the use of the political process. *Social policy* is policy that is intended to promote the welfare of the general public (Leavitt & Mason, 1998). *Health care policy* is a defined set of principles

Competencies for Policy Development

- Ability to mobilize constituencies
- Organizational leadership skills
- Program planning capabilities
- Skills in data collection and analysis
- Understanding of health care finance
- Coalition-building and negotiation skills
- Skill in interpersonal communication
- Consensus-building skills
- Information dissemination skills

used to guide activities to safeguard and promote the health of the public. Health policies may be allocative or regulatory. *Allocative policies* direct the distribution of resources among members of a society. *Regulatory policies*, on the other hand, are designed to control the actions or decisions of specific people.

Public policy is a direction or course of action undertaken by a government or an official governmental agency (Milio, 1998). A public policy is a decision made by a society or its elected representatives that has material effects on members of the public. Public policies determine the parameters for individual and collective social behavior in allocating and distributing resources. A *public health policy*, then, is the way a society or its elected representatives allocate and distribute political and economic resources to meet the health needs of the populace.

All policies are values based; values determine the policy issues that arise, how they are resolved, and by whom. When the values held by different groups in a society vary, the need for politics arises. *Politics* is the process of exerting influence over events or the actions of others (Leavitt & Mason, 1998).

Policy can be made in any setting or organizational system where values are at issue, and policy formation takes place at many levels in society: family, community, institution, state, nation, even the international level. Institutional goals and purpose shape policy decisions at the level of the health care agency or institution. Examples of institutional policy related to community health would be decisions to create new programs or to expand or discontinue current ones. Decisions by local health departments to charge fees for previously free services such as immunizations are another example of institutional policy that affects the health of the public. Community health nurses need to be involved in the development of these and similar institutional policies to safeguard the interests of the public.

Health care policy decisions at the community level may be reflected in budget allocations for health care pro-

grams, disaster preparation, and housing codes. At the state level, health care policies focus on provision of health care and may include health programming decisions as well as policies related to licensure of health care professionals and regulation of health care institutions. At both the state and local levels, policies may also be formulated in legislation that regulates health-related behaviors by citizens. State laws and local ordinances that limit smoking in public places are examples of such policies.

National policy focuses on issues of concern to the society at large and is exemplified by health-related legislation and regulations that are developed by federal agencies. Although there are a number of health-related policies generated by the federal government, there is, at present, no single coherent policy that directs provision of health care across the country. National health care policy at this level is called *macropolicy*, policy that shapes the entire health care delivery system, either by controlling funding resources or by controlling the actions of key groups or individuals (e.g., insurers or providers) (Longest, 1994).

Health-oriented organizations such as the American Public Health Association (APHA) have long campaigned for a well-defined national health care policy. APHA's landmark call for a national health program was first made more than 50 years ago. Since that time, the federal government has periodically made tentative efforts to develop a national health care policy (the most recent being the failed Health Securities Act in 1994). Such efforts have not been sustained, and each tentative effort has been lost in the priority changes of successive administrations.

Business and industry, consumers, and, recently, Congress have recognized that the United States is experiencing a health care crisis that can no longer be tolerated. Although efforts have been unsuccessful to date, nurses and other providers must continue their efforts to promote a meaningful national health care policy.

AVENUES FOR POLICY DEVELOPMENT

Health policy formation may take one of four major forms in the public sector: legislation and health programs created by legislation, rules and regulations for implementing legislation, administrative decisions, and judicial decisions (Hanley, 1998).

Legislation

Laws are public policy decisions generated by the legislative branch of government at the federal, state, or local level. Laws are created in a social system to express the collective values, interests, and beliefs of the society that generates them. As a society develops, so do its beliefs, values, and interests. Some laws enacted in earlier periods of a society's evolution eventually become obsolete. Sometimes laws are created or revised to address new problems that surface as society changes. Modifications or changes in laws are legislative attempts to correct discrepancies that may have arisen between past and current social practices. Although this description of the function of legislation is highly simplified, the point is that laws reflect societal needs and values and are subject to revision.

Policy formation via the legislative process is very similar at the federal and state levels. Figures 4–1 ■ and 4–2 ■ depict the typical progress of a bill through the state and federal legislative processes. The asterisks in each of the figures indicate points in the process at which community health nurses might influence legislation.

Legislative proposals are statements of beliefs or interests that have been brought to the attention of a legislator. These interests may come to the legislator's attention through his or her constituents, personal experiences, or involvement on a legislative subcommittee dealing with specific issues. Community health nurses can influence the legislative process at this point by making lawmakers aware of the need to develop policy or to modify existing policies. After due consideration, constituents' beliefs or interests are drafted in a *bill,* which is a formally worded statement of the desired

Federal legislation is only one way in which the political context influences health and health care services. (Photo courtesy of the White House Photo Office)

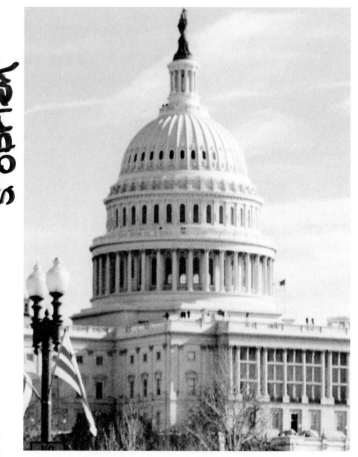

policy. Once a bill has been drafted, the sponsoring legislator submits it for identification, meaning that the bill will carry the legislator's name as sponsor. It is not unusual for a proposed bill to have multiple sponsors. Approximately 10,000 bills are introduced in Congress each year; only about 600 of them ever become law (Mittlestadt & Hart, 1993).

At the congressional level, the bill is assigned a number and listed by the House or Senate clerk and sent to a general committee for review. The committee may revise the language of the bill or amend it. In the normal course of events, the bill would then be sent on to the House or Senate floor for its "first reading." A first reading usually consists of a reference to the bill by number and title. The title may address the bill's content or the name(s) of its sponsor. The entire bill is not read at this time.

After its first reading, the bill might be referred to the appropriate committee for hearings. Some bills are sent to multiple committees. For example, the Health Security Act was assigned to five separate standing committees, one of the factors that assisted in its demise (Reagan, 1999). At the congressional level, there are six committees that deal with most health-related legislation: (a) the Senate Finance Committee, which establishes policy related to health programs supported by taxes and trusts, such as Medicare and Medicaid; (b) the House Ways and Means Committee, which oversees similar legislation for the House of Representatives; (c) the Senate Labor and Human Resources Committee; (d) the House Energy and Commerce Committee, both of which address matters related to programs administered by the Department of Health and Human Services; (e) the House Appropriations Committee; and (f) the Senate Appropriations Committee. The first four of these committees are enabling committees that deal with legislation establishing, modifying, or discontinuing health care programs. The House Appropriations and Senate Appropriations committees are responsible for allocating the funds for the various federal programs. Similar committees exist at the state level.

Community health nurses can influence the legislative process at this point by contacting lawmakers and making their views known on legislation pending before them. The Resource List included on the companion Web site for this book provides information on some congressional committees and other agencies and organizations that may assist nurses in influencing health care policy.

Committee members considering a particular piece of legislation can either review and modify a bill or decide not to report the bill out of committee, thus effectively killing it. Legislation can also bypass assignment to a standing committee and be assigned to a specially created ad hoc committee or advance directly to a second reading on the House or Senate floor. The bill may then proceed to a third reading, be referred back to committee, or be sent to another committee for review and

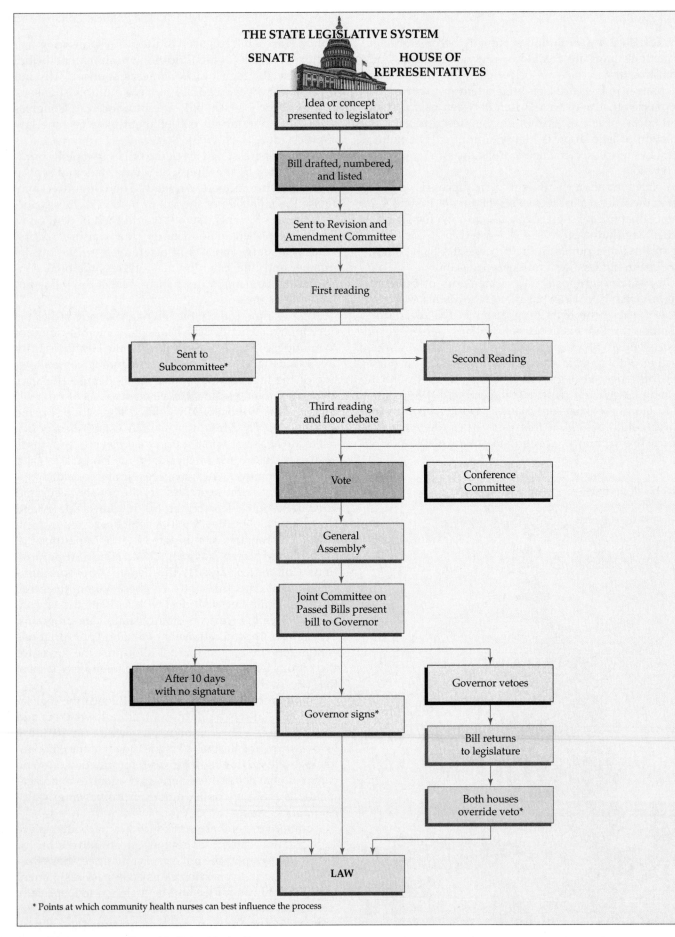

THE STATE LEGISLATIVE SYSTEM

SENATE   **HOUSE OF REPRESENTATIVES**

Idea or concept presented to legislator*

Bill drafted, numbered, and listed

Sent to Revision and Amendment Committee

First reading

Sent to Subcommittee*

Second Reading

Third reading and floor debate

Vote

Conference Committee

General Assembly*

Joint Committee on Passed Bills present bill to Governor

After 10 days with no signature

Governor signs*

Governor vetoes

Bill returns to legislature

Both houses override veto*

LAW

* Points at which community health nurses can best influence the process

FIGURE 4–1 ■ *A Typical State Legislative Process*

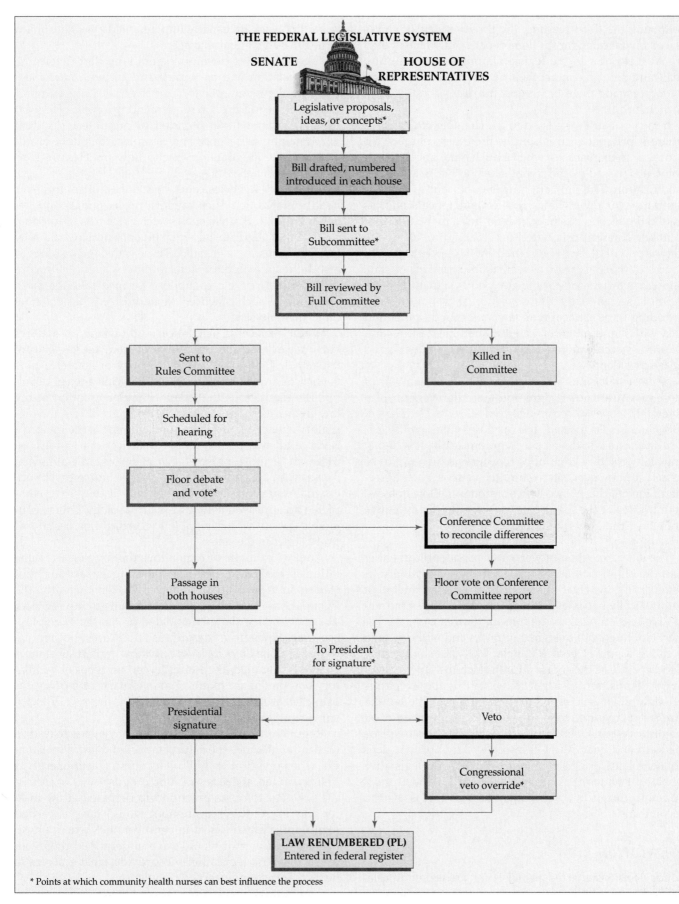

FIGURE 4-2 ■ *The Federal Legislative Process*

revision before advancing to the third and final reading. Following the third reading, the proposed legislation is placed on the calendar for floor debate and, finally, voted on. At this point in the legislative process, community health nurses can contact their own representatives and try to persuade them to support nursing's position on a particular bill.

If the legislation is passed in the chamber of Congress where it originated, it is sent to the other chamber for approval. In many cases, when a bill has advanced to this point, it is passed by the second chamber without further modification. The bill can, however, be sent to another committee for review and modification. Once a bill has passed the second chamber, it is returned to the house or chamber where it originated for final approval. At the state level, a bill must be signed by the leaders of both houses of the legislature as well as the secretary of state before it is forwarded for the governor's signature. After the bill is signed by the governor, it is renumbered according to the appropriate lawbook code number and filed with the secretary of state, and becomes law. A similar process occurs at the federal level after a bill is signed by the president.

In most states and in Congress, if the two chambers of the legislature cannot agree on a similar version of a given bill, a special committee composed of members of both chambers is formed. The purpose of this *joint conference committee* is to develop a compromise bill. It is highly unusual for a joint committee recommendation not to be passed. If, however, the committee cannot reach agreement, the bill dies. Once the compromise bill has passed both houses of the legislature, it is sent to the executive branch of the government (governor or president) for final approval.

The chief executive (governor or president) can either sign the bill or hamper its progress by not signing it or vetoing it. If the chief executive does not sign the bill, it automatically becomes law after ten days, unless the legislative session ends in the interim. In that case, the bill dies. Holding a bill unsigned until the end of the session is called a *pocket veto* (Longest, 1994). Lobbying may also be used at this point to influence the chief executive's disposition of a particular bill. If the executive vetoes a bill, it is returned to the legislature. The legislature is then required to meet a constitutionally prescribed majority vote (usually a two-thirds majority) to override the veto and enact the bill into law. Any bill that does not complete the legislative process during the legislative session in which it is introduced is dead, and it must be reintroduced in a subsequent session if it is ever to become law.

Regulation

Policy decisions enacted as legislation are usually implemented by regulatory agencies charged with implementing specific types of legislation. For example, federal policies related to environmental issues are implemented by the Environmental Protection Agency (EPA); state health-related policies are usually implemented by a state board of health or a comparable agency.

These agencies develop regulations that determine how legislation will be implemented. A *regulation* is a rule or order having the force of law that deals with procedures to be followed in implementing a piece of legislation. Regulations are intended to promote individual accountability for actions and to protect the public health and welfare. Regulations specify how policies are realized in actual behavior.

Regulatory agencies exert a great deal of control over health-related activities by both professionals and the general public. State agencies such as boards of nursing, for example, regulate who may practice nursing and how nursing licensure is granted. These same agencies might also be responsible for determining which health care providers can write prescriptions for medication in those states where such practices are authorized for personnel other than physicians.

When a piece of legislation authorizing an activity such as prescription writing is passed, the legislature usually designates an existing agency or creates a new agency to implement the legislation. This agency develops the regulations that govern implementation of the law. In the case of prescription writing privileges, the regulatory agency would determine who can write prescriptions and what additional qualifications might be required of those persons. For example, in California, nurses who are certified by the state as nurse practitioners may write prescriptions, but only if they have completed an approved course in pharmacology. Other regulations specify who is eligible for certification as a nurse practitioner in the state.

Another example of regulations that implement legislation is the procedures for handling hazardous substances in the workplace, which were developed by the Occupational Safety and Health Administration (OSHA). The enabling legislation mandated protection of employees from exposure to hazardous substances, but regulations developed by OSHA specify how certain substances should be handled. For example, certain types of ventilatory equipment are required in manufacturing processes using hazardous aerosols to minimize the risk of exposure to employees.

Regulations instituted by various agencies may dramatically influence the actual impact of a law. For example, when prescription writing by nurse practitioners was first instituted in Tennessee, one proposal was to restrict the privilege to nurse practitioners prepared at the master's level. As this requirement would have excluded many nurse practitioners in rural counties where physicians were scarce, it would have undermined the intent of the enabling legislation—to provide greater access to health care for underserved populations.

Community health nurses can have input into regulations that affect their professional practice as well as into the legislation that shapes public health policy.

When a regulatory agency is in the process of formulating regulations, the public is informed that the process is being initiated. Generally, the agency formulates some preliminary regulations that are published for public review and comment. At the federal level, proposed regulations are published in the *Federal Register* as a *Notice of Proposed Rulemaking (NPRM)*; similar registers exist in each state. Interested parties are then allowed to comment on the proposed regulations and suggest changes.

When regulations deal with particularly sensitive areas, the regulatory body involved may hold public hearings to solicit input from interested parties. Community health nurses may either comment on proposed regulations in written communications to the regulatory agency or provide testimony at public hearings. The regulatory agency can then use the input received to refine the regulations. Regulations are published in the appropriate state or federal publication and promulgated among individuals affected by them. For example, schools of nursing in California were informed in writing of changes requiring educational content on child abuse for public health nursing certification in the state. Once regulations are published and go into effect, they have the force of law (Abood & Mittlestadt, 1998).

Administrative and Judicial Decisions

Health policy development can also occur by means of administrative or judicial decisions. Administrative decisions are those made by an individual or agency that affect the implementation of health care policies or programs. One specific type of administrative decision is an executive order. *Executive orders* are additions to legislation that an executive officer (president or governor) can make as long as they do not contravene the provisions of the legislation or contradict other existing laws (Reagan, 1999). Former President Clinton, for example, used executive orders for achieving a number of health policy changes that were not originally included in legislation, such as instituting programs to promote Medicaid enrollment for eligible children. *Judicial decisions* are decisions within the court system regarding how laws are to be interpreted.

⑥THINK ABOUT IT

What legislators in your area are sympathetic to nursing's position on health-related issues? What could you, as a nurse, do to elicit the support of other legislators who are not currently sympathetic to nursing initiatives?

THE POLICY DEVELOPMENT PROCESS

Community health nurses can influence health-related policies at all levels. To do so, however, they must be conversant with the political process and its use. The ability of community health nurses to influence policy development is affected by their skill in assessing the policy situation, planning and implementing health care policy, and evaluating the effects of health policy development and the resulting health policies and by their ability to use two types of information: science-based information and nonscience-based information (Milio, 1998).

Science-based information is derived from research and is used to assist in identifying problems and for assessing and evaluating policy options. Nonscience-based information is less verifiable and arises from stakeholders' informed judgments and personal experiences. This type of information is used to legitimize the social problem as a policy issue and to promote public support for its resolution. The information on which policy decisions are made is invariably incomplete, but policy makers, including community health nurses, must make the best use of the available information within the context of other relevant considerations to make the most effective policy decisions (Savitz, Poole, & Miller, 1999).

ASSESSING THE POLICY SITUATION

Nurses must be adept at assessing policy situations. This involves identifying and defining a policy issue, examining the policy environment, and identifying stakeholders in a particular policy situation.

Societal problems form the basis for policy issues. Identification and resolution of policy issues requires involvement of multiple levels of the population, including both policy makers and those who will be affected by the policies made (Kesler, 2000). Community health nurses must be able to collect and analyze large amounts of data to identify health problems that present policy issues. Agreement must be reached that integrates multiple perceptions of what the problem is and how the issue is to be defined. For example, a community may differentially define the same problem or policy issue as adolescent sexual activity or lack of access to contraceptive services. How the issue is defined has a great deal of influence on potential policy options. If the policy is defined as adolescent sexual activity, the focus of policy development will be on preventing sexual intercourse by teenagers. If, however, the community defines the issue as a lack of contraceptive services, policy development will focus on providing adolescents with needed services.

Community health nurses and other policy makers must also identify factors in the environmental context that are impinging on the policy issue. This might include social values and attitudes surrounding the issue, economic factors, ethical considerations, and political and legal factors that may influence the issue or the potential for developing effective policy to resolve it. For example, a policy issue that has serious economic implications, either in the cost of the underlying problem to society or the potential costs of its resolution, may gain or lose support based on these implications. Other considerations in the policy situation might be the history of the issue, the degree of public acceptance and support of the issue, other issues that may take priority among policy makers, and so on (Cohen, Leavitt, Leonhardt, & Mason, 1998).

Finally, in assessing the policy situation, policy makers must identify the stakeholders involved. *Stakeholders* are those who are involved in the development of a policy or who will be affected by the policy (Hanley, 1998). Stakeholders may either support policy initiatives or oppose them, and policy makers need to differentiate between the two groups of stakeholders. Stakeholders may be overt or indirect in their relationship to the policy issue (Cohen, Leavitt, et al., 1998). For example, the state agency responsible for licensure of health professionals is an overt stakeholder in policy changes related to licensure as are the licensed professionals. Indirect stakeholders are those who could become stakeholders based on their values and interests. For example, a parent group could become stakeholders in a licensure issue if the issue is presented to them as either safeguarding or jeopardizing the health of their children.

PLANNING HEALTH CARE POLICY

Planning health care policy involves a number of activities in which community health nurses can be involved. These activities include setting priorities and goals, defining the appropriate political arena, defining and evaluating policy options, outlining the policy, and strategic management of the policy development process.

Setting Priorities and Goals

There are many policy issues on which community health nurses may wish to have input, including issues related to the needs of the profession as well as those of the public. Choices among these issues must be made carefully and priority given to those issues that are most relevant to improving the health of the public. As noted previously, early community health nursing leaders chose to champion some issues over others rather than jeopardize their credibility or lessen their impact on what they considered the most important issues.

Community health nurses and other policy makers must also set achievable goals for policy development. Goals will be closely related to the way in which the issue has been defined. Using the previous example, if the issue is adolescent sexual activity, the goal will be to decrease the extent of sexual intercourse among teenagers. If, on the other hand, the issue is defined as lack of contraceptive services, the goal will be to provide these services in venues that are accessible and acceptable to the adolescent population. Again, both problem definition and the resulting goals provide direction for policy development.

⑥THINK ABOUT IT

Why are nurses not more active in policy formation? What strategies could facilitate their involvement in policy making?

Defining the Political Arena

A second consideration in planning health care policy is determining the appropriate political arena for the effort.

assessment tips assessment tips assessment tips

ASSESSING THE POLICY SITUATION

- What is the health problem or issue to be addressed? Why has the need for policy development or change arisen? What are the data related to the problem or issue?

- What is the appropriate policy arena? Where does jurisdiction lie?

- Are there strongly held values that will be supported or threatened by the proposed policy?

- Who will be affected by the policy? Who will support the policy? Who might be in opposition? Why? What influence does the opposition wield?

- Who should be involved in policy development? Implementation?

- Does the proposed policy adequately address the issue?

- Does the policy safeguard individual rights as much as possible?

- Are proposed implementation strategies fair and equitable?

- How easy or difficult will it be to implement the proposed policy?

- What will be the cost of policy implementation? What resources will be needed? How will these resources be obtained?

This involves identifying who has jurisdiction regarding the policy issue. Appropriate political arenas may be institutional, professional, or legislative, or may involve local, state, or federal policy makers. For example, a local health care institution should determine the degree of its involvement in health promotion and education activities within the community, but should not make decisions related to the educational preparation of health care professionals, which is more properly the purview of professional organizations. Other policy issues can be solved only through legislative efforts, but, again, the appropriate political arena should be identified. Is this an issue that can be resolved by a local ordinance, or will it require legislation at the state or federal government level?

Defining and Evaluating Choices

To influence health care policy decisions, community health nurses must be able to define and evaluate policy alternatives. Many avenues can be taken in the development of health care policies. Community health nurses have a responsibility to identify and evaluate alternative directions for health policy and to make policy makers aware of potential advantages and disadvantages of various alternatives. This means that community health nurses must keep abreast of issues and developments that affect the health of the public as well as potential approaches to dealing with health-related issues.

A number of policy vehicles have been identified that could be incorporated into the resolution of a particular policy issue. For example, regulation and enforcement of some particular health-related behavior (e.g., prohibiting smoking in public places) is one approach to dealing with the health effects of tobacco use. Some other potential vehicles that may be appropriate in a given policy situation include incentives to engage in desired behaviors, education, direct service provision, or investment in organizational infrastructure to support health services (Milio, 1998).

Policy options should be assessed in terms of identified criteria. Some possible criteria for evaluating multiple policy options include complexity, cost, and feasibility of the alternative; the extent to which the alternative supports clients' rights; the equitability of the policy in its effects; and its effects on provider autonomy. Specific criteria used to evaluate policy options in a given situation will be determined by the situation itself and the contextual factors that surround the situation. For example, the Health Security Act proved not to be a viable policy option for health care reform because it was perceived by the public as a potential loss of health services and because the public was still generally comfortable with the existing system (Leavitt & Mason, 1998). With changes in these aspects of the contextual situation, similar legislation might have a greater likelihood of success.

Outlining the Policy

Once policy options have been evaluated and the most viable alternative or combination of alternatives selected, policy makers must develop a well-thought out plan for

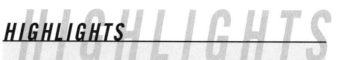

its implementation. The program or plan should be made as clear and simple as possible. One of the other reasons suggested for the failure of the Health Security Act was its complexity and the inability of the general public, as well as legislators, to understand it (Reagan, 1999). In addition, many details of the policy and its implementation, particularly with respect to program funding, had not been fully developed, leaving legislators with too many questions regarding the potential effectiveness of the program in addressing the need for health care reform.

An important consideration in outlining the details of the selected policy option is the identification of needed resources and their potential availability. What will be required to implement the planned policy? Is there a need for specially trained personnel? For equipment? Where will these resources be obtained, and how will they be financed? Where will funding for policy implementation be derived?

Strategic Management

Strategic management of policy development requires the establishment of an organizational structure to monitor and direct the development process. Strategic management involves choosing and adjusting tactics to target groups whose support is critical to approval of the policy. It also means setting up mechanisms for data collection and dissemination as well as monitoring public attitudes related to the policy issue. Other aspects of strategic management involve funding media coverage, selecting media appropriate to the audiences involved, and developing targeted media messages. Finally, strategic management involves tracking and responding to opposition tactics and strategies. All of these activities require operating funds and mechanisms for generating and controlling those funds.

STRATEGIES FOR IMPLEMENTING POLICY

Community health nurses and other policy makers can adopt a variety of strategies for implementing selected policy options. Some of these include creating support for the policy, and traditional activities such as voting, campaigning, and holding office.

Creating Support

Community health nurses alone cannot assure the development and implementation of effective health care policies. While they may be actively involved in policy development, achieving policy approval and implementation usually requires broad-based support in many segments of society. Nurse policy makers can use a variety of strategies to create support for desired policy options. These include coalition building, creating media support, community organizing, lobbying, and providing testimony.

Coalition Building

Coalitions are alliances of individuals or groups who unite to address a common interest. There are several important considerations or guidelines for community health nurses seeking to form coalitions. These guidelines include the following:

- Identify the goal that members are to align around and potential means to that goal.
- Project the expected time frame for the existence of the coalition and the target date for goal achievement.
- Identify resources needed by and available to the coalition.
- Identify potential supporters and opposition forces that the coalition must combat.
- Decide who will be invited to join the coalition, selecting influential parties who can assist in goal achievement.
- Identify hidden agendas and reasons for participating that may jeopardize goal achievement.
- Determine the organizational structure and ground rules for participation in the coalition.
- Identify leadership roles and who will fill them.
- Identify and communicate the benefits of participation to coalition members.

When the coalition's goal has been achieved, identify "next steps" (dissolution, new focus, etc.) (Leavitt & Pinsky, 1998).

⑥THINK ABOUT IT

What coalitions exist between nursing and other groups in your community interested in policy issues? What coalitions might enhance nursing's position on specific issues?

Creating Media Support

Much of the information regarding policy issues received by the general public is transmitted by the media. In order to create public support for a policy initiative, com-

munity health nurses must carefully select and orchestrate media coverage. Again, this was one of the flaws in the campaign to pass the Health Security Act. The news media focused more on the politics behind the legislation than on its content, diminishing the U.S. public's understanding of the proposed program and thereby diminishing their support (Leavitt & Mason, 1998; Milio, 1998). Another problem was the well-organized media campaign mounted by the opposition (Reagan, 1999).

Nurses need to help assure that policy debate is framed in the interests of the public's health while accounting for contextual factors that influence the policy situation. For example, a policy should not be perceived to unduly advantage one segment of the population to the disadvantage of others. Policy makers should seek out media that are favorable to the particular issue and media messages should be targeted to specific audiences to create support for a given policy initiative. Media messages should be designed not only to inform the public, but to encourage them to mobilize to support the initiative. Public support is only effective when it is visible to policy makers through organized efforts such as contacting legislators, and so on (Milio, 1998).

Community Organizing

Another way community health nurses create support for policy directions is community organizing. *Community organizing* is the process of mobilizing community resources in support of planned change within the community. It is a systematic process of assessment, analysis, and planning, conducted within the context of the political process. Steps in the community organization process include establishing legitimacy, defining the problem to be addressed, assessing and analyzing the problem, selecting goals, planning to obtain these goals, marketing, and evaluating.

Members of the community are involved in each step of the process and provide the motivating force behind the movement. The first step, however, is probably the most critical in creating support for health policy. Legitimizing the project requires development of authority to act. This may involve requesting officials to create a special task force to address a problem or including government officials in the planning body of the community organization structure. Subsequent steps of the community organization process are similar to those of the nursing process and need not be reiterated here. It should be remembered, however, that the steps are carried out by members of the community rather than by the nurse.

Community organization can create a mechanism to influence policy makers in several of the ways discussed earlier in this chapter. Community groups can generate and evaluate policy alternatives and can collect data for presentation to policy makers. In addition, the organization provides avenues to educate voters and motivate their participation in policy decisions affected by voting.

Lobbying

Lobbying is a concerted effort to influence legislators to take certain positions on prospective bills, and it is another means of creating support for policies promoted by community health nurses. Individuals may lobby independently, or groups of people with common interests may also engage in organized lobbying efforts. For example, health-related organizations, such as the American Public Health Association, and professional organizations, such as the American Nurses Association and the American Medical Association, employ lobbyists at both federal and state levels. Their function is to acquaint legislators with the position of the organization on a particular issue and to attempt to persuade them to support that position.

Individuals who lobby do so by contacting a legislator and making their position on an issue known. The position should be supported by data that persuade the legislator to adopt a similar position. Whether lobbying is done by individuals acting on their own or with an organized group, there are strategies that influence the effectiveness of lobbying. These strategies, as well as approaches to be avoided, are summarized in Table 4–1 ■.

It is important for community health nurses to know both the legislative process and the legislators involved. Legislators can be observed and their statements studied to determine their positions on issues influencing community health. Their voting records on significant issues can also be examined.

Once legislators' positions are known, they and their staff can be contacted to establish influential interpersonal relationships. Personal contact through visits followed by telephone calls and follow-up letters or telegrams has been found to be an effective means of influencing lawmakers. Some observers believe that one should not focus exclusively on legislators from one's own political party, but should contact members of both parties. Legislators who support one's position can be encouraged in that support, and those who do not may be persuaded to change their position.

In addition to knowing a legislator's position on specific issues, nurses should be aware of which legislators serve on committees that deal with health care issues.

■ **TABLE 4–1   Effective and Ineffective Lobbying Techniques**

Effective	Ineffective
Become familiar with the legislative process	Make threats about loss of votes
Become familiar with legislators	Make promises that cannot be kept
Know the issues	Pretend to have influence
Know your lobbying power	Repeat the message too frequently
Work through your own representatives	

CULTURAL CONSIDERATIONS

The voices of many members of ethnic groups in the United States are not heard in the policy-making process. What might community health nurses do to make sure that these voices are heard? What culturally appropriate strategies might be used to promote political involvement among these groups?

These legislators, along with one's own elected representatives, are appropriate candidates for lobbying efforts. Knowledge of the legislative structure and committee assignments can assist nurses to target lobbying efforts in areas where they will be most effective.

Community health nurses also need to be conversant with the issues they are addressing and with arguments on both sides of particular issues. Research related to health policy issues can be presented to lawmakers and can be persuasive in promoting their support of a position. In discussing an issue, one should acknowledge the nature, source, and extent of possible opposition to one's position. The community health nurse should present the legislator with brief, factual, and documentable data related to the issue. It is usually preferable to provide legislators or their staff members with these data in written form and to include documentation.

Generally speaking, individuals who lobby on their own should focus their efforts on legislators elected from their own districts. Legislators are usually more inclined to listen to constituents than to nonconstituents. Nurses need to network with each other so that several legislators are contacted by their own constituents regarding nursing's position on an issue.

Approaches to legislators that should be avoided when trying to exert influence include making threats regarding loss of voter support and making promises of support; pretending to have influence; repeating one's message too frequently; and demanding a commitment from a legislator before an issue has been completely explored. Such tactics can result in a loss of credibility and decrease one's ability to influence a legislator's behavior.

It is important to acknowledge a legislator's support or lack of support for a given piece of legislation. This action helps legislators realize that their actions are indeed monitored. When a legislator does not support nursing's position on a particular bill, a note indicating regret for that nonsupport and the hope that "perhaps, next time we can work together" is more appropriate than a threat of nonsupport in the next election.

Presenting Testimony

Policy makers sometimes hold public hearings or meetings to gather background information on an issue before attempting to draft legislative proposals or regulations. On occasion, such meetings are held by legislative subcommittees to explore the potential impact of a proposed piece of legislation. Writing and presenting testimony in a public hearing is another method community health nurses can use to influence policy makers.

Testimony presented by community health nurses should specifically address the issue in question and be brief, factual, and well documented. Legislative representatives are not usually health care providers, so testimony should avoid medical jargon and be clearly understandable. A copy of the testimony should be given to the legislative representatives and staff either immediately preceding or at the time of the hearing. Documentation of sources of data permits later verification by legislators or their staff members.

For an excellent example of the use of these and other methods for creating support for a policy initiative visit the companion Web site for this book.

Traditional Political Activities

Community health nurses can also influence policy development and implementation through more traditional political activities. These activities influence the selection of policy makers and issues to be addressed and include voting, campaigning, and holding office.

Voting

Voting is perhaps the easiest means of influencing health care policy formation at governmental levels. Nurses can themselves vote and motivate others to vote to support policy directions that enhance public health. One vote alone may not seem important, but it may be a key factor in determining the outcome on an important issue. Because lawmakers in the United States are elected, they are susceptible to the power their constituents hold through the ballot box. Thus, voting is a vital component of the political process in which all nurses can participate.

In addition to voting, nurses can educate others regarding the need to vote. Legislative networks among nurses are intended to keep members informed of health-related issues and the need for support or lack of support of certain policy directions. Nurses can also educate the general public on legislative issues that come up for public vote. Finally, nurses can participate in voter registration programs that motivate the general public to exercise their constitutional right to influence policy formation.

Campaigning

Campaigning is a process designed to influence the public to vote in a particular way on an issue or a candidate. An issue or candidate is presented in a favorable light with the intent of influencing voters. Campaigning can be implemented via media presentations, in group meetings or rallies, or in face-to-face contacts with the public.

Campaigning for an issue involves presenting information related to the issue that persuades people to support nursing's position. Campaigning for a specific candidate can help ensure election of policy makers

who support nursing's position on important issues. Campaigning is an opportunity for nurses to become personally known to a candidate and other campaign workers. It is also an opportunity to become known as a reliable source of information about health and health care issues. Campaigning for a candidate also creates a debt on the part of an elected official that may result in future support for a position promoted by community health nurses.

Much of the work of political action committees (PACs) is designed to support the candidacy of specific individuals. The American Nurses Association Political Action Committee (ANA-PAC) was created in response to nursing's perceived lack of influence in the formulation of health care policy. The purpose of ANA-PAC is to promote constructive national health care legislation through the political "electioneering" process. *Electioneering* is the active process of endorsing candidates and contributing time and money to their campaigns. ANA-PAC and similar political action committees supported by nurses seek to enhance the political influence of nurses by supporting the election of candidates who back the profession and its position on significant health-related issues.

There are some constraints on campaign involvement for certain groups of nurses. For example, nurses employed by government agencies (whether part time or full time, permanently or temporarily) are prohibited by the Hatch Act from soliciting campaign contributions (even anonymously by telephone) or engaging in campaign activities while on duty, in uniform, or using an agency vehicle. They are also prohibited from running for office in a partisan election. Similar prohibitions are in force for military nurses (Chaffee, 1998).

ETHICAL AWARENESS

The resolution of ethical issues often requires political action. Conversely, policy development frequently has ethical ramifications or implications. Community health nurses engaged in policy development should analyze the ethical aspects of policy options. Aroskar (1998) has suggested a framework for ethical analysis in policy development and evaluation. Considerations in ethical analysis should include the following:

- Identification of the goals of policy development. Do the intended goals pose any ethical dilemmas?

- Examination of the involvement of those affected in policy development. Does lack of involvement infringe on rights to self-determination?

- Examination of mechanisms for policy implementation. Does policy implementation result in inequities, infringement of personal rights, and so on?

- Examination of the direct and indirect consequences of a policy. Do the outcomes of policy development and implementation pose ethical dilemmas?

TABLE 4-2 Strategies for Developing and Implementing Policy

STRATEGY	DESCRIPTION OF STRATEGY
Creating support	
Coalition building	Creating a temporary alliance among individuals or groups to work toward common goals
Creating media support	Selecting appropriate media and designing targeted media messages for specific audiences
Community organizing	Mobilizing community resources in favor of planned change or a proposed policy
Lobbying	Engaging in personal communications with policy makers in an attempt to influence their actions in policy decisions
Presenting testimony	Providing information on an issue to policy makers at a public hearing
Traditional political activity	
Voting	Exercising one's personal right to vote
	Encouraging others to vote
	Participating in voter registration drives
Campaigning	Providing endorsements or monetary support for specific policy proposals or candidates with the intent of influencing voters' responses
Holding office	Assuming a position as a policy maker by virtue of election or appointment to a specific office

Holding Office

A final means of creating support for policy directions promoted by community health nurses is to become a policy maker oneself. This may involve running for elective office or being appointed to a specific position. In either case, the community health nurse must first become politically active in some of the other ways described in this chapter to be sufficiently well known to be elected or appointed to a policy-making position.

One may also work in the background in policy making by becoming a legislative staff person or a lobbyist for an organized group. Again, such positions require familiarity with the political process and well-developed interpersonal relationships with legislators and other policy makers. Strategies to influence policy development and implementation are summarized in Table 4–2 ■.

EVALUATING POLICY DEVELOPMENT

Community health nurses should be involved in the evaluation of the policy development process. In evaluating the process itself, the nurse would consider the extent to which all stakeholders, including those affected by a given policy, have been involved in policy development. In addition, the nurse would assess the adequacy of strategic management of the policy development process, gaining insights into what worked and what did not for application in future policy development efforts.

Community health nurses should also evaluate the adequacy of health policies developed. Criteria for evaluating health policies include their adequacy in meeting the health needs of the public, safeguards for the rights of individuals, equitable allocation of resources, their capacity for implementation, and the effects of the policy on the target population.

Health policies must be developed that effectively address the health needs of the affected population and identification of needs must derive from population-based data (Aday, Begley, Lairson, & Slater, 1998). For example, a local government policy allowing homeless persons to sleep in city-owned buildings addresses only one small part of the plight of the homeless population. In this case, a more comprehensive policy that addresses both short-term and long-term solutions to the problems of homelessness is needed.

Safeguarding individual rights is another criterion for sound health care policy development. As an example, a policy that would require homeless individuals to surrender personal belongings to meet communal needs when admitted to a shelter would violate their property rights. There are circumstances, however, in which the good of society supersedes individual rights. For example, homeless persons may be prohibited from smoking in a shelter to prevent exposure of others to smoke or to prevent a fire. Whenever possible, though, health policies should be written so that they do not violate the rights of individuals affected by them.

Health care policies should also promote equitable distribution of health care resources. This means that policies should not discriminate against certain subgroups within the population. For example, open housing policies in homeless shelters may inadvertently discriminate against women and children who may be subjected to force to make them give way to adult males who desire shelter. Sex-segregated shelters that ensure access for both males and females provide for a more equitable allocation of resources.

For a specific health policy to be effective in promoting health or preventing illness, it must be capable of being implemented or enforced. For example, a local government might adopt a policy encouraging houses of worship to provide overnight shelter for homeless individuals. But, unless the houses of worship are willing to cooperate, the policy cannot be implemented.

Community health nurses planning to influence health care policy formation should assess proposed policies or modifications of existing policies in light of these five criteria. Policies that do not meet the criteria should be redesigned, if possible, before they are presented to policy makers. If a proposed policy continues not to meet

HIGHLIGHTS
HIGHLIGHTS

Criteria for Evaluating Proposed Policies

• Adequacy in meeting identified health needs
• Safeguards for individual rights
• Equitability of resource allocation
• Capacity for implementation
• Effects on the target population

one or more criteria, its supporters should be prepared to justify the need for the policy. For example, nurses should be prepared to convince policy makers that a smoking ban in shelters for the homeless is warranted despite the violation of the individual's personal freedom of choice.

Community health nurses may also be actively involved in assessing the effects of health care policies on meeting the needs of the particular target group. Community health nurses could assist in collecting data related to the outcomes of programs put into operation. For example, data might be gathered on the incidence of health problems among the homeless to evaluate the effects of policies designed to promote primary and secondary prevention activities in this population. In addition, information could be collected regarding the number of persons who continue to be homeless despite assistance from established programs. For additional

CRITICAL THINKING IN RESEARCH

In the past, nurses as a professional group were less politically active than members of other groups. In today's society, political astuteness and involvement are critical to the development of health care delivery systems that support the primary goal of community health nursing: improved health for the public.

• What contribution might research make to understanding nursing's traditional lack of political involvement?
• What is the role of research in policy making?
• How would you go about determining what factors promote political activity by community health nurses?
• If you wanted to conduct a study of the extent of political activity among certain groups of students on your campus, what groups would you include? Why? How would you design your study?

resources related to health care policy development, consult the Web addresses listed on the companion Web page to this book.

Effective community health nurses use the political process to enable them to attain their primary objective, enhancing the health of the populations with which they work. Political activity by community health nurses may occur at the institutional or societal level and often involves efforts to influence legislation related to health issues.

APPLYING YOUR KNOWLEDGE IN PRACTICE

CASE STUDY
Influencing Health Policy Development

In focus groups conducted to determine health care needs, residents of a low-income culturally diverse neighborhood repeatedly voiced concerns about intimidation of tenants by landlords. Because of housing shortages, many tenants were (justifiably) worried that reporting inadequacies to landlords would result in evictions. With limited low-income housing available, people were not willing to take the risk of making complaints about needed repairs or noisy neighbors.

Lack of tenants' facility with English, cultural differences, and the fact that most owners of rental units are absentee landlords complicate the situation. More

than half of the residents in the community are members of ethnic cultural groups, including many relatively recent refugees from Southeast Asia and the Middle East. Long-time area residents are primarily older persons on fixed incomes who also cannot afford to antagonize landlords.

There is a fledgling Landlord/Tenant Association in the neighborhood, but few of the absentee landlords are active participants. There is also a neighborhood collaborative that has been successful in mounting some initiatives to improve conditions for residents, including decreasing drug dealing in selected areas of the neighborhood and putting up anti-tobacco bill-boards. The collaborative has developed relatively close relationships with city council members and county supervisors in the wider community, but recently several political positions have been filled by new electees. One or two long-time residents are particularly influential with local politicians. The nearby university law school provides landlord/tenant mediation services to individuals in the community. Other agencies and associations active in the neighborhood include local schools, the community center, Boys and Girls Club, the community health center, the local health department office, the university school of nursing, a Lao-Hmong Association and the Vietnamese Federation, and several programs geared toward children and the elderly.

- What steps might the local community health nurses take to address the problem of intimidation by landlords?
- What community groups might be appropriate coalition partners in resolving this problem? Why?
- What approaches might be taken in terms of policy development to deal with intimidation?
- Are there particular government agencies that should become involved?
- How might local residents become actively involved in resolving the issue?
- What cultural considerations have relevance for this situation and its resolution?

✎ TESTING YOUR UNDERSTANDING

- What potential contributions can nurses make to policy development? (pp. 62–63)
- What competencies are required of community health nurses engaged in policy development? (p. 63)
- Identify at least three levels at which health care policy formation takes place. (p. 64)
- Outline the legislative process at the state and federal levels. Identify strategies by which community health nurses might influence the process and points at which those strategies might be most effective. (pp. 64–68)

- Describe the regulatory process. How might community health nurses influence this process? (pp. 68–69)
- Describe aspects of the policy development process. How might community health nurses be involved in each? (pp. 69–74)
- Identify four criteria for evaluating health policy development. (pp. 75–76)

REFERENCES

Abood, S., & Mittlestadt, P. (1998). Legislative and regulatory processes. In D. J. Mason & J. K. Leavitt (Eds.), *Policy and politics in nursing and health care* (3rd ed.) (pp. 384–396). Philadelphia: Saunders.

Aday, L. A., Begley, C. E., Lairson, D. R., & Slater, C. H. (1998). *Evaluating the healthcare system: Effectiveness, efficiency, and equity.* Chicago: Health Administration Press.

Aroskar, M. A. (1998). Ethical issues: Politics, power, and policy. In D. J. Mason & J. K. Leavitt (Eds.), *Policy and politics in nursing and health care* (3rd ed.) (pp. 241–248). Philadelphia: Saunders.

Brydoff, C. (January 8, 1996). Nurses can make a difference by becoming politically active. *NurseWeek, 1,* 7, 26.

Chaffee, M. (1998). Political activity and government-employed nurses. In D. J. Mason & J. K. Leavitt (Eds.), *Policy and politics in nursing and health care* (3rd ed.) (pp. 704–707). Philadelphia: Saunders.

Cohen, S. S., Leavitt, J. K., Leonhardt, M. A., & Mason, D. J. (1998). Policy analysis and strategy. In D. J. Mason & J. K. Leavitt (Eds.), *Policy and politics in nursing and health care* (3rd ed.) (pp. 139–159). Philadelphia: Saunders.

Cohen, S., Mason, D., Kovner, C., Leavitt, J., Pulcini, J., & Sochalski, J. (1996). Stages of nursing's political development: Where we've been and where we ought to go. *Nursing Outlook, 44,* 259–266.

Fritz, K. (1995). *A history of the concept of creativity in western nursing: A cultural feminist perspective.* Unpublished doctoral dissertation, University of San Diego.

Gebbie, K. M., Wakefield, M., & Kerfoot, K. (2000). Nursing and health policy. *Journal of Nursing Scholarship, 32,* 307–315.

Hanley, B. (1998). Policy development and analysis. In D. J. Mason & J. K. Leavitt (Eds.), *Policy and politics in nursing and health care* (3rd ed.) (pp. 125–138). Philadelphia: Saunders.

Kesler, J. T. (2000). Healthy communities and civil discourse: A leadership opportunity for public health professionals. *Public Health Reports, 115,* 238–242.

Leavitt, J. K., & Mason, D. J. (1998). Policy and politics: A framework for action. In D. J. Mason & J. K. Leavitt (Eds.), *Policy and politics in nursing and health care* (3rd ed.) (pp. 3–17). Philadelphia: Saunders.

Leavitt, J. K., & Pinsky, J. B. (1998). Coalitions for action. In D. J. Mason & J. K. Leavitt (Eds.), *Policy and politics in nursing and health care* (3rd ed.) (pp. 180–187). Philadelphia: Saunders.

Longest, B. B. Jr. (1994). *Health policy making in the United States.* Ann Arbor, MI: AUPHA Press.

Milio, N. (1998). Priorities and strategies for promoting community-based prevention policies. *Journal of Public Health Management Practice, 4*(3), 14–28.

Mittlestadt, P. C., & Hart, M. A. (1993). Legislative and regulatory processes. In D. J.

Mason, S. W. Talbot, & J. K. Leavitt (Eds.), *Policy and politics for nurses* (2nd ed.) (pp. 399–411). Philadelphia: Saunders.

Reagan, M. D. (1999). *The accidental system: Health care policy in America*. Boulder, CO: Westview Press.

Roberts, J. I., & Group, T. M. (1995). *Feminism and nursing: An historical perspective on power, status, and political activism in the nursing profession*. Westport, CT: Praeger.

Salmon, M. E. (1995). Public health policy: Creating a healthy future for the American public. *Family and Community Health, 18*(1), 1–11.

Savitz, D. A., Poole, C., & Miller, W. (1999). Reassessing the role of epidemiology in public health. *American Journal of Public Health, 89*, 1158–1161.

Secretary's Commission on Nursing. (1988). *Final Report, Volume 1*. Washington, DC: Department of Health and Human Services.

THE ECONOMIC CONTEXT

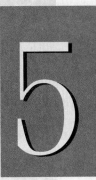

Chapter Objectives

After reading this chapter, you should be able to:

- Describe interrelationships among economic conditions, health care services, and health status.
- Discuss factors contributing to escalating health care costs.
- Discuss the effects of economic factors on the provision of public health services.
- Distinguish among selected mechanisms for financing health care services.
- Describe the effects of selected health care financing mechanisms.

KEY TERMS

access 83
block grant 92
categorically needy 92
consumer price index 82
cost containment 81
cost shifting 82
diagnosis-related groups (DRGs) 84
economics 81
entitlement 92
health maintenance organization (HMO) 86
independent practice association (IPA) 87
managed care organizations (MCOs) 86
medically needy 92
medigap insurance 85
Medigrant program 92
per capita expenditures 81
point of service plan (POS) 87
preferred provider organization (PPO) 87
prospective reimbursement 84
Resource-Based Relative Value Scale (RBRVS) 84
retrospective reimbursement 84
uncompensated care 82

Media Link

http://www.prenhall.com/clark

Additional interactive resources for this chapter can be found on the companion Web site. Click on Chapter 5 and "Begin" to select the activities for this chapter.

Economic factors influence the health of clients as well as the delivery of health care services. For individuals and their families, economic factors affect the ability to obtain necessities, such as food and shelter. One's income also influences the ability to obtain health care. The general economic climate also influences health at the aggregate level. For example, a declining economy contributes to high levels of unemployment. Unemployment, in turn, leads to reduced incomes and a reduced tax base to finance government-supported health and welfare programs. In addition, unemployment is usually accompanied by loss of employer-provided health insurance benefits. Finally, economic factors that contribute to inflation further impair the ability of the public to obtain necessities and health care.

Relationships between economic factors and health (Figure 5–1 ■) are of concern to community health nurses because they influence the health of individuals, families,

FIGURE 5–1 ■ *Relationship of Selected Economic Factors to Health*

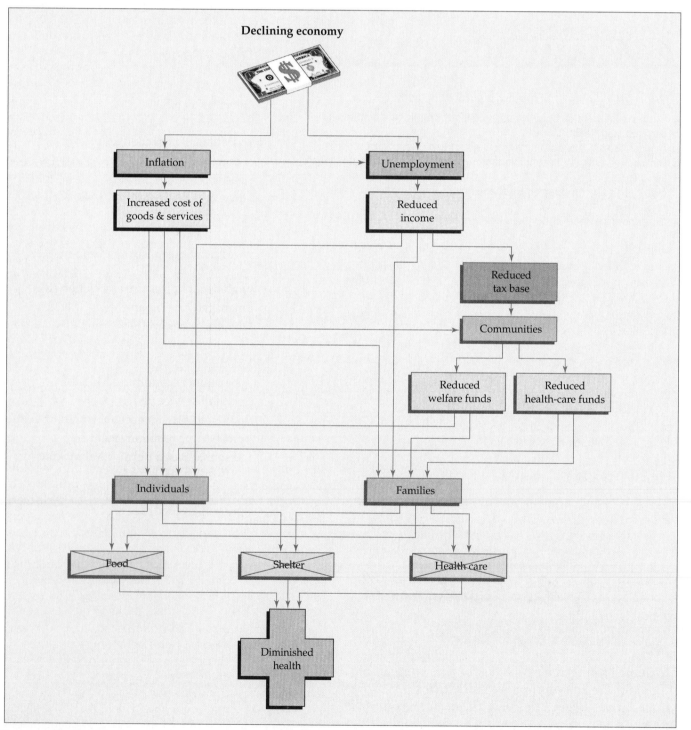

and communities. Although community health nurses cannot significantly influence the overall economic climate, they can help to mitigate its adverse effects. For example, nurses can assist clients to budget their resources effectively or make referrals to financial assistance programs. Or the community health nurse can engage in the political process to influence policies related to economic issues, particularly funding for health care services. To do so, some understanding of the economic context as it affects health and health care services is essential.

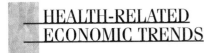

HEALTH-RELATED ECONOMIC TRENDS

Economics is the social science that addresses the production, distribution, and consumption of goods and services. Three fundamental economic principles must be considered in examining the effects of economic conditions on health and health care services. The first principle is that resources are always more limited than what is needed for desired levels of consumption. Second, resources have alternative uses, and, third, different people will have differing ideas as to what those uses should be. Based on these principles, the basic question related to health care economics is how limited resources should be used. What types of health services should consume the resources available? Two related questions relate to the methods by which those services should be produced and how they should be distributed within the population (Price, Pfoutz, & Chang, 2001).

Understanding of the effects of economic factors on health care delivery and the health status of the population requires examination of several health-related economic trends. These trends include the rising costs of health care services, a shift to for-profit status among many health care institutions, funding of public health services, and welfare reform.

Rising Health Care Costs

Despite cost containment efforts over the last decade, health care costs have continued to rise at an alarming rate. *Cost containment* refers to action designed to slow this rise. Although cost containment measures have had some effect on the level of health care inflation, the measures employed are by no means completely successful. In 1960, for example, the United States spent $26.9 billion on health, including medical research and facility construction. This amount represented 5.1% of the gross domestic product (GDP) (U.S. Census Bureau, 1996). From 1960 to 1990, health care spending grew by an average 6% per year, twice the rate of growth of the rest of the economy (Lasker, 1997). Although the rate of growth slowed somewhat from 1995 to 1997, total health care expenditures in 1997 had increased to $1.1 trillion, con-

suming 13.5% of the GDP (Price et al., 2001). It is estimated that expenditures will reach $2.2 trillion or 16.2% of the GDP by 2008 (Smith, Heffler, Freeland, & the National Health Expenditures Projection Team, 1999).

Many factors contribute to increasing costs for health care in the United States. The most obvious is population changes over time. Population growth leads to increased demand for and total cost of services. From 1970 to 1995, for example, the U.S. population increased by more than 29%. Increase in the number of people receiving health care, however, does not explain the rise in per capita expenditures. *Per capita expenditures* reflect the average amount spent on health care per person per year. In 1960, per capita spending for health amounted to $143 per person (U.S. Census Bureau, 1996). By 1997, this figure had increased to $4,000 per person (Price et al., 2001).

Part of the increase in per person spending is due to the increasing proportion of elderly in the population. Older persons use proportionally more health care resources than younger persons because of infirmities related to age and long-standing chronic diseases. Persons over the age of 65 years constituted 11.3% of the population in 1980; by 1998, they constituted 12.4% and by 2050 they are expected to constitute 20% of the U.S. population. Similarly, in 1980, persons over 85 years of age constituted less than 1% of the U.S. population. By 1998, the size of this subpopulation had increased by 50%, and by 2050 this group is expected to comprise 4.6% of the population (U.S. Census Bureau, 1999). The need for long-term care, as well as other personal health services, in this fragile group will greatly add to health care costs.

Health care costs for the elderly population are growing at a faster rate than the growth in the GDP. In fact, at current rates of growth, it is estimated that by 2020, 10% of the GDP will be expended on health care services for this group alone and will amount to $25,000 per person per year (Fuchs, 1999). Medicare spending by that time is anticipated to reach $14,000 per person (McClellan & Skinner, 1999).

One reason for the growth in the elderly population is the ability of "high-tech" medicine to prolong life. Advanced technology is expensive and is estimated to account for approximately 50% of increases in health care costs (Bryce & Cline, 1998). In addition, specialized technology contributes to specialization among health care providers, which also adds to cost. In many instances, care provided by highly specialized providers at high cost could be provided as effectively by other providers, particularly nurse practitioners, at lower costs (Federwisch, 1999).

Advanced technology contributes, in part, to overuse, and thus waste, of health care resources. High-tech medical equipment tends to be used more frequently than necessary to justify its cost. Consequently, more expensive diagnostic and treatment procedures may be chosen when less expensive ones might be equally effective. Overuse of high-tech procedures may also be explained as "defensive medicine" in a society where health care providers feel a need to protect themselves from malpractice litigation.

A related factor in rising health care costs is the use of prescription drugs. The availability of newer, frequently more expensive drugs, leads to increased use and, thereby, increased cost. For example, U.S. drug prices have risen 2.4 times faster than the consumer price index (Tone, 1999). The *consumer price index* is the estimated cost of all goods and services purchased by a typical household (Chang, 2001b). In 1997, prescription drugs cost nearly $79 billion, with an increase of more than 14% over 1996 expenditures. In addition to increased drug prices, the number of medications prescribed has also escalated. For example, the number of prescriptions increased by 6% in 1995 and 4.2% in 1996 and 1997 (Levit et al., 1998). Again, the growing number of elderly persons in the population contributes to this growth in medication use. Persons over 65 years of age take approximately one third of all prescription drugs used in the United States, at an average of 14 prescriptions per person. It is estimated that as much as 25% of these prescriptions are inappropriate and needlessly add to health care costs in this country (Whitelaw & Warden, 1999).

Another factor that contributes to the high cost of health care is the emphasis on cure rather than prevention of illness. Greater attention to prevention could lead to marked reductions in health care costs.

Paradoxically, both availability and lack of health insurance have contributed to increased health care costs. When both providers and clients can be assured of payment for health care services by private or government insurance programs, neither has any incentive to contain costs. On the other hand, a large segment of the population is uninsured or underinsured (approximately 42.5 million people in the United States in 1999) (U.S. Census Bureau, 2000), resulting in large amounts of "uncompen-sated care" provided by health care institutions and providers. *Uncompensated care* is that proportion of care for which the provider receives no reimbursement. Uncompensated care leads to a phenomenon known as *cost shifting*, the passing on of the cost of uncompensated care to those who do pay for care, either those who pay out-of-pocket or those covered by health insurance. Cost shifting leads, in turn, to higher insurance premiums and higher overall costs for health care. A final source of increased health care costs lies in fraudulent claims for reimbursement for services not provided or provided but not needed.

For-Profit Shift

Another economic trend in health care delivery that is of concern to community health nurses is the absorption of many nonprofit organizations, particularly community hospitals, by large for-profit companies. Since the 1970s, for example, more than 800 public and nonprofit hospitals have closed or changed to a for-profit status (Reagan, 1999). The emphasis on profit has led some insurance companies to target only the healthiest persons, a practice known as "cherry picking." Pharmaceutical companies are accused of charging higher prices for drugs to Americans than to foreign consumers and of putting a higher percentage of revenues into profit than into research and development activities. There are significant differences in drug prices charged to some recipients and payers than to others. For example, Medicare is charged 15% to as high as 1,600% more for some drugs than the Veterans Administration or some managed care organizations (Tone, 1999). Profit motives may also lead managed care organizations to undertreat clients with verifiable health needs.

Funding Public Health Services

Poor funding of public health services is another longterm trend that affects the health of the population. In 1997, for example, total health care expenditures in the United States amounted to more than $1 trillion, yet only $38.5 billion (3.5%) was spent for public health services (Price, Pfoutz, & Chang, 2001). Federal government spending on public health services amounted to $4.1 billion, while $34 billion was expended by state governments (U.S. Census Bureau, 1999).

Many public health agencies have relied on government funding sources for personal care services to subsidize other traditional health services as well as care for uninsured populations, with public health agencies serving as safety-net providers. As we will see later in this chapter, there is a growing emphasis on shifting Medicaid and Medicare recipients into mainstream managed care organizations which may significantly decrease the revenue on which many public agencies have come to depend. In 1997, 60% of Medicaid managed care safety-net organizations lost money (Gray & Rowe, 2000). The loss of revenues as more Medicaid enrollees move to

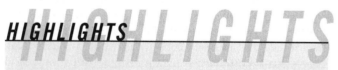

HIGHLIGHTS

Factors Contributing to Rising Health Care Costs

- Population growth
- Increasing longevity
- Overuse of expensive technology
- Specialization of health care providers
- Increased use of prescription drugs
- Lack of emphasis on prevention
- Access to health insurance
- Lack of health insurance
- Uncompensated care and consequent cost shifting
- Fraudulent reimbursement claims

managed care plans may jeopardize the abilities of public agencies to meet their public health obligations (Holahan, Zuckerman, Evans, & Rangarajan, 1998). Curtailment of services by safety-net agencies will also result in the loss of services to clients who have no other source of health care and are not eligible for publicly funded insurance programs.

ETHICAL AWARENESS

Some health care policy makers have proposed that government funding should be used to provide health promotion and illness and injury prevention services rather than to treat existing health problems. What are the ethical implications of such proposals? What approaches to ethical decision making would support such proposals? What approaches would argue against them?

Welfare Reform

Welfare reform is the last economic trend affecting health to be addressed here. In 1996, welfare reform terminated the Aid to Families with Dependent Children (AFDC) program and replaced it with Temporary Assistance for Needy Families (TANF). This change has several ramifications for eligibility for health care assistance. Children in families receiving AFDC were automatically eligible for Medicaid, but the welfare reform provisions divorced welfare assistance from health care assistance. In addition, the new program places time limits on eligibility for assistance (Levit et al., 1998). The intent of the new program was to move people from the welfare rolls and have them become involved in gainful employment. Research indicates, however, that a large portion of those affected by welfare reform are single women with children who have chronic health problems that necessitate a variety of services. The time away from work necessitated by the health care needs of these children will make it difficult for their mothers to sustain employment, putting them at greater risk for poverty as well as health complications (Heymann & Earle, 1999).

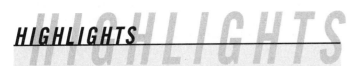

HIGHLIGHTS

Economic Trends Affecting Health

- Increasing health care costs
- For-profit shift
- Lack of funding for public health services
- Welfare reform

ECONOMIC EFFECTS ON HEALTH

Economic factors affect client health status in two primary ways. The first mechanism of influence is a direct effect of poverty on health and the second is economic influences on one's ability to obtain needed health care services.

Poverty and Health

Poverty has long been known to contribute to poor health status. Poverty affects one's ability to procure housing and food necessary for survival and for good health. The poor also tend to be less well educated than the nonpoor and, therefore, have less knowledge of self-care and behaviors that promote health. Research has indicated that the "medically vulnerable," those who have limited income for meeting health care needs, such as the poor, the elderly, and the uninsured, have higher levels of disability and poorer health status than those who are not vulnerable and are less likely to have visited a health care provider within the last year (Broyles, McAuley, & Baird-Holmes, 1999).

Diminished Access to Care

Poverty also affects health indirectly by limiting one's access to necessary health care services. *Access* is defined as "the timely use of needed, affordable, convenient, acceptable, and effective personal health services (Chang, 2001a, p. 336). Generally speaking, there are two kinds of access problems: access for special population groups and general access problems related to the inability of the health care system to meet consumer demands (Chang, 2001a). Both types of problems affect the poor. The poor constitute a special population that has diminished access to care directly because of their poverty and the consequent inability to afford the cost of health care services. One study indicated that as many as 8% of U.S. adults aged 55 to 64 years delayed getting needed care due to cost. Percentages are even higher for members of ethnic groups who also tend to have higher levels of poverty (Janes et al., 1999). Cost is also the most frequent reason given by pregnant women who do not receive prenatal care (National Center for Health Statistics, 2000). Poor children are also less likely than their richer agemates to receive necessary mental health services (Cunningham & Freiman, 1996).

Much of health care is financed by insurance. The poor are significantly less likely than the nonpoor to be insured. For example, 22% to 23% of poor children are uninsured compared to 8.6% of children in middle-income families and 4.2% of those in high-income families (Chang, 2001a). In 1999, 42.5 million people in the United States (15.5% of the population) were without health insurance. Figures are even higher for the poor, among whom 32.4% are uninsured (U.S. Census Bureau, 2000). Research has indicated that the uninsured are less likely than others to have a regular source of health care, are more likely to report difficulty obtaining needed health care services, and have fewer visits to health care providers than those with insurance (Berk & Schur, 1998).

In addition, the poor are disproportionately disadvantaged by general problems of access such as long waits or lack of transportation and other "wraparound" services that are needed to be able to obtain care. For example, a poor client may not be able to take the time from work to make or keep an appointment even if they are financially eligible for care. Similarly, a mother with several small children may be hindered from taking advantage of services if she cannot afford child care. General access problems lead to greater use of emergency departments and hospital out-patient departments, contributing to the high cost of health care services (Pina, 1998).

It would seem obvious from the figures cited here that current economic mechanisms for funding health care services are inadequate. Community health nurses can be influential in bringing about changes in funding policies, but first they must have some understanding of the mechanisms for financing health care services.

REIMBURSEMENT MECHANISMS

Payments to providers of health care services, whether professionals or institutions, may take one of two forms, retrospective payment or prospective payment. Traditional means of funding health care have been retrospective in nature. **Retrospective reimbursement** is payment for services rendered based on the cost of those services; cost is determined after the fact. Forms of retrospective reimbursement include fee-for-service payment, discounted fee-for-service payment, and per diem payments. Figure 5–2 ■ displays the mechanism of retrospective payment directly from client to provider.

FIGURE 5–2 ■ *Retrospective Client Payment*

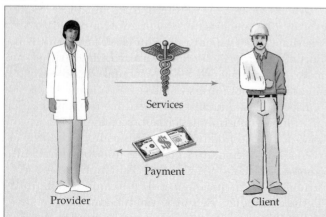

Services

Payment

Provider   Client

In a fee-for-service system, providers are paid for each service rendered after that service has been provided (Chang, Price, & Pfoutz, 2001). Fee-for-service payment is based on the unit of service as a single visit to a provider or a single procedure. Payment may either come from the recipient of services or from another source such as insurance. As we will see later, some managed care organizations (MCOs) have attempted to reduce costs for services to their enrollees by contracting with providers who agree to provide services at discounted fee-for-service rates. Per diem payment is a similar arrangement in which an inpatient facility is paid retrospectively, at a flat rate per day, for the number of days a client was hospitalized (Ling, 2000). Per diem reimbursement is usually used for institutional providers such as hospitals, skilled nursing facilities, and long-term care facilities.

Retrospective reimbursement has the disadvantage of encouraging health care providers to give services that may not be necessary, merely because they are reimbursable. A provider who can be reimbursed for each office visit may be tempted to see a client three times when two visits would suffice. Or tests and treatments may be given that are not strictly necessary. For example, a surgeon might suggest a hysterectomy to a woman when other less expensive measures would be equally effective.

In 1983, prompted by increasing costs, the federal government instituted prospective reimbursement for services provided under Medicare. **Prospective reimbursement** is payment at a predetermined, fixed rate for a specific health care program or set of services (Chang et al., 2001). Forms of prospective payment include diagnosis-related groups (DRGs), the Resource-Based Relative Value Scale (RBRVS), and capitation. Both the DRG and RBRVS systems are based on payment for each episode of illness.

Prospective payment for services provided under the Medicare program is based on clients' diagnoses, with set fees for care of clients who fall into specific diagnosis-related groups. **Diagnosis-related groups (DRGs)** are categories of client diagnoses for which typical costs of care have been calculated, based on the cost of specific services required. In the DRG system, providers are paid a set fee based on clients' diagnoses and the typical costs of care for someone with that diagnosis.

A similar prospective payment system, the **Resource-Based Relative Value Scale (RBRVS),** was initiated in 1992 for physician services provided to Medicare clients. In this system, the typical costs of a given health service have been calculated based on the prevailing cost for that service in a particular locale. Physicians providing a given service are paid a flat fee based on the estimated cost of the service. Costs are categorized into more than 7,000 Current Procedural Terminology (CPT) codes that are used for Medicare billing purposes (Reagan, 1999).

In a capitation system, health care providers receive a lump sum payment for each client enrolled in the program. The net effect is a fixed budget for the program that must cover all services provided. Three approaches may be taken to set capitation rates: (a) administrative rate setting, (b) negotiated rates, and (c) competitive bidding (Holahan et al., 1998). In administrative rate setting, capitation rates are based on discounted fee-for-service rates in the area. Insurers who set negotiated capitation rates negotiate specific rates of reimbursement per enrollee with each group of providers that provide fee bids above an upper payment limit based on fee-for-service costs. Finally, insurers may accept competitive bids from potential contracting groups and accept the lowest bid that covers agreed upon services. As we will see later, capitation is a prominent feature of many managed care plans, and in 1997, 36% of physicians had some capitated contracts, which contributed 23% of their income (Levit et al, 1998).

Prospective reimbursement eliminates the incentive to overtreat clients. Because providers are paid at a fixed rate, extending the services provided to a client does not result in additional revenue. Indeed, continued service may be to the provider's disadvantage if the costs of service exceed the fixed rate paid for them. Providers, then, have an incentive to minimize the costs of care. Implementation of DRGs has led to shorter hospital stays and movement of many services to outpatient settings to cut costs (Abood, 2000).

Prospective payment systems also have disadvantages. Health care institutions may attempt to avoid caring for the very sick or provide inadequate care to minimize costs. For example, under the DRG system, a hospital would be paid the same rate for Medicare recipients hospitalized for diabetes, whether their hospital stays were 3 days or 30 days. Those who are very ill and who require more than the average stay for their diagnostic group may be discharged from services before they are actually ready for discharge. In the long run, such practices may lead to subsequent readmissions and to increased health care costs.

Prospective reimbursement has also been criticized as detrimental to provider–client relationships. Because providers may be pressured by hospitals and other institutions to minimize the cost of clients' care and maximize revenues, they may put the needs of the institution before those of the client and discharge clients before they are really ready for discharge. Or physicians may mislabel clients' diagnoses to put them into groups with higher reimbursement rates. Methods of provider reimbursement are summarized in Table 5–1 ■.

⑥THINK ABOUT IT

If you were going to receive direct reimbursement for community health nursing services, would retrospective or prospective payment be more advantageous for you? Why?

■ **TABLE 5–1 Methods of Provider Reimbursement, Units of Service, and Characteristic Features**

METHOD	UNIT OF SERVICE	CHARACTERISTIC FEATURES
Fee for service	Visit or procedure	Retrospective, based on actual cost of services
Episode	Illness episode	Prospective, includes all services rendered in the care of a single episode of illness, based on type of episode
Per diem	Day	Retrospective or prospective, usually used for institutional services, flat rate
Capitation	Person enrolled	Prospective, lump sum payment for all covered services, flat rate

FINANCING HEALTH SERVICES

Funds for health care services arise from two basic sources: client payment and third-party payment.

Client Payment

Payments from clients may take several different forms. These include direct payments to providers, insurance premiums, cost sharing, and other out-of-pocket expenses. In 1997, the U.S. public spent more than $187 billion dollars out-of-pocket. Much of this expenditure was in direct payments to providers for health care services and some was in the form of copayments or deductibles, but a significant portion (nearly $23 billion) was spent on prescription drugs (Levit et al., 1998). By 2008, it is expected that out-of-pocket expenses will consume more than $355 billion (Smith et al., 1999).

Approximately 60% of consumer outlay ($348 billion) in 1997 was for insurance premiums (Levit et al., 1998). This figure is expected to rise to $715 million by 2008 (Smith et al., 1999). The cost of employment-based insurance more than doubled from 1977 to 1996 (Gabel, 1999), while premiums for *medigap insurance,* supplemental insurance to cover costs not covered under Medicare, increased 35% from 1994 to 1999 (Update, 1999). In 1998, premiums for managed care plans increased an average of 7.8% from $128 per month to $138 (Matisoff, 1999). Unfortunately, an estimated 40% to 50% of insurance premiums goes toward administrative costs and industry profit rather than into health care services for covered populations (McGuire & Anderson, 1999).

Clients also assist in funding health care services through cost sharing. Cost sharing is payment of a portion of the cost of health care services with the rest paid by some form of health insurance. Two approaches to cost sharing are deductibles and copayments. A *deductible* is a fixed amount that the client must pay before the insurance plan begins to pay for any care. The amount of the deductible may be several hundred dollars and must usually be paid each year before insurance benefits begin. Another term for this is coinsurance.

A *copayment* is a fixed amount or percentage that the client pays for each visit or service provided (Chang, Price, & Pfoutz, 2001). Until recently, copayments have been relatively small, at $5 to $10 per office visit or prescription. In 1993, for example, only 34% of managed care plans had copayment requirements of $10 or more. By 1997, however, more than 70% of plans had copayments of at least $10 (Levit et al., 1998), and in some plans copayment for prescriptions has doubled in the last year. There is some evidence to suggest that cost sharing has a negative influence on utilization of preventive services such as mammograms and preventive counseling and that this practice should be abandoned for certain preventive services to increase their use (Solanki, Schauffler, & Miller, 2000).

Third-Party Payment

Third-party payment mechanisms were designed to protect the average citizen from the financial devastation of serious illness and to supplement client payment. In a third-party reimbursement system, payment for health care services is made by someone or some agency other than the individual receiving service, usually some form of public or private insurance.

TYPES OF HEALTH INSURANCE

There are basically two types of health insurance plans, indemnity plans and managed care plans. To "indemnify" means to protect against hurt or loss. Indemnity health insurance is intended to protect the policy holder against financial loss due to illness or injury and was originally developed to cover the hospital costs of serious illness. When health insurance first became a common employment benefit, indemnity plans were the major type of coverage offered. In fact, as recently as 1977, the majority of job-based insurance was indemnity based, and only 11% of workers had other health insurance options. By 1998, only 14% of insured employees carried traditional indemnity insurance (Gabel, 1999).

Indemnity insurance operates on a retrospective, fee-for-service basis. Most plans cover hospitalization costs, but some also cover the services of professional providers. Only a few indemnity plans offer coverage for preventive services. Because reimbursement is retrospective, there is a high incentive to overtreat clients to increase revenues. Figure 5–3 ■ depicts the mechanism of third-party payment through privately purchased indemnity insurance. The broken lines in the figure indicate that in some plans, clients must pay the provider themselves and then be reimbursed by the insurance company. In addition,

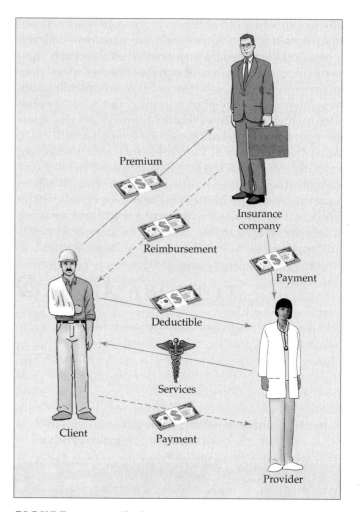

FIGURE 5–3 ■ *Third-Party Reimbursement—Individual Private Indemnity Insurance*

clients pay a deductible amount to the provider before insurance payments are activated.

Managed care plans combine both the financing and provision of health care services. Indemnity plans, on the other hand, pay for services but do not provide them. Managed care plans or *managed care organizations (MCOs)* are "delivery systems or health-care entities that are willing to be clinically and financially accountable for the health outcomes of a group of individuals for predetermined capitation payments" (Chang et al., 2001, p. 302). They are characterized by integration of funding and delivery systems and a comprehensive array of services.

There are several types of MCOs available, including health maintenance organizations, preferred provider organizations, and point of service plans. A *health maintenance organization (HMO)* is an organized health care delivery system providing a wide range of health services to a voluntarily enrolled population for a fixed prepaid fee. Under the Health Maintenance Organization Act of 1973, federally designated HMOs were required to exhibit four characteristics:

1. An organized system to provide health care in a particular geographic area

2. An agreed-on set of services for health maintenance and treatment

3. A voluntarily enrolled membership

4. Rates based on those for similar services in the surrounding community

These attributes remain characteristic of most MCOs.

Several different models of HMO organization are based on the arrangement between the HMO and health care providers. The types of arrangements include the staff, group, and network models, independent practice associations, and direct contract models (Chang et al., 2001). In the staff-model HMO, providers are salaried employees and provide services only to plan members (Chang et al., 2001). This type of provider relationship is becoming more common. In fact, in 1996, 43% of physicians were employed rather than self-employed as in the past (Levit et al., 1998).

In the group model, the HMO develops an exclusive contract with a multispecialty group of providers to obtain care for plan enrollees (Chang et al., 2001). The network-model HMO contracts for services with several provider groups. In this and the independent practice association, providers may also see clients from outside the HMO. In fact, in 1997, 92% of physicians had at least some managed care contracts, and managed care provided approximately 49% of physician income (Levit et al., 1998).

An *independent practice association (IPA)* is a group of independent health care providers who join together to contract with an HMO to provide services for enrollees. The IPA negotiates and administers the contract. The HMO pays the IPA a capitated amount based on the number of enrollees involved. The IPA, in turn, reimburses individual providers also usually on a capitated basis (Grumbach, Coffman, Blick, & O'Neil, 1998). Finally, in the direct contract model, the HMO enters contractual agreements with multiple independent providers to obtain services for enrollees (Powell, 1996).

A *preferred provider organization (PPO)* is a negotiated association between a funding source (usually an employer, although the source may also be an insurance company) and health care providers, whereby providers give discounted services to a defined group of people (e.g., employees). The discount may be as much as 15% to 20% of the usual fee for services (Chang et al., 2001). When employees use these "preferred" providers, the employer usually covers the bulk of charges. When someone chooses to use other providers, their out-of-pocket costs are higher than if they choose a preferred provider.

For providers to remain on the preferred list, they must provide quality services at a reasonable cost, thus encouraging efficiency, but not at the risk of quality. In a PPO, providers are paid for specific services on a per case basis at a predetermined fee, and providers are independent of the reimbursement system. PPOs decrease the per visit cost of health care, but, if the number of visits increases, may not reduce the overall cost of health care to the employer or to society.

Consumer choice exists both within and outside of the PPO. Consumers enrolled in the plan have a choice among several providers within the plan and can also choose between in-plan and out-of-plan providers. The final characteristic of PPOs is more expeditious reimbursement of providers than is often the case with other forms of third-party payment.

A *point of service plan (POS)* is a combination of an HMO and traditional insurance coverage in which the client chooses whether to use an in-plan provider or another provider. This choice can be made with each episode of health service. For example, a client might elect to see an in-plan provider for gynecologic services, but continue to see an out-of-plan pediatrician liked by her children. Out-of-plan provider use, however, may require a deductible and a 20 to 50% copayment. Specialist referrals must be made by the primary provider to be covered, whether the specialist is a part of the plan or not. POS plans generally operate on a fee-for-service payment basis (Chang et al., 2001).

MCOs provide a number of advantages over indemnity insurance plans. Some of these include less of an incentive for overtreatment than under indemnity plans, more comprehensive care, better patient information systems and, consequently, better access to aggregate data for program evaluation, emphasis on primary versus specialty care, and greater emphasis on preventive and health-promotive services. Additional advantages include greater emphasis on cost-effectiveness with a concomitant use of midlevel practitioners (e.g., nurse practitioners and physician assistants) to decrease the cost of care and an impetus for strategic planning. A further recent advantage is the development of the Health Plan Employer Data and Information System (HEDIS) which provides employers and consumers with quality of care and client satisfaction data on major MCOs, permitting them to make more well-informed choices among programs (Reagan, 1999).

MCOs also have several disadvantages. Among these are incentives to undertreat clients to save money and to recruit the healthiest clientele, leaving sicker clients and those with chronic diseases to other providers. MCOs may also place constraints on provider practice and client access to specialty services with requirements for prior authorization for many procedures and services. Higher client volumes typical of MCOs may also create waits for and difficulty in arranging appointments as well as less individual attention from a provider. Finally, MCOs have created more paperwork for providers (Reagan, 1999).

Despite growing awareness of these disadvantages, the number of MCO enrollees has continued to increase. For example, enrollments increased by 300% from 1988 to 1994 (Pulcini & Mahoney, 1998), and by 1998, 86% of persons with job-based insurance were enrolled in MCOs (Gabel, 1999). Advantages and disadvantages of managed care approaches are compared to those of fee-for-service and indemnity insurance approaches in Table 5–2 ■.

⑥THINK ABOUT IT

Would prospective or retrospective reimbursement for community health nursing services be more advantageous to clients if they were paying for services themselves? Why?

SOURCES OF HEALTH INSURANCE

Health insurance may be privately purchased by the individual, employment based, or supported by any of several public insurance programs. In 1997, 5.6% of people 45 to 60 years of age purchased health insurance for themselves. Among those 61 to 64 years of age, a slightly higher percentage of the U.S. population had privately purchased insurance (Glied & Stabile, 1998). In 1998, roughly 8% of the total population was covered by privately purchased insurance policies (U.S. Census Bureau, 2000).

EMPLOYMENT-BASED INSURANCE   Employment-based health insurance is far more common than privately purchased policies, but there has been a steady decline in the percentage of those covered by employment-based plans. In 1977, 70% of the U.S. population received insurance through their employers (Gabel, 1999). By 1998, however, job-based coverage had dropped to 62.8% of the population (U.S. Bureau of Census, 2000). In part, this decline is the result of increased cost of health insurance premiums, which increased 260% from 1977 to 1996, with employee contributions increasing 350% over the same period (Gabel, 1999). Higher costs are causing some employees to reject health care insurance when it is offered to them. In one study, slightly over 11.4 million workers in firms that offered health insurance benefits elected not to accept them. Of this group, 2.5 million remained uninsured, while the others had other sources of health care insurance. Most employees indicated that cost was the major factor in declining health insurance (Thorpe & Florence, 1999).

Many small employers do not offer health insurance benefits. Compared to firms with more than 200 employees, 99% of which offer health insurance to their employees, only 46% of small businesses provide health insurance (Ginsburg, Gabel, & Hunt, 1998). Forty percent of employees in these small firms do not have any form of health insurance. Other employees may work for employers who offer health insurance for which they are not eligible. This group includes approximately 10.1 million U.S. workers, more than a third of whom remain uninsured (Thorpe & Florence, 1999). Figure 5–4 ■

■ TABLE 5–2   Advantages and Disadvantages of Selected Approaches to Health Care Financing

APPROACH	ADVANTAGES	DISADVANTAGES
Fee-for-service	Unlimited choice of providers	Personal responsibility for all costs No quality control mechanisms except licensure No external review process
Indemnity insurance	Wide choice of providers No gatekeeper	Deductibles, coinsurance Potential for excessive use High cost premiums No quality control of providers except licensure No external review except state insurance board
Managed care (general)	"Credentialed" providers promote quality control External review process (e.g., HEDIS) promotes quality	
HMO	Comprehensive care No deductible or coinsurance Lower premiums than indemnity insurance	Gatekeeper Restricted to plan providers Copayment Potential for lower quality care to minimize costs
PPO	Greater selection of providers than HMO Expedited provider reimbursement Lower premiums than indemnity insurance	Gatekeeper Additional cost for out-of-plan provider use Potential for lower quality care to minimize costs
POS	Most flexibility Comprehensive services within plan	Deductible and 20 to 50% coinsurance for out-of-plan provider use Referral by primary provider required for services to be covered

depicts third-party payment from employment-based indemnity insurance plans. Again, the broken lines indicated the route reimbursement may take with clients sometimes paying providers directly and then being reimbursed by the insurer. Figure 5–5 ■ depicts a capitated funding mechanism arising from employment-

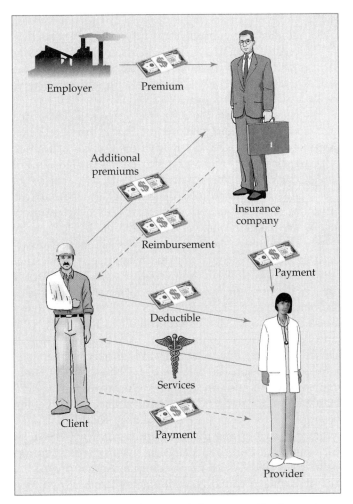

FIGURE 5–4 ■ *Third-Party Reimbursement—Employment-Based Group Indemnity Insurance*

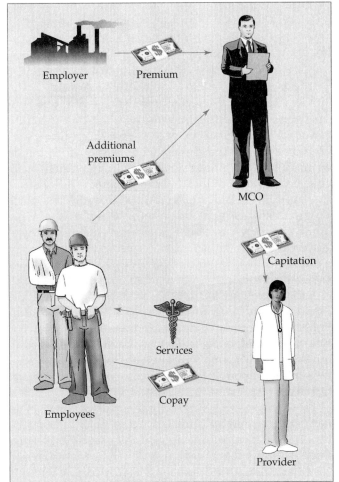

FIGURE 5–5 ■ *Capitated Funding in Employment-Based Managed Care Plan Enrollment*

based enrollment in a managed care plan. The MCO reimburses providers for services, but clients make a small copayment.

PUBLIC INSURANCE PROGRAMS   Publicly funded insurance programs are the third source of health insurance in the United States. In 1998, nearly a quarter of the U.S. population was covered under some form of government insurance program (U.S. Census Bureau, 2000). The public component of the third-party system consists of the Medicare and Medicaid programs, programs for active duty and retired military personnel and dependents, and the Children's Health Insurance Program (CHIP).

Medicare   Medicare is part of the social insurance program arising from provisions of the Social Security Act. Under Medicare, people over 65 years of age who are eligible for Social Security benefits receive partial coverage of health services. Certain other individuals, such as the disabled, are eligible for Medicare coverage before age 65. At its inception in 1965, Medicare was intended to protect the elderly against expensive hospitalizations. The optional Medicare Part B was added to cover physician expenses. More recently, Medicare has begun to

CRITICAL THINKING IN RESEARCH

There is considerable research that indicates that economic factors have a direct effect on access to and use of health care services. There is also some research, however, suggesting that even when economic factors are equalized, some subpopulations have lower utilization rates for health care services and poorer health status. This is particularly true of ethnic cultural groups (Tarver, 2000).

- How would you design a study to separate economic from noneconomic factors influencing use of health care services?
- What subpopulations might you want to study? Why? How would you recruit members of that population for participation in your study?
- How might you go about gathering information from your study participants? What information would you want to gather? What data collection methods might you use?

provide for some preventive services such as influenza and pneumonia immunization and mammography (Fox, Etheredge, & Jones, 1998). Medicare Part C, or Medicare+ Choice, was instituted in 1997 to provide beneficiaries with a choice of options among traditional fee-for-service practices and MCOs (Pulcini & Mahoney, 1998).

Medicare pays the greatest percentage of the federal investment in health care services. Projected expenditures for 2000 were in excess of $252 billion, and Medicare payments are expected to climb to $356 billion by 2005. In 1997, more than 38 million individuals were covered by Part A of the Medicare program (U.S. Census Bureau, 1999). Medicare Part A, the Hospital Insurance Program, covers inpatient services, hospice, and some home care services. Part B is a Supplemental Medical Insurance Program that covers services by a physician or a nurse or other health care professional working under the direction of a physician or other outpatient services.

Part A coverage is available to all participants in the Social Security program and is provided without additional premiums. Funding for Medicare Part A is derived from nonvoluntary Social Security payroll taxes on one's income with a matching payment from the employer. Information about Part A services, costs, and requirements is presented in Table 5–3 ■.

Part B coverage is optional and entails payment of an additional premium similar to that paid for private health insurance, but much less costly. In 2001, the premium for Part B coverage was $50 per month (Health Care Financing Administration, 2001). Medicare Part B is also supported by general federal revenues. Approximately 95% of persons eligible for Part A Medicare bene-fits also receive Part B benefits (U.S. Census Bureau, 1999). Under both components of the program, the client is responsible for a deductible and also pays a percentage of the cost of care (usually 20%) for services provided under Part B. Part B of Medicare is summarized in Table 5–4 ■.

As noted earlier, the Medicare program instituted prospective payment systems for Part A (the DRG system) and Part B (RBRVS). RBRVS also places a limit on total Medicare revenue a provider may earn. This limit is called the Volume Performance Standard (Reagan, 1999).

Because of escalating Medicare costs, the federal government has been encouraging enrollees to select managed care plans in place of the traditional fee-for-service Medicare benefits package (Tone, 1999). A managed care option has been in place in the Medicare system since 1985; however, initially few enrollees chose this option. By 1993, 1.8 million Medicare beneficiaries were enrolled in managed care plans. From 1994 to 1996, use of managed care among Medicare enrollees increased by 81%, and by 1998, approximately 15% of Medicare recipients (more than 5 million persons) were enrolled in managed care plans (Tudor, Riley, & Ingber, 1998). Unfortunately, many MCOs are not finding the Medicare market as profitable as anticipated and are discontinuing coverage. For example, a 1998 Families USA survey found that of 90 managed care plans discontinuing Medicare services, 60% were doing so because of insufficient earnings (Update, 1999). As another example, Aetna, one of the major managed care organizations involved in Medicare, anticipated terminating coverage for a significant portion of its 670,000 Medicare enrollees following termination of

■ **TABLE 5–3**   **Medicare Part A Benefits, Deductibles, Copayments, and Requirements, 2001**

BENEFIT	DEDUCTIBLE	COPAYMENT	REQUIREMENTS FOR CARE
Hospital services (150-day maximum) Semiprivate room/meals Hospital services/supplies Nursing services Inpatient psychiatric care (190-day lifetime maximum)	$792/benefit period	None until day 61 Days 61–90, $198/day Days 91–150, $396/day All costs beyond 150 days	Hospital admission
Blood transfusion	None	Cost of replacing first three pints	More than three pints needed
Skilled nursing (100-day maximum/benefit period)	None	None until day 21 Days 21–100, $99/day	Hospitalized minimum three days
Home health care	None	20% of approved charge for medical equipment	Medicare-certified agency; client is homebound and requires intermittent skilled nursing, physical, speech, or occupational therapy; care is ordered and reviewed periodically by physician
Hospice care	None	$5 for outpatient prescription drugs 5% of approved inpatient respite care	Terminal illness

■ **TABLE 5–4**   Medicare Part B Benefits, Deductibles, Copayments, and Requirements, 2001

BENEFIT	DEDUCTIBLE	COPAYMENT	REQUIREMENTS FOR CARE
Physician's services	$100/year for all Part B services	Monthly premium $50 20% of approved charges	Physician accepts Medicare
Outpatient hospital services Emergency services	No additional*	Coinsurance or fixed payment based on service needed	Medical emergency
Blood transfusion		Cost of replacing first three pints, then 20% of approved charges	
Physical and occupational therapy	No additional*	20% of approved charges	Physician-prescribed treatment plan with periodic physician review
Outpatient psychiatric services	No additional*	50% of charges	
Laboratory fees	No additional*	None for approved tests	Use of Medicare-certified laboratory
Ambulance services	No additional*	20% of approved charges	Medical need, other forms of transport could endanger client's life
Home health care: home health aide and durable medical equipment	No additional*	20% of approved medical equipment charges	Receiving Medicare-covered home health services under Part A
Bone mass measurement	No additional*	20% of approved charges	Risk of bone mass loss
Colorectal cancer screening			Age 50 and over
Fecal occult blood every 12 months	No additional*	None	
Flexible sigmoidoscopy every 48 months	No additional*	20% of approved charges or 25% if performed in an ambulatory surgery center or hospital outpatient department	
Colonoscopy every 24 months Barium enema (in place of fecal occult blood or sigmoidoscopy)	No additional*		High risk of colon cancer
Diabetes services			Diagnosed diabetes
Glucose monitoring supplies	No additional*	20% of approved charges	
Diabetes self-care training	No additional*	20% of approved charges	
Mammogram every 12 months	None	20% of approved charges	Women age 40 and over
Pelvic examination and Pap smear	None	20% of approved charges	All women with Medicare
Prostate cancer screening			Men age 50 and over
Digital rectal examination every 12 months	No additional*	20% of approved charges	
Prostate-specific antigen (PSA) test every 12 months	None	None	
Immunization			
Influenza every year	None	None	All Medicare recipients
Pneumonia	None	None	All Medicare recipients
Hepatitis B	No additional*	20% of approved charges	Medium to high risk for hepatitis B

* If provided by a Medicare-approved facility.

Source: Health Care Financing Administration. (2001). *Medicare and you.* Retrieved January 27, 2001, from the World Wide Web: *www.medicare.gov.*

17,000 and 67,000 enrollees in the two prior years. Managed care executives indicate that almost every managed care plan is dropping Medicare recipients in at least some markets (Mitchell, 2000).

Medicare has provided access to health care for many older and disabled persons who could otherwise not have afforded care; however, Medicare deductibles and increasing premiums for Part B and Part C coverage still make health care unaffordable for some older persons. All Medicare enrollees pay the same deductibles and

premiums, whatever their income. The original premium when Part B coverage was instituted was $3 per month (Miller, 1995). For 2001, the cost of Part B premiums was $50 per month, while Part A deductibles increased to $792 for each benefit period (Health Care Financing Administration, 2001). A benefit period begins with hospitalization and ends 60 days after discharge from all covered institutions, so a beneficiary could be responsible for more than one deductible payment during a calendar year (Powell, 1996). Medicare

Part C premiums have increased by 41% since 1994, and annual Part B premiums are expected to more than double from $526 in 1998 to $1,172 by 2006. Many Medicare recipients who have not opted for managed care enrollment carry additional insurance policies, called medigap policies, to supplement Medicare coverage. Premiums for these policies, however, have also increased by 34% since 1994, and nearly one fourth of Medicare recipients do not have supplemental insurance (Update, 1999). Because of the increased expenses associated with Medicare, approximately 16% of low-income elderly Americans are considered "dual eligible" and qualify for assistance under the Medicaid program (Kenney, Rajan, & Soscia, 1998).

Medicaid   The Medicaid program was established in 1965 to provide health care services to a large segment of the population who could not otherwise afford care. Its original purpose was to integrate the indigent into mainstream health care services. In 1999, Medicaid provided insurance coverage for just over 10% of the U.S. population (U.S. Census Bureau, 2000). Medicaid expenditures for the year 2000 were expected to be $188 billion, rising to more than $283 billion by 2005 (U.S. Census Bureau, 1999; Kenney et al., 1998). Despite these growing expenditures, Medicaid covers only about half of the U.S. population with incomes below the poverty level (Reagan, 1999).

Medicaid is a means-tested *entitlement* program based on financial eligibility. Under the program, the federal government pays half of the costs of health care for Medicaid enrollees, with matching funds from the states. The federal government previously established eligibility criteria for the *categorically needy,* those who because of membership in certain categories (e.g., recipients of AFDC) were automatically eligible for Medicaid, and the *medically needy,* persons whose health care needs are beyond the scope of their income, but who are otherwise able to maintain themselves financially. As noted earlier, welfare reform initiatives have divorced Medicaid eligibility from welfare eligibility and dismantled the AFDC program, replacing it with TANF. This move has decreased the number of persons eligible for Medicaid and limited the length of eligibility for those who remain eligible (Heymann & Earle, 1999).

The Medicaid program is administered by the states, but state programs must provide a minimum set of federally defined benefits. This mandatory benefits package includes the following services:

- Inpatient and outpatient hospital services
- Prenatal care (including nurse midwifery services)
- Childhood immunizations
- Primary provider services (from physicians or family or pediatric nurse practitioners)
- Nursing home care

- Family planning services and supplies
- Rural health services
- Home health care for those eligible for skilled nursing care
- Laboratory and x-ray services
- Early and Periodic Screening, Diagnosis, and Treatment (EPSDT) services, a preventive program for children under age 21 years (Rovner, 2000)

Recent federal policy changes have initiated a move from entitlement status for Medicaid to a block grant type of program in an effort to shift responsibility for social action from the federal government to the states (Hosek & Levine, 1996). A *block grant* is a lump sum made available to the states by the federal government to be used as each state sees fit within certain broadly defined parameters. The *Medigrant program,* as the block grant program to cover welfare, health, and training funds is being called, would provide the states with a specified sum of money for use to meet these three social needs. Reconfigured as a block program, there would no longer be any categorical eligibility and the states would have the ability to define eligibility criteria, services to be provided, and how services would be financed. Funds received from the federal government would be less than in the past Medicaid program, but the states would have greater latitude in how that money would be spent. In 1998, categorical eligibility was reinstated for the following groups:

- Pregnant women, infants, and children in families with incomes less than 133% of the federal poverty level
- Children aged 6 to 15 in families with incomes less than 100% of the poverty level
- Adults and children in families who would have met AFDC eligibility guidelines in 1996
- Recipients of Supplemental Security Income, an assistance program for low-income Social Security recipients (reinstated in most states)
- Adoptive or foster care children receiving assistance under Title IV of the Social Security Act
- Children and adults who lose cash assistance due to increased incomes (Medicaid coverage is for a transitional period only)
- Medicare beneficiaries with incomes less than 100% of the poverty level (Rovner, 2000)

States have the option to expand both the eligible populations and the services provided. Approximately three fourths of Medicaid enrollees are low-income children and adults, but the elderly and disabled account for two thirds of Medicaid expenditures (Montoya & Bell, 1998). One of the major cost categories for this population group is home health care, which increased fourfold from 1987 to 1995 and has continued to climb. Medicare home health costs increased tenfold over the same period, making a significant contribution to governmental health care costs (Kenney et al., 1998).

Similar to the Medicare program, Medicaid enrollees have been encouraged to select managed care options rather than traditional fee-for-service providers. The reasons for this shift are twofold: to provide a cost-effective alternative to emergency department care used by many Medicaid recipients and to move Medicaid enrollees into mainstream health care organizations that focus on preventive activities (Pina, 1998). The number of managed care plans involved in Medicaid has grown steadily, increasing by 22% per year from 1992 to 1996 (McCue, Hurley, Draper, & Jurgensen, 1999). By 1997, 47.5% of Medicaid recipients were enrolled in managed care plans (U.S. Census Bureau, 1999).

There is some concern that managed care practices developed for higher-income populations may not be as effective with the Medicaid population. Private managed care plans have little understanding of the relationship of poverty to health and do not offer some of the wraparound services previously provided by public Medicaid safety net providers. Loss of these services may make it more difficult for enrollees to obtain health care services. Managed care plans may need to add "enabling services" such as home visits, health education, and social services to permit Medicaid enrollees to make effective use of health services (Lillie-Blanton & Lyons, 1998).

⑥THINK ABOUT IT

Would prospective or retrospective reimbursement for community health nursing services be more advantageous to insurers if services were reimbursed by a third-party payer? Why?

CHAMPUS/TRICARE The Civilian Health and Medical Program of the Uniformed Services (CHAMPUS) is a program that provides payment for civilian medical services for active-duty and retired military personnel and their dependents. CHAMPUS is usually used to pay for inpatient services not available through a uniformed services medical facility (e.g., a naval hospital or an army medical center). CHAMPUS may also be used to finance nonhospital services provided in the civilian health care sector. In 1997, 3.8% of adults aged 45 to 60 years and 4.6% aged 61 to 64 years were insured under the CHAMPUS program (Glied & Stabile, 1998). Dependent children may also be covered under CHAMPUS.

Although care provided through a uniformed services medical facility is free (except for a small daily fee

for inpatient services), there is a deductible for outpatient services provided under CHAMPUS. Under CHAMPUS, civilian hospitals and providers are reimbursed for services at DRG rates. Like other government-funded health care programs, however, CHAMPUS costs have escalated significantly, rising 15% from 1981 to 1987. For this reason, the Department of Defense initiated a pilot project in 1988 that permitted CHAMPUS recipients to choose between traditional fee-for-service care and enrollment in managed care. The project demonstrated better access to care and better client satisfaction than the standard CHAMPUS program, but slightly higher costs due to increased utilization (Zwanziger et al., 2000).

The CHAMPUS managed care project was chosen as the prototype for a replacement program called TRICARE. TRICARE offers recipients three options: a low-cost HMO-like program, a provider network with low cost sharing but no enrollment requirement, and a program similar to the original CHAMPUS program (Zwanziger et al., 2000).

CHIP Despite the fact that Medicaid covered more than 14 million children under the age of 18 in 1999, an estimated 10 million children remained uninsured (U.S. Census Bureau, 2000). The Children's Health Insurance Program (CHIP) is a federally funded program intended to provide health care for children who are not eligible for Medicaid or other forms of insurance. In 1997, Congress authorized the expenditure of $48 billion over a 10-year period to meet this goal. Like Medicaid funding, federal money is granted to states, which may choose either to expand their Medicaid programs to include previously ineligible children or develop separate CHIP programs. If the former option is chosen, states must provide the usual complement of Medicaid services to the additional children. If a separate CHIP program is established, the state may determine the extent of services provided.

CHIP is intended to assist children in families with incomes less than 200% of the federal poverty level or 150% of the state's Medicaid eligibility criteria, whichever is higher. In addition, CHIP must provide outreach services to determine Medicaid eligibility and assist Medicaid-eligible children to obtain coverage. It is anticipated that CHIP will extend insurance coverage to 2.8 million previously uninsured children and that an additional 600,000 Medicaid-eligible children will be identified and assisted to obtain Medicaid (Rosenbaum, Johnson, Sonosky, Markus, & DeGraw, 1998).

As noted in previous chapters, the federal government also provides direct care services that are not associated with the publicly funded health insurance programs described here. These services are provided through the Department of Defense, the Veterans Administration, the Indian Health Service, and the National Institutes of Health.

assessment tips assessment tips assessment tips

ASSESSING THE ECONOMIC STATUS OF A POPULATION

- What is the average income of the group?
- What proportion of the group has incomes at or below poverty level?
- What subpopulations are included in the low-income group?
- What proportion of low-income families receive some form of public assistance? Are all those eligible for assistance receiving it? If not, why not?
- What is the level of unemployment in the population? For those who are employed, what are the typical salaries?

- What proportion of the population receives employment-based health insurance benefits? Why do others not receive benefits (e.g., part-time employment, cannot afford premiums, etc.)?
- How are most health care services for the population funded?
- What revenue sources fund public health services for the population? Are these revenues adequate to provide needed services?

EFFECTS OF FINANCING MECHANISMS

What effects do various financing mechanisms have on the health status of the population? Current research is limited and provides no clear-cut answers to this question, but there are some general conclusions that can be drawn regarding the relative effectiveness of various means of funding health care.

Public insurance programs such as Medicare and Medicaid have accomplished, in part, their intended purposes of providing health care services for selected vulnerable populations, particularly the elderly and the poor. However, it is clear that these programs are not meeting the entire need. For example, Medicaid enrollees have been found to be more likely than those without insurance to have a regular source of health care but have less favorable outcomes in this respect than clients with private insurance. Similarly, Medicaid recipients have less difficulty obtaining care than the uninsured, but more difficulty than the privately insured (Berk & Schur, 1998). Medicaid has also been credited with an increase in the number of pregnant women getting prenatal care (National Center for Health Statistics, 2000).

Looking at Medicare, even though preventive practices such as mammograms, immunizations, and eye examinations for diabetics are now covered by the program, relatively few Medicare enrollees may receive them. For example, during 1995–1996, only 28.3% of women aged 65 to 69 years received a mammogram, and 12% of enrollees received one preventive test. Immunization rates for pneumonia vaccine varied from 9% to a high of only 38% in various states, and the percentage of diabetics who received an eye examination ranged from 25% to 60% (*The Nation's Health,* 1999).

Prospective payment and managed care have had some effect in slowing the rise in health care costs.

However, there is some concern that this has occurred at the expense of desirable health outcomes. For example, 49% of cases referred to the Medicare Rights Center Hotline in 1997 and 1998 involved MCO noncompliance with Medicare rules (Update, 1999). Some MCOs also engage in "carve-out" practices, removing costly services from the service plan for Medicaid enrollees when services are not contractually defined by the state. These carved-out categories of service can then be provided only at an additional charge to the client (Holahan et al., 1998).

Medicaid enrollees and the poor enrolled in MCOs have also been found to engage in greater use of emergency departments than those in fee-for-service arrangements (Lillie-Blanton & Lyons, 1998). This behavior may be a result of inability to obtain appointments or the absence of wraparound services that enable clients to take advantage of services in less expensive settings. Depressed Medicaid recipients have been shown to receive fewer new antidepressant drugs and less psychotherapy than clients in fee-for-service practices (Melfi, Croghan, & Hanna, 1999).

Other potential problems in the area of Medicaid and Medicare managed care include the potential for poor-quality services due to low reimbursement rates, possible inability of enrollees to maintain existing provider relationships if they move into managed care plans, and less provider time available to clients. Medicaid MCO clients have also experienced longer waits for services than Medicaid recipients in fee-for-service practices. They also express less satisfaction with access to care and with relationships with providers (Pina, 1998). Fee-for-service care has demonstrated lower mortality rates for colorectal cancer than those found among Medicaid recipients, MCO enrollees, or the uninsured (Roetzheim et al., 2000). Other studies also demonstrate better access and fewer barriers to care among fee-for-service clients than for those enrolled in HMOs (Shi, 2000). In one review of several studies, MCOs performed better than fee-for-service practices on a variety of measures in only four studies, with equal effectiveness in 19 studies and worse in 21 studies (Sullivan, 1999).

Medicare and Medicaid enrollment in MCOs may also have negative consequences for the organization. For example, financial declines seem to be greater for MCOs with large Medicaid populations than for other MCOs. These declines do not seem to be related to excess medical expenses for Medicaid enrollees, but to low capitation rates and greater administrative requirements (McCue et al., 1999). Home health agencies that provide services under Medicare also experience difficulties with reimbursement, never knowing until afterward whether services will be approved for payment. Home care managers have suggested that this uncertainty may lead to more conservative treatment plans that address clients' needs less effectively (Whitelaw & Warden, 1999).

On the positive side, inclusion of mental health benefits in managed care programs has been shown to reduce the number of outpatient sessions and admissions, as well as length of stay for clients who are admitted to inpatient facilities, with lower costs (Goldman, McCulloch, & Sturm, 1998). Similarly, Medicare recipients enrolled in MCOs were more satisfied with the costs of care and obtaining care at a single location than those in fee-for-service arrangements (Tudor et al., 1998).

Some studies have mixed findings. For example, in general, managed care recipients and fee-for-service clients provide similar ratings on most access and satisfaction measures, but MCO enrollees again report more difficulty obtaining services. This is even more true for Blacks and Hispanics and those in poor health than among other MCO enrollees (Leigh, 1999). HEDIS data also show mixed results from managed care plans. For example, in 1997, 61% of MCOs advised smokers to quit, 70% provided screening for breast and cervical cancer, and 84% provided prenatal care in the first trimester of pregnancy. Results for childhood immunization and diabetic eye examinations were less favorable, at 65% and

38%, respectively (Thompson, Bost, Ahmed, Ingalls, & Sennett, 1998). It seems clear from the findings presented here that the question of the relative effectiveness of different forms of health insurance is yet to be answered and that additional research is needed in this area.

FUTURE DIRECTIONS

Future directions for health care financing are not yet clear. It is obvious that there needs to be continued attention to rising health care costs and to access to health care services for the U.S. population. Some authors suggest that there are a limited number of strategies available. Some options focus on controlling costs and others on finding new means of paying for care (Fuchs, 1999). Options for controlling costs include paying less for health care goods and services, using less, and finding more effective ways to provide care. The first two options have decided limits. Society can reduce payments to providers only to a certain limit before the number of people entering health care professions drops drastically, further reducing access to care. Similarly, the growing number of elderly with multiple chronic diseases suggests that there will be a need for more health care services rather than less (Federwisch, 1999). Viable approaches to diminishing the need for care that are of particular interest to community health nurses include health promotion and illness prevention and education of clients for self-care. Provision of these services, however, will require funding mechanisms under which they are reimbursable.

Use of nurse practitioners might be one approach to more effective provision of care, maintaining quality while lowering costs. Case management is another approach to more cost-effective care while still maintaining optimal outcomes. Some authors also suggest that standardized disease management protocols and group clinical services might be effective means of providing care. Similarly, provision of enabling services might improve access to and use of less costly modes of care (Fox et al., 1998).

Approaches suggested for developing new payment mechanisms include additional taxes, devoting more of the GDP to health care, increased working years, and greater retirement savings (Fuchs, 1999). The latter two approaches are primarily targeted toward increased health care funding available for care of the elderly under Medicare. Another suggested approach that might improve funding sources for working age citizens is increasing tax subsidies for insurance coverage. Currently, insurance is partially subsidized in four ways. The portion of insurance premiums paid by employers is considered nontaxable income for employees. In addition, people who spend more than 7.5% of their income on health expenses can deduct these expenses from their taxable income. Workers in firms

CULTURAL CONSIDERATIONS

Members of ethnic cultural groups have been shown to have poorer health care outcomes than others in the U.S. population. In part, this is due to lack of access to care due to financial constraints. Even when members of these groups have health insurance, however, their health outcomes tend to be less favorable than among Caucasian members of the population with similar forms of health care coverage. What other factors might be contributing to these differential outcomes? Which of these factors arise out of ethnic cultures and which arise out of the dominant culture or the culture of the health care system?

with group insurance that qualify under Section 125 of the IRS code can make before-tax insurance premium contributions, and, finally, those who are self-employed can deduct a portion of insurance premiums from their taxable income. Proposed tax credit strategies would provide for deduction of a greater portion of insurance premiums for all employees making job-based health insurance of greater benefit and less net cost (Gruber & Levitt, 2000).

Whatever approaches are taken to controlling the costs of health care and developing new payment mech-anisms, community health nurses should be actively involved in relevant policy decisions. Community health nurses may also be involved in research to determine the outcomes and cost-effectiveness of various modes of health care delivery. Future financing mechanisms must support a balance between cost control and access to and quality of health care services, and community health nurses must help to assure that such a balance is main-tained. For more information about health care financ-ing, visit the Web destination provided on the compan-ion Web page for this book.

APPLYING YOUR KNOWLEDGE IN PRACTICE

✖ CASE STUDY
Financing Care for the Underserved

You have been appointed to the mayor's task force on health care in the midsize community in which you work as a community health nurse. The assessment of community health and economic status conducted by the task force indicates that most of the population's health care needs are adequately met at all three levels of prevention. The exception to this, however, is the population of the migrant farm camp at the edge of town.

This group consists of primarily male Mexican workers who have entered the United States on legal work visas. Very few of the workers have brought their families with them. Most of this population receive no health care except for treatment in the emer-gency room of the community hospital. Usually, this care is provided for work-related injuries or serious ill-ness. Members of this group receive no primary pre-ventive care and do not seek care for minor illnesses because of their inability to pay.

Because most of these people are in the United States legally, they would be eligible for county med-ical assistance; however, very few have applied for this program because of language barriers, lack of trans-portation to the social services office, and inability to afford to take the time off work to submit an applica-tion. Even if they did receive assistance, they would be unlikely to find a regular health care provider who has a contract with the county to provide services under Medicaid reimbursement. Only one community clinic and one independent nurse practitioner, in addition to the community hospital, have county contracts. Local physicians receive adequate income from private pay-ing clients and those with private health insurance. Because of the extended time between provision of services and receipt of reimbursement, these physi-cians no longer accept county assistance clients.

The rest of the population is well off compared with average state and national incomes. With the excep-tion of the migrant workers, most residents are employed by three large industries and receive salaries that are quite adequate to meet the cost of liv-ing. Because of the industry present in the community, the local tax base is more than adequate. The commu-nity does not budget any public funds for health care as the majority of the population are adequately served by private providers. There is no local health department, but the county offers public health ser-vices in a town 50 miles away.

- What factors are influencing the health status of the migrant group?
- How would you finance health care for this popu-lation group?
- Would fee-for-service care or managed care arrangements be more appropriate for providing care to the migrant population? Why?

🐾 TESTING YOUR UNDERSTANDING

- How do economic factors influence health? What effects do economic factors have on health care delivery? (pp. 80–84)
- What are some of the factors contributing to escalating health care costs? What effects do escalating costs have on access to care? (pp. 81–82)
- What effects have economic factors had on the provision of public health services? (pp. 82–83)
- What is the difference between prospective and retrospective reimbursement? What are the advantages and disadvantages of each? (pp. 84–85)

- What characteristics do managed care programs have in common? How do types of managed care plans differ? (pp. 86–88)
- What are the advantages and disadvantages of fee-for-service care and managed care? (pp. 85–88)
- What effects has managed care had on public insurance programs? (pp. 90, 93–95)

REFERENCES

Abood, S. (2000). Why care about Medicare reimbursement? *American Journal of Nursing, 100*(6), 70–72.

Berk, M. L., & Schur, C. L. (1998). Access to care: How much difference does Medicaid make? *Health Affairs, 17*, 169–180.

Broyles, R. W., McAuley, A. J., & Baird-Holmes, D. (1999). The medically vulnerable: Their health risks, health status, and use of physician care. *Journal of Health Care for the Poor and Underserved, 10*, 186–200.

Bryce, C. L., & Cline, K. E. (1998). The supply and use of selected medical technologies. *Health Affairs, 17*, 213–224.

Chang, C. F. (2001a). Access to health care. In C. F. Chang, S. A. Price, & S. K. Pfoutz (Eds.), *Economics and nursing: Critical professional issues* (pp. 335–363). Philadelphia: Davis.

Chang, C. F. (2001b). Why does health care cost so much? In C. F. Chang, S. A. Price, & S. K. Pfoutz (Eds.), *Economics and nursing: Critical professional issues* (pp. 68–96). Philadelphia: Davis.

Chang, C. F., Price, S. A., & Pfoutz, S. K. (2001). The impact of managed care. In C. F. Chang, S. A. Price, & S. K. Pfoutz (Eds.), *Economics and nursing: Critical professional issues* (pp. 297–334). Philadelphia: Davis.

Cunningham, P. J., & Freiman, M. P. (1996). Determinants of ambulatory mental health services use for school-age children and adolescents. *HRS: Health Services Research, 10*, 409–427.

Federwisch, A. (1999). Runaway costs: How can we rein in healthcare expenses? *NurseWeek, 12*(4), 1, 10.

Fox, P. D., Etheredge, L., & Jones, S. B. (1998). Addressing the needs of chronically ill persons under Medicare. *Health Affairs, 17*, 144–151.

Fuchs, V. R. (1999). Health care for the elderly: How much? Who will pay for it? *Health Affairs, 18*, 11–21.

Gabel, J. R. (1999). Job-based health insurance, 1977–1998: The accidental system under scrutiny. *Health Affairs, 18*, 62–74.

Ginsburg, P. B., Gabel, J. R., & Hunt, K. A. (1998). Tracking small-firm coverage, 1989–1996. *Health Affairs, 17*, 167–171.

Glied, S., & Stabile, M. (1999). Covering older Americans: Forecast for the next decade. *Health Affairs, 18*, 208–213.

Goldman, W., McCulloch, J., & Sturm, R. (1998). Costs and use of mental health services before and after managed care. *Health Affairs, 17*, 40–52.

Gray, B. H., & Rowe, C. (2000). Safety-net health plans: A status report. *Health Affairs, 19*, 185–193.

Gruber, J., & Levitt, L. (2000). Tax subsidies for health insurance: Costs and benefits. *Health Affairs, 19*, 72–85.

Grumbach, K., Coffman, K. V., Blick, N., & O'Neil, E. H. (1998). Independent practice association physician groups in California. *Health Affairs, 17*, 227–237.

Health Care Financing Administration. (2001). *Medicare and you.* Retrieved January 27, 2001, from the World Wide Web, *www.medicare.gov.*

Heymann, S. J., & Earle, A. (1999). The impact of welfare reform on parent's ability to care for their children's health. *American Journal of Public Health, 89*, 502–505.

Holahan, J., Zuckerman, S., Evans, A., & Rangarajan, S. (1998). Medicaid managed care in thirteen states. *Health Affairs, 17*, 43–63.

Hosek, J., & Levine, R. (1996). An introduction to the issues. In J. Hosek & R. Levine (Eds.), *The new fiscal federalism and the social safety net* (pp. 1–17). Santa Monica, CA: RAND.

Janes, G. R., Blackman, D. K., Bolen, J. C., Kamimoto, L., et al. (1999). Surveillance for use of preventive health-care services by older adults, 1995–1996. *Morbidity and Mortality Weekly Report, 48*(SS-8), 51–88.

Kenney, G., Rajan, S., & Soscia, S. (1998). State spending for Medicare and Medicaid home care programs. *Health Affairs, 17*, 201–212.

Lasker, R. D., & the Committee on Medicine and Public Health. (1997). *Medicine and public health: The power of collaboration.* New York: New York Academy of Medicine.

Leigh, W. A. (1999). Managed care in three states: Experiences of low-income African Americans and Hispanics. *Inquiry, 36*, 753–757.

Levit, K., Cowan, C., Braden, B., Stiller, J., Sensenig, A., & Lazenby, H. (1998). National health expenditures in 1997: More slow growth. *Health Affairs, 17*, 99–119.

Lillie-Blanton, M., & Lyons, B. (1998). Managed care and low-income populations: Recent state experiences. *Health Affairs, 17*, 238–247.

Ling, C. (2000). Managed care: Its origins, today's picture—and what's ahead. *NurseWeek, 13*(14), 20–21.

Matisoff, A. (1999). Premium prospects. *NurseWeek, 12*(10), 32.

McClellan, M., & Skinner, J. (1999). Medicare reform: Who pays and who benefits? *Health Affairs, 18*, 48–62.

McCue, M. J., Hurley, R. E., Draper, D. A., & Jurgensen, M. (1999). Reversal of fortune: Commercial HMOs in the Medicaid market. *Health Affairs, 18*, 223–230.

McGuire, M. T., & Anderson, W. H. (1999). *The US health care dilemma: Mirrors and chains.* Westport, CT: Auburn House.

Melfi, C. A., Croghan, T. W., & Hanna, M. P. (1999). Access to treatment for depression in a Medicaid population. *Journal of Health Care for the Poor and Underserved, 10*, 201–215.

Miller, D. F. (1995). *Dimensions of community health* (4th ed.). Dubuque, IA: Brown.

Mitchell, S. (2000). Left in the dust: Aetna leads HMOs in exodus from Medicare markets. *NurseWeek, 13*(13), 25.

Montoya, I. D., & Bell, D. C. (1998). Implications of managed care in a publicly funded health care delivery system. *Journal of Public Health Management Practice, 4*(1), 45–51.

National Center for Health Statistics. (2000). Entry into prenatal care—United States, 1989–1997. *Morbidity and Mortality Weekly Report, 49,* 393–398.

The Nation's Health. (1999, July). Many Medicare patients do not receive preventive care. p. 16.

Pina, D. L. (1998). Medicaid beneficiaries' experiences in HMO and fee-for-service health care. *Journal of Health Care for the Poor and Underserved, 9,* 433–447.

Powell, S. K. (1996). *Nursing case management: A practical guide to success in managed care.* Philadelphia: Lippincott-Raven.

Price, S. A., Pfoutz, S. K., & Chang, C. F. (2001). The economics of nursing and health care. In C. F. Chang, S. A. Price, & S. K. Pfoutz (Eds.), *Economics and nursing: Critical professional issues* (pp. 3–36). Philadelphia: Davis.

Pulcini, J., & Mahoney, D. (1998). Health care financing. In D. J. Mason & J. K. Leavitt, (Eds.), *Policy and politics in nursing and health care* (3rd ed.) (pp. 80–99). Philadelphia: Saunders.

Reagan, M. D. (1999). *The accidental system: Health care policy in America.* Boulder, CO: Westview Press.

Roetzheim, R. G., Pal, N., Gonzales, E. C., Ferrante, J., Van Durme, D. J., & Krischer, J. P. (2000). Effects of health insurance and race on colorectal cancer treatments and outcomes. *American Journal of Public Health, 90,* 1746–1754.

Rosenbaum, S., Johnson, K., Sonosky, C., Markus, A., & DeGraw, C. (1998). The children's hour: The state Children's Health Insurance Program. *Health Affairs, 17,* 75–89.

Rovner, J. (2000). *Health care policy and politics A to Z.* Washington, DC: CQ Press.

Shi, L. (2000). Type of health insurance and the quality of the primary care experience. *American Journal of Public Health, 90,* 1848–1855.

Smith, S., Heffler, S., Freeland, M., & the National Health Expenditures Projection Team. (1999). The next decade of health spending: A new outlook. *Health Affairs, 18,* 86–95.

Solanki, G., Schauffler, H. H., & Miller, L. S. (2000). The direct and indirect effects of cost-sharing on the use of preventive services. *Health Services Research, 34,* 1331–1350.

Sullivan, K. (1999). Managed care plan performance since 1980: Another look at two literature reviews. *American Journal of Public Health, 89,* 1003–1008.

Tarver, J. M. (2000). Non-economic barriers to health care utilization by African Americans. Unpublished doctoral dissertation, University of San Diego.

Thompson, J. W., Bost, J., Ahmed, F., Ingalls, C. E., & Sennett, C. (1998). The NCQA's quality compass: Evaluating managed care in the United States. *Health Affairs, 17,* 152–158.

Thorpe, K. E., & Florence, C. S. (1999). Why are workers uninsured? Employer-sponsored health insurance in 1997. *Health Affairs, 18,* 213–218.

Tone, B. (1999). Drugs and money: Paying for prescriptions for seniors. *NurseWeek, 12*(20), 1, 8.

Tudor, C. G., Riley, G., & Ingber, M. (1998). Statisfaction with care: Do Medicare HMOs make a difference? *Health Affairs, 17,* 165–176.

Update. (1999). Publications and reports. *Health Affairs, 18,* 264.

U.S. Census Bureau. (1996). *Statistical abstract of the United States, 1996* (116th ed.). Washington, DC: Government Printing Office.

U.S. Census Bureau. (1999). *Statistical abstract of the United States, 1999* (119th ed.). Washington, DC: Author.

U.S. Census Bureau. (2000). *Health insurance coverage: 1999.* Retrieved November 17, 2000, from the World Wide Web, *http://www.census.gov/hhes/hlth.*

Whitelaw, N. A., & Warden, G. L. (1999). Reexamining the delivery system as part of Medicare reform. *Health Affairs, 18,* 132–143.

Zwanziger, J., Kravitz, R. L., Hosek, S. D., Hart, K., et al. (2000). Providing managed care options for a large population: Evaluating the CHAMPUS reform initiative. *Military Medicine, 165,* 403–410.

THE CULTURAL CONTEXT

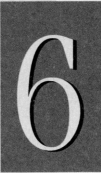

6

Media Link

http://www.prenhall.com/clark

Additional interactive resources for this chapter can be found on the companion Web site. Click on Chapter 6 and "Begin" to select the activities for this chapter.

Every day community health nurses interact with people from multiple cultural backgrounds, both clients and other people with whom they collaborate. Given the demographic changes occurring in the United States and elsewhere in the world, this interaction can only increase. For example, it is estimated that by 2050 the Hispanic population in the United States will triple, rising from 31.4 million in 1999 to 98.2 million. Similarly, the African American population will increase from 34.9 million to 59.2 million; the Asian/Pacific Islander population is expected to triple; and the Native American population will increase by approximately 17%. During this same time period, the non-Hispanic white population is only expected to grow by an estimated 9% (Henderson, 2000).

Within each of these groups are multiple different ethnic cultures which community health nurses may encounter in their practice. Nurses, themselves, come from a personal cultural background and have assimilated a culture specific to nursing. This chapter, for example, is written from the perspective of the scientific health care culture, in which ethnic cultural practices may be considered "alternatives" to the dominant health care culture. While it is not possible for a particular nurse to be conversant with every culture encountered, he or she must have a good general understanding of the effects of culture on health and on the interactions between nurse and client and between nurses and other providers.

Culture has been described as the socially transmitted beliefs, values, and behaviors that define the worldview of a group of people and direct decision making (Purnell & Paulanka, 1998b) or as ways of living developed by a group and transmitted from one generation to another (Ferran, Tracy, Gany, & Kramer, 1999). In this book, *culture* is defined as the ways of thinking and acting developed by a group of people that permit them to interact effectively with their environment and to address concerns common to the human condition. A group's *worldview* is their way of looking at the universe and their relationship to that universe.

Culture is characterized by universality, largely unconscious influence, uniqueness, stability as well as dynamism, and internal variability. Culture is a universal experience. All people engage in culturally prescribed behavior patterns. Examples of *cultural universals*—areas addressed by all cultures—are family, marriage, parenting roles, education, health, work, and modes of communication. Although culture affects virtually every aspect of life, its influence is largely unconscious. The influence of culture is rarely consciously noted, unless one purposefully undertakes a study of one's own culturally determined behavior. As aptly noted by one author, "Culturally learned assumptions control our lives, with or without our permission" (Pedersen, 1995).

⑥THINK ABOUT IT

How has your own culture influenced your health-related behavior? Have these influences been positive or negative?

Moreover, the culture of any particular group is unique. Although several cultures may exhibit certain commonalities, no two cultures, like no two individuals, are exactly alike. The beliefs and behaviors that constitute a particular culture arise from the unique constraints faced by a given group of people in dealing with problems common to humanity. These unique situational constraints are the source of cultural variation among groups of people. For example, exposure to periodic drought and famine in India may have resulted in the Hindu prohibition on killing cattle (Harris, 1989). Because the cow was a source of milk and assistance in plowing the farmer's fields, killing and eating the family's only cow in a time of deprivation would decrease the family's chances of long-term survival and also jeopardize the survival of the society. In this instance, the environmental constraints imposed on Hindu society led to the development of a specific cultural practice that ensured society's survival in times of drought or famine.

Another characteristic of culture is its stability. Cultural characteristics tend to endure across generations. Culture, however, is neither static nor immutably fixed; it is dynamic and subject to change. Although the superficial aspects of culture can change relatively easily, basic cultural values and beliefs change slowly and may provide the basis for strong resistance to change.

Finally, the degree to which members of a cultural group adhere to cultural beliefs, values, and customs varies considerably. Cultural adherence is affected by many factors. Among these are an individual's education level, social status, facility with the dominant language, length of exposure to the culture of the larger society, and residence in an urban or rural setting in the country of origin. Often, a person's education level is associated with greater use of the dominant language. It cannot always be assumed, however, that use of the dominant language is indicative of an individual's identification with the culture of the larger society or that an individual adheres less to subcultural norms. Adherence to the values and behaviors of one's culture of origin is negatively related to the degree of acculturation to the dominant culture. *Acculturation* or cultural assimilation is the acquisition of at least some of the beliefs, values, and behaviors of the dominant culture, and usually occurs because such adaptation is required for survival in a new environment (Munet-Vilaro, Folkman, & Gregorich, 1999). Characteristics of culture are summarized on page 101.

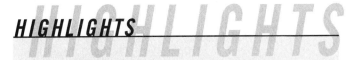

Characteristics of Culture

- *Universality*
  Culture is a pervasive phenomenon that involves all human populations.
- *Unconscious influence*
  Expression of cultural meanings through behaviors and symbols often occurs without conscious awareness.
- *Uniqueness*
  All cultures are unique and, although similarities may exist among cultural groups, no two cultures are exactly alike.
- *Stability*
  Culture is lasting and endures through generations.
- *Dynamism*
  Culture changes over time. Superficial aspects of culture change more readily than deeply held beliefs and values.
- *Variability*
  The degree of adherence to cultural beliefs, values, and behaviors varies with individual members of the culture and depends on a variety of factors.

RACE, CULTURE, AND ETHNICITY

Two terms that are frequently confused with culture are race and ethnicity. *Race* is an attribute that allows classification of human beings on the basis of certain biological and genetic characteristics, such as color of skin, eyes, or hair; hair texture; and shape of eyes, nose, and lips (Flaskerud, 2000). Such distinctions, however, are unreliable as scientific classifications because there are few people who fit exclusively into one racial category. A case in point is the racial admixture found among Latinos, whose forebears may have included non-Hispanic whites, Native Americans, African Americans, and Asians.

Simply put, *ethnicity* involves belonging to a particular ethnic group or a "shared sense of peoplehood" (Flaskerud, 2000). Ethnicity is characterized by some or all of several shared features. These features include a common geographic origin; language; religious tradition; and shared traditions, values, and symbols. Other common features that may be shared by members of an ethnic group are their literature, folklore, and music; food preferences; group institutions; and common settlement and employment patterns. Ethnicity also involves internal and/or external identification with a particular group. Internal identification means that the person considers him or herself a member of the ethnic group. In external identification, persons outside the group perceive the person as a group member (Spector, 2000b). Culture may contribute to ethnic distinctions, but is not equivalent to ethnicity.

CULTURE AND HEALTH

Culture has both direct and indirect effects on health. Direct effects stem from specific culturally prescribed practices related to diet and food or to health and illness. For example, all cultures have prescribed practices intended to promote health and prevent illness or to restore health when illness occurs. Similarly, all cultures have particular dietary practices that contribute to the nutritional status and, thereby, to the health status of their members.

Culture also affects health indirectly. Some of these indirect effects result from cultural definitions of health and illness, acceptability of health care programs and providers, and cultural influences on compliance with suggested health or illness regimens. Cultural definitions of health and illness determine what kinds of health problems are considered worthy of attention and what conditions are likely to be disregarded. If, for example, certain behaviors that are perceived as evidence of mental illness by the larger society are considered normal in the client's culture, then the client is unlikely to take any action to deal with those behaviors. Similarly, minor illnesses may be ignored if health is defined in terms of one's ability to work or to perform other social roles. In general, people are likely to disregard any type of condition that is not defined as illness in their own culture. This cultural propensity can lead to serious health consequences.

Cultural factors may also determine the acceptability of both health programs and health providers. For example, cultures that eschew scientific medicine in favor of healing based on faith in God may view immunization programs as inimical to their beliefs. In other cultures, health care providers may be considered lower-class persons not to be associated with, effectively preventing people from taking advantage of many health opportunities. For example, nursing has been considered a lower-class occupation in India, and nurses have had limited opportunity to influence the health of their clients for the better because of their low social status.

Cultural factors often determine whether clients will comply with recommendations when they do seek professional help. Culture gives rise to certain expectations regarding treatment. If health care providers' recommendations are too far removed from these expectations, the provider loses credibility, and the client is unlikely to comply with those recommendations (Flaskerud, 2000). For example, clients may have a cultural expectation that illnesses are to be treated with multiple medications.

When the provider prescribes a single drug, credibility may be lost and compliance will suffer.

⑥THINK ABOUT IT

What are some aspects of the culture of professional nursing? How might nursing's professional culture interfere with effective interaction with clients?

NURSING AND CULTURE

The interface between community health nursing and culture occurs in one of three arenas: one's personal culture, the professional culture of nursing, and care of clients from a culture different from one's own. All of us are the products of our own cultural heritage. Many nurses adhere to the major tenets of the dominant American culture, but maintain many beliefs, values, and practices derived from familial culture and our cultures of origin. We have attitudes toward time, cleanliness, the value of religious affiliation, "proper behavior" and so on that may enhance or impede our interactions with others. Community health nurses should become aware of these cultural influences in their own lives and their impact on interactions with others.

Nursing, as a profession, also has a distinct culture as do other health care professionals and people with whom community health nurses collaborate in their practice. Differences between these cultures may give rise to as much misunderstanding or conflict as differences between nurse and client. For example, a cultural emphasis on cure among physicians may hamper their ability to understand the motivations of a nurse who advocates for termination of life support in keeping with a client's or family's wishes. In this instance, the cultural values of cure and advocacy, arising out of the medical and nursing cultures, respectively, are in conflict. Similarly, nursing has its own language, which may or may not be understood by persons from another culture (ethnic or professional). In addition to the general professional culture, subcultures exist in specific health care settings that may make it difficult even for two nurses to understand each other (Andershed & Ternestedt, 1999).

The final aspect of the interface between nursing and culture lies in our interactions with clients. In this interaction, we may need not only to address the differences between the client's ethnic culture and our cultural heritage, but we must examine the effects of differences between professional and lay cultures on effective health care.

Community health nurses should cultivate an awareness of their own cultural beliefs, values, and attitudes

and their potential interactions with the cultures of clients and other health care providers. To do this, nurses may explore their own cultures using the cultural assessment tips presented on page 135. Introspection, interviews with family members, and discussions of changes from "my day" to now with older family members may uncover previously unrecognized cultural influences on the nurse's behavior.

Attention to cultural issues related to clients can be traced to Florence Nightingale, who was interested in the health of indigenous groups in Australia. Early public health nurses in the United States and Canada devoted their efforts to improving the health status of immigrant groups. More formalized attention to cultural issues in nursing is seen in nursing documents. Although cultural sensitivity is implicit in *Nursing's Social Policy Statement,* it is explicitly noted as a required feature of nursing practice in the American Nurses Association's *Position Statement on Cultural Diversity in Nursing Practice* (Poss, 1999). As noted earlier, it is increasingly important for community health nurses to be prepared to care for a highly culturally diverse population.

Community health nurses employ knowledge of culture and culturally sensitive health care with populations as well as with individual clients. At the level of the individual, the nurse devises health care interventions congruent with the client's culture, being sensitive to cultural influences affecting health and incorporating cultural health beliefs and practices whenever possible. At the population level, community health nurses must be involved in the development of culturally sensitive health care delivery systems and programs.

CULTURAL COMPETENCE

In order to interact effectively with clients, health professionals, or other people from cultures different from their own cultures of origin, community health nurses must develop cultural competence. The United States Health

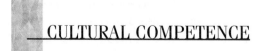

Resources and Services Administration (2000) described cultural competence as the possession of academic and personal skills that enable one to understand cultural differences and similarities. Others add to this definition an understanding of the total client context including cultural factors (Spector, 2000a) as well as acceptance and respect for cultural differences and the ability to adapt care to incorporate cultural values, beliefs, and behaviors whenever possible (Purnell & Paulanka, 1998b). At the organizational level, cultural competence incorporates behaviors, attitudes, and policies that allow the agency to work effectively in cross-cultural situations whether these involve clients or staff (Ferran et al., 1999). In this chapter, *cultural competence* is defined as the knowledge, willingness, and ability to adapt health care to enhance its acceptability to and effectiveness with clients from cultures other than that of the nurse.

More than knowledge of other cultures, the nurse's attitude toward the beliefs, values, and behaviors of others is the crucial element of cultural competence. Knowledge must be acted upon, and action must be guided by attitudes of acceptance and respect for other cultures. Some authors have suggested that "cultural humility" might be the goal in professional education, rather than competence. Competence connotes mastery of a finite body of knowledge regarding another culture and may contribute to the development of cultural stereotypes. A *stereotype* is an assumption that all members of a particular group will always act in accord with specific cultural expectations. Stereotypes may have their basis in fact or fiction. But, even when the stereotypical notion conforms to an actual cultural norm, expecting that all members of the group accept that norm can be as detrimental to nurse–client interactions as ignoring cultural differences.

Cultural humility, on the other hand, suggests an awareness that we never know as much about a cultural group as its members. Cultural humility incorporates ongoing self-evaluation and self-critique, attention to power imbalances between clients and providers, and development of partnerships with clients (Tervalon & Murray-Garcia, 1998). Using the definition of cultural competence presented above, we can subsume the concept of cultural humility in one's willingness to respect other cultures and to examine the effects of one's own attitudes, values, and beliefs on interactions with clients and professionals from other cultural backgrounds.

Characteristics of Cultural Competence

Cultural competence is characterized by recognition of similarities as well as differences between cultural groups. Some values seem to be universal among cultures. For example, in one study, Hispanic, African American, and non-Hispanic white family members of clients in intensive care all had similar expectations of the nurses, including equity, dignity, and respect for the client (Waters, 1999). Expectations of how these values are implemented may differ among groups, however.

Other characteristics of cultural competence include recognition of culture as a predominant force influencing behaviors and values of clients as well as those of providers and institutions, and an acceptance of cultural differences and their impact on health and health care delivery. Cultural competence is also characterized by respect for the unique culturally defined needs of clients and by recognition of the existence of diversity within, as well as among, cultures. Other critical features of cultural competence are the capacity for cultural self-assessment, an awareness of the dynamic nature of the interaction between cultures, and the ability to incorporate cultural considerations in practice. Finally, cultural competence includes a realization that health care services are most effective when delivered by those who are part of or fully understand a client's culture (Bureau of Primary Care, 2000; Ferran et al., 1999; Health Resources and Services Administration, 2000). The characteristics of cultural competence are summarized below.

Barriers to Cultural Competence

Some authors have noted that, in spite of the emphasis on including cultural content in nursing education, cultural competence is largely lacking in nursing practice (Poss, 1999). In part, this lack of cultural competence in the profession can be explained by several barriers to cultural competence, many of which arise out of our societal background and are not easily undone in the educational process. These barriers include ethnocentrism, cultural blindness, cultural shock, cultural conflict, xenophobia, and stereotyping. Other barriers include racism, prejudice, discrimination, and cultural imposition.

HIGHLIGHTS

Characteristics of Cultural Competence

- Recognition of culture as a predominant force influencing values and behaviors of both clients and health care providers
- Realization of the need for cultural competence in health care
- Recognition of cultural similarities as well as differences
- Acceptance of cultural differences and their impact on health
- Respect for the unique culturally-defined needs of others
- Recognition of diversity within cultures
- Awareness of the dynamic nature of culture
- Capacity for cultural self-assessment
- Ability to incorporate cultural considerations in practice

Ethnocentrism is a conviction that one's own way of life, values, beliefs, and customs are superior to those of others (Spector, 2000b). A related concept, which is often displayed by nurses, is *medical centrism,* a belief that medicine (or nursing) is always correct and that scientific medical practices are superior to alternative health practices (Flaskerud, 2000). **Cultural blindness** involves ignoring or denying cultural differences, behaving as if these differences do not exist. **Cultural shock** occurs when the nurse is only too aware of cultural differences and is stunned and immobilized by the "shocking" aspects of the alien culture. Cultural shock is most likely to occur in response to behaviors approved in one culture that are disapproved in another. The stronger the taboos against the behavior in the disapproving culture, the greater the shock when that behavior is accepted, or even encouraged, in the other. Clients, as well as nurses, experience cultural shock. In fact, clients from other cultural groups may experience two levels of culture shock—one in response to exposure to the dominant U.S. culture and the other in response to exposure to the health care culture which may be quite alien to them (Dreher, 1996).

In *cultural conflict,* the nurse is aware of cultural differences and is threatened by them. This threat arises when recognition of cultural differences causes the nurse to doubt the validity of personal beliefs and values, threatening self-esteem. In response to this perceived threat, the nurse may actively seek to support personal beliefs and behaviors by denigrating those of others. *Stereotyping* is attributing a cultural pattern to all members of a group on the basis of prior opinions, attitudes, and interactions. Stereotyping or unwarranted generalization fails to recognize that cultures are not homogeneous, nor are they static. There is also a need to differentiate between generalizations about the "rules" espoused by a cultural group and how people actually behave (Papadopoulos, 1999). For example, many people in the United States value honesty, but have no qualms about taking pens or other items home from work. *Xenophobia* is an irrational fear of strangers (Spector, 2000b), particularly those who are significantly different from oneself in appearance or behavior.

⓺THINK ABOUT IT

What effect, if any, do you think cultural differences have on racial conflict?

The negative attitudes discussed thus far can lead to other negative responses by nurses and others caring for members of another cultural group. *Racism* is the belief that people can be classified on the basis of biophysical traits into groups that differ in terms of mental, physical,

and ethical capabilities, with some groups being intrinsically superior or inferior to other groups. **Prejudice** is a set of attitudes unfavorable to a given group of people based on preconceptions rather than fact. Both racism and prejudice may lead to discrimination. **Discrimination** is differential treatment of an individual or group based on unfavorable attitudes toward the group.

Cultural imposition is another potential barrier to culturally competent care. **Cultural imposition** refers to the nurse's expectation that everyone should conform to the nurse's cultural practices, whatever their own personal beliefs. This response to cultural differences is an extension of ethnocentrism in that the nurse not only believes that other practices are inferior, but expects them to be abandoned and those of the nurse's culture assumed. For example, an Asian American nurse might be appalled when a European American adolescent challenges his parent's opinion and expect the parent to chastise the son. Barriers to cultural competence are summarized above.

ASSESSING CULTURAL INFLUENCES ON HEALTH AND HEALTH CARE

As noted earlier, community health nurses must incorporate cultural concepts into the care of individuals and their families as well as the development and implementation of health care programs for population groups. To accomplish this, nurses must have knowledge of the cultural groups with which they are likely to come in contact. Such knowledge is derived from cultural assessments: assessments of the group to determine typical beliefs, values, and behaviors and assessments of individuals in terms of their adherence to those beliefs, values, and behaviors.

Principles of Cultural Assessment

Four basic principles should guide nurses engaged in the study of another culture. First, view all cultures in the context in which they developed. As noted earlier, cultural practices arise out of a need to meet common human problems in a particular human setting. That setting must be considered in exploring another culture.

Second, examine the underlying premise of culturally determined behavior. What was the intended purpose for the behavior when it originated? Does the behavior still fulfill this purpose? When one knows the underlying reason for behaviors that seem strange, the behaviors may not seem quite so strange after all. The nurse should also examine the meaning of the behavior in the cultural context. The meaning of certain behaviors from the perspective of the nurse's culture may be very different from the behavior's meaning in the context of the client's culture. For example, resistance to having one's head shaved for a cranial surgical procedure may be interpreted as vanity from a European American nurse's perspective. When the nurse understands that some clients view the head as the home of the soul, however, such resistance is more understandable.

Finally, recognize the existence of intracultural variation. Not every member of any given cultural group displays all of the beliefs and behaviors typical of that culture. There may be several subgroups within one cultural group with different behavior patterns. Or individual clients may be more or less acculturated to the dominant U.S. culture. The nurse who expects to find intracultural variation tends to avoid stereotyping and responding to clients as if they were typical representatives of their cultural group. Principles of cultural assessment are summarized at right.

Obtaining Information About Another Culture

How does one become knowledgeable about another culture? Perhaps the best way to begin is to become conversant with one's own culture, recognizing the influences of culture on one's life and behavior. Personal insights regarding culture will enable the nurse to accept cultural beliefs and behaviors that may differ from his or her own. Once familiar with his or her own cultural heritage, the nurse can begin to read literature related to other cultures of interest. In reading, the community health nurse should examine the qualifications of the authors writing. Was the book or article written by a member of the culture? Is it based on empirical data derived from research, on per-

Principles of Cultural Assessment

- View all cultures in the context in which they developed.
- Examine underlying premises for culturally determined beliefs and behaviors.
- Interpret the meaning and purpose of behavior in the context of the specific culture.
- Recognize the potential for intracultural variation.

sonal experience with a particular culture, or on stereotypes?

A second means of acquainting oneself with another culture is to interview colleagues who are members of that culture. Explore with them their concepts of health and illness and attitudes and practices affecting health. Discover how these concepts may differ from those held by previous generations or other members of their family. Health care professionals, by virtue of their knowledge of health matters, are likely to have achieved a greater degree of acculturation and conformity with the dominant U.S. culture with respect to health practices than nonprofessionals from the same group. These individuals, however, remain a valid source of information regarding cultural health beliefs and practices.

One of the best ways to become familiar with a particular culture is to spend time living within it. This approach, however, is not always feasible. Alternatives include home visits to families within the group to observe daily living in the cultural context and questioning clients and families regarding health-related beliefs and practices. Another possible approach is observing activities and interactions at health facilities and community or religious functions.

When assessing another culture directly, the community health nurse should follow a few general guidelines. First, look and listen before asking questions or taking action. Observation aids in asking pertinent and timely questions and forestalls actions that may be inappropriate. Second, explore how the group feels about being studied. Explain that your reasons for studying the culture are practical and do not arise out of idle curiosity. Third, discover any special protocols. Should one speak to a local leader before beginning to observe a group? Is there a council or leadership group who should grant permission for participation in group activities? Fourth, foster human relations, putting them before the need to obtain information. Information will not assist the nurse to provide care if he or she alienates members of the group. Social amenities are very important in many cultures and should be attended to before the "business" of

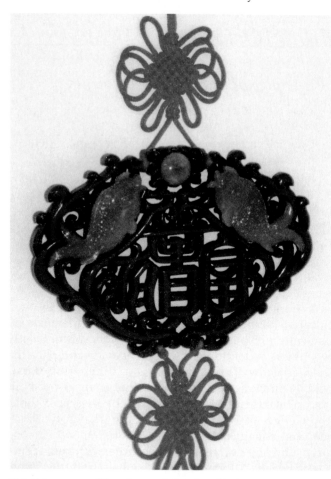

This Taiwanese wall hanging symbolizes good luck.

information gathering begins in earnest. In fact, information about social amenities is part of the data needed by the nurse.

Many people, in exploring another culture, look for differences from their own culture. The nurse, however, should also look for cultural similarities to use as a foundation in aiding clients to accept and use health care services. Cultural differences should be accepted as normal.

Locate group leaders and respected residents, those considered wise, "ordinary" group members, and clients who can converse knowledgeably about another culture. Critics of the traditional aspects of the culture may also be interviewed to provide a balanced picture.

Participate as well as observe. The nurse must assess each situation as it occurs to determine whether participation or observation is the more appropriate activity. Participation conveys an openness to cultural differences and a willingness to engage in culturally prescribed activities rather than ridicule them. Some activities, however, are closed to outsiders, and the community health nurse's participation would not be welcomed.

When exploring another culture, the nurse should also consider the feelings of group members about questions asked. The nurse should ascertain what types of questions are acceptable or offensive in a particular culture. For example, U.S. Peace Corps Volunteers in India found it difficult to adjust to frequent questions about their salary or how much their clothes cost. Such questions were perfectly acceptable in Indian society, but considered impolite or "nosy" in the United States.

A little forethought as to the phrasing and timing of questions can prevent serious mistakes. Ask questions positively without implying value judgments. For example, "I notice you put garlic on a string around the baby's neck; can you tell me what it's used for?" is far more acceptable than "Why in the world do you hang garlic around the baby's neck?" Nurses might ask the same questions of themselves and gauge their own emotional reaction to the questions. A nurse can also try out questions on colleagues who are members of the culture being explored. Suggested modes of cultural exploration are summarized below. General areas to be considered in a cultural assessment include biological factors influencing the cultural group, psychosocial considerations, life experiences, and health system interactions.

Biological Factors

Biological factors are those intrinsic to the individual that influence life. As noted earlier, because of racial characteristics, different cultural groups may display biophysical variations in their anatomic and physiologic makeup (Spector, 2000b). Groups may differ in terms of body build and structure, skin color and texture, genetic structure, enzyme activity, disease susceptibility, and so on. Many African American and Asian clients, for instance, experience lactose intolerance, and so do not consume large amounts of milk products. Another example of biological variation is the large stature and bone structure common to many African Americans compared to the small stature of many Asians.

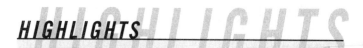

HIGHLIGHTS

Modes of Cultural Exploration

- Become conversant with your own culture and its influences on your life.
- Review the existing literature on beliefs, values, and behaviors of specific cultural groups.
- Interview colleagues who are members of the cultural group in question.
- Immerse oneself in the culture to be studied.
- Observe members of specific cultural groups.
- Interview members of cultural groups, particularly group leaders.
- Interview other persons who are conversant with the culture.

Genetic inheritance may also play a part in the types of health problems commonly seen in members of some ethnic and cultural groups. For example, the prevalence of diabetes among Latinos is estimated to be two to four times that among non-Hispanic whites (Black, Ray, & Markides, 1999). Diabetes is a common problem among many Native American tribes as well (National Center for Chronic Disease Prevention and Health Promotion, 1998), whereas sickle cell disease is a genetically transmitted disease particularly prevalent among African Americans. Ethnic and racial groups also differ in their abilities to metabolize drugs.

In addition to differences in body structure and function present in some ethnic groups, members of different cultures may also display differential attitudes to bodily functions and specific parts of the body. Care of one's body and attention to basic physiologic functions often differ from one group to another. A particular cultural group may employ specific hygiene practices (e.g., applying oil to the hair) that the nurse may need to incorporate into the client's personal care.

Special significance may be attached to certain body parts in a particular culture. For instance, in some cultures, the head is considered sacred and is to be treated with respect. In these cultures, bumping someone's head is considered an insult. Among many Vietnamese and Hmong, for example, touching the head is thought to cause loss of the soul or vital force (Geissler, 1994).

In some cultures, certain body parts are believed to be responsible for functions and conditions that are not in accordance with scientific knowledge of physiology. In many Asian folk medicine systems, for example, the heart is thought to be responsible for insomnia, dreams, forgetfulness, insanity, and delirium. The kidneys, on the other hand, are believed to control water, birth, development, reproduction, and maturation (Cargill, 1994). Beliefs and attitudes toward body parts and physiologic functions may influence acceptance of such scientific medical procedures as transfusions, venipuncture, transplantation, and autopsy.

Exposure of certain body parts is appropriate in some cultures and not in others. In some regions of the world, neither men nor women cover their breasts, yet for the U.S. female, exposing the breasts is generally unacceptable. In India, many village people consider uncovering the shoulders and upper arms indecent.

Differences also exist between cultures in terms of what body parts may appropriately be touched and who may touch them. Touching members of the opposite sex or members of the same sex may be restricted. For example, it would be unusual for adult members of the same sex to hold hands or to kiss in public in the United States. In other cultures, same-sex touching or kissing may be perfectly acceptable, whereas similar behavior toward members of the opposite sex is thought to be inappropriate.

Another consideration to be addressed relative to physiologic function is privacy. Cultures differ in terms of what physiologic functions may be performed in public and those for which privacy is required. Latinos and other cultural groups, for instance, exhibit a great deal of modesty regarding urination and defecation as well as bathing and dressing. Similarly, people from some cultural groups may have difficulty accepting the presence of the husband or father during delivery. In others, multiple family members, including children, may be present.

In exploring cultural attitudes toward physiologic function, the nurse should also determine whether there are periods during which individuals are considered ritually unclean. In some cultures, for example, postpartum or menstruating women are considered unclean, and their activities and interactions with others are restricted (Snow, 1998).

Age is another biological factor and is relevant to cultural assessment in two respects. First community health nurses should be aware of attitudes to age in the cultural groups with which they work. In many cultural groups, older persons tend to be highly respected and influential. Children are highly valued, although boy children may be more highly valued than girls by some groups (e.g., some Asian and Arab populations). In most cultural groups, children are expected to be quiet and respectful of their elders and do not participate in family decisions. In some other cultures, however, children are active participants in decision making.

The nurse also considers the age composition of the cultural group because this information will help to identify potential age-related health concerns and health service needs. Statistical data on group composition by age is available from census figures for Native Americans, African Americans, Asian Americans, and Latinos, but is not readily available for other cultural groups. Many ethnic groups have a higher proportion of children under five years of age than the general population. They also frequently have larger adolescent populations and fewer elderly than the general population. These facts suggest that some cultural groups have higher proportions of young people subject to a variety health problems common among the young than the general population and help to guide health care planning at the aggregate level.

Psychosocial Considerations

Many of the visible effects of culture occur in the psychosocial realm. Specific behaviors in this area are the product of cultural attitudes and values. Two general considerations in assessing the psychosocial aspects of culture are perceptions of one's place in the cosmos and cultural responses to common life experiences.

One's Place in the Cosmos

Cultural groups differ in their perceptions of relationships between people and the environment, among people, and between people and the supernatural world. With respect to environmental relationships, typical American culture seeks mastery over the environment.

Many traditional cultures, on the other hand, seek harmonious relationships with the external physical environment. For example, traditional African American cultural groups have often perceived a need for cooperation with a powerful natural environment in order to promote survival. Similarly, a number of cultural groups also view seasonal changes as directly affecting human health and behavior. Signs of the zodiac and tidal rhythms, for example, are believed to affect blood flow and initiation of labor in pregnant women (Snow, 1998).

Other aspects of relationships to the external environment include perceptions of space and time. With respect to time, some cultural groups, such as the dominant culture in the United States and African American culture, are future oriented, while others are past or present oriented. Many Asian cultures, for example, attach great importance to the past and are considered past oriented. Native American and Latino groups, on the other hand, tend to be oriented to the present moment (Ferran et al., 1999). Both past- and present-oriented cultural groups may have difficulty in long-range planning for future events.

Other perceptions related to time may also be of importance in planning nursing care for individual clients or for population groups. Care of a Muslim client, for example, may need to be planned to prevent interference with specified times for prayer (Hughes, 1998). At the group level, effective health programs targeted to Jewish clients or Seventh Day Adventists would not be scheduled on Saturday. Similarly, many cultural groups have fluid concepts of time that make appoint-based health care delivery less effective (Bankston, 1995).

Cultural groups also have differing attitudes to space. Most community health nurses in the United States subscribe to European American notions of acceptable personal space in certain situations. Preferred distance between people in European American culture can be described as follows:

- Public distance: greater than 12 feet
- Social distance: 4 to 12 feet
- Personal distance: 1½ to 4 feet
- Intimate distance: within 1½ feet (Spector, 2000b)

European Americans are frequently uncomfortable when their perceived personal space is invaded by another person. Among other cultural groups, however, there is considerable variation in what is perceived as one's personal space, leading to the potential for discomfort and conflict.

INTERPERSONAL RELATIONSHIPS   Another aspect of one's perceived place in the world lies in one' interactions with other people. All cultures have attitudes and behaviors that shape interpersonal relationships. In part, these attitudes and behaviors are influenced by social organization and family structure. Some cultural groups, such as the dominant U.S. culture, have loose social ties to multiple groups. Others have strong ties to family, church, and neighborhood. African Americans and Latinos typically fall into the latter group, although not every member of these groups will have similar levels of affiliation to social groups within the culture (Watson, 1998c). In many Asian cultures, as well, social organization is specifically prescribed. For example, traditional Hmong social organization is based on clan membership (Bankston, 1995), and social organization among traditional Native American groups is based on tribal affiliation. The Japanese have a strong tradition of *miushi-ishiki*, in which the needs of the individual are submerged in favor of the common good (Okuno, Tagaya, Tamura, & Davis, 1999). A similar orientation to group welfare over personal considerations is characteristic of several traditional cultural groups.

Family structure and expected roles also influence interactions among people. In most traditional ethnic cultures, the extended family is the typical family structure. Extended family, however, may not always be restricted to blood kin. For example, Latino families often include *compadres,* and African American extended families may include "adopted" children or adults. Similarly, in the Hmong clan structure, many people may be referred to as "aunt" or "cousin" without the usual familial interpretation of such titles in European American culture (Mattison, Lo, & Scarseth, 1994).

Many traditional cultures maintain hierarchical family structures in which the father is the head of the household and primary decision maker. Others, such as many Native American tribes, are matriarchal in nature. In all cultures, there are gender specific roles for males and females as well as specific familial roles for parents, children, and other family members. For example, filial piety, or respect of children for their parents, is a strongly held value in traditional Chinese culture as well as among other Asian groups. While respect for one's parents is also a primary

This example of traditional Hmong embroidery and appliqué depicts village life in Laos.

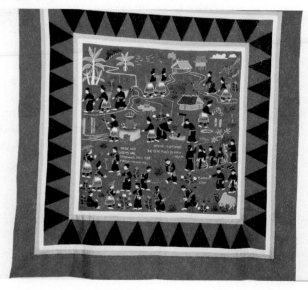

value in U.S. society, its operationalization may be quite different (Dai & Dimond, 1998). Table 6–1 ■ presents some of these differences in perceptions of filial piety.

Family roles may also differ with respect to responsibility for child care and socialization (Niska, 1999; Um & Dancey, 1999). In some cultures, both care of children and their socialization is the responsibility of women. In others, women are responsible for child care, but discipline and socialization are the purview of the father (Keenan, El-Hadad, & Balian, 1998). In still others, responsibility may be shared by both parents. Similar distributions of roles and responsibilities with respect to health care and health decisions may exist within cultures. It is important for community health nurses to be aware of these role expectations in order to promote effective use of health care services by individuals or by groups. If, for example, the mother is responsible for health care decisions and their implementation, the nurse will need to work with her to assure adequate immunization of young children. At the group level, the input of male elders in a particular ethnic group may need to be sought in the design of effective health care programs. Some examples of culturally defined family roles and responsibilities are presented in Table 6–2 ■ .

Another aspect of family roles that should be assessed by the nurse is the role of the family in health care. In many

traditional ethnic cultures, care of the sick is a family responsibility, and family members expect to be included in decisions about therapy and in the care of family members (Andershed & Ternestedt, 1999; Flaskerud, 2000). Some nurses, particularly in inpatient situations, have

■ **TABLE 6–1   Perceptions of Filial Piety in Traditional Chinese and Dominant U.S. Cultures**

TRADITIONAL CHINESE CULTURE	DOMINANT U.S. CULTURE
Obedience, submissiveness to parents' wishes	Egalitarian relationship, confrontation and challenge are acceptable
Son is responsible for care	Sons and daughters are equally responsible for care
Unlimited responsibility for care, self-sacrifice	Limited responsibility for care, not required to oversacrifice
Legitimate support includes meeting all needs	Legitimate support includes assistance with basic needs and maintaining elders' independence

■ **TABLE 6–2   Examples of Traditional Culturally Defined Family Structures and Roles**

CULTURAL GROUP	FAMILY STRUCTURE	FAMILY ROLES
African American	Traditionally matriarchal, now egalitarian, extended	Collaborative family roles
Appalachian	Patriarchal, extended	Father is head of household, decision maker, provider Woman cares for home and family and provides health care Grandparents may care for children
Chinese	Patriarchal, extended	Father is head of household Women make health decisions Sons are responsible for care of older parents Children are obedient to parents
Filipino	Egalitarian, extended	Parents hold equal roles in decision making Older children may support education for younger siblings
Hmong	Patriarchal, clan	Father is head of household Women care for home and children Children are obedient to parents Husband may have several wives
Korean	Patriarchal, extended	Father is bread winner, decision maker Wife's role is to nuture husband and children
Mexican American	Patriarchal, extended	Father is authority figure Mother cares for home and children All family members socialize children
Middle Eastern	Patriarchal, extended	Father is authority, disciplinarian Woman cares for home
Navajo	Matriarchal, tribal extended	Men care for livestock Women care for home and family Elderly women make health care decisions

been resistant to the incorporation of family members into the care of clients. When care occurs in the home or other community settings, incorporation of family caregivers may occur more easily.

Communication is another psychosocial consideration influencing relationships between people in cultural groups. The most obvious, though by no means the only, aspect of communication affecting nurse–client relationships is language. Language has been identified as one of the most significant barriers to health care access (Torres, 1998). In 1990, 32 million people in the United States spoke a language other than English in the home (Chang & Fortier, 1998). There are two general approaches to dealing with language as a factor in health care delivery: provision of care by bilingual providers and the use of interpreters. Unfortunately, fewer than 10% of nurses in the United States are from cultural minority groups (Poss, 1999), and not all of those are bilingual.

When nurse and client do not speak the same language or have varying degrees of fluency in each other's language, the services of an interpreter may be warranted. Several issues arise, however, when one employs an interpreter. These include issues of confidentiality, lack of health care background and familiarity with medical terminology, and potential unwillingness of clients to confide in an interpreter (Morris, Ogilvie, Fung, & Lau, 1999). Other concerns in the use of interpreters include the proficiency of the interpreter in English and/or the language of the cultural group, his or her understanding of the culture as well as the language, and potential impediments to the development of rapport between client and provider (Bureau of Primary Health Care, 2000; Chang & Fortier, 1998; Torres, 1998). Several suggestions for the use of interpreters are provided at right.

Interpretation is used for verbal communication in another language. Health messages are often communicated in writing as well. *Translation* is the process used to produce a written message as close as possible in intended meaning to the original message (Chang & Fortier, 1998). Unfortunately, many foreign-language materials related to health are literal translations of materials originally written in English and may not be comprehensible to the client. Translated educational materials should make use of native idioms whenever possible.

The words used are only one aspect of communication. Another aspect is the context in which the message is conveyed (Purnell & Paulanka, 1998a). In a "low-context" culture such as that of the United States, the essence of a message is conveyed in the *words* used. In a "high-context" culture, on the other hand, much of the message is communicated by the *context* in which the message is relayed rather than in the words used. Suppose, for example, that the nurse asks a mother when she plans to follow up on an immunization referral. In some cultures, it is polite to respond with the answer that one believes is expected, and the client might reply that she plans to get the immunizations that week. When the nurse visits the following week and finds that the

HIGHLIGHTS

Suggestions for the Use of Interpreters in Health Care Organizations

- Employ interpreters who are knowledgeable regarding the culture as well as the language.
- Provide training for interpreters regarding health issues and medical language, their role as interpreters, legal and ethical issues (e.g., confidentiality), and interpersonal skills.
- Stress the confidential nature of client interactions.
- Select an interpreter who will be acceptable to the client.
- Make arrangements for interpretation prior to the client visit if possible.
- Schedule additional time for the visit.
- Meet with the interpreter prior to the visit to discuss issues likely to be addressed and to review unfamiliar terms.
- Have the interpreter sit slightly behind or beside the client.
- Speak to the client rather than to the interpreter.
- Speak in a normal voice, pausing frequently to permit translation.
- Express yourself clearly but not in an overly simple manner.
- Avoid idioms that may not be easily translated.
- Have the interpreter assist you in understanding cultural beliefs, values, and practices.
- Avoid long discussions in English with the interpreter.
- Provide for periodic evaluation of the quality of interpretation.

mother has not yet had the child immunized, the nurse may interpret the client's previous statement as a lie. Yet, in the context of the client's culture, she was giving the appropriate response. If the nurse is aware of this cultural context, he or she is more likely to interpret correctly the mother's response as meaning that she will get the immunizations in the not-too-distant future.

Conflict can occur between individuals from high-context and low-context cultures primarily as a result of misinterpretation of communications. Those from the high-context culture may be reading into the message contextual considerations that might not exist. At the same time, the low-context person may be missing a large portion of the content of the message through neglect of contextual considerations.

Contextual considerations might include the need to observe certain social amenities before directing the conversation to the area of interest. For example, Puerto Ricans, as well as members of other cultures, might expect to learn something about the nurse as a person before getting down to the business at hand.

Culturally prescribed reticence, courtesy titles, epithets, and gestures are other culturally determined aspects of communication. Culturally prescribed reticence refers to the degree of openness about personal matters expected in casual encounters with others. Asians, for example, display a high degree of reticence. They traditionally consider it impolite to ask personal questions and are uncomfortable discussing personal matters with casual acquaintances, including health care professionals. Native Americans are also socialized to little self-disclosure. Reticence may be particularly problematic in therapy in which participants are expected to share intimate information with virtual strangers (LaFramboise, Trimble, & Mohatt, 1998). Latinos are also frequently reluctant to discuss personal matters with strangers (Zuniga, 1997).

Gestures are another important contextual factor. Gestures, like words, can convey totally different meanings in different cultures. In the dominant U.S. society, for example, one apologizes for accidentally bumping into someone else, but thinks nothing of pointing the sole of one's shoe at another. Some clients from India would be highly insulted to have the soles of one's shoes directed toward them or, worse yet, to be touched by someone's shoe. Footwear is considered dirty and contaminated in India, and the implications of intentionally touching someone with your shoe would be comparable to spitting in someone's face in the United States.

Other gestures, even if not insulting, may convey different meanings in different cultures. For instance, in the dominant U.S. culture, one indicates agreement by nodding the head, whereas in India one says yes by tilting the head toward the shoulder. In Vietnamese culture, it is unacceptable to crook one's finger to beckon another person, as that is how Vietnamese call dogs.

Cultures also differ with respect to their use of first or last names and courtesy titles. As with any client, it is wise to ask how a client from another culture wishes to be addressed. Often, the use of a first name is restricted to close friends or children. Adults may be referred to by last name with or without the appropriate title (e.g., "Gordon" versus "Mrs. Gordon"). In Korean culture, family members are addressed in terms of their relationship to the youngest child in the family (e.g. "Sung's grandmother"). As other children are born into the family constellation, the individual's relationship changes and forms of address change. Such practices may pose some difficulties for health record keeping (Nowak, 1998).

Some epithets are considered insulting in different cultures. An epithet is a word or phrase used in place of the correct designation and may or may not be derogatory in nature. When cultural differences intervene, generally innocent words may take on the character of

CRITICAL THINKING IN RESEARCH

One fairly common approach to qualitative research is the use of focus group interviews in which participants voice their thoughts and feelings about topics of specific interest to the researcher. The idea is that thoughts voiced by one participant may spark related comments from other participants in ways that do not occur in individual interviews, thus providing a richer description of a phenomenon from the perspective of the participants. Strickland (1999) noted, however, that the communication patterns of different cultural groups may lead to different outcomes than those usually provided by focus groups. For example, Strickland noted that Native Americans tended to use a traditional talking circle mode in focus groups rather than the interactive mode anticipated. Participants each spoke in turn about the topic or another area of interest with little interactive discussion among participants. Participants were also noted to ignore direct questions asked by the group facilitator, a technique often used in research focus groups. Another potential barrier to open communication was the fact that many of the participants were known to each other because of the close tribal structure. Similarly, obtaining information from focus groups composed of members of some Asian cultures has been difficult because of the cultural expectation that one should say what the listener wants to hear rather than what one really thinks.

- In what other ways might communication styles within cultural groups influence research? Give some examples related to cultural groups with which you are familiar.
- How might a community health nurse researcher incorporate cultural communication patterns effectively into the research design? How might the nurse circumvent barriers to data collection posed by cultural communication patterns?

---

insults. Most nurses are sensitive enough to refrain from calling an African American male "boy." Some Mexican Americans may or may not be offended by being referred to as *chicano* depending on what part of the United States they are from and their level of acculturation. Again, ask the individual client the preferred form of address.

Another aspect of interpersonal relationships within a specific culture that is of particular concern to community health nurses is the demeanor or behavior expected in one's interactions with others. In every culture, certain behaviors are acceptable and others are not. If community health nurses are to work effectively with clients from other cultures, they must engage in acceptable behaviors and avoid behaviors that might give offense.

Behaviors acceptable in one culture are not necessarily acceptable in another. For example, it is not unusual in some cultures for men to embrace or for women to hold hands while walking down the street. In the United States, however, such behavior might be interpreted as homosexuality. Members of the opposite sex, however, holding hands in public is acceptable in the United States and unacceptable in other parts of the world. Community health nurses need to consider how their behavior is perceived by clients as well as how clients' behavior should be interpreted. Community health nurses should be aware of and validate their interpretations of client behavior. They must also recognize that clients are using a similar process to assign meaning to the behavior of the nurse. Therefore, it is important to understand the usual meaning of a given behavior in the client's culture to avoid misunderstanding or giving offense. Table 6–3 ■ presents examples of acceptable and unacceptable behaviors for several cultural groups.

■ **TABLE 6–3   Selected Examples of Culturally Unacceptable Behavior**

UNACCEPTABLE BEHAVIOR	RECOMMENDED APPROACH
Disrespect for elders and others in authority, especially men (Asian, African American, Latino, Appalachian, Native American, Gypsy, Arab)	Show respect for elders and those in authority, incorporate in treatment decisions Give things to elders with both hands (Hmong)
Using informal forms of address inappropriately (Asian, Latino, African American, European American)	Use appropriate forms of address (e.g., using formal mode of speech with older persons), ask about preferred form of address Use last name with Mexican American clients Use first name only with close African American friend
Using the titles of "Miss" or "Mrs." for women (dominant United States)	Use title "Ms."
Direct eye contact (Native American, Latino, Appalachian, Arab—sexual overture between sexes, Navajo—may cause soul loss, Asian—implies equality, St. Helena Island black—implies disrespect of elder)	Look at the ground or to the side when speaking to others
Not maintaining eye contact (European American)	Maintain eye contact when speaking to others
Asking someone their name (Hmong)	Ask a third party, "Whose son (daughter, wife, etc.) is this?"
Assuming authority over others (Appalachian)	Avoid conflict Mind your own business
Arguing with authority figures (Asian, Latino, Appalachian)	Show respect and acceptance Avoid conflict
Competing with others (Native American, Appalachian)	Cooperate with others
Causing others to "lose face" (Asian)	Prevent others from losing face
Strong hand clasp (Native American)	Moderate grasp when shaking hands Lightly touch hand (Native American)
Weak hand clasp (European American)	Firm hand shake
Writing a "life story" (Native American)	Display modesty and respect for privacy
Self-disclosure (Native American, Asian, Latino, Appalachian, Gypsy, Arab)	Use tact in obtaining health history Use trusted interpreters from family Provide for physical privacy
Overt discussion of sexuality (Asian, Latino, Arab, Hmong)	Discuss sexual matters without members of opposite sex present; ensure availability of same sex health care provider
Aggressiveness or self-assertion (Native American, Latino, Asian, Appalachian)	Display humility and self-effacement
Lack of motivation or initiative (European American)	Display initiative in task accomplishment
Drawing attention to oneself (Native American, Asian)	Display humility and self-effacement
Expressing personal opinions (Asian)	
Ridiculing others, teasing (Asian, Appalachian)	Direct humor at self (especially with Appalachian clients)
Dependence on others, being a burden (Asian, Appalachian, European American)	Display self-reliance
Complaining (Asian)	Accept without complaining
Displaying emotion (Asian, Native American, Appalachian)	Control emotions

UNACCEPTABLE BEHAVIOR	RECOMMENDED APPROACH
Accepting things when first offered (Asian)	Repeat offers of food, pain medication
Giving negative information or disagreeing (Asian, Arab)	Give a polite response (whether true or not)
Giving misinformation (European American)	Tell the truth, however hurtful
Putting personal needs before family needs (Asian, Latino, Appalachian, Vietnamese)	Try to incorporate personal needs into family goals
Physical contact by opposite sex (Asian, Appalachian, Latino)	Avoid physical contact when possible
Physical contact with same sex (dominant United States)	Avoid physical contact when possible
Touching the head (Hmong, Vietnamese)	Avoid touching the head if possible
Pointing at others, especially with feet (Vietnamese, Indian, Native American)	Avoid pointing objects at others
Being more successful than one's husband (Navajo, Arab)	Help with role conflict
Interrupting, chattering (Native American)	Maintain silence, do not interrupt
	Allow time to formulate answers
Failure to understand others (Asian—causes loss of face for teacher)	Validate client's understanding of information
Getting right down to business (Asian, Latino, Native American, Appalachian)	Observe social amenities before business
Wasting time (European American)	Come to the point immediately
Saying no, refusing a request (Asian)	Graciously accept requests
Refusing hospitality (Asian, Appalachian, Arab, European American)	Graciously accept hospitality
Being late for an appointment or social event (European American)	Arrive on time

RELATIONSHIPS WITH THE SUPERNATURAL   The third aspect of determining one's place in the cosmos reflects relationships between people and the supernatural. In general, these relationships take one of two forms: religion and magic.

Religion is an organized system of beliefs, values, and practices reflecting a relationship with supernatural powers or a deity (Spector, 2000b). Religion is one aspect of a cultural group's attempt to explain the unexplainable. The nurse exploring another culture may encounter religious practices that enhance or detract from health. Most people are familiar with the prohibition against blood transfusions among some religious groups and the position of the Roman Catholic Church against artificial forms of birth control. Either of these practices can be detrimental to health in situations where a transfusion is indicated or where pregnancy is medically contraindicated. On the other hand, Jewish and Muslim proscriptions against pork probably originated as a measure designed to promote health by preventing infestation with trichinosis (Harris, 1989).

A community health nurse needs to examine several cultural aspects of religion. First, one would explore the extent to which religion is involved in health care. Are there specific religious beliefs regarding the cause of illness or appropriate treatments? Do members of religious groups play a role in the diagnosis and treatment of illness? For example, belief in faith and prayer as healing interventions is strong among Latinos and other cultural groups (Mehl-Medrona, 1999; Zapata & Shippee-Rice,

1999). In faith healing, religion takes on a direct curative aspect in the treatment of illness. The healer is believed to have been "called by God" and exercises healing powers through divine intervention. In some instances, providers of scientific medicine are seen as an extension of God's will (Rehm, 1999).

Second, one should explore the influences of religion on the health of a cultural group's members and on the health care system. Are certain religious practices detrimental to health? Examples of potentially dangerous religious practices are snake handling in some parts of Appalachia (Covington, 1995) and views of illness as punishment for sin, which may inhibit care-seeking behaviors or justify abusive behaviors, particularly toward the mentally ill (Morrison & Thornton, 1999). Another related area of inquiry is determining the degree to which religious and health care systems either conflict with or complement each other.

A third aspect of the impact of religion on health is the effect of religious sponsorship on the use of health services. Does this sponsorship enhance or detract from the acceptability of health programs? For example, if the only hospital in the community is a Roman Catholic hospital, are Protestant Appalachian clients reluctant to obtain services there? The fourth consideration is the relationship of religious leaders and healers to health care personnel. Is this a cooperative relationship, or are they in competition with each other?

Religion and magic are closely intertwined in many cultures. Distinctions between the two are based on the

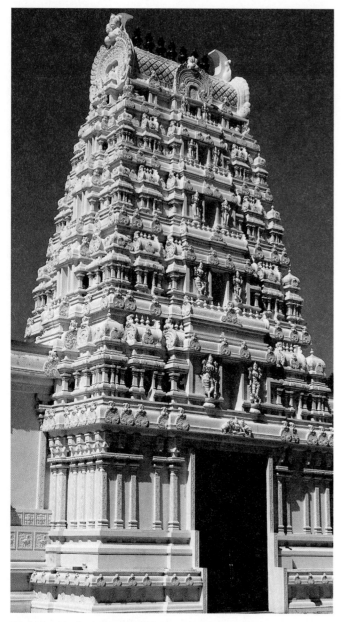

Traditional houses of worship help to maintain a group's culture.

agent of action. Religion is viewed as supplicative; the person typically conciliates personified supernatural powers, requesting specific action on their part. For example, a particular client may make an offering to gods or spirits or pray for a cure for his or her illness or relief from suffering. Magic, on the other hand, is considered manipulative. In using magic, an individual manipulates impersonal powers to achieve a desired result (Watson, 1998a). Beliefs in magic as a means of causing or curing disease are common in many traditional ethnic cultures, including African American (Snow, 1998; Watson, 1998a), Latino (Zapata & Shippee-Rice, 1999), Asian (Mattison et al., 1994), and Native American cultures (Still & Hodgins, 1998), as well as in a variety of European cultures (Spector, 2000b).

Knowledge of beliefs regarding the influence of magic on health and health practices is useful to community health nurses. If a nurse determines that the client or family attributes illness to witchcraft, he or she can encourage consultation with a practitioner of folk medicine *in addition* to compliance with a medically prescribed regimen. Understanding and acceptance of such beliefs also enable the nurse to contribute to the client's emotional health by promoting expression of fears and anxieties.

Life Experiences

The second major consideration in assessing psychosocial considerations in a group's culture is that of life experiences. Although all cultural groups deal with these common life experiences, cultural beliefs and behaviors related to life experiences can vary considerably. Life experiences that will be addressed here include experiences related to sexuality and reproduction, health and illness, and death.

SEXUALITY AND REPRODUCTION Cultural groups vary in their beliefs about, attitudes toward, and behaviors related to human sexuality and reproduction. Some groups, (e.g., fundamentalist Muslims and Christians) perceive sexual activity as inherently sinful and to be tolerated only within the bounds of marriage (Pope & Chung, 1999). Other groups are more tolerant of sexual activity outside of marriage, but may differ in terms of their application of this norm to men and women. For example, among Latinos, extramarital sexual activity is accepted for men but not women. "Good" women are not sexually experienced or knowledgeable and may not be willing to discuss sexual issues with their partners for fear of being thought prostitutes (Organista & Organista, 1997). These cultural attitudes place Latinas at risk for sexually transmitted diseases and cervical cancer since sexual beliefs have been found to influence willingness to obtain Pap smears.

Female genital mutilation (FGM) is an extreme mode of controlling sexuality and reproduction among women in which portions of the female genitalia (clitoris and possibly the labia) are excised. This practice is sometimes associated with the Muslim religion, but it is practiced by multiple cultural and religious groups throughout the world. Some authors suggest that immigrant women may be at greater risk for FGM in resettlement areas than in their country of origin due to attempts of the group to maintain their cultural identity. Although FGM is illegal in the United States, an estimated 168,000 girls were considered victims or at risk for FGM in 1990, most often in large metropolitan areas such as New York, Los Angeles, Atlanta, and Washington, D.C. (Compton & Chechile, 1999). Community health nurses should be alert to the possible practice of FGM in client populations with whom they work because of the serious physical and psychological health effects, including infection and difficulties with fertility, pregnancy, and delivery.

Attitudes toward homosexuality are another area that should be explored by the community health nurse engaged in a cultural assessment of a group of people. Homosexuality may be defined differently in some cultures than in the dominant U.S. culture. For example, Latino, Middle Eastern, and Greek men who have sex with other men are considered homosexual only if they assume a receptor role, whereas for Haitians, intercourse with other men is not homosexual if it is done for money (Gropper, 1996; Organista & Organista, 1997). Attitudes toward homosexual activity also differ among cultural groups. Again, Muslims and Christians generally consider homosexuality sinful. In Asian cultures, homosexuality can be considered as expressing disdain for societal norms that include expectations for marriage and children, and brings shame to the family of the homosexual individual. China is particularly repressive of homosexual behavior and such attitudes may accompany recent immigrants (Pope & Chung, 1999).

Cultural groups also vary with respect to attitudes and behaviors related to contraception. In societies where childbearing is an expectation, contraception is not approved and abortion is not to be considered. Nonetheless, even in these cultures, there may be a variety of methods employed to induce abortion, some of which can be extremely dangerous. For example, poisoning with pennyroyal, a common abortifacient that is highly toxic, occurs on a fairly regular basis in the United States (Anderson et al., 1996). Many cultural groups also engage in a variety of behaviors designed to prevent conception, some of which are based on traditional explanatory models for conception. For example, some African Americans believe that one is more apt to get pregnant if one has intercourse during menses and is "safe" at midcycle or that it is impossible to become pregnant until one has had a menstrual period following delivery of a baby. Cultural beliefs regarding menstruation and the reproductive cycle may likewise interfere with use of contraceptive devices. One such belief among some African Americans is that a regular menstrual flow indicates health, and that the heavy flow induced by intrauterine devices and scanty flow resulting from use of oral contraceptives are unhealthy (Snow, 1998). Members of cultural groups may also engage in a variety of behaviors to promote conception. Selected cultural beliefs and behaviors related to menstruation, conception, and contraception are presented in Table 6–4 ■.

All cultural groups have prescribed and proscribed behaviors to be performed when pregnancy does occur as well as during labor and delivery. Some authors have noted the relatively positive birth outcomes among immigrant women compared to other low-income women, suggesting that healthful behaviors arising out of cultural beliefs about pregnancy should be emulated by other groups (Guendelman, 1995).

Birth rituals, which occur in some form in all cultures, are intended to protect both mother and baby. This protection may be against natural events, such as the effects of exposure to cold, or against supernatural events. It has been noted that some of these rituals closely parallel activities in a modern obstetrical setting. For example, cultural practices of watching closely over mother and baby parallel the obstetrical nurse's monitoring of the mother for postpartum hemorrhage (Spector, 2000b). Selected cultural beliefs and behaviors related to the perinatal period are presented in Table 6–5 ■.

HEALTH AND ILLNESS   Health and illness are also life experiences common to all cultural groups. Cultural responses to health and illness vary widely, however. Some of the major areas of variation with which community health nurses should familiarize themselves are cultural definitions of health and illness and explanatory models of disease causation, as well as behaviors performed to promote health and prevent illness or restore health.

Perceptions of Health and Illness and Disease Causation
All cultures have concepts of health and illness and theories of disease causation, although these may differ widely from group to group.

It has been suggested that each culture has "explanatory models" of illness that define the etiology or cause of the illness, the time and characteristics of symptom onset, the pathophysiology involved, the course of the illness, and the appropriate treatment. When the client's explanatory model differs from that of the health care provider, conflicting expectations occur that may lead to noncompliance with recommendations and dissatisfaction with care (Allan, 1998). Nurses who wish to understand clients' conceptions of health and illness must investigate the explanatory models found in each client's culture.

Many cultural groups have multiple theories of disease causation that usually fall into three categories: (a) natural diseases, (b) occult diseases, and (c) behavioral diseases. Natural diseases are those that result from a physical cause, for example, exposure to cold, wind, dampness, and so on. Occult diseases are caused by purposeful malign interventions, either by another person or by evil spirits. Behavioral diseases are those that result from inappropriate behaviors—violation of either sound principles of healthful living or of the precepts of religion (e.g., sin).

Cultural groups also differ in the ways in which they define health and illness. Among Native Americans, for example, health is viewed in terms of the life cycle, which encompasses birth, life, and death. Health is the result of harmony and order between man and universe, congruence with other people, the environment, and supernatural forces (Spector, 2000b).

The Asian concept of health involves achieving a state of *Qi* (pronounced "chee"), which is a balance of Yin and Yang (Morris et al., 1999). An imbalance between *Yin* and *Yang* (or *Am* and *Duong* among Vietnamese) results in disharmony or illness. Most Asian cultures believe that all components of the universe, including humans, are

■ **TABLE 6–4**   Selected Beliefs and Behaviors Regarding Menstruation, Conception, and Contraception

FOCUS	BELIEF OR BEHAVIOR
General	The uterus is the center of female energy. (Hmong) Sexuality should not be discussed between men and woman. (Asian, Latino, Arab)
Menstruation	Menstrual cramping can be alleviated by avoiding hot spicy food. (Appalachian, Latino) Menstruation is a "hot" condition, so "cold" foods should be eaten. (Appalachian) Menstruation opens one to infection. (African American) Burning menstrual pads prevents them from being used to lay a hex. (African American) Avoid sex during menstruation and wear shoes to prevent poisons entering the body. (African American) A normal menstrual flow indicates health. Increased or decreased flow is not healthy. (African American) The presence of a menstruating woman pollutes the environment and endangers living things, especially strong males and vulnerable persons (e.g., infants). (African American) Exposure of an infant to a menstruating woman may cause an umbilical hernia. (African American, Latino)
Contraception	Herbal preparations can be used to prevent pregnancy. They may be given as teas, suppositories, or douches; applied topically; or inhaled. (Latino) Pregnancy should be prevented by abstinence. (Chinese, Filipino, Latino, Roman Catholic) Oral contraceptives cause birth defects and ill health for the mother. (Appalachian) Oral contraceptives cause decreased menstrual flow which is not healthy. (African American) Abortion can be caused by drinking ginger root tea, jumping from a height, or stepping over a rail fence. (Appalachian) A wife who asks her husband to use a condom marks herself as a prostitute. (Latino) Nine drops of turpentine taken nine days after intercourse will prevent conception. (Appalachian) Charms and ceremonies may prevent conception. (Native American) Contraception challenges the will of God. (Latino, Arab) An ice water and vinegar douche slows sperm and kills them (African American) Holding one's breath during orgasm, standing up immediately after intercourse, or holding one's nose and blowing forcefully through the mouth can expel semen from the vagina and prevent pregnancy. (African American)
Conception	Herbs can be used to "heat" the womb to promote conception. (Latino) The fertile period for a woman is a few hours of a "heat cycle" midway between menstrual periods. (Appalachian) The child's sex is determined by the side the mother turns to after intercourse. (Appalachian) The right ovary produces "girl seeds"; the left produces "boy seeds." (Appalachian) Pregnancy is more apt to occur during one's menses. (African American)[b] One cannot conceive until after the first menses following delivery. (African American)[b] Infertility may be perceived as failure to fulfill family role expectations (Chinese)[b]

[b] Potentially harmful beliefs or practices.

composed of a *Yin* and a *Yang*. The *Yin* is the negative female force, characterized by darkness, cold, and emptiness. The *Yang* is the positive male force producing light, warmth, and fullness. An overabundance of either *Yin* or *Yang* is thought to trigger illness. Other recognized causes of illness in some Asian cultures include soul loss or theft, spirit possession, breach of taboo, and object intrusion in which a magical foreign object enters the body. Similar causes of disease are also noted among some Native American tribes.

African Americans tend to classify illnesses as natural or unnatural. In traditional African American culture, all illnesses are thought to be curable, and the concept of chronic disease is difficult to accept (Gropper, 1996). The belief in a cure for every illness is derived from the principle that for everything, including disease, there exists its opposite. African Americans tend not to separate mental and physical illness.

In some Latino subgroups, illness is viewed as more than a mere biological occurrence and is seen in terms of its spiritual and social ramifications. Health is seen as balance among the social, spiritual, physical, and psychological aspects of life (Higgins & Learn, 1999). Illness, on the other hand, is defined in terms of limitation of activity and imbalance (Zapata & Shippee-Rice, 1999). Other examples of definitions of health arise from Russian culture, absence of symptoms (Ferran et al., 1999), and that of Greek Cypriots who define health as being able to do what you want without suffering (Papadopoulos, 1999). Selected cultural beliefs regarding disease causation are presented in Table 6–6 ■.

Promoting Health and Preventing Illness   In addition to culturally defined concepts of health and illness and disease causation, cultural groups differ widely in practices designed to promote health and prevent or cure illness. All of us employ such practices whether or not we identify them as cultural behaviors. In early America, such practices included use of patent medicines and a variety of home remedies. Some authors have commented

■ **TABLE 6–5**   **Selected Beliefs and Behaviors Regarding the Perinatal Period**

FOCUS	BELIEF OR BEHAVIOR
Pregnancy	Childbirth is a natural event. (Appalachian)[a]
	Children are a sign of a man's virility. (Latino)
	Wives should become pregnant as soon as possible after marriage. (Latino, Korean)
	A visible double pulse in the neck, dreaming of fish, or change in skin color indicates pregnancy. (African American)
	A pregnant woman is considered ill or weak. (Latino)
	Pregnancy is a time of danger for mother and child, but is not an illness. (Asian)
	Pregnant women should eat a balanced diet and avoid sweets and snacks. (Appalachian)[a]
	Pregnancy is a "hot" condition so meat should be avoided and sodium intake increased. (African American)[b]
	"Hot" foods including protein foods should be avoided in pregnancy. (Latino)[b]
	"Cold" foods (many vegetables) should be avoided in pregnancy. (Chinese)[b]
	Red meat should be avoided during pregnancy to prevent "high blood." (African American, Appalachian)[b]
	Iron in the prenatal diet causes hardening of the bones and a difficult labor. (Asian)[b]
	Milk during pregnancy may result in a large baby and a hard labor. (Latino)[b]
	Soy sauce and shellfish should be avoided during pregnancy. (Asian)
	Unclean foods should be avoided during pregnancy. (Asian)
	Cravings should be satisfied to prevent a defect related to the food craved. (Appalachian, Latino)
	Ginseng tea will strengthen the pregnant woman. (Asian)
	Strong emotions during pregnancy will leave a mark on the baby. (Appalachian, Latino)
	Fright or surprise during pregnancy can injure the baby. (Latino, Appalachian)
	A pregnant woman's workload should be reduced. (Native American)
	Pregnant women should avoid raising their arms or hanging laundry to prevent knots in the umbilical cord. (Latino)
	Sitting cross-legged will cause knots in the umbilical cord. (Latino)
	Bathing should be encouraged during pregnancy. (Latino)[a]
	Pregnant women should sleep on their backs. (Latino)
	Pregnant women should keep active. (Latino)[a]
	Nausea and vomiting can be treated with a mixture of flour and water, lemon and water, or chamomile tea. (Latino)
	Violent purging herbs can be used for constipation in pregnancy. (Latino)[b]
	Prenatal care and delivery by a woman is preferred. (Appalachian, Asian)
	Pregnant women should be accompanied to the doctor by husbands or female family members. (Latino)
	Periodic massage during pregnancy can help fix the uterus in the correct position for delivery. (Latino)
	Baby showers should be held close to the time of delivery to prevent envy and the "evil eye." (Latino)
	Planning for the baby prior to delivery defies God's will. (Arab)
	Sexual activity should be continued throughout pregnancy to keep the birth canal lubricated. (Latino)
Delivery	There is a correlation between the hour of conception and time of delivery. (Appalachian)
	Labor can be stimulated by the use of herbal preparations. (Latino)
	Tea made of winter fat leaves and roots will enhance contractions. (Hopi)
	Wrapping warm cloths around the mother's ankles will speed delivery. (Appalachian)
	The presence of the father or an article of his clothing will speed delivery. (Appalachian)
	The father or one of his relatives should deliver the child. (Hmong)
	Husbands should not be present during labor and delivery. (other Asian, Latino, Arab)
	Husbands should be present during delivery. (dominant United States)
	Children should be excluded from delivery. (dominant United States)
	Physical exertion will initiate labor in women who go over term. (European American)
	The pregnant woman's mother-in-law should attend her during delivery. (Chinese)
	Birth attendants should be female. (Native American)
	Changes in the moon's phase may trigger labor. (African American)
	The person who delivers and "breathes life into" the baby has a special bond with the baby. (Native American)
	Pain speeds delivery so pain relief is to be avoided. (African American)
	It is inappropriate to exhibit pain during labor. (Asian, many European Americans)
	Emotional expression is expected during labor. (Arab, Italian)
	Labor pains can be "cut" by placing a sharp implement under the bed. (Appalachian)
	Aspirin given for pain will thin the blood and cause increased bleeding. (Appalachian)[a]
	Recitation of certain biblical passages will stop hemorrhage. (Appalachian)
	Delivery should take place in a squatting position. (Asian)
	Delivery causes a loss of body heat that must be replaced. (Asian)
	Delivery is a "hot" condition, so no pork (a hot food) should be eaten afterward, also no penicillin, which is a hot medicine. (Latino)
	Delivery is a "cold" experience that may allow spirits to leave the body. (Hmong)
	Spinal anesthesia/epidural is dangerous. (Arab)

(continued)

■ **TABLE 6–5 Selected Beliefs and Behaviors Regarding the Perinatal Period** *(continued)*

FOCUS	BELIEF OR BEHAVIOR
Postpartum	Castor oil or paregoric should be given to the woman after delivery. (Appalachian)[b]
	Boiled cedar tea should be drunk to cleanse the mother after delivery. (Native American)
	Cleansing rituals including washing, incense, or burning sage may be used after delivery. (Native American)
	Fresh fruit and other "cold" foods should not be eaten after delivery. (Appalachian, Asian, Hmong, Mexican)
	Incompatible "hot" and "cold" foods should be avoided during hospitalization after delivery. (Arab)
	A postpartum diet should include chicken, soup, nonsticky rice, and special herbs to "wash out" the uterus. (Hmong)
	Warm or hot fluids should be drunk after delivery. (Hmong)
	Ginseng tea should be drunk after delivery to build the blood. (Chinese)
	Salads and sour foods cause postpartum incontinence. (Asian)
	Postpartum fluid intake should be decreased to prevent stretching the stomach. (Asian)[b]
	Beef and seafood cause itching at the episiotomy site. (Asian)
	Alcohol in rice wine causes bleeding. (Asian)
	Prolonged bed rest and avoidance of strenuous activity prevent complications after delivery. (Appalachian, Asian, Hmong, Chinese)[b]
	Bathing should be avoided after delivery. (Mexican)
	Outside visitors should be discouraged after delivery. (Korean)
	Strangers after delivery may steal the mother's milk. (Hmong)
	Postpartum pain can be relieved by whiskey or by hanging the husband's pants over the bedpost. (Appalachian)
	Herbal preparations can relieve afterpains. (Latino)
	Burning, burying, or salting the placenta will prevent harm to mother and child. (Appalachian, Hmong, African American)
	The placenta should be disposed of in the Rio Grande with a prayer ceremony. (southwestern Native American)
	Drinking cold water should be avoided after delivery. (Asian)
	No water should be drunk for four months after delivery; then water from the Rio Grande should be drunk. (southwestern Native American)
	Intercourse should be avoided two to three months after delivery to prevent disease. (Asian)
	Women are unclean after delivery due to nine months accumulation of menstrual blood during pregnancy. (African American)
Infant	Infants should not be fussed over or cuddled or evil spirits may steal them. (Vietnamese)
	A beautiful baby may provoke envy and the evil eye so praise should be given to the mother for her performance in delivery rather than to the baby. (Arab)
	Wearing of amulets and not mentioning the number 5 will protect against the evil eye. (Arab)
	Massage of the newborn by the mother promotes bonding. (Native American)[a]
	Infants do not join human society until the third day after birth. No funeral is held if death occurs prior to the third day. (Hmong)
	The Shaman invokes a soul to be reborn in the infant. The infant should be given a silver necklace to prevent the soul from wandering. (Hmong)
	The infant should not be named until it is brought home. (Vietnamese)
	An Indian name may be given at a traditional naming ceremony and a saint's name at baptism. (Native American)
	An infant's name may be given by an older relative or tribal leader. (Native American)
	An infant's name may be selected on the basis of his or her horoscope or personal characteristics. (Asian)
	Colostrum is "bad milk" and may make the infant ill; breast-feeding should not start until actual milk comes in. (Latino)
	Castor oil will seal the umbilical stump. (Appalachian)[b]
	A raisin on the umbilical stump will prevent air from entering the infant's body. (Latino)[b]
	Kohl should be put on the umbilical stump. (Arab)[b]
	Cob webs or animal manure will seal the cord stump. (African American)[b]
	A belly band on the infant will prevent umbilical hernia or protruberant umbilicus. (Latino)
	Infants should be given a purge or tonic (may contain lead). (Asian, African American)[b]
	A second stillbirth can be prevented by placing a dead infant face down in the coffin. (Appalachian)
	Infants should be warmly clothed and wrapped. (European American)
	Infants should not be cuddled too much to avoid spoiling them. (European American)
	Infants should be kept wrapped on a cradle board provided by the father. (Native American)[a]
	The child should be kept physically close to the mother for the first year. (Mexican)
	Breast-feeding may continue for several years. (Asian)
	Males do not do child care. (Middle Eastern)

[a] Beliefs or practices consistent with scientific health care.
[b] Potentially harmful beliefs or practices.

that "today's population medicine is, in a sense, commercial folk medicine" (Spector, 2000b, p. 28).

Generally speaking, the practices used to promote health and prevent illness are of two types: natural practices and magico-religious practices (Spector, 2000a). Natural practices include the ordinary ways that people attempt to stay well such as diet, exercise, safety precautions, and so on. Magico-religious practices include use of charms, religious or magical rituals, prayer, and other approaches to supplication or manipulation of supernatural powers.

■ **TABLE 6–6   Selected Cultural Beliefs Regarding Disease Causation**

FOCUS	BELIEF
General	Illness can result from either natural or supernatural causes. (Native American, Asian, Appalachian, African American, Latino, Vietnamese)
Natural illness	Illness can result from violation of a natural law. (Native American)
	Natural phenomena such as storms, lightning, and other disturbances may cause disease. (Native American)
	Germs may cause disease. (Appalachian, Vietnamese)
	Environmental hazards (e.g., bad air, water) may result in illness. (African American, Vietnamese, Mexican)
	Imbalance among person, nature, and God may cause illness. (Latino)
	Imbalance between "hot" and "cold" forces may cause illness. (Arab, Appalachian, Vietnamese, Puerto Rican, Mexican, Hmong, Chinese)
	Natural illnesses may result from insect bites, bruises, or injuries that cause fractures. (Zuni)
	Bad blood may cause disease. (African American, Hmong)
	Illness may be due to inharmonious relationships or inappropriate behavior by client, relatives, and/or neighbors. (Southeast Asian, Chinese, Native American, Mexican, African American)
	Natural diseases occur when one confronts the forces of nature without adequate protection. (African American)
	Poor health habits and bad hygiene may cause disease. (African American, Appalachian)
	Irregular bowel habits might bring on illness. (African American, Appalachian)
	"Nerves" can cause illnesses such as depression, gastrointestinal upset, weight loss, and headache. (Appalachian)
	Disease may result from dislocation of a body part. (Latino)
	Being deprived of certain foods may cause illness. (Saudi)
	Cutting one's hair may result in weakness or illness. (Native American)
	Fright may cause soul loss and illness. (Latino, Hmong)
	Exposure to cold weather may cause illness. (European American)
Supernatural illness	"Bad" illnesses are caused by the evil action of people or spirits. (Otomi)
	"Airs" or wandering ghosts of those who met violent ends may cause illness. (Otomi)
	Disease may result from spirit intrusion or object intrusion. (Otomi, Zuni, other Native American, Asian)
	Breach of taboo may result in disease. (Zuni, Asian)
	Germs must be activated by a sorcerer before they can cause disease. (Thai)
	Evil spirits cause disease. (Hmong, African American, Latino, Zuni, Navajo)
	Illness may be punishment for sins or a test of faith. (African American, Appalachian, Latino, Vietnamese)
	Soul loss may cause disease. (Hmong, Lao, Native American, Latino)
	Illness may be due to witchcraft. (African American, Latino, Asian, Appalachian, Vietnamese, Native American)
	Disease may result from exposure to an "evil eye." (Scot, Latino, Asian, Jewish, Italian, Iranian, Indian, Greek, Central American, Mediterranean, Middle Eastern, African American, Filipino)
	Illness may be the will of God. (Latino, Filipino, Muslim, African American, Appalachian)
	Having blood drawn may cause disease. (Hmong)

Knowledge of dietary practices is particularly important for community health nurses working with people from other cultural groups because of the pervasive influence of diet on health. The nurse will want to obtain information regarding the typical daily diet of group members as well as special uses of foods to promote health and prevent or cure illness.

Generally, cultural groups classify foods in five types of systems: food versus nonfood items, sacred versus profane foods, parallel foods, social foods, and foods used as medicine (Helman, 1994). What is considered food may vary considerably among cultural groups. For example, dogs and snails are considered delicacies by members of some cultures, but are repulsive to others. Sacred foods are those used for religious purposes (e.g., corn for many Native Americans or bread and wine for Christians). Profane foods are unclean and forbidden. For example, pork and pork products are forbidden to Jews and Muslims. Many cultures classify foods (and other substances such as medications) in a parallel system of "hot" and "cold," although cultures differ significantly in what is considered hot or cold. Social foods are those that signify relationships, gender, occupation, or group identity. For example, grandma's homemade fudge cake may be a family tradition on special social occasions. A great deal of symbolism is attached to food in every culture. Food can function as a focus of emotional association, a channel for interpersonal relationships, or as a means of communicating love, disapproval, or discrimination.

Methods of food preparation should also be assessed since these can affect the nutritional status of many foods.

For example, the rapid cooking of vegetables by many Asians helps to retain the vegetables' vitamin content, whereas overcooking by other groups causes loss of nutrients. Frying foods in animal fats, a common practice among many southern blacks, increases their cholesterol consumption and dietary fat content. Another area to be considered is meal patterns exhibited by group members. How many meals are eaten per day? Is caloric intake relatively evenly distributed among meals or are some meals more substantial than others?

As is the case with other culturally determined behavior, dietary practices vary with the extent to which an individual client has adopted the culture of the larger society. Pressures to change food practices arise from two sources: the environment and demands for acculturation. The environment affects the availability of particular food items as well as their suitability to the new environment. Demands for acculturation, or a desire not to be "different," can lead to either positive or negative changes in eating habits. For instance, the desire to fit Western cultural norms has led to decreased breast-feeding among Southeast Asian women, a negative result of acculturation.

Food items can also be used for preventive and therapeutic purposes by members of cultural groups. For example, ginseng preparations as well as other special foods may be given to pregnant Asian women to provide strength and prevent complications. African Americans, on the other hand, may avoid red meat to prevent "high blood." Among both Latinos and Asians, maintenance of a balance between "hot" and "cold" foods is used to prevent illness. Avoidance of specific items may also promote health or prevent illness. For example, both whites and African Americans in the southern United States may avoid consuming fish and milk in the same meal (Snow, 1998).

Another consideration in investigating behaviors that promote health or contribute to illness is use of tobacco, alcohol, and other substances. With the exception of the use of tobacco for religious purposes among Native Americans, much tobacco use among minority cultural groups is an adverse result of acculturation to Western cultural practices. Due to acculturation, use of tobacco is prevalent among Asian and Latino groups. Similarly, alcohol intake increases with acculturation in many cultural groups, particularly among Native Americans and Alaskan Natives. Many Asian cultural groups, on the other hand, use alcohol only moderately, if at all, possibly due to the high value placed on self-control. Among African Americans and Latinos, use of alcohol is considered part of the male adult image, but is proscribed among Muslim Arabs.

The use of herbal and other medicinal preparations is another common preventive strategy in a number of cultures. For example, many European Americans take large doses of vitamins C or E to prevent illness. Herbal teas are widely used among Native Americans and Asians as well as other cultural groups, although the herbs used may vary from one group to another.

Many cultural groups also use religious or magical amulets or charms to prevent disease or misfortune. For example, many European American and Latino Catholics wear medals of patron saints or the Virgin Mary. Similarly, Arab Americans may use amulets to ward off evil spirits or the evil eye (AbuGarbieh, 1998). Among some Native American tribes, a medicine bundle, or *gist*, is carried to ensure blessing. Charms and amulets are common among Asian cultural groups as well.

Cleansing is another health promotion strategy that may be employed either figuratively or literally. Sweat baths are used by several Native American tribes to remove impurities. Ritual cleansing is also employed by Muslim Arabs. African Americans and Appalachians, on the other hand, may engage in internal cleansing of impurities through the use of laxatives.

Some cultural groups also engage in measures designed to limit the transmission of communicable diseases. Interestingly, African American slaves practiced smallpox inoculation well before the acceptance of this practice in the larger society (Spector, 2000b). Similarly, some Native American tribes developed a number of precautions for communicable diseases without benefit of knowledge of pathogenic organisms. Some of these practices included isolation, burning or washing of contaminated articles, and burning of refuse. Meditation and massage are other primary prevention practices used in some cultural groups.

Protection from illness may also involve environmental measures related to the supernatural. For example, some African Americans will add red pepper and urine to soapy water used to scrub floors in order to protect a house against evil spirits. Others may believe that plants in a home protect against evil, since hexes and spells will cause plants to sicken first, giving warning to residents (Snow, 1998). Table 6–7 ■ presents examples of cultural practices related to health promotion and illness prevention.

Restoring Health   Approaches to restoring health when illness occurs generally take one of three forms: home remedies to restore physical health, procedures to restore mental health, and those to restore spiritual health (Spector, 2000b). Many similarities exist between cultures in such practices. Table 6–8 ■ includes selected cultural beliefs and practices related to diagnosis and treatment of illness.

Several diagnostic techniques are used in different cultures. For example, some Native American and Asian cultural groups use dreams as diagnostic tools. Seers or prophets within some Native American tribes may be responsible for interpreting dreams. Other types of Native American diagnosticians include the "hand trembler" and "crystal" or "star gazers" who identify the locale and cause of disease.

Asian medicine employs four diagnostic techniques: (a) glossoscopy, (b) osphretics, (c) anamnesis, and (d) sphygmopalpation (Spector, 2000b). *Glossoscopy* involves primarily inspection of the tongue; *osphretics* assesses sounds and odors. *Anamnesis*, or questioning, addresses

■ **TABLE 6–7** Selected Cultural Beliefs and Behaviors Related to Health Promotion and Illness Prevention

FOCUS	BELIEF OR BEHAVIOR
General	Moving in a clockwise direction in the home maintains balance with the environment. (Navajo)
	A variety of herbal preparations can be used to promote health and prevent illness. (Asian, Latino, African American, Native American, Appalachian, European American)
	Periodic purges keep the system open and prevent disease. (African American)
	Silver or copper bracelets worn by young girls warn of impending illness by turning the surrounding skin black. (African American)
	A *limpia* or cleansing ceremony may be used as a general preventive measure. (Otomi)
	Herbal remedies must be gathered at appropriate times to be effective. (Chinese, Appalachian)
	Avoid water after engaging in a "hot" activity. (Mexican)
	Sulfur and molasses rubbed on the back provides a spring tonic. (African American)
	Hanging garlic or onions in the home can prevent illness. (Native American)
	Burning refuse will prevent disease. (Native American)[a]
	Dressing warmly can prevent illness (European American)
	Red pepper and urine in scrub water can protect the home against evil. (African American)
Diet	Children, pregnant women, convalescents, and the elderly should avoid red meat to prevent "high blood." (African American, Appalachian)[b]
	Pork, cabbage, instant coffee, "store tea," fish with scales, round-hoofed animals, oysters, potatoes, plums, grapefruit, cherries, cranberries, graham crackers, salt, and saccharin lead to waste buildup and illness and should be avoided. (Appalachian)
	A balance of "hot" and "cold" foods should be eaten. (Asian, Latino, Appalachian, Arab)
	"Hot" foods include beef, pork, potatoes, and whiskey. "Cold" foods include chicken, fish, fruit, and beer. (Pakistani)
	Eating three meals, including breakfast, promotes health. (African American, dominant United States)
	Eating a 1,000-year-old egg can prevent illness. (Chinese)
Lifestyle	Excess in food, drink, and activity should be avoided. (African American)
	Keeping the body clean inside and out will prevent illness. (African American)
	Rest promotes health. (African American)
	Staying active promotes health. (Appalachian)
Prayer and magic	Carrying a printed prayer on one's person will prevent mishap. (African American, Appalachian)
	Prayer and veneration of the relics of saints can prevent illness. (Latino, and other Roman Catholic)
	Blessing throats on St. Blaise's feastday (Feb. 3) can prevent choking. (Latino and other Roman Catholic)
	Wearing garlic on one's person wards off evil spirits. (African American)
	Charms made of the fat of a person who died a violent death can scare away evil spirits. (Lao)
	Amulets, chains, and tattoos prevent spirit invasion. (Khmer)
	A string on the wrist or neck protects the infant from evil spirits. (Hmong)
	Charms and fetishes will ward off evil. (Native American)
	Wearing religious medals or displaying religious statues in the home can prevent misfortune. (Latino, and other Roman Catholic)
	Carrying or wearing a medicine bundle can prevent illness. (Native American)
	Placing a red ribbon on a child can prevent illness. (Mexican)
	Prevent evil spirits by wearing amulets in the hair or in a red bag pinned to clothing or hanging them over doors, on walls, or on curtains. (Chinese)
	Jade charms bring health. If the charm dulls or is broken, misfortune follows. (Chinese)
	Tying a string on an arm, leg, or around the neck controls spirits. (Vietnamese)
	A gold ring on a red ribbon around the neck will prevent anxiety. (Latino)
	Keeping a black animal will prevent witchcraft. (Mexican)
	Wearing coral around the neck or wrist will prevent depression and "evil eye." (Latino)
	Touching a child while admiring him or her will prevent evil eye. (Mexican)
	Moistening a finger with saliva and tracing a cross in a child's forehead can prevent evil eye. (Filipino)
	Charms can prevent the evil eye. (Mediterranean)
	Wearing copper or silver bracelets, necklaces, or anklets prevents soul loss by locking the soul into the body. (Hmong)
Specific prevention	Eating onions or baking soda will prevent "flu." (Appalachian)[b]
	Avoiding tomatoes will prevent cancer. (Appalachian)
	Immunization prevents smallpox. (ancient Chinese)[a]
	Asafetida, or rotten flesh, worn in a bag around the neck prevents communicable disease. (African American)
	Avoiding cutting infants' fingernails will prevent heart disease. (Asian, dominant United States)
	Nosebleeds can be prevented by not becoming overheated. (Latino)
	Prevent chills by not eating or drinking cold things when hot. (Latino)
	Not cutting ones hair will prevent loss of strength. (Native American)
	Avoid writing one's story to prevent loss of life spirit. (Native American)

(continued)

■ **TABLE 6–7   Selected Cultural Beliefs and Behaviors Related to Health Promotion and Illness Prevention (continued)**

FOCUS	BELIEF OR BEHAVIOR
Specific prevention *(continued)*	Isolation will prevent the spread of communicable diseases. (Native American)[a]
	Isolating ill persons will prevent their condition from becoming worse. (Native American)[a]
	Not going barefoot will prevent tonsillitis. (Latino)
	Chachayotel, a seed, tied around the waist will prevent arthritis. (Mexican)
	Cod liver oil prevents colds. (African American)
	Avoid sitting under a mango tree when hot to prevent kidney infection and back problems. (Puerto Rican)
	Avoid baby formula for infants because it causes rashes. (Puerto Rican)
	Avoid going into the coffee fields when hot to prevent respiratory illness. (Puerto Rican)
	Avoid drinking cold water when hot to prevent colds. (Puerto Rican)

[a] Belief or practice consistent with scientific health care.
[b] Potentially harmful belief or practice.

many of the same areas covered in a routine health history. In *sphygmopalpation,* the practitioner examines several pulses. One other diagnostic approach that may be used by some practitioners is *iridology,* or examination of various parts of the iris that reflect the condition of specific body parts (Holl, 1999). Some African Americans and traditional Appalachians may consult the signs of the zodiac in diagnosing illness.

Treatment modalities also vary among cultural groups, but certain categories of treatments are found among several groups. These include diet and herbal remedies, prayer and magical interventions, massage and other treatment techniques involving the skin, and sophisticated treatment systems such as acupuncture, acupressure, and reflexology.

Special foods are often used to treat illness. For example, chicken soup is used as a restorative in many cultures and jello water is often given to people with diarrhea. In many cultural groups, dietary interventions are used to restore the balance of "hot" and "cold" or Yin and Yang. "Hot" foods should be taken to treat "cold" illnesses and vice versa. What is considered hot or cold, however, may vary considerably from culture to culture. For example, fruits and vegetables are considered cold foods in some cultures, while many meats are considered hot foods.

A variety of herbal preparations and other medicinals are also used. For example, goldenrod tea is used for colds, sore throat, and cough among the Zuni, and sassafras for lung fever, ulcers, and gout among Appalachians. Ginseng is widely used among Asian cultural groups. Catnip tea or baking soda may be used by some African Americans and Native Americans to relieve babies of gas (Snow, 1998), and Georgia Sea Islanders may use moss in the shoes to treat hypertension (Blake, 1998).

Some medicinal preparations may have adverse health effects. For example, the relatively common practice in the dominant U.S. culture of taking baking soda for gastric upset may lead to electrolyte imbalance or mask the symptoms of myocardial infarction. Other folk remedies contain contaminants and toxic substances, frequently heavy metals such as lead, mercury, and arsenic. Similarly, a number of herbal medicines contain ephedrine and have been respon-

sible for approximately 500 adverse events since tracking of such occurrences was initiated in 1994 (Devine, 2000). Types of dangers posed by certain herbal remedies include:

*   Allergic reaction
*   Toxicity
*   Potentiation of desired effects (frequently in combination with prescription medications)
*   Mutagenesis
*   Drug interactions with prescription medications
*   Contamination with infectious organisms or toxic substances
*   Mistaken plant identity (inadvertent or purposeful to save on costs) (Ernst, 1998).

Potentially harmful folk remedies are presented in Table 6–9 ■.

Community health nurses should be aware that many cultural groups have different orientations to medication use. Many European Americans, for example, believe that there is a pill to cure every ill, others prefer not to take medications at all if they can possibly avoid doing so. Chinese clients may believe that one dose of an herbal preparation should cure the condition and are confused by multiple-dose therapies. Laotians, on the other hand, may take several doses of medication in the belief that if one is good, more is better.

Religious or magical rituals are frequently used in many cultures to treat illness. Among the Navajo, for example, "sings" are major healing rituals performed by a medicine man or singer, with different chants or songs used for different types of health problems. Religious treatment rituals are also used by many Roman Catholics as well as Protestants and Muslims, and magical treatments may be employed in several cultural groups. Among some African Americans, for example, remedies used may include reading Scripture, prayer, and sleeping with a Bible open to the Twenty-third Psalm under one's mattress (Snow, 1998).

A number of external treatments may also be employed. These may include techniques such as massage, cupping, pinching, coining, moxibustion, and the

■ **TABLE 6–8 Selected Cultural Beliefs and Practices Related to Diagnosis and Treatment of Illness**

FOCUS	BELIEF OR BEHAVIOR
Diagnosis	Diagnosis is by means of dreams, "hand tremblers," "star gazers," or "crystal gazers." (Native American)
	Diagnosis is made using techniques of inspection, listening, questioning, and palpation. (Chinese)
	Diagnosis of women should be made on the basis of pulses only. (Asian)
	Women may point to areas on an alabaster figure to indicate areas of complaint. (Chinese)
	Diagnosis is made by iridology, the condition of the iris. (Asian)
	Susceptibility to certain illnesses is determined by signs of the zodiac. (Appalachian)
General treatment	Exercise may be suggested as a remedy for illness. (Asian)[a]
	Herbal preparations are used to treat illness. (Asian, Native American, Latino, African American, Appalachian)
	Sweat baths may be used to treat illness. (Native American, Lao, Khmer)
	Massage may be used to treat illness. (Zuni, Otomi, Lao, Hmong, Chinese)
	Onions placed on the wall of a sickroom will absorb illness. (Appalachian)
	Signs of the zodiac should be consulted when planning surgery. (African American)
	Pressure on specific points on the foot (reflexology) may relieve illness. (Japanese)
	Medication should be discontinued when symptoms disappear. (Lao, other Asian, African American)
	Wounds should be covered to keep them clean. (Lao)[a]
	Medicines are usually prepared by boiling herbs in a prescribed amount of water and taking all of the preparation. (Chinese, other Asian)[b]
	Scientific medicines are considered "hot" and may not be taken for a "cold" illness. (Otomi, Asian)[b]
	Scientific medicines are considered very strong so clients may take only half the prescribed dose. (Vietnamese)[b]
	Everything has an opposite; every disease has a cure. (African American)
Diet	"Hot" foods should be taken to treat "cold" illnesses and "cold" foods taken to treat "hot" illnesses. (Asian, Latino, Appalachian)
	Treat "cold" illnesses like diarrhea and fever with "hot" foods like sweets, candies, and spices. Treat "hot" illnesses like pimples, boils, and skin problems with "cold" foods like vegetables and fruits and water. (Vietnamese)
	"Cold" foods used to treat "hot" illnesses include tropical fruit, dairy products, goat, fish, chicken, honey, cod, raisins, bottled milk, and barley water. "Hot" foods used to treat "cold" illnesses include chocolate, cheese, temperate-zone fruits, eggs, peas, onions, aromatic beverages, oils, beef, waterfowl, mutton, goat's milk, cereals, and chili peppers. (Mexican)
	Eating snake flesh improves vision. (Chinese)
	Use green vegetables and onions to treat respiratory disease. (Otomi)
	Use cooked onions to gain weight, raw onions to lose weight. (Otomi)
	Avoid spices, salt, and garlic when ill and eat plain food and soup. (Hmong)
	Treat constipation with vegetables, tea, honey, or prunes. (Chinese)[b]
	Karo syrup added to the bottle will help constipation in an infant (dominant United States)[b]
	Chicken soup stimulates recovery from illness (Jewish, dominant United States)
	Jello water or flat soft drinks should be given to persons with diarrhea (dominant United States)
Prayer and magic	Prayer may bring about cure of illness. (Latino, Native American, Filipino)
	Promises, visiting shrines, offering medals or candles, and prayer may help cure illness. (Mexican)
	Gather bark from the east side of a tree to appease the Gods (Native American) or for greater potency. (Appalachian)
	Use cornmeal in healing rituals. (Native American)
	Gist, or medicine bundles, are used in healing rituals. (Native American)
	Like cures like. (African American, Appalachian)
	Use invocations to spirits accompanied by rattle or drum in healing rituals. (Native American)
	Prayers and laying-on-of-hands may cure illness. (African American, Appalachian)
	Songs or chants amplify the forces of good in their battle with evil. (Otomi, other Native American)
	A *limpia*, or cleansing of evil, may be accomplished by passing an object over the body to pick up evil spirits. (Otomi, Latino)
	Recital of the Twenty-third Psalm, reading Scripture, prayer, and positive reminiscences may cure illness caused by a hex. (African American)
	A *baci* ceremony may be used to placate spirits causing illness. (Lao)
	Small spirit cures (chants) may be used for minor problems. For major problems, large spirit cures are required to release demons. (Hmong)
	After releasing evil spirits in a place away from home, a chant should be sung to prevent the spirits following the healer home (Hmong)
Herbal treatments	"Hot" herbs or medicines used for "cold" illnesses include ginger, garlic, cinnamon, anise, penicillin, tobacco, vitamins, iron, cod liver oil, castor oil, and aspirin. "Cold" herbs or medicines include orange flower water, linden, sage, milk of magnesia, and sodium bicarbonate. (Mexican)

(continued)

▥ **TABLE 6–8   Selected Cultural Beliefs and Practices Related to Diagnosis and Treatment of Illness** *(continued)*

FOCUS	BELIEF OR BEHAVIOR
Herbal treatments *(continued)*	Herbal teas may be used for fatigue, cold, sore throat, cough, chest ailments, and other conditions. (Appalachian)
	Sassafras is used for agues, lung fever, ulcers, stomach problems, skin conditions, sore eyes, catarrh, gout, dropsy, syphilis, and anemia (Appalachian) or for colds. (African American)
	Use goldenseal (an herb) for weak stomach, liver, or intestinal problems, hemorrhages, poor circulation, and "nerves". (Appalachian)
	Use ginseng for stomach and female problems, aging, sore eyes, asthma, poor appetite, rheumatism, longevity, and luck (Appalachian) or for anemia, colic, depression, indigestion, impotence, rheumatism, or as a sedative (cannot be prepared in any metal container). (Chinese)
	Any plant root or plant with a yellow cast can be used to treat jaundice. (Appalachian)
	A hot moist tea bag held in the mouth relieves canker sores. (European American)
	Oil of clove is good for a toothache. (European American)
	Whiskey rubbed on the gums will soothe a teething baby. (European American)[b]
	Honey and lemon are effective for sore throat. (dominant United States)
	Vicks Vaporub is useful for chest congestion and cough or stuffy nose. (dominant United States)[b]
	Use yellow root tea for sore throat, stomach upset, high blood pressure, canker sores, or tonic. (Appalachian)
	Treat diarrhea with boiled green persimmons. (Appalachian)
	Treat indigestion with chrysanthemum, crystal, ginseng, or other teas. (Chinese)
	Smoke jimson weed for asthma. (Appalachian)
	Use ginger to strengthen the heart and treat nausea and dyspepsia. (Asian)
	Grind up guava and put in the mouth to treat sores. (Otomi)
	Boiled banana peel or stems will stop heavy or prolonged menstrual bleeding. (Otomi)
	A tamarind bath can be used for the chronically fatigued child. (Otomi)
	Chopped garlic, onion, parsley, and water can be used as an expectorant. (African American)
	Onions applied to the feet wrapped in warm blankets will cure fever. (African American)
	Goldenrod tea is used for colds, sore throat, and cough. (Zuni)
	Thistle concoctions can be used for fever, gastrointestinal problems, or genitourinary infections (Zuni) or to treat worms. (Hopi)
	Blanket flower can be used to treat painful urination. (Hopi)
	A tea made from painted cup can be used for menstrual pain. (Hopi)
	Witch hazel or sweet flag is used for colds. (Oneida)
	Elderberry flowers can be used for diarrhea. (Oneida)
	Dried raspberry leaves can be used for mouth sores. (Oneida)
	Mustard plant can be used to treat headache or sunburn. (Zuni)
	Use sage to treat burns (Zuni) or on boils. (Hopi)
	Tansy and sage can be used to treat headache. (Oneida)
	Use a sunflower water bath for spider bites. (Hopi)
	Chew the root of a bladder pod plant and put it on a snake bite. (Hopi)
	Fleabane can be bound to the head or used in a tea for headache. (Hopi)
	Yucca stem can be used as a laxative.
	Raw potato soaked in vinegar may be placed on the forehead to treat headache. (Latino)
	Treat skin conditions with grated potato or tomato. (Latino)
	Oregano tea may be used for cough. (Latino)
	Earache is treated with a preparation of rue on cotton placed in the ear. (Latino)
	Hot tea or a dock (weedy plant) or saline gargle can be used to treat sore throat. (Latino) Or use comfrey. (Oneida)
	Fever may be treated with an enema of "malva leaves." (Latino)
	Chamomile tea (Latino) or garlic (Vietnamese) is good for high blood pressure.
	High blood pressure may be treated by eating pears, being tranquil, and eating garlic (to prevent stroke). (Latino)
	Put globe mallow on cuts and wounds. Chew the root for broken bones. (Hopi)
	Use cliff rose to wash wounds. (Hopi)
	Swab a baby's mouth with its own diaper to treat thrush (African American)[b]
External treatments	Coining is used to treat pain, colds, vomiting, and headache (Khmer); heatstroke, indigestion, and colic (Chinese); colds, flu, and wind entering the body. (Vietnamese)
	Pinching is used for headache and sore throat. (Vietnamese)
	Cupping is used to treat headache and bodyache by removing noxious elements (Khmer); to treat arthritis, abdominal pain, abscess, and stroke paralysis (Chinese); to treat joint or muscle pain. (Vietnamese, also some Europeans)
	Moxibustion is used to treat mumps, convulsions, and nosebleed, and during labor and delivery. (Chinese)
	Balms and medicated plasters can be applied to the skin for bone and muscle problems. (Vietnamese)
	Treat pain with acupuncture, acupressure, blowing in the ear, painting with a purple spot, pinching, cupping, or coining. (Asian)
	Acupuncture may also be used to treat any "hot" illness. (Chinese)

FOCUS	BELIEF OR BEHAVIOR
	Sweatbaths are useful for childbirth, opium withdrawal, mental disorder, and psychosomatic illness. (Lao) Warts can be removed with water from the rotted stump of a chestnut tree. (Appalachian)
Other treatments	Treat object intrusion with massage to draw the object up; then suck over the area. (Otomi, other Native American) Use "bluestone" powder in open wounds or for poison ivy. (African American) Use stale bread or sour milk or salt pork on lacerations. (African American) Use the skin from inside the shell of a raw egg for boils. (African American) Pinon sap is used to treat ulcers. (Zuni) Pinon gum may be used as an antiseptic and to keep air from wounds. (Zuni, Hopi, Navajo) Tape treated with camphor balm can be placed over the temples to treat headache. (Lao) Poultices may be used to treat heart pain (Otomi); inflammation. (African American) Deer antler strengthens bones, improves potency, and eliminates nightmares. (Chinese) Rhino horn can be used for pus boils and snakebite. (Chinese) Turtle shell can be used to stimulate the kidneys and cure gallstones. (Chinese) Seahorses can be used to treat gout. (Chinese) Use quicksilver (mercury) to treat venereal disease. (Chinese)[b] Dissolve certain tree insects in the mouth to treat sores or drink the juice of the insect. (Otomi) Take sugar and turpentine by mouth to treat worms. (African American) Purgatives should be used for "poison." (Otomi) Drink sugar and turpentine for worms; rub it for backache. (African American) Clay in a dark leaf can be wrapped around a sprained ankle. (African American) For stiff neck, place crossed pieces of silverware over the area. (African American) Fluid intake should be decreased with fever. (Khmer)[b] Anemia may be treated with blood pudding. (Latino) Greta or azarcon can be used to treat *empacho* (both have high lead content). (Latino)[b] Rattlesnake capsules may be used for a variety of chronic conditions. (Latino)[b] Use warmth to treat fever. (Japanese, other Asian, Latino, African American)

[a] Belief or practice consistent with scientific health care.
[b] Potentially harmful belief or practice.

use of poultices or rubs. Massage is widely used in Asian cultures and may be combined with medicinal preparations to improve its effectiveness. Similar healing through massage is performed by *sobadores* (Ferran et al., 1999).

Cupping involves burning an alcohol swab in a cup and placing the heated cup over a painful area to draw out noxious elements (Spector, 2000b). Pinching, believed to bring out wind (Frye, 1995), produces bruises or welts and is commonly done on the neck and over the bridge of the nose. Coining or rubbing is performed on lubricated skin with the edge of a coin or spoon and leaves ecchymotic strips in symmetrical rows. Moxibustion consists of the application of pulverized and heated wormwood or moxa plant over specific meridians or areas that indicate points of entry to channels leading into the body and may produce characteristic burn marks on the skin

(Spector, 2000b). Each of these treatment modalities is widely used in many Asian cultural groups and the resulting skin lesions are often mistaken for evidence of child abuse. The community health nurse working with Asian populations should be aware of these practices and their beneficial intent and should not view them as abuse.

Poultices are another externally applied treatment measure and may be used for a variety of conditions in different cultures. Sea Islanders off the coast of Georgia, for example, make a poultice of oil leaves to draw the pain from a sore limb (Blake, 1998). Cucumber poultices have been used in many cultures for removing freckles.

Acupuncture makes use of small needles inserted into specific points that control the flow of *Qi* along the body's meridians. Acupressure, a related Japanese technique, makes use of pressure rather than needles to stimulate

■ **TABLE 6–9 Potentially Harmful Alternative Remedies and Herbals**

REMEDY/HERBAL	USE	POTENTIAL HARMFUL EFFECT
Alarcon		May cause lead poisoning
Alfalfa	Nutritive, arthritis	Potentiates hormone therapy
Alkohl		May cause lead poisoning
Azarcon	*Empacho*	May cause lead poisoning
Bajiaolian		May cause liver toxicity
Bali goli		May cause lead poisoning
Bint al dhahab		Lead, antimony, or cadmium encephalitis

(continued)

■ **T A B L E   6 – 9**   **Potentially Harmful Alternative Remedies and Herbals** *(continued)*

REMEDY/HERBAL	USE	POTENTIAL HARMFUL EFFECT
Black cohosh	Diuretic, antidiarrheal, anti-inflammatory	Potentiates hormone therapy
Borage (star flower)	Melancholy, common cold, anti-inflammatory	Interferes with anticonvulsants
Chamomile	Stomach upset, sleep	Inhibits iron absorption; may cause allergic reaction
Chapparal	Bronchitis, cancer, skin disorders, pain	May lead to liver toxicity
Chromium		Affects blood glucose
Coral		May cause lead poisoning
Danshen	Cardiovascular problems	Leads to anticoagulation; decreases warfarin elimination
Deshi Dewa	Fertility drug	May cause lead poisoning
Devil's claw	Antiarthritic, appetite stimulant	Affects blood glucose
Dong quai	Gynecologic disorders	Potentiates hormone therapy
Echinacea	Immune stimulation	Use for more than eight weeks may lead to hepatotoxicity; interferes with immunosuppressants
"Eternal life tea"		Causes dermatitis
Evening primrose oil	Sedative, asthma, breast pain, multiple other uses	Interferes with anticonvulsants
Fenugreek	Constipation, anorexia, GI disorders	Affects blood glucose
Feverfew	Migraine, antipyretic	Use with nonsteroidal anti-inflammatory drugs (NSAIDs) may diminish effectiveness, allergic reaction in those allergic to ragweed, chamomile, yarrow Increases clotting time
Garlic	Reducing serum lipids Multiple other uses	Increases clotting time; affects blood glucose
Germander	Weight control, antiseptic	May lead to acute liver failure
Ginger	Prenatal nausea	Increases clotting time, may cause mutagenesis of *E. coli*; affects blood glucose
Ginko	Dementia	Increases clotting time; neurotoxic in seizure disorder; may combine with tricyclic antidepressants to lower seizure threshold
Ginseng	Multiple uses	Increases clotting time; may cause headache, tremors, and mania in combination with phenylzine sulfate; may cause hypertension, insomnia, vomiting, headache, epistaxis, and vaginal bleeding; may be addictive in combination with estrogens or corticosteroids; interferes with digoxin effects and monitoring; potentiates monoamine oxidase inhibitors (MAOIs), phenelzine; affects blood glucose
Gliasard		May cause lead poisoning
Goldenseal	Diuretic, anti-inflammatory, antispasmodic	May interfere with diuretics
Gossypol	Contraception, easing labor, menstrual difficulty	Inhibits sperm cells and interferes with implantation; may lead to irreversible hypokalemia; GI upset; inhibits iron absorption
Greta	*Empacho*	May cause lead poisoning
Gun powder	Worms	Toxicity
Hai gen fen (clamshell powder)		May cause lead poisoning
Hawthorn	Cariovascular problems	Interferes with digoxin effects and monitoring; Inhibits iron absorption
Horseradish	Edema, joint inflammation	May depress thyroid function
Jin Bu Huan	Pain, insomnia	May cause liver toxicity
Karela		Improves glucose tolerance, do not use with diabetics

REMEDY/HERBAL	USE	POTENTIAL HARMFUL EFFECT
Kava	Seizures, antipsychotic	In combination with benzodiazepam leads to coma; may also lead to Kawaism
Kelp	Iodine supplement, abortion, hypertension, anticoagulant	May interfere with thyroid replacement and lead to edema, may also pose dangers in combination with stimulants (amphetamines, ephedrine)
Kohl	Cosmetic	May cause lead poisoning
Kombucha "mushroom"		Causes dermatitis
Koo Sar or *Koo So* pills	Menstrual cramps	May cause lead poisoning
Kyushin		Interferes with digoxin effects and monitoring
Licorice	Peptic ulcer, cough	Interferes with digoxin effects and monitoring, interferes with spironolactone and may lead to hypertension; affects blood glucose; potentiates hormone therapy
Liga		May cause lead poisoning
Ma huang (ephedrine)	Diet pills, energy supplement	Adverse response/death; affects blood glucose
Nettle	Rheumatism, antispasmodic, hypertension, asthma	Inhibits iron absorption, affects blood glucose
Nutmeg	Worms, antiemetic, GI upset	Toxicity
Pay-loo-ah	Tonic	May cause lead poisoning
Pennyroyal	Abortion	Toxicity
Plantain	Dermatitis, diarrhea, cough, bulk laxative	Interferes with digoxin effects and monitoring; inhibits iron absorption
Red clover	Estrogen replacement, whooping cough	Potentiates hormone therapy
Rueda		May cause lead poisoning
Sage	Antispasmodic, diarrhea, dysmenorrhea, GI upset	Interferes with anticonvulsants; affects blood glucose
Saw palmetto	Benign prostatic hypertrophy (BPH)	Inhibits iron absorption; may have addictive effect in combination with estrogens and oral contraceptives
Shankapulshpi		Decreases phenytoin anticonvulsant activity
Shitake mushroom		Causes dermatitis
Skullcap	Anticonvulsant, lower cholesterol, spasticity	May lead to liver toxicity
Soy bean		Potentiates hormone therapy
St. John's wort	Depression, anxiety, and multiple other uses	Reduced effectiveness of HIV-protease inhibitors, cyclosporin; may lead to photo-sensitivity; may interact with MAOIs and ephedrine
Surma		May cause lead poisoning
Syo-saiko-to		May cause liver toxicity
Tannic acid	BPH	Inhibits iron absorption
Tobacco smoke	Blow in baby's face for gas	Secondhand smoke
Uzara root		Interferes with digoxin effects and monitoring
Valerian	Sedative, antispasmodic	Use with barbiturates or alcohol produces excessive sedation; inhibits iron absorption; may lead to liver toxicity
Vitamin E		Causes anticoagulation, discontinue prior to surgery
Wormwood	Sedative, antipyretic, worms	Interferes with anticonvulsants
Zinc	Immune stimulation	Interferes with immunosuppressants; in excess, depresses immune system

Sources: Bloch, A. S. (2000). Pushing the envelope of nutrition support: Complementary therapies. *Nutrition, 16,* 236–239; Devine, N. (2000). Dangerous combinations: Understanding the risks of mixing herbal products and drugs. *NurseWeek, 13*(8), 26; Ernst, E. (1998). Harmless herbs? A review of the recent literature. *American Journal of Medicine, 104,* 170–178; Fetrow, C. W., & Avila, J. R. (1999). *Professional's handbook of complementary and alternative medicines.* Springhouse, PA: Springhouse; Izzat, M. B., Yim, A. P. C., & El-Zufari, M. H. (1998). A taste of Chinese medicine. *Annals of Thoracic Surgery, 66,* 941–942; Miller, L. G. (1998). Herbal medicines: Selected clinical considerations focusing on known or potential drug–herb interactions. *Archives of Internal Medicine, 158,* 2200–2211; and National Institute for Occupational Safety and Health. (1999). Adult lead poisoning from an Asian Remedy for Menstrual Cramps—Connecticut, 1997. *Morbidity and Mortality Weekly Report, 48,* 27–29.

the flow of *Qi* (Phillips & Gill, 1995). Both acupressure and acupuncture have demonstrated effectiveness in treating a variety of conditions. Reflexology is another related technique in which certain points on the hand and foot are stimulated with pressure to achieve specific therapeutic effects in related parts of the body (Spector, 2000b).

Death   All cultural groups have beliefs and practices related to death and dying that may vary considerably from those of the community health nurse. Culture influences attitudes toward death and dying in a number of ways. One area of influence is the need for comfort experienced by the dying client. In those cultures in which death is seen as a normal part of life, there may be less need to comfort the dying and his or her family; conversely, in cultures in which death is feared, comfort may be needed and appreciated.

The community health nurse should assess whether those he or she is dealing with have a cultural belief in an afterlife. Some non-Western religions, including Hinduism, believe in reincarnation until the soul has achieved perfection and passes to Nirvana. Do religious beliefs regarding death and afterlife offer a source of comfort to clients and families or do they engender fear and anxiety?

Culture also influences the selection and perception of health care providers when death is imminent. People from some cultures, including a growing body of mainstream Americans, believe that death should occur at home and are, therefore, unlikely to seek medical care for a dying client for fear that he or she will be removed from the home and placed in a hospital to die. For many people, going to the hospital means that death is inevitable. For example, Asian, Native American, African American, and Appalachian clients may equate hospitalization with imminent death.

Care of the body following death, and funeral and burial practices, are also influenced by culture, as are expectations regarding grief and mourning and practices to be observed during this period. Mourning is a cultural expression of grief following death, and mourning practices may vary from group to group.

Finally, culture influences communication regarding death, particularly with respect to children and their knowledge of and participation in the rites that accompany a death. For example, for African Americans on the Sea Islands, preparation for death involves holding a "prewake" for several months before an anticipated death during which friends and family discuss the person's life and contributions to society (Blake, 1998). Appalachians are usually quite open in their communication about death, and Native American and Latino children help with the care of the dying family member and participate in funeral and grieving practices. Despite this participation, members of many cultural groups may resist telling the client or others regarding imminent death.

Similarly, some cultural groups may resist the discussion or use of advance directives for fear that such a discussion implies a belief that death is near and may cause the ill client to lose hope. For these groups, discussion of death is avoided. Use of advance directives may also be resisted in some cultures because of a perceived lack of need for them. For example, Japanese clients and African Americans traditionally rely on family members to make decisions and do not see the need of a legal document for them to do so (Okuno et al., 1999; Waters, 2000).

Other questions relate to who should attend the dying client. The eldest son of a Chinese client should be present with his dying parent, whereas in some Native American tribes, the maternal aunt is the more important figure. Members of other tribes believe that the spirit cannot leave the body until family members are present.

Nurses should be familiar with the death rites of specific cultural groups so they can assist the family through their time of grief. Should the nurse wash and prepare the body or is a family member responsible for this? Should personal belongings be left with the body or given to the family? The nurse should learn the answers to such questions when working with clients from other cultures. Death rites and presence of family members may violate institutional policies in some health care settings, and nurses may need to function as advocates for culturally competent care in these instances (*Minority Nurse*, 1998).

Members of many Native American tribes see the body as a "seed to be planted" and believe that the body must be disposed of in its entirety. Thus, family members may request amputated limbs to be kept until death and disposal of the body. They may also resist having an autopsy performed. In a similar view, some Native Americans may request the return of hair or nail clippings from hospitalized clients to prevent their use by witches. Disposal of the body can vary among tribes. For example, cremation is traditionally practiced by the Tlingit and Quechan tribes, whereas the Sioux place the dead on elevated platforms, and members of Pueblo tribes bury their dead. Among many tribes, such as the Navajo, the body is dressed in fine clothes and jewelry and wrapped in new blankets. The Tlingit fear to touch a dead body, so the client may be dressed in funeral clothes several days before death.

Mourning can be very emotional in some cultural groups and very subdued in others and may last for varying periods of time. For instance, following four days of mourning, the Cheyenne and Quechan cease grieving, as do members of some other tribes. In some tribes, the name of the deceased is never spoken again, and memory of the deceased is actively suppressed. Among Hmong clans, mourning may last until the following new year celebration (which usually occurs in late December), when the deceased is invited to participate in a "final release" ceremony that releases the soul for reincarnation (Mattison et al., 1994).

Clothing may assume special meanings in relationship to death. The clothing of a deceased Chinese person, for instance, is believed to contain evil spirits. Family members of hospitalized clients should be encouraged to take clothing home until the client is discharged. If the client should die, the family may be reluctant to accept the deceased's personal effects. Clothing is also used to symbolize mourning, and mourning garments are worn for varying lengths of time in different cultures. The color of mourning can also vary. For example, black is the color of mourning for many cultures, but among the Hmong and Vietnamese, white signifies mourning and black is worn for weddings and other celebrations.

Non-Anglo cultural groups often celebrate death in a way that is foreign to many U.S. nurses. Traditional American culture, on the other hand, is more likely to try to defy death. (*Minority Nurse*, 1998). In traditional African American culture, death is perceived as a passage from one realm of life to another. Funerals are generally occasions for celebration despite the grief of family members left behind. Some African Americans also practice passing a child over the dead body to carry away any illness the child may have. As is true in the larger society, funerals and wakes are seen as a psychosocial mechanism that facilitates grieving. Funerals for many Latinos are evidence of their deep religious belief in an afterlife. Among the Hmong, funerals are very elaborate functions that may last for several days and incorporate different major participants depending on the age and sex of the deceased (Mattison et al., 1994).

As we have seen, beliefs and behaviors regarding death and dying vary among different cultures. Table 6–10 ■ presents selected cultural behaviors related to death and dying.

■ TABLE 6–10   Selected Cultural Beliefs and Behaviors Regarding Death and Dying

FOCUS	BELIEF OR BEHAVIOR
General	Death is a normal part of life. (Native American, Asian) Death is passage from one realm of life to a better one. (African American, Appalachian) Death is passage into the next life. (Asian) No belief in an afterlife. (Native American) Flowers should not be given to the living because they are reserved for the dead. (Vietnamese) Visitation by a clergy member may be perceived as indicating imminent death. (Vietnamese)
Violent death	Violent death provokes stronger emotional outbursts than does a normal death. (African American) Violent death is punishment for misdeeds. (Lao) Violent death creates a ghost to wander forever. (Navajo, Cheyenne)
Suicide	Suicide should be concealed because of its shameful nature. (Latino, Filipino) Suicide may be used to restore family honor. (other Asian)
Time and place of death	Hospitalization means death is imminent. (African American, Asian, Native American, Appalachian) Death should occur at home. (Hmong, Vietnamese) Removal of life support should be postponed until an "auspicious" time.
Preparation and disposal of body	Touching a dead body may bring misfortune. (Navajo, Tlingit) Touching an animal struck by lightning can bring misfortune. (Navajo) Passing an ill child over a dead body may cure illness. (African American) Entire body must be disposed of together. Autopsy may be resisted. (Native American, Vietnamese) Bodies should be cremated. (Tlingit, Quechan) Bodies should be buried. (Pueblo tribes) Bodies should be exposed to air on a funeral platform. (Sioux) The dying person should be dressed in funeral clothes before death. (Tlingit) Family members should prepare the body for disposal. (Sioux) Bodies are prepared for burial by commercial mortuary. (Latino, European American) Bodies should be richly dressed and wrapped in new blankets. (Navajo) Clothing of a dead person may contain evil spirits. (Chinese) The hair of the dead person should be unraveled. (Navajo) The home of a dead person may contain evil spirits and should be sealed to prevent its future use. (Navajo) Touching articles belonging to a dead person may bring misfortune. (Navajo) The dead should be buried in family graveyards when possible. (Appalachian) Graveyards should be placed on hilltops to prevent the graves from being covered by water. (Appalachian)

(continued)

■ **TABLE 6–10** Selected Cultural Beliefs and Behaviors Regarding Death and Dying *(continued)*

FOCUS	BELIEF OR BEHAVIOR
Preparation and disposal of body *(continued)*	If a body is exhumed and reburied, the person will not go to heaven. (Appalachian) The body should be buried facing Mecca. (Arab) Organ donation is prohibited. (Arab)
Grief and mourning	Emotional grieving lasts 4 days, after which the name of the dead is never spoken. (Cheyenne, Quechan, Navajo) White should be worn during the mourning period. (Hmong) Black should be worn during the mourning period. (Latino, European American) Social activities should be restricted during the mourning period. (Latino) The dead should be included in rituals commemorating ancestors. (Vietnamese) Homage paid to ancestral spirits will prevent illness. (Hmong, Vietnamese) The funeral and wake are a time to rejoice for the dead and comfort the living. (African American) Funeral Mass is preceded by saying the Rosary. (Latino) The first Monday after death begins 9 days of evening prayer for the dead. (Latino) Funerals should be followed by food (European American, African American, Hmong) Condolences should be offered with a handshake and special phrases of consolation. (Arab) Bits of colored paper should be burned at the funeral to provide the deceased with money in the spirit world. (Hmong) Food and drink should be offered to the spirit of the deceased at the funeral. (Hmong) Gifts brought to the grieving family should include whiskey, a basket of lunch, and the liver of a pig or chicken. (Hmong)
Participation and knowledge	Dying clients should be protected from knowledge of impending death. (Latino, Chinese, Japanese, Arab, African American) Bad news should be mixed with an element of hope. (Hmong) Children should participate in the care of dying family members, funerals, and mourning. (Native American, Latino) The eldest son should be present at the death of a parent. (Chinese) Family members must be present for the spirit to leave the body. (Native American)

Health System Considerations

As noted earlier, members of all cultural groups engage in a variety of practices related to promoting and restoring health. Often, these activities take place in the home, but they may also be performed by or at the direction of folk practitioners who are part of the alternative health system. Community health nurses should become conversant with these practitioners as well as with the practices they employ for several reasons. When appropriate, the nurse may wish to refer individual clients to folk practitioners or invite practitioners to become part of the health team addressing the client's needs. At the population level, effective health program development may require the endorsement and cooperation of cultural providers of care. For example, incorporation of traditional African American midwives into prenatal care programs in the southern United States is viewed as one of the factors in successfully decreasing infant and maternal mortality rates (Smith, 1994).

In other circumstances, community health nurses may need to be aware of potentially harmful cultural health practices occurring in the community (e.g., the practice of FGM) and take steps to educate the public and folk health providers regarding the dangers involved. Knowledge of folk health systems will also help community health nurses incorporate traditional health practices into health care delivery programs or to explain these practices to other providers.

Alternative Health Systems

In addition to prescribed practices to promote and cure health, cultural groups also develop one or more social systems or "health cultures." These health cultures encompass the group's traditional ways of addressing health concerns (Snow, 1998). Scientific medicine or health care constitutes one health culture, and community health nurses would do well to recognize that this culture influences their beliefs, values, and behaviors in the same way that ethnic health cultures may influence members of the cultural group.

Health cultures or systems can be categorized into two general types: allopathic and homeopathic systems. The allopathic system involves conventional scientific health care and espouses a mind–body dualism in which the mind and body operate independently of each other. Homeopathic systems focus on balance among multiple facets of the person. Homeopathic systems can be further divided into alternative therapy systems, those not a part of one's own cultural heritage, and traditional or ethnocultural systems, which are derived from one's personal cultural tradition (Spector, 2000b). Ethnocultural systems are the focus of the discussion here, while alternative systems are addressed later in this chapter.

A variety of ethnocultural health systems have developed and flourished in different cultural groups, and one ethnic or cultural group may encompass more than a single system. For example, voodoo and shango are two systems found among some African Americans (Watson, 1998a). *Voodoo* is a syncretic religion based on a combination of African and French Catholic beliefs and is named for the Yoruban god Vodu. Magical powers possessed by Voodoo practitioners (primarily female priestesses) can be used to cause or cure disease, and belief in hexes and their removal by these practitioners is strong among some African Americans. Shango is similarly derived from African and Catholic beliefs but is symbolized by the Nigerian god of thunder and lightning. Practitioners of Shango specialize in healing illness and protection from evil (Watson, 1998a).

Ethnocultural health systems found among Latinos include *Santeria*, which is common in Cuba and Puerto Rico and may also be seen among some African Americans, and *curanderismo*, encountered most frequently among those of Mexican descent. *Santeria* is a combination of African and Cuban Catholic cultural heritages in which Nigerian gods or *orishas* have been associated with Roman Catholic saints as beings with healing powers. These *orishas*/saints come to practitioners and assist them with healing, but must be worshipped and propitiated by the practitioner (Grossman, 1998). *Curanderismo* is derived from both Spanish Catholicism and the practices of people indigenous to Mexico and deals primarily with natural illness (Purnell, 1998). In the southwestern United States, *curanderismo* has incorporated many African beliefs and values as well (Watson, 1998a).

Chinese medicine, which is the basis for many other Asian cultural health systems, is based on the concepts of *yin* and *yang*. When these two forces, which make up all living beings, are in balance, health results. Conversely, illness is the consequence of imbalance. Therapeutic practices in this system are designed to restore the balance of *yin* and *yang*. *Shamanism* is both religion and health system for Asian groups like the Hmong. The Hmong see the world as composed of two parts, one visible and the other invisible. Components of the invisible world include the souls of the living, spirits of the dead, caretaker spirits, and evil spirits among others. *Shamanism* is directed toward intervention with the spirit world on behalf of humankind and may involve propitiation or battle with spirits (Bankston, 1995).

Ayurveda is another cultural health system arising in India. Ayurveda employs diet, herbs, and other natural therapies to promote health and cure illness (Spector, 2000b). Many Native American tribes have well-developed cultural health systems as well. The Zuni, for example, have a system of medicine societies that incorporate 12 different specialist practitioners. Characteristics of selected cultural health systems are presented in Table 6–11 ■.

■ **TABLE 6–11 Health Systems Found in Some Cultural Groups**

CULTURAL GROUP	CULTURAL HEALTH SYSTEMS
African American	Faith healing: Divine intervention channeled through a healer, but based on the faith of practitioner and client. Herbalism: Use of herbs to promote health and prevent and cure disease. *Santeria:* Use of magical healing powers conferred by saints or orishas. *Shango:* Use of drums, herbs, and medications mixed with ghee (animal lard), palm oil, or nut oil to heal illness and ward off evil. *Voodoo:* Use of magical powers to cause or cure illness.
Amish	*Brauche* or *powwow:* Use of sympathetic manipulation to cure illness.
Appalachian	Faith healing: See above. Herbalism: See above.
Asian Indian	*Ayurveda:* Use of herbs, diet, natural therapies to promote and restore health.
Chinese	Chinese medicine: Based on maintenance of the balance between *yin* and *yang*.
Hmong	*Shamanism:* Health care based on abilities to manipulate the spirit world.
Latino	*Curanderismo:* Use of herbs, cleansings, and spiritual interventions to cure disease. *Espiritualism:* Use of prayer and religious rituals to cure diseases of magical origin. Herbalism: See above. Practiced by yerberos. *Santeria:* See above.
Roman Catholic	Charismatic healing: Healing based on faith in Divine intervention.
Vietnamese	Chinese medicine (*thuoc bac*): See above. *Thuoc nam:* Use of diet, herbs, hygiene, and other practices to maintain or regain balance between *am* and *duong*.

Alternative Health Practitioners

Every culture has its own alternative health practitioners. Alternative practitioners may come to their calling in several ways including inheritance, family position, birth portents, revelation, apprenticeship, and self-study. Healing skills are sometimes believed to be passed down in families from generation to generation. Among the Hmong, for example, healers may inherit a *neng*, or healing spirit from another clan member (Bankston, 1995). One's position within the family may also indicate special abilities, for instance, a seventh or ninth child or a child born after twins. In some cultures, the elderly are also considered to have special powers due to their closeness to death. Unusual occurrences during pregnancy or at birth, such as being born with a "caul" or amniotic membrane over the face, may also herald healing skills. Other alternative practitioners may be called in a dream or vision or after recovering from a life-threatening illness themselves. Others show an aptitude for healing and may be apprenticed to an experienced healer (Snow, 1998). Finally, some alternative practitioners learn their calling on their own due to personal interest.

There is wide variation in the types of alternative healers found in different cultural groups, from the family member or friend with expertise in dealing with illness to the specialist practitioner. Many people first seek advice on health from these knowledgeable family members or friends before seeking more professional assistance. These family members and friends practice what may be called "domestic medicine" (Zapata & Shippee-Rice, 1999). In less serious illnesses, for example, Hmong family members may act as "soul callers" to recall the wandering soul of the ill person. For more serious illness, however, the professional skills of a *shaman* are sought (Bankston, 1995).

Professional assistance may be sought from a variety of different practitioners depending on one's cultural background. There is also a growing tendency among the general public to seek health care from providers of other cultural groups. Many clients with AIDS, for example, are seeking relief of symptoms through acupuncture, and the use of chiropractic services for back pain is also increasing. In fact, some health insurance plans are even beginning to cover some more traditional alternative healing practices, and there is a growing body of scientific research attesting to the efficacy of many traditional forms of healing.

Some cultural groups include a wide array of health providers, many of them highly specialized. Zuni healers, for example, are divided into 12 highly secret medicine societies, each of which specializes in the treatment of specific conditions (Hultkrantz, 1992). Navajo healers or singers may also specialize in the kinds of songs they are qualified to perform. Asian practitioners are often divided into the categories recognized in Chinese medicine including acupuncturists and herbalists. Herbalists are also found among African American, Latino, and Appalachian cultural groups.

Religious healers, faith healers, or spiritualists are found among many cultural groups, including Asians, Latinos, African Americans, and Appalachians. Religion as a source of healing is common, and prayer and other religious rituals may accompany more scientific forms of healing for many of us. The charismatic healing tradition of the Roman Catholic Church is another example of the use of religious practices in healing. Other cultural groups embrace the practice of psychic healers (Cavender, 1996) thought to possess healing energy that can be transmitted to others, usually by some form of touch. Belief in this transfer of energy underlies the practice of therapeutic touch as a nursing intervention.

Practitioners of healing magic may also be found in a number of cultural groups. For example, the *abolarios* in the Latino alternative health tradition of *curanderismo* specialize in the treatment of illness due to witchcraft (Weaver, 1994). Two levels of healers exist among the Hmong, *shamans* of the red veil and those of the black veil. Red-veiled shamans have a higher bridge to the spirit world and have better access than black-veiled shamans. The two shamanist groups also differ slightly in their practices, with red-veiled shamans standing on a bench to effect their cures (Mattison et al., 1994). The voodoo priest or priestess found among some African American groups is another example of magic used in healing. Other African American practitioners with powers to heal unnatural illness include spiritualists (Snow, 1998).

A number of specialty healers may also be found among some African American groups. For example, "blood stoppers" have the power to stop bleeding by reciting magical verses, while a "fire drawer" removes the pain of a burn by drawing the fire away or blowing on the burn three times and reciting a verse. Another African American practitioner that originated in German alternative health systems is the "wart talker" (Snow, 1998.)

Another group of health practitioners found in many cultures specializes in massage and is exemplified by the *sabador* in some Latino cultures. Also in some Latino cultures, *hueseros* or bone therapists care for injuries to bones (Ferran et al., 1999). Finally, many cultural groups include midwives as recognized health practitioners. In fact, midwifery as a specialized practice is a growing phenomenon in nursing that is gaining in popularity throughout the United States.

In assessing any cultural group, the nurse explores several areas related to alternative health practitioners. Among these are the types of practitioners recognized by the group, the health-related services provided, and the methods employed. Who and where are the practitioners? Is there a recognized hierarchy among practitioners? Who uses the alternative practitioner and what is the prevailing attitude of community members toward alternative practitioners? Finally, the nurse explores the expectations involved in the client–practitioner relationship.

Nurses should also be alert to the potential for chicanery. Most alternative healers are sincere and legitimate practitioners of their arts. Others, however, may exploit illness for personal gain (Watson, 1998c). This same dichotomy between legitimate and exploitive healers may also be found among practitioners of scientific medicine.

Recognized Folk Illnesses

Another significant area of difference in alternative and scientific health care systems lies in the types of health problems that are recognized. Many cultural groups recognize recurrent patterns of behavior or symptoms that lie outside the conventional diagnostic system of scientific medicine. These culturally recognized illnesses are referred to as **culture-bound syndromes** (Ng, 1999). They are often unique to a given culture, although similar conditions may be seen in several cultural groups. Culture-bound syndromes are also noted in the dominant American culture. For example, anorexia nervosa is a recognized illness in Western cultures that is not seen in many other cultural groups (Flaskerud, 2000).

African American and Appalachian alternative medicine systems recognize a number of similar conditions related to the character of the blood. Among these are high blood, low blood, thin blood, bad blood, and poison blood. Hypertension, a diagnosis recognized in scientific medical circles, may signify nervousness or hyperactivity to some African Americans (Snow, 1998). Some of the recognized alternative illnesses among Latino cultural groups include *susto, empacho, caida de mollera, mal de ojo* (evil eye), *mal puesta, serena,* and *coraje.* Belief in the evil eye as a cause of illness is fairly widespread and may be encountered among people of Jewish, Italian, German, Greek, Arab, Asian, and Filipino origin among others (Geissler, 1994; Spector, 2000b). Other culture-bound syndromes found in Latino cultures include *mal de cerebro ode la mente,* and *ataque de nervios.*

Culture-bound syndromes can be found among some Asian groups as well. *Toa* is a culture-bound syndrome experienced by Khmer women after childbirth and is a condition of extreme cold that causes physical collapse and death if not treated. *Hwa Byung, latah, koro,* and *amok* are other Asian culture-bound syndromes that result in psychiatric rather than physical symptoms (Kwan, 1999; Ng, 1999). These and other culture-bound syndromes are described in Table 6–12 ■.

■ **TABLE 6–12** Selected Examples of Culture-Bound Syndromes

CONDITION	CULTURAL GROUPS	DESCRIPTION
High blood	African American, Appalachian	An excess of blood in the body or too much blood high in the body (not related to hypertension), or excessive sweetness in the blood
Low blood	African American, Appalachian	Too little blood (comparable to anemia), or excessive bitterness in the blood
Thin blood	African American, Appalachian	Increased susceptibility to illness
Bad blood	African American, Appalachian	Sexually transmitted disease acquired through sexual promiscuity (not necessarily related to bacterial or viral infection) or contaminated blood due to disvalued behavior
Poison blood	African American, Appalachian	Septicemia or illness due to witchcraft
Susto	Latino	Magical fright resulting in soul loss
Empacho	Latino	Adherence of a bolus of food to the walls of stomach or intestine
Caida de mollera	Latino	A depressed fontanel resulting from an infant being bounced too vigorously or having a nipple suddenly or forcefully withdrawn from the mouth
Mal de ojo (evil eye)	Latino, Arab, Asian, Italian, Greek, Scottish, German, Jewish, Filipino	Disease caused by someone with the evil eye looking at, admiring, or envying the victim (may not be intentional)
Mal de cerebro ode la mente	Latino	Bad in the brain
Mal puesta	Latino	Unusual behavior caused by magic, voodoo
Ataque de nervios or *Ataque*	Latino, Puerto Rican, Mediterranean Carribean	An attack of nerves, hyperkinetic activity, aggression, or stupor due to tension, stress, grief, uncontrollable shouting, crying, trembling, and heat in the chest
Bilis, colera, or *muina*	Latino	Rage resulting in tension, headache, trembling, screaming
Serena	Latino	Upper respiratory symptoms caused by dampness, draft, or evil spirits
Coraje (rage)	Latino	Hyperactivity, screaming, or crying due to an extreme emotional reaction
Espanto	Latino	Severe fright caused by witnessing supernatural beings or events
Pujos	Latino	Umbilical protrusion and grunting in an infant exposed to a menstruating woman

(continued)

■ **TABLE 6–12**   **Selected Examples of Culture-Bound Syndromes** (*continued*)

CONDITION	CULTURAL GROUPS	DESCRIPTION
Locura	Latino	Psychosis due to inherited vulnerability, incoherence, agitation, hallucinations, possible violence
Pasmo	Puerto Rican	Paralysis due to an imbalance of hot and cold forces
Toa	Khmer	Extreme cold after childbirth leading to physical collapse
Koucharang	Cambodian	Preoccupation with distressing thoughts and memories due to "thinking too much"
Latah	Siberian, Thai, Japanese, Filipino	Trancelike behavior due to hypersensitivity to sudden fear
Koro or Suk-yeong	Chinese, Assam, Thai, East Asian	Intense anxiety over genitals retracting into the body and causing death
Amok	Malaysian, other Asian	Isolation and withdrawal followed by violence and aggression
Dhat or *Shen-kuei*	Indian, Sri Lankan, Chinese, Taiwanese	Anxiety and hypochondria associated with discharge of semen, whitish urine, weakness and exhaustion
Hwa-Byung	Korean	Anger or fire illness with epigastric pain due to a mass in the throat or upper abdomen
Shin-Byung	Korean	Anxiety and dissociation, somatic complaints due to possession by ancestral spirits
Taijin kyofusho	Japanese	Intense fear that bodily parts or functions displease or anger others
Qi-gong	Chinese	Psychotic reaction after practicing "exercise of vital energy" (time-limited)
Brain fag	West African	Brain fatigue resulting in poor memory, concentration, pain/pressure in the head, blurred vision, and feeling of "worms" in the head due to the stress of school
Falling out	Southern African American, Bahamian, Haitian	Sudden collapse, loss of vision with eyes open, inability to move, dizziness
Boufee delirante	East African, Haitian	Agitated aggressive behavior and confusion
Zar	North African, Middle Eastern	Spirit possession causing shouting, laughing, head banging
Ghost sickness	Native American	Preoccupation with death, bad dreams, fear, fainting, appetite loss, hallucinations
Pibloktoq	Eskimo	Physical and verbal violence followed by convulsions and coma

⑥THINK ABOUT IT

Why is it important to assess the degree to which a particular client conforms to the norms of his or her cultural group?

Alternative Therapies

The use of alternative therapies is not unique to ethnic cultural groups, and their use has been increasing in various segments of the U.S. population in recent years. However, because many alternative therapies originated in cultural health systems, they will be addressed here. *Alternative therapies* are those that do not fit the standards of practice in the scientific medical community and are not generally available in the professional health care system (Spector, 2000b). Approximately one in three Americans use some form of alternative therapy, and use is higher among persons with chronic diseases (Fetrow & Avila, 1999). There are several reasons why people choose alternative therapies over or in addition to scientific medicine. These include a fear of harm or intrusion due to more invasive scientific therapies, desires to use "natural" substances, and easier access and lower cost in many instances. Additional reasons include lack of success of medical treatment and disinterest of the medical community in some conditions (Donley, 1998).

The National Center for Complementary and Alternative Medicine in the National Institutes for Health has classified alternative therapies into several types:

- Mind/body interventions that are aimed at controlling physiologic function through mental activity such as meditation, yoga, and imagery
- Alternative practice systems such as acupuncture, ayurveda, homeopathy, and naturopathic medicine
- Manual healing techniques such as acupressure, massage, chiropractic, and reflexology
- Herbal medicine

- Diet, nutrition, and lifestyle change
- Bioelectromagnetic applications such as magnetoresonance, electroacupuncture, and use of electromagnetic fields
- Pharmacologic and biologic treatments such as chelation and cell treatment (Wolfe, 1999)

Many alternative therapies have been shown to have positive health effects, and research supports use of some treatments in some conditions. For example, acupuncture has been shown to be effective in the control of chronic pain. Many herbal remedies also have demonstrated therapeutic effects. In fact, nearly 25% of conventional drugs are plant derivatives (Fetrow & Avila, 1999). Some alternative therapies, however, particularly herbal med-

ications and other ingested substances, pose potential dangers. Some of the possible problems include toxicity related either to the components themselves or to the manufacturing process, improper use, and delay in obtaining needed medical care. Some over-the-counter remedies, such as laxatives and those with high alcohol content, also have the potential for addiction or abuse (Primm, 1998).

Community health nurses working with clients using alternative therapies should encourage them to disclose this use to their health care providers. Nurses should also educate clients regarding the benefits and risks of alternative therapies, the interactions of medicinal substances with prescription drugs, and product quality, as well as monitor clients for adverse effects.

assessment tips assessment tips assessment tips

ASSESSING CULTURAL INFLUENCES ON HEALTH

Biological Factors

- What is the age composition of the cultural group? What attitudes toward age and aging are prevalent in the culture? At what age are members of the culture considered adults? Are there cultural rituals associated with coming of age?

- Do members of the cultural group display genetically determined physical features or physiologic differences? Do group members display differences in normal physiologic values (e.g., hematocrit, height)? What genetically determined illnesses, if any, are prevalent in the cultural group?

- What are the cultural attitudes to body parts and physiologic functions?

Psychosocial Considerations

Relationships

- What are the attitudes of members of the group toward the environment? Do environmental hazards hold particular risk for members of the cultural group (e.g., potential for pesticide exposure)?

- What is the typical family structure within the culture? What roles are typically performed by family members? How interchangeable are these roles? How congruent are family roles with those of the dominant culture? What are the attitudes of group members toward children? What childrearing practices are typical of the cultural group?

- What is the typical social organization of the group? Are group or individual goals given priority? Who has influence in the social group? How is that influence exercised? What are group members' attitudes toward authority? What is the cul-

tural group's attitude toward change? What is the character of interaction between the cultural group and the dominant society?

- What is the primary language spoken by members of the culture? How important is context to communication? Are there formal and informal modes of address within the cultural group? In what circumstances is each used? Is a certain degree of personal reticence expected by group members? What courtesy titles are used and for whom? What gestures are considered appropriate or inappropriate?

- What behaviors are expected in interactions with others? What behaviors are considered unacceptable by members of the cultural group?

- What is the typical religious affiliation of group members, if any? Does religion influence health? If so, how is this influence exerted? Are religious leaders or groups involved in health care? What is the effect of religious sponsorship on use of health services? Are religious beliefs and practices incorporated in health care? Do members of the group express belief in magical causes or treatments for illness?

Life Events
Sexuality and Reproduction

- What are the attitudes of members of the cultural group toward heterosexual activity? Homosexual activity? Do group members engage in any specific sexual practices? Do group members practice female genital mutilation?

- What are the attitudes of members of the cultural group toward conception and contraception? Is conception expected early in marriage? Are there special cultural practices to promote or prevent conception?

- Are there certain behaviors expected during pregnancy? Are there behaviors or circumstances that should be avoided during pregnancy? What is the attitude of group members toward prenatal care?

- Are there special cultural practices related to labor and delivery? Who should be present during labor and delivery? Where should labor and delivery occur? Are there special practices related to disposal of the placenta? What behaviors are expected of the mother during the postpartum period? What does cultural care of the newborn entail? Who provides this care? What are the cultural attitudes toward breast-feeding?

Health and Illness

- How do members of the cultural group define health and illness?

- Do group members hold specific theories of disease causation?

- What cultural health practices are used to promote health and prevent illness? What health practices are used to restore health when illness occurs? To what extent are these practices used by the population group? Are any of the cultural practices used by group members potentially harmful?

Death and Dying

- What are the attitudes of the cultural group toward death? Do group members believe in an afterlife?

- Is death a topic discussed by members of the cultural group? By whom? Do group members wish to be informed of terminal illness? What is the group's attitude toward advance directives?

- Where should death occur? Who should be present at the time of a family member's death? Who should be involved in preparation of the body after death? What is the typical mode of disposal of the body after death?

- Are there special practices related to grief and mourning in the culture? Who should participate in rituals and practices related to death?

Health System Considerations

- What alternative health systems are operant within the culture? What are the characteristic aspects of those systems?

- Are there specific culture-bound syndromes recognized by the group? How are they manifested? What approaches are used to resolve these problems?

- Are there recognized alternative practitioners within the cultural group? How do they learn their craft? What health-promotive, diagnostic, and treatment measures do they employ? To what extent do members of the group use the services of alternative health providers?

- What is the relationship of alternative and scientific health care systems within the cultural group? What is the attitude of practitioners within each system to those of the other system? To what extent do group members use both systems? What are their reasons for using one system or another? What are the health implications of use of both systems?

PLANNING CULTURALLY COMPETENT CARE AND CARE DELIVERY SYSTEMS

Three strategies assist community health nurses in planning culturally competent care for other cultural groups. These include incorporating cultural beliefs and practices in care whenever possible, promoting interaction between the alternative and scientific health care systems, and assisting clients with cultural adaptation as needed.

Incorporating Cultural Beliefs and Practices

Community health nurses can incorporate cultural beliefs and practices into the care of individual clients and families. For example, a diabetic diet can be designed to incorporate desired ethnic foods and eating patterns as much as possible. Similarly, the nurse can determine the extent of desired family involvement in client care and include culturally designated family members as caregivers. Nurses

can also demonstrate an attitude of acceptance of cultural health practices and actively encourage these if they are not harmful to clients. For instance, nurses may incorporate alternative healers into the plan of care, encouraging the *curandero*, medicine man, or elderly female practitioner to attend the client at home or in the health care facility. A nurse may choose to participate in healing rituals if comfortable with this role and if the client has grown to accept and trust the nurse. When appropriate, the nurse may make referrals to an alternative healer in place of or in conjunction with the usual plan of care. This may be warranted particularly when the client considers his or her condition to be the result of magical intervention.

Community health nurses can also incorporate cultural elements into health care systems designed to provide care to culturally diverse clients. For example, in working with cultures with differing perceptions of time, health services may be designed on a walk-in, rather than an appointment, basis.

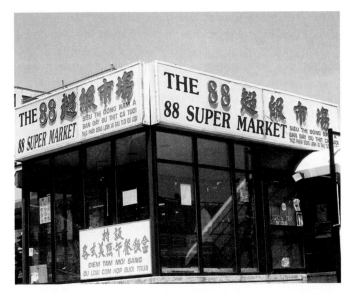
Ethnic markets support cultural food preferences.

Use of health promoters or community outreach workers from the specific cultural group can also enhance provision of culturally sensitive care (Poss, 1999). These individuals can help bridge the gap between clients and the scientific health care system as well as assist health care professionals to design culturally relevant health care delivery systems. Cultural outreach workers can also motivate use of services more effectively than media campaigns, since many cultural groups rely more heavily on recommendations by persons known to them than on media information (Watson, 1998c).

Promoting Interaction Between Alternative and Scientific Health Care Systems

Community health nurses can also be actively involved in promoting interactions between alternative and scientific health care systems. At the level of the individual client or family, this may involve encouraging clients to make providers aware of their use of both systems and alerting both alternative and scientific practitioners to their use of alternative and conventional therapies. Another strategy in this area is to make referrals to alternative health care providers and to establish relationships in which they make referrals to scientific providers when needed. Implementation of this strategy will require development of trust and rapport based on acceptance of other providers and their approaches to health care.

At the population level, nurses can examine the extent of current interaction between alternative and scientific health care systems and practitioners. Large segments of the U.S. population use both systems, often without making the practitioner of either aware of the overlapping practice arena. Clients often have different reasons for using different practitioners. For example, they may see scientific practitioners for physical healing and alternative practitioners for emotional or spiritual healing (Watson, 1998b). The basis for this differential use of alternative or scientific practitioners lies in basic differences between the two systems.

Alternative and scientific practitioners differ in their theories of illness as well as in their approach to the client. For example, even when personally religious, scientific practitioners usually divorce their religious beliefs from their practice, whereas alternative practitioners frequently incorporate spiritual aspects into their interventions (Snow, 1998). In addition, causation may be perceived to be upward in the scientific system, with mental activity derived from brain chemistry, and downward in alternative systems, with thoughts and emotions affecting physiologic function (Wolfe, 1999). Health professionals address decisions regarding therapeutic intervention on the basis of medical and health effects. Alternative practitioners, on the other hand, consider the effects of intervention on social priorities and the client's life as well as on health (Langer, 1999).

There are several other differences between alternative and scientific health care systems. Scientific care tends to be standardized by diagnostic category, whereas alternative system care is individualized. The former is physician centered and the latter is client centered. The expectation of client participation in therapy also varies between the two systems. In the scientific system, clients are expected to be receptive and passive; in the alternative system, they are viewed as having a primary responsibility for their own healing.

Practitioners in both systems utilize various healing substances and medications; however, their purpose is somewhat different. For example, scientific practitioners use substances to ward off pathogens, whereas alternative practitioners use them to enhance the body's natural healing processes. Similarly, scientific practitioners focus on symptom suppression, whereas alternative practitioners view symptoms as manifestations of an underlying imbalance and gear therapy to restoring balance. Scientific practitioners also tend to employ multiple pharmacologic agents, while alternative practitioners rely more heavily on diet, rest, and exercise in curing illness (Wolfe, 1999).

Scientific medicine makes a definite distinction between mental and physical illness, whereas many folk health systems do not. Alternative medicine is community oriented, whereas scientific medicine is more oriented to the individual client. Alternative medicine also tends to take place in familiar surroundings, whereas care in the scientific system is frequently provided in a distinctly foreign environment.

Other differences have also been noted between alternative and professional health care systems. Alternative health care is primarily humanistic, whereas scientific care is impersonal. Emphasis is placed on familiar, practical, and concrete facts in the alternative system and on unfamiliar and more abstract concepts in the scientific system. The alternative system is holistic in its orientation; the scientific system tends to be more fragmented. Generally speaking, the focus is on *caring* in the alternative system and on *curing* in the scientific system. The alternative system stresses prevention of illness; the scientific system emphasizes diagnosis and treatment. There is also less emphasis on cultural support systems in the scientific system than in the alternative system.

Finally, scientific and alternative practitioners differ greatly in their fees, with alternative practitioners providing free or low-cost care rather than the high-priced care of scientific providers. For example, Hmong healers usually accept only enough payment to "keep the healer's spirit happy" and may often accept only half of what is offered by the client (Mattison et al., 1994).

There are also similarities in alternative and scientific health care systems. Both employ similar diagnostic skills such as listening and observation, and both make use of verbal and nonverbal communication skills. As noted earlier, both systems use medicinal substances, and both engage in some forms of laying on of hands or massage. Finally, both the alternative and scientific systems are based on an unequal relationship in which one party is an expert and one is a layperson. Differences and similarities between alternative and scientific health care systems are summarized in Table 6–13 ■.

Once community health nurses have an idea of the differences between alternative and scientific health care systems, the extent to which each is used by members of the population, and the reasons why each may be used, they can engage in activities designed to acquaint practitioners in each with the beliefs and practices of the other. They can also present research, particularly to scientific practitioners, on the effectiveness of cultural remedies and practices.

■ **T A B L E   6 – 1 3**   **Differences and Similarities Between Alternative and Scientific Health Care Systems**

DIFFERENCES

The Alternative Health Care System	The Scientific Health Care System
Incorporates religious/spiritual aspects into care	Divorces religious belief from practice
Stresses downward causation in which thoughts and emotions affect physical status	Stresses upward causation in which mental activity arises from physical chemistry
Bases therapeutic decisions on the effects on the client's life	Bases therapeutic decisions on medical and health effects
Provides individualized therapy	Provides standardized therapy
Is client centered	Is provider centered
Expects client participation in the healing process	Expects a passive, receptive client
Uses substances to enhance natural healing processes	Uses substances to ward off pathogens
Emphasizes dealing with underlying imbalances	Emphasizes symptom suppression
Relies heavily on diet, rest, and exercise	Relies heavily on pharmacologic agents
Emphasizes mind–body interactions	Distinguishes between mind and body
Is oriented to the community	Is oriented to the individual
Takes place in familiar surroundings	Takes place in unfamiliar surroundings
Emphasizes humanistic care	Emphasizes impersonal care
Emphasizes familiar, practical, and concrete facts	Emphasizes abstract concepts
Provides holistic care	Provides fragmented care
Emphasizes caring	Emphasizes curing
Stresses prevention	Stresses diagnosis and treatment
Emphasizes cultural support	Does not emphasize cultural support
Is of moderate cost	Is of high cost

SIMILARITIES: BOTH SCIENTIFIC AND ALTERNATIVE HEALTH CARE SYSTEMS

Employ similar diagnostic techniques including observation and listening	Use medicinal substances and employ listening and some form of laying on of hands in the care of the sick
Use verbal and nonverbal communication	Based on asymmetric relationships between experts and laypersons
Engage in naming of illnesses and creation of positive expectations	Provide an explanation of disease, a rationale for treatment, and a rationale for social and moral norms
Employ suggestion, interpretation, emotional support, and manipulation of the environment as therapeutic modalities	

Assisting Cultural Adaptation

In addition to incorporating cultural beliefs and behaviors into scientific health care, community health nurses can assist clients from other cultures to adapt to the dominant American culture where necessary. For example, nurses may need to help clients understand how to access care in the scientific health care system. Or community health nurses may be involved in developing care systems for non–English-speaking clients. Some strategies that can be used to improve access to care for clients who speak languages other than English are summarized below.

As noted earlier, nurses may also need to educate individual clients and population groups regarding potentially harmful cultural health practices. For example, community health nurses can assist groups who are accustomed to having older siblings care for smaller children to understand the concepts of parental supervision and neglect. There are also many safety issues that may need to be addressed when members of immigrant groups are introduced to areas with heavy motor vehicle traffic patterns or other liv-

ETHICAL AWARENESS

You are a community health nurse working with clients in a predominantly Asian Indian community. In India, young children are frequently given the responsibility of watching even younger siblings while parents work, and it is not uncommon to find an 8-year-old girl supervising two or three younger children. In your community, both parents in most Indian families work in order to meet the high cost of living, and you have encountered a number of children under the age of 10 left home alone with younger siblings. Your nursing supervisor recently issued a directive indicating that such incidents are to be reported to the local Child Protective Services as child neglect and endangerment. What will you do about this situation?

ing conditions with which they are not familiar. For instance, many Hmong attempt to continue traditional cooking practices with open barbecues that pose fire and other safety hazards in U.S. residences.

EVALUATING CULTURAL COMPETENCE

Evaluation of care provided to clients from another cultural group should focus on both the outcomes of care and the delivery processes employed. In terms of outcomes, nurses should examine indicators of health status for individual clients and for subcultural groups. For example, has the nurse been able to improve the client's nutritional status without changing the client's cultural dietary pattern? Has a woman from another cultural group had a successful pregnancy outcome? Have parents ceased giving potentially harmful tonics to their children? The health status of selected cultural populations, as addressed in *Healthy People 2010: Goals for the Population* (U.S. Department of Health and Human Services, 2000), is summarized on page 140.

Health care delivery systems should also be examined in terms of their cultural competence. Organizations or health care agencies may be in one of five stages in relation to cultural competence. At stage zero, the agency is involved in no action related to culturally competent care. In stage one, the organization begins to take some action that acknowledges the diversity of clients and staff. Stage two, the stage of formal internal activities, involves recognition of the need for cultural competence and training to foster competence among staff members. At stage three, the agency engages in internal and external diversity initiatives. Internal initiatives are directed toward improving diversity among agency personnel; external initiatives involve targeting services to specific cultural groups, improving interpretation services, and efforts to meet with members of the cultural community. A stage four organization is described as a diverse learning

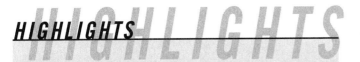

HIGHLIGHTS

Strategies to Promote Access to Care for Non–English-Speaking Groups

- Develop organizational policies that promote access to care for non–English-speaking clients.
- Commit organizational funds to developing resources to support non-English-speaking client groups.
- Recruit and train multilingual/multicultural staff whenever possible.
- Make use of bilingual community outreach workers.
- Employ professional interpreters who are not pulled away from other responsibilities to interpret for clients.
- Establish training and standards for interpreters.
- Develop protocols for developing accurate translations of written materials.
- Create written materials that are culturally sensitive, as well as linguistically correct, that consider literacy levels among the population. Share translated materials with other organizations and agencies serving similar cultural groups.
- Do not attempt to use translated written materials to replace verbal communication with clients.
- Coordinate activities and develop partnerships with cultural groups in the community.

Source: Riddick, S. (1998). Improving access for limited English-speaking consumers: A review of strategies in health care settings. *Journal of Health Care for the Poor and Underserved, 9*(Suppl.), S40–S61.

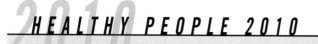
HEALTHY PEOPLE 2010

GOALS FOR THE POPULATION

Population Health Status

Physical Activity
▪ Objective 22-2. Increase the percentage of adults with daily moderate physical activity for 30 minutes to 30%.

	1997 Status
Native American	13%
Asian/Pacific Islander	15%
African American	10%
Latino	11%
White	15%

Tobacco Use
▪ Objective 27-1a. Reduce adult cigarette smoking to 12%.

Native American	34%
Asian/Pacific Islander	16%
African American	26%
Latino	20%
White	25%

Substance Abuse
▪ Objective 26-10a. Increase no use of alcohol and illicit drugs in the past month among adolescents to 89%.

Native American	45%
Asian/Pacific Islander	86%
African American	80%
Latino	78%
White	76%

▪ Objective 26-10c. Reduce adult illicit drug use in the past 30 days to 3%.

Native American	11.3%
Asian/Pacific Islander	3.4%
African American	7.1%
Latino	5.1%
White	5.7%

▪ Objective 26-11c. Reduce adult binge drinking in the past 30 days to 6%.

Native American	22%
Asian/Pacific Islander	7%
African American	12%
Latino	18%
White	17%

Injury and Violence
▪ Objective 15-15. Reduce deaths due to motor vehicle accidents to 9 per 100,000 population.

Native American	31.5
Asian/Pacific Islander	10.6
African American	17.0
Latino	15.2
White	15.8

■ Objective 15-32. Reduce homicides to 3.2 per 100,000 population.

	1997 Status
Native American	10.4
Asian/Pacific Islander	4.1
African American	25.2
Latino	9.9
White	4.3

Immunization
■ Objective 14-24. Increase the proportion of children with complete immunizations to 80%.

Native American	65%
Asian/Pacific Islander	73%
African American	66%
Latino	69%
White	74%

Access to Health Care
■ Objective 1-1. Increase the proportion of persons with health insurance to 100%.

Native American	79%
Asian/Pacific Islander	83%
African American	84%
Latino	70%
White	87%

■ Objective 1-4a. Increase the proportion of persons with a regular source of health care to 96%.

Native American	88%
Asian/Pacific Islander	89%
African American	85%
Latino	78%
White	87%

■ Objective 16-6a. Increase the proportion of pregnant women who receive prenatal care in the first trimester to 90%.

Native American	68%
Asian/Pacific Islander	82%
African American	72%
Latino	74%
White	85%

Source: U.S. Department of Health and Human Services. (2000). *Healthy people 2010* (Conference edition, in two volumes). Washington, DC: Author.

organization in which cultural considerations are integrated into the organization's daily operation (Andrulis, 1999). The stages of cultural competence in organizations are summarized on page 142.

Community health nurses working with agencies and organizations within the community can assist these groups to identify the extent of their cultural competence both in terms of the stages of development and in terms of specific guidelines developed by the U.S. Health Resources and Services Administration (2000) for assessing cultural competence in organizations. These guidelines include:

- The organization's history of involvement with the target population
- The extent of staff training for cultural competence in general and in relation to cultural patterns exhibited by local populations
- The degree to which members of cultural groups are represented in organizational planning bodies
- The availability of multilanguage resources required by the populations served
- The cultural appropriateness of materials disseminated by the organization

- The extent to which evaluation of agency programs is congruent with the cultural norms of the populations served
- The extent to which the organization demonstrates understanding of the cultural aspects of the community served

⑥THINK ABOUT IT

Using the references cited in this chapter, explore a culture with which you are not familiar. Do a similar cultural assessment of your own culture. How are the two cultures similar? How do they differ? How might those differences and similarities affect your care if you were the client and your nurse was from the other culture?

Community health nurses can assist existing health care agencies and organizations to assess and improve their cultural competence. They can also assist in the planning of health care delivery systems and programs that exhibit the characteristics of culturally competent organizations. Additional resources for community health nurses working to incorporate cultural variables into their practice can be obtained from the agencies and organizations referenced on the companion Web page for this book.

Community health nurses work with individuals, families, and groups of people with diverse cultural backgrounds. An understanding of the possible influences of culture on health will allow these nurses to provide culturally competent health care and to assist the members of these groups to improve their health status.

HIGHLIGHTS

Stages of Cultural Competence in Organizations

Stage 0, Inaction: The organization does not recognize the need for cultural competence or take any action to develop competence in its operations.

Stage 1, Symbolic action and initial organization: The organization takes initial action to recognize and address diversity among staff and clients.

Stage 2, Formalized internal activity: The organization recognizes the need for cultural competence and provides training for staff.

Stage 3, Diversity initiatives: The organization engages in both internal and external initiatives. Internal initiatives are directed toward increasing diversity among staff; external initiatives are directed toward improving the cultural sensitivity of services to targeted cultural groups (e.g., providing interpretation services, meeting with community members to plan relevant programs).

Stage 4, Culturally diverse learning organization: The organization integrates cultural considerations into its everyday operation.

Source: Andrulis, D. P. (1999). Cultural competence assessment of practices, clinics, and health care facilities. In E. J. Kramer, S. L. Ivey, & Y. Ying (Eds.), *Immigrant women's health: Problems and solutions* (pp. 330–335). San Francisco: Jossey-Bass.

APPLYING YOUR KNOWLEDGE IN PRACTICE

✄ CASE STUDY
Culture and Care

Apple Valley is a rural agricultural community approximately 100 miles from the U.S.–Mexico border. Because of the mild climate, there are crops to be tended and harvested much of the year, and many Latino migrant workers are involved in this work. Although there is work for a significant portion of the year, many of the laborers have extended families still in Mexico. They frequently work for several months, then return to Mexico to share their earnings and visit with family members. When they return to the United

States, they often come as nuclear family groups and both parents work in the fields. Children may or may not attend school while in Apple Valley.

There are high infant and maternal mortality rates among this group as the women do not usually receive care during their pregnancies. In part, this is because of the high cost of care, but also results from lack of facility with English and inability to take time from work to receive care. Although most of the workers are legal immigrants, they are not eligible for financial assistance or care at the local health department prenatal clinic. Complicated deliveries often take place in the local hospital, however, and contribute to the burden of "uncompensated care" since the migrant families are usually unable to pay the hospital bills. According to some of the workers, there is a Latino woman living year-round in Apple Valley who serves as a midwife for some of the women.

- What cultural factors are operating in this situation? What other circumstances, not necessarily cultural in origin, complicate the situation?
- What interventions by the community health nurse could help to reduce the infant and maternal mortality rates?
- Who else should be involved in efforts to resolve the problem? Why?
- How could the community health nurse motivate involvement by other segments of the population?

✖ TESTING YOUR UNDERSTANDING

- How does culture differ from race and ethnicity? (p. 101)
- How does culture influence health? Give some examples of cultural influences on the health of individuals of populations. (pp. 101–102)
- Define cultural competence. What are some barriers to cultural competence? How can these barriers be overcome? (pp. 102–103)
- Describe four principles of cultural assessment. Give an example in which each principle has been violated. (p. 105)
- What are some of the similarities and differences between alternative and scientific health care systems? What are some strategies for integrating elements of alternative and scientific health care systems? (pp. 137–138)

REFERENCES

AbuGharbieh, P. (1998). Arab-Americans. In L. D. Purnell & B. J. Paulanka (Eds.), *Transcultural health care: A culturally competent approach* (pp. 137–162). Philadelphia: Davis.

Allan, J. D. (1998). Explanatory models of overweight among African American, Euro-American, and Mexican American women. *Western Journal of Nursing Research, 20(1),* 45–66.

Andershed, B., & Ternestedt, B. (1999). Involvement of relatives in care of the dying in different care cultures: Development of a theoretical understanding. *Nursing Science Quarterly, 12(1),* 45–51.

Anderson, I. B., Mullen, W. H., Meeker, J. E., Khojasteh-Bakht, et al. (1996). Pennyroyal toxicity: Measurement of toxic metabolite levels in two cases and review of the literature. *Annals of Internal Medicine, 124,* 726–734.

Andrulis, D. P. (1999). Cultural competence assessment of practices, clinics, and health care facilities. In E. J. Kramer, S. L. Ivey, & Y. Ying (Eds.), *Immigrant women's health: Problems and solutions* (pp. 330–335). San Francisco: Jossey-Bass.

Bankston, C. L. III. (1995). Hmong Americans. In J. Galens, A. Sheets, & R. V. Young (Eds.), *Gale encyclopedia of multicultural America* (pp. 670–681). Detroit, MI: Gale Research.

Black, S. A., Ray, L. A., & Markides, K. S. (1999). The prevalence and health burden of self-reported diabetes in older Mexican Americans: Findings from the Hispanic established populations for epidemiologic studies of the elderly. *American Journal of Public Health, 89,* 546–552.

Blake, J. H. (1998). "Doctor can't do me no good": Social concomitants of health care attitudes among elderly blacks in isolated rural populations. In W. H. Watson (Ed.), *Black folk medicine: The therapeutic significance of faith and trust* (pp. 33–40). New Brunswick, NJ: Transaction.

Bureau of Primary Health Care. (2000). Cultural competence: A journey. Retrieved May 22, 2000, from the World Wide Web, *www.bphc.hrsa.gov.*

Cargill, M. (1994). *Acupuncture: A viable medical alternative.* Westport, CT: Praeger.

Cavender, A. (1996). Local unorthodox healers of cancer in the Appalachian south. *Journal of Community Health, 21,* 359–373.

Chang, P. H., & Fortier, J. P. (1998). Language barriers to health care: An overview. *Journal of Health Care for the Poor and Underserved, 9*(Suppl.), S5–S20.

Compton, K. M., & Chechile, D. (1999). Female genital mutilation. In E. J. Kramer, S. L. Ivey, & Y. Ying (Eds.), *Immigrant women's health: Problems and solutions* (pp. 194–204). San Francisco: Jossey-Bass.

Covington, D. (1995). *Salvation on Sand Mountain.* Reading, MA: Addison-Wesley.

Dai, Y., & Dimond, M. F. (1998). Filial piety: A cross-cultural comparison and its implications for the well-being of older parents. *Journal of Gerontological Nursing, 24*(3), 13–18.

Devine, N. (2000). Dangerous combinations: Understanding the risks of mixing herbal products and drugs. *NurseWeek, 13*(8), 26.

Donley, R. Sr. (1998). The alternative health care revolution. *Nursing Economics, 16,* 298–301.

Dreher, M. (1996). Nursing: A cultural phenomenon. *Reflections* (fourth quarter), 4.

Ernst, E. (1998). Harmless herbs? A review of the recent literature. *American Journal of Medicine, 104,* 170–178.

Ferran, E., Tracy, L. C., Gany, F. M., & Kramer, E. J. (1999). Culture and multicultural competence. In E. J. Kramer, S. L. Ivey, & Y. Ying (Eds.), *Immigrant women's health: Problems and solutions* (pp. 19–34). San Francisco: Jossey-Bass.

Fetrow, C. W., & Avila, J. R. (1999). *Professional's handbook of complementary and alternative medicines.* Springhouse, PA: Springhouse.

Flaskerud, J. H. (2000). Ethnicity, culture, and neuropsychiatry. *Issues in Mental Health Nursing, 21,* 5–29.

Frye, B. A. (1995). Use of cultural themes in promoting health among Southeast Asian refugees. *American Journal of Health Promotion, 9,* 269–280.

Geissler, E. M. (1994). *Pocket guide: Cultural assessment.* St. Louis: Mosby.

Gropper, R. C. (1996). *Culture and the clinical encounter: An intercultural sensitizer for the health professions.* Yarmouth, ME: Intercultural Press.

Grossman, D. (1998). Cuban-Americans. In L. D. Purnell & B. J. Paulanka (Eds.), *Transcultural health care: A culturally competent approach* (pp. 189–215). Philadelphia: Davis.

Guendelman, S. (1995). Immigrants may hold clues to protecting health during pregnancy: Exploring a paradox. *1995 Wellness Lecture Series.* Berkeley, CA: California Wellness Foundation.

Harris, M. (1989). *Cows, pigs, wars and witches: The riddles of culture.* New York: Random.

Health Resources and Services Administration. (2000). Guidelines to help assess cultural competence in program design, application, and management. Retrieved May 22, 2000, from the World Wide Web, *www.bphc.hrsa.gov.*

Helman, C. G. (1994). *Culture, health, and illness* (3rd ed.). Oxford: Butterworth-Heinemann.

Henderson, G. (2000). Race in America: Dreams realized and deferred. *National Forum, 80*(2), 12–15.

Higgins, P. G., & Learn, C. D. (1999). Health practices of adult Hispanic women. *Journal of Advanced Nursing, 29,* 1105–1112.

Holl, R. M. (1999). Iridology: Another look. *Alternative Health Practitioner, 5*(1), 35–43.

Hughes, M. (1998, summer/fall). The graying of minority America. *Minority Nurse,* 20–23.

Hultkrantz, A. (1992). *Shamanic healing and ritual drama: Health and medicine in native North American religious traditions.* New York: Crossroads.

Keenan, C. K., El-Hadad, A., & Balian, S. A. (1998). Factors associated with domestic vio-

lence in low-income Lebanese families. *Image: Journal of Nursing Scholarship, 30,* 357–362.

Kwan, K. K. (1999). Assessment of Asian Americans in counseling: Evolving issues and concerns. In D. S. Sandhu (Ed.), *Asian and Pacific Islander Americans: Issues and concerns for counseling and psychotherapy* (pp. 229–249). Commack, NY: Nova Science.

LaFramboise, T. D., Trimble, J. E., & Mohatt, G. V. (1998). Counseling intervention and American Indian tradition: An integrative approach. In D. R. Atkinson, G. Morten, & D. W. Sue (Eds.), *Counseling American minorities* (5th ed.) (pp. 159–182). Boston: McGraw-Hill.

Langer, N. (1999). Culturally competent professionals in therapeutic alliances enhance patient compliance. *Journal of Health Care for the Poor and Underserved, 10*(1), 19–26.

Mattison, W., Lo, L., & Scarseth, T. (1994). *Hmong lives from Laos to LaCrosse.* LaCrosse, WI: The Pump House.

Mehl-Medrona, L. E. (1999). Native American medicine in the treatment of chronic illness: Developing an integrated program and evaluating its effectiveness. *Alternative Therapies, 5*(1), 36–44.

Minority Nurse. (1998, summer/fall). Cultures in mourning. p. 12.

Morris, H. M., Ogilvie, L., Fung, M., Lau, A., et al. (1999). Cultural brokering in community health. *Canadian Nurse, 95*(6), 28–32.

Morrison, E. F., & Thornton, K. A. (1999). Influence of Southern spiritual beliefs on perceptions of mental illness. *Issues in Mental Health Nursing, 20,* 443–458.

Munet-Vilaro, F., Folkman, S., & Gregorich, S. (1999). Depressive symptomatology in three Latino groups. *Western Journal of Nursing Research, 21,* 209–224.

National Center for Chronic Disease Prevention and Health Promotion (1998). Prevalence of diagnosed diabetes among American Indians/Alaskan Natives—United States, 1996. *Morbidity and Mortality Weekly Report, 47,* 901–904.

Ng, A. T. (1999). Culture-bound syndromes. In E. J. Kramer, S. L. Ivey, & Y. Ying (Eds.), *Immigrant women's health: Problems and solutions* (pp. 249–256). San Francisco: Jossey-Bass.

Niska, K. J. (1999). Mexican American family processes: Nurturing, support, and socialization. *Nursing Science Quarterly, 12,* 138–142.

Nowak, T. T. (1998). Vietnamese-Americans. In L. D. Purnell & B. J. Paulanka (Eds.), *Transcultural health care: A culturally competent approach* (pp. 449–477). Philadelphia: Davis.

Okuno, S., Tagaya, A., Tamura, M., & Davis, A. J. (1999). Elderly Japanese people living in small towns reflect on end-of-life issues. *Nursing Ethics, 6,* 308–315.

Organista, P. B., & Organista, K. C. (1997). Culture and gender sensitive AIDS prevention with Mexican migrant laborers: A primer for counselors. *Journal of Multicultural Counseling and Development, 25,* 121–129.

Papadopoulos, I. (1999). Health and illness beliefs of Greek Cypriots living in London. *Journal of Advanced Nursing, 29,* 1097–1104.

Pedersen, P. B. (1995). Culture-centered counseling skills as a preventive strategy for college health services. *Journal of American College Health, 44,* 20–25.

Phillips, K., & Gill, L. (1995). The use of simple acupressure bands reduces post-operative nausea. *Complementary Therapies in Medicine, 2,* 158–160.

Pope, M., & Chung, Y. B. (1999). From Bakla to Tongzhi: Counseling and psychotherapy with gay and lesbian Asian and Pacific Islander Americans. In D. S. Sandhu (Ed.), *Asian and Pacific Islander Americans: Issues and concerns for counseling and psychotherapy* (pp. 283–300). Commack, NY: Nova Science.

Poss, J. E. (1999). Providing culturally competent care: Is there a role for health promoters? *Nursing Outlook, 47*(1), 30–36.

Primm, B. J. (1998). Poverty, folk remedies, and drug misuse among the black elderly. In W. H. Watson (Ed.), *Black folk medicine: The therapeutic significance of faith and trust* (pp. 67–70). New Brunswick, NJ: Transaction.

Purnell, L. D. (1998). Mexican-Americans. In L. D. Purnell & B. J. Paulanka (Eds.), *Transcultural health care: A culturally competent approach* (pp. 397–421). Philadelphia: Davis.

Purnell, L. D., & Paulanka, B. J. (1998a). Purnell's model for cultural competence. In L. D. Purnell & B. J. Paulanka (Eds.), *Transcultural health care: A culturally competent approach* (pp. 7–51). Philadelphia: Davis.

Purnell, L. D., & Paulanka, B. J. (1998b). Transcultural diversity and health care. In L. D. Purnell & B. J. Paulanka (Eds.), *Transcultural health care: A culturally competent approach* (pp. 1–6). Philadelphia: Davis.

Rehm, R. S. (1999). Religious faith in Mexican-American families dealing with chronic childhood illness. *Image: Journal of Nursing Scholarship, 31,* 33–38.

Smith, S. L. (1994). White nurses, black midwives, and public health in Mississippi, 1920–1950. *Nursing History Review, 2,* 29–49.

Snow, L. F. (1998). *Walkin' over medicine.* Detroit: Wayne State University Press.

Spector, R. E. (2000a). *Cultural care: Guidelines to heritage assessment and health traditions.* Upper Saddle River, NJ: Prentice Hall Health.

Spector, R. E. (2000b). *Cultural diversity in health and illness* (5th ed.). Upper Saddle River, NJ: Prentice Hall Health.

Still, O., & Hodgins, D. (1998). Navajo Indians. In L. D. Purnell & B. J. Paulanka (Eds.), *Transcultural health care: A culturally competent approach* (pp. 423–447). Philadelphia: Davis.

Strickland, C. J. (1999). Conducting focus groups cross-culturally: Experiences with Pacific Northwest Indian people. *Public Health Nursing, 16,* 190–197.

Tervalon, M., & Murray-Garcia, J. (1998). Cultural humility versus cultural competence: A critical distinction in defining physician training outcomes in multicultural education. *Journal of Health Care for the Poor and Underserved, 9,* 117–125.

Torres, R. E. (1998). The pervading role of language on health. *Journal of Health Care for the Poor and Underserved, 9*(Suppl.), S21–S25.

Um, C. C., & Dancey, B. L. (1999). Relationships between coping strategies and depression among employed Korean immigrant wives. *Issues in Mental Health Nursing, 20,* 485–494.

U.S. Department of Health and Human Services. (2000). *Healthy people 2010* (Conference edition, in two volumes). Washington, DC: Author.

Waters, C. M. (2000). End-of-life care directives among African Americans: Lessons learned—A need for community-centered discussion and education. *Journal of Community Health Nursing, 17*(1), 25–37.

Waters, C. M. (1999). Professional nursing support for culturally diverse family members of critically ill adults. *Research in Nursing and Health, 22,* 107–117.

Watson, W. H. (Ed.). (1998a). *Black folk medicine: The therapeutic significance of faith and trust.* New Brunswick, NJ: Transaction.

Watson, W. H. (1998b). Central tendencies in the practice of folk medicine. In W. H. Watson (Ed.), *Black folk medicine: The therapeutic significance of faith and trust* (pp. 87–97). New Brunswick, NJ: Transaction.

Watson, W. H. (1998c). Folk medicine and older blacks in the southern United States. In W. H. Watson (Ed.), *Black folk medicine: The therapeutic significance of faith and trust* (pp. 53–66). New Brunswick, NJ: Transaction.

Weaver, T. (1994). The culture of Latinos in the United States. In T. Weaver (Ed.), *Handbook of Hispanic cultures in the United States: Anthropology* (pp. 15–38). Houston: Arte Publico Press.

Wolfe, K. (1999). Integrating complementary health practices into managed care. *Alternative Health Practitioner, 5*(1), 9–17.

Zapata, J., & Shippee-Rice, R. (1999). The use of folk healing and healers by six Latinos living in New England: A preliminary study. *Journal of Transcultural Nursing, 10,* 136–142.

Zuniga, M. E. (1997). Counseling Mexican American seniors: An overview. *Journal of Multicultural Counseling and Development, 25,* 142–155.

THE ENVIRONMENTAL CONTEXT

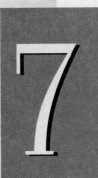

7

Chapter Objectives

After reading this chapter, you should be able to:

- Describe three ecological issues and their influence on human health.
- Discuss four environmental public health issues and their implications for population health.
- Identify the health effects of selected environmental conditions.
- Analyze the role of the community health nurse with respect to environmental health issues at the individual/family and population levels.
- Identify at least five primary prevention measures for environmental issues that affect population health.
- Identify secondary and tertiary prevention measures for individuals affected by environmental diseases.

Media Link

http://www.prenhall.com/clark

Additional interactive resources for this chapter can be found on the companion Web site. Click on Chapter 7 and "Begin" to select the activities for this chapter.

During much of history, human beings have been subjected to the effects of the natural environment. Earthquakes, famines, floods, droughts, and other environmental calamities have created upheavals in human society. Human progress has, to a certain extent, been measured in terms of capabilities for controlling the environment. Environmental factors, however, continue to exert an impact on human health and welfare. Air, water, noise, radiation, and waste present a variety of hazards to human health.

Community health nurses are concerned with the effects of environmental factors on the health of individuals, families, and communities. Interventions related to environmental concerns may occur at any of these levels. For example, a community health nurse may teach a family how to reduce the indoor air pollution in the home or work for legislation to promote safe disposal of hazardous wastes. To engage in effective action at all levels, community health nurses must have an understanding of environmental influences on health.

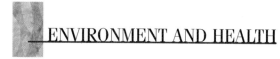

ENVIRONMENT AND HEALTH

Environmental health is defined as freedom from illness or injury due to exposure to factors in the physical environment that are potentially detrimental to human health (U.S. Environmental Protection Agency, 2000b). The *physical environment* is the set of factors beyond the individual's choice or control that can have either positive or negative effects on health (Lipschutz, 1995). The physical environment excludes those elements of the environment that involve interactions with other human beings.

The importance of environmental factors in health was recognized by Hippocrates in his treatise *On Airs, Waters, and Places* written in about 400 B.C. Attention to environmental factors waned, however, with the advent of evidence for specific causation in disease. Although environmental factors were recognized as playing a part in the transfer of microorganisms causing infectious diseases, other aspects of the environment and its effects on health were largely ignored. More recently, however, greater attention is being given to environmental issues by the scientific community and by the general public. In a 1999 survey of the U.S. public, 85% of those responding indicated that environmental factors were important determinants of health. Areas of concern demonstrated by the public include drinking water contamination, toxic wastes, air pollution, bacterial contamination of food, and pesticides in food (Pew Charitable Trusts, 2000). Many other environmental health problems remain largely unrecognized by the public.

Public Health and Ecological Perspectives

Environmental health and protection is defined as the "art and science of protecting against environmental factors that may adversely impact human health or adversely impact the ecological balances essential to long-term human health and environmental quality" (Gordon, 1997). As this definition indicates, there are both public health and ecological perspectives relevant to environmental concerns. The public health perspective concerns itself with the effects of the environment on human health, for example, the effects of lead exposure on child growth and development. The ecological perspective is one of concern for the preservation of the environment, for example, preventing species extinction. In the past, nursing in general has subscribed to an egocentric perspective in which the needs of the individual are paramount. Community health nursing, on the other hand, has focused on the public health perspective, which is homocentric in nature. In a homocentric perspective, the emphasis is on the good of the group, but still exclusively focused on concern for humanity. More recently, nursing has become more attuned to the ecological, or ecocentric, perspective in which the concern is with the cosmos, the total environment. This ecological perspective includes a concern for a variety of global changes that may not be directly related to human health, but may cause indirect health effects as well as effects on the environment itself.

Ecological Issues

Issues from the ecological perspective that are of concern include several global changes that are affecting the balance of the environment and its ability to maintain itself. Some of these issues include deforestation, desertification, loss of biodiversity, global warming, ozone depletion, planetary toxification, and overpopulation.

DEFORESTATION, DESERTIFICATION, AND LOSS OF BIODIVERSITY

Deforestation, desertification, and loss of biodiversity are interrelated issues that are affecting the face of the earth more intensely each year. *Deforestation* refers to loss of the earth's crown cover of trees to less than 10% of its original extent (Nadakavukaren, 1995). Deforestation may involve cutting trees, but is more efficiently accomplished by burning. In addition to eliminating natural habitats for many plant and animal species, deforestation contributes to soil erosion and changes in climatic and hydrologic cycles. The method of burning forest lands also contributes to the vast quantities of pollutants in the air. Deforestation also contributes to global warming through the release of greenhouse gases (by-products of the burning of fossil fuels such as coal and oil) that trap heat close to the earth. Thus far, one third to one half of the earth's forests have already been transformed by human activity (Herring & Kaufman, 1999).

Desertification is the conversion of fertile land into desert. In part, desertification occurs as a result of deforestation and the subsequent climate changes achieved by altering the rain cycle. Desertification also results from poor land management, overgrowth of crops that deplete essential nutrients from soil, and climatic changes. Desertification prohibits effective use of land for crops needed to feed the world's population as well as reducing the amount of water available for human consumption.

Loss of biodiversity refers to the extinction of certain species of plants and animals, which may result from loss of natural habitat as well as desertification, overhunting, and reproductive changes related to other environmental changes. Another contributing factor is the accidental or purposeful introduction of exotic species into local ecologies. More than half of the extinct species known to man have disappeared since 1900 as a result of human activity. In 1990, approximately 12% of existing mammals and 11% of birds were considered to be threatened with extinction, and it is estimated that tropical rain forests are losing three species per hour, many of them as yet unknown to humans (Nadakavukaren, 1995). California condors and timber wolves are only two of the species threatened with extinction in the United States. Loss of raptors such as the condors inhibits the natural cleansing function performed by carrion eaters, contributing to breeding grounds for microorganisms that may affect human health.

GLOBAL WARMING

Global warming is an overall increase in temperature throughout the world. One suggested contributing factor to global warming is the *greenhouse effect* in which gases resulting in large part from the use of fossil fuels collect in the atmosphere and reflect heat back to the earth rather than letting it dissipate. It is estimated that the atmospheric concentration of carbon dioxide in 1994 was 760 billion tons compared to 590 billion tons present prior to industrialization. This increase is believed to increase the earth's energy absorption by 1%. The resulting climatic changes have other effects on the environment and on health. Increasing warmth has been associated with increased growth rates for insects and parasites, leading to crop destruction and infectious disease. Global warming also results in the melting of the polar ice cap and rising sea levels, posing dangers of flood for some island areas (Ashton & Laura, 1998). Other health effects linked to increasing temperature and humidity include heat-related mortality (National Center for Environmental Health, 1998).

OZONE DEPLETION

The protective stratospheric layer of ozone is gradually being destroyed. This destruction is a result of chemical interactions between air pollutants, primarily chlorofluo-rocarbons (CFCs), and ozone. As we will see later, ozone is itself an air pollutant in ambient air. In the stratosphere, however, the ozone layer performs a filtering function that reduces the extent of ultraviolet radiation that reaches the earth. Without the ozone layer, it is estimated that skin cancer incidence rates would increase significantly. Depletion of the ozone layer also contributes to the phenomenon of global warming discussed above. Efforts to decrease the production of ozone-depleting substances, arising from the Montreal Protocol initiated in 1987 and the U.S. Clean Air Act in 1990, have had some positive effect, and since 1996, concentrations of these chemicals in the stratosphere have declined (U.S. Environmental Protection Agency, 2000a).

PLANETARY TOXIFICATION

Planetary toxification refers to the accumulation of a variety of wastes on the planet, with their consequent environmental effects. Some of those effects, such as air and water pollution and acid rain, will be addressed later in this chapter. Other aspects of planetary toxification include the accumulation of solid, liquid, and hazardous wastes. In 1997, 217 million tons of solid wastes were generated in the United States, amounting to 4.4 pounds per person per day. Only about 28% of this amount was recovered for reuse, while 55% was deposited in landfills and other disposal sites. Solid wastes consist of paper, glass, metal, and plastic products; rubber and leather; textiles; food and yard wastes; and other wastes (U.S. Census Bureau, 1999). Table 7–1 ■ provides a breakdown of the relative contribution of each of these forms of solid waste to the total amount generated.

Liquid wastes also present hazards that affect environmental quality as well as health. One of the primary contributors to liquid waste is sewage. Only 65% to 70% of U.S. households are connected to municipal sewage treatment systems; the remaining third of residences use household treatment systems, most of which are septic systems. Septic systems employ settling of sediment,

■ **TABLE 7–1** **Proportion of Solid Waste Generation by Type of Waste**

MATERIAL	PERCENTAGE
Paper and paperboard	38.6%
Yard wastes	12.8%
Food wastes	10.1%
Plastics	9.9%
Metals	7.5%
Glass	5.5%
Wood	5.3%
Textiles	3.8%
Other	3.3%
Rubber and leather	3.0%

filtration of the remaining liquid, and release into adjacent soil. Unfortunately, only about one third of the soil in the United States is appropriate for absorption of septic runoff, so septic systems may lead to contamination of ground water sources. In addition, about 25% of septic systems malfunction, contributing to the potential for sewage contamination of fresh water. Agricultural runoff and industrial liquid wastes also pose potential health hazards. In fact, it is estimated that agricultural runoff contributes to 40% of the pollution in U.S. rivers (Moeller, 1997).

The United States also produces millions of tons of toxic or hazardous wastes. *Hazardous wastes* include discarded materials that may pose a threat to human health or to the environment. The majority of hazardous wastes are generated by a few industries, most notably chemical and metal-related industries and those producing and using petroleum and coal products (Nadakavukaren, 1995). In fact, in 1997, industries released 2.4 billion pounds of toxic chemicals. Nearly 60% of these chemicals were released into the air, 7% into surface water, 8% to underground injection, and nearly 13% to land. Hazardous waste management is expensive and in 1998 cost $5.7 billion in the United States alone (U.S. Census Bureau, 1999). Solid, liquid, and toxic wastes contribute to a variety of health problems including cancers, heavy metal poisoning, and infectious diseases.

OVERPOPULATION

Overpopulation is another area of environmental concern from an ecological perspective. Despite efforts in many parts of the world, most notably China, to achieve zero population growth, the world's population continues to increase rapidly, and the rate of increase is growing. If one thinks in terms of the amount of time required for the world's population to double, that period is becoming shorter and shorter. For example, from approximately 8000 B.C. to 1650 A.D., the world's human population doubled only every 1,500 years. Doubling occurred again in the next 200 years to a total population of 1 billion people in 1850. The next doubling required only 80 years to 2 billion people in 1930 and then 45 years to 4 billion in 1975 (Nadakavukaren, 1995). For the United States alone, total population increased from 180.6 million people in 1960 to 270.5 million in 1998, with a projected growth to almost 394 million people by 2050 (U.S. Census Bureau, 1999).

Sources of population growth include birth rates, which range from 1.2 children per family in Hong Kong to 7.6 children in Yemen, and declining death rates. The combination of these two factors leads to the *growth rate* or *rate of natural increase* (Nadakavukaren, 1995). Population growth, combined with economic and environmental factors, is expected to result in food shortages in many parts of the world. These shortages will be the result of actual insufficiency rather than maldistribution of food because of the diminishing technologic ability to increase food yields commensurate with population growth. Water will also be in short supply if population growth continues

unabated. Other social effects include growing unemployment, illiteracy, insufficient housing, poverty, and political unrest. Ecological effects of population growth include continued overgrazing, soil erosion, deforestation, desertification, and further loss of biodiversity.

Environmental Public Health Issues

In recent years, greater attention has been given to the health risks posed by environmental conditions. This attention is evident in the number of national health objectives for the year 2010 that focus on environmental health issues. Sixteen objectives related to environmental health were included in the objectives for the year 2000 (U.S. Department of Health and Human Services, 1991), and an additional 14 objectives were added to the current objectives (U.S. Department of Health and Human Services, 2000a). These objectives can be found at the Healthy People Web site, which can be reached through the link provided on the companion Web page for this book.

Many environmental forces influence human health. Microorganisms such as bacteria, viruses, and fungi cause communicable diseases, and animals contribute to the spread of these diseases. Plants may contribute to accidental poisoning or to allergic reactions. Industry, vehicles, and buildings add to air and water pollution and excess noise. Climate and terrain contribute to natural disasters, which are discussed in Chapter 27. In addition, climate and terrain add to air and water pollution that have long-term effects on health. All of these facets of the environment give rise to environmental hazards that affect human health. Some of the environmental components that produce health hazards are presented in Figure 7–1 ■. Health hazards arising from environmental conditions fall into five categories: physical hazards, biological hazards, chemical and gaseous hazards, mechanical hazards, and psychosocial hazards. Mechanical and psychosocial hazards are addressed elsewhere in this book and are not dealt with here except as they influence the other categories.

PHYSICAL HAZARDS

Physical hazards are those conditions related to the physical objects and conditions that surround human beings. Physical hazards to be addressed here include radiation, lead and other heavy metals, and noise.

RADIATION   *Radiation* is energy in motion that occurs in the form of waves or particles. Two forms of radiation can be health hazards: ionizing radiation and nonionizing radiation. *Ionizing radiation* is the transfer of energy through electromagnetic waves or subatomic particles that cause ionization. *Ionization* is a process in which atoms gain or lose electrons to become electrically charged (Diehl, 1995). When ionizing radiation passes through human tissue, atoms are ionized, creating

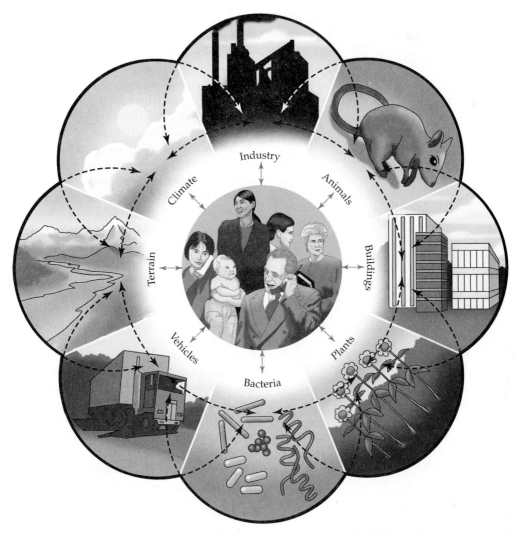

FIGURE 7–1 ■ *Selected Environmental Components That Produce Health Hazards*

a variety of health effects. Ionizing radiation is created when radioactive elements break up. Ionizing radiation occurs naturally in the soil and rock, and humans are exposed to this form of radiation daily. In fact, more than 80% of human exposure to ionizing radiation arises from natural sources (MacIntyre & Saha, 1995). Exposure to natural ionizing radiation is greater in some parts of the country than in others, depending on the extent of radioactive elements found. Exposure to artificial ionizing radiation may occur as a result of some forms of technology. X-ray procedures, for example, are a form of ionizing radiation. Ionizing radiation also results from a variety of industrial processes and processes used to create nuclear power.

Radon, a radioactive gas created by the breakdown of radium occurring naturally in the soil and in many building materials, is one source of exposure to ionizing radiation. Radon is also found in some well water and may be expelled into household air through seepage from cracks in foundations or during showers and baths. Radon gas can be inhaled in free form or attached to dust particles. After inhalation, the radioactive gas continues to decom-

pose, releasing alpha particles that damage lung tissue and may result in lung cancer. Radon exposure has been indicated as a significant contributing factor in 7,000 to 30,000 deaths each year in the United States (Ford, Kelly, Teutsch, Thacker, & Garbe, 1999). Radon exposure has also been implicated in 10% to 14% of lung cancer deaths. Despite efforts to increase the number of households tested for radon, from 1993 to 1994 only 6.4% of U.S. households had been tested (National Center for Health Statistics, 1999).

Cosmic radiation comes from outer space, whereas terrestrial radiation arises from radioactive substances found in the earth. Internal radiation sources include radioactive substances ingested or inhaled and deposited in body tissues. Dietary potassium isotopes, for example, emit small amounts of ionizing radiation. Radium is also found in some well water and in Brazil nuts (Moeller, 1997).

Medical and dental x-ray procedures are the source of approximately 11% of human exposure to ionizing radiation, and nuclear medicine treatments account for another 4% (MacIntyre & Saha, 1995). There is some

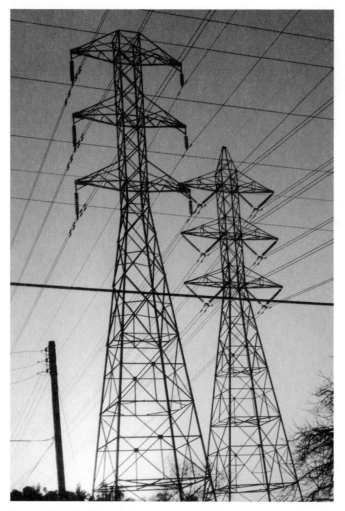

Potential health effects of electomagnetic fields are not yet fully known.

type of acute radiation exposure over a short period, adverse health effects can be expected to begin at exposures of 25 rem or 0.25 Sievert (Sv). (A rem is a measure of the biological damage produced in human tissue by radiation; an mrem is one-thousandth of a rem. The Sievert, a more recent measurement term, equals 100 rem.) When acute exposures reach 300 to 600 rem (3 to 6 Sv), there is a 50% fatality rate within weeks of exposure. Death may occur within hours at exposures of 5,000 rem (50 Sv) or greater (Moeller, 1997). Barring nuclear accidents, however, nuclear fallout and power sources generally account for less than 0.4% of ionizing radiation exposures; occupational exposures account for another 0.3% (MacIntyre & Saha, 1995).

The vast majority of people are not exposed to high levels of ionizing radiation. However, evidence reveals that long-term exposure to low levels of ionizing radiation may have cumulative health effects. Because little can be done about most natural sources of ionizing radiation, minimizing human exposure to radiation focuses primarily on control of exposure to artificial radiation.

Nonionizing radiation passes through matter without any transfer of energy and does not result in ionization. Forms of nonionizing radiation include electromagnetic fields, ultraviolet radiation, visible light, infrared radiation, and microwaves. Electromagnetic fields (EMFs) are created in the generation of electricity, and occur around power lines, electrical wiring, and electrical equipment and appliances. Video display terminals (VDTs) also create electromagnetic fields.

The health effects of this type of radiation are not yet fully known, but there is some evidence to suggest that chronic exposure may result in immunologic or endocrine changes, leading to disease (Moeller, 1997).

Ultraviolet radiation consists of waves of light energy beyond the capability of the human eye to see. Ultraviolet radiation occurs naturally in sunlight and is created by fluorescent lights and sunlamps. Ultraviolet radiation has several positive uses, including destroying pathogenic microbes and producing light that is less harsh and uses less energy than incandescent lighting. Ultraviolet light is also involved in producing vitamin D when human skin is exposed to sunlight. Unfortunately, ultraviolet light also results in sunburn, and exposure contributes to the incidence of basal and squamous cell carcinomas and malignant melanomas. The potential for skin cancer due to exposure to ultraviolet radiation is increased by the destruction of the protective stratospheric layer of ozone discussed earlier. Exposure to ultraviolet radiation also contributes to the formation of cataracts (Mood, 2000).

LEAD AND OTHER HEAVY METALS Other physical hazards to health arise from the presence of lead and other heavy metals in the environment. Lead may be present in soil, in water, and in the air, as well as in dust or paint chips in older dwellings painted with lead-based

question of the health effects of medical irradiation. Some studies have found no relationship between diagnostic x-rays and diseases such as leukemia and non-Hodgkin's lymphoma, whereas others have found relationships with multiple myeloma and breast cancer. The uncertainty in this area underscores the need for keeping medical exposures to ionizing radiation to a minimum. In addition to client exposures, health care providers who work with radiologic treatments or who care for clients who have radioactive implants are at risk for exposure (Worthington, 2000).

Some consumer products such as smoke detectors using americium, some tinted glasses, and glazes on some dentures and "fiesta-ware" china are also sources of ionizing radiation. Tobacco is another consumer product commonly containing radioactive material (MacIntyre & Saha, 1995).

The health hazards of nuclear power were demonstrated by the effects of the bombing of Japanese cities that occurred at the close of World War II. These effects were demonstrated more recently in the morbidity and mortality that occurred as the result of the nuclear accident at Chernobyl, in the former Soviet Union. In this

paint. Sources of lead in the air include vehicle emissions, stationary source fuel combustion (e.g., burning coal to generate electrical power), industrial processes, and decomposition of solid wastes. Lead in vehicle emissions was significantly reduced with the introduction of unleaded gasoline (Block & Rosenblum, 2000).

Use of lead-based paint in residential units was prohibited in 1977. These efforts have resulted in lower blood lead levels (BLLs) in children and the absence of overt signs of lead toxicity in most pediatric practices. Blood lead levels of 10 to 25 µg/dL, however, do not produce symptomatic lead poisoning and an estimated 4.4% of all children in the United States under age 5 have blood lead levels high enough to cause declining intelligence and retarded development (Bloch, Rosenblum, & Guthrie, 2000). As noted in Chapter 6, another source of lead for some children is traditional folk remedies. Prenatal lead exposure may also occur and result in lead poisoning in infants (Wolfe, 2000).

Young children are particularly at risk for lead poisoning because of their propensity to place objects that may be contaminated with lead-bearing dust in their mouths. Children may also ingest paint chips from peeling walls in deteriorating buildings. In addition, children absorb and retain higher levels of lead than adults. Infants may also develop high lead levels through formula mixed with lead-contaminated water.

Abatement procedures to remove lead-based paint in older homes traditionally consist of open-flame burning or sanding techniques with minimal cleanup of the resulting dust. This dust is heavily contaminated with lead and may present subsequent exposure risks, so community health nurses working in older residential areas may still encounter clients with lead poisoning.

Exposure to lead and other heavy metals can also occur through drinking water. These metals enter water as it passes through soils containing lead, nickel, mercury, arsenic, cadmium, and other metals. This process is facilitated if water is acidified as a result of acid rain caused by chemical air pollution. Metals are also leached into the water system from improper solid waste disposal. Finally, lead and copper may be leached from lead and copper pipes in older homes. Again, acidification of water due to acid rain enhances leaching of metals from pipes.

Lead interferes with red blood cell production and may cause damage to the brain, liver, and other vital organs. Typical symptoms of lead poisoning include headache, irritability, weakness, abdominal pain, vomiting, and constipation. In later stages, victims may exhibit convulsions, coma, and paralysis. Low-level exposure to lead in children can result in mental retardation as well as behavior problems (American Academy of Pediatrics, 1998). Mildly elevated blood lead levels have also been associated with a two- to three-point decline in IQ for every 10 µg/dL increase in blood lead. Elevated blood lead levels may also contribute to hearing loss, dental cavities, learning disability, and school dropouts (Wolfe,

2000). Treatment for lead exposure involves correcting dehydration and electrolyte imbalances and using chelating agents to facilitate urinary excretion of lead. Prevention and treatment activities, particularly the elimination of lead in gasoline, have resulted in declining blood lead levels in children. For example, BLLs greater than 10 µg/dL in children declined from 10.6% in 1996 to 7.6% in 1998 (National Center for Health Statistics, 2000).

Mercury poisoning manifests initially as listlessness and irritability. Recurrent rashes, photophobia, and a pinkish coloration of fingertips, toes, nose, hands, and feet are characteristic of the disease. Severe perspiration, pruritus, desquamation of hands and feet, and a burning sensation of hands and feet are also typical. Neurologic symptoms include neuritis, mental apathy, and loss of deep tendon reflexes. Chelating agents and maintenance of nutrition and fluid and electrolyte balances are the key to therapy. Prior to 1991, mercury could be found in some interior and exterior paints.

Arsenic is used in both pesticides and herbicides and is found in water contaminated by runoff in agricultural areas. Arsenic is also found in the home in over-the-counter ant poisons and may be a source of accidental poisoning. Symptoms of acute arsenic poisoning include nausea, vomiting, diarrhea, severe burning of the mouth and throat, and acute abdominal pain. Chronic poisoning may manifest as weakness, prostration, muscle aches, desquamation and hyperpigmentation of the trunk and extremities, and linear pigmentation of fingernails.

Cadmium poisoning can occur when acidic foods are prepared in cadmium-lined containers (e.g., mixing lemonade in metal cans) or from contaminated drinking water. Another source of cadmium contamination of water supplies is decomposition of rechargeable batteries in landfills. Cadmium filters through into groundwater. Symptoms of cadmium poisoning include nausea, vomiting, diarrhea, and prostration within 10 minutes of ingestion. Cadmium fumes can also be produced by some industrial processes and, when inhaled, cause a severe pneumonitis.

NOISE In addition to the physiologic effect of noise on hearing, evidence suggests that prolonged exposure to noise contributes to increased anxiety and emotional stress that may manifest as nausea, headaches, and sexual impotence. Other effects include insomnia, skin problems, swollen ankles, increase in the incidence of minor accidents, heart trouble and hypertension, cardiac dysrhythmias, and drug use. The psychological effects of noise can include irritability, depression, and diminished work productivity (Nadakavukaren, 1995).

Hearing loss due to noise exposure is a serious problem in industry. Exposure to noise outside the work environment is also a problem. Approximately 20 million people are exposed to hazardous noise levels in the United States. Examples of noise sources that exceed the

CRITICAL THINKING IN RESEARCH

Kegler et al. (1999) conducted a study with parents of Native American children with increased potential for exposure to environmental lead. Parents were interviewed prior to an intensive campaign to mobilize community response to the lead problem. They were asked about preventive behaviors to minimize children's exposure to lead such as handwashing, promoting play in grassy areas rather than on dirt, using a damp cloth when dusting, obtaining BLL screening tests, and so on. Participation in these behaviors was minimal, and parent interviews indicated a number of barriers to performing them such as being too busy to remember to wash the child's hands, children's preference for playing in the dirt, not wanting to see the child hurt during a blood test, and so on.

- What other factors might be influencing parents' use of preventive behaviors?
- How might you identify these factors? How would you test the extent of their influence in the situation?
- What interventions might improve the use of these behaviors?
- How would you test the effectiveness of these interventions?

hearing impairment threshold include buses; trucks; motorcycles; garbage trucks; trains; subways; recreational and off-road vehicles such as snowmobiles; motor boats; airplanes; and loud music. The health effects of noise are a function of both the intensity of sound (decibels) and the duration of exposure. Exposure to daily average noise levels of 85 decibels can produce mild, but irreversible, hearing loss, and many everyday noises are above this level. For example, a crying baby, a lawnmower, and city traffic all exceed this level (Nadakavukaren, 1995).

BIOLOGICAL HAZARDS

Biological hazards are those caused by living organisms in the environment. Biological hazards of concern to community health nurses include infectious agents, insects and animals, and plants.

INFECTIOUS AGENTS   Many infectious agents are transmitted by means of contact with an infected person. Others are transmitted by environmental means. Water is a primary means for environmental transmission of infectious agents. Approximately 20% of people worldwide do not have access to safe water (Mood, 2000). In the United States, sanitation and water treatment have limited the extent of waterborne infectious diseases, but transmission via contaminated water still occurs. In fact, in 1999, an estimated 10% of the U.S population received drinking water that violated federal standards (U.S. Department of Health and Human Services, 2000c). From 1997 to 1998, 17 waterborne disease outbreaks occurred in the United States related to drinking water, resulting in illness in more than 2000 people, and 32 outbreaks were related to recreational water use. More than 12% of the illness due to recreational water outbreaks was fatal (Barwick, Levy, Craun, Beach, & Calderon, 2000).

In large part, contamination of drinking water supplies occurs via improper sewage treatment and improper solid waste disposal. Septic tanks may have leach lines that are too short to permit adequate filtration of water contaminated with human wastes before it enters the groundwater supply. Approximately 30% of the population use septic tanks to dispose of wastes, and 3.5 billion gallons of human waste are introduced into the soil and portions of it into groundwater each day. Sewer systems prevent this sort of occurrence, but because of population expansion in many parts of the country, sewage treatment plants are inadequate to meet the demand for services. In some areas, untreated sewage contaminates water supplies. In San Diego, for example, untreated sewage from neighboring Tijuana, Mexico, contaminates both ground and surface water supplies, thus creating a biological health hazard.

Biological contamination of water supplies also occurs when solid wastes are improperly handled and rain water is contaminated as it flows through waste disposal sites that breed bacteria, viruses, and other disease-producing microorganisms. There is also potential for contamination of both drinking water and food supplies through the use of reclaimed water. Increased demands for water have led to an upsurge in wastewater recycling. This is particularly true in some parts of the country such as southern California, where wastewater reclamation programs are being developed or are already in operation in many communities. Most of this water is used for crop irrigation, a use that not only provides needed water, but recharges groundwater basins and provides a nitrogen-rich fertilizer for crops. Because of its high nitrogen content, however, recycled wastewater could contaminate drinking water supplies. Use of wastewater to irrigate food crops must be closely monitored to prevent contamination of fruits and vegetables with organic wastes.

Chlorination assists in reducing the hazards of bacterial contamination of water, but water systems are occasionally recontaminated after chlorination due to surface water leaking into faulty pipes. In addition, chlorination is not effective against newer pathogens such as *Cryptosporidium* or *Giardia lamblia* (U.S. Department of Health and Human Services, 2000b). Chlorination also produces its own hazards when it reacts with organic compounds that may be present in water to create carcinogenic compounds. Currently, however, chlorination remains the most widely used mode of water treatment in the United States.

An increasing number of pathogens are also found in foods, and as many as 9,000 deaths and 6.5 to 33 million cases of illness may be attributed to contaminated food each year. The cost of these foodborne pathogens is approximately $35 billion a year. The most common contributor to foodborne disease is *Salmonella* (often found in undercooked eggs and chicken), with the elderly, young children, and persons with immunosuppression at greatest risk for illness and death. In fact, 85% of deaths attributed to *Salmonella* occurred among nursing home residents (U.S. Department of Health and Human Services, 1998).

Increased risk of exposure to foodborne pathogens in the United States occurs for a number of reasons. People engage in less food preparation at home, and the use of fast food restaurants and prepared foods increases the potential for exposure to pathogens. In the complex food processing industry, the potential for contamination can exist anywhere along the production/distribution system. In addition, there is an increased reliance on foreign-grown produce, which may be imported from countries with less rigid safety standards.

Biological hazards also occur with improper disposal of medical wastes such as needles, syringes, and other objects contaminated with human blood or other secretions and excretions. Although disposal of biological hazards from medical facilities is supposed to be strictly controlled, medical wastes have been found on beaches, apparently washed ashore from ocean dumping. Contaminated medical wastes have also surfaced among ordinary solid wastes where they pose risks to waste industry workers as well as contribute to the potential for biological contamination of water through solid waste disposal sites.

Finally, infectious agents can be transmitted through the air. This transmission is enhanced by technology when improperly cleaned air-conditioning units and heating systems provide breeding grounds for disease-causing microorganisms. For example, contaminated heating, cooling, and water systems have been implicated in the spread of Legionnaires' disease.

⑥THINK ABOUT IT

What type of hazardous wastes do you generate? How could you cut down on the amount of hazardous waste generated?

INSECTS AND ANIMALS   Insects and animals serve as reservoirs and vectors for a variety of communicable diseases that affect human beings. Insects such as flies, cock-

roaches, and mosquitoes and animals such as rats transmit communicable diseases. Again, improper solid waste disposal can provide a breeding ground for these and other insect and animal vectors.

The presence of large numbers of wild animals such as skunks, foxes, bats, coyotes, bobcats, and raccoons increases the potential for transmission of rabies to humans. Large numbers of unimmunized domestic animals such as dogs and cats also present a biological health hazard for the human population. In addition, animal feces provide breeding grounds for flies and other insects that transmit disease.

Insects and animals also cause significant crop destruction, limiting food supplies for human consumption, particularly in developing nations. For example, it is estimated that rats destroy 20% of the world's crops each year and are responsible for $1 billion in losses in the United States alone (Moeller, 1997).

Another way in which insects and animals affect health is in terms of their contribution to the exacerbation of conditions such as asthma. Research data supports a significant contribution to asthma from cat dander, roaches, mites, and dogs as well as plant sources such as molds and fungi. The role of these factors in the development, as opposed to exacerbation, of asthma is as yet unknown, but may prove equally significant (Pew Environmental Health Commission, 2000b).

PLANTS   Plants can pose biological health hazards in two ways. First, many plants are poisonous and present the opportunity for accidental poisoning among small children. A variety of plants commonly found in homes and yards are potential poisons. Several of these common plants are listed on page 156. Plants also pose a biological hazard to those individuals who are allergic to pollen. Allergic responses to plant pollens, molds, and fungi may include mild to severe hay fever symptoms or irritants that trigger asthma (Pew Environmental Health Commission, 2000a). Other plants such as poison ivy and poison oak produce severe dermatologic symptoms.

CHEMICAL AND GASEOUS HAZARDS

The environment also provides opportunities for human contact with a variety of *chemical and gaseous hazards*. These hazards are created by the effect of certain chemicals and gases on human tissue, and can involve poisons and air and water pollution.

POISONS   Chemical poisons include insecticides, herbicides, fungicides, and rodenticides as well as a variety of household and industrial chemicals. The use of pesticides has been a primary factor in the increased agricultural production experienced in the United States, but it has also contributed to the occurrence of a number of health-related effects. Pesticide poisoning occurs through massive exposures such as when several thousand peop died as a result of exposure to methyl isocyanate resulting from a leak at a chemical plant in Bhopal, India, in 1984. Poisoning also occurs with single exposures or with cumulative exposures over a period of time. In 1996, for example, pesticide exposures among adults generated 40,000 calls to local poison control centers, with twice as many calls related to child exposures. As a result of these exposures, 60% of adults and 25% of the children developed symptoms related to pesticide poisoning. Most exposures (85%) result in mild illness, but 14% cause moderate illness, and 1% have major or fatal outcomes (U.S. Environmental Protection Agency, 2000b).

Pesticide exposures can occur as a result of working with the chemicals or servicing and repairing equipment used to apply them. Approximately 76% of pesticide use occurs in agricultural settings, placing pesticide handlers and agricultural workers at greatest risk for occupational exposures. Other groups who may be subjected to occupational exposures include nursery workers and pest control personnel (U.S. Environmental Protection Agency, 2000b).

Indirect pesticide exposure occurs through contamination of food and water ingested by humans and by animal sources of human food. In particular, DDT is absorbed in body fat and is found in animals that consume treated vegetation. These animals, in turn, serve as a food source for humans, who are thus exposed to the stored DDT. It is estimated that eating one fish taken from contaminated waters provides toxic exposure equivalent to drinking 1,000 gallons of water from the same source (U.S. Department of Health and Human Services, 2000c).

Chemical poisoning can also result from several household and industrial products and medications. Generally, such poisoning occurs in young children who ingest chemical compounds or medications improperly stored in the home. In 1996, the rate of accidental poisoning due to drugs and medicines among all age groups was 3.2 per 100,000 persons (U.S. Census Bureau, 1999). Accidental poisoning is addressed in more detail in Chapters 16 and 29.

AIR POLLUTION   Chemicals and gaseous materials add to air pollution, thus presenting additional hazards to human health. Both volatile chemicals and particulate matter contribute to the problem, and air pollution occurs in both indoor and outdoor, or "ambient," air. Pollution of the ambient air is measured in terms of the Pollutant Standards Index (PSI). PSI ratings between 100 and 200 are considered "unhealthful," ratings from 200 to 300 "very unhealthful," and levels over 300 "hazardous" to health. Specific pollutants that are routinely monitored include carbon monoxide, ozone, sulfur oxides, volatile organic compounds, nitrogen oxides, lead, and particulates (U.S. Census Bureau, 1999).

Some progress has been made in controlling pollutants in the ambient air. From 1980 to 1999, the amount of particulate matter in ambient air declined by 18%, and the level of sulfur dioxide decreased by 50%. Declines were noted for carbon monoxide and nitrogen oxides (57% and 25%, respectively), as well as for lead (94%) and ozone (20%). In spite of these gains, however, in 1999 more than 62% of the U.S. population lived in areas with air quality below federal standards for at least some part of the year (U.S. Environmental Protection Agency, 2000a).

Social factors such as widespread automobile use contribute to air pollution. Unfortunately, although vehicles produced today emit fewer hazardous and polluting substances than in the past, the number of autos on U.S. roads has doubled from that of 20 years ago. Each vehicle also travels more miles than ever before and spends more time idling in traffic. Automotive engineering appears to have made the greatest contribution to clean air possible without a complete revolution in the type of engine built.

Sources of ambient air pollution include technological processes used to manufacture consumer goods required to maintain the U.S. standard of living. The level of emissions permissible by large industries is controlled under Clean Air Act standards, but contributions to air pollution are made by numerous small businesses such as dry cleaning and other processes and the use of nail polish remover, paints, aerosols, and other household products that are not controlled.

Pollutant emissions have a cumulative effect compounded by geographic features in some parts of the country. For example, in Los Angeles a persistent inversion layer, or increase in air temperature with increasing altitude, results in decreased dispersion of pollutants that would normally occur with air movements. The effect of the inversion layer is further compounded by the barrier to air movement presented by nearby mountains. In addition, sunlight interacts with particulate and gaseous matter to produce a photochemical smog (Blewett & Embree, 1998).

Health effects of air pollution include respiratory symptoms, eye irritation, fatigue, and headache. Occasionally, air pollution causes death. Air pollution–related mortality generally occurs in the elderly and those with chronic respiratory diseases. Air pollution can also result in increased nonfatal respiratory illness, particularly in children and the elderly.

Air pollution causes acid rain, which contributes to chemical pollution of both groundwater and surface water supplies. As noted earlier, acid rain enhances leaching of a variety of compounds from soil and solid waste disposal sites and from lead and copper pipes. Air pollution also produces a chemical reaction that depletes the stratospheric ozone layer and reduces the extent of atmospheric filtering, contributing to the adverse health effects of ultraviolet radiation.

Indoor air pollution is also a cause for concern to community health nurses. Indoor air pollution tends to be most severe in newer buildings that have been designed, for reasons of energy conservation, to reduce air exchange with the outdoors.

Sources of indoor air pollution include contaminants such as formaldehyde, asbestos, organic dust, and fibrous glass particles released by structural components of buildings or by furnishings. Other sources of pollution indoors include smoking, cooking, heating, cleaning with a variety of household products, and the use of personal hygiene products such as aerosol deodorants. The high cost of energy has also resulted in a shift to new forms of home heating that increase the number and types of pollutants present in dwellings. For example, the use of wood stoves or kerosene heaters, particularly in poorly ventilated areas, leads to the buildup of combustion products in the air.

Indoor air pollution is particularly serious since most people spend more than 90% of their time indoors. Those at particular risk for health effects of this type of pollution (children, the elderly, and the infirm) spend an even greater portion of their day inside. Health effects of indoor air pollution range from nose, throat, and eye irritation to respiratory impairment, heart disease, central nervous system damage, and a variety of cancers. For example, smoking in the household has been shown to increase hospitalization for respiratory illness by 55%, and secondhand smoke is implicated in more than 350,000 cases of bronchitis, 430,000 episodes of asthma, and 152,000 cases of pneumonia in children each year (Blewett & Embree, 1998). Indoor air pollution may also result in fatality as in the case of more than 1,500 deaths each year due to unintentional carbon monoxide poisoning (Epidemiology Program Office, 1999).

WATER POLLUTION Only 2.5% of the earth's water is fresh water and two thirds of that amount comprises glaciers and polar ice caps, leaving less than 1% of the earth's water for human consumption (Moeller, 1997). Because of increased world population, water consumption increases each year. Per capita withdrawal in the United States, for example, has risen from 1,000 gallons per day in 1940 to 1,600 gallons per day in 1990, and then declined to 1,500 gallons per day in 1995 (U.S. Census Bureau, 1999). Daily personal water use typically includes 15 to 20 gallons for bathing, 2 quarts for cooking and drinking, and 15 to 25 gallons for flushing toilets. It takes approximately 250 gallons of water to carry 1 pound of fecal material through a sewer system. An additional 140 billion gallons are used each day for irrigation purposes, and 36 billion gallons are used for industrial purposes (Moeller, 1997). Given this level of water use and the limited availability of water, it is not surprising that water pollution is of serious concern.

⑥THINK ABOUT IT

To what extent does your educational institution recycle materials? What interventions by nursing students might promote recycling?

As noted earlier, acid rain is one source of water pollution, but other sources exist as well. The U.S. Environmental Protection Agency (EPA) currently regulates some

Industrial processes may contribute to water pollution.

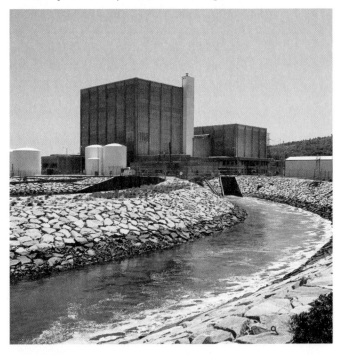

CULTURAL CONSIDERATIONS

CULTURAL CONSIDERATIONS

Members of several ethnic cultures hold beliefs and attitudes toward human/environment relationships that differ from those of the dominant U.S. culture. What are some of the environmental beliefs and attitudes of cultural groups in your area? Would these beliefs and attitudes enhance or hinder community efforts to deal with environmental health issues? Why?

90 drinking water contaminants (U.S. Department of Health and Human Services, 2000b), and the World Health Organization provides guidelines for more than 100 chemical water pollutants (Reckhow & Olin, 1999).

Manufacturing industries are major sources of chemical pollution of the water, but pollution also arises from mining operations, underground storage of chemicals, septic tanks, and the use of salt and deicing chemicals on highways. Another source of contamination is the 7 million tons of sewage sludge containing both organic and inorganic chemicals produced in the United States each year. In 1995, 35% of U.S. rivers and streams violated fecal coliform bacteria standards (U.S. Census Bureau, 1999), and 2,500 bodies of water in the United States have fish consumption advisories related to chemical contamination (U.S. Environmental Protection Agency, 2000a). Pesticides and fertilizers also find their way into the water supply to create chemical pollution.

Even measures taken to prevent air pollution have contributed to water pollution. For example, methyl tertiary butyl ether (MTBE) has been added to gasoline to increase its oxidation and decrease air pollutant emissions, but MTBE is now contaminating ground water sources. In 2000, for example, 10% of wells tested in the United States were found to be contaminated with MTBE (U.S. Department of Health and Human Services, 2000c).

Health effects of water pollution include bladder and colorectal cancers, central nervous system effects, skin irritation, alopecia, peripheral neuropathies, seizures, hepatitis and cirrhosis, infertility, congenital anomalies, developmental disabilities, anemia, renal failure, esophagitis, gastritis, stomach cancer, and heart disease. These effects occur through ingestion, inhalation of vapors and aerosols formed during use in showers, cooking, and so on, and through dermal absorption during direct contact with contaminated water (Weisel, 1999).

COMMUNITY HEALTH NURSING AND ENVIRONMENTAL HEALTH

Because of their consistent presence in the community, community health nurses are some of those most likely to become aware of environmental health problems, yet they are often unprepared to recognize and deal with them. The Institute of Medicine has recommended that environmental health should be given new emphasis in nursing education, practice, and research and that nurses become actively involved in environmental protection efforts at both the individual and aggregate levels (Pope, Snyder, & Mood, 1995). Protection of the environment is one of the core functions of public health, and community health nurse participation in this function is essential (Josten, Clarke, Ostwald, Stoskopf, & Shannon, 1995). Community health nursing activity related to environmental health issues occurs at both the level of the individual/family client and at the population level.

ASSESSING ENVIRONMENTAL HEALTH IN COMMUNITIES

The first step in ameliorating environmental health problems is an assessment of the factors contributing to them and their effects on human health. In addition to identifying environmental factors in the community that may affect health, community health nurses assess the population for factors that may increase the risk or severity of the health effects of environmental conditions. The age composition of the population is one such factor. For example, children's higher metabolic rate increases the rate of absorption of toxins, and very young children are closer to the floor, where air pollutants, in particular, accumulate. In addition, the rapid rate of growth and cell differentiation in children fosters genetic alteration and carcinogenesis. Older adults, because of changes in cardiovascular, renal, pulmonary, and immune systems, are less able to detoxify environmental toxins, placing them at increased risk of adverse health effects.

Existing genetic and physiologic conditions may also increase the potential for health effects of environmental factors. For example, levels of environmental toxins that might not harm an adult may be harmful to the fetus in a pregnant woman. Increased prevalence of chronic respiratory conditions such as asthma increases the adverse health effects of plant pollens and air pollution.

Community health nurses also assess individual clients and population groups for evidence of environmentally caused disease. Air pollution, for example, affects the respiratory system primarily, but may also produce cardiovascular, central nervous system, or hematopoietic effects. Air pollution also irritates the eyes and mucous membranes of the respiratory system. Water pollution can affect the gastrointestinal system, skin, liver, and reproductive, hematopoietic, lymphatic, cardiovascular, and genitourinary systems. Pesticides can adversely affect the central nervous system and produce kidney damage, a variety of cancers, and chromosomal changes. Radiation can cause skin cancer, visual impairment, cataracts, and genetic mutations, as well as lung and other cancers. Lead poisoning damages the central nervous system as well as the gastrointestinal system and can impair growth and development. Other metals and hazardous chemicals may cause cancers or central nervous system, gastrointestinal, and metabolic damage. Finally, high levels of noise not only compromise human hearing, but can contribute to gastrointestinal, dermatologic, central nervous system, cardiovascular, and psychological problems. Some of the effects of these environmental hazards are presented in Figure 7–2 ■.

Occupational settings give rise to multiple opportunities for exposure to environmental hazards, and community health nurses should assess the potential for occupational exposure to hazardous environmental conditions posed by local occupations and industries. For example,

miners may be exposed to high levels of radon, and sawmill workers are at higher risk for lymphomas (Hertzman et al., 1997). Other social factors, such as socioeconomic status, may influence exposure to environmental hazards. For example, children in families with lower income levels are at higher risk for lead poisoning (National Center for Health Statistics, 2000).

Certain personal behaviors prevalent in the population may interact with elements of the physical environment to cause or exacerbate health problems. Smoking, for example, increases lead absorption levels for both

FIGURE 7–2 ■ *Human Health Effects of Environmental Hazards*

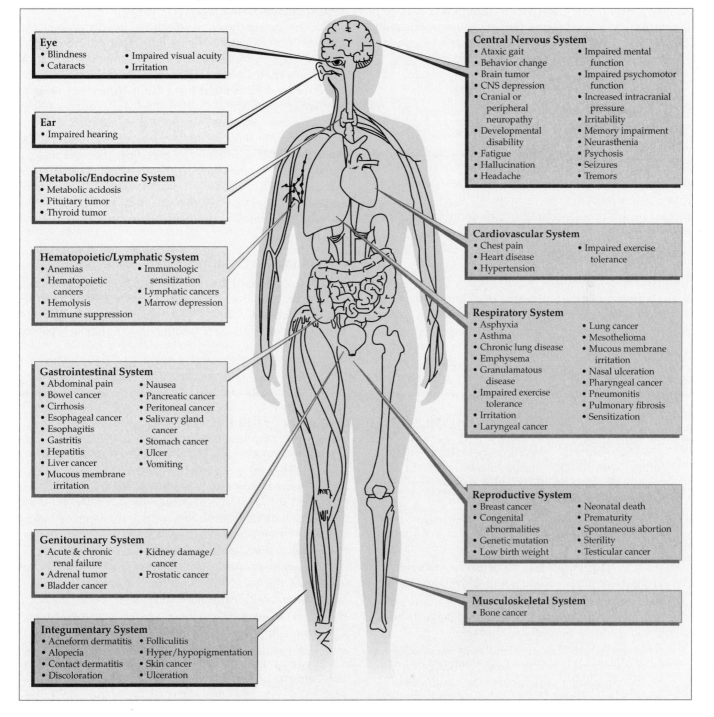

smokers and their children, and similar findings have been noted for cocaine users. In addition, inadequate calcium intake may further enhance lead absorption (American Academy of Pediatrics, 1998). Recreational activities may also contribute to environmental exposures. For example, campers have been found to be at particularly high risk for carbon monoxide (CO) poisoning due to the use of propane heaters or charcoal grills in enclosed areas (Epidemiology Program Office, 1999).

Finally, health system factors may contribute to or exacerbate environmental health problems. For example, despite a federal mandate for routine lead screening for all children on Medicaid, 81% of Medicaid enrolled children under age five were not screened (Bloch et al., 2000). Similarly, health care providers have little knowledge of the manifestations or treatment of many environmentally caused diseases. Tips to assist you in your assessment of environmental health issues are presented below.

PLANNING TO IMPROVE ENVIRONMENTAL HEALTH

Community health nurses assess for environmental hazards present in the community, the factors contributing to them, and the health effects that result. They then use this information to plan interventions to address environmental health problems affecting the population. These interventions can occur at the primary, secondary, or tertiary level of prevention.

Primary Prevention

Primary preventive measures are directed toward modifying or eliminating environmental hazards or reducing the potential for exposure to them. Primary prevention can occur with individuals and their families or with groups of people. For instance, the community health nurse might discourage the use of industrial paints that may still contain lead for painting surfaces in a family's home. Or the nurse may suggest that the family run the tap for a while before getting water for drinking or cooking and to use only cold water. The effects of acidified water in leaching lead from pipes in older homes are enhanced by heat, so warm water or water that has been standing in sun-heated pipes for some time contains higher levels of lead or copper than cold water that has been allowed to run. Another primary preventive measure directed toward the health of individuals and families would be education on the safe storage of medications and household chemicals to prevent accidental poisonings.

At the group level, community health nurses can engage in political efforts to minimize environmental hazards. For example, a nurse might campaign for a local ordinance that requires landlords to engage in safe and effective lead abatement procedures (processes used to remove environmental sources of lead) in older dwellings or a law that prevents improper disposal of hazardous wastes. Community health nurses can also educate the public regarding preventive measures. For example, a nurse might be involved in developing a campaign to educate people on the appropriate disposal of hazardous household chemicals. Other primary preventive measures for individuals, families, and populations are listed in Table 7–2 ■.

Secondary Prevention

Secondary prevention with individuals and their families would be geared to identifying and resolving existing health problems caused by environmental conditions. For example, community health nurses might be involved

assessment tips assessment tips assessment tips

ASSESSING ENVIRONMENTAL INFLUENCES ON POPULATION HEALTH

- What environmental conditions have the potential to influence the health of the population? How do these conditions affect health? What is the extent of their influence on health at the present time?

- What segments of the population are most likely to be adversely affected by environmental conditions? Why?

- What factors contribute to the presence and influence of environmental conditions within the population?

- To what extent do environmental conditions arise from or are influenced by individual behavior (e.g., smoking, use of aerosols and cleaners)?

- What are the attitudes of members of the population to environmental health issues? What priority is given to resolution of environmental health issues?

- What barriers exist to improving environmental conditions?

- What is the potential for eliminating hazardous environmental conditions? What is the potential for limiting human exposure if hazardous environmental conditions cannot be eliminated?

- What actions will be required to address environmental health concerns within the population?

- Does the health care system contribute to environmental health hazards? If so, how?

- Is the health care system adequate to address environmentally caused disease in the population?

- Are health care providers prepared to recognize and treat environmentally caused diseases in individual clients?

■ **TABLE 7–2**   **Primary Preventive Measures for Selected Environmental Hazards for Individuals, Families, and Populations**

ENVIRONMENTAL HAZARD	INDIVIDUAL/FAMILY	POPULATION
Radiation	Refer for assistance with testing and sealing a home against radon leaks.	Educate the public on the hazards of radon exposure and preventive measures. Encourage targeted screening of homes for high radon levels.
	Encourage spending most of one's time in higher levels of the home.	Engage in political activity to promote building standards that safeguard occupants in areas with high levels of natural radiation.
	Discourage overuse of diagnostic x-rays.	Educate public about the hazards of overuse of diagnostic x-rays.
	Encourage adequate cleaning of door seals on microwave ovens and maintenance of safe distance while microwave is in operation.	Engage in political activity to promote and enforce safety standards for nuclear reactors.
	Discourage sunbathing. Encourage use of sunscreen and protective clothing when outdoors	Educate the public about the hazards of exposure to ultraviolet radiation.
	Discourage smoking in home, refer for smoking cessation assistance.	Promote availability of smoking cessation services.
Lead and heavy metals	Encourage families to remove lead-based paint from older homes. Encourage covering peeling paint surfaces. Encourage families to wash small children's hands as well as toys to remove lead-contaminated dust. Encourage close supervision of small children.	Encourage communities to remove lead-based paint from older homes.
	Encourage calcium intake to limit lead absorption.	Promote legislation to ban air pollution and acid rain to prevent pollution of water with heavy metals.
	Encourage families to use cold water to drink and cook with and to allow the tap to run for a few minutes.	Encourage policy makers to set and enforce standards for solid waste sites to prevent metal contamination in waters.
Noise	Encourage families to limit noise in the home. Encourage use of ear protection in high-noise areas.	Promote noise abatement ordinances.
Infectious agents	Promote routine immunization for all ages.	Educate the public on the need for immunizations. Encourage policy makers to provide low-cost immunization services.
	Encourage good hygiene. Encourage washing fruits and vegetables before eating. Encourage adequate refrigeration of food.	
		Encourage enforcement of regulations for food processing and food handlers.
	Encourage susceptible individuals to boil water for cooking and drinking in areas with unsafe water.	Promote adequate sanitation, waste disposal, and water treatment.
Insects and animals	Encourage immunization of family pets.	Encourage development and enforcement of immunization and leash laws.
	Refer for assistance in eliminating insects, rats, and other pests from the home. Encourage use of insect repellent and protective clothing when outdoors.	Promote ordinances controlling insect breeding areas.
Plants	Eliminate poisonous houseplants. Eliminate poisonous plants from the yard. Eliminate other hazardous plants (e.g., poison ivy, plant allergens) from home environment. Encourage close supervision of small children.	Eliminate poisonous plants from recreation areas.

(continued)

■ **TABLE 7–2   Primary Preventive Measures for Selected Environmental Hazards for Individuals, Families, and Populations** (*continued*)

ENVIRONMENTAL HAZARD	INDIVIDUAL/FAMILY	POPULATION
Poisons	Educate families on proper use and storage of household chemicals and medications.	Educate public on hazards of household chemicals and medication.
	Encourage close supervision of children.	Promote legislation to limit use of hazardous chemicals in home and industry.
	Encourage proper disposal of hazardous wastes.	Promote hazardous waste disposal services.
Air pollution	Encourage limiting physical activity on days	Promote legislation to prevent air pollution. with high air-pollutant levels.
	Encourage carpooling.	Promote incentives for carpooling.
	Discourage use of space heaters in poorly ventilated areas.	Promote legislation to develop safety standards for home heating devices.
	Encourage frequent cleaning of heater and air-conditioning filters.	Promote building standards that ensure adequate ventilation.
	Encourage opening doors and windows to permit air exchange.	Promote replacement of hazard producing industrial processes.
	Encourage replacing asbestos insulation as needed.	
	Encourage installation of CO monitors in home.	
	Educate for use of household products with adequate ventilation.	
Water pollution	Encourage use of bottled water by high-risk persons in areas with heavily polluted water.	Promote legislation to prevent water pollution.
	Encourage use of fewer polluting products.	Promote replacement of hazard producing industrial processes.
		Promote filtration of water sources for newer pathogens, etc.

in screening for elevated lead levels or for hearing loss. They might also make referrals for testing of water supplies for clients who are concerned about potential contamination. When possible environmentally caused health conditions are identified, community health nurses might make referrals for medical diagnosis and treatment as needed. They might also make referrals for assistance with eliminating environmental hazards. For example, the nurse might be aware of lead-based paint in dwellings in some parts of town. He or she can screen young children in the area for elevated blood lead levels and make referrals for treatment for children with positive test results. The nurse might also make a referral for assistance in removing lead-based paint from the homes of affected children. Finally, the nurse might monitor children's responses to therapy and potential for continued exposure to lead.

Another important consideration in the care of individual clients with toxic exposures is protection of health care providers from exposure. Earlier, we noted the importance of protecting health care providers from radiation in caring for clients with radioactive implants. Another source of exposure for health care providers is clients who have been exposed to organophosphates and other toxic chemicals (National Center for Environmental Health, 2001).

At the population level, community health nurses might promote targeted screening programs to identify the prevalence of risk factors in the community. For

example, although the 2010 objective sets a goal of radon testing in 20% of all U.S. homes (U.S. Department of Health and Human Services, 2000a), cost-effectiveness analyses have indicated that targeted screening and mitigation in the homes of smokers is far less expensive ($80,000 per cancer death prevented) than universal screening ($520,000 per death prevented) (Ford et al., 1999). Community health nurses can encourage policy makers to adopt targeted screening practices for appropriate populations in the community.

Political activity might also be used to influence health care policy makers to provide adequate access to diagnostic and treatment facilities for people with health problems caused by environmental conditions. Or a nurse might campaign for stricter standards for pollutant emissions in air and water. Potential secondary preventive measures for individuals, families, and populations are listed in Table 7–3 ■.

⑥THINK ABOUT IT

What health hazards are present in your campus environment? What actions could be taken to minimize the health risks of environmental hazards on campus?

■ **TABLE 7–3** **Secondary Preventive Measures for Selected Environmental Hazards for Individuals, Families, and Populations**

ENVIRONMENTAL HAZARD	INDIVIDUAL/FAMILY	POPULATION
Radiation	Look for signs of health problems that may be caused by radiation among clients and members of their families. Refer for diagnosis and treatment as needed. Monitor effectiveness of treatment.	Monitor incidence of health problems caused by radiation. Promote accessibility of diagnostic and treatment facilities. Monitor longevity to determine effects of treatment in groups of people.
Lead and heavy metals	Screen for elevated blood levels of heavy metals in persons at risk. Observe for signs of heavy metal poisoning. Refer for diagnosis and treatment as needed. Monitor effects of treatment.	Promote accessibility of screening services. Promote compliance with Medicaid lead screening guidelines. Promote adequate reimbursement for lead screening services. Monitor incidence of heavy metal poisoning. Promote accessibility of diagnostic and treatment facilities. Monitor prevalence of complications due to heavy metal poisoning.
Noise	Screen for hearing loss in persons at risk. Refer for diagnosis and treatment as needed. Monitor effects of treatment.	Promote accessibility of screening services. Promote accessibility of diagnostic and treatment services.
Infectious agents	Screen for selected communicable diseases in high-risk persons. Observe for signs of communicable diseases.	Promote accessibility of screening services. Monitor incidence of communicable diseases.
Insects and animals	Educate families about first aid for insect and animal bites. Observe for signs and symptoms of diseases caused by insects or animals. Refer for medical assistance as needed.	Promote accessible treatment facilities for animal bites. Monitor the incidence of diseases caused by insects or animals. Promote accessibility of diagnostic and treatment services for diseases caused by insect and animal bites.
Plants	Inform families of poison control center activities. Refer families for poison control center services as needed. Refer for treatment of allergies and other conditions caused by plants.	Educate the public about poison control activities. Promote community support of poison control centers.
Poisons	Educate families about first aid for poisoning. Observe for signs and symptoms of poisoning. Refer families for poison control services as needed.	Educate the public about first aid for poisoning. Monitor the incidence of accidental poisoning. Promote access to poison control center services.
Air pollution	Observe for signs and symptoms of diseases caused by air pollution. Refer for diagnosis and treatment as needed.	Promote legislation to reduce pollutant emissions. Promote access to diagnostic and treatment services.
Water pollution	Observe for signs and symptoms of water-related diseases. Refer for diagnosis and treatment of water-related diseases.	Promote legislation to control water pollution. Promote availability of diagnostic and treatment services for water-related diseases.

Tertiary Prevention

Community health nurses may need to work with individuals or families to prevent recurrence or complications of environmentally caused health problems. For example, a community health nurse might assist a family to find housing where exposure to lead is not a problem. Or the nurse might provide parents with referrals for assistance in coping with the mental effects of long-standing lead poisoning in their children. Another tertiary preventive measure might involve suggestions for decreasing noise levels in the home to prevent further impairment of hearing.

Tertiary prevention might also be needed to deal with environmental problems at the aggregate or group level.

ETHICAL AWARENESS

Legislation aimed at preventing exposure to second-hand smoke in public places has been criticized because it infringes on the rights of individuals to decide for themselves whether, when, and where they will smoke. What approaches to ethical decision making would support such legislation? What approaches would support the rights of smokers to self-determination? Which position would you support? Why?

An example of tertiary control measures at this level might include political activity to mandate standards that prevent the recurrence of a leak at a nuclear power plant or to pass a bond issue to renovate a water treatment plant and prevent recontamination of drinking water with sewage. Other possible tertiary preventive interventions by community health nurses are presented in Table 7–4 ■.

In addition to political activity and other measures that help to protect the environment, community health nurses can also model environmentally conscious behaviors in their personal and professional lives. Some of these measures are summarized below.

EVALUATING ENVIRONMENTAL MEASURES

Community health nurses are also involved in evaluating the effectiveness of environmental control measures.

Evaluation would focus on the effectiveness of primary, secondary, and tertiary preventive measures related to individuals, families, and population groups. For example, the nurse might monitor blood lead levels of children in housing with lead-based paint to determine whether primary preventive measures have prevented initial elevation. For those children who already have elevated blood lead levels, evaluation would focus on the effects of chelating agents in reducing blood levels and the prevention of symptoms of lead poisoning. Evaluation of tertiary measures would be aimed at the effectiveness of abatement procedures in preventing

HIGHLIGHTS

Personal and Professional Environmental Protection Strategies

Personal Strategies

- Avoid unnecessary driving or gasoline consumption by combining trips or carpooling.
- Install water-conserving bathroom and kitchen fixtures.
- Reduce power use to minimum requirements by turning off appliances, computers, and so on when not in use; engage in family activities in one room to decrease use of lights; run major appliances during off-peak use hours; replace worn-out appliances with energy-conserving models; use cold water to wash clothes; wash full loads of clothing and hang them to dry; wash dishes by hand or run the dishwasher only when full.
- Use grass clippings and fallen leaves as mulch rather than burning them or taking them to a landfill.
- Dispose of hazardous wastes appropriately.
- Recycle materials whenever possible.
- Use nontoxic, environmentally safe household cleaners and other products.
- Refrain from use of aerosol sprays.
- Purchase recyled goods.
- Refrain from smoking.

Professional Strategies

- Encourage health care institutions and agencies to use recyclable materials where possible.
- Promote recycling in the work setting.
- Promote appropriate disposal of hazardous medical wastes.
- Promote use of nontoxic, environmentally safe cleaning products in health care settings.
- Promote carpool programs among fellow employees.
- Promote a smoke-free workplace.

■ **TABLE 7–4   Tertiary Preventive Measures for Selected Environmental Health Hazards for Individuals, Families, and Populations**

INDIVIDUAL/FAMILY	POPULATION
Monitor for long-term effects of environmentally caused illnesses.	Monitor effects of environmental changes on incidence of environmentally caused disease.
Promote adjustment to the long-term effects of environmentally caused illness.	Promote availability of services for members of the population affected by environmentally caused illness.
Refer families to personal or environmental health services for dealing with consequences of adverse environmental conditions.	
Promote changes in environmental conditions to prevent reoccurence of environmentally caused disease.	Promote environmental policies to prevent recurrence of environ mental health problems

blood lead levels from rising again after treatment. Similar approaches to evaluation of primary, secondary, and tertiary preventive interventions could be used for each of the environmental health problems addressed in this chapter. Evaluation at the aggregate level would focus on the extent to which national objectives for environmental health have been achieved. Possible foci for evaluating primary, secondary, and tertiary preventive measures for other environmental hazards are listed in Table 7–5 ■. The status of national health objectives related to the environmental health of the U.S. population is summarized on page 166.

Although community nurses will not be able to single-handedly change environmental influences on health, their role in protecting and promoting the health of the public requires that they be alert to environmental conditions and their potential effects on health. Community health nurses may identify the existence of hazardous environmental conditions and bring these conditions to the attention of those who can address them. In addition, community health nurses can educate the public to prevent adverse effects of environmental conditions until they can be ameliorated or eliminated.

■ **T A B L E 7 – 5** **Sample Questions for Evaluating Primary, Secondary, and Tertiary Prevention of Environmental Hazards**

ENVIRONMENTAL HAZARD	PRIMARY PREVENTION	SECONDARY PREVENTION	TERTIARY PREVENTION
Radiation	Have exposures to radiation been eliminated or reduced? Has the incidence of radiation-related illness been reduced?	Have those with radiation-related diseases received adequate treatment? Have the effects of radiation exposure been minimized?	Have reexposures to radiation been reduced or prevented altogether?
Lead and heavy metals	Have environmental sources of exposure to heavy metals been eliminated? Has the incidence of heavy metal poisoning decreased?	Have blood levels for heavy metals decreased after treatment? Have long-term effects of heavy metal poisoning been prevented?	Has reexposure to heavy metals been prevented? Have lowered blood levels for heavy metal been maintained after treatment?
Noise	Have noise levels been reduced to prevent hearing loss? Has the incidence of hearing loss been reduced?	Have persons with hearing impairment received needed services? Has hearing been restored by means of hearing aids or other devices?	Has further deterioration of hearing been prevented?
Infectious agents	Has the incidence of communicable disease declined? Has the proportion of persons immunized against immunizable diseases increased?	Have individuals with diseases been adequately treated?	Have recurrent cases of communicable diseases been prevented?
Insects and animals	Has the incidence of diseases spread by insects and animals decreased? Have insect and animal vectors been eliminated?	Have individuals with diseases spread by insects and animals been adequately treated?	Have recurrent episodes of diseases caused by insects and animals been prevented?
Plants	Have poisonous plants been removed from the environment? Has the number of cases of plant-related poisonings declined?	Has mortality due to plant poisonings been prevented?	Have recurrent plant poisonings been reduced?
Poisons	Has the incidence of poisoning decreased? Are hazardous substances disposed of appropriately?	Has poisoning mortality decreased?	Have recurrent episodes of poisoning been prevented?

(continued)

■ **TABLE 7–5** Sample Questions for Evaluating Primary, Secondary, and Tertiary Prevention of Environmental Hazards *(continued)*

ENVIRONMENTAL HAZARD	PRIMARY PREVENTION	SECONDARY PREVENTION	TERTIARY PREVENTION
Air pollution	Has the level of pollutants in ambient or indoor air been reduced? Has the incidence of diseases due to air pollution declined?	Have individuals with diseases due to air pollution received adequate diagnostic and treatment services?	Has further contamination of ambient or indoor air been prevented?
Water pollution	Has the number of exposures to polluted water been reduced? Has the incidence of diseases due to polluted water declined?	Have individuals with diseases due to water pollution been adequately treated?	Have recurrent episodes of diseases due to water pollution been prevented? Has recontamination of water by pollutants been prevented?

HEALTHY PEOPLE 2010

GOALS FOR THE POPULATION

Status of Selected National Objectives Related to Environmental Health

Objective	Target	Status
■ 8-1. Reduce the proportion of people exposed to harmful air pollutants (1997)		
Ozone	0%	43%
Particulate matter	0%	12%
Carbon monoxide	0%	18%
Nitrogen dioxide	0%	5%
Sulfur dioxide	0%	2%
Lead	0%	<1%
■ 8-5. Increase the proportion of people receiving safe drinking water from community water systems (1995)	95%	73%
■ 8-6. Reduce waterborne disease outbreaks (1987–1996 average)	2	6
■ 8-7. Reduce daily per capita water withdrawals (1995)	90.9 gal	101 gal
■ 8-11. Eliminate elevated BLLs in children (1991–1994)	0	4.4%
■ 8-13. Reduce pesticide exposures resulting in visits to health care facilities (1997)	13,500	27,156
■ 8-15. Increase recycling of municipal solid waste (1996)	38%	27%
■ 8-18. Increase the proportion of homes tested for radon (1998)	20%	17%
■ 8-22. Increase the proportion of pre-1950s homes tested for lead-based paint (1998)	50%	16%
■ 8-23. Reduce the proportion of substandard homes (1995)	3%	6.2%
■ 8-29. Reduce the global burden of disease deaths due to poor water quality, sanitation, and personal/domestic hygiene (1990)	2.1 mil	2.6 mil

Source: U.S. Department of Health and Human Services. (2000). *Healthy people 2010.* (Conference edition, in two volumes). Washington, DC: Author.

APPLYING YOUR KNOWLEDGE IN PRACTICE

✎ CASE STUDY
Environmental Advocate

Janice Wu, a community health nurse, is visiting a new client in a nursing home in an inner-city area in Los Angeles. As she enters the nursing home, she notices that several of the residents are doing calisthenics in the yard. Some of the residents are sitting on the sidelines and appear quite short of breath. When Janice checks to be sure they are all right, they tell her that they usually have a hard time breathing when they exercise on smoggy days like today. The residents say that they usually try to continue their exercises because it is one of the few activities that gets them out of the building. They also enjoy the social aspects of the exercise sessions. Many of them state that they have always been active and want to maintain their strength and mobility as long as possible. They express fears of being bedridden and unable to care for themselves.

After Janice is sure that all of the residents will be alright, she goes on to see her client. When she enters the building, she notices that it is quite hot inside, even though all of the windows and doors are open. Although it is only 10 A.M., it promises to be one of L.A.'s scorching summer days. After seeing her client, Janice talks to the director about the heat in the build-

ing. The director tells her that the building is always hot and that the air conditioning has never worked properly. The last time the repairmen came to fix the air-conditioning unit, they said it could not be repaired and would have to be replaced. The nursing home is run by a large national corporation, and the director says she has been told that they will have to wait until the next budget year (October) before money will be available for a new air conditioner. Fortunately, the heating system is separate, so there will be heat when the colder weather starts. The director says that staff members have been particularly careful about maintaining hydration in the residents during the hot weather, but many of the residents seem fatigued and listless with the heat.

- What environmental hazards are present in this situation? What health effects, if any, are these hazards causing?
- What factors are interacting with environmental hazards to contribute to problems?
- What level(s) of prevention is (are) warranted in this situation? What might Janice do to intervene?

✎ TESTING YOUR UNDERSTANDING

- Why should community health nurses be concerned with both the public health and ecological perspectives on environmental issues? (pp. 148–158)
- What are three physical hazards to health arising from the environment? Give an example of the effects of each on human health. (pp. 150–154)
- Describe three types of biological hazards that may be present in the environment. Discuss how each might adversely affect health. (pp. 154–155)
- What three types of hazards to human health are posed by chemical or gaseous materials? Give an example of the effect of each type of hazard. (pp. 155–158)

- Describe at least two health effects of environmental conditions on each of six human target organs or body systems. (pp. 158–160)
- What primary, secondary, and tertiary prevention actions might community health nurses take with respect to the effects of environmental conditions on the health of individual/family clients? (pp. 160–164)
- What primary, secondary, and tertiary prevention activities might be appropriate at the population level? (pp. 160–164)

REFERENCES

American Academy of Pediatrics. (1998). *Lead screening and prevention: Guidelines for parents.* Elk Grove Village, IL: Author.

Ashton, J., & Laura, R. (1998). *Perils of progress: The health and environment hazards of modern technology and what you can do about them.* Sydney, Australia: University of New South Wales Press.

Barwick, R. S., Levy, D. A., Craun, G. F., Beach, M. J., & Calderon, R. L. (2000). Surveillance for water-borne disease outbreaks—United States, 1997–1998. *Morbidity and Mortality Weekly Report, 49*(SS-4), 1–35.

Blewett, S. E., & Embree, M. (1998). *What's in the air: Natural and man-made air pollution.* Ventura, CA: Seaview.

Bloch, A. B., & Rosenblum, L. R., & Guthrie, A. M. (2000). Recommendations for blood lead screening of young children enrolled in Medicaid: Targeting a group at high risk. *Morbidity and Mortality Weekly Report, 49*(RR-14), 1–13.

Diehl, J. F. (1995). *Safety of irradiated foods* (2nd ed.). New York: Marcel Dekker.

Epidemiology Program Office. (1999). Carbon monoxide poisoning deaths associated with camping—Georgia, March 1999. *Morbidity and Mortality Weekly Report, 48,* 705–706.

Ford, E. S., Kelly, A. E., Teutsch, S. M., Thacker, S. B., & Garbe, P. L. (1999). Radon and lung cancer: A cost-effectiveness analysis. *American Journal of Public Health, 89,* 351–357.

Gordon, L. J. (1997). Environmental health and protection. In F. D. Scutchfield & C. W. Keck (Eds.), *Principles of public health practice* (pp. 300–317). Albany, NY: Delmar.

Herring, D. D., & Kaufman, Y. J. (1999). Assessing the role of biomass burning in global climate change. *National Forum, 79*(2), 19–22.

Hertzman, C., Teschke, K., Ostry, A., et al. (1997). Mortality and cancer incidence among sawmill workers exposed to chlorophenate wood preservatives. *American Journal of Public Health, 87,* 71–79.

Josten, L., Clarke, P. N., Ostwald, S., Stoskopf, C., & Shannon, M. D. (1995). Public health nursing education: Back to the future for public health sciences. *Family and Community Health, 18*(1), 36–48.

Kegler, M. C., Malcoe, L. H., Kegler, S. R., Lynch, R. A., & Tolliver, R. (1999). Caregiver beliefs and behaviors in the prevention of childhood lead poisoning. *Family Community Health, 22*(1), 50–65.

Lipschutz, R. D. (1995). Healthy environment, healthy community: Promoting community health in California through effective environmental protection, regulation, and education. *1995 wellness lectures.* San Francisco: California Wellness Foundation.

MacIntyre, W. J., & Saha, G. B. (1995). Sources of ionizing radiation and their effects on humans. In E. M. Cordasco, S. L. Demeter, & C. Zenz (Eds.), *Environmental respiratory diseases* (pp. 337–348). New York: Van Nostrand Reinhold.

Moeller, D. W. (1997). *Environmental health* (Revised ed.). Cambridge, MA: Harvard University Press.

Mood, L. (2000). Deep in the roots of nursing comes a search for harmful sources. *Reflections on Nursing LEADERSHIP, 26*(2), 21–25.

Nadakavukaren, A. (1995). *Our global environment: A health perspective* (4th ed.). Prospect Heights, IL: Waveland.

National Center for Environmental Health. (1998). Heat-related mortality—United States, 1997. *Morbidity and Mortality Weekly Report, 47,* 473–476.

National Center for Environmental Health (2001). Nosocomial poisoning associated with emergency department treatment of organophosphate toxicity—Georgia, 2000. *Morbidity and Mortality Weekly Report, 49,* 1157–1158.

National Center for Health Statistics. (1999). Radon testing in households with a residential smoker—United States, 1993–1994. *Morbidity and Mortality Weekly Report, 48,* 683–686.

National Center for Health Statistics. (2000). Blood lead levels in young children—United States and selected states, 1996–1999. *Morbidity and Mortality Weekly Report, 49,* 1133–1137.

Pew Charitable Trusts. (2000). Public opinion about public health—United States, 1999. *Morbidity and Mortality Weekly Report, 49,* 258–260.

Pew Environmental Health Commission. (2000a). *Attack asthma.* Baltimore, MD: Author.

Pew Environmental Health Commission. (2000b). *Attack asthma: Report with technical appendices.* Baltimore, MD: Author.

Pope, A. M., Snyder, M. A., & Mood, L. H. (Eds.). (1995). *Nursing, health, and environment: Strengthening the relationship to improve the public's health.* Washington, DC: National Academy Press.

Reckhow, D. A., & Olin, S. S. (1999). Contaminant characteristics. In S. S. Olin (Ed.), *Exposure to contaminants in drinking water: Estimating uptake through the skin and inhalation* (pp. 7–30). New York: CRC Press.

U.S. Census Bureau. (1999). *Statistical abstract of the United States, 1999* (119th ed.). Washington, DC: Author

U.S.. Department of Health and Human Services. (1991). *Healthy people 2000: National health promotion and illness prevention objectives.* Washington, DC: Government Printing Office.

U.S. Department of Health and Human Services. (1998). Government and private sectors join forces for food safety. *Prevention Report, 12*(4), 1–5.

U.S. Department of Health and Human Services. (2000a). *Healthy people 2010* (Conference edition, in two volumes). Washington, DC: Author.

U.S. Department of Health and Human Services. (2000b). Safe drinking water is fundamental to public health. *Prevention Report, 15*(1), 1–3.

U.S. Department of Health and Human Services. (2000c). Safe ground water: Who's minding the wells? *Prevention Report, 15*(1), 1, 5.

U.S. Environmental Protection Agency. (2000a). *Latest findings on national air quality control: 1999 status and trends.* Washington, DC: Author. Retrieved October 16, 2000, from the World Wide Web *http://www.epa.gov/airtrends.*

U.S. Environmental Protection Agency. (2000b). *Pesticides and national strategies for health care providers.* Washington, DC: Author.

Weisel, C. P. (1999). Developing exposure estimates: Introduction/overview. In S. S. Olin (Ed.), *Exposure to contaminants in drinking water: Estimating uptake through the skin and inhalation* (pp. 86–89). New York: CRC Press.

Wolfe, C. A. (2000). Assess for lead. *RN, 63*(8), 26–30.

Worthington, K. (2000). Guarding against radiation exposure. *American Journal of Nursing, 100*(5), 104.

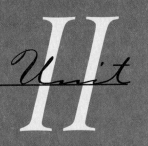

Unit II

COMMUNITY HEALTH NURSING AND ITS THEORETICAL FOUNDATION

SNOWBOUND

So we are snowbound
in a snowbound city
where only "essential" employees
reported to work.

Surely we are essential,
or at least I am,
to one or two if not to all

    to Sadie perhaps
    or Sultana or Nellie
    Alma
    Alberta
    or Herman.

Invalids, they are homebound
not just today but all year round.

Who will dress their wounds if not we?
Who will bring them their pills?
Who will hear their frail hearts
    and scarred lungs
    and night fears
    if not we—or me?

But we are snowbound.
On the telephone
we agonize over the fact
that we're frozen in place.

Surely it is essential
to get to them, isn't it?
To one or two if not to all?

    Yet all have survived
    except Herman who died
    quietly
    this morning
    in his chair.

Reprinted with permission from V. Masson (1999),
Rehab at the Florida Avenue Grill. *Washington,*
DC: Sage Femme Press.

nowbound reflects the commitment of community health nurses to the individuals and populations they serve.

COMMUNITY HEALTH NURSING

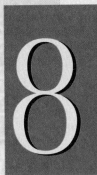

Chapter Objectives

After reading this chapter, you should be able to:

- Define community health nursing.
- Distinguish between community health nursing and community-based nursing.
- Differentiate between district and program-focused community health nursing.
- Identify at least five attributes of community health nursing.
- Summarize the standards for community health nursing practice.
- Distinguish among client-oriented, delivery-oriented, and population-oriented community health nursing roles.
- Describe at least five client-oriented roles performed by community health nurses.
- Describe at least three delivery-oriented roles performed by community health nurses.
- Describe at least four population-oriented roles performed by community health nurses.

KEY TERMS

Media Link

http://www.prenhall.com/clark

Additional interactive resources for this chapter can be found on the companion Web site. Click on Chapter 8 and "Begin" to select the activities for this chapter.

In his 1916 address to Johns Hopkins Hospital Training School graduates, William H. Welch noted that America had "made at least two unique contributions to the cause of public health—the Panama Canal and the public health nurse" (Krampitz, 1987). According to a 2000 survey of registered nurses conducted by the Division of Nursing (2001), public health and community health nurses constituted 18.3% of employed registered nurses in the United States. They practice in state and local health departments, home health agencies, community health centers, and student and occupational health services as well as other settings. Who are they and what makes their practice unique? In this chapter, we explore the features that set community health nursing apart from other nursing specialties and examine the roles and functions performed by community health nurses.

POPULATION-FOCUSED NURSING

There is considerable debate about what we should call this specialty area of nursing practice. Some of the terms that have been used include *public health nursing, community health nursing, community-driven nursing* (Bellack, 1998), and *community-oriented health care* (Chen, Ervin, Kim, & Vonderheid, 1999). This confusion regarding terminology characterizes the field in the United States as well as other parts of the world (Hamer, 2000; Murashima, Hatono, Whyte, & Asahara, 1999).

In 1996, the Public Health Nursing Section of the American Public Health Association (APHA) defined public health nursing as "the practice of promoting and protecting the health of populations using knowledge from nursing, social, and public health sciences." The section further described public health nursing as a systematic process of assessing populations to identify groups in need of health promotion or at risk for disease, planning for community intervention, implementing the plan, evaluating outcomes, and using the resulting data to influence health care delivery.

The American Nurses Association (ANA) (1986) presented a similar definition, but used the term *community health nurse*, in the introduction to *Standards of Community Health Nursing Practice*. More recently, the Quad Council of Public Health Nursing Organizations (1999), a coalition composed of the American Nurses Association (ANA) Council for Community, Primary, and Long-Term Care Nursing Practice; the Public Health Nursing Section of the American Public Health Association; the Association of Community Health Nurse Educators (ACHNE); and the Association of State and Territorial Directors of Nursing, reinstated the term *public health nursing* and defined the specialty as follows:

Public health nursing is the practice of promoting and protecting the health of populations using knowledge from nursing, social, and public health sciences (American Public Health Association, Public Health Nursing Section, 1996). Public health nursing is population-focused, community-oriented nursing practice. The goal of public health nursing is the prevention of disease and disability for all people through the creation of conditions in which people can be healthy (pg. 2).

Both the terms *public health* and *community health* nursing leave room for misinterpretation. Critics of the term *public health nursing* note that it implies the clientele of official public health agencies, who are often the underserved sick poor, as the primary recipients of care (Baldwin, Conger, Abegglen, & Hill, 1998). In fact, the specialty addresses the needs of whole populations, including those who are well and affluent as well as those who are poor and sick. Although the Quad Council (1999) specifies that public health nursing can occur in either public or private agencies, the term *public health nurse* is often used for those nurses employed by official government health agencies such as state and local health departments. This is somewhat ironic since the term itself was coined by Lillian Wald, whose Henry Street Settlement, which gave birth to this nursing specialty in the United States, was certainly not an official government agency (Kuss, Proulx-Girard, Lovitt, Katz, & Kennelly, 1997).

Community health nursing, as a name for the specialty, also has the potential for inappropriate connotations. The term *community health nursing* was coined by the American Nurses Association as a general term for all nurses who worked outside of institutional settings such as hospitals (Kuss et al., 1997). Unless these nurses are engaged in population-focused nursing, however, they are not true community health nurses, but are nurses providing sick care in community settings. These nurses might be more appropriately described as engaged in "community-based" nursing (Baldwin et al., 1998).

"Community-driven" care terminology has the potential for limiting the focus of practice to those health needs identified by members of the community or population group. Although community involvement in the identification and resolution of health needs and issues is important, it is also true that part of community health nursing practice is raising community consciousness levels to the point where community members recognize the existence of health needs that they may have previously ignored. Similarly, "community-oriented" care can be somewhat limiting, focusing program development on small aggregates while potentially ignoring health issues that affect larger population groups.

Despite the disagreement regarding labels, there is basic agreement that the defining characteristic of the specialty is population-focused nursing care directed toward the health of communities or population systems as the recipients. Some authors have suggested that the most appropriate title for the specialty is, indeed, "population-focused nursing" (Baldwin et al., 1998). At this time, however, there appears to be considerable resistance within the specialty to such a major change in terminology, so we will use the term *community health nursing* throughout this book.

Community health nursing is a synthesis of nursing knowledge and practice and the science and practice of public health, implemented via systematic use of the nursing process and other processes, designed to promote health and prevent illness in population groups. The focus of care is the aggregate. The goal of care is the promotion of health and the prevention of illness. Health promotion and illness prevention in the population may be achieved through interventions directed at the total population or at the individuals, families, and groups that constitute its members.

TRENDS IN COMMUNITY HEALTH NURSING PRACTICE

Some trends in community health nursing are worth noting as a basis for describing the current practice of community health nurses. When community health nursing began with groups like the Henry Street Settlement in the United States, district nursing in England, and the Victorian Order of Nurses (VON) in Canada, community health nurses worked toward improvements in the health of the population both through services to individuals and families and through political activism at the aggregate level. This dual-service level was most often accomplished through *district nursing,* a mode of service delivery in which each community health nurse was responsible for addressing all the health needs of a given population. Services included health promotion and education, and often illness care, to all the people residing in the nurse's "district" whatever their age, ethnicity, or economic level. Because of the broad spectrum of services provided across the age span, these nurses were required to engage in generalist practice and to have a broad knowledge base regarding a variety of community health problems from prenatal diet to treatment for tuberculosis to substance abuse. A district nursing approach sometimes encouraged nurses to become focused on the needs of specific individuals and families who made up their caseloads, losing sight of the bigger picture of health of the total population and the need for involvement in policy development as well as service delivery.

As funding sources for public health services became more categorical, community health nursing tended to adopt a program-focused approach. *Program-focused nursing* is a service delivery system in which nurses focus their activities and efforts on specifically designated health problems or specific target populations. In program-focused nursing, community health nurses became specialists in a single program area, for example, tuberculosis screening and treatment or promotion of child development (Rafael, 1999a). Emphasis shifted from involvement with all segments of the population to specifically targeted high-risk groups (Chalmers, Bramadat, & Andrusyszyn, 1998).

Program-focused nursing also tended to place emphasis on group work with fewer services to individuals and families and was characterized by distance from clients. Community health nurses were no longer intimately involved in all health-related aspects of clients' lives but dealt only with their specialty areas (Rafael, 1999a).

In the wake of the Institute of Medicine report (1988), *The Future of Public Health,* which identified the core functions of public health, community health nursing groups have moved even more toward a focus on populations, with less emphasis on direct care to individuals and families within those populations. Lack of emphasis on direct services, however, has resulted in the loss of connection with the community that was experienced by prior generations of community health nurses. This loss of connectedness, in turn, has made it more difficult for community health nurses to carry out the core functions. When community health nurses were intimately connected with community members, they were aware of the needs and problems faced by members of the population. They also had access to data that allowed them to carry out their assurance function and to evaluate the effectiveness of health care delivery systems (Rafael, 1999a).

The point in discussing the dichotomous approaches to community health nursing exemplified by district nursing and program-focused nursing is to emphasize that community health nursing is not an either/or proposition. It is not a question of *either* providing direct services to individuals and families *or* engaging in population-focused activities, but a synthesis of the two. Services are provided to individuals and families as a means of improving the health of the overall population. The improvement of the health status of individuals and families is an admirable goal in itself, but appropriate to community health nursing only if it also leads to improved health of the total population. This perspective may lead to ethical dilemmas related to resource allocation when the good of the larger group is best served by denying certain services to individuals and families (Billings, 1998). Community health nursing in the future must address this dual mission of service to individuals and families and population health rather than dichotomize these two levels of service.

The community health nursing literature has often debated the related question of whether adequately prepared community health nurses should be generalists or specialists. It would seem that connectedness to communities requires visibility on the part of community health nurses that is served by multiple interactions with different types of clients with a wide array of health problems. These interactions would seem to necessitate a generalist background through which the community health nurse deals with multiple kinds of issues and problems. However, community health nursing also requires specialist preparation not possessed by nurses in other fields. This specialist preparation lies in the population skills required for population-focused practice. We will discuss some of these specialized skills needed by community health nurses later in this chapter.

TENETS OF COMMUNITY HEALTH NURSING

As noted earlier, the defining characteristic of community health nursing is its focus on the health of population groups. Community health nursing is also defined by its adherence to eight tenets of practice as delineated by the Quad Council (1999). Although other nursing specialties may incorporate one or more of these tenets in their practice, public health nursing is distinguished from these other specialty areas by incorporation of all of them in practice. These defining tenets are presented below.

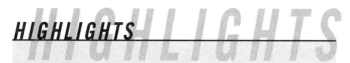

HIGHLIGHTS

Tenets of Public Health Nursing

- Population-based assessment, policy development, and assurance are systematic and comprehensive.
- All processes must include partnering with representatives of the people.
- Primary prevention is given priority.
- Intervention strategies are selected to create healthy environmental, social, and economic conditions in which people can thrive.
- Public health nursing practice includes an obligation to actively reach out to all who might benefit from an intervention or service.
- The dominant concern is for the greater good of all the people or the population as a whole.
- Stewardship and allocation of available resources supports the maximum population health benefit gain.
- The health of the people is most effectively promoted and protected through collaboration with members of other professions and organizations.

Reprinted with permission from: Quad Council of Public Health Nursing Organizations. *Scope and Standards of Public Health Nursing Practice,* © 1999, American Nurses Publishing, American Nurses Foundation/American Nurses Association.

STANDARDS FOR COMMUNITY HEALTH NURSING PRACTICE

One of the hallmarks of a profession is the establishment of standards of practice. Nursing, like other health-related professions, has set up standards for nursing practice and nursing service. The standards for nursing practice are further delineated in standards established for each of several specialty areas in nursing. Among these, and of particular interest to community health nurses, are the Quad Council's *Scope and Standards of Public Health Nursing Practice* (1999).

The standards of care for community health nursing practice have been developed within the framework of the nursing process and the core functions of public health. They relate to the areas of assessment, diagnosis, outcomes identification, planning, assurance, and evaluation. Additional standards address expected levels of professional performance and deal with quality of care, performance appraisal, education, collegiality, ethics, collaboration, research, and resource utilization. Measurement criteria have been developed for each of the two sets of standards. The standards of care and performance standards for community health nursing are summarized below.

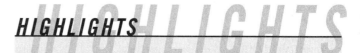

HIGHLIGHTS

Standards for Public Health Nursing

Standards of Care

Standard I. Assessment: The public health nurse assesses the health status of populations using data, community resources, identification, input from the population, and professional judgment.

Standard II. Diagnosis: The public health nurse analyzes collected assessment data and partners with the people to attach meaning to those data and determine opportunities and needs.

Standard III. Outcomes Identification: The public health nurse participates with other community partners to identify expected outcomes in the populations and their health status.

Standard IV. Planning: The public health nurse promotes and supports the development of programs, policies, and services to provide interventions that improve the health status of populations.

Standard V. Assurance: The public health nurse assures access and availability of programs, policies, resources, and services to the population.

Standard VI. Evaluation: The public health nurse evaluates the health status of the population.

Standards of Professional Performance

Standard I. Quality of Care: The public health nurse systematically evaluates the availability, accessibility, acceptability, quality, and effectiveness of nursing practice for the population.

Standard II. Performance Appraisal: The public health nurse evaluates his or her own nursing practice in relation to professional practice standards and relevant statutes and regulations.

Standard III. Education: The public health nurse acquires and maintains current knowledge and competency in public health nursing practice.

Standard IV. Collegiality: The public health nurse establishes collegial partnerships while interacting with health care practitioners and others, and contributes to the professional development of peers, colleagues, and others.

Standard V. Ethics: The public health nurse applies ethical standards in advocating for health and social policy, and delivery of public health programs to promote and preserve the health of the population.

Standard VI. Collaboration: The public health nurse collaborates with representatives of the population and other health and human service professionals and organizations in providing for and promoting the health of the population.

Standard VII. Research: The public health nurse uses research findings in practice.

Standard VIII. Resource Utilization: The public health nurse considers safety, effectiveness, and cost in the planning and delivery of public health services when using available resources, to ensure the maximum possible health benefit to the population.

Reprinted with permission from: Quad Council of Public Health Nursing Organizations. *Scope and Standards of Public Health Nursing Practice,* © 1999, American Nurses Publishing, American Nurses Foundation/American Nurses Association.

ATTRIBUTES OF COMMUNITY HEALTH NURSING

In addition to adherence to the tenets discussed earlier, community health nursing is characterized by a constellation of attributes that make it a unique field of nursing practice. These attributes include population consciousness, orientation to health, autonomy, creativity, continuity, collaboration, intimacy, and variability.

Population Consciousness

Community health nurses must have a consciousness beyond the needs of and services to individual clients and families. The nurse must develop an awareness of how information related to individual clients relates to the health status of the total population. Are this family's needs characteristic of the population or unique to the family? Are the factors impinging on a particular client's health impinging on the health of the community at large?

Community health nurses must also have an awareness of what is taking place in the general population (Salmon, 1998). What changes in the economic situation will affect the health of the population? What effect will closure of a major health care system have on community health? In short, community health nurses must see the big picture and be aware of the interactive nature of factors that influence health and well-being.

Orientation to Health

The 1988 Institute of Medicine report noted that the mission of public health is that of "fulfilling society's interest in assuring conditions in which people can be healthy." Promotion of health has also been a nursing function from the inception of district nursing with Florence Nightingale (Erickson, 1996), and was actively supported by Lillian Wald and the founders of the VON (Rafael, 1999b).

In other nursing specialties, health promotion is a facet of care, but one that is, of necessity, frequently given lower priority than health restoration needs. In community health nursing, on the other hand, the emphasis is on health promotion and maintenance rather than the cure of disease or disability. Although community health nurses frequently help clients resolve existing health problems, their major goal is to promote clients' highest level of physical, emotional, and social well-being. Health promotion as practiced by community health nurses encompasses both promotion of self-care behaviors by clients and advocacy for social and environmental conditions that promote health. For example, the health orientation of a community health nurse may lead to assistance with smoking cessation for individual clients as well as political activism to promote safe water supplies.

Autonomy

Autonomy, or self-direction, is a twofold attribute of community health nursing. Both the community health nurse and the client tend to be more self-directed than either might be in an institutional health care setting. Although all clients have the right and responsibility to

ETHICAL AWARENESS

Your state is considering restricting the bulk of state health funding for health promotion and illness prevention services. This means that very little money would be available for assisting low-income clients with major health care expenditures (e.g., liver transplants). What would be your position on this issue? Why? To what extent is your position congruent with the standards for community health nursing practice?

make decisions about their health care, their autonomy in this regard tends to be undermined by the way health care institutions operate. Because community health nursing care is typically provided in the client's home or neighborhood, the client is more likely to demand an active role in health care decision making, a situation the community health nurse should anticipate and foster.

Community health nurses also exercise a considerable degree of professional autonomy. In some situations, community health nurses may be the only providers of health care available. They must then rely on their own judgment to choose an appropriate course of action, frequently without consultation from other providers (Rafael, 1999a). In this sense, the community health nurse is more autonomous in practice than is the institution-based nurse.

Creativity

Community health nurses deal with increasingly complex problems both at the individual/family and population levels. Considerable creativity is required to develop solutions that fit within the constraints posed by client and community situations. Competition for resources by acute care delivery systems leaves little in the way of funding available for community health nursing activities, and that little must be used in ever more creative ways to achieve maximum benefit (Chalmers et al., 1998). Marla Salmon, former Director of the Division of Nursing within the United States Health Resources and Services Administration, noted that an effective community health nurse will "constantly scan the environment for new insights, ideas, and ways of enhancing action" (1998, p. 12).

Continuity

Continuity of care is another hallmark of community health nursing. Whatever the setting in which community health nurses work, relationships between nurse and client tend to be of relatively long duration. Community health nurses often have the flexibility to work with most clients until both feel that services are no longer needed. Because of the extended nature of the relationship, community health nurses are able to evaluate long-term as well as short-term effects of nursing interventions. They are also able to provide care for a wider range of client needs than is usually possible in acute care nursing. Problems not addressed today can be dealt with in subsequent meetings, and changing circumstances can be evaluated over time.

Collaboration

Because of the autonomy discussed earlier and the fact that interaction occurs in settings familiar to clients, nurse and client interact on a more equal footing than might otherwise be the case. This equality increases the potential for a truly collaborative relationship between nurse and client.

There is also greater opportunity for interaction and collaboration with other providers of client services

linked directly or indirectly to health. In the acute care setting, nurses frequently interact with other health and social services providers. Nurse historians have noted that community health nurses always maintained collaborative relationships with other providers, particularly physicians, and never assumed a subservient or "handmaiden" posture (Anglin, 1990). Collaboration in community health nursing is described as both *intersectoral* and *multisectoral* (Kuss et al., 1997). It is intersectoral in that collaboration occurs with persons outside of the health care system. It is multisectoral in that community health nurses must usually collaborate with multiple other sectors of the population at the same time. For example, other sectors of society with which community health nurses might collaborate in addressing the problem of adolescent substance abuse might include police, school systems, and so on.

This multisectoral collaboration characteristic of community health nursing requires what have been referred to as *multilingual* and *multiperspectival* skills on the part of nurses (Diekemper, SmithBattle, & Drake, 1999a). Community health nurses must speak the languages, not only of different ethnic groups, but also of other segments of society. They must be able to communicate in understandable terms with policy makers, funders, educators, and others with whom they collaborate. In addition, they must have an understanding of the multiple perspectives these groups bring to community health issues.

Intimacy

Another difference between community health nursing and other areas of nursing practice is the sphere of intimacy that typifies community health practice settings. Hospitals and other institutional health care environments often modify a client's behavior, thus affecting the accuracy of the nurse's observations of clients, their families, and their problems. Practicing in the community setting, however, the nurse can get a more accurate picture of the factors that affect the client's health. The community health nurse may also become more intimately aware of everyday details of the client's normal life and environment. For example, the community health nurse might discover evidence of spouse abuse that might not be uncovered in other health care settings. Intrusion into the client's sphere of intimacy may provoke hostility, particularly in instances when care has not been sought but is mandated by circumstances (e.g., child abuse). Effective community health nurses also become intimately involved with the community. More often than not, community health nursing is not circumscribed by specific working hours, and community activities may impinge on other aspects of the nurse's life.

Variability

The last characteristic of community health nursing, one that is highly valued by practicing community health

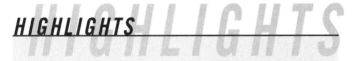

HIGHLIGHTS

Attributes of Community Health Nursing

Population consciousness	Awareness of factors that impinge on the health of populations as well as that of individuals
Health orientation	Emphasis on health promotion and disease prevention rather than cure of illness
Autonomy	Greater control over health care decisions by both nurse and client than in other settings
Creativity	Use of innovative approaches to health promotion and resolution of health problems
Continuity	Provision of care on a continuing, comprehensive basis rather than a short-term, episodic basis
Collaboration	Interaction between nurse and client as equals; greater opportunity for collaboration with other segments of society
Intimacy	Greater awareness of the reality of client lives and situations than is true of other areas of nursing
Variability	Wide array of clients at different levels, from different ethnic backgrounds, and in different settings

nurses, is variability. Community health nurses deal with diverse clients of different levels (individual, family, or population group) and ethnic backgrounds in a wide variety of settings. This variability necessitates a broad knowledge base and provides an exciting area of practice for those willing to accept the challenge.

All of these attributes are evidence of the unique status of community health nursing, which uses principles of both nursing and public health to prevent or alleviate health problems of groups of people as well as individual members of society. Attributes characteristic of community health nursing are summarized above.

CULTURAL CONSIDERATIONS

How would you describe the culture of community health nursing? How does this culture differ from that of nurses in the acute care setting? What cultural features in both arenas might make communication difficult? How does the culture of community health nursing interface with that of client populations?

SKILLS FOR COMMUNITY HEALTH NURSING

As noted earlier, community health nurses require broad knowledge and patient care skills to allow them to address the myriad health problems and needs of individuals and families in the population. They also require specialized knowledge and skills for addressing the needs of the population. Specialized knowledge includes content related to epidemiology, infection control, ethical decision making, cultural diversity, and information management (Chen et al., 1999; Fahrenwald, Fischer, Boysen, & Maurer, 1999).

Like nurses in all areas of practice, community health nurses need excellent interpersonal communication skills. These skills are incorporated in their care of individuals and families and include skills in counseling and health education. They also need communication skills directed toward populations including advocacy, negotiation, coalition-building, and group facilitation skills (Gebbie & Hwang, 2000; Reder, Gale, & Taylor, 1999). Additional population-focused communication skills include social marketing skills (Rafael, 1999a).

Community health nurses also need other skills related to population-based practice, including community assessment and development skills, leadership and change agency, grant-writing capabilities, and skills in financial and program management. Additional skills required for effective community health nursing practice include capacities for data collection and data analysis and program evaluation. Many of these skills will be discussed in the context of the community health nursing roles addressed later in this chapter and in subsequent chapters.

ROLES AND FUNCTIONS OF COMMUNITY HEALTH NURSES

In their practice, community health nurses engage in a variety of roles and perform multiple functions. Although the emphasis on specific roles and functions varies from one practice setting to another, most community health nurses engage in some way in the roles described below. These roles are categorized on the basis of the primary focus of nursing care as client-oriented, delivery-oriented, or population-oriented roles.

Client-Oriented Roles

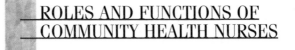

Client-oriented roles involve direct provision of client services to individuals, families, and occasionally groups of people. As noted earlier, community health nursing does not entail exclusive provision of population-focused services, but instead uses services to individuals and families as one means of improving population health. Population-focused nursing is thus grounded in individual/

family-focused care (Diekemper, SmithBattle, & Drake, 1999b). In fact, position statements by community health nurses have indicated their understanding "that a community's health is inextricably linked with the health of its constituent members and is often reflected first in individual and family health experiences (Community Health Nurse's Interest Group, 1998). Client-oriented community health nursing roles include those of caregiver, educator, counselor, referral resource, role model, advocate, primary care provider, and case manager.

CAREGIVER

The caregiver role involves applying the principles of epidemiology and the nursing process to the care of clients at any level—individual, family, group, or community. Some of the functions entailed in this role are assessing client needs, deriving nursing diagnoses, and planning appropriate nursing intervention. Implementing the plan of care may involve performing technical procedures or assuming one or more of the other client-oriented roles. Evaluating nursing care and its outcomes is another function performed in the caregiver role. This role is basic to all client encounters, and its functions are performed whether or not any of the other community health nursing roles are assumed.

Community health nurses also engage in the caregiver role with populations as the recipients of care. Just as in the care of individuals and families, the community health nurse assesses the health status of the population, develops nursing diagnoses, and plans, implements, and evaluates care for the population. This usually entails the development of health care delivery programs to meet identified needs. The use of the nursing process with populations as clients is discussed in more detail in Chapter 15.

EDUCATOR

Education is the process of facilitating learning that leads to positive health behavior (Keller, Strohschein, Lia-Hoagberg, & Schaffer, 1998). In the educator role, the community health nurse provides clients and others with information and insights that allow them to make informed decisions on health matters. The educator role may be performed at any client level. Community health nurses often provide educational services to individuals, families, and groups, and are frequently involved in the development of population-based health education programs. Community health nurses, for example, educate individuals and their families about adequate nutrition. At the same time, they may educate the general public regarding the harmful effects, say, of a high-cholesterol, low-fiber diet.

Focus group interviews with community health nurses have indicated that changes in the health care delivery system have made the role of educator of even greater importance. Short hospital stays limit the amount of time available for client education in institutional settings and increase the amount of education required of

community health nurses. Unfortunately, this increase in need has not usually been factored into time allocations for community health nurse visits to clients (Chalmers et al., 1998).

In the educator role, the nurse assesses the client's need for education and motivation for learning, develops and presents a health lesson, and evaluates the effects of health education. We discuss these functions in greater detail in Chapter 11.

Although the educator role is primarily a client-oriented role, the community health nurse may also serve as an educator for his or her peers or other professionals, in keeping with the community health nursing performance standard for collegiality. The nurse may be involved, for example, in educating student nurses or students in other health-related disciplines. On occasion, the nurse may be called on to educate other health professionals as well. For example, it has been the responsibility of community health nurses in some jurisdictions to assist in educating private physicians regarding appropriate diagnostic, treatment, and reporting procedures for sexually transmitted diseases.

COUNSELOR

Although many people do not distinguish between counseling and education, they *are* different. **Counseling** is the process of helping the client to choose viable solutions to health problems. In educating, one is presenting facts and developing attitudes and skills. In counseling, one is *not* telling people what to do but helping them to employ the problem-solving process and to decide on the most appropriate course of action. In the role of counselor, community health nurses explain the problem-solving process and guide clients through each step. In this way, the nurse is not only helping the client to solve the immediate problem but also assisting in the development of the client's problem-solving abilities. This is true whether the client is an individual, a family, or a population group. Community health nurses have indicated that the increased complexity of problems encountered by clients make their counseling role particularly important in the provision of care (Chalmers et al., 1998).

Counseling involves several steps on the part of the community health nurse. The first step is to assist the client to identify and clarify the problem to be solved. The nurse and client together examine the factors that contribute to a problem and those that may enhance or impede problem resolution.

At the second step of the counseling process, the community health nurse helps the client identify alternative solutions to the problem. If, for example, a large proportion of pregnant women in the population do not receive prenatal care, one could suggest an educational campaign, outreach efforts by lay health promoters, financial subsidies for care by available providers, or promoting the use of nurse midwives.

Assisting the client to develop criteria for an acceptable solution to the problem is the third step in the counseling

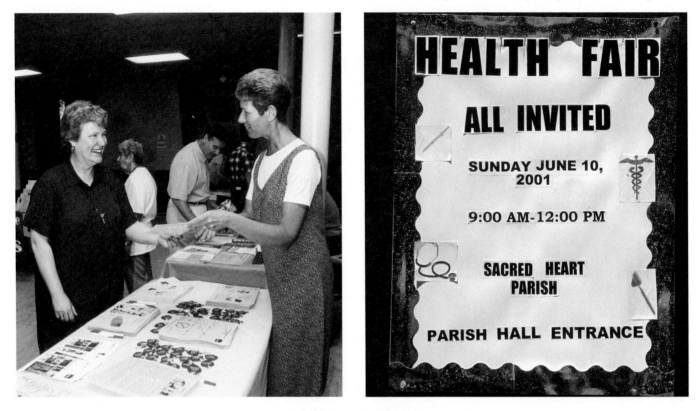

Community health fairs are excellent opportunities for health activities by community health nurses.

process. For example, an acceptable solution to the problem of poor nutrition among family members would need to fit the family's budget and might need to conform to cultural dietary preferences.

Next, the community health nurse would assist the client to evaluate each of the alternative solutions in terms of criteria established for an acceptable solution. The most appropriate alternative is one that best meets the acceptability criteria. This alternative is then implemented. Evaluation is the fifth step of the problem-solving process. If the alternative selected solves the problem, fine! If not, the process begins again. The problem-solving process is depicted in Figure 8–1 ■.

REFERRAL RESOURCE

Referral is the process of directing clients to resources required to meet their needs. These resources may be other agencies that can provide necessary services or sources of information, equipment, or supplies that the client needs and the community health nurse cannot supply. Referral is one of the key functions of community health nurses. In fact, in one study, community health nurses estimated that approximately 80% of their time was spent in arranging and coordinating referrals for service (Chalmers et al., 1998).

A distinction must be made, however, between the functions of referral and consultation. In a referral, the client is directed toward another source of services. On the other hand, in *consultation,* the nurse may seek assistance or information needed to help the client, but the client does not receive services directly from the consultant. Community health nurses also provide consultation to other professionals and to policy-making bodies.

Referral is an important part of the role of the community health nurse in any practice setting. It is the nurse's responsibility to explore available resources and direct clients to them as appropriate. The degree of intervention required in a specific referral varies with the type of referral and the client situation. Sometimes it is sufficient to let a client know that a certain resource exists. On other occasions, the particular agency may require a written referral from the nurse or from a physician.

In some instances, the client may not be capable of following through on a referral. For example, the depressed client may not have the energy to phone for an appointment at the local mental health center, but may be able to keep an appointment made by the nurse. The nurse must determine in each situation the degree of dependence or independence needed by that client at that time, with the goal, of course, of gradually increasing the client's ability to function independently. Specific functions of the community health nurse in the referral role include determining the need for referral, identifying the appropriate referral resources, and making and following up on the referral. The referral process is discussed in more detail in Chapter 12.

ROLE MODEL

A *role model* is someone who consciously or unconsciously demonstrates behavior to others who will perform

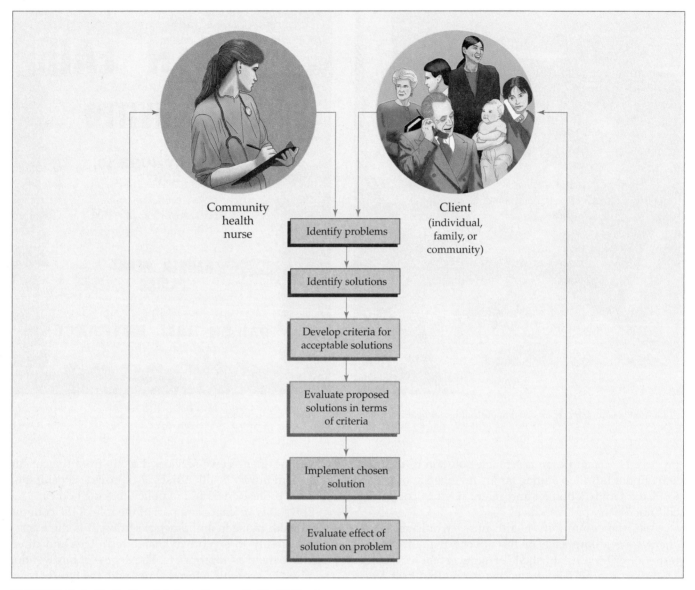

FIGURE 8–1 ■ *Problem Solving in Community Health Nursing*

a similar role. Community health nurses serve as role models for a variety of people with whom they come in contact. Through their own behavior, nurses influence the behavior of others. For instance, the community health nurse's ability to deal with crisis without panic provides guidance for clients to do the same.

The community health nurse's role as a model is not confined solely to influencing the health-related behavior of clients. The nurse also serves as a role model for other health care professionals. One of the areas in which the role-modeling function is of primary importance is in the educational preparation of student nurses. The way the community health nurse treats clients, the type of activity in which the nurse engages, and the level of competence displayed may all influence students' attitudes and practice. This influence can be either positive or negative.

ADVOCATE

Advocacy has been defined as speaking for people who cannot speak for themselves (Clark, unpublished raw data, 2001) or acting on their behalf (Keller et al., 1998). Client advocacy is another of the roles of the community health nurse that may take place at the individual, family, or population level. The nurse may serve as an advocate for the individual client in explaining the client's needs to the family or to other health care providers. For example, the parents of a handicapped child may tend to be overprotective, refusing to allow the child to engage in normal activities out of fear for the child's safety. The nurse can serve as an advocate for the child by explaining to the parents that their behavior is actually detrimental to the child's development. The nurse is intervening here to prevent the child from developing a further handicap, a psychological one, and is speaking for the child who cannot speak for himself or herself.

Community health nurses also engage in advocacy when they act to resolve difficulties encountered by clients in dealing with the health care system. Insisting that a case worker reevaluate a family's application for food stamps because their financial status has changed is an example of advocacy at the family level.

Advocacy also takes place at the population level. Helping communities organize and present grievances to the city council is an example of advocacy for aggregates in today's world. Other forms of advocacy at this level, as noted in Chapter 4, include nurses' involvement in political activity at local, state, and national levels. Population advocacy is viewed as a form of "emancipatory nursing," which empowers groups to change societal forces that contribute to health problems rather than attempt to adapt to them (Erickson, 1996).

As an advocate, the community health nurse engages in a number of activities or functions. The first of these is determining the need for advocacy and the factors that prevent clients from acting on their own behalf. Such factors can be quite varied. Some clients, for example, may not know how to go about making their needs known. Fear of reprisal might be another reason why clients do not speak for themselves. Other factors include apathy, feelings of hopelessness, and even language barriers.

A second function of the nurse as advocate is determining the point at which advocacy will be most effective. For example, should the nurse raise concerns of safety violations in rental housing with the landlord, with the housing authority, or with the media? Answers to such questions might be derived from knowledge of what has been tried previously and the effects of prior action. Related questions involve how the case should be presented. Should one ask, for example, for a meeting with interested parties or stage a demonstration?

Collecting facts related to the problem is another advocacy-related function. An advocate is considerably less effective when he or she does not have all the facts about a situation. A community health nurse advocate should get a detailed chronological account of events related to the problem for which advocacy is needed. The nurse should also try to validate or verify the information obtained to support the claim that a problem exists and action is needed.

The fourth task in advocacy is presenting the client's case to the appropriate decision makers. This function requires tact and interpersonal skills. Threatening or confrontational behavior should be avoided whenever possible, as both can set up an adversarial relationship, rather than a collaborative one, which may be detrimental to the client's cause. When other avenues fail, threats may have to be employed, but nurse and client must be committed to acting on them. For example, if the nurse threatens to report a landlord for safety code violations unless action is taken to remove hazards, he or she should actually be prepared to make the report.

The final function of the nurse as an advocate is to prepare clients to speak for themselves. The activities and functions of advocacy should not be carried out by the nurse alone, but should be a collaborative effort between nurse and client. In this way, clients learn how to develop and present a forceful argument for their own needs and may, in the future, be able to act without nursing intervention.

Advocacy necessitates involvement and commitment. The effective community health nurse cannot be content with the attitude that "I'd like to help, but my hands are tied." Advocacy is not a popular concept. It frequently means frustration and argument. It is the antithesis of complacency and is essential to the practice of effective community health nursing. Community health nurses must speak for those who cannot speak for themselves and articulate their needs to those in power. Nurses must also assist members of the community to learn how to speak for themselves rather than remain dependent on the nurse. Advocacy is a twofold obligation to take the part of others and, in time, to prepare them to stand alone.

A final comment is necessary with respect to advocacy. Because advocacy promotes clients' right to self-determination, community health nurses must be prepared to support clients' decisions even when they run counter to health interests. For instance, the nurse may need to accept a client's unwillingness to agree to cancer therapy and then support the client's decision in interactions with family members or other health care providers.

PRIMARY CARE PROVIDER

Many community health nurses have assumed roles as nurse practitioners providing primary care to a variety of clients. *Primary care* is defined as essential health care services made universally accessible to all. It consists of initial care provided to clients at their point of entry into the health care system. The primary care function of most community health nurses involves health-promotive and illness-preventive interventions such as routine prenatal assessments, well-child care, and immunizations. Community health nurses also routinely deal with minor health problems such as constipation and diarrhea.

Other community health nurses, with advanced educational preparation, provide primary care as nurse practitioners. These nurses have assumed diagnostic and treatment services that were once the exclusive province of physicians. There has been some concern that incursions into medical practice by nurse practitioners might detract from the emphasis placed by community health nurses on health promotion and illness prevention. Although this is sometimes the case early in a nurse practitioner's career, most practitioners regain their nursing perspective fairly rapidly and provide both curative and health-promotive services.

Performance of the primary care role by community health nurses and other advanced practice nurses (APNs) enhances the accessibility and comprehensiveness of health care services available to the general public. APNs have been shown repeatedly to provide equal or better quality care than physicians in a cost-effective manner (Boyd, 2000).

CASE MANAGER

Although case management is a new concept for many nurses, it has long been an integral component of community health nursing. Indeed, *case manager* may be seen as a comprehensive role that encompasses many of the other client-oriented roles described here. A *case manager* is a health professional who coordinates and directs the selection and use of health care services to meet client needs, maximize resource utilization, and minimize the expense of care.

The Case Management Society of America (1995) defined case management as "a collaborative process which assesses, plans, implements, monitors, and evaluates options and services to meet an individual's health needs through communication and available resources to promote quality cost-effective outcomes." The aims of case management include identifying high-risk clients or those with the potential for high-cost service needs, selecting appropriate choices among available services and providers, controlling costs, and coordinating care to achieve optimal client outcomes.

Case management has been shown to be cost effective and to result in enhanced health outcomes in many settings (Bedell, Cohen, & Sullivan, 2000). Given this fact and community health nursing's long association with case management, it would seem appropriate to retain case management as an essential part of the community health nursing role. The process of case management will be addressed in more detail in Chapter 12.

Nursing functions in the case manager role and other client-oriented roles are summarized in Table 8–1 ■.

Delivery-Oriented Roles

The *delivery-oriented roles* of community health nurses are those designed to enhance the operation of the health care delivery system, resulting in better care for clients. Roles in this category include coordinator or care manager, collaborator, and liaison.

COORDINATOR/CARE MANAGER

Community health nurses frequently care for clients who are receiving services from a variety of sources. Because of their awareness of the needs of the client as a whole being, community health nurses are in an ideal position to serve as coordinators of care. *Coordination* is the process of organizing and integrating services to best meet client needs in the most efficient manner possible. Unlike the case manager, the coordinator does not plan the care to be carried out by other health care professionals, but organizes that care to meet clients' needs as effectively as possible. At the population level, coordination may be referred to as *care management* or the grouping of

■ TABLE 8–1   Client-Oriented Community Health Nursing Roles and Related Functions

ROLE	FUNCTION
Caregiver	Assess client health status Derive nursing diagnoses Plan nursing intervention Implement the plan of care Evaluate the outcome of nursing intervention
Educator	Assess client's need for education Develop health education plan Present health education Evaluate outcome of health education
Counselor	Identify and clarify problem to be solved Help client identify alternative solutions Assist client to develop criteria for solutions Assist client to evaluate alternative solutions Assist client to evaluate effects of solution Make client aware of problem-solving process
Referral resource	Obtain information on community resources Determine the need for and appropriateness of a referral Make the referral Follow up on the referral
Role model	Perform the behavior to be learned by clients or others
Advocate	Determine the need for advocacy Determine the appropriate avenue for advocacy Obtain facts related to the situation Present the client's case to decision makers Prepare clients to stand alone
Primary care provider	Assess client health status and identify problems Plan and provide interventions for problems Introduce other supportive services as needed Teach and supervise others Modify care plan as required Teach clients self-care Coordinate health care services Serve as liaison between client and system
Case manager	Identify need for case management Assess and identify client health needs Design plan of care to meet needs Oversee implementation of care by others Evaluate outcome of care

people with similar needs in order to meet those needs more cost effectively (Michaels, 1997). This may involve the development of networks of providers and payers who combine efforts to provide services for specific population groups in a way that maximizes use of resources. Population care management provides a continuum of services to the designated population and facilitates information transfer between and among providers as well as easing client transfers between agencies (Williams, 2000). Community health nurses may be actively involved in initiating such systematic interorganizational coordination.

For individual clients, it is the community health nurse who most frequently enters the home or community and sees firsthand how the client is responding to a physical therapy program or how effective a roach-control program has been. She or he is also in the best position to transmit to other providers information regarding client needs, attitudes, and progress. The community health nurse is also best able to interpret to the client, in language he or she can understand, the purposes and procedures involved in programs instituted by other health care providers.

The community health nurse serving as a coordinator of client care performs a variety of functions. The first function involves determining who is providing care to the client, where services overlap, and where gaps in care may be occurring. The second function is to communicate with other providers regarding the particulars of the client situation and needs. Communication includes informing providers of other persons and agencies dealing with the client. Except in certain circumstances (e.g., child abuse or threat of harm to self or others), communication should be undertaken *only* with the consent of the client.

A simple example of coordinating services for an individual client might involve arranging for appointments in a prenatal clinic and a child health clinic on the same day, when both services are provided at the same location. Coordinating appointments in this way assists a pregnant woman with a 2-year-old and limited transportation to obtain needed health care for herself and her child without a second bus trip.

One additional function of the community health nurse in a coordinator role might be arranging a case conference to include nurse, client, and other providers of services. For example, the school nurse might arrange a meeting that would include not only the nurse, but also the child, parents, teachers, and school psychologist to discuss the child's behavior problems in school.

COLLABORATOR

Collaboration is "a dynamic, transforming process of creating a powersharing partnership" (Sullivan, 1998, p. 19), or, put more practically, a process of shared decision making by two or more people. As a collaborator, the community health nurse engages in joint decision making regarding action to be taken to resolve client health problems. Collaboration should always take place between nurse and client or a significant other. Collaborative efforts, however, may also include other providers.

Collaboration is frequently confused with the nurse's coordination role. Coordination is essentially a management function, and involves making sure that efforts to provide services are consistent and occur without gaps or overlaps. Collaboration, on the other hand, entails joint decision making. Both collaboration and coordination, of course, necessitate working with clients and other professionals (and nonprofessionals) who contribute to the health care of clients. This contribution by others may be directly related to the client's (or population's) health status, as in the case of physicians, physical therapists, nutritionists, and other health care personnel. It may also be indirectly related, as are the services of police and firefighters, sanitation engineers, and city officials.

Collaboration is not a matter of each health care worker designing and providing a program in his or her area of expertise with a certain amount of coordination between efforts. Rather, it is a joint effort on the part of health care providers *and clients* to set mutual goals and to arrive at a mutually acceptable plan to achieve them. Collaboration is a relatively new function for most nurses and cannot take place without a mutual feeling of respect and collegiality among health team members.

The two primary functions of the community health nurse in a collaborative role are communication and joint decision making. In communicating, the nurse conveys to other team members his or her perceptions of client needs, factors influencing those needs, and ideas for problem resolution. In decision making, the community health nurse participates in joint problem-solving efforts, using the problem-solving process with the health care team to identify and evaluate alternative solutions to client problems and to select an appropriate alternative. Collaboration may also extend to joint activity to implement solutions selected and to evaluate the outcome.

LIAISON

The liaison role of the community health nurse incorporates facets of the coordinator and referral resource roles and may even incorporate the advocacy role depending on the client situation. A *liaison* provides a connection, relationship, or intercommunication. The community health nurse working with clients dealing with multiple health and social agencies may serve as that connection or liaison. In the referral resource role, the community health nurse may function as the initial point of contact between client and agency. The liaison role might involve continued communication between client and other providers via the nurse. Sometimes this communication includes the additional function of interpretation and reinforcement of provider recommendations to the client or advocacy for the client with the provider agency. A summary of delivery-oriented roles and related functions is presented in Table 8–2 ■.

Population-Oriented Roles

The client-oriented and delivery-oriented roles of community health nurses usually relate to the care of specific individuals or families. At times these roles may be extended to the care of communities or populations. As noted throughout this text, community health nurses are concerned primarily with the health of the population, and they perform a number of roles that are exclusively group oriented.

Population-oriented roles include those of case finder, leader, and change agent. Additional population-oriented

■ **TABLE 8–2** **Delivery-Oriented Community Health Nursing Roles and Related Functions**

ROLE	FUNCTION
Coordinator	Determine who is providing care to client
	Communicate with other providers regarding client situation and needs
	Arrange case conferences as needed
	Assist in development of care networks
Collaborator	Communicate with other health team members
	Participate in joint decision making
	Participate in joint action to resolve client problems
	Participate in joint activities to evaluate the outcome of care
Liaison	Serve as initial point of contact between client and agency
	Facilitate communication between client and agency personnel
	Interpret and reinforce provider recommendations
	Serve as client advocate as needed

roles are community developer, coalition builder, and researcher. Population-oriented roles are essential because the health of the population cannot be accomplished merely by changes in individual or family health status or behaviors, but also rests on changes in larger social and environmental factors that affect health (SmithBattle, Diekemper, & Drake, 1999).

CASE FINDER

Case finding has been described as basic to community health nursing. *Case finding* by the community health nurse involves identifying individual cases or occurrences of specific diseases or other health-related conditions requiring services. Why, then, is this considered a population-oriented role? Despite the fact that case finding involves location of individual cases of a condition, the primary intent is the assessment and protection of the health of the general public. As we will see in Chapter 28, case finding is an important strategy in preventing the spread of communicable diseases in large population groups. Case finding is also a means of monitoring the health status of a group or community. For example, identifying more instances of child abuse may be an indication of a community health problem.

Community health nurses have a relatively close and often prolonged association with clients and have the opportunity to detect changes in health status or early signs of health problems. During a visit to a hypertensive client, for example, the community health nurse may discover that the client's teenage daughter is pregnant and in need of prenatal care. Or the nurse may observe that members of a number of families who obtain water from a common source have had recent episodes of vomiting and diarrhea. If the nurse is dealing with clients as unified entities (whether individuals, families, or communities), he or she is in a position to detect potential or actual health problems early and intervene rapidly. The ability of community health nurses to conduct physical examinations has further enhanced their case-finding ability by giving them another avenue for detecting the presence of disease or disability.

Case-finding responsibilities include developing an index of suspicion, identifying instances of disease or other health-related conditions, and providing follow-up services. An *index of suspicion* is an estimation of the likelihood that a disease or problem may exist and is based on a broad foundation of knowledge of the signs and symptoms of a variety of health problems and their contributing factors. For example, to identify a potential case of tuberculosis (TB), the nurse must be familiar with the signs and symptoms of TB. The nurse should also be aware of the factors associated with TB. The community health nurse who encounters a client from Asia (where the incidence of TB is relatively high) complaining of a chronic cough with hemoptysis, weight loss, and night sweats suspects TB.

The case-finder role necessitates use of the diagnostic reasoning process to identify potential cases of disease or instances of other health-related conditions (such as pregnancy or the need for immunizations) based on relevant cues. This diagnostic processing of relevant signs and symptoms into a probable diagnosis of the disease is the second function of the community health nurse as case finder.

The third community health nursing function related to case finding is the provision of follow-up care to the person or population with the identified condition. This usually entails referral of individual clients for further diagnostic services and for treatment if needed or initiation of population-based efforts to address the problem.

LEADER

Leadership in the community health nursing context is a requisite skill for community health nurses. The leadership role of the community health nurse may be enacted both with individual clients or families and with communities and populations; however, because this role demands knowledge of group dynamics as well as interpersonal skills, we deal with leadership as a population-oriented role.

Leadership is the ability to influence the behavior of others. Community health nurses may assume a leadership role with a variety of individuals, including clients, other health care professionals, members of other disciplines, public officials, and the general public. Because of the number of different types of followers that may be involved, the community health nurse as leader must be able to adapt a leadership style to fit the needs of the moment.

Community health nurse functions in the leadership role include identifying the need for action and leadership, assessing the leadership needs of followers, and selecting and executing a style of leadership appropriate to both the followers and the situation. The leadership process and the functions involved are discussed in greater detail in Chapter 13.

⑥THINK ABOUT IT

Which of the three categories of community health nursing roles do you think are most crucial to achieving the goals of community health nursing? Why?

CHANGE AGENT

Community health nurses also fill the role of change agent. A *change agent* is one who initiates and brings about change. Frequently, this role is performed in conjunction with the leadership role. Change is an unavoidable part of human existence, but when change is systematically planned, it can be controlled and used to enhance rather than undermine health. Specific functions of the community health nurse in the change agent role include recognizing the need for change, making others aware of the need for change, motivating others to change, and initiating and directing the desired change.

Community health nurses may serve as change agents working with individuals, families, groups, and communities or in health care delivery. For example, change may be required in the dietary patterns of individual clients or families. Or there may be a need to alter the way a community deals with the homeless or approaches sex education in its schools. Similar changes might be needed in the health care system. For example, services might need to be redesigned to meet the needs of ethnic minority groups moving into the area. Efforts to bring about changes in health care delivery to meet evolving societal needs have historically been an area of strength of community health nursing in the United States. If we are to continue to fulfill our role as community health nurses and achieve our purpose of improved health for all, we must renew our efforts as change agents at the population level. The change process and its implications for community health nursing are discussed in greater detail in Chapter 13.

COMMUNITY DEVELOPER

Community development is a planned process of mobilizing groups of people to take action to accomplish identified goals (Keller et al., 1998) and is part of the historical heritage of community health nursing (Rafael, 1999b). Studies of community health nurses indicate that they spend considerable amounts of time engaging in community development activities, but that these activities have become more difficult with the loss of direct contact with

community members as a result of decreasing services to individuals and families (Chalmers et al., 1998).

Community development promotes the participation of members of population groups in the control of their own lives and gives them the power to enact changes in circumstances that affect their health (Kuss et al., 1997). Functions of the community health nurse in the community developer role include assisting communities to identify health issues of concern and to collect data related to the issue, mobilizing members to action, and assisting with coalition development within the community. Additional functions related to this role include helping community members to identify goals, assisting in the determination of plausible strategies to meet those goals, and participating in strategy implementation. Community development will be discussed in more detail in Chapter 15.

⑥THINK ABOUT IT

What kinds of clinical learning experiences would best equip community health nurses to carry out the full spectrum of roles in this practice specialty?

COALITION BUILDER

As we saw in Chapter 4, coalition building is a strategy often used in political activism. *Coalition building* is the process of creating temporary or permanent alliances of individuals or groups to achieve a specific purpose. Considerations in developing coalitions have already been addressed (see Chapter 4). Functions of community health nurses as coalition builders include identifying potential coalition members, presenting the mutual benefit to be derived from alliance to potential coalition members, helping to delineate the goals of the coalition, assisting in the development of operating guidelines for the coalition, and participating in the selection and implementation of means to accomplish the goals of the alliance.

⑥THINK ABOUT IT

Should some of the community health nursing roles discussed in this chapter be the focus of practice in specific educational levels in nursing (e.g., ADN prepared nurse, BSN, MSN, etc.)? If so, which roles should be performed by nurses at which educational levels? Why?

RESEARCHER

A *researcher* explores phenomena observed in the world with the intent of understanding, explaining, and ultimately controlling them. The research role of the community health nurse is sometimes seen as a relatively recent one; however, even at the beginnings of community health nursing in the United States, Lillian Wald and her contemporaries made use of carefully documented data to identify societal needs and fuel social reforms. The community health nurse's current research role may be carried out at several levels. Responsibilities of the community health nurse related to research include critically reviewing relevant research and its application to practice, identifying researchable problems, designing and conducting research studies, collecting data, and disseminating research findings. Functions related to the role of researcher and other population-oriented community health nursing roles are summarized in Table 8–3 ■.

Community health nursing has as its primary goal the improvement of the health of the total population. This specialty area of nursing practice is characterized by population consciousness, orientation to health, autonomy, creativity, continuity, collaboration, intimacy, and variability. Community health nurses engage in client-oriented, delivery-oriented, and population-oriented roles. The degree of emphasis placed on the roles in each category, however, will vary from setting to setting.

♋CRITICAL THINKING IN RESEARCH

One of the needs in community health nursing practice is research to support the effectiveness of community health nursing interventions. Select one of the community health nursing roles discussed in the chapter and describe how you would conduct a study to evaluate the effectiveness of nursing interventions in that role. For example, you might study the effectiveness of nursing interventions in the referral resource role.

- What aspects of the role would you want to study? Why?
- What kind of study would you design? Why?
- How would you measure role effectiveness? What variables would you examine? How would you collect data related to those variables?
- How useful would information derived from your study be to community health nurses? Why?

■ **TABLE 8–3 Population-Oriented Community Health Nursing Roles and Related Functions**

ROLE	FUNCTION
Case finder	Develop knowledge of signs and symptoms of health-related conditions and contributing factors Use diagnostic reasoning process to identify potential cases of disease or other health-related conditions Provide follow-up care to identified cases
Leader	Identify the need for action Assess situation and followers to determine appropriate leadership style Motivate followers to take action Coordinate group member activities in planning and implementing action Assist followers to evaluate the effectiveness of action taken
Change agent	Recognize the need for change Alert others to the need for change Motivate others for change Initiate and direct change
Community developer	Assist community members to identify health issues of concern Participate in data collection relevant to issues of concern Mobilize community members to take action Assist with coalition development to foster community action Assist community members to identify achievable goals Participate in the development of strategies to accomplish identified goals Participate in the implementation of community strategies to achieve goals
Coalition builder	Identify potential coalition members based on common interest, assets available, etc. Present potential coalition members with the benefits to be achieved through alliance Participate in the delineation of coalition goals Assist in the development of operating guidelines for the coalition Participate in the selection and implementation of strategies to accomplish coalition goals
Researcher	Critically review research findings Apply research findings to practice as appropriate Identify researchable problems Design and conduct nursing research Collect and analyze data Disseminate research findings

assessment tips assessment tips assessment tips

ASSESSING COMMUNITY HEALTH NURSING PRACTICE

Assess the performance of community health nursing roles in several agencies in your area.

- To what extent are community health nurses in each agency engaged in client-oriented, delivery-oriented, and population-oriented roles?
- Looking at the full array of roles performed by community health nurses in your area, are the core func-

tions of public health being met? Is there an imbalance in the emphasis placed on the three categories of roles? Where does that imbalance lie?

- What actions might serve to correct an imbalance, if one exists? Would some agencies have greater responsibility for correcting the imbalance than others? Why or why not?

APPLYING YOUR KNOWLEDGE IN PRACTICE

✄ CASE STUDY
Improving Population Health Through Family Care

Ms. Brown, a community health nurse, has received a request to visit Mrs. Jones to inform her of a class II Pap smear from her last visit to the family planning clinic. On her record, Ms. Brown notes that Mrs. Jones is 45 years old, married, and has three children. When Ms. Brown arrives at the home and explains the reason for her visit, Mrs. Jones tells her that Mr. Jones is unemployed and they have no health insurance. She does not know how she will be able to afford to have a repeat Pap smear now.

Mrs. Jones is also concerned because she has not had a period for 2 months. She has been on birth control pills for several years and has had no problems with missed periods until now. Her periods have become rather scanty in the last few months. She has no complaints of urinary frequency or breast tenderness.

Mrs. Jones states that tensions have been high in the house because she and her husband suspect that their

15-year-old daughter is taking some kind of drugs. Her performance in school has dropped sharply and she has become withdrawn and moody. As far as Mrs. Jones knows, she has not had any problems with her friends or an argument with her boyfriend. Mrs. Jones tells you that she has heard that there is considerable drug use among the students at her daughter's high school.

- What client-oriented and delivery-oriented community health nursing roles will Ms. Brown probably perform in caring for Mrs. Jones and her family? Why are these roles appropriate to this situation?
- Give examples of some specific activities that Ms. Brown might carry out in performing each role.
- Is Ms. Brown likely to engage in any population-oriented roles in relation to this situation? If so, which ones is she likely to perform?

✄ TESTING YOUR UNDERSTANDING

- What is community health nursing? How does it differ from community-based nursing? (pp. 172–173)
- How does district nursing differ from program-focused nursing? How do both relate to population-focused nursing? (p. 173)

- Describe at least five attributes of community health nursing. Give an example of each attribute. (pp. 175–177)
- Describe the standards of care for community health nursing practice. How do they differ from

the standards of professional performance? (pp. 174–175)

- Distinguish among client-oriented, delivery-oriented, and population-oriented community health nursing roles. (pp. 177–186)
- What are the client-oriented roles of community health nurses? Give an example of the performance of each role. (pp. 177–182)

- Describe the three delivery-oriented roles performed by community health nurses. What functions are involved in each? How might you enact these roles with a family client? (pp. 182–183)
- What are the population-oriented roles of community health nurses? Give an example of the performance of each role. (pp. 183–186)

REFERENCES

American Nurses Association. (1986). *Standards of community health nursing practice.* Kansas City, MO: American Nurses Association.

American Public Health Association, Public Health Nursing Section (1996). *The definition and role of public health nursing: A statement of the APHA Public Health Nursing Section.* Washington, DC: American Public Health Association.

Anglin, L. T. (1990). The roles of nurses: A history, 1900 to 1988. Doctoral dissertation, Illinois State University.

Baldwin, J. H., Conger, C. O., Abegglen, J. C., & Hill, E. M. (1998). Population-focused and community-based nursing—Moving toward clarification of concepts. *Public Health Nursing, 15,* 12–18.

Bedell, J. R., Cohen, N. L., & Sullivan, A. (2000). Case management: The current best practices and the next generation of innovation. *Community Mental Health Journal, 36,* 179–194.

Bellack, J. P. (1998). Community-based nursing practice: Necessary but not sufficient. *Nurse Educator, 37*(3), 99–100.

Billings, J. (1998). Public health: A long time coming. *Nursing Times, 94*(28), 30–31.

Boyd, L. (2000). Advanced practice nursing today. *RN, 63*(9), 57–62.

Case Management Society of America. (1995). *Standards of practice for case management.* Little Rock, AR: Author.

Chalmers, K. I., Bramadat, I. J., & Andrusyszyn, M. (1998). The changing environment of community health practice and education: Perceptions of staff nurses, administrators, and educators. *Journal of Nursing Education, 37*(3), 109–117.

Chen, S. C., Ervin, N. E., Kim, Y., & Vonderheid, S. C. (1999). Competency in community-oriented health care: Instrument development. *Evaluation & the Health Professions, 22,* 358–370.

Clark, M. J. (2001). Voicing their voice: The structure of advocacy. Unpublished raw data.

Community Health Nurse's Interest Group. (1998). *Public Health Nursing Position Statement.* Toronto, Ontario: Author.

Diekemper, M., SmithBattle, L., & Drake, M. A. (1999a). Bringing the population into focus: A natural development in community health nursing practice. Part I. *Public Health Nursing, 16*(1), 3–10.

Diekemper, M., SmithBattle, L., & Drake, M. A. (1999b). Sharpening the focus: An intentional community health nursing approach. Part II. *Public Health Nursing, 16,* 11–16.

Division of Nursing. (2001). *The registered nurse population: National sample survey of registered nurses—March 2000.* Washington, DC: Author.

Erickson, G. (1996). To pauperize or empower: Public health nursing at the turn of the 20th and 21st centuries. *Public Health Nursing, 13,* 163–169.

Fahrenwald, N. L., Fischer, C., Boysen, R., & Maurer, R. (1999). Population-based clinical projects: Bridging community-based and public health concepts. *Nurse Educator, 24*(6), 28–32.

Gebbie, K. M., & Hwang, I. (2000). Preparing currently employed public health nurses for changes in the health system. *American Journal of Public Health, 90,* 716–720.

Hamer, S. B. (2000). Public health nursing: Identifying priorities. *Nursing Standard, 14*(30), 31–32.

Institute of Medicine. (1988). *The future of public health.* Washington, DC: National Academy Press.

Keller, L. O., Strohschein, S., Lia-Hoagberg, B., & Schaffer, M. (1998). Population-based public health nursing interventions: A model from practice. *Public Health Nursing, 15,* 207–215.

Krampitz, S. D. (1987). The Yale experiment: Innovation in nursing education. In C. Maggs (Ed.), *Nursing history: The state of the art* (pp. 60–73). London: Croom Helm.

Kuss, T., Proulx-Girard, L., Lovitt, S., Katz, C., & Kennelly, P. (1997). A public health nursing model. *Public Health Nursing, 14,* 81–91.

Michaels, C. (1997). Leading beyond traditional boundaries: A community nursing perspective. *Nursing Administration Quarterly, 22*(1), 30–37.

Murashima, S., Hatono, Y., Whyte, N., Asahara, K. (1999). Public health nursing in Japan: New opportunities for health promotion. *Public Health Nursing, 16,* 133–139.

Quad Council of Public Health Nursing Organizations. (1999). *Scope and standards of public health nursing practice.* Washington, DC: American Nurses Publishing.

Rafael, A. R. F. (1999a). From rhetoric to reality: The changing face of public health nursing in Southern Ontario. *Public Health Nursing, 16,* 50–59.

Rafael, A. R. F. (1999b). The politics of health promotion: Influences on public health promoting nursing practice in Ontario, Canada from Nightingale to the nineties. *Advances in Nursing Science, 22*(1), 23–39.

Reder, S., Gale, J. L., & Taylor, J. (1999). Using the dual method needs assessment to evaluate the training needs of public health professionals. *Journal of Public Health Management Practice, 5*(6), 62–69.

Salmon, M. E. (1998, fall). Guest editorial—The future of public health nursing: A state of mind. *Public Health Nursing Section Newsletter, 3,* 12.

SmithBattle, L., Diekemper, M., & Drake, M. A. (1999). Articulating the culture and tradition of community health nursing. *Public Health Nursing, 165,* 215–222.

Sullivan, T. J. (1998). Concept analysis of collaboration: Part I. In T. J. Sullivan (Ed.), *Collaboration: A health care imperative* (pp. 3–42). New York: McGraw-Hill.

Williams, D. B. (2000). Population care management: What's in it for your organization? *Nursing Case Management, 5,* 1.

THEORETICAL FOUNDATIONS FOR COMMUNITY HEALTH NURSING

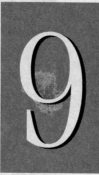

9

Chapter Objectives

After reading this chapter, you should be able to:

- Identify the need for a theoretical foundation for community health nursing.
- Describe the components of selected theoretical models for community health nursing.
- Apply selected theoretical models to community health nursing practice with individuals, families, and populations.

KEY TERMS

conceptual model 190
metaparadigm 190

Media Link

http://www.prenhall.com/clark

Additional interactive resources for this chapter can be found on the companion Web site. Click on Chapter 9 and "Begin" to select the activities for this chapter.

One of the hallmarks of a scientific profession is the unique body of knowledge that it uses to direct professional practice. This body of knowledge is the result of systematic, scientific inquiry involving the formulation and testing of theory. As is the case with other scientific disciplines, professional nursing practice needs a sound theoretical foundation that describes the interrelationships among key concepts. These concepts form the metaparadigm for the discipline. A *metaparadigm* is a global overview or explanation of a discipline. The metaparadigm for nursing traditionally encompasses the four related concepts of person, health, environment, and nursing (Parker, 2001).

Nurse theorists have developed unique perspectives on the relationships among the concepts of the nursing metaparadigm to create different conceptual models. A *conceptual model* is a schematic or verbal picture of the interrelationships that exist among concepts. A number of conceptual models have been developed to guide nursing practice and several of them are applicable to community health nursing.

Effective nursing practice is facilitated when nurses use a systematic approach to clients, their health status, and the nursing interventions needed to promote, maintain, or restore health. Conceptual or theoretical models provide such an approach. If used consistently, a theoretical model assists the nurse to evaluate the client's health and to plan, implement, and evaluate effective nursing care to improve health. The model directs the nurse's attention to relevant aspects of the client situation and to interventions that are apt to be most effective in that situation.

To direct practice, nursing models must incorporate three basic components: the client, the goal of nursing intervention, and the activities involved in nursing intervention. A nursing model must define the client or recipient of nursing action. Is the nursing client always someone who is ill or can the client be a healthy individual? Can the recipient of care be a family or a population rather than an individual? The model must also specify the expected outcome of nursing intervention. Different nursing models use different terms to express outcomes, for example, *adaptation, reconstitution,* and *self-care.* The final requisite for a nursing model is a description of the nurse's activities in providing care. Again, depending on the nursing model, these activities may be educative, curative, restorative, supportive, preventive, and so on.

THEORETICAL MODELS ADAPTED FOR COMMUNITY HEALTH NURSING

All of the initial theoretical models for nursing were developed to assist nurses in the care of individual clients. Some of these models were adapted by community health nurses for use with families and communities or population groups. For example, previous community health nursing texts examined several of the traditional nursing conceptual models and demonstrated their application to community health nursing (Clark, 1984, 1992, 1996, 1999; Hanchett, 1988). Other authors have applied a single conceptual model in community health nursing practice (Dixon, 1999; Jaarsma, Halfens, Senten, Saad, & Dracup, 1998) or research (Gigliotti, 1999; Hart & Foster, 1998; Levesque, Ricard, Ducharme, Duquette, & Bonin, 1998).

More recently, one of the traditional nursing models has been specifically revised for use by community health nurses. Anderson and McFarlane (1996) based their community-as-partner model on Neuman's Health Systems model. Both the original model and the revised model will be discussed briefly.

Neuman's Health Systems Model

Neuman's health systems model involves a client system striving to prevent "penetration" or disruption of the system by a variety of stressors. A *stressor* is a problem or condition capable of causing instability in the system. The client's state of health is dependent on the degree of success achieved in preventing penetration of the client system by stressors or in effecting "reconstitution" of the system after penetration by stressors. Nursing intervention is indicated whenever the client is unable to prevent penetration or accomplish reconstitution without assistance (Aylward, 2001).

In Neuman's model, the client is viewed as a composite of a basic structure, lines of resistance, and normal and flexible lines of defense (Neuman, 1994). These elements of the client are depicted in Figure 9–1 ■. The client system is protected from penetration by the flexible line of defense. The *basic structure* is the inner core of the client that must be maintained to ensure survival. Penetration of the basic structure results in death.

The *normal line of defense* is the client's usual state of wellness or the normal range of response to stressors. The *flexible line of defense* is a dynamic state of wellness that changes over time and is composed of factors that fluctuate. The flexible line of defense provides a protective cushion that prevents stressors from penetrating the normal line of defense (Freese et al., 1998).

When the flexible line of defense is incapable of protecting the system, penetration of the normal line of defense occurs. The extent of penetration and the degree of reaction to penetration are influenced by physiological, psychological, sociocultural, developmental, and spiritual variables in the client situation. *Lines of resistance* are internal factors that act to return the client to a normal or improved state of health and protect against stressor penetration of the basic structure (Freese et al., 1998).

Once stressor penetration of the client system occurs, the system engages in activities aimed at reconstitution. *Reconstitution* involves stabilization of the system and movement back toward the normal line of defense. The normal line of defense may be stabilized at a level either

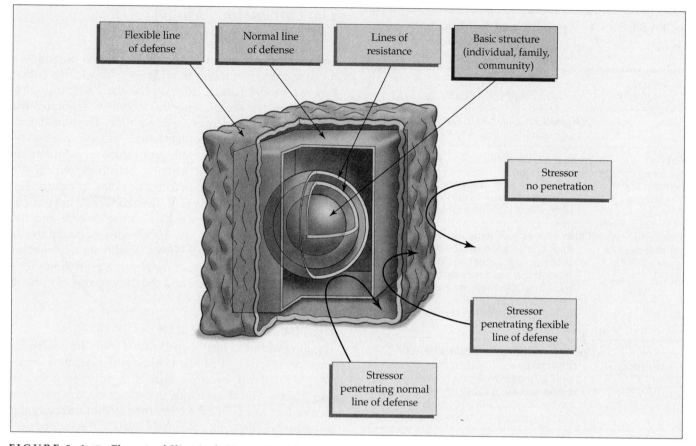

FIGURE 9–1 ■ *Elements of Client in the Neuman Model*
Adapted from Neuman, B. (1994). The Neuman systems model. In B. Neuman (Ed.), *The Neuman systems model* (3rd ed.). Norwalk, CT: Appleton & Lange.

higher or lower than that prior to penetration. For the client system to survive stressor penetration, reconstitution must take place before penetration of the basic structure can occur. Nursing intervention is indicated whenever a client system is unable to prevent penetration by a stressor or to accomplish reconstitution on its own. Nursing intervention occurs at the three levels discussed in Chapter 1: primary, secondary, and tertiary prevention.

Community-as-Partner Model

Anderson and McFarlane (1996) based their community-as-partner model (originally the community-as-client model) on Neuman's health systems model and the nursing process. In the community-as-partner model, the client for nursing care is the community or population group. The inner core consists of the people who make up the community along with their beliefs, values, and history. The core is surrounded by eight community subsystems that affect community members and are, in turn affected by them. These subsystems include those related to the physical environment, education, safety and transportation, politics and government, health and social services, communication, economics, and recreation. Factors in these subsystems may affect the flexible line of defense or the community's lines of resistance.

The normal line of defense in this model represents the community's usual level of wellness and its problem-

solving or coping capacities. The flexible line of defense is a changing level of community health in response to stressors. As in the Neuman model, the client possesses lines of resistance or internal capacities to deal with stressor penetration.

The community health nurse using the community-as-partner model participates with members of the community to assess the health status of the community core and factors in the eight subsystems that affect health as well as the strength of the normal and flexible lines of defense and the lines of resistance. The nurse and community also assess for potential stressors occurring from within or outside the community and the degree of community reaction when stressor penetration has occurred. Nurse and community together develop community health diagnoses and plan, implement, and evaluate interventions at the appropriate level of prevention (Anderson & McFarlane, 1996). Table 9–1 ■ applies concepts of the community-as-partner model to the community health problem of increased tobacco use among adolescents.

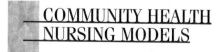

COMMUNITY HEALTH NURSING MODELS

Although Neuman's health systems model and its adaptation in the community-as-partner model have utility in

■ **TABLE 9–1**   Application of the Community-as-Partner Model to the Problem of Adolescent Tobacco Use

MODEL CONCEPT	APPLICATION
Core	Adolescent population in the community; community attitudes to tobacco use
Stressor	Increased tobacco use among adolescents
Normal line of defense	Community's usual response to tobacco use, prior history of ability to cope with similar problems
Flexible line of defense	Other factors impinging on the community's ability to deal with the problem (e.g., recent loss of local recreational resources for teens—recreational subsystem; current government instability due to recent political scandals—governmental subsystem)
Lines of resistance	Limited education on health effects of tobacco use—education subsystem; media images fostering tobacco use—communication subsystem; failure of police to enforce laws regarding tobacco sales to minors—safety subsystem
Primary prevention	Educational campaigns targeted to social perceptions of tobacco use aimed specifically at adolescents; enforcement of tobacco sales laws; initiation of adolescent social activities that preclude tobacco use (e.g., smoke-free rock concerts); removal of tobacco vending machines from public places
Secondary prevention	Identification and referral of adolescent tobacco users to smoking cessation programs

community health nursing practice, models designed specifically for community health nursing practice may be more useful. Such models have been slow in coming (Clarke, 1998), but there are now several models developed specifically for population-based practice in community health nursing. Five such models will be presented here including the dimensions model of community health nursing, the Florida Atlantic University community nursing model, Pender's health promotion model, and the public health nursing interventions and public health nursing models.

⑥ THINK ABOUT IT

Why has community health nursing been slow to develop its own theoretical models?

The Dimensions Model of Community Health Nursing

The dimensions model of community health nursing is a revision of the previously titled Epidemiologic Prevention Process Model (Clark, 1996). Like the community-as-partner model, the dimensions model incorporates the nursing process and levels of prevention. The model also, however, includes an epidemiologic perspective on the factors that influence health and illness in populations and addresses relevant nursing activities within the dimensions of nursing that affect population health. The dimensions model consists of three elements: the dimensions of health, the dimensions of health care and the dimensions of nursing. The dimensions of health guide the nurse's assessment of clients' health status, whether the client is an individual, a family, or a population. The dimensions of health care and the dimensions of nursing guide nursing interventions.

THE DIMENSIONS OF HEALTH

The dimensions of health are derived from the epidemiologic perspective of public health, which acknowledges the interaction of multiple factors in population health and illness. The dimensions consist of six categories of factors that can be used to organize a community health assessment. These six categories include the biophysical dimension, the psychological dimension, the physical environmental dimension, the sociocultural dimension, the behavioral dimension, and the health system dimension.

THE BIOPHYSICAL DIMENSION   The biophysical dimension includes factors related to human biology that influence health. These factors may be related to age and developmental level, genetic inheritance, and physiologic function. Age can affect one's susceptibility to illness or the potential for exposure to other risk factors. Genetic inheritance encompasses gender and racial/ethnic characteristics as well as the specific gene pattern transferred by one's parents. Certain health problems are more frequently associated with some gender or racial/ethnic groups than with others. The presence of certain genetically transmitted traits also increases one's risk of developing some health problems.

Factors related to physiologic function include one's basic state of health as it affects the probability of developing other health problems. Considerations in this area would include the presence or absence of other disease states. For example, obesity is a physiologic factor that contributes to a variety of health problems including heart disease, diabetes, and stroke. Immunity is another aspect of physiologic function that affects susceptibility to disease. The concept of immunity is discussed in more detail in Chapter 10.

When assessing populations, rather than individuals, the age, gender, and racial/ethnic composition of the groups would be determined. Other information related to the components of the biophysical dimension include the prevalence of genetic traits for specific health conditions, the prevalence of specific physiologic conditions in the population (e.g., pregnancy, diabetes), and population levels of immunity.

THE PSYCHOLOGICAL DIMENSION The psychological dimension encompasses the health effects of both internal and external psychological environments. Depression and low self-esteem are two factors in one's internal psychological environment that contribute to a variety of health problems including suicide, substance abuse, family violence, and obesity. External psychological factors can also influence the development of health problems. For example, a person who has a great deal of emotional support in a crisis is less likely to attempt suicide than a person who faces a crisis without such support. Stress is another factor in the external psychological environment that is associated with a variety of health problems. The ability to cope with stress, on the other hand, is a factor in one's internal psychological environment.

Psychological dimension determinants at the population level would include the incidence and prevalence of psychiatric disorders, the amount of stress experienced by members of the population, and the extent of coping behaviors among individual members of the population. Another important factor to be assessed in the population is the capacity to deal with adverse events. For example, is the community able to cope with increased numbers of homeless individuals or with increasing unemployment?

THE PHYSICAL ENVIRONMENTAL DIMENSION While the psychological dimension addresses aspects of one's psychological environment, the physical environmental dimension encompasses the health effects of factors in the physical environment. The physical environment consists of weather, geographic locale, soil composition, terrain, temperature and humidity, and hazards posed by poor housing and unsafe working conditions. Additional elements of the physical environment that affect health include light and heat, exposure to pathogens and allergens, radiation, pollution, and noise. The health effects of physical environmental factors were addressed in detail in Chapter 7. Using the dimensions model, the community health nurse would assess the population for the presence of environmental conditions detrimental to health.

THE SOCIOCULTURAL DIMENSION The sociocultural dimension consists of those factors within the social environment that influence health, either positively or negatively. Elements of the social structure such as employment, economics, politics, ethics, and legal influences all fall within this dimension of health. The sociocultural dimension also includes societal norms and culturally accepted modes of behavior. Another important factor in the sociocultural dimension is prevailing attitudes toward specific health problems. For example, the fear and stigma attached to HIV infection may seriously hamper efforts to control the spread of disease. Substance abuse, mental illness, family violence, and adolescent pregnancy are other examples of health problems in which social attitudes contribute to the problem or hinder the solution.

Societal action with respect to health behaviors also falls within this dimension. For example, legislative actions to increase cigarette taxes have been shown to lead to reduced smoking in the populations affected. The sociocultural dimension can also influence health in other ways. Congregating in large groups, particularly indoors during the winter, enhances the spread of certain diseases such as colds and influenza. Media portrayals of a variety of healthy and unhealthy behaviors are another way in which the sociocultural dimension influences health and illness. Occupation is another aspect of the sociocultural dimension that may influence health. Many of the factors in the sociocultural dimension were addressed in the chapters related to economics, politics, and culture.

Community health nurses using the dimensions model with populations would assess the effects of sociocultural dimension factors on the health of the public. For example, the nurse might examine the unemployment rate in the population and the consequent effects on access to health care services.

THE BEHAVIORAL DIMENSION The behavioral dimension consists of personal behaviors that either promote or impair health. Behavioral factors are often those most amenable to change in efforts to prevent disease and promote health and, so, are of particular importance in community health nursing practice. Health-related behaviors include dietary patterns, recreation and exercise, substance use and abuse, sexual activity, and use of protective measures.

Dietary habits can either enhance or undermine health, and both leanness and obesity can predispose one to other health problems. Exercise patterns also influence health status as do smoking, drinking, and drug use. Recreational activities may pose health risks, but may also improve both physical and emotional health. Sexual activity poses risks related to pregnancy and sexually transmitted diseases. Failure to use protective measures such as contraceptives or barrier devices during intercourse can also increase one's chances of health problems. Similarly, not wearing seat belts or motorcycle helmets increases the potential for serious injury.

THE HEALTH SYSTEM DIMENSION The final dimension to be considered is the health system dimension. The way in which health care services are organized and their availability, accessibility, affordability, appropriateness, adequacy, acceptability, and use influence the health of individual clients and population groups. Availability refers to the type and number of health services present in a community, and accessibility reflects the ability of clients to make use of those services. Affordability, the ability to pay for services, also influences health outcomes. Service appropriateness refers to a health care system's ability to provide those services needed and desired by its clientele. The adequacy of health services refers to the quality and amount of service provided relative to need, and acceptability reflects the level of congruence between services provided and the expectations, values, and beliefs of the target population. Finally, the extent to which members of the population actually make use of available health care services will influence health status.

Health system factors can influence health status either positively or negatively. For example, immunization services that are available and easily accessible to all community members promote control of communicable diseases such as measles, polio, and tetanus. Conversely, the failure of health professionals to take advantage of immunization opportunities contributes to increased incidence of these diseases.

As we saw in Chapter 5, some health care system contributions to health problems stem from the economics of health care delivery. The high cost of health services limits the ability of many individuals to take advantage of them. In other instances, inappropriate actions on the part of health care providers may actually contribute to health problems. For example, inappropriate use of antibiotics has contributed to the development of antibiotic-resistant strains of gonorrhea and syphilis. Elements of the dimensions of health are summarized at right.

The community health nurse uses the dimensions of health to collect and organize data regarding client health status. Factors in each of the six dimensions may apply to clients at multiple levels, including individuals, families, groups, communities, and populations. From the data, the community health nurse derives community health diagnoses that guide the planning of nursing interventions.

THE DIMENSIONS OF HEALTH CARE

Nursing interventions for identified health needs in the population are planned within the dimensions of health care. The dimensions of health care include primary prevention, secondary prevention, and tertiary prevention.

Primary prevention was defined by the originators of the term as "measures designed to promote general optimum health or . . . the specific protection of man against disease agents" (Leavell & Clark, 1965, p. 20). Primary prevention involves action taken prior to the occurrence of health problems and encompasses aspects of health promotion and protection. In its health promotion aspect, primary prevention focuses on improving the overall health of individuals, families, and population groups. Health protection is aimed at preventing the occurrence of specific health problems. For example, immunization is a protective measure for certain communicable diseases. The health protection aspect of primary prevention may also involve reducing or eliminating risk factors as a means of preventing disease.

HIGHLIGHTS

The Dimensions of Health

Biophysical Dimension

- Age
- Genetics
- Physiologic function

Psychological Dimension

- Internal psychological environment
- External psychological environment

Physical Environmental Dimension

- Physical environment
- Environmental hazards

Sociocultural Dimension

- Social structure
- Societal norms
- Societal attitudes
- Social action

Behavioral Dimension

- Dietary practices
- Recreation and exercise
- Substance use and abuse
- Sexual activity
- Use of protective measures

Health System Dimension

- Availability
- Accessibility
- Affordability
- Appropriateness
- Adequacy
- Acceptability
- Use

Secondary prevention focuses on the early identification and treatment of existing health problems and occurs after the health problem has arisen. In community health practice at this stage, the major emphasis is on resolving health problems and preventing serious consequences. Secondary prevention activities include screening and early diagnosis, as well as treatment for existing health problems.

Tertiary prevention is activity aimed at returning the client to the highest level of function and preventing further deterioration in health. In community health nursing, tertiary prevention also focuses on preventing recurrences

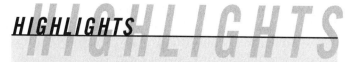

HIGHLIGHTS

The Dimensions of Health Care

Primary Prevention
- Prevention of the occurrence of a condition or problem
- Health promotion
- Illness and injury prevention

Secondary Prevention
- Screening
- Diagnosis
- Treatment

Tertiary Prevention
- Prevention of consequences
- Treatment of consequences
- Prevention of recurrence

and willing to act for the benefit of clients rather than for personal gain. Willingness to advocate for clients is another element of the ethical dimension of community health nursing. Aspects of the ethical dimension influence all of the other dimensions of nursing.

The skills dimension of community health nursing encompasses both manipulative and intellectual skills which are common to all areas of nursing practice. Manipulative skills include the ability to perform such activities as giving immunizations, providing tuberculin skin tests, conducting hearing examinations and physical assessments, and so on. Intellectual skills include capacities for critical thinking as well as abilities to examine data and draw inferences.

Community health nurses employ knowledge, attitudes, and skills in the application of several specific processes when providing care to individuals, families, and

of the problem. A particular nursing intervention may be viewed as a primary, secondary, or tertiary preventive measure depending on its relationship to the occurrence of a problem. If the intervention is designed to prevent the problem from occurring, it is primary prevention. For example, regular exercise can promote health. If the intent is to resolve an existing problem, the intervention involves secondary prevention. Exercise for the obese client as a way of losing weight would be secondary prevention. When the intervention is intended to prevent long-term consequences of an existing or former problem, it is tertiary prevention. For example, exercise after a broken leg is tertiary prevention designed to prevent muscle atrophy and contractures. The dimensions of health care are summarized above.

THE DIMENSIONS OF NURSING

The dimensions of nursing include the cognitive, interpersonal, ethical, skill, process, and reflective dimensions. The cognitive dimension of community health nursing practice encompasses the knowledge needed for the nurse to identify client health needs and to plan and implement care to meet those needs. This knowledge includes concepts drawn from multiple disciplines in addition to nursing. The interpersonal dimension includes affective elements and interaction skills. Affective elements consist of the attitudes and values of the community health nurse that influence his or her ability to practice effectively with a variety of different people. Interaction skills and the abilities to collaborate and communicate effectively with others are additional elements of the interpersonal dimension.

In the ethical dimension, the community health nurse acts in accord with moral and ethical principles. Community health nurses must be able to make ethical decisions

HIGHLIGHTS

The Dimensions of Nursing

Cognitive Dimension
- Knowledge

Interpersonal Dimension
- Affective elements
- Interaction skills

Ethical Dimension
- Ethical decision making
- Advocacy

Skills Dimension
- Manipulative skills
- Intellectual skills

Process Dimension
- Nursing process
- Epidemiologic process
- Health education process
- Home visit process
- Case management process
- Change process
- Leadership process
- Group process
- Political process

Reflective Dimension
- Theory development
- Research
- Evaluation

population groups. The most fundamental of these processes is, of course, the nursing process. Other processes used by community health nurses in their practice are the epidemiologic process, the health education process, the home visit process and the case management process. Community health nurses also use change, leadership, group, and political processes in their care of clients. These processes and others compose the process dimension of community health nursing. Many of these processes are addressed in greater detail in later chapters of this book.

The reflective dimension is the final dimension of nursing in the model. In the reflective dimension, community health nurses reflect on their care through theory development, research, and evaluation. The creation of the dimensions model is, itself, an example of theory development in community health nursing. The importance of the other elements of the reflective dimension, research and evaluation of practice, is emphasized in each chapter of this book. The dimensions of nursing are summarized on page 195.

In the dimensions model, nursing actions occur in the context of the nursing process, as depicted in Figure 9–2 ■. The dimensions of health, for example, are used to guide assessment of the client's health status and to derive nursing diagnoses. The dimensions of health care direct the planning, implementation, and evaluation of nursing interventions. For instance, the nurse may plan and implement a community immunization fair as a primary preventive measure and then evaluate the effects of the fair in terms of the resulting increase in community

immunization levels and subsequent decrease in incidence rates for immunizable diseases.

The dimensions of nursing are also employed in the context of the nursing process. For example, the nurse uses intellectual skills and cognitive knowledge of causative factors in health problems to assess health and derive nursing diagnoses. Similarly, the nurse might need to use interpersonal skills in collecting assessment data as well as in engaging members of the community in planning and implementing strategies to resolve identified health problems. Elements of the process dimension such as the health education process and the leadership process may also be required in implementing a plan of care. Finally, elements of the reflective dimension of nursing are used in the evaluation of nursing interventions and in the development of theory that provides the knowledge base for the cognitive dimension. Table 9–2 ■ summarizes the application of the dimensions of health to the problem of high incidence and prevalence of obesity in a university population.

Florida Atlantic University Community Nursing Model

The community health nursing model developed by the faculty of the Florida Atlantic University (FAU) (Parker & Barry, 1999) was designed to guide community health nursing practice in school-based nursing centers, but could be applied in a variety of settings and populations. The model consists of a central core of essential services surrounded by three concentric circles as depicted in

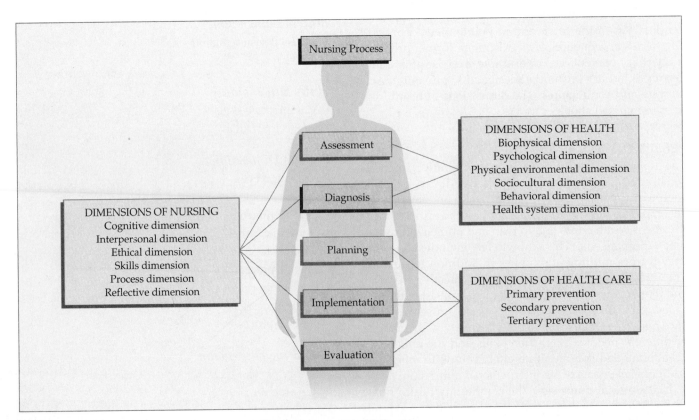

FIGURE 9–2 ■ *Elements of the Dimensions Model of Community Health Nursing*

■ **TABLE 9–2   Application of the Dimensions of Health to the Problem of Obesity in a University Population**

MODEL CONCEPT	APPLICATION
Biophysical dimension	Age composition of the population; prevalence of obesity in the population
Psychological dimension	Population attitudes to obesity, stress of college life; extent of use of food as stress reliever; extent of exposure to stressful circumstances; prevalence of eating disorders on campus
Physical environmental dimension	Weather conducive to outdoor exercise; facilities available for obese members of the population (e.g., size of classroom chairs)
Sociocultural dimension	Use of eating and drinking as social activities; extent of peer support for healthy life styles; availability of education for healthy lifestyles
Behavioral dimension	Dietary practices in campus population; availability of healthy foods in campus dining facilities; availability of recreational activities and equipment; extent of participation in physical activity among campus population; sedentary nature of university life
Health system dimension	Health center staff attention to weight problems among campus community members; availability of weight/diet counseling programs; availability of stress-reduction/counseling programs

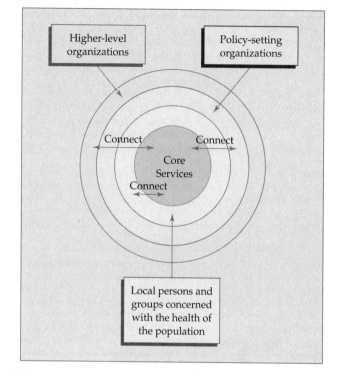

FIGURE 9–3 ■ *Elements of the Florida Atlantic University Community Nursing Model*

Figure 9–3 ■. The central core includes nursing services provided to enhance, promote, and protect health and enhance safety. These core services are based on essential values of respect for person, caring, and wholeness. Core services include design and coordination of care, health education, screening, services to protect well-being (e.g., immunizations), primary care services, and services to nurture wholeness (e.g., mentoring, self-care).

The first circle in the model involves persons and groups in the setting that have a common interest in the health of the population in that setting. Service activities within the first circle include consultation and collaboration services (including community assessment and community development activities) and evaluation and further development of services to the population. The second circle contains local organizations and groups that are concerned with the health of similar groups in related settings (e.g., in the case of a school population, the second circle might include the school district, local health department, and so on). Organizations in the second circle develop policy for the settings that comprise the first circle. Community health nursing activities in this circle

involve consultation and collaboration in policy development, staff development activities, and research and evaluation with application of research findings to the setting. The third circle represents agencies and organizations at higher societal levels (e.g., state, region, and nation) that influence health in the target setting.

Connections between the core and the circles are also depicted in the model. The primary connection between the core services and the first circle lies in assessing the needs of constituencies in the setting and designing nursing services to address those needs. This assessment is conducted by the authors of the model primarily through the use of community-based inquiry groups that identify health care needs in the population. Inquiry groups also participate in evaluation of program services (Parker, Barry, & King, 2000). Connections to the second circle lie in collaborative activities with policy making bodies that influence the design and implementation of services. The primary connection between the service core and the third circle involves the dissemination of findings related to the effects of services provided in the core and support for continuation of services (e.g., legislative funding bills). Table 9–3 ■ presents an application of the FAU community nursing model to the population of pregnant women in a community.

Pender's Health Promotion Model

Nola Pender has developed a nursing model that directs nursing intervention for health promotion. Because health promotion is a major emphasis in community health nursing, Pender's model is presented here even though it

MODEL CONCEPT	APPLICATION
Core	Pregnancy-related services available in the community; prenatal services; nurse midwifery services; birthing centers; delivery services; childbirth preparation classes; financial assistance for pregnancy-related services
First circle	Demographics of pregnant women in the community: age distribution, ethnicity, parity; cultural beliefs and practices related to pregnancy and childbirth; economic status; extent to which pregnancies are planned/desired; service needs and desires among the population; providers of prenatal, labor, and delivery services; local hospitals, clinics, and private providers; availability of transportation to needed services
Connections	Core services are designed to meet the needs and desires of the population involved; core services are also designed to assure an acceptable income for providers to assure ability to continue to provide care; core services address ancillary needs (e.g., transportation and child care needs of pregnant women)
Second circle	Groups responsible for policy related to pregnancy services: county social service agencies; local hospitals, local health department
Connection	Core service providers participate in policy development to assure provision of optimal services to pregnant women in the population; second circle agencies develop policies that facilitate core services provision
Third Circle	State health department, federal/state Medicaid programs, foundation funding sources
Connection	Third circle organizations develop policies and funding mechanisms that support provision of core services; providers of core services conduct and report on research that informs policy development

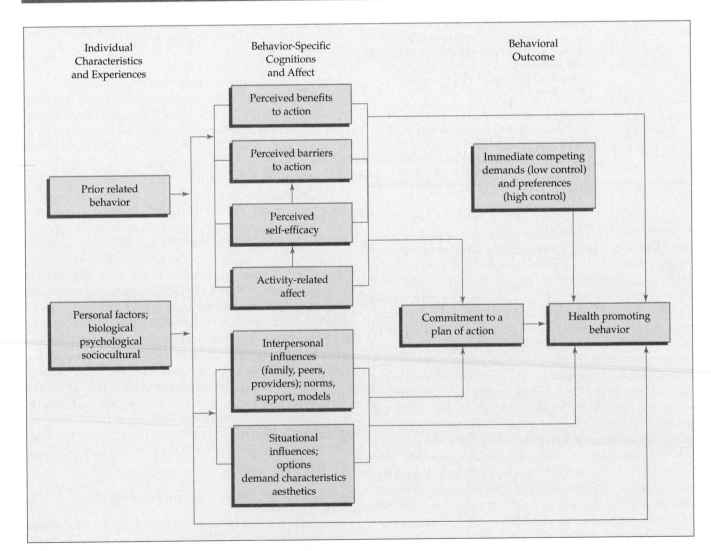

FIGURE 9–4 ■ *Elements of Pender's Health Promotion Model*

Reprinted by permission of Pearson Education, Inc. Upper Saddle River, NJ. Pender, N. J. (1996). *Health promotion in nursing practice* (3rd ed.) Stamford, CT: Appleton & Lange.

addresses only one aspect of community health nursing. Components of the model are depicted in Figure 9–4 ■. In the health promotion model, behavior is influenced by individual characteristics and behavior-specific cognitions and affect that result in a commitment to action. Commitment to action results in actual behavior but may be modified by competing demands and preferences (Pender, 1996). Individual characteristics include personal biological, psychological, and sociocultural factors that are relevant to the behavior involved. Prior behavior in this area is another individual characteristic that influences health-promoting behavior. For example, a client who was physically active prior to pregnancy will be more likely to engage in exercise after delivery than one who was not.

Behavior-specific cognitions and attitudes include the perceived benefits of and barriers to health-promoting activity as well as one's perceived self-efficacy. For example, the community that does not perceive itself as able to cope with the problem of inadequate housing will probably not take any action to resolve the problem. Activity-related affect or feeling states related to the behavior, to oneself, or to the situation are also important in motivating health-promoting behavior. Interpersonal and situational influences are additional factors related to cognition and affect that influence behavior. For example, if family members support weight loss, a client is more likely to stick to a diet. Conversely, low income, a situational influence, might adversely affect the client's weight loss options.

Individual characteristics and behavior-specific cognitions and affect may lead to a commitment to health promoting activity. Commitment includes both the intention to act and a specific plan of action. Commitment to action should lead to performance of the actual health-promoting behavior unless there is interference from competing demands and preferences. For example, the client's intention to diet may be subverted by a family member's serious illness and the need to eat in fast food restaurants near the hospital.

Although Pender's model was developed to be used to enhance health promoting behavior with individual clients, it can also be applied to population groups. Community health nurses can use the model to predict the likelihood that communities or population groups will take desired health promoting actions. Table 9–4 ■ depicts the application of Pender's model to a commnity experiencing a high incidence of adolescent pregnancy.

■ **TABLE 9–4**   **Application of Pender's Health Promotion Model to a Community Problem of Adolescent Pregnancy**

MODEL CONCEPT	APPLICATION
Individual Characteristics	
Prior related behavior	If prior proposals to initiate school-based clinics were met with community furor, community action related to adolescent pregnancy is unlikely to occur.
Biological factors	A concomitant outbreak of Ebola virus disease and related mortality may receive greater priority for community action than the problem of adolescent pregnancy.
Psychological factors	Denial by community members of widespread sexual activity among adolescents will not lead to community action related to adolescent pregnancy.
Sociocultural factors	If the community views pregnancy as a fitting consequence of adolescent sexual activity, action is unlikely.
Cognitions and Affect	
Perceived benefit	If the community perceives prenatal care for pregnant adolescents as less expensive than possible maternal and infant complications, the potential for action is enhanced.
Perceived barriers	If community politicians see supporting contraceptive services for adolescents as jeopardizing their chances of reelection, action is unlikely.
Self-efficacy	If the community was able to successfully initiate sex education at all grade levels, the probability of taking action related to adolescent pregnancy is enhanced.
Activity-related affect	If the community fears contraceptive availability will promote adolescent sexual activity, action is unlikely.
Interpersonal influences	If the state mandates pregnancy-related services for adolescents, community action is likely.
Situational influences	If closure of a major local industry has adversely affected the local tax base, funds may not be available for programs to deal with adolescent pregnancy.

CRITICAL THINKING IN RESEARCH

Select a proposition suggested by one of the models discussed in the chapter. For example, you might select a proposition from the dimensions model that suggests that health system factors can actually contribute to health problems as well as resolve them or a proposition from Pender's model that competing demands may affect action even when people intend to engage in health promoting behaviors.

- What is the proposition that you have derived from the model?
- How might you go about testing the validity of your proposition?
- What variables would you measure? Where might you obtain your data and how would you go about collecting it?
- What implications might the findings of your study have for community health nursing practice? Who should be apprised of the results of your study?

THINK ABOUT IT

What features in a model do you think would be useful in community health nursing practice? Which of the models presented in the chapter, if any, have these features?

The Public Health Nursing Interventions Model

The public health nursing interventions model was developed by the Minnesota Department of Health, Section of Public Health Nursing and is based on input from expert community health nursing consultants and practicing public health nurses (Keller, Strohschein, Lia-Hoagberg, & Schaffer, 1998). The model, as depicted in Figure 9–5 ■, consists of 17 identified community health nursing interventions that cross over three levels of population-based practice: individual-focused, community-focused, and systems-focused practice. According to the authors, the core functions of public health, assessment, policy development, and assurance are incorporated to some degree in each of the interventions at each level of practice.

Interventions are defined as categories of action by community health nurses in the care of individuals, families, and communities or population groups. Population-based individual-focused interventions are those that nurses provide to individuals and families within a designated population. Population-based community-focused interventions are directed toward communities or population groups and are designed to change community norms, attitudes and behaviors. Population-based systems-focused interventions are directed at policy and program development within health care systems (Keller et al., 1998).

Categories of interventions in the model include advocacy, case management, coalition building, collaboration, community organizing, consultation, counseling, delegated medical treatment and observation, disease investigation, and health teaching. Additional interventions are related to outreach and case finding, policy development, provider education, referral and follow-up, screening, social marketing, and surveillance. Many of these interventions were discussed in the context of the community health nursing roles presented in Chapter 8. Others are addressed in more detail in later chapters in this book. Table 9–5 ■ applies the interventions to the three levels of community health nursing practice.

THINK ABOUT IT

Are some of the models described in this chapter more useful for guiding community health nursing practice than others? If so, which ones and why?

Public Health Nursing Model

The public health nursing model developed by Kuss and associates (Kuss, Proulx-Girouard, Lovitt, Katz, & Kennelly, 1997) provides a means of conceptualizing public health or community health nursing rather than as a guide for practice. In this respect, it is more philosophical and less practical than the models described previously. In the model, community health nursing is pictured as a flowering tree depicted in Figure 9–6 ■. The grass surrounding the base of the tree represents community empowerment, participation of community members and groups in action to support their own health. The roots of the tree lie in the history of community health nursing and the education that provides a foundation for practice. The tree trunk symbolizes the cadre of

ETHICAL AWARENESS

Community health agencies may provide services within the context of a particular model that the agency has adopted. All of the nursing personnel who work at the agency are expected to use that model as the basis for practice. What might be the ethical arguments for such requirements? What ethical arguments might be raised against them?

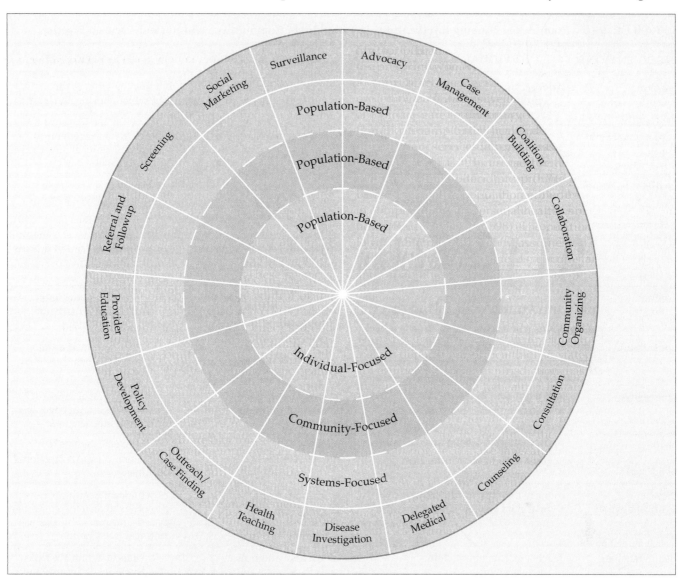

FIGURE 9–5 ■ *Elements of the Public Health Nursing Interventions Model*

From Keller, L.O., Strohschein, S., Lia-Hoagberg, B., & Schaffer, M. (1998). Population-based public health nursing interventions: A model from practice. *Public Health Nursing, 15,* 207–215. Reprinted by permission of Blackwell Science, Inc.

community health nurses and the core competencies they possess. These core competencies are similar to the intervention categories described above. Like the trunk of a tree, community health nurses support and nurture other aspects of the tree and permit the accomplishment of population health goals. This support and nurturance often involves interdisciplinary collaboration.

The bifurcation of branches from the tree trunk represents community empowerment at another level, that of taking power to produce change with the assistance of community health nurses. Tree branches symbolize the levels of clients served by community health nursing in

⑥THINK ABOUT IT

Are there other nursing models that could be adapted for use in community health nursing practice? Could they be used with all three levels of client (individual, family, and community)?

CULTURAL CONSIDERATIONS

Nursing theoretical models developed in the United States have often been adopted wholesale in other countries. Many times these adoptions have not been a good fit for the countries in which they were used. Why do you think this would be true? Which of the community health nursing models described here might be applicable in other cultures and countries? Where might they be most applicable? Why?

■ **TABLE 9–5   Examples of Nursing Interventions in Individual-, Community-, and System-Focused Practice**

INTERVENTIONS	INDIVIDUAL-FOCUSED	COMMUNITY-FOCUSED	SYSTEM-FOCUSED
Advocacy	Advocacy for preschool enrollment for the child of a depressed mother	Advocacy for recreation activities for teenagers	Advocacy for services for substance abusing adolescents
Case management	Arrange home care for an elderly client	Develop a case management program for pregnant adolescents	Develop case management standards for local government agencies
Coalition building	Develop a family coalition to enact an intervention with a substance abusing member	Build a coalition of police, school, and health personnel to prevent gang violence	Build a coalition to promote enforcement of local laws against tobacco sales to minors
Collaboration	Collaborate with church to provide transportation for client	Collaborate with local churches to provide homeless shelters	Collaborate in the development of a single application process for all forms of county assistance
Community organizing	Not relevant	Organize community members to request fee discounts from local health care providers	Develop a group to facilitate community organizing in several communities
Consultation	Assist a family in developing a nutritious diet	Provide assistance to local schools in developing school nutrition programs	Provide information to a state legislator on a health-related issue
Counseling	Assist a pregnant woman to explore prenatal care options	Help develop an eating disorders counseling program in high schools	Engage in political activity to mandate insurance coverage for counseling services
Medical treatment	Provide directly observed therapy to a client with TB	Develop protocols for TB treatment services	Develop policies for TB treatment in local correctional facilities
Disease investigation	Identify the source of infection in a child with TB	Advise nursing home coordinators on influenza prevention measures	Work with local health care providers to develop computer-based communicable disease notification system
Health teaching	Teach a mother about child development	Work with school and police officials to develop an antidrug education campaign in local schools	Develop a local health Web site to address health questions
Outreach/case finding	Identify a pregnant family member on a home visit to a woman with hypertension	Arrange a referral system for school nurses who identify pregnant mothers of students	Develop a notification system for immunizations
Policy development	Promote multilingual provider employment in area health agencies	Participate in policy development in relation to dispensing medications in schools	Engage in agency policy analysis and revision as needed
Provider education	Offer online information on treatment guidelines to providers	Provide immunization updates to school nurses	Promote agency policy on continued education for employees
Referral	Refer a family for financial help	Establish criteria for social service referrals	Develop a community referral network for prenatal care
Screening	Screen an adolescent for sexually transmitted disease	Arrange a community screening program for hypertension	Develop systems for community screening, follow-up, and treatment for HIV infection
Social marketing	Distribute no smoking buttons in local elementary school	Develop a teen theater campaign to address issues of conflict resolution	Write a grant to fund a media campaign to support smoke-free public spaces

INTERVENTIONS	INDIVIDUAL-FOCUSED	COMMUNITY-FOCUSED	SYSTEM-FOCUSED
Surveillance	Follow up on family members exposed to TB	Collect data on instances of family violence	Establish data systems that incorporate information on disease prevalence from private providers

graduated representations, with large branches representing populations and communities, smaller ones symbolizing families, and the smallest branches representing individuals. The leaves of the tree are the designated outcomes of community health practice: health promotion, health protection, illness and injury prevention, and access to health care services. The flowers represent the ultimate objective of community health nursing activity—health.

Surrounding the tree is the environment or the collection of forces that impinge on and influence community health nursing. Aspects of the environment include social,

cultural, political, economic, and ecological factors that were discussed in Unit I.

In this chapter, we have explored several theoretical models that can be applied to community health nursing practice. Readers may choose to employ one of the models presented here or another model that is appropriate to community health nursing practice, or the reader may construct a personal model of practice. Whatever the option chosen, community health nursing is most effective when some kind of theoretical model is used as an organizing framework for care.

FIGURE 9–6 ■ *Elements of the Public Health Nursing Model*

From Kuss, T., Proulx-Girouard, L., Lovitt, S., Katz, C., & Kennelly, P. (1997). A public health nursing model. *Public Health Nursing, 14,* 81–91. Reprinted by permission of Blackwell Science, Inc.

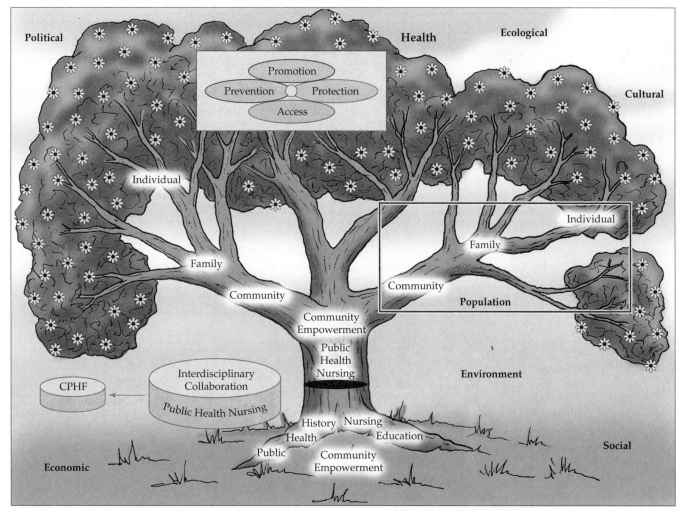

APPLYING YOUR KNOWLEDGE IN PRACTICE

❧ CASE STUDY
Using Theory in Population-Focused Care

Sandville is a small community in Texas situated five miles from the U.S.-Mexico border. The primary industry in the area is cattle ranching. Most of the Anglo residents are descendants of the western cattle barons who make up about 40% of the town's population of 3000. Another 25% of the population are long-time Latino residents descended from wranglers who worked on the ranches in the past. Now many work in service occupations. About 10% are Mexican immigrants who cross the border (legally or illegally) to obtain work, but return frequently to Mexico where extended family members continue to reside. The remainder of the town's population includes a group of newly arrived Asian engineers and their families who have come to staff the electronics plant that opened recently and a small group of African Americans who have lived in the area since the end of the Civil War.

Most young people do not stay long in the area and those who do have few children, so the population (with the exception of the Asian families) is aging. Cardiovascular disease and motor vehicle accidents on the two-lane highway passing through town create a booming business for the small local hospital. There are three primary care physicians in the community, one dentist, one pediatrician, and two family nurse practitioners. The county health department maintains a branch office in the town that is staffed by a public health nurse and sanitation engineer two days a week.

Community health problems, in addition to cardiovascular disease and accidents, include arthritis and anemia. There is also a high rate of tuberculosis among the Mexican immigrants.

- Select one of the models presented in the chapter and apply it to this case situation.
- What elements of the model are exemplified by the information provided in the case study?
- What problems might be present in the community other than those specified? What information in the case study led you to suspect the presence of these problems?
- What nursing interventions would you employ as the community health nurse assigned to this community? Why?

❧ TESTING YOUR UNDERSTANDING

- Why should community health nursing be based on a model or theory? (p. 190)
- What are the major components of Neumans' health systems model? How have they been adapted for community health nursing practice in the community-as-partner model? How might you apply this model to the care of a family? (pp. 190–191)
- What are the three elements of the dimensions model of community health nursing? What are the dimensions included in each element? Give an example related to the dimensions in each element that addresses the health of a population group. (pp. 192–196)
- Describe the major concepts in the FAU community nursing model. How would you apply the model to a specific population group? (pp. 196–197)

- What are the elements of Pender's health promotion model? Apply the elements of the model to the problem of poor immunization rates in a community. (pp. 197–199)
- How do the nursing interventions presented in the public health nursing interventions model differ across levels of community health nursing practice? Give several examples of interventions at different levels. (p. 200)
- What are the elements of public health/community health nursing represented in the tree figure of the public health nursing model? (pp. 200–203)

REFERENCES

Anderson, E. T., & McFarlane, J. (1996). A model to guide practice. In E. T. Anderson and J. McFarlane (Eds.), *Community as partner: Theory and practice in nursing* (2nd ed.) (pp. 165–176). Philadelphia: Lippincott.

Aylward, P. D., (2001). Betty Neuman: The Neuman systems model and global applications. In M. Parker (Ed.), *Nursing theories and nursing practice* (pp. 329–342). Philadelphia: Davis.

Clark, M. J. D. (1984). *Community nursing: Health care for today and tomorrow*. Reston, VA: Reston.

Clark, M. J. (1992). *Nursing in the community*. Norwalk, CT: Appleton & Lange.

Clark, M. J. (1996). *Nursing in the community* (2nd ed.). Stamford, CT: Appleton & Lange.

Clark, M. J. (1999). *Nursing in the community: Dimensions of community health nursing* (3rd ed.). Stamford, CT: Appleton & Lange.

Clarke, P. N. (1998). Nursing theory as a guide for inquiry in family and community health nursing. *Nursing Science Quarterly, 11*, 47–48.

Dixon, E. L. (1999). Community health nursing practice and the Roy adaptation model. *Public Health Nursing, 16*, 290–300.

Freese, B. T., Beckman, S. J., et al. (1998). Betty Neuman: Systems model. In A. M. Tomey & M. R. Alligood (Eds.), *Nursing theorists and their work* (4th ed.) (pp. 267–299). St. Louis: Mosby.

Gigliotti, E. (1999). Women's multiple role stress: Testing Neuman's flexible line of defense. *Nursing Science Quarterly, 12*, 36–44.

Hanchett, E. S. (1988). *Nursing frameworks and community as client*. Norwalk, CT: Appleton & Lange.

Hart, M., & Foster, S. N. (1998). Self-care agency in two groups of pregnant women. *Nursing Science Quarterly, 11*, 167–171.

Jaarsma, T., Halfens, R., Senten, M., Saad, H. H. A., & Dracup, K. (1998). Developing a supportive-educative program for patients with advanced heart failure within Orem's general theory of nursing. *Nursing Science Quarterly, 11*, 79–85.

Keller, L. O., Strohschein, S., Lia-Hoagberg, B., & Schaffer, M. (1998). Population-based public health nursing interventions: A model from practice. *Public Health Nursing, 15*, 207–215.

Kuss, T., Proulx-Girouard, L., Lovitt, S., Katz, C., & Kennelly, P. (1997). A public health nursing model. *Public Health Nursing, 14*, 81–91.

Leavell, H. R., & Clark, E. G. (1965). *Preventive medicine for the doctor in his community: An epidemiologic approach* (3rd ed.). New York: McGraw-Hill.

Levesque, L., Ricard, N., Ducharme, F., Duquette, A., & Bonin, J. (1998). Empirical verification of a theoretical model derived from the Roy adaptation model: Findings from five studies. *Nursing Science Quarterly, 11*, 31–39.

Neuman, B. (1994). The Neuman systems model. In B. Neuman (Ed.), *The Neuman systems model* (3rd ed.). Norwalk, CT: Appleton & Lange.

Parker, M. (2001). Introduction to nursing theory. In M. Parker (Ed.), *Nursing theories and nursing practice* (pp. 3–13). Philadelphia: Davis.

Parker, M., & Barry, C. (1999). Community practice guided by a nursing model. *Nursing Science Quarterly, 12*, 125–131.

Parker, M., Barry, C., & King, B. (2000). Use of inquiry method for assessment and evaluation in a school-based community nursing project. *Family and Community Health, 23*(2), 54–61.

Pender, N. J. (1996). *Health promotion in nursing practice* (3rd ed.). Stamford, CT: Appleton & Lange.

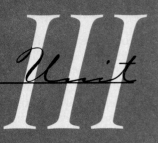

Unit III

PROCESSES USED IN COMMUNITY HEALTH NURSING

THE PROMISE

If you could just lose weight
your blood pressure would go down
your diabetes would clear up
you could get off all those pills you take
your joints wouldn't ache
you could climb the stairs
run after the bus
carry the groceries
pick up the baby
the swelling in your legs would go down
you could reach all the way to your aching
  feet
you could breathe again

You could find clothes to fit
get out of those slippers and into real shoes
who knows but your old man would come
  back
you'd get more respect from your children

a decent job
your son would kick drugs
your daughter wouldn't get pregnant again
you'd live to see your last one grown

Your neighbors wouldn't talk about you
the toilet would flush
the roof wouldn't leak
there'd be food enough at the end of the
  month
they wouldn't cut off your check
jack up the rent
you'd hit the number
go off for two weeks in Aruba

Jesus would save the world from sin
those who mourn would be comforted
the poor would enter the Kingdom of God
your hunger would be filled.

Reprinted with permission from V. Masson (1999),
Rehab at the Florida Avenue Grill. *Washington,*
DC: Sage Femme Press.

he Promise provides insights into the myriad problems encountered in community health nursing practice. We deal with more than physical health, but with all of the parameters that affect the health of our clients.

EPIDEMIOLOGY AND HEALTH PROMOTION

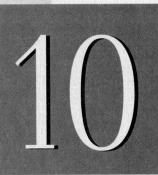

10

Chapter Objectives

After reading this chapter, you should be able to:

- Describe at least two theories of disease causation.
- Identify at least three criteria for determining causality in a relationship between two events.
- Define risk.
- Distinguish between morbidity and mortality rates.
- Identify six steps of the epidemiologic process.
- Differentiate among descriptive, analytical, and experimental epidemiology.
- Identify the three major elements of the epidemiologic triad.
- Describe advantages and disadvantages of the web of causation model.
- Describe the four major components of Dever's epidemiologic model.
- Identify two foci for health promotion programs.

Media Link

http://www.prenhall.com/clark

Additional interactive resources for this chapter can be found on the companion Web site. Click on Chapter 10 and "Begin" to select the activities for this chapter.

The epidemiologic process is one of the key processes used in community health nursing. Epidemiology is a health-related discipline that provides a systematic framework for examining states of health in terms of factors contributing to their development. The primary concern of epidemiology, like community health, is the health of groups of people; however, epidemiologic principles can also direct community health nurses in assessing health-related conditions experienced by both individuals and families. The nursing process indicates the need for client assessment, and the epidemiologic process suggests the types of data to be collected and how they can be organized to facilitate nursing intervention. In this chapter, we explore the major elements of an epidemiologic perspective in community health nursing and apply epidemiologic methods to health promotion.

BASIC CONCEPTS OF EPIDEMIOLOGY

Epidemiology is the study of the distribution of health and illness within the population and the factors that determine the population's health status (Friis & Sellers, 1999). This definition encompasses two broad concepts: control of health problems through an understanding of their contributing factors, and application of epidemiologic techniques to health-related conditions other than acute communicable disease.

The purposes of epidemiology are twofold: to search for causal relationships in health and illness, and to control illness through the resultant understanding of causality. The ultimate concern of epidemiology in any of its uses is preventing disease and maintaining health. Specific uses of the epidemiologic process include:

- Identifying causative factors and risk factors for health conditions affecting populations
- Diagnosing the health status of population groups
- Describing signs and symptoms and the course of a disease
- Evaluating the effectiveness of existing and proposed interventions and modes of health care delivery
- Providing a basis for health policy development (Gordis, 2000)

The study of factors contributing to communicable diseases was the initial focus of epidemiologic investigation. As the incidence of many communicable diseases declined, epidemiologists directed their attention to chronic disease as a focus of investigation. More recently still, epidemiologic methods have been used to identify factors that promote health.

Three basic concepts underlie epidemiologic investigation of health and illness: causality, risk, and rates of occurrence. Each of these concepts finds direct application in community health nursing.

Causality

To control health problems, epidemiologists and community health nurses must have some idea of causality. The concept of *causality* is based on the idea that one event is the result of another event. Theories about the cause of disease have evolved over time.

THEORIES OF CAUSATION

The first recognized attempt to attribute a cause to illness occurred during the "religious era," which extended from roughly 2000 B.C. through the age of the early Egyptian and Greek physicians to around 600 B.C. During this period, disease was thought to be caused directly by divine intervention, possibly as punishment for sins or as a trial of faith.

Subsequent to the religious era, disease was often attributed to various physical forces, such as miasmas or mists. A rudimentary environmental theory of disease was developed by Hippocrates in his treatise, *On Airs, Waters, and Places,* about 400 B.C. The primary belief at that time was that disease was caused by harmful substances in the environment (Friis & Sellers, 1999).

The bacteriologic era commenced in the late 1870s with the discovery of specific organisms as etiologic (causative) agents for specific diseases. One of the classic epidemiologic studies demonstrating the probability of some causative organism in communicable diseases was that of John Snow, who deduced that the cause of a cholera epidemic was contaminated water from a specific London well. Subsequently, actual bacteria were isolated and found to be the source of this and other infectious diseases. These discoveries gave rise to theories of a single cause for any specific disease. Single-cause theories were further supported by the identification of other specific agents as causative elements for certain health problems. For example, lack of vitamin C was found to result in scurvy. The discovery of specific agents responsible for particular diseases did not, however, explain why one person exposed to an agent developed the disease, while another did not, so the evolution of disease theory entered the current era of multiple causation.

The hallmark of the era of multiple causation is the recognition of the interplay of a variety of factors in the development of health or illness. Epidemiology examines this interplay of factors with an eye toward control of a particular health condition. Prevention or control of any disease within population groups depends on knowledge of these factors and determination of the point at which intervention will be most feasible and most effective.

The historical development of theories of disease causation is summarized in Table 10–1 ■. It should be noted that, although the scientific community has accepted the current idea of multiple causation, each of the preceding theories continues to have support among members of the lay population.

All of these theories are considered "sufficient-component" causal models because they assist in identifying factors

■ **TABLE 10–1** **Historical Development of Theories of Disease Causation**

ERA	PERIOD	THEORY OF CAUSATION PREVALENT
Religious era	2000–600 B.C.	Disease caused by divine intervention, possibly as punishment for sins or test of faith
Environmental era	Circa 400 B.C.	Disease caused by harmful miasmas, or mists, or other substances in the environment
Bacteriologic era	1870–1900	Disease caused by specific bacteriologic or nutritive agents
Era of multiple causation	1900 to present	Disease caused by interaction of multiple factors
Amalgam of sufficient component and population model theories	Future	Disease caused by interaction of individual risk factors and population exposure patterns

required for the development of adverse health conditions in individuals. Recent authors have noted a need to combine the sufficient component perspective with population systems models of causation that address population level characteristics and patterns of exposure to causative factors (Koopman & Lynch, 1999). For example, a specific level of exposure to lead is known to cause lead poisoning in children (sufficient-component model), but population patterns of lead exposure are also important. How much of the exposure to lead in the population occurs as a result of lead-based paint in the home and how much can be attributed to parental work in lead-based industries where lead particles are brought home on shoes and clothing? Knowing the potential for various sources of exposure within a population will help to direct control efforts.

CRITERIA FOR CAUSALITY
With the advent of single-cause/single-effect theories of disease causation, the scientific community began to look for specific causes for all health problems. Now, however, the concept of causality has become more complicated in view of the recognized interplay of a variety of factors in the development of illness. A factor may be considered causative if the health condition is more likely to occur in its presence and less likely to occur in its absence. Even when these conditions are met, however, a specific factor may not necessarily cause a particular condition. Various authors identify anywhere from four to ten criteria to be used in determining causality (Friis & Sellers, 1999; Harkness, 1995). Generally, however, they agree on five basic criteria that can be used to attribute causation in both infectious and noninfectious conditions. These criteria are the consistency and the strength of the association, its specificity, the temporal relationship between events, and coherence with other known facts (Valanis, 1999).

CONSISTENCY The first criterion for establishing a causal relationship is consistency. The association between the factor in question and the problem must be consis-

tent. The condition in question must occur when the factor is present, not when it is absent. For example, people cannot develop measles without being exposed to measles virus. In addition, the association must always occur in the same direction. Exposure cannot result in disease in one instance, and disease result in exposure to the virus in another.

STRENGTH OF ASSOCIATION The second criterion for establishing causality is the strength of the association. The greater the correlation between the occurrence of the factor and the health condition, the greater the possibility that the relationship is one of cause and effect. For example, not every susceptible person who is exposed to measles virus develops the disease, but most of them do. The association between exposure and disease, in this instance, is quite strong and supports the idea that the measles virus causes measles. The strength of the association may reflect a *dose-response gradient* in which the greater the exposure to the presumed cause, the greater the likelihood of developing the problem (Gordis, 2000). For example, the fact that people who smoke two packs of cigarettes a day are more likely to develop lung cancer than those who smoke one pack is strong evidence for a causal relationship between smoking and lung cancer.

SPECIFICITY Specificity is the third criterion for causality. Specificity is present when the factor in question results in one specific condition. For instance, exposure to measles virus results only in measles, not mumps, chickenpox, or any other communicable disease. Specificity is the weakest of the criteria with respect to noninfectious conditions. For example, smoking not only causes lung cancer, but also contributes to stomach and bladder cancers and heart disease.

TEMPORAL RELATIONSHIP The fourth criterion for establishing causation is the time (or temporal) relationship between the factor and the resulting condition. The factor thought to be causative should occur before the condition appears. For example, one is always exposed to measles virus before, not after, one gets measles.

COHERENCE   Coherence with the established body of scientific knowledge is the last criterion for determining causality. The idea that one condition causes another must be logical and congruent with other known facts. For example, it is known that alcohol consumption increases the time required for voluntary muscles to react to stimuli. Therefore, it is reasonable to consider alcohol consumption as a causative factor in many accidents because this interpretation is consistent with the idea of a slowed response to changing driving conditions.

Only the criterion of a correct temporal relationship is absolutely required for attributing causation; however, the greater the number of criteria met, the more credible the idea that the factor in question causes the condition of interest. Criteria for determining causality are summarized in Table 10–2 ■.

Risk

In addition to establishing the causes of health-related conditions, epidemiologists are interested in estimating the likelihood that a particular condition will occur. *Risk* is the probability that a given individual will develop a specific condition. One's risk of developing a particular condition is affected by a variety of physical, emotional, environmental, lifestyle, and other factors. When epidemiologists speak of *populations at risk,* they are referring to groups of people who have the greatest potential to develop a particular health problem because of the presence or absence of certain contributing factors.

The basis for risk may lie in one's susceptibility to a condition or potential for exposure to causative factors. *Susceptibility* is the ability to be affected by factors contributing to a particular health condition. For example, very young unimmunized children are susceptible to,

and constitute the population at risk for, pertussis (whooping cough). In this case, the basis for increased risk lies in the increased susceptibility of this group. Persons over the age of 10 and children who have been immunized against pertussis are less likely to develop the disease and so are not part of the population at risk. Another example of risk based on susceptibility is found in the population of sexually active women of childbearing age who are at risk for pregnancy. Men, children, and older women are not susceptible to pregnancy and, therefore, are not considered part of the population at risk.

Exposure potential is another factor in one's risk of developing a particular condition. *Exposure potential* is the likelihood of exposure to factors that contribute to the condition. For example, those most at risk for sexually transmitted diseases are adolescents and young adults. In this instance, the basis of risk is not increased susceptibility, as in the case of pertussis, but an increased potential for exposure because of more frequent and less selective sexual activity. Another population at risk through increased chance of exposure includes individuals whose occupation brings them in contact with toxic substances.

Members of a population at risk have a greater probability of developing a specific condition than those who are not affected by factors known to contribute to the condition. This difference in the probability of developing a given condition is known as the *relative risk ratio* (Coggon, Rose, & Barker, 1997). This ratio is derived by comparing the frequency of occurrence of the condition in a group of people with known risk factors to that among individuals without these factors. For example, if 50% of smokers develop heart disease versus only 5% of nonsmokers, smokers have a relative risk of 10:1, or have a 10 times greater risk of heart disease than their nonsmoking counterparts. The relative risk ratio is useful in identifying those areas where preventive interventions will have the greatest impact on the occurrence of disease.

When the relative risk is greater than 1:1, there is a positive association between factor and condition, suggesting that eliminating the factor may prevent the condition. Similarly, a negative association in which the relative ratio is less than 1:1 (e.g., 1:5) suggests that enhancing the factor or causing it to be present may prevent the condition. For example, smoking has a positive relationship with heart disease and regular exercise has a negative relationship, so preventing smoking and promoting exercise should both decrease the incidence of heart disease.

The population at risk becomes the target group for any intervention designed to prevent or control the problem in question. The *target group* includes those individuals who would benefit from an intervention program and at whom the program is aimed. Using one of the previous examples, the target group for an immunization campaign against pertussis would include unimmunized children under the age of 10.

■ **TABLE 10–2**   Criteria for Determining Causality

CRITERION	DESCRIPTION OF CRITERION
Consistency	The association between the supposed cause and its effect is consistent and always occurs in the same direction.
Strength of association	The greater the correlation between supposed cause and effect, the greater the possibility the relationship is a causal one.
Specificity	The supposed cause always creates the same effect.
Temporal relationship	The supposed cause always occurs before the effect.
Coherence	The supposition of one event causing another is coherent with other existing knowledge.

Rates of Occurrence

The rate of occurrence of a health-related condition is also of concern to community health nurses. *Rates of occurrence* are statistical measures that indicate the extent of health problems in a group. Rates of occurrence allow comparisons between groups of different sizes with respect to the extent of a particular condition. For example, a community with a population of 1,000 may report 50 cases of syphilis this year, whereas another community of 100,000 persons may report 5,000 cases. On the surface, it would seem that the second community has a greater problem with syphilis than the first; however, both communities have experienced 50 cases per 1,000 population. In other words, both have a problem with syphilis of comparable magnitude.

Computing the statistical rates of interest in community health nursing involves dividing the *number of instances of an event* during a specified period by the *population at risk* for that event and *multiplying by 1,000* (or 100,000 if the numbers of the event are so small that the result of the calculation using a multiplier of 1,000 would be less than 1). The basic formula for calculating statistical rates of interest to community health nurses is presented below.

Both morbidity and mortality rates are of concern in community health nursing. *Mortality* is the ratio of the number of deaths in various categories to the number of people in a given population, whereas *morbidity* is the ratio of the number of cases of a disease or condition to the number of people in the population. Mortality rates describe deaths; morbidity rates describe cases of health conditions that may or may not result in death. For example, the number of people in a particular group who die as a result of cardiovascular disease is reflected in the mortality rate; however, the number of people experiencing cardiovascular disease is indicated by the morbidity rate.

MORTALITY RATES

Mortality rates of interest in community health nursing include the overall or "crude" death rate, cause-specific death rates, infant and neonatal mortality rates, fetal and perinatal mortality rates, and the maternal death rate. Each rate is calculated from the number of events during a specified period and the average population at risk during that same period. Formulas for calculating some specific rates of interest are presented below.

HIGHLIGHTS

Formulas for Calculating Selected Mortality Rates

$$\text{Crude death rate} = \frac{\text{Total number of deaths during year}}{\text{Total population at midyear}} \times 1{,}000$$

$$\begin{array}{c}\text{Cause-specific}\\\text{annual death}\\\text{rate}\end{array} = \frac{\text{Number of deaths from specific cause during year}}{\begin{array}{c}\text{Total population at}\\\text{midyear}\end{array}} \times 1{,}000$$

$$\begin{array}{c}\text{Annual infant}\\\text{mortality rate}\end{array} = \frac{\begin{array}{c}\text{Number of deaths during}\\\text{year (birth to 1 year of age)}\end{array}}{\begin{array}{c}\text{Number of live births}\\\text{during year}\end{array}} \times 1{,}000$$

$$\begin{array}{c}\text{Annual neonatal}\\\text{mortality rate}\end{array} = \frac{\begin{array}{c}\text{Number of deaths during}\\\text{year (birth to 28 days of age)}\end{array}}{\begin{array}{c}\text{Number of live births}\\\text{during year}\end{array}} \times 1{,}000$$

$$\begin{array}{c}\text{Annual fetal}\\\text{death rate}\end{array} = \frac{\begin{array}{c}\text{Number of fetal deaths}\\\text{during year (20 to 28}\\\text{weeks' gestation)}\end{array}}{\begin{array}{c}\text{Number of live births plus}\\\text{fetal deaths during year}\end{array}} \times 1{,}000$$

$$\begin{array}{c}\text{Annual perinatal}\\\text{death rate}\end{array} = \frac{\begin{array}{c}\text{Number of perinatal deaths}\\\text{during year (20 weeks'}\\\text{gestation to 1 week of age)}\end{array}}{\begin{array}{c}\text{Number of live births plus}\\\text{fetal deaths during year}\end{array}} \times 1{,}000$$

$$\begin{array}{c}\text{Annual maternal}\\\text{death rate}\end{array} = \frac{\begin{array}{c}\text{Number of maternal}\\\text{deaths during year}\end{array}}{\begin{array}{c}\text{Number of live births}\\\text{during year}\end{array}} \times 100{,}000$$

HIGHLIGHTS

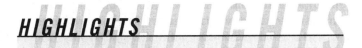

Basic Formula for Calculating Statistical Rates

$$\text{Rate} = \frac{\text{Number of events over a period of time}}{\text{Population at risk at that time}} \times \begin{array}{c}1{,}000 \text{ (or}\\100{,}000)\end{array}$$

For example, in a community with a population of 10,000 females aged 13 to 18 years, there were 200 teenage pregnancies in 1998. What is the rate of teenage pregnancy?

$$\begin{array}{c}\text{Rate of}\\\text{teenage}\\\text{pregnancy}\end{array} = \frac{\begin{array}{c}200 \text{ pregnancies in}\\\text{females } 13–18\\\text{during } 1998\end{array}}{\begin{array}{c}10{,}000 \text{ females}\\\text{aged } 13–18 \text{ in the}\\\text{population at}\\\text{midyear}\end{array}} \times 1{,}000 = \begin{array}{c}20\\\text{pregnancies}\\\text{per } 1{,}000\\\text{females}\end{array}$$

Rates are reported in terms of the multiplicative factor used to calculate them. For example, cancer deaths occur in fairly large numbers, so a cause-specific death rate for cancer would be calculated using 1,000 as the multiplier. If Community A, with a population of 50,000, had 100 cancer-related deaths, the cause-specific death rate for cancer would be reported as 2 deaths per 1,000 population. Deaths from pancreatic cancer, on the other hand, occur relatively infrequently, so 100,000 would be the multiplier used to calculate the pancreatic cancer death rate. For instance, if there were 6 deaths from pancreatic cancer in Community B last year, and Community B has a population of 500,000 people, the annual pancreatic cancer mortality rate would be reported as 1.2 deaths per 100,000 population. Sample calculation of rates with different multipliers is presented below.

Age-adjusted mortality rates can be calculated to account for differences in age distribution between groups. This allows one to make more accurate comparisons of mortality between groups with widely different age distributions. For example, Community A might have a considerably higher crude death rate for influenza than Community B. If, however, Community A also has a higher proportion of elderly persons in the population, more influenza deaths would be expected, because older people are more vulnerable to this condition. Age-adjusted mortality rates for influenza, on the other hand, allow the community health nurse to compare the effects of influenza on Communities A and B as if they had similar proportions of elderly in the population. If Community A's influenza death rate remains higher when adjusted for age, the nurse would look for other factors in the community to explain this difference.

MORBIDITY RATES

Morbidity rates reflect the number of cases of particular health conditions in a group or community. Morbidity is described in terms of incidence or prevalence rates. *Incidence* rates are calculated on the basis of the number of *new* cases of a particular condition identified during a specified period. *Prevalence* is the *total number* of people affected by a particular condition at a specified point in time.

To illustrate the concepts of incidence and prevalence, consider a town with a population of 30,000 in which 15 new cases of hypertension were diagnosed in June. This is an indication of the incidence of hypertension. People who were diagnosed as hypertensive prior to June and who continue to live in the town still have hypertension. These additional cases of hypertension, however, are not reflected in the hypertension incidence rate for June, but are included in the prevalence, the total number of people in the community affected by hypertension. The formulas below are used to calculate annual incidence and prevalence rates. Again, the results of the calculations are reported in terms of the rate per 1,000 population.

Case fatality rates and survival rates are also of concern in community health. The *case fatality rate* for a particular condition reflects the percentage of persons with the condition who die as a result of it. For example, at present, many people infected with Ebola virus die because of the lack of an effective treatment. Very few people die of mumps, on the other hand, so mumps has a low case fatality rate.

The converse of fatality is the *survival rate*, the proportion of people with a given condition remaining alive after a specific period (usually five years). For example, the five-year survival rate for women with breast cancer is relatively high compared with the survival rate of those with pancreatic cancer. A related concept is *survival time*, or the average length of time from diagnosis to death. For example, given current medical technology, the survival time for children with Down syndrome is much longer

HIGHLIGHTS

Sample Mortality Rate Calculations Using Multipliers of 1,000 and 100,000

Community A

$$\text{Cancer mortality rate} = \frac{\text{100 deaths due to cancer, 1999}}{\text{50,000 population at midyear}} \times 1{,}000 = \text{2 cancer deaths per 1,000 population}$$

Community B

$$\text{Pancreatic cancer mortality rate} = \frac{\text{6 deaths from pancreatic cancer, 1999}}{\text{500,000 population at midyear}} \times 100{,}000 = \text{1.2 deaths due to pancreatic cancer per 100,000 population}$$

HIGHLIGHTS

Formulas for Calculating Annual Incidence and Prevalence Rates

$$\text{Annual incidence rate} = \frac{\text{Number of new cases of a condition last year}}{\text{Total population at risk at midyear}} \times 1{,}000$$

$$\text{Annual prevalence rate} = \frac{\text{Total number of cases of a condition last year}}{\text{Total population at risk at midyear}} \times 1{,}000$$

today than at the turn of the century. Caution should be used in interpreting both survival rate and survival time information. Diagnostic technology has permitted earlier diagnosis of many conditions, increasing the time from diagnosis to death, but not appreciably lengthening one's life (Gordis, 2000). Other rates that may be of interest to community health nurses include marriage and divorce rates, illegitimacy rates, employment rates, utilization rates for health care services and facilities, and rates for alcohol and drug use and abuse.

Community health nurses use morbidity and mortality data in assessing the health status of a community. Community morbidity and mortality rates that are generally high or higher than state or national rates indicate health problems that require intervention. For example, the nurse may note that local morbidity rates for childhood illnesses such as measles and rubella are twice those of the rest of the state. These differences indicate that a significant portion of the local child population is unimmunized. The nurse then uses these data to begin an investigation of the factors involved in the problem and to plan a solution. Is it a matter of inaccessibility of immunization services, lack of education on the need for immunization, or poor surveillance of immunization levels in the schools? The solution to the problem must be geared to the cause. Statistical data merely serve to indicate the presence of a problem; they do not delineate its specific nature.

Low morbidity and mortality rates do not indicate the absence of health problems in the community, as biostatistics are only one indicator of health status. Many health problems are not reported statistically, and their presence in the community is not reflected in morbidity and mortality rates. The nutritional status of the population is one area not addressed by biostatistics such as morbidity and mortality rates. Other indicators that the community health nurse employs in assessing a community's health status are discussed in Chapter 15.

THE EPIDEMIOLOGIC PROCESS

Epidemiologists use a systematic process, similar to the nursing process, to study states of health and illness in an effort to control disease and promote health. The steps of this *epidemiologic process* are:

- Defining the condition
- Determining the natural history of the condition
- Identifying strategic points of control
- Designing control strategies
- Implementing control strategies
- Evaluating control strategies

Determining the natural history of the condition is analogous to the assessment and diagnosis phases of the nursing process. Identifying strategic points of control

and designing control programs reflect the planning aspects of the nursing process, and the implementation and evaluation steps are equivalent to similar steps in the nursing process.

Defining the Condition

The first step in the epidemiologic process is defining the health condition requiring intervention. As we will see later, the epidemiologic process can be applied to health as well as illness. In either case, it is necessary to define the state or condition for which intervention is required. Taking a health promotion focus, one needs to define health. With respect to a specific disease or health problem, one must clearly define what is and is not an instance of the problem. For example, to study the factors contributing to suicide, one must be able to differentiate suicide from accidental death. Similarly, one must be able to differentiate cases of measles from cases of rubella to study and control either of these diseases.

Determining the Natural History of the Condition

The natural history of a disease or condition is a description of the events that precede its development and occur during its course, as well as its outcomes. Determining the condition's natural history involves identifying factors that contribute to its development, its signs and symptoms, its effects on the human system, and its typical outcomes and factors that may affect those outcomes. For example, crowded living conditions, lack of immunization, and exposure to influenza virus are some factors involved in the development of influenza. The typical course of influenza includes a short incubation period and the rapid onset of respiratory and/or gastrointestinal symptoms. Most cases of influenza resolve after several days, but the eventual outcome depends on such factors as the individual's overall health, age, nutritional status, and personal habits such as smoking. All of these bits of information are part of the natural history of influenza.

The description of the natural history also incorporates information on the frequency of occurrence, severity of outcomes, and geographic distribution of the condition. Information is obtained on time relationships and trends related to the condition. Time relationships refer to the occurrence of the condition at specific times or during particular seasons. For example, influenza occurs primarily in the winter, and the incidence of suicide rises around holidays. Trends refer to patterns of occurrence for the condition. Incidence of hepatitis A, for example, is declining, while patterns of occurrence for family violence indicate increasing incidence.

The natural history of a condition is usually divided into four stages: preexposure, preclinical, clinical, and resolution. In the *preexposure stage,* factors contributing to the development of the condition are present. When exposure to causative factors has occurred, but no symptoms have appeared, the condition is in the *preclinical stage.* The *clinical stage* begins with the onset of signs and symptoms characteristic of the disease or condition. In the *resolution stage,* the condition culminates in a return to health, death, or continuation in a chronic state. These stages are depicted in Figure 10–1 ■.

Determining the factors involved in the natural history of a condition is usually undertaken using a specific epidemiologic model. Three such models are discussed later in this chapter. The dimensions of health in the dimensions model of community health nursing discussed in Chapter 9 also provide an epidemiologic perspective for examining the natural history of a health condition.

⑥THINK ABOUT IT

Trace the natural history of a specific health condition. What factors would affect the outcome of this condition? How could these factors be altered to achieve a better outcome?

Identifying Strategic Points of Control

Knowledge of the natural history of a disease or condition allows epidemiologists to identify strategic points of

control. One might, for example, design interventions to eliminate or modify factors contributing to a condition to prevent its occurrence. Similarly, knowledge of factors affecting a condition's course may lead to interventions designed to minimize its effects.

Strategic points of control may involve interventions at the primary, secondary, or tertiary level of prevention. Primary prevention takes place before the problem occurs, during the preexposure and preclinical stages of its natural history. Secondary prevention occurs once the problem appears, during the clinical stage; tertiary prevention may be required during the resolution stage either to prevent lasting effects or to prevent a recurrence of the problem. Figure 10–1 depicts the relationship of levels of prevention to the stages of the natural history of a health-related condition.

Designing, Implementing, and Evaluating Control Strategies

Once strategic points of control for a specific condition have been identified, health care programs can be designed to prevent it or minimize its effects on the health of the population. Programs are then implemented and evaluated in terms of their effects on the occurrence of the particular condition. These steps of the epidemiologic process parallel similar components of the nursing process and are discussed in relation to population health care in Chapter 15.

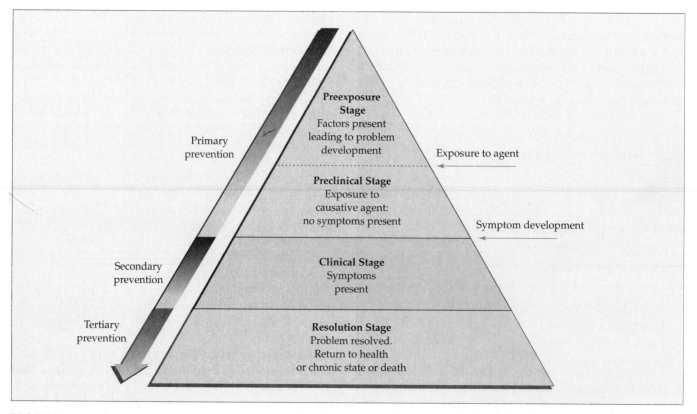

FIGURE 10–1 ■ *Stages in the Natural History of a Condition and Their Relationship to Primary, Secondary, and Tertiary Levels of Prevention*

EPIDEMIOLOGIC INVESTIGATION

The basic requirement for using the epidemiologic process to control health and illness is information on contributing factors as well as on effective control strategies. Information on any given condition is usually obtained over time from multiple epidemiologic investigations. Epidemiologic studies are of three general types: descriptive, analytic, and experimental.

Descriptive Epidemiology

Descriptive epidemiology is the study of the distribution of a given health state in a specified population in terms of person, place, and time. The person element identifies those affected by the condition. For example, who develops arthritis and what features are characteristic of these people? The element of place examines where the condition occurs. Does arthritis occur more frequently in some parts of the country than others? What features of those parts of the country might explain these differences? Finally, the time element reflects when the condition occurs. For example, measles occurs primarily in the winter. What factors account for this seasonal variation? Information in each of these areas suggests possible causative factors and potential control strategies for arthritis or measles.

Descriptive epidemiology is useful for several purposes. These include evaluating trends in the occurrence of a condition within a given population and comparing occurrences between populations. Descriptive epidemiology also provides a basis for planning health services and allocating resources. Finally, descriptive epidemiology identifies problems for analytic epidemiologic investigations.

Analytic Epidemiology

Analytic epidemiology is the study of factors contributing to health states. Its purposes are to (1) suggest mechanisms of causation, (2) generate etiologic hypotheses, and (3) test etiologic hypotheses. Analytic epidemiology can be divided into three categories of investigations: ecological studies, case-control studies, and cohort studies (Friis & Sellers, 1999).

Ecological studies compare rates of disease occurrence among several population groups, usually 10 or more. Ecological studies are useful when the level of exposure of specific individuals is unknown, but there is information about the general level of exposure in the population; ecological studies can be used to assess relationships between exposure rates and disease rates in different populations. Ecological studies also provide information on trends in exposures as compared to trends in disease.

Case-control studies involve comparisons between persons with a specific condition and those without it.

Differences in characteristics of members of these two groups may suggest causative or preventive factors related to the health condition. Cohort studies, also called prospective or longitudinal studies, follow people exposed to a supposed causative factor, but without disease, over time to determine the proportion of people who actually develop the condition of interest.

Experimental Epidemiology

Experimental studies involve manipulation of exposure to the supposed causative factor and look for differences in the incidence of the supposed effect. Experimental studies are used to test the effectiveness of interventions. Application of an intervention by the researcher is called a *trial. Clinical trials* apply interventions to individuals; *community trials* test interventions with population groups (Friis & Sellers, 1999). Trials can involve removal of a risk factor or addition of some other factor and can be either prophylactic or therapeutic in nature depending on the timing of the intervention.

In prophylactic trials, the intervention is designed to prevent the occurrence of a health problem. Interventions designed to promote health are also tested in prophylactic trials. Therapeutic trials, on the other hand, investigate the effects of secondary preventive interventions. In these studies, the researcher exposes a group of subjects to an intervention designed to resolve an existing health problem. The intervention may be either positive or negative. Positive interventions add a factor to the situation being studied, whereas negative interventions reduce or eliminate causative factors. For example, one might explore the effects of teaching parenting techniques (a positive intervention) or reducing environmental stressors (a negative intervention) on the incidence of child abuse by parents who are already abusive.

The relationships among the types of epidemiologic investigations presented here are depicted in Figure 10–2 ■. The selection of a particular investigative approach depends on the purpose of the study to be conducted and the extent of previous research in the area. For example, descriptive studies are appropriate in studying conditions about which little is known. In other areas where there is already evidence of possible relationships between variables, analytic or experimental studies might be more appropriate. Choice of an analytic or experimental approach depends primarily on whether the situation permits manipulation of variables of interest by the researcher. In some instances, manipulation of variables is not possible; in others, manipulation of the variables involved would be unethical.

Community health nurses may be actively involved in epidemiologic investigations. Some agencies and organizations that support epidemiology and epidemiologic research are provided on the companion Web site for this book. 🌐

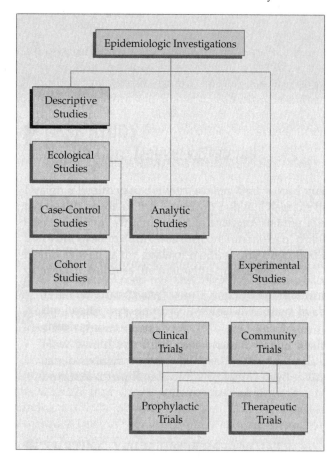

FIGURE 10–2 ■ *Approaches to Epidemiologic Investigation*

EPIDEMIOLOGIC MODELS

Both nurses and epidemiologists use the epidemiologic process and epidemiologic research findings to direct interventions to control health-related conditions. Determining the natural history of a health condition and identifying control strategies involve collecting large amounts of data about multiple factors that may be contributing to the condition. For this reason, it is helpful to have a model or framework to direct the collection and interpretation of these data. We explore three such models: the epidemiologic triad, the web of causation model, and Dever's epidemiologic model. The dimensions model of community health nursing discussed in Chapter 9 can also be used in epidemiologic investigations.

The Epidemiologic Triad

Traditionally, epidemiologic investigation has been guided by the epidemiologic triad. In this model, data are collected with respect to a triad of elements: host, agent, and environment. The interrelationship of these elements results in a state of relative health or illness. The relationships among host, agent, and environment and specific considerations under each are depicted in Figure 10–3 ■.

HOST

The *host* is the client system affected by the particular condition under investigation. Community health nursing is concerned with the health of human beings, so, for our purposes, the host is a human being. A variety of factors can influence the host's exposure, susceptibility, and response to an agent. Host-related factors include intrinsic factors (e.g., age, race, and sex), physical and psychological factors, and the presence or absence of immunity. These factors are addressed in more detail in the discussion of Dever's epidemiologic model.

AGENT

The *agent* is the primary cause of a health-related condition. The causes of some health problems may be so complex that no single agent can be identified. The concept of agent, however, remains useful for exploring many health problems.

Agents can be classified into six types: physical agents, chemical agents, nutritive elements, infectious agents, genetic agents, and psychological agents (Valanis, 1999). Physical agents include heat, trauma, and radiation. Chemical agents include various substances to which people may develop untoward reactions. Some plants such as poison ivy and ragweed can be considered chemical agents because they cause a chemical reaction resulting in an allergic response.

An absence or an excess of a variety of nutritive elements is known to result in disease, as does the presence of and exposure to a number of infectious agents that cause communicable diseases. Genetic agents arise from genetic transmission from parent to child. Finally, psychological agents such as stress can produce a variety of stress-related conditions. The types of agents and examples of health conditions to which they contribute are listed in Table 10–3 ■.

An agent's characteristics influence whether a given individual develops a particular health-related condition. These characteristics vary somewhat depending on the type of agent involved.

CHARACTERISTICS OF INFECTIOUS AGENTS   Characteristics that influence the effects of infectious agents include the extent of exposure to the agent and the agent's infectivity, pathogenicity, and virulence. Additional characteristics of infectious agents include toxigenicity, resistance, and antigenicity (Friis & Sellers, 1999). The *extent of exposure* to a disease-causing microorganism, or the *infective dose*, affects the outcome of the exposure. For example, the person exposed to a few *Mycobacterium tuberculosis* organisms is unlikely to develop tuberculosis (TB). The greater the number of these microorganisms inhaled, however, the greater the likelihood of developing TB.

Infectivity is the ability of an agent to invade the host system. Infectivity is determined, in part, by the agent's portals of entry and exit. The *portal of entry* is the means by which the agent invades the host; the *portal of exit* is the avenue by which the agent leaves the host. The portals

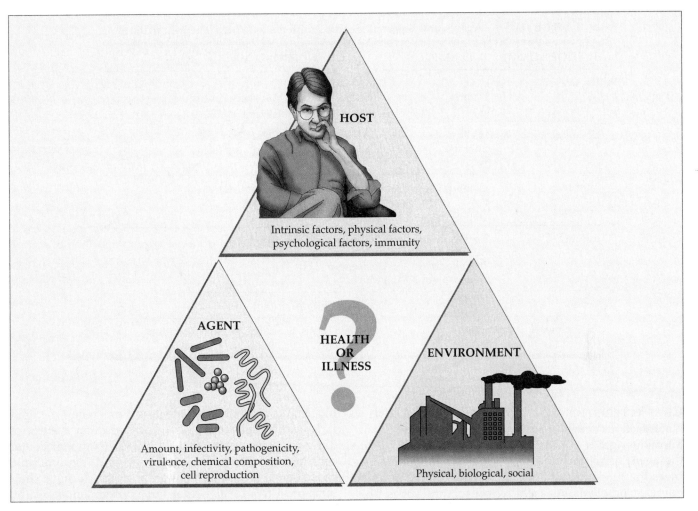

FIGURE 10–3 ■ *Elements of the Epidemiologic Triad Model*

of entry and exit also influence the *mode of transmission,* or means by which the agent is transmitted from one host to another. Modes of transmission are addressed in greater detail in Chapter 28. Measles virus, for example, has a higher infectivity than does tetanus bacillus. The measles virus enters the body quite easily through the respiratory system, whereas tetanus gains entry through a break in the skin, usually a deep puncture wound. Similarly, variola virus, the causative organism for smallpox, is usually inhaled and can be transmitted from person to person or by means of an aerosol cloud, making it a possible weapon of biological terrorism. *Pathogenicity* is the ability of the agent to cause disease. In terms of infectious agents, measles virus causes disease in most susceptible infected individuals. *M. tuberculosis,* on the other hand, produces disease in only a small portion of individuals infected. Therefore, the measles virus has a higher pathogenicity than *M. tuberculosis*. Smallpox, if reintroduced into the population by terrorism, would also have high pathogenicity, with an attack rate of about 50% in unvaccinated individuals (Chinn, 2000).

Another epidemiologic concept closely related to pathogenicity is that of *attack rate,* which is the proportion of those exposed to the agent who develop the disease. As is

the case with pathogenicity, measles has a high attack rate, whereas tuberculosis has a low attack rate.

Virulence is a term used to describe the severity of the health problem caused by the agent. Rubeola or measles has a low virulence because uncomplicated measles is not a serious illness. Tetanus, on the other hand, is extremely virulent because it results in fatality unless treatment is instituted. The virus that causes AIDS is another infectious agent with a very high virulence. Virulence is frequently confused with pathogenicity, but the two terms refer to different agent characteristics. For example, cold viruses that cause disease in infected individuals are highly pathogenic, but have a low virulence because the diseases caused are relatively minor. Virulence is closely related to case fatality rates.

The *toxigenicity* of an infectious agent refers to its ability to produce toxins that are harmful to the human body. The primary effect of tetanus is due to the effects of the toxin produced by tetanus bacilli on the human nervous system. *Resistance* refers to the ability of the infectious agent to survive in adverse conditions, including exposure to antibiotics, but also including heating, drying, and so on. *Antigenicity* is the ability of the agent to cause immunity and is the basis for immunization practices.

■ **TABLE 10–3   Agents and Selected Health Problems to Which They Contribute**

TYPE OF AGENT	EXAMPLE	PROBLEMS
Physical	Heat	Burns, heat stroke
	Trauma	Fractures, concussion, sprains, contusions
	Genetic changes	Down syndrome, Turner's syndrome
Chemical	Medications	Accidental poisoning, suicide
	Chlorine	Poisoning, asphyxiation (in gas form)
	Poison ivy	Rash and pruritus
Nutritive	Vitamin C	Scurvy (in absence of vitamin C)
	Iron	Anemia (in absence of iron)
	Vitamin A	Poisoning (in excess)
Infectious	Measles virus	Measles, measles encephalitis
	HIV	AIDS
	Varicella virus	Chickenpox
	Influenza virus	Influenza
Genetic	Genetic tendency	Sickle cell disease
Psychological	Stress	Ulcerative colitis, heart disease, suicide, asthma, alcoholism, drug abuse, violence

CHARACTERISTICS OF NONINFECTIOUS AGENTS
Noninfectious agents share some of the characteristics of infectious agents. For example, the extent of exposure to the agent affects its ability to cause health problems. Ingesting moderate amounts of alcohol or aspirin does not cause problems, but excessive consumption does. The amount of stress to which one is exposed can also affect the development of stress-related illness.

The concept of infectivity can also be applied to other types of agents, although the term was developed in relation to communicable diseases. For example, asbestos, which can be inhaled, has a higher "infectivity" than an overdose of aspirin, which must be ingested. Stress, as an agent of illness, also has a high infectivity because it is an everyday factor impinging on people. All of us are "infected" by stress.

Stress can also be viewed in terms of its ability to cause disease. Although everyone experiences some degree of stress, not all people develop stress-related illnesses. Stress, therefore, has a relatively low pathogenicity. Noninfectious agents may vary in terms of their virulence as well. Stress can produce a mild stomach upset in some individuals and drive others to suicide. In the first instance, stress has a low virulence, and in the second, a high virulence.

ENVIRONMENT
The third element of the epidemiologic triad includes factors in the physical, biological, and social environments that contribute to health-related conditions. The physical environment consists of such factors as weather, terrain, and buildings. A variety of physical environment factors can influence health. For example, air pollution contributes to respiratory disease as well as other physi-ologic and psychological effects in human beings. Similarly, excessive heat exposure resulted in an average of 371 deaths per year from 1979 to 1997 (National Center for Environmental Health, 2000), and hypothermia caused an average of 699 deaths per year during a similar period (National Center for Environmental Health, 2001).

The biological environment, in the triad model, consists of all living organisms other than humans. Components of the biological environment include plants and animals as well as microorganisms, all of which can influence health.

The social environment includes factors related to social interaction that may contribute to health or disease. For example, cultural factors, which are part of the social environment, can influence health behaviors. In a similar fashion, social norms may influence health and illness. For example, societal views of alcoholism and drug abuse as character weaknesses have hampered efforts to control these problems.

The Web of Causation Model

The "web of causation" is a second model for understanding the influence of multiple factors on the development of a specific health condition. In this model, factors are explored in terms of their interplay, and both direct and indirect causes of the problem are identified. The web of causation approach allows the epidemiologist to map the interrelationships among factors contributing to the development (or prevention) of a particular health condition. This approach also assists in determining areas where efforts at control will be most effective.

Some of the factors in the web of causation for the problem of adolescent tobacco use are depicted in Figure 10–4 ■. It is obvious from the complexity of Figure 10–4 that multiple factors contribute to adolescent tobacco use. The interplay of these factors determines whether or not the problem occurs. The most direct causes are those linked directly to tobacco use, purchase of tobacco products and the decision to use them. Numerous other factors, however, contribute to the adolescent's decision to engage in the use of tobacco.

Factors influencing tobacco use by adolescents include perceptions of tobacco use as grown up or "cool," peer pressure, and easy access to tobacco products. Perceptions of tobacco use are influenced by media messages and adult role models as well as by peer perceptions. Easy access to tobacco products is influenced by poor enforcement of laws regarding sale of tobacco products to minors, which is in turn influenced by public acceptance of tobacco use. Other contributing factors and their interrelationships are depicted in the figure.

Dever's Epidemiologic Model

Dever's epidemiologic model provides a third approach to conceptualizing the interplay of factors involved in the development of a particular condition. The model, based on prior work by Lalonde and on the work of Blum, was developed as an approach to formulating health care pol-

icy for the State of Georgia. The model has been used extensively in Georgia to determine health care priorities and to design programs to address those priorities. G. Alan Dever was a health policy analyst with the Georgia State Department of Health at the time of the model's development. The model itself consists of four basic elements: human biology, environment, lifestyle, and the health care system (Dever, 1991). The elements of Dever's model and specific considerations related to each are depicted in Figure 10–5 ■.

It should be noted that, although this model has been extensively used as a basis for health policy formation, epidemiologic data alone are not sufficient for this purpose. In addition to information about factors contributing to disease, policy makers must consider other elements in policy decisions (Savitz, Poole, & Miller, 1999). As we saw in Unit I, economic, cultural, and ethical considerations must also enter into deliberations about health care policy.

HUMAN BIOLOGICAL FACTORS

Human biological factors in Dever's model are similar to the host-related factors of the epidemiologic triad and the biophysical dimension of health in the dimensions model. Biological factors include genetic inheritance, the functioning of complex physiologic systems, and maturation and aging.

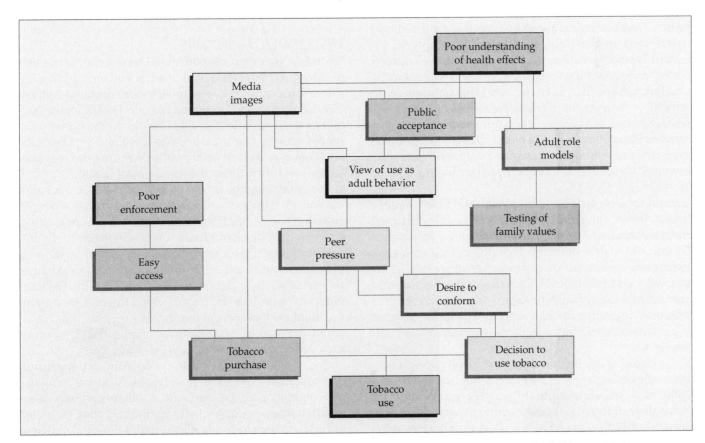

FIGURE 10–4 ■ *The Web of Causation for Adolescent Tobacco Use, Indicating the Interplay Between Multiple Direct and Indirect Causative Factors*

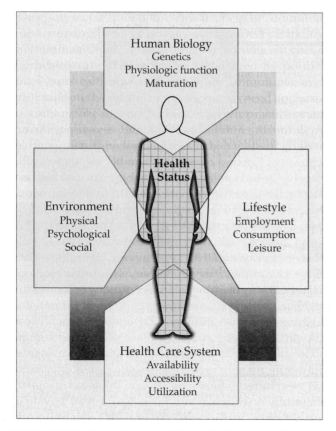

FIGURE 10–5 ■ *Elements of Dever's Epidemiologic Model*

GENETIC INHERITANCE   Genetic inheritance encompasses the influence of human features that are genetically determined such as race, gender, and predisposition to certain types of health problems. As noted in Chapter 9, some health conditions are more prevalent in some racial or ethnic groups than in others, and some occur more frequently in men than in women. Genetic predisposition to disease is seen in a variety of conditions including several cancers, heart disease, and diabetes. There is also growing evidence that genetic factors may be operating in some mental illnesses and in other types of conditions.

COMPLEX PHYSIOLOGIC FUNCTION   One's state of health and physiologic functional status also influences the development of other health problems. For example, fatigue and malnutrition are both physiologic states that may predispose one to developing illnesses such as influenza and tuberculosis. Preexisting disease may also contribute to other health problems. For example, depression may be a factor in child neglect in the same way that hypertension contributes to cardiovascular disease and stroke.

Immunity is another element of one's physiologic state that influences susceptibility to disease. *Immunity* is a state of nonsusceptibility to a disease or condition. Physiologic immunity is based on the presence of specific antibodies to disease and is described as passive or active depending on the role of the host in developing those antibodies. In *active immunity*, the host is exposed to the antigen, either through having the disease or via immunization with active antigens (e.g., diphtheria/tetanus/pertussis [DTaP] vaccine). Active immunity is relatively long lasting, waning over several years if at all. In *passive immunity,* externally produced antibodies are provided to the host by way of immunization (e.g., hepatitis immune globulin) or transfer (e.g., from mother to fetus across the placenta).

Cross-immunity occurs when immunity to one agent also confers immunity to a related agent. This type of immunity was operating when Edward Jenner inoculated people with material from cowpox lesions to prevent smallpox. Another concept related to physiologic immunity that has relevance for groups of people is herd immunity. *Herd immunity* is generalized resistance to disease within a population that arises because most of the people have specific immunity to the condition. Herd immunity decreases the potential for exposure among those few people who do not have immunity.

MATURATION AND AGING   The third element of Dever's human biology component is the influence of maturation and aging on the development of health problems. The very young and the very old, for example, are often more vulnerable to the effects of abuse than other age groups because of their dependence on the abuser. Similarly, adolescent development, which is characterized by a sense of personal invulnerability, may lead to risk-taking sexual and drug use behaviors contributing to the development of health problems.

ENVIRONMENTAL FACTORS

The environmental component of Dever's model consists of physical, psychological, and social environments. These categories are comparable to the concepts of physical and social environment and host psychological factors in the epidemiologic triad model. In the dimensions model, environmental categories identified by Dever are subsumed within the physical environmental, psychological, and sociocultural dimensions of health.

Environmental factors have a variety of effects on population health status. For example, lack of space in crowded homes has been reported as a deterrent to physical activity (Nies, Vollman, & Cook, 1999). Similarly, animal hoarding or the keeping of more pets that an individual is capable of caring for may arise from psychiatric problems such as dementia, but poses health risks for individuals and for the population at large. Although little attention has been given to this problem, it is anticipated that 700 to 2,000 cases of animal hoarding occur each year in the United States (Patronek, 1999).

Social environmental factors also influence the health of populations. We have already discussed the influence of economic, political, and cultural factors as they affect health. Other examples include findings that increased population density is associated with rehospitalization in persons with mental illness (Husted & Jorgens, 2000) and that longer exposure to low socioeconomic status has a cumulative effect on health with health effects arising at younger ages than in more affluent populations (Power, Manor, & Matthews, 1999). Similarly, unsafe neighborhoods and lack of child care affect the extent of physical activity in some populations (Nies et al., 1999).

Social factors influencing health also include the effects of political activities by special-interest groups. For instance, tobacco lobbyists mounted extensive media campaigns in attempts to delay implementation of California's smoke-free bars legislation. These efforts were only overcome by a sustained effort by local public health interest groups (Magzamen & Glantz, 2001).

LIFESTYLE FACTORS

Dever (1991) contended that lifestyle factors are the greatest contributors to most health problems and provide the best avenue for control of those problems. Lifestyle factors include employment, consumption patterns, and leisure activity and associated risks. Employment or occupation may influence health in several ways including the potential for exposure to hazardous conditions. One occupational factor that affects many nurses is shift work. Approximately 17% of all U.S. workers are involved in shift work, and research indicates increased potential for injury and mistakes due to loss of concentration in this population. These effects are believed to be the results of poor sleep patterns displayed by many people who engage in shift work (Erwin, 1998). In addition, the fact of being employed (or unemployed) may influence access to survival necessities as well as to health care.

Consumption patterns include dietary and exercise patterns as well as the use or abuse of substances like tobacco, caffeine, and alcohol and other drugs. Finally, recreational aspects of lifestyle may influence health either in their presence or absence. Absence of recreational opportunities or leisure activities may influence the effects of stress on health. Certain types of recreation, on the other hand, may contribute to health problems. For example, use of hot tubs and swimming pools has been linked to cases of dermatitis and otitis externa (Epidemiology Program Office, 2000), and the popularity of unpowered scooters resulted in more than 27,000 injuries requiring emergency care from January to October of 2000 (National Center for Injury Prevention and Control, 2000).

HEALTH SYSTEM FACTORS

Factors within the health care system and the attitudes and activities of health care providers also contribute to health and illness. For example, use of a specific protocol in prenatal care increased detection of abuse of women from 0.8% to 7% of clients served (Wiist & McFarlane, 1999). Studies also indicate that specific messages from personal health providers influence clients' health-promotive behaviors (Centers for Disease Control and Prevention, 2000). Factors in the health care system may also exert negative effects on health. Invasive medical

procedures, for example, may increase the risk of HIV or hepatitis infection, or health care providers may miss, or even ignore, evidence of spouse, elder, or child abuse.

Health system factors may interact with other categories of factors to limit care. For example, adults with physical disabilities have been found to receive fewer health promotive services than those without disabilities. Reasons for this difference have been identified as short appointment times that do not accommodate limited mobility, physically inaccessible services, and equipment (e.g., mammography equipment) that cannot accommodate clients who cannot stand (Iezzoni, McCarthy, Davis, & Siebens, 2000).

Each of the three epidemiologic models presented here can be used to organize information related to client health status, to identify health problems, and to direct interventions. The epidemiologic triad is the most extensively used of the three models, but may be somewhat difficult to use in describing health problems that have no identifiable agent or that arise from the complex interaction of multiple factors. The web of causation model addresses the complexity of factors influencing health and illness, but its very complexity may limit its utility. In using the model, one could potentially go on at length examining causative factors. This model is useful, however, in identifying points at which intervention is likely to eliminate or control a health problem. Neither of these two models acknowledges the influence of the health care system on the health of populations, nor do they highlight lifestyle factors that are some of the greatest influences on health and illness. Dever's model incorporates these elements, but fails to address other aspects of health behavior, such as use of safety measures, that may influence health. For these reasons, the dimensions model, which incorporates the dimensions of health as outlined in Chapter 9, will be used to provide an epidemiologic perspective throughout the remainder of this book.

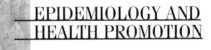

EPIDEMIOLOGY AND HEALTH PROMOTION

Thus far, epidemiology has been discussed primarily in relation to problems of ill health. In addition to considering factors that contribute to or prevent specific problems, community health nurses should investigate and identify those factors that promote health. It has been suggested that the health care professions should focus on an "epidemiology of health."

From its beginning, community health nursing has been engaged in health promotion, and this should remain a primary focus of community health nursing practice. Recently, other health care providers have become aware of the need for promoting health in addition to treating or even preventing specific diseases. This recognition is coming slowly, however, and community health nursing has the advantage of already being the forerunner in this area.

Interest in health promotion has occurred as a result of the shift from infectious to chronic disease as the major cause of death. This shift has been accompanied by increased cost for medical care, changes in payment sources, and research indicating that individual behavior may contribute to chronic illness. These factors have encouraged consumers and funders of health care services to turn to health promotion and behavior modification as means of decreasing costs.

Health promotion has been defined by the World Health Organization (WHO) (1986) as the "process of enabling people to increase control over and to improve their own health" (p. iii). This enabling process has two primary foci: changes in lifestyle behaviors by individuals and changes in structural elements that influence health (Benson & Latter, 1998).

Structural elements that influence health involve the creation of environments that are conducive to healthy behaviors and that promote health. Several levels of influence on health behaviors can be identified. The first level includes the intrapersonal factors that influence each of us, and the second encompasses interpersonal factors and the degree of support provided by one's social network. The third level involves institutional factors that may impinge on health behavior, for example, a no-smoking policy in the work environment. At the fourth level community factors influence health-promoting behavior. We noted earlier, for example, that unsafe neighborhoods influence people's willingness to engage in physical activity. The final level of influence is that of public policy and includes such factors as ordinances and legislation, resource allocation, regulation, and enforcement (Baker & Brownson, 1998; Schneider, 2000). The levels of influence in health promotion activities are summarized below.

CULTURAL CONSIDERATIONS

The concept of group learning activities is not a cultural norm in some ethnic cultures, such as the Hmong. For this reason, they are unlikely to attend community health education presentations designed to promote health. How might you design health promotion programs to be more consonant with cultural behavior patterns? Conversely, what might you do to attract them to health education sessions?

ASSESSING THE HEALTH PROMOTION SITUATION

In order to provide effective health promotion to individual clients, families, and populations, community health nurses must assess the factors operating in the health promotion situation. One key element for the nurse to assess is population attitudes to and perceptions of health and health promotion (Zhan, Cloutterbuck, Keshian, & Lombardi, 1998). Community health nurses should also consider health promotion strategies already employed by the population. What are they? To what extent are they employed? Who employs them?

Another consideration in assessing the health promotion situation is the factors present in the environment that either promote healthy behaviors or impede them. Community health nurses should consider not only

Health promotion campaigns may make use of media advertising.

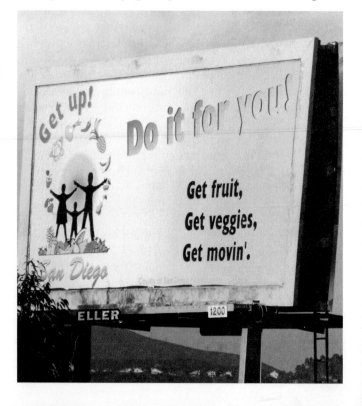

HIGHLIGHTS

Levels of Influence in Health Promotion

Intrapersonal factors: Factors intrinsic to the individual that enhance or deter health-promoting behavior

Interpersonal factors: Social support networks that facilitate or impede health promotion

Institutional factors: Factors within an organization that enhance or deter health promotion

Community factors: Factors in the larger environment that influence health promotion

Public policy: Legislative and other societal policy initiatives that influence health promotion

Sources: Baker, E. A., & Brownson, C. A. (1998). Defining characteristics of community-based health promotion programs. *Journal of Public Health Management Practice, 4*(2), 1–9; and Schneider, M. J. (2000). *Introduction to public health.* Gaithersburg, MD: Aspen.

facilitators and barriers to personal health behaviors, but other environmental factors that may facilitate or impede health promotion (Raphael, 1998). Barriers to health promotion arise from multiple sources, including clients, health care providers, and health care systems and settings (U.S. Department of Health and Human Services, 1998). Identified barriers related to clients include lack of knowledge or motivation, anxiety regarding specific activities and their effects, cost, inconvenience, and unrealistic expectations regarding the effects of certain health-promoting behaviors. Barriers may also exist with respect to health care providers, including lack of training in health promotion and preventive services, lack of confidence in the effects of interventions, lack of time, and confusion regarding conflicting recommendations. The existence of these barriers is further supported by findings that education in health promotion was one of the training needs most often identified by public health professionals (Reder, Gale, & Taylor, 1999). Additional provider-related barriers include inadequate reimbursement for health promotion activities, liability concerns, and client demands and expectations. Finally, barriers to health promotion and prevention activities arise from health care systems, particularly in their emphasis on cure rather than prevention and the absence of systems for tracking and monitoring health promotion activities.

⑥THINK ABOUT IT

What health promotion activities could be used to modify social factors contributing to disease in the general population?

Given the recent growth of managed care organizations (MCOs) as a mode of health care delivery, community health nurses may also want to assess the contribution of local MCOs to population-based health promotion activities. Research has indicated a continuum of models of involvement of MCOs in population-based health promotion (Stoil & Hill, 1998). These models are summarized at right. A summary of an article describing health promotion activities in MCOs is available on the companion Web site for this book.

Nurses should also assess other resources for health promotion in the community including specific programs and personnel as well as the presence of community health problems (e.g., high injury incidence) that suggests the need for health promotion activities. Tips for assessing a health promotion situation are presented on page 226.

HIGHLIGHTS

Models of Managed Care Organization (MCO) Involvement in Health Promotion

Revenue center model: MCO contracts with specific populations to provide health promotion services that generate revenue for the MCO.

Prevention subcontract model: MCO subcontracts with an out-of-network community agency to provide a specific package of health promotion services determined by the MCO.

Prevention carve-out model: MCO supports certain designated providers who provide a package of services determined by a government agency or buying cooperative. MCO involvement may be limited to contributing a portion of funds per enrolled client.

Case referral model: MCO refers clients as needed to outside agencies for health promotion services without compensation.

Community patron model: MCO employees donate time and energy for health promotion services as a charitable project. MCO may provide in-kind materials, supplies, and so on.

Strategic investment model: MCO views health promotion activities as providing a long-term return. Specific activities are frequently selected for visibility.

Collaborative model: MCO engages in full cooperative effort with public sector or nonprofit organizations to provide health promotion services. Again, projects may be selected on the basis of their visibility for public relations.

Integrated services model: Prevention and promotion services are an integral component of MCO clinical services.

Source: Stoil, M. J., & Hill, G. A. (1998). Survey results on behavioral health promotion in managed primary health care. *Journal of Public Health Management Practice, 4*(1), 101–109.

PLANNING AND IMPLEMENTING HEALTH PROMOTION STRATEGIES

Generally speaking, there are two broad types of health promotion programs: those that are intended to prevent specific diseases or promote specific health outcomes and those that focus on improving a population's capacity to promote health (Mittelmark, 1999). Both may employ five general strategies for health promotion identified in the *Ottawa Charter for Health Promotion.* These strategies include:

assessment tips assessment tips assessment tips

ASSESSING THE HEALTH PROMOTION SITUATION

- What are the expectations of the population with respect to health and health promotion? What is the attitude of health care providers to health promotion activities? What is the level of motivation for health promotion among various segments of the population?
- What factors in the population affect the ability of its members to promote their health? To what extent are these factors related to personal behavior? To environmental factors?
- What facilitates health promotion in the population? What barriers to health-promoting activities exist?

- What health-promoting behaviors do members of the population currently use? What additional health promotion activities are needed?
- What resources are available within the health system to support health promotion?
- Who determines health promotion policies and priorities?
- What societal changes are needed to create an environment conducive to health and health promotion? What barriers exist to these changes?

- Development of public policy that supports health
- Creation of environments conducive to health
- Strengthening community action with respect to health issues
- Developing personal health-related skills
- Reorienting health services to a focus on health promotion (Green, Poland, & Rootman, 2000).

Although each of the two foci for health promotion programs may make use of these general strategies, they may differ considerably in terms of the specific interventions employed. Preventing specific health conditions or promoting specific health outcomes frequently relies on interventions with individual clients including health education, behavior modification, and so on. Enhancing the capacity of populations to promote health is more likely to involve policy development and societal change, although there may be a certain amount of cross-over in strategies that accomplish these two purposes.

In planning specific health promotion programs at either level, community health nurses should incorporate interventions that have been shown to be effective in population studies. The Centers for Disease Control and Prevention (2000) has suggested a systematic approach for identifying interventions that may be used in health promotion. First, the community health nurse should use a systematic approach to selecting and grouping interventions to be reviewed. For example, the nurse may be interested primarily in interventions that enhance immunization levels within the population and may group them in terms of those directed toward recipients of care and those directed toward providers. The nurse then systematically searches for and retrieves research related to the selected intervention categories, summarizing data on the effectiveness of these interventions. The nurse will also attend to data related to other

aspects of the interventions, for example, the types of populations to which they have been applied, their cost-effectiveness, potentially harmful effects, barriers to implementation, and so on. From this review, nurses and other health promotion program developers can select one or more health promotion strategies most likely to be effective with a given population in a specific situation. These strategies can then be developed and implemented, incorporating the scientific data derived as well as the expectations of the population to be served.

Motivating individuals, populations, or policy makers to take actions that will promote health can be a difficult aspect of program implementation. The health promotion matrix model has been suggested as a means of assisting to motivate action at varying levels (Gorin & Arnold, 1998). The model begins with the client's creation of an idealized image of health. The nurse then assists the client (whether family, community, or policy-making group) to examine current health status in light of that idealized image, identifying discrepancies and factors that contribute to them. Nurse and client proceed to identify strategies to minimize health-depleting patterns and maximize health-promoting patterns, eventually, if successful, internalizing these strategies and creating movement toward the ideal image. This model is depicted in Figure 10–6 ■.

Implementation of health promotion strategies frequently makes use of media messages and images. Mass media has certain advantages as a vehicle for health promotion information and advocacy because of its wide audience, its ability to reach otherwise hidden audiences, and its ability to create an awareness of public health issues in the general public as well as among policy makers. For some purposes, media also have the disadvantages of not being able to target interventions to specific groups and the potential for unintended effects (Wellings & Macdowall, 2000).

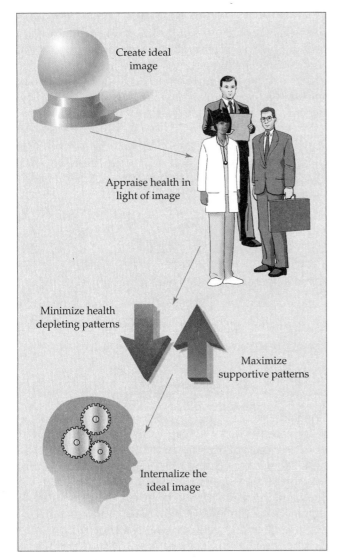

FIGURE 10–6 ■ *Matrix Model of Health Promotion*

⑥THINK ABOUT IT

How can community health nurses engage representatives of mass media in health promotion activities?

Community health nurses and others involved in health promotion activities may employ media campaigns for a variety of purposes. These include agenda setting and consciousness raising, interpreting meaning of events and information in ways that are favorable to health action, and conferring legitimacy on health-related issues. Media can also be used to promote understanding of issues and to disseminate health-related information as well as to promote a particular public health stance (Finnegan & Viswanath, 1999). Most use of media for health promotion occurs in the form of specific health-related messages. Although not

fully developed, there is considerable potential for the use of entertainment media to promote health as well. Nurses engaged in planning and implementing health promotion programs may access additional resources through the links provided on the companion Web site for this book. 🌐

■ EVALUATING HEALTH PROMOTION ACTIVITIES

Community health nurses should also be involved in the evaluation of the outcomes and effectiveness of health promotion efforts. In this evaluation, it is important to evaluate both the achievement of outcomes and the processes designed to accomplish them. Evaluating health promotion programs can lead to better design, promote informed choices among program options, assist with funding decisions, and test new ideas in practice. In addition, program evaluation can assist in determining the transferability of interventions to other populations (Wright, 1999).

In order to truly assess the effectiveness of population-based programs, their effects must be examined both in light of those who participated as well as those who did not (Pirie, 1999). One approach to doing this comparative evaluation involves the use of the RE-AIM framework for evaluating health promotion effectiveness. The acronym RE-AIM stands for reach (R), efficacy (E), adoption (A), implementation (I), and maintenance (M) (Glasgow, Vogt, & Boles, 1999).

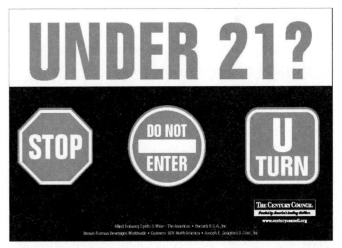

Media campaigns are designed to make a point obvious with few words. (Photo courtesy of The Century Council, Washington DC.)

⤳CRITICAL THINKING IN RESEARCH

Several authors have noted that it is difficult to evaluate the effects of population-based health promotion programs because the programs are not evenly applied to all members of the population. In programs designed for individuals, on the other hand, one can compare persons who were exposed to the health promotion intervention to a matched group of people who were not. Population-based programs are usually targeted to large segments of the population, and any given individual may or may not have been exposed to the program.

- How might you design a study to evaluate the effects of a population-based media campaign to prevent family violence that would address this type of difficulty?
- What outcome measures would you use?
- Who would your study population include? How would you recruit them?
- What kind of data would you collect? How and when might you collect it?

Reach refers to program participants and their characteristics and risk factors as compared to members of the target population who do not participate. *Efficacy* reflects program outcomes, both positive and negative and intended and untended. These outcomes occur for program recipients, staff, and payers or purchasers of services and should consider behavioral outcomes, quality of life, and satisfaction measures as well as biological outcomes and participation measures.

⑥THINK ABOUT IT

How might an individual's level of risk for a specific condition differ from that of the population at large for the same condition? Give several examples.

ETHICAL AWARENESS

Keeping people healthy is a more cost-effective use of limited resources than treating them once they develop health problems. This type of thinking has led some policy makers to redesign resource allocation strategies so that the majority of public health care funding is directed toward health promotion, with less money devoted to care of those who are ill. This generally means that public funds are not used for expensive "high-tech" procedures such as cardiac bypass and so on. One result is that people who have money can afford such procedures and those who do not are often denied needed care. What do you think of the ethical implications of such policies? What ethical points of view would support such policies? From what perspectives might they be attacked?

Outcomes may occur at several levels: immediate, intermediate, and ultimate. Immediate outcomes may occur at the level of individual program participants and could include such measures as reduction in risk behaviors or improved coping abilities. Intermediate outcomes can be initial health-related results such as increased productivity in the occupational setting or reductions in health services utilization. Ultimate outcomes for community-based health promotion programs usually occur at the population level and may include reduced incidence of disease or an extended healthy life span (as opposed to mere longevity) (Gillis, 1995).

⑥THINK ABOUT IT

Why is it inappropriate to "blame the victim" when individuals do not engage in health-promoting behaviors (e.g., when they resist physical activity in spite of knowledge of the adverse health effects of inactivity)?

Adoption refers to the extent to which the health promotion intervention or policy has been implemented in a variety of populations and settings. For example, one might examine the extent to which occupational settings have adopted no-smoking policies in the absence of state legislation mandating such policies. Assessment of this element of the framework would also address barriers to adoption in certain settings (e.g., revenue from vending machine sales in the work setting).

Implementation reflects the degree to which a particular program, policy, or strategy has been implemented as planned. Assessment of implementation involves both program recipients and providers. Implementation can be said to have failed if participants drop out of the program before completion or if staff fail to implement it as designed. Finally, the *maintenance* aspect of the framework addresses the extent to which program outcomes have been maintained (for recipients) and the degree to which the program or policy has been incorporated into the daily operation of the organization (Glasgow et al., 1999). Potential evaluation questions related to each of the components of the RE-AIM framework are presented at right.

The RE-AIM framework does not specifically address economic assessment of health promotion programs, but this is an important aspect of their evaluation to justify the use of limited resources (Wonderling & Karnon, 2000). Three approaches to economic assessment, their general purposes, and a brief description of the method are summarized in Table 10–4 ■. Information from health promotion program evaluation can be used to improve program performance and to facilitate health promotion in population groups.

■ **TABLE 10–4   Approaches to Economic Evaluation of Health Promotion Programs**

APPROACH	TYPICAL USE	DESCRIPTION
Cost-effectiveness analysis	Choice between program alternatives to achieve the same ends	Comparison of cost per unit of outcome (preferred choice is program with lowest cost per unit)
Cost-utility analysis	Choice among different types of programs to meet different ends	Comparison of programs in terms of improvements in life expectancy and quality of life versus cost (preferred choice is program with lowest cost per weighted quality unit)
Cost-benefit analysis	Comparison between health- and non–health-related programs	Comparison of monetary value of outcomes achieved versus cost of resources used to achieve them (preferred choice is program that achieves highest value outcome for lowest cost in resources)

From their early history, community health nurses have been actively involved in health promotion. This involvement has occurred at the level of both the individual or family client and at the societal level. Contact information for agencies and organizations that support health promotion activities and that can be of assistance to community health nurses in their efforts are provided on the companion Web site for this book.

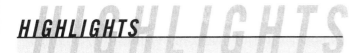

HIGHLIGHTS

Evaluation Questions Related to Components of the RE-AIM Framework

Reach: Is the program reaching those for whom it was intended? Who is participating in the program and how do they differ from those who are not?

Efficacy: What are the intended and unintended, positive and negative outcomes of the program for participants, staff, and payers?

Adoption: To what extent has the program, strategy, or policy been adopted in relevant settings? What barriers to adoption have been identified?

Implementation: To what extent has the program or policy been implemented as designed? Have participants completed the program?

Maintenance: To what extent have program effects been maintained? Has the program or policy been institutionalized as a part of the normal operation of the agency?

APPLYING YOUR KNOWLEDGE IN PRACTICE

✂ CASE STUDY
Promoting Population Health

New state legislation has mandated that the majority of funds allocated for public health efforts be devoted to health promotion activities rather than to care of clients with existing health problems. Some of the major health problems encountered in the state at this time include heart disease, family violence, and social isolation among the elderly.

• Which of these issues would be most amenable to health promotion efforts? Why?

• What additional information would you want regarding risk factors for each of these conditions prior to designing health promotion programs for addressing them? Where might you obtain the needed information?

- Choose one of the three problems and design a set of strategies to address it. What factors would need to be addressed at the intrapersonal, interpersonal, institutional, community, and public policy levels of influence in order to promote health in the area chosen? What community health nursing activities might promote action at those levels?

❦ TESTING YOUR UNDERSTANDING

- Compare and contrast at least two of the theories of disease causation discussed in the chapter. How does each of the theories compare with today's understanding of causation? (pp. 210–211)
- Describe a cause and effect relationship with which you are familiar. Describe how the relationship does or does not exemplify the criteria for causality presented in the chapter. (pp. 211–212)
- What is meant by the term *risk*? How is the concept of risk used in community health nursing? (p. 212)
- What is the difference between morbidity and mortality? (p. 213)
- What are the steps in the epidemiologic process? How do they relate to those of the nursing process? (pp. 215–216)

- How do analytic and experimental epidemiologic investigations differ? In what ways are they similar? How do they differ from descriptive epidemiology? (p. 217)
- What are the three elements of the epidemiologic triad? (pp. 218–220)
- What are some of the advantages and disadvantages of the web of causation model as compared to the epidemiologic triad and Dever's model? (pp. 220–223)
- What are the major components of Dever's epidemiologic model? (pp. 221–223)
- What are the two major foci of health promotion activities? How do they differ in terms of the types of strategies that might be used? (p. 224)

REFERENCES

Baker, E. A., & Brownson, C. A. (1998). Defining characteristics of community-based health promotion programs. *Journal of Public Health Management Practice, 4*(2), 1–9.

Benson, S., & Latter, S. (1998). Implementing health promoting nursing: The integration of interpersonal skills and health promotion. *Journal of Advanced Nursing, 27,* 100–107.

Centers for Disease Control and Prevention. (2000). Strategies for reducing exposure to environmental tobacco smoke, increasing tobacco-use cessation, and reducing initiation in communities and health-care systems. A report on recommendations of the Task Force on Community Preventive Services. *Morbidity and Mortality Weekly Report, 49*(RR-12), 1–11.

Chinn, J. (2000). *Control of communicable diseases manual* (17th ed.). Washington, DC: American Public Health Association.

Coggon, D., Rose, G., & Barker, D. J. P. (1997). *Epidemiology for the uninitiated* (4th ed.). London: BMJ.

Dever, G. E. A. (1991). *Community health analysis: A global analysis at the local level* (2nd ed.). Gaithersburg, MD: Aspen.

Epidemiology Program Office. (2000). *Pseudomonas* dermatitis/folliculitis associated with pools and hot tubs—Colorado and Maine, 1999–2000. *Morbidity and Mortality Weekly Report, 49,* 1087–1091.

Erwin, J. (1998). Staying alert: How shift work affects nurses' health. *NurseWeek, 11*(21), 13.

Finnegan, J. R., & Viswanath, K. (1999). Mass media and health promotion: Lessons learned with implications for public health campaigns. In N. Bracht (Ed.), *Health promotion at the community level* (2nd ed.), (pp. 119–126). Thousand Oaks, CA: Sage.

Friis, R. H., & Sellers, T. A. (1999). *Epidemiology for public health practice* (2nd ed.). Gaithersburg, MD: Aspen.

Gillis, A. (1995). Exploring nursing outcomes for health promotion. *Nursing Forum, 30*(2), 5–12.

Glasgow, R. E., Vogt, T. M., & Boles, S. M. (1999). Evaluating the public health impact of health promotion interventions: The RE-AIM framework. *American Journal of Public Health, 89,* 1322–1327.

Gordis, L. (2000). *Epidemiology* (2nd ed.). Philadelphia: Saunders.

Gorin, S. S., & Arnold, J. (1998). *Health promotion handbook.* St. Louis: Mosby.

Green, L. W., Poland, B. D., & Rootman, I. (2000). The settings approach to health promotion. In B. D. Poland, L. W. Green, & I. Rootman (Eds.), *Settings for health promotion: Linking theory and practice* (pp. 1–43). Thousand Oaks, CA: Sage.

Harkness, G. A. (1995). *Epidemiology in nursing practice.* St. Louis: Mosby.

Husted, J., & Jorgens, A. (2000). Population density as a factor in the rehospitalization of persons with serious and persistent mental illness. *Psychiatric Services, 51,* 603–605.

Iezzoni, L. I., McCarthy, E. P., Davis, R. B., & Siebens, H. (2000). Mobility impairments and use of screening and preventive services. *American Journal of Public Health, 90,* 955–961.

Koopman, J. S., & Lynch, J. W. (1999). Individual causal models and population systems models in epidemiology. *American Journal of Public Health, 89,* 1170–1174.

Magzamen, S., & Glantz, S. A. (2001). The new battleground: California's experience with smoke-free bars. *American Journal of Public Health, 91,* 245–252.

Mittelmark, M. B. (1999). Health promotion at the communitywide level: Lessons from diverse perspectives. In N. Bracht (Ed.), *Health promotion at the community level* (2nd ed.), (pp. 3–27). Thousand Oaks, CA: Sage.

National Center for Environmental Health. (2000). Heat-related illnesses, deaths, and risk factors—Cincinnati and Dayton, Ohio, 1999, and United States, 1979–1997. *Morbidity and Mortality Weekly Report, 49,* 470–473.

National Center for Environmental Health. (2001). Hypothermia-related deaths—Suffolk County, New York, January 1999–March 2000, and United States, 1979–1998. *Morbidity and Mortality Weekly Report, 50,* 53–57.

National Center for Injury Prevention and Control. (2000). Unpowered scooter-related injuries—United States, 1998–2000. *Morbidity and Mortality Weekly Report, 49,* 1108–1110.

Nies, M. A., Vollman, M., & Cook, T. (1999). African American women's experiences with physical activity in their daily lives. *Public Health Nursing, 16,* 23–31.

Patronek, G. J. (1999). Hoarding of animals: An under-recognized public health problem in a difficult-to-study population. *Public Health Reports, 114,* 81–87.

Pirie, P. L. (1999). Evaluating community health promotion programs: Basic questions and approaches. In N. Bracht (Ed.), *Health promotion at the community level* (2nd ed.), (pp. 127–134). Thousand Oaks, CA: Sage.

Power, C., Manor, O., & Matthews, S. (1999). The duration and timing of exposure: Effects of socioeconomic environment on adult health. *American Journal of Public Health, 89,* 1059–1065.

Raphael, D. (1998). Emerging concepts of health and health promotion. *Journal of School Health, 68,* 297–300.

Reder, S., Gale, J. L., & Taylor, J. (1999). Using a dual method needs assessment to evaluate the training needs of public health professionals. *Journal of Public Health Management Practice, 5*(6), 62–69.

Savitz, D. A., Poole, C., & Miller, W. C. (1999). Reassessing the role of epidemiology in public health. *American Journal of Public Health, 89,* 1158–1161.

Schneider, M. J. (2000). *Introduction to public health.* Gaithersburg, MD: Aspen.

Stoil, M. J., & Hill, G. A. (1998). Survey results on behavioral health promotion in managed primary health care. *Journal of Public Health Management Practice, 4*(1), 101–109.

U.S. Department of Health and Human Services. (1998). Put prevention into practice: Teamwork improves CPS delivery. *Prevention Report, 13*(1), 1–2, 4.

Valanis, B. (1999). *Epidemiology in health care* (3rd ed.). Stamford, CT: Appleton & Lange.

Wellings, K., & Macdowall, W. (2000). Evaluating mass media approaches. In M. Thorogood & Y. Coombes (Eds.), *Evaluating health promotion: Practice and methods* (pp. 113–128). New York: Oxford University Press.

Wiist, W. H., & McFarlane, J. (1999). The effectiveness of an abuse assessment protocol in public health prenatal clinics. *American Journal of Public Health, 89,* 1217–1221.

Wonderling, D., & Karnon, J. (2000). Economic evaluation of health promotion programmes. In M. Thorogood & Y. Coombes (Eds.), *Evaluating health promotion: Practice and methods* (pp. 70–83). New York: Oxford University Press.

World Health Organization. (1986). Ottawa charter for health promotion. *Health Promotion, 1*(4), iii–v.

Wright, L. (1999). Evaluating health promotion: The proof of the pudding? In E. R. Perkins, I. Simnett, & L. Wright (Eds.), *Evidence-based health promotion* (pp. 393–403). New York: John Wiley & Sons.

Zhan, L., Cloutterbuck, J., Keshian, J., & Lombardi, L. (1998). Promoting health: Perspectives from ethnic elderly women. *Journal of Community Health Nursing, 15*(1), 31–44.

HEALTH EDUCATION

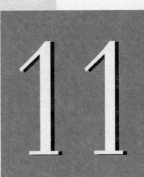

Chapter Objectives

After reading this chapter, you should be able to:

- Describe three types of health-related decisions facilitated by health education.
- Describe at least two barriers to effective health education.
- Assess learning needs in terms of factors related to the six dimensions of health.
- Identify five levels of educational diagnosis.
- Distinguish between process and outcome learning objectives.
- Classify learning objectives according to the domains of learning involved.
- Define a focusing event.
- Describe the use of formative evaluation in a health education encounter.

Media Link

http://www.prenhall.com/clark

Additional interactive resources for this chapter can be found on the companion Web site. Click on Chapter 11 and "Begin" to select the activities for this chapter.

Much of the practice of community health nursing involves educating people about health and health promotion. *Health education* is a participatory learning process that enables people to make informed decisions about health. Recent authors have noted a shift in the rhetoric of health education from an emphasis on providing information and motivating clients to comply with suggested health behaviors to a focus on equipping clients with the knowledge and skills to make their own decisions related to health and health-related behaviors even if these decisions run counter to professional advice. The first approach is the "patient information" model, whereas the second is referred to as a "patient empowerment" model (Piper & Brown, 1998). In the patient information model, the nurse or other health professional is an expert providing objective knowledge; the second model is client-focused and is based on both objective knowledge and the subjective health knowledge and experiences of the client.

When population groups are the client, the information model becomes a "structural change" model in which the nurse still functions as an expert emphasizing objective knowledge on which the population group is expected to act. The more client-centered model at this level becomes a "collective action" model, wherein the community or population has the expertise and chooses to take one or more courses of action (Piper & Brown, 1998).

PURPOSES OF HEALTH EDUCATION

The primary purpose of health education is to assist clients in making health-related decisions. Health education may equip clients to make any of three types of health-related decisions: decisions about self-care, decisions about the use of health resources, and decisions about societal health issues. The latter two types of decisions are, however, related to self-care decisions.

Self-Care

Clients engage in four types of self-care: regulatory, preventive, reactive, and restorative self-care (Barofsky, cited in Hibbard, Greenlick, Jimison, Kunkel, & Tusler, 1999). Decisions related to regulatory self-care reflect attention to normal human processes, such as the foods to be eaten, amount of rest one will obtain, and so on. Preventive self-care involves decisions regarding preventive behaviors such as obtaining immunizations, wearing a seat belt, or exercising. People engage in reactive self-care when they experience symptoms of ill health. Reactive self-care activities may involve getting more rest or using over-the-counter or home remedies. Finally, clients make decisions regarding restorative self-care designed to restore function after illness. For example, one may decide to gradually resume one's usual routine after an episode of illness or eat yogurt after a bout of diarrhea to restore the normal intestinal flora. Restorative self-care may also involve adaptations to the presence of chronic health problems, such as deciding to take an antihypertensive as directed.

Resource Use

The second type of health decision that people make relates to their use of health resources. Health education designed to promote self-care is anticipated to reduce the need and demand for health care services at several levels. Preventive self-care should assist people to remain healthier, while reactive and restorative health care practices may allow clients, even those with chronic diseases, to deal with the consequences of their disease, lessening their dependence on health professionals for illness management (Kramer, Bucher, Glassman, & Siu, 1999). In fact, health education for self-care in the management of chronic illness has been found to decrease health services use by 7% to 17% (Fries, Koop, Sokolov, Beadle, & Wright, 1998). However, when self-care is not sufficient to address client health problems, health education should equip clients to make the most effective use of available health care services, assisting them to select the most appropriate services to meet their needs, preferably at the lowest cost to society.

Health Issues

The third type of decision that can be influenced by health education includes decisions related to societal health issues. Health-related decisions at this level can also be conceptualized as self-care, but self-care for communities or populations rather than individuals. Self-care at this level addresses actions by population groups to safeguard the environment and protect the health of the population (Lipson & Steiger, 1996). Health education, for example, can help people determine whether they should vote for or against mandatory screening for AIDS in the general population, or whether they should contribute funds to the local heart association. Health education can also aid in decisions regarding the merits of motorcycle helmet laws, banning of smoking in public places, or development of a nuclear power plant. Health education can create an informed public prepared to make thoughtful decisions on major health issues.

ETHICAL AWARENESS

Children are sometimes punished by their parents for behaviors enacted "when they know better." Some people have suggested similar sanctions for people who "know better" but continue to engage in unhealthful behaviors. For example, it has been suggested that smokers should be ineligible for public assistance for health problems related to smoking or that motorcycle riders who fail to wear helmets should bear responsibility for the consequences of their actions. Are such attitudes justified? Why or why not?

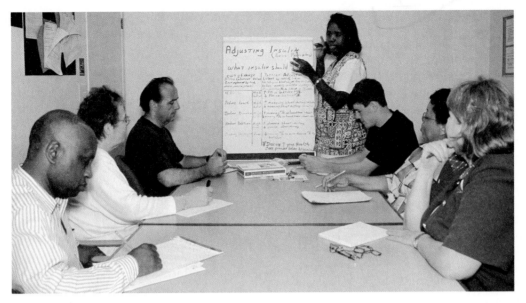

Educational settings are ideal places to present health education messages.

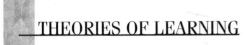

BARRIERS TO LEARNING

Prior to planning health education, the community health nurse must recognize that barriers to learning need to be overcome if health education is to be effective. Barriers may be internal or external. Internal barriers can be physical, social, or psychological. Physical barriers such as pain, fever, and visual disturbances, could interfere with the client's abilities to focus on concepts presented. Social barriers to learning may include the client's education level, language barriers, and incongruence of client beliefs and values with those of the health system. Psychological barriers include anxiety, depression, denial, and inability to accept or, occasionally, overacceptance of the sick role. Other psychological barriers might be previous negative experiences with illness or the health care system and lack of readiness to learn.

External barriers to learning may arise from the learning environment (e.g., noise, distractions) or from the learning situation. Factors related to the learning situation that may create barriers include the timing of educational efforts, the method of teaching used, the level of material presented, or the quality of interaction between nurse and client. In using the education process, the community health nurse identifies potential barriers in a given client situation and circumvents these barriers by planning appropriate interventions.

THEORIES OF LEARNING

An understanding of how learning occurs helps the community health nurse educator to facilitate learning and promote health-related decision making by clients or populations. Learning theories provide that understanding. There are two major types of learning theories, conditioning theories and cognitive theories. In conditioning theories, learning is thought to occur when the learner has made an association between a specific stimulus and a response as a result of repeated exposure to both. When the stimulus is presented, the learner automatically performs the conditioned response without benefit of conscious thought processes. In cognitive theories, on the other hand, learning is believed to result from cognitive processes that involve thinking and problem solving (Coates, 1999). Some theoretical perspectives combine aspects of both types of theory. The theoretical perspectives addressed here include behavioral, cognitive, social, psychodynamic, and humanistic theories (Braungart & Braungart, 1997).

Behavioral Learning Theory

In the behavioral perspective, learning is the result of conditioning in which the learner's behavior is reinforced, either positively or negatively, until the desired behavior becomes the habitual response. Teaching, from this perspective, is a matter of arranging stimuli to elicit the desired response and then reinforcing that response. For example, a group of young children may be presented with a set of pictures of different foods spread on a table and asked to select foods that contain vitamins. Each correct selection is verbally approved and the child gets to put the picture in the "vitamin" box. A negative verbal comment is made each time a child selects an incorrect food item, and the child is told to replace the picture on the table. Through repeated performances and reinforcement, the children should learn to correctly distinguish vitamin-rich foods from other foods.

Cognitive Learning Theory

According to cognitive learning theory, learning involves a complex process of information recognition, classification, coding, storage, and retrieval for use at the appropriate time (Braungart & Braungart, 1997). Operating from this perspective, the educator presents content in a fashion that allows it to be easily integrated into the learner's existing network of information after determining how that network is organized and what prior information it contains. As an example, the community health nurse educator might determine what a group of high school students knows about communicable diseases in general and then introduce content related to HIV infection by comparing and contrasting the new content with prior knowledge.

Social Learning Theory

Social learning theory, developed by Bandura, combines aspects of behavioral and cognitive learning theories (Redman, 2000). The learner attends to new behaviors as modeled by others, including the consequences of the behavior (reinforcing factors), integrates the observations into an existing network, stores and retrieves information to reproduce the behavior, and receives reinforcement through experiencing the expected and valued consequences (Braungart & Braungart, 1997). Returning to the example of the children learning about vitamin-rich foods, children in the group would learn not only from the results of their own food selections, but from observing the outcomes of classmates' selections as well.

Psychodynamic Learning Theory

In the psychodynamic perspective, emotional motivations influence learning. These emotions are derived from past experiences. Suppose, for example, that a nursing student was forced as a child to eat some food he or she abhorred. He or she may later have difficulty learning about the nutritional content of that food. Conversely, fear of becoming a burden to family members may motivate a client to relearn self-care skills following a stroke.

Humanistic Learning Theory

Humanistic learning theories focus on internal motivation for learning rather than on external consequences that figure in behavioral, cognitive, and social theories. One of the most well known of these theories is probably already familiar to you and is based on Maslow's hierarchy of human needs (Braungart & Braungart, 1997). From this perspective, learning is motivated from within by one's need to become self-actualized. In this perspective, both cognitive (informational) learning and affective (attitudinal) learning are important (Gleit, 1998). Teachers operating from this perspective encourage learners to identify and pursue their own needs for learning. Thus, the role of the teacher becomes one of responding to learner's requests. As an example, a nurse educator might ask a group of clients enrolled in a parenting class what aspects of parenting are most problematic for them and what areas they would like the class to address.

PRINCIPLES OF LEARNING

Each of the theories of learning presented here conveys some understanding of how learning occurs and what kinds of activities influence learning. This understanding in turn gives rise to several principles of learning or statements about conditions that facilitate learning. The community health nurse educator uses these principles to create situations and experiences conducive to learning. Five general principles influence the effectiveness of health education. These principles are summarized below and include relevance, individualization, facilitation, feedback, and reinforcement (Coates, 1999).

These five general principles lead to several more specific principles that can guide the design of health education programs. These guiding principles are presented in Table 11–1 ▪. The first few principles relate to the learner. People vary with respect to their need for information and their perception of its relevance. This variability results in differing levels of motivation or willingness to learn which, in turn, influences learning. People also vary in the modes by which they learn best and in the rate at which they learn. For example, some people learn what they see (visual learners), whereas others learn what they hear (auditory learners). Still others learn kinesthetically, by physical manipulation of objects, for example, writing down what they see and hear. Learners may also differ in terms of the time of day at which they learn best and their modes of processing information. For example, some

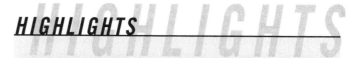

HIGHLIGHTS

General Principles of Learning

Relevance: People are motivated to learn content perceived to be relevant to their lives.

Individualization: People learn differently and the constraints of learning situations differ, so health education encounters must be tailored to the learners and the learning situation.

Facilitation: Learning can be facilitated by pairing a new desired behavior with the client's usual routine.

Feedback: Learning is enhanced when the learner receives feedback that corrects misinformation or inadequate performance and reinforces effective performance.

Reinforcement: Praise for goal achievement increases motivation to learn and facilitates learning and retention of content.

■ **TABLE 11–1   Principles Guiding Health Education**

LEARNER

People learn best what they perceive to be most relevant.

Motivation to learn enhances learning.

People learn in different ways.

Learning can be influenced by clients' physical or emotional states.

LEARNING SITUATION

The context of the learning situation influences learning.

Distractions in the learning situation impede learning.

PRESENTATION OF CONTENT

Individualization of presentation to the learner promotes learning.

Multiple modes of presenting content enhance learning.

Focusing the learner's attention facilitates learning.

Content presented first is learned best.

Logical organization of content facilitates learning.

Progression from simple content to more complex content and from known to unknown information promotes learning.

Association of new material with previous learning enhances learning.

Presentation of positive, rather than negative, behaviors facilitates behavior change.

Active participation by the learner facilitates learning.

Imitation promotes learning.

REINFORCEMENT AND RETENTION

Repetition enhances learning.

Positive reinforcement is more effective than negative reinforcement.

Prompt and accurate feedback enhances learning.

Recency of learning influences retention.

Application of information in several contexts promotes generalization of learning.

learners prefer to engage in active experimentation, while others employ reflective observation to process information (Kitchie, 1997).

Learner differences are one aspect of the context of the learning situation that affects learning. Other factors within that context may include psychological factors, such as the degree of trust the learner has in the teacher, or aspects of the physical environment that affect the learning situation. Distractions present in the learning situation can impede learning.

Variability among learners and learning situations means that various modes of presenting health-related materials will be more effective with some people than with others. Despite this variability, however, there are some general concepts related to the way in which material is presented that apply to most health education encounters. These are included under Presentation of Content in Table 11–1. Because of the differences among learners, the more a health-related presentation is tailored to the needs and capabilities of individual learners, the more effective it will be. People learn in a variety of ways, so presenting content in several ways creates greater opportunity for learning. First, however, learners must attend to the presentation, so the nurse educator attempts to focus their attention. Because people tend to learn best what is presented first, the educator may want to present the most important material immediately after gaining the learner's attention.

Content that is logically organized and that associates new material with prior learning facilitates the integration of new concepts into learners' existing cognitive frameworks. Progressing from simple concepts to more complex content and from the known to the unknown creates a sense of mastery that increases the motivation to learn. Similarly, focusing on desirable behaviors facilitates behavior change more effectively than focusing on behavior to be eliminated. For example, a health education message to "use condoms" encourages a positive behavior, whereas the negatively worded message "don't have unprotected sex" leaves learners wondering what they should do.

People learn from doing. From this perspective, it is easy to see why it is important for learners to participate actively in a learning encounter. One form of participation is imitation of the desired behavior which also promotes learning.

Once a behavior has been learned, it needs to be reinforced before it becomes a habitual response for the learner. Principles of learning related to reinforcement and retention of learning are listed last in Table 11–1. Both repetition and reinforcement enhance learning. In this regard, positive reinforcement is more effective than negative reinforcement. Negative reinforcement can create psychological effects such as anxiety that may impede learning. Prompt and accurate, rather than delayed, feedback on the learner's performance also reinforces learning whether the feedback is positive or negative. Positive feedback creates a sense of success and increases motivation to learn; negative feedback, if it includes suggestions for improving performance, can allay anxiety by providing direction.

Material learned recently is more easily retrieved from stored memory than material learned some time ago. This suggests that if current content is to build on prior learning, a review of prior content may be helpful to reinforce that prior learning and provide readily accessible associations for integrating new material. In a similar way, application of learning in several contexts reinforces learning at the same time it promotes generalization to new situations (Breckon, 1998).

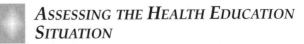

ASSESSING THE HEALTH EDUCATION SITUATION

The health education process begins with an assessment of the audience, their health education needs, and the learning environment. When the client is a group or a community, the first task in assessment is to identify the target audience. Selection of the target audience may be based on level of need, resources available, or probability of success. Assessment then proceeds to identifying characteristics of the audience that influence the learning situation. The assessment can be conducted in terms of the six dimensions of health and addresses biophysical, psychological, physical environmental, sociocultural, behavioral, and health system factors influencing the health education situation.

Biophysical Considerations

Human biology influences both the learning needs and the learning capabilities of individual clients or populations. Areas for consideration include skills and needs related to maturation level and physiologic function.

Skills and Needs Related to the Level of Maturation

To learn effectively, clients need to have the skills appropriate to their level of maturation. In educational terms this is called developmental readiness. For example, small children who have not yet developed abilities for abstract thought will need concrete examples of concepts to be learned. Similarly, a child who still has poorly developed eye–hand coordination will have difficulty learning insulin injection techniques, so teaching will most likely involve parents as well. Changes associated with aging may lead to sensory impairment that influences health education with older populations (Duffy, 1998).

Age or maturation level also affects the client's need for education. For instance, preschool children do not need information about menstruation, but preadolescent girls do. In addition, clients' maturational levels may influence existing knowledge of a particular subject. For example, a group of third graders will probably have a broader knowledge of nutrition concepts than preschoolers.

Physiologic Function

Assessing aspects of physiologic function in the population may reveal special needs for health education or impediments to learning. For example, a high prevalence of diabetes in the population suggests a need for diabetes self-care education, while high incidence rates for sexually transmitted diseases among adolescents indicate other health education needs. Inadequate physiologic function can also give rise to impediments to learning. For example, a group of hearing-impaired youngsters or visually impaired older people require specialized approaches to health education to facilitate their ability to learn. Another aspect of physiologic function that the nurse should consider is the effect of pain on learning abilities (Kramer et al., 1999). For example, pain may distract the client and limit the attention given to an educational presentation.

Psychological Considerations

Elements of the psychological dimension can profoundly influence willingness and ability to learn. Attitudes toward health and health behaviors can either enhance or detract from the motivation to learn. Among clients attending a series of parenting classes, for example, those parents who attend only because of a court mandate related to child abuse usually benefit less than those who attend because they perceive a need for help.

Psychological factors such as stress and anxiety can also impede learning, even for those who are motivated to learn. Nurses can limit the negative effects of the psychological dimension by actions designed to decrease stress and anxiety. For example, the nurse can create a climate in which clients do not feel threatened and in which the nurse educator is seen as a source of support rather than a threat. The nurse who has children and who teaches parenting classes for abusive parents might create such a climate by beginning the first session with a description of the frustration the nurse sometimes feels as a parent.

Other psychological factors that motivate healthy behaviors in the population can be reinforced to enhance learning. For example, educational campaigns to enhance adult car seat belt use can focus on safety and role modeling for children.

⑥THINK ABOUT IT

Do you think that a certain level of stress and anxiety promotes learning? Why or why not?

Physical Environmental Considerations

The physical environment should also be considered in terms of its effects on learning. Is there adequate lighting for the tasks to be accomplished? Is there too much noise? Will clients be distracted by other activities occurring in the learning environment? During a home visit, for example, it might be wise to turn off the television before attempting to educate a hypertensive client about his or her medication.

Physical environmental factors may also give rise to the need for health education. For example, population groups affected by natural disasters may need assistance in preventing communicable diseases. Similarly, health education efforts might be targeted to persons with chronic respiratory conditions in areas with significant air pollution.

Sociocultural Considerations

The sociocultural dimension is particularly influential in shaping attitudes about health and health-related behaviors. Examples and attitudes of those around us influence our willingness to engage in self-care behaviors as well as affecting our attitudes to health issues at the societal level.

Elements of the sociocultural dimension also influence one's exposure to health-related information. People with lower education levels are less likely than those with more formal education to have been exposed to prior health education. The education level of the population and of specific target audiences necessarily influences the nurse's choice of teaching strategies and content to be presented.

Cultural influences on health education with population groups include typical communication styles, concepts of time and personal space, values, and perceptions of environmental control (Davidhizar, Dowd, & Giger, 1998). Client life roles and role expectations, which are culturally defined, are other factors that may affect interest in health education and motivation to learn. When content is perceived to be relevant to the roles one is expected to fulfill, one's motivation to learn is likely to be high. Roles may also influence one's ability to attend to health messages. For example, if members of the audience are responsible for the care of children, they are unlikely to be able to attend educational presentations unless child care is arranged (Duffy, 1998).

Culture may also influence the effectiveness of health education in terms of the trust placed in health professionals. Many culturally diverse audiences may distrust health professionals as a result of past experiences or cultural misunderstandings (Breckon, 1998).

Language is another sociocultural factor that might hamper learning abilities unless the nurse allows for language differences in planning health education. In conducting the client assessment, the nurse determines the group's fluency in the dominant language (usually English in the United States) as well as the languages usually spoken. When educating clients who speak other languages, community health nurses should keep in mind that educational materials translated directly from English may not convey the intended message or may be unintelligible to the client. Interpreters can be used, but again it is important to use interpreters who speak a form of a language familiar to the particular client. The general principles regarding the use of interpreters discussed in Chapter 6 apply to health education situations as well.

Occupation is another social dimension factor that can give rise to health education needs. Trash collectors, for example, might require education related to body mechanics and techniques for lifting heavy objects, whereas nurses require information about how to handle contaminated needles and other equipment.

Behavioral Considerations

Behavioral factors influence needs for health education. For example, the extent of obesity in the United States suggests the need for intensive dietary education. Other health-related behaviors prevalent in the population may also give rise to health education needs. Smokers may need help with smoking cessation and education on alternative ways to meet needs satisfied by smoking. Similarly, sexually active clients may need education regarding contraceptives and safe sexual practices.

Health System Considerations

In the health system dimension, health care recommendations may precipitate a need for health education. For example, clients may need to be educated on the correct use of medications or how to keep a sprained ankle immobilized to promote healing. Elements of the health care regimen may also influence clients' abilities to learn. For example, pain medication may make a client drowsy and inhibit the ability to learn material presented. In such a case, the community health nurse can plan to provide educational interventions at times pain is sufficiently controlled to prevent distractions, but the client is alert enough to attend to the lesson, or education may be provided to a family member along with or instead of the client.

The degree of emphasis placed on health education by health care providers and providers' expertise in using the health education process are health care system factors that influence client's health-related knowledge and attitudes. Health care providers who engage in health education need a strong background in both educational principles and health content. Community health nurses involved in health education should assess their ability to employ principles of education and take the steps needed to enhance that ability.

Tips for assessing a health education situation are presented on page 240. In addition, an assessment tool such as the Educational Planning and Implementation Guide (available on the companion Web site for this book) can be used to direct the community health nurse's assessment of the client and the learning situation. Completing the tool also documents assessment findings. In addition, the tool can be employed to document the other elements of the health education process discussed later in this chapter. 🕸

DIAGNOSTIC REASONING IN HEALTH EDUCATION

Several years ago, noted health educator Lawrence Green and his colleagues (Green & Kreuter, 1991) developed the PRECEDE model for educational diagnosis. The acronym PRECEDE stands for predisposing, reinforcing, and enabling causes in educational diagnosis and evaluation and addresses five levels of educational diagnosis:

1. Social diagnosis: Assessment of quality of life in the population
2. Epidemiologic diagnosis: Identification of health problems contributing to reduced quality of life

assessment tips assessment tips assessment tips

ASSESSING THE HEALTH EDUCATION SITUATION

Biophysical Considerations

- What is the age composition of the target audience? What learning needs arise from the age and developmental level of the audience? How will the developmental level of the audience affect the ability to learn? How will the developmental level of the audience influence teaching strategies and methods?
- Do physical health problems in the population give rise to the need for health education?
- Does physiologic function pose any impediments to learning? Will teaching strategies need to be modified to accommodate sensory deficits or other physical limitations of the target audience?

Psychological Considerations

- Is the target population aware of the need for health education? Will population attitudes toward health and health behaviors enhance or detract from learning ability?
- What is the level of motivation to learn? What factors will motivate clients to learn healthful behaviors?
- Does the target audience exhibit levels of stress or anxiety that are likely to interfere with learning?

Physical Environmental Considerations

- Are there conditions in the physical environment that give rise to a need for health education? What effects, if any, will the physical environment have on learning? Are there elements of the physical environment that will distract learners?

Sociocultural Considerations

- What effects will the learners' peers have on motivation to learn?

- What is the current education level of the learners? What prior exposure to health information has the population received? How will the group's education level influence teaching strategies and content?
- What is the primary language spoken by members of the target audience?
- Are there cultural beliefs and practices that are likely to influence learning?
- Do the occupations of group members give rise to a need for health education?
- Are there other facets of the social situation that may influence health education (e.g., needs for child care)?

Behavioral Considerations

- Do health behaviors prevalent in the population (e.g., unprotected sexual activity, smoking, lack of seat belt use) give rise to the need for health education?

Health System Considerations

- Do local health care providers emphasize health education?
- Does the population have a need for education regarding the use of health care services?
- Do health care recommendations give rise to a need for health education? Are there elements of the health care regimen that may influence learning abilities (e.g., medications)?
- Will attitudes to health care services and providers influence the ability to learn?

---

3. Behavioral and environmental diagnosis: Identification of behavioral and environmental risk factors resulting in population health problems
4. Educational diagnosis: Identification of predisposing, reinforcing, and enabling factors that influence health-related behavior
5. Administrative and policy diagnosis: Assessment of administrative and organizational resources and capabilities

In the first level of diagnosis, the community health nurse educator assesses the quality of life experienced by individual clients or members of the population, problems encountered, and clients' priorities for resolving those problems. Diagnoses at this level are derived both from subjective perceptions of group members and social indicators such as rates of violent crime, illegitimacy, and so on (Breckon, 1998). Epidemiologic diagnosis, the second level, consists of identifying health-related problems that are contributing to diminished quality of life and the extent of those problems in the population. Third-level diagnosis addresses the environmental and behavioral risk factors underlying these health problems. Change in these risk factors then becomes the objective of the health education initiative.

The educational diagnosis level involves identifying predisposing, reinforcing, and enabling factors that facilitate change to the desired health behavior (Maltby & Robinson, 1998). *Predisposing factors* are factors internal to the client that influence motivation for healthy behavior. These factors include knowledge, attitudes, and values related to the target behavior. *Reinforcing factors* are external forces that affect the client's motivation to act in a healthy way. Reinforcing factors include perceived rewards resulting from the behavior and feedback from significant others about the behavior. When the consequences of the behavior are perceived favorably and feedback from others is positive, the behavior in question is reinforced (Breckon, 1998). For example, when peers express positive attitudes and values toward condom use as a means to prevent such diseases as HIV/AIDS, use of condoms as a healthy behavior is fostered. *Enabling factors* are also external to the client and include other factors in a given situation that influence clients' abilities to act in a healthy manner. Using the previous example, the accessibility of condoms to sexually active adolescents is an enabling factor that influences condom use.

The final level of educational diagnosis in the PRECEDE model is administrative and policy diagnosis. At this level, the health educator assesses administrative and organizational resources and capabilities for developing a health education program to promote the targeted behavior. Diagnosis at this level may also include identification of policies that impede healthy behavior or that are needed to enhance such behaviors. Incorporating all five levels of educational diagnosis, the community health nurse would develop a diagnostic statement expressing the client's learning needs. Such a diagnosis would be based on information derived from the assessment of the learner and learning setting. A sample diagnosis might be "Need for education to modify community attitudes toward bicycle helmet use." Reflected in this diagnosis are the social problem of accidental injury and the underlying factors contributing to failure to use bicycle helmets. Subsumed in the diagnosis is the nurse's assessment of his or her organizational capability to address this need.

Since its development, the PRECEDE model has been linked to a PROCEED model in which the community health nurse educator proceeds to develop, implement, and evaluate a health education program related to the desired health behavior. PROCEED stands for *p*olicy, *r*egulatory, and *o*rganizational *c*onstructs for *e*ducational and *e*nvironmental *d*evelopment. The PROCEED model consists of four steps, the first being implementation of the educational plan and the last three reflecting process, impact, and outcome evaluation of the educational encounter (Richards, 1997). Execution of each of these steps in the health education process is guided by the educational assessment and diagnosis and is addressed in detail in the remainder of this chapter.

PLANNING THE HEALTH EDUCATION ENCOUNTER

Planning health education encounters is similar to planning any nursing intervention and follows a similar planning process. There are, however, some general princi-

ples of planning that should be considered in a health education situation. These principles are summarized below.

HIGHLIGHTS

General Principles for Health Education Planning

- *Plan the process.* Give thought to who should be involved in planning and program implementation.
- *Plan with people.* It is particularly important to include potential participants, implementers, and other relevant groups of people.
- *Plan with data.* Base the plan on data regarding the need identified, existing programs, existing social and environmental supports for the program, and the anticipated target population.
- *Plan for permanence.* Plan for continued health education efforts to resolve identified problems rather than a single program or event.
- *Plan for priorities.* Identify the most effective use of staff time and other resources and discard non-priority activities.
- *Plan for measurable outcomes in acceptable formats.* Identify and plan activities to achieve specific expected outcomes in such a way that their accomplishment can be evaluated.
- *Plan for evaluation.* Design the evaluation plan at the same time the program is being designed.

Source: Breckon, D. J. (1998). *Community health education: Settings, roles, and skills for the 21st century.* Gaithersburg, MD: Aspen.

Several tasks are to be accomplished in planning a health education encounter. These tasks include establishing priorities for health education, identifying goals and the level of prevention involved, developing and classifying objectives, and selecting content and teaching strategies. Reviewing or developing educational materials and planning for evaluation are two additional tasks in planning a health education encounter.

Prioritizing Learning Needs

The first task in planning health education is prioritizing learning needs. A population group may exhibit several unrelated learning needs. Because learners can assimilate only a certain amount of information at a time and because resources are finite, the community health nurse and other members of the community need to decide which learning needs should be addressed first. Other needs can be addressed later, as time and resources permit.

Prioritization involves determining the relative effects of behaviors and risk factors present in the population and the benefits to be achieved by changing them.

Another consideration in prioritizing health education needs is the ease with which contributing factors can be changed. For example, members of the population may not use seat belts, get too little exercise, and not conduct monthly breast self-examinations. A change to using seat belts would result in the most immediate and dramatic benefit to the community and be the easiest of the three behaviors to change. For these reasons, the community health nurse might first begin with health education efforts in this area.

Identifying Goals and Levels of Prevention

Goal identification involves specifying the broad purpose of the health education encounter. The goals of HIV education, for instance, might be to broaden the population's understanding of HIV infection and to decrease fears of contagion. For an educational program on parenting, the goal would be the development of good parenting skills.

Identifying goals for an educational encounter also enables the community health nurse to identify the level of prevention to be addressed. For example, a goal of reducing the incidence of adolescent pregnancy indicates that education will be directed toward preventing teenage girls from becoming pregnant and involves primary prevention. The goal of preparing members of the population to provide cardiopulmonary resuscitation (CPR) in emergency situations, on the other hand, reflects secondary prevention—dealing with an existing problem—whereas an educational program directed at preventing further abuse of children by abusive parents reflects tertiary prevention.

Developing Specific Learning Objectives

Developing specific learning objectives is the next activity in planning health education. Learning objectives are statements of specific behaviors expected in the health education encounter.

Objectives for learning encounters are of two types: process objectives and outcome objectives. *Process objectives* are statements that define the process of client education and describe the actions to be taken by the nurse in educating clients. *Outcome objectives* are statements of behaviors or attitudes the audience is expected to demonstrate as a result of the health education encounter.

Outcome objectives should be stated in measurable terms that allow one to evaluate whether or not the expected results have been achieved. Evaluability of outcomes also requires that they be specific. For example, an outcome objective such as "reduce adolescent tobacco use" is somewhat nebulous. If one adolescent smoker stops smoking, have we met our objective? Similarly, an objective to "stop adolescent tobacco use" is not particularly realistic. No matter what interventions are employed, it is unlikely that we will ever prevent all adolescents from using tobacco. A more realistic, and more measurable, objective for tobacco education might be to "reduce

the prevalence of tobacco use among high school seniors by 50% within one year." As stated, the objective provides a target measure for accomplishment (a 50% decline in the number of seniors who use tobacco) as well as a time frame for expected accomplishment (one year from program initiation).

Classifying Objectives

It is sometimes helpful to classify outcome objectives according to the learning domain to which they relate and the level of task within the domain (Bastable & Sculco, 1997). A *learning domain* is a category or type of learning desired as a result of the health education encounter. The four domains of learning developed thus far are the cognitive, affective, perceptual, and psychomotor domains (Bloom, Englehart, Furst, Hill, & Krathwohl, 1956). The cognitive domain encompasses intellectual skills related to factual information and its application (Kramer et al., 1999). In the affective domain, the focus of learning is on attitudes and values. Emphasis in the psychomotor domain is on the learning of physical manipulative skills (Coates, 1999). Finally, in the perceptual domain, emphasis is on learning to perceive and extract information from stimuli. Another, as yet undeveloped, domain of learning that may be of concern to community health nurses is the social skills domain (Bloom et al., 1956).

Taxonomies of learning tasks classify tasks within each of the established domains in a hierarchical fashion. In the cognitive and psychomotor domains, learning tasks are arranged in order of increasing complexity of intellectual or physical skill involved. For example, it requires greater intellectual skill to apply a fact to a particular decision-making situation than simply to recall the fact. Similarly, less skill is required to follow printed knitting instructions than to create one's own pattern. Hierarchies of learning tasks in the cognitive and psychomotor domains are presented in Table 11–2 ■.

Tasks in the affective domain are organized in terms of the degree to which an attitude or value has been internalized by the learner (Krathwohl, Bloom, & Masia, 1964). For example, the student who consistently displays empathy for clients is operating at a higher level of internalization than one who merely discusses the importance of empathy in nursing. The taxonomy of the affective domain is also presented in Table 11–2.

Finally, learning tasks in the perceptual domain are arranged in terms of the extent to which the learner is able to extract information from a situation by way of perceptual skills. For example, a nursing student might notice a few salient characteristics of a client during a preliminary encounter, whereas an experienced community health nurse would derive much more information from the same encounter. The levels of a proposed taxonomy for the perceptual domain are listed in Table 11–2.

■ **TABLE 11–2** **Taxonomy of Learning Tasks in Established Domains**

COGNITIVE DOMAIN

Knowledge	Recall of facts, methods, or processes
Comprehension	Basic understanding of the meaning of facts
Application	Use of abstractions in concrete situations
Analysis	Breakdown into constituent parts
Synthesis	Combination of parts into a new pattern or whole
Evaluation	Judgment about the value of information and processes for specific purposes

PSYCHOMOTOR DOMAIN

Perception	Awareness of objects and relationships among them
Set	Physical, mental, and emotional readiness to act
Guided response	Performance of an action with instructor input and guidance
Mechanism	Performance of the task as a habit
Complex overt response	Performance of task with a high degree of skill
Adaptation	Adjustment of the skill to meet the needs of the situation
Origination	Creation of new acts or ways of manipulating materials

AFFECTIVE DOMAIN

Receiving	Sensitization to the existence of a phenomenon
Responding	Low level of commitment to behaviors embodying a value, performance of the behavior because of outside constraint
Valuing	Ascribing worth to a thing, behavior, or value accompanied by fairly consistent performance of related behaviors
Organization	Organization of values in hierarchical relationships
Characterization	Person can be characterized by consistent behavior in keeping with a specific set of values

PERCEPTUAL DOMAIN

Sensation	Awareness of differences, or change, in stimuli
Figure perception	Awareness of an object or phenomenon as a distinct entity
Symbol perception	Identification of pattern or form, ability to name or classify an object or phenomenon
Perception of meaning	Awareness of significance of symbols, ability to interrelate symbols
Perceptive performance	Complex decisions with multiple factors, ability to change behavior based on its effectiveness

⑥THINK ABOUT IT

What types of learning tasks did your nursing instructor expect you to accomplish in relation to this chapter?

It is helpful to classify the outcome objectives developed for a specific health education encounter in terms of the domain of learning and the level of task involved (Redman, 2000). This classification helps to refine the precision of outcome objectives and ensure that objectives are realistic. Generally speaking, if an objective cannot be classified according to domain and level, it is not precise enough and needs to be reworded. For example, an objective regarding the ability of the population to list at least three mechanisms by which HIV is transmitted is clearly a cognitive objective at the rudimentary level of knowledge recall. It would be difficult, however, to classify an objective such as, "The audience will list three modes of HIV transmission and identify the most effective means of preventing transmission." As written, this objective contains some elements related to the knowledge level of the cognitive domain and some related to the evaluation level (using criteria to judge which means of prevention is "best"). The objective would be better written as two separate objectives dealing with each level of behavior independently.

Classifying objectives by domain and taxonomic level also allows them to be compared with current levels of performance and aids in the development of more realistic objectives. If the population lacks factual knowledge, the health education encounter should focus on presentation of facts, and outcome objectives should reflect their acquisition. Education at the evaluation level can provide a focus for later sessions. For example, if you are just learning about different communication techniques (knowledge acquisition), you are yet not capable of critically evaluating the communication techniques employed by staff nurses in your clinical site (evaluation). That skill will be developed at a later time.

Finally, classifying objectives by level of difficulty within taxonomic domains can help to identify unrealistic expectations of learners. Generally speaking, objectives for a health education encounter should all be at a similar level. If your objectives address too many different levels within the domain, they may not be realistic given the audience's current capabilities in that area. For example, your instructors would not realistically expect you to learn research terminology (knowledge acquisition level) and develop the ability to critique a research article (evaluation level) during the same class session.

Selecting and Sequencing Content

The next task in planning the health lesson is selecting and sequencing the content to be presented. Because the nurse usually has greater knowledge of a particular topic than can or should be presented in a health education encounter, the nurse needs to select content that is most appropriate and relevant to clients' needs and that is most likely to result in accomplishing the stated learning objectives. Once content has been selected, it must be organized in a logical sequence so that new learning is based on previous learning. Content may be sequenced from simple to complex, from most important to least important, or from familiar to less familiar.

Selecting Teaching Strategies

Selection of teaching strategies depends on the characteristics of the target audience, the characteristics of the nurse, the type of learning tasks and content involved, and the availability of resources needed to implement specific strategies. The effectiveness of any given strategy depends on its appropriateness to the situation. Several general principles guide selection of teaching strategies (Anspaugh & Ezell, 1994). First, the strategies chosen should contribute to total learning, not just knowledge acquisition. Second, strategies should foster learner participation in the encounter. Third, the more complex the content, the greater the number and variety of activities needed to learn it. Application of this third principle also permits adaptation of the lesson to a variety of learning styles. The fourth principle is that the strategies chosen should reflect simple activities at first, followed by more complex activities. Finally, audiovisual aids should be used whenever possible to promote learning. These principles are summarized in Table 11–3 ■. The teaching strategies selected should be appropriate to the age, developmental level, and educational level of the audience and should reflect preferred learning styles, and the constraints of the situation (Duffy, 1998). Strategies should be chosen that maintain the interest of the learner and adequately address the content to be presented.

⑥THINK ABOUT IT

What effects do the media have on health education for the general public? What role should the media play in health education, if any?

Certain learning tasks lend themselves to particular teaching strategies (Fitzgerald, 1997). For example, discussion and role playing are effective methods for creating awareness of personal values, whereas lecture is more appropriate to knowledge acquisition. Problem-solving skills, on the other hand, are best learned through exercises in problem resolution. Table 11–4 ■ presents several commonly used teaching strategies and the learning tasks for which they are best suited.

■ **TABLE 11–3** General Principles for Selecting Teaching Strategies

- Strategies should contribute to total learning.
- Strategies should incorporate learner participation.
- The more complex the content, the more activities needed.
- Strategies should graduate from simple to complex.
- Strategies should incorporate audiovisuals whenever possible.

Preparing Materials

Any materials needed for the health education encounter must be either developed or obtained. Materials selected should be appropriate to the client audience and to the content presented. For example, if the target audience is young children, a coloring book might be an effective teaching aid for nutrition education. A coloring book would not be appropriate for adolescents, but comic book-style materials might be. Some sources of materials and resources for designing health education presentations are available on the companion Web site for this book. 🌐

Nurses planning health education may use existing materials and teaching aids. This is appropriate when these materials have been thoroughly reviewed and found to be appropriate to the target audience. Materials used need to convey information at a level that can be understood by clients. They should also be sensitive to client cultural beliefs, attitudes, and values. For example, materials on sexually transmitted diseases (STDs) that picture only persons from minority groups imply that only members of these groups get STDs. Such an implication is not only erroneous but also discriminatory and offensive to members of minorities who might be part of the client audience.

Problems with written materials occur when members of the client audience have low literacy skills. Recent studies of written information on a variety of health topics, for example, indicate that most are written at reading levels above that of many clients. Studies indicate that approximately 25% of the U.S. population have rudimentary reading skills and another 25% have limited skills, resulting in 40 to 44 million people who are unable to understand written materials that require only basic reading proficiency (National Work Group on Literacy and Health, 1998). In one study of English-speaking clients, 27% were unable to read their appointment slips and 42% could not read the instructions on medication bottles (Stein, 2000).

An estimated 20% of the U.S. population is considered "functionally illiterate," meaning that they cannot read beyond the fourth or fifth grade level (Habel, 2000); many health-related messages are written at considerably higher levels. For example, studies have shown the mean

■ **TABLE 11–4**   **Commonly Used Teaching Strategies**

STRATEGY	DESCRIPTION	LEARNING TASK APPLICABILITY
Case study	Use of a detailed account of an actual or hypothetical situation to help learners apply principles learned or to make them aware of attitudes and values and enhance the potential for change	Application, analysis Responding, valuing Perception
Computer-assisted instruction	Use of computers to present content	Knowledge Analysis Perception
Demonstration	Teacher performance of a skill or process to be learned, usually followed by a return demonstration (see below)	Motor skills development
Discussion	Verbal exploration of an idea or concept, attitude, value, etc., with participation by learners and teacher	Application, analysis Synthesis, evaluation Valuing Perception of meaning
Lecture	Formal oral presentation of information by teacher	Knowledge Comprehension
Media	Use of auditory or visual media presentations (e.g., audiotapes, filmstrips) to present content	Knowledge Comprehension Analysis Valuing, perception Motor skills development
Readings	Presentation of content in written form, frequently followed by discussion	Knowledge Comprehension Valuing
Return demonstration	Learner performance of a learned skill or process	Motor skills development
Role modeling	Teacher performance of a behavior to be adopted (e.g., sensitivity to the needs of others)	Valuing
Role playing	Acting out the role of another to get a different perspective, usually followed by discussion	Valuing
Supervision	Teacher-guided performance of desired behavior by learner	Motor skills development Analysis Evaluation
Visual aids	Use of visually oriented materials (e.g., pictures, posters) to present content	Knowledge Comprehension Motor skills development

readability of asthma literature to be at a grade level of 8.6, while cancer literature has a mean readability level of nearly 12th grade (Horner, Surratt, & Juliusson, 2000). The American Medical Association estimates that more than 90 million people in the United States lack basic health literacy, or the ability to "read, understand, and act correctly on health information, (Stein, 2000, p. 10).

Many people get much of their health-related information from non-written sources. For example, an estimated 97% of persons over age 65 get the bulk of their health information from television. Similarly, many non-English speakers get most of their information from oral rather than written communication (National Work Group on Literacy and Health, 1998).

Poor readers are apt to misrepresent the extent of their reading ability because of the stigma attached to the inability to read. For example, as many as two thirds of the poorest readers have been found to report that they read "well" or "very well". In addition to the inability to read many health messages, which are often written at levels beyond the sixth grade, poor readers have been shown to process information differently from good readers. For example, poor readers tend to take instructions literally, and fail to interpret them within the context of the situation. They also tend to skip uncommon or unfamiliar words and may miss important inferences (Habel, 2000). For clients with low literacy levels or those attuned to oral sources of information, pictorial materials, videotapes, or filmstrips can be used in place of or to complement written materials.

Several general principles have been established for the design of written health education materials for persons with low literacy levels. These principles are summarized below.

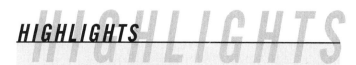

HIGHLIGHTS

Developing Health Education Materials for Groups with Low Literacy Levels

- Write in conversational style using short words and short sentences.
- Write in active voice.
- If health terminology must be used, define terms in understandable language.
- Organize information in related "chunks" with headings that emphasize key concepts.
- Organize content from simple to more complex concepts.
- Limit content to three to five important points relevant to the reader.
- Provide examples that are relevant to the reader and that clarify concepts.
- Eliminate gender and racial biases.
- Use a large, easy-to-read type font and maintain consistency in the fonts used.
- Use lowercase letters as much as possible since they are easier to read than uppercase.
- Leave the right margin ragged rather than justifying it.
- Make points stand out with judicious use of "white space."
- Select pictures and graphics relevant to the audience and the content and place them appropriately in the text of the message.
- Pilot test your materials with members of the target audience.

Problems also arise for audiences who are literate in other languages when materials written in English are translated literally. Translated materials should be reviewed for their consistency with local idiomatic lan-

guage. English and other language translations can be placed side by side on a page rather than on separate pages or back and front of the page. This placement allows for readers skilled in English to assist non-English speakers to understand the content of the material more fully (Horner et al., 2000).

Other considerations in selecting teaching aids and other materials to be used include the need for special equipment (e.g., projector and screen for filmstrips), currency of content, and ease of use. Constraints may be imposed by the type of setting in which the learning occurs. For example, if a class is to be conducted outdoors, filmstrips are inappropriate, or if education is being provided to a family who lack a television set, a videotape will not be useful. A final consideration in selecting visual aids is the ability of the audience to see the materials. If overhead transparencies are used, for example, the print must be large enough to be read by all those in the back of the room. Similarly, when demonstration is used, all clients in the group need to be able to see what is being demonstrated.

Planning Evaluation

The last task in planning health education is developing a plan to evaluate its effects. Criteria for evaluating the outcomes of health education are derived from the outcome objectives. Criteria for evaluating the performance of the nurse and the educational process itself arise from process objectives. The nurse also plans mechanisms for *formative evaluation,* which involves assessing the effects of the presentation as it is given. Formative evaluation includes determining whether clients understand what is being presented and whether the presentation maintains their interest. The nurse would also be alert to cues that indicate response to the content presented. For example, the nurse might note that description of discrimination against a person with AIDS generates anger in the listeners. If the nurse was trying to make clients aware of attitudes toward AIDS, such a response would indicate success.

Formative evaluation also reflects the quality of the presentation. For example, frenzied note taking by learners would indicate that content is being presented too rapidly. The tasks involved in planning a health education encounter are summarized on page 247.

CULTURAL CONSIDERATIONS

In many Asian cultural groups, it is considered polite to give the person to whom you are speaking the answer they wish to hear, whether or not this answer reflects your true beliefs or feelings. Similarly, a student who does not learn reflects poorly on the teacher and causes him or her to "lose face." How might these cultural values and expectations affect a health education situation? How might you overcome any adverse influences on the effectiveness of health education?

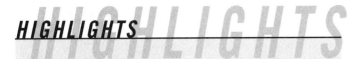

HIGHLIGHTS

Tasks Involved in Planning a Health Education Encounter

Identifying the Goal
Specifying the broad purpose to be accomplished

Developing Objectives
Stating specific behavioral outcomes expected as a result of the encounter

Classifying Objectives
Identifying the learning domains to be addressed

Selecting and Sequencing Content
Determining what will be taught and the order in which it will be presented

Selecting Teaching Strategies
Determining approaches to be used in presenting content

Preparing Materials
Developing any teaching aids to be used in the presentation

Planning Evaluation
Determining criteria and processes to be used for formative, outcome, and process evaluation

IMPLEMENTING THE HEALTH EDUCATION ENCOUNTER

Several key points must be kept in mind in implementing a health education encounter. The first is to speak the client's language. This refers not only to using a foreign language or an interpreter for non–English-speaking clients, but also eliminating medical and nursing jargon. The second recommendation is to be specific; the third is to keep the message short. Key points should be presented early in the lesson for emphasis and to enhance recall. Verbal headings will help clients keep track of material presented and recognize transitions from one topic to another. Finally, repetition—particularly of important points—will enhance learning and recall.

The Focusing Event

The lesson itself begins with a *focusing event,* which is a specific strategy designed to gain the attention of the audience and to focus that attention on the material to be presented. A focusing event in a presentation on child abuse might involve showing several slides of abused

children or giving statistics on the incidence of child abuse in the community.

ⓒTHINK ABOUT IT

Content Presentation

Following the focusing event, the lesson is presented as planned with formative checks during the course of the lesson to determine the need for on-the-spot revisions. The presentation of content should include audience participation whenever possible. Learning theory indicates that the greater the learner's involvement with the material, the greater the learning that results. Client participation can be facilitated by such activities as group discussion, case studies, and role playing. The nurse can also encourage participation by asking thought-provoking questions or questions that serve to summarize and synthesize previous content.

Lesson Summary

The lesson should close with a summary that reinforces pertinent points. In summarizing, the community health nurse recaps and highlights the major concepts covered. He or she should also attempt to synthesize content in a few major themes that the client needs to remember. General considerations in implementing health education are summarized below.

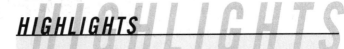

HIGHLIGHTS

Considerations in Implementing a Health Education Encounter

Focusing Event
A teaching strategy designed to attract attention to the topic

Presentation of Content
Actual presentation of planned content, encouraging learner participation as much as possible

Summary
Restatement and reinforcement of the most important points of the presentation

CRITICAL THINKING IN RESEARCH

You and your classmates have noticed that a large percentage of the drivers on campus fail to wear seat belts. As a class project, you decide to conduct a campus-wide education campaign to promote seat belt use on campus.

- How would you go about designing a study to evaluate the effectiveness of your education campaign?
- How would you measure the outcomes of your intervention?
- What other competing explanations might there be for changes in seat belt use on campus? How would you control for these other variables?

EVALUATING THE HEALTH EDUCATION ENCOUNTER

As noted earlier, evaluation takes place throughout the presentation and as the last step of the educational process. Three types of evaluation are done: formative, outcome, and process.

Formative Evaluation

During presentation of the lesson, the community health nurse periodically assesses the lesson and its effects as it is being presented. The nurse uses client feedback to determine whether the content of the lesson is being effectively communicated. For example, if clients' facial expressions indicate confusion, the nurse might infer that they do not understand the material being presented. Similarly, the nurse might ask questions on material offered earlier in the lesson as a formative evaluation strategy. If clients are able to answer these questions correctly, the lesson has been effective thus far. Again, formative evaluation might also include assessing client emotional responses to content presented.

Formative evaluation can also be used for health education that takes place by other means. For example, if health information is presented on billboards around the community, one aspect of formative evaluation might be evaluating the placement of the billboards. Are they easily seen? Or, are they hidden by tree limbs or behind buildings?

Outcome Evaluation

After the lesson, the nurse evaluates the presentation in terms of its effects. Effects can best be measured in terms of the degree to which the outcome objectives were met. Were the learners able to perform the stated behaviors at the expected level of performance?

In evaluating outcomes, the nurse should remain alert to other outcomes of the educational program in addition to the intended outcomes or objectives. Health education may result in serendipitous outcomes. These results should not be overlooked or underestimated and may be reason for continuing a program even when intended objectives are not accomplished.

Process Evaluation

The nurse also evaluates the presentation in terms of the use of the educational process. Were the process objectives established for the encounter met? Was one as well prepared as desired? Did the lesson maintain the interest of the audience? Were the teaching strategies, materials, and content selected appropriate to the learning needs of the clients? The answers to such questions allow the nurse to make any necessary modifications in the lesson plan for future use. Considerations in evaluating the health education encounter are summarized below.

HIGHLIGHTS

Considerations in Evaluating a Health Education Encounter

Formative Evaluation
An evaluation conducted periodically during the presentation to detect a need for immediate modification

Outcome Evaluation
Evaluating the encounter to determine whether stated outcome objectives have been met

Process Evaluation
Evaluating the performance of the community health nurse in the light of established process objectives

Health education is an effective tool for promoting health in population groups. It is also one of the community health nurse's most frequently used tools, whether with individuals, families, or groups of clients. To provide effective health education, however, nurses should engage in systematic planning as described here. Additional sources for information about health education are provided on the companion Web site for this book.

APPLYING YOUR KNOWLEDGE IN PRACTICE

❧ CASE STUDY
Educating for Health

You have been asked by a private high school principal to give a presentation on date rape to the Parent/Teacher Group and, afterward, to make a presentation to junior and senior students on the same topic. The school is run by a nondenominational Christian foundation. Students in the school come from an upper-middle-class neighborhood and most of their parents are professional people. The students are above the national average in all areas of standardized testing, and English is the primary language spoken by both parents and students.

Recently, the news media have highlighted several cases of date rape in the local community. So far, no known instances of date rape have occurred in this school, but school officials are interested in avoiding potential problems. Parents of children in this school have already begun to ask about supervision at school-sponsored social activities.

- Using the Educational Planning and Implementation Guide provided on the companion Web site for this text, document the assessment data available to you. What additional assessment data might you want to obtain? How would you obtain these data?
- What are your goals for the two presentations?
- What learning domains are involved in the presentations? Would the learning tasks involved differ between the student and parent groups? Why or why not?
- Develop two or three specific outcome objectives that you would expect learners to accomplish as a result of your presentation.
- Would content presented differ between your two audiences? What would you present and why? Would you sequence content any differently? Why or why not?
- What teaching strategies might be most effective with each group? What type of teaching aids or materials would you need? Where might you obtain these teaching aids?
- What type of focusing event would you use for the student group? For the parent group?
- How would you encourage learner participation in the two groups? Would you use similar or different approaches to stimulate learner participation?
- What key points would you include in a summary of your presentation? Would these be the same or different for the two groups of learners?
- How would you conduct formative evaluation during your presentation? How would you evaluate the presentation in terms of client outcomes and your performance?

❧ TESTING YOUR UNDERSTANDING

- What three types of health-related decisions can be facilitated by health education? How is the concept of self-care central to each type of decision? (p. 234)
- What are some of the barriers to effective health education? Give an example of each and describe how a community health nurse might avoid them. (p. 235)
- What is the difference between process and outcome objectives in a learning encounter? (p. 242)
- What are the four established domains of learning? Give an example of a learning task related to health education within each domain. (pp. 242–243)
- What is a focusing event? What is the purpose of the focusing event? (p. 247)
- How is formative evaluation used in a health education encounter? (p. 248)

REFERENCES

Anspaugh, D. J., & Ezell, G. (1994). *Teaching today's health* (4th ed.). Boston: Allyn & Bacon.

Bastable, S., & Sculco, C. (1997). Educational objectives. In S. B. Bastable (Ed.), *Nurse as educator: Principles of teaching and learning* (pp. 237–260). Boston: Jones & Bartlett.

Bloom, B. S., Englehart, M. D., Furst, E. J., Hill, W. F., & Krathwohl, D. R. (1956). *Taxonomy of educational objectives: The classification of educational goals: Handbook 1: The cognitive domain.* New York: David McKay.

Braungart, M. M., & Braungart, R. G. (1997). Learning theory and nursing practice. In S. B. Bastable (Ed.), *Nurse as educator: Principles of teaching and learning* (pp. 31–52). Boston: Jones & Bartlett.

Breckon, D. J. (1998). *Community health education: Settings, roles, and skills for the 21st century.* Gaithersburg, MD: Aspen.

Coates, V. E. (1999). *Education for patients and clients.* New York: Routledge.

Davidhizar, R., Dowd, S. B., & Giger, J. N. (1998). Educating the culturally diverse healthcare student. *Nurse Educator, 23*(2), 38–42.

Duffy, B. (1998). Get ready—Get set—Go teach. *Home Healthcare Nurse, 16,* 597–602.

Fitzgerald, K. (1997). Instructional methods: Selection, use, and evaluation. In S. B. Bastable (Ed.), *Nurse as educator: Principles of teaching and learning* (pp. 261–286). Boston: Jones & Bartlett.

Fries, J. F., Koop, C. E., Sokolov, J., Beadle, C. E., & Wright, D. (1998). Beyond health promotion: Reducing need and demand for medical care. *Health Affairs, 17*(2), 70–84.

Gleit, C. J. (1998). Theories of learning. In M. D. Boyd, B. A. Graham, C. J. Gleit, & N. I. Whitman (Eds.), *Health teaching in nursing practice* (3rd ed.). Stamford, CT: Appleton & Lange.

Green, L. W., & Kreuter, M. W. (1991). *Health promotion planning: An educational and environmental approach* (2nd ed.). Mountain View, CA: Mayfield.

Habel, M. (2000). Get your message across to low-literacy patients. *NurseWeek, 13*(12), 14–15.

Hibbard, J. H., Greenlick, M., Jimison, H., Kunkel, L., & Tusler, M. (1999). Prevalence and predictors of use of self-care resources. *Evaluation and the Health Professions, 22*(1), 107–122.

Horner, S. D., Surratt, D., & Juliusson, S. (2000). Improving readability of patient education materials. *Journal of Community Health Nursing, 17*(1), 15–23.

Kitchie, S. (1997). Determinants of learning. In S. B. Bastable (Ed.), *Nurse as educator* (pp. 55–89). Boston: Jones and Bartlett.

Kramer, E. J., Bucher, J. A., Glassman, K. S., & Siu, S. (1999). Strategies for patient teaching: How to seize the teachable moment. In W. B. Bateman, E. J. Kramer, & K. S. Glassman (Eds.), *Patient and family education in managed care and beyond: Seizing the teachable moment* (pp. 19–36). New York: Springer.

Krathwohl, D. R., Bloom, B. S., & Masia, B. B. (1964). *Taxonomy of educational objectives: The classification of educational goals: Handbook 1: The affective domain.* New York: David McKay.

Lipson, J. G., & Steiger, N. J. (1996). *Self-care nursing in a multicultural context.* Thousand Oaks, CA: Sage.

Maltby, H. J., & Robinson, S. (1998). The role of baccalaureate nursing students in the matrix of health promotion. *Journal of Community Health Nursing, 15,* 135–142.

National Work Group on Literacy and Health. (1998). Communicating with patients who have limited literacy skills. *The Journal of Family Practice, 46,* 168–176.

Piper, S. M., & Brown, P. A. (1998). The theory and practice of health education applied to nursing: A bi-polar approach. *Journal of Advanced Nursing, 27,* 383–389.

Redman, B. K. (2000). *The process of patient education* (9th ed.). St. Louis: Mosby.

Richards, E. (1997). Motivation, compliance, and health behaviors of the learner. In S. B. Bastable (Ed.), *Nurse as educator: Principles of teaching and learning* (pp. 124–144). Boston: Jones & Bartlett.

Stein, T. (2000). Unhealthy mismatch: Major gaps in Americans' understanding of medical concepts. *NurseWeek, 13*(11), 10.

CASE MANAGEMENT

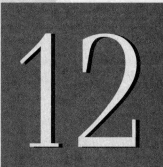

Chapter Objectives

After reading this chapter, you should be able to:

- Identify five goals of case management.
- Discuss the standards of case management practice.
- Describe legal and ethical issues related to case management.
- Identify criteria for selecting clients in need of case management.
- Assess the need for case management and factors influencing the case management situation.
- Discuss two basic aspects of developing a case management plan.
- Describe at least three considerations in delegation.
- Describe the benchmarking process and its use in case management.

Media Link

http://www.prenhall.com/clark

Additional interactive resources for this chapter can be found on the companion Web site. Click on Chapter 12 and "Begin" to select the activities for this chapter.

Case management is the recent focus of a great deal of attention, primarily because of its effects on reducing health care expenditures as managed care becomes a growing emphasis in health care delivery. Recent interest notwithstanding, community health nurses have been doing case management since the beginning of their practice more than a century ago. What is case management? What are the elements of the case management process? What is its relationship to community health nursing? These questions are the focus of this chapter.

DEFINING CASE MANAGEMENT

A variety of definitions of case management can be found in the literature of several disciplines, including nursing and social work. These definitions are often based on a particular model of case management and so may appear remarkably different (Powell, 2000). A recent review of definitions of case management, however, found several common themes. These areas of agreement include the concepts that case management addresses management of clinical services, effective resource utilization, quality of care, and cost-effectiveness (Tahan, 1999).

The most commonly found definition for case management is that developed by the Case Management Society of America (CMSA) (1995). CMSA defined case management as "a collaborative process which assesses, plans, implements, coordinates, monitors and evaluates options and services to meet an individual's health needs through communication and available resources to promote quality cost-effective outcomes" (pg. 8). *Case management,* as practiced by community health nurses, is a process of identifying needs for and arranging, coordinating, monitoring, and evaluating quality, cost-effective primary, secondary, and tertiary prevention services to achieve designated health outcomes.

The case management process is employed at two levels, that of the individual or family and that of population groups. The latter is sometimes referred to as *population care management* or *population management* (Schroeder, Trehearne, & Ward, 2000; Williams, 2000). Individual or family case management is a one-to-one endeavor in which the case manager develops a relationship with a particular client and his or her family (Michaels, 1997). *Population case management* is the development of systems of care, across multiple agencies, for specific groups of people with similar needs (Williams, 2000). Population case management may address episodes of illness or cut across the wellness/illness continuum (Schroeder et al., 2000). Epidemiologic findings can be used by community health nurses and others to provide a foundation for the development of systems of care that meet the health needs of a given population (Schmidt et al., 1999). For example, knowing that a large percentage of clients with uncontrolled hypertension live in certain areas of a com-

munity can help target case management services directed toward hypertension control to those areas.

THINK ABOUT IT

Why are community health nurses better prepared to be client case managers than physicians or social workers?

THE IMPETUS FOR CASE MANAGEMENT

Why is the concept of case management of such interest in today's health care delivery system? The answer to this question lies in the advantages posed by a case management approach for both the client and the health care industry. For the client, case management assures effective coordination of care and helps to reduce the confusion and complexity of the health care system. The case manager can assist the client to obtain needed services in the most acceptable and affordable settings. Case management, if effectively performed, should also result in improved client health outcomes in most instances. Effective case management also results in attention to all of the client's health needs to minimize the development of other health problems. In addition, case management provides clients with continuity of care and a regular and consistent source of assistance with health needs (Blaha, Robinson, Pugh, Bryan, & Havens, 2000).

At the health system level, case management also emphasizes service delivery in the least expensive setting possible, thereby limiting the overall costs of health care. Effective case management minimizes hospitalization for needs that can be dealt with in community practice settings. For those clients who do need hospitalization, case management may shorten the length of stay and prevent subsequent readmissions by adequately addressing continuing health care needs after discharge. The cost of health care is also minimized when case management eliminates duplication of services. Population case management arrangements among several agencies provide a consistent flow of clients as well as limiting overlapping services. In addition, transfer of clients, ease of access to services, and communication between providers are also facilitated by population case management arrangements. When payers are included in the design of population case management systems, paperwork and waits for authorization for services are also reduced (Williams, 2000). Benefits that create an impetus for case management are summarized in Table 12–1 ■.

Evidence of these effects of case management is found in the research literature, although findings do not equivocally support positive outcomes. For example, no change in patient outcomes and higher service costs were found

■ **TABLE 12–1**   Benefits of Case Management for Clients and Health Care Delivery Systems

BENEFICIARY	BENEFITS
Client	Better coordination of care
	Assistance in negotiating a complex health care system
	Access to acceptable and affordable health care services
	Attention to multiple health care needs
	Improved health outcomes
	Continuity of care and consistent assistance
Health care delivery systems	Reduced cost of care
	Minimization of hospitalization
	Prevention of rehospitalization
	Elimination of service duplication
	Ease of transfer among agencies
	Better communication among agencies and providers
	Increased access to services
	Decreased paper work
	Reduced time for authorization of services

for case management programs for clients with renal insufficiency (Harris, Luft, Rudy, Kesterson, & Tierney, 1998). Similar findings were noted for older clients (Gagnon, Schein, McVey, & Bergman, 1999). Other studies, however, have found significant positive effects of case management for clients with chronic illnesses. Three such studies reported a 58% decline in in-patient visits, a 50% decline in emergency department use, a decrease in average length of stay of seven days, and a 61% cost savings (reported in Taylor, 1999). Some studies have shown improvement in client outcomes, but at higher costs than routine care. For example, one study of case management with schizophrenic clients indicated improved thought processes, better functional ability, and better client satisfaction among clients provided with case management services. Unfortunately, the cost of case management was approximately $900 per year more per client than routine follow-up care. The authors pointed out that health policy makers may need to determine if improved client outcomes in some situations outweigh increased costs (Chan, Mackenzie, & Jacobs, 2000).

⑥THINK ABOUT IT

What is the role of the community health nurse case manager with respect to other health care providers?

CASE MANAGEMENT MODELS

Some of the findings on the effectiveness of case management have been found to relate to the type of case management model used. For example, case management models have been characterized as full-service models, broker models, and hybrid models (Bedell, Cohen, & Sullivan, 2000). Full-service models provide most of the services needed by a given client within the organization. Broker models, on the other hand, provide very few direct client services, referring clients to other agencies for care. Hybrid models provide some direct services, but refer clients for others. Research with psychiatric clients has indicated that full-service models demonstrated consistent positive effects on treatment compliance, hospital readmissions, cost of care, symptom management, and client satisfaction, but had little effect on client quality of life and functional level and actually increased the use of community-based services. Patient outcomes were consistently better in full-service models than in broker models. Hybrid models that more closely resembled full-service models were more effective than those that incorporated more elements of broker models (Bedell et al., 2000).

Case management models can also be categorized in terms of their focus as either client-focused or system-focused models or social service models (Taylor, 1999). Client-focused models are usually disease specific and focus on the care of individuals and their families through a disease episode. Client-focused models have been criticized for their tendency to transfer client dependence to less costly providers rather than promoting independence. System-focused models emphasize the service environment, organizational structure, and resource base within the system. System models address population case management, but continue to focus on specific health conditions. Social service models, on the other hand, focus on health and wellness and promoting client independence.

Another type of case management model is advanced practice nursing models in which case management is viewed as an advanced practice role executed by nurses with specific educational preparation for the role. Examples of advanced practice nursing models include the differentiated model in which the case manager develops, and is responsible for, the plan of care but care is provided by care associates or staff nurses; the Star model in which the case manager integrates activities between clients, providers, and payers; and the professional nurse case management model in which the case manager integrates services over the continuum of care across settings (Taylor, 1999). This last model is a longitudinal model because case management services extend beyond the hospital setting to management of client care in the community as well (Blaha et al., 2000).

The final way of categorizing case management models is based on the setting for practice. Hospital-based models address case management needs during hospitalization and shortly after discharge. Community-based models focus on care after hospital discharge. Combination hospital- and community-based models are again longitudinal in nature in that they provide a continuum of care across settings (Stanton, Walizer, Graham, & Keppel, 2000).

GOALS OF CASE MANAGEMENT

The overall purpose of case management is to create a balance between quality of care and cost containment (Stanton et al., 2000). This dual focus leads to the twofold role of the case manager; one aspect focused on improving the health status of clients and providing access to needed services, the other focused on organizational needs to cut costs and make efficient use of available resources. This twofold role leads, in turn, to multiple client-centered and system-focused goals for case management services.

Client-centered goals include ensuring access to quality health care needed to address identified health needs, attaining positive health outcomes, promoting independent function, assisting with adjustment to illness, and improved quality of life. System-focused goals include reducing health care costs, eliminating duplication or inappropriate care, promoting effective resource allocation, promoting early discharge, and integrating delivery services. Additional system-focused goals include increased client satisfaction, decreased fragmentation of services, improved professional satisfaction, and support of the organization's financial viability (Davidson, 1999; Tahan, 1999).

☉THINK ABOUT IT

What do you think is the most important goal of case management? Why?

Simultaneous achievement of these multiple goals often requires a delicate balance. The community health nurse must attempt to provide clients with the type and quantity of services that meet their needs to achieve optimal health outcomes in the most cost-effective manner possible. Client-centered and system-focused goals of case management are summarized at right.

HIGHLIGHTS

Goals of Case Management

Client-Centered Goals

- Access to quality sources of needed care
- Attainment of positive health outcomes
- Ability to function independently
- Adjustment of client and family to illness states
- Improved quality of life

System-Focused Goals

- Cost containment
- Reduced duplication of services
- Elimination of inappropriate care
- Effective resource allocation
- Earlier discharge
- Integrated service delivery
- Increased client satisfaction
- Decreased fragmentation of services
- Increased professional satisfaction
- Financial viability

STANDARDS OF CASE MANAGEMENT PRACTICE

Standards of case management practice have been developed by the Case Management Society of America (1995) and are currently under revision. Measurement criteria have been identified for each standard. The standards of practice are similar to those for community health nursing presented in Chapter 8. They include standards related to case identification and assessment, problem identification, planning, monitoring implementation of the case management plan, evaluating the effects of intervention, and modifying the plan to achieve appropriate, cost-effective outcomes.

LEGAL AND ETHICAL ISSUES IN CASE MANAGEMENT

Although many of the legal and ethical issues in case management are common to other aspects of community health nursing, there are some that warrant special attention. These issues include confidentiality, denial of services, breach of contract, negligence, failure to follow clinical pathways or, conversely, to individualize care, and reportable events. The issue of confidentiality has two aspects in case management. The first is the need for client permission to make contacts and arrangements for services on the client's behalf. The case management plan should be presented to and agreed upon by the client before any further action is taken. The second aspect of confidentiality relates to unauthorized disclosure of information about the client (Powell, 2000). To avoid a breach of confidentiality in this area, the community health nurse case manager should inform clients of the need to share information with others and obtain client authorization before doing so.

Denial of services includes failure to initiate needed services and abandonment. Wrongful denial of services involves decisions not to provide care that are arbitrary and are not based on medical information related to need (Ling, 1998). *Abandonment* occurs when the case manager terminates services to a client with continuing needs without notifying the client or arranging for services from another provider (Nichols, 1996). Although community health nurse case managers may encounter situations in which services need to be terminated (e.g., in the face of client failure to comply with the treatment plan), the nurse should make every effort to avoid abandonment. It may be helpful to develop a contract with clients indicating both case manager and client responsibilities with respect to the case management plan. In addition, the case manager should carefully document both positive and negative aspects of the client's response to case management services and continued efforts to enlist client cooperation.

Breach of contract occurs when a managed care organization drops a client from the plan without adequate justification or when the system fails to pay for care that should be covered by a plan (Ling, 1998). Several types of negligence also pose legal and ethical issues in case management. *Negligence* is the failure to act in a situation as a reasonable person would if faced with the same situation. Wrongful denial of services could be considered a form of negligence on the part of the system (Williams, 2000). Other types of negligence include negligent actions on the part of the case manager or other providers and negligent referrals.

Although designed to promote standardization of patient care and limit legal liability, legal issues can arise from the use of or failure to use clinical pathways. A *clinical pathway* is an established sequence of operational activities designed to achieve designated outcomes in specific health problems. Clinical pathways are frequently used as standards against which actions may be judged in a malpractice or negligence suit. Failure to adhere to a clinical pathway can be considered as negligence if the clinical pathway is appropriate to the client situation. Conversely, case managers and other care providers may be found negligent for failing to take the individual client situation into account and deviating from the clinical pathway as needed. Deviations from the typical path are called *variances* (Berry, Cranston, & Fox, 2000). Legal challenges can be avoided with careful documentation of implementation of the clinical pathway and client variance that warrants deviation from the path. Periodic update of clinical pathways based on new best practices information can also forestall legal action (Forkner, 1996). Clinical pathways are discussed in more detail later in this chapter.

Nurse case managers may also be held legally liable for negligent referrals. A *negligent referral* may be (a) a referral that results in harm or injury to the client because the case manager has not adequately assessed the competency of the provider or (b) a failure to make a referral when one is warranted (Williams, 2000). Case managers can prevent negligent referrals by investigating the providers or agencies to which they refer clients in terms of licensure and relevant accreditation, client outcomes data, billing practices, insurance coverage, and malpractice information. A second tactic to prevent negligent referrals is to provide the client with several provider options rather than making a single referral. Finally, the case manager should follow up on the outcomes of referrals made.

The last legal issue to be addressed here is reportable events. Like all nurses, nurse case managers have a legal mandate to report the occurrence, or even the suspicion, of certain kinds of events. These include child and elder abuse, and in some jurisdictions, spouse abuse. Other reportable events include violent injuries, specific communicable diseases, and coroners' cases. Nurse case managers should be aware of what events (particularly what communicable diseases) are considered reportable in their area and should also let clients know of the need to report such events if they should occur.

ETHICAL AWARENESS

Clients may reach the limits of their health insurance coverage of certain types of services before their health needs have been fully met. When this occurs, health care providers may terminate services provided if the client does not have another means of paying for them. Obviously, this is not in the client's best interests. Continuing to provide uncompensated services, however, may lead to failure of the health organization, jeopardizing care to many other clients. What ethical arguments can be brought to bear for either action (continuing services without payment or discontinuing services)? What might the role of the nurse case manager be in such an ethical dilemma?

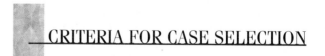

CRITERIA FOR CASE SELECTION

Not all of the clients encountered by community health nurses will need case management services, so the nurse must identify those clients who do need services and can benefit most from them (Fox, Etheredge, & Jones, 1998).

Case selection may involve identifying certain population groups for whom case management systems should be developed (population case management) and identifying individual clients and families in need of case management services (Ling, 1998). Both population groups and individual clients can be identified on the basis of several indicators. Indicators for population groups needing case management services include those with high-cost diagnoses, high-volume diagnoses, and those with the greatest potential for positive effects of case management (Ling, 1998). An example of a population group with a high-cost diagnosis is members of a community who are HIV positive. Community epidemiologic data might indicate a high incidence of uncontrolled diabetes, a high-volume diagnosis that may warrant development of case management services. Similarly, case management services might be developed for pregnant women or children with asthma for whom case management has been shown to have significant positive effects at both client and health system levels.

⑥THINK ABOUT IT

Is case management more appropriate for some clients than others? Why or why not? If so, what categories of clients should be targeted for case management?

Individual client indicators can be categorized as personal indicators, health-related indicators, and social indicators. Personal indicators may include diminished functional status, a history of substance abuse or mental illness, poor cognitive abilities, prior noncompliance with treatment plans, age over 65 years, experience of a major life change or significant change in self-image, potential for severe emotional response, or unrealistic expectations of potential outcomes of care. Health-related factors include the presence of specific medical conditions or diagnoses (e.g., Alzheimer's disease, AIDS, eating disorders, severe burns, trauma), multiple diagnoses, history of prolonged recovery or increased potential for complications, recent or frequent hospital readmissions or emergency department use, intentional or unintentional drug overdose, and involvement of multiple health care providers, agencies, or funding sources. Social indicators are living alone or with a person who is disabled, being uninsured, evidence of family violence, homelessness or an unhealthy home environment, lack of support systems or financial resources, single parenthood, or living in an area where services are lacking (Ling, 1998; Powell, 2000). Presence of one or more of these indicators does not necessarily mean that the client is in need of case management services, but should alert the community health nurse to that possibility. The nurse would then further explore the client situation to determine an actual need for services. Population and client indicators of the need for case management services are summarized below.

HIGHLIGHTS

Population and Client Indicators of the Need for Case Management Services

Population Indicators
- Populations with high-cost diagnoses
- Populations with high-volume diagnoses
- Populations that will experience significant benefit from case management services

Individual Client Indicators

Personal Indicators
- Reduced functional status that will impede self-care
- History of substance abuse or mental illness that may interfere with self-care or compliance
- Poor cognitive abilities that may interfere with understanding of and compliance with treatment recommendations
- A history of prior difficulty in compliance with treatment plans
- Age over 65 years
- A recent major life change or change in self-image (e.g., due to mastectomy)
- Potential for severe emotional response (e.g., depression over a miscarriage)
- Unrealistic expectations regarding prognosis and probable outcomes of care

Health-Related Indicators
- Specific targeted medical diagnoses requiring complex or prolonged care
- Multiple diagnoses
- History of prolonged recovery or increased potential for complications
- History of frequent hospitalization or emergency department use
- History of intentional or unintentional drug overdose
- Involvement of multiple providers, agencies, or funding sources necessitating careful coordination

Social Indicators
- Living alone or with someone who is disabled
- Lack of health insurance
- Instances of, or potential for, family violence
- Homelessness or unhealthy home environment

- Lack of social support or social isolation
- Inadequate financial resources
- Single parenthood or significant change in family roles
- Living in an area lacking in needed services

ASSESSING THE CASE MANAGEMENT SITUATION

In order to develop an effective case management plan, the community health nurse case manager must assess the client's health status and identify factors in the client situation that affect health and are likely to affect the case management plan and achievement of planned health outcomes. Assessment of these factors involves considerations in each of the six dimensions of health: biophysical, psychological, physical environmental, sociocultural, behavioral, and health system dimensions. The assessment should also validate the need for case management services.

Biophysical Considerations

Biophysical factors of age and physiologic function influence case management needs and the case management plan. The client's age may be a factor in eligibility for services as well as the appropriateness of specific services. For example, a younger person with a traumatic injury may do better in a rehabilitation unit that serves a variety of age groups than one that serves primarily older clients. Similarly, an adolescent with a new baby is likely to need more intensive post-discharge follow-up than a more mature woman.

Physiologic function can profoundly influence the level and types of care needed by the client. The nature of medical diagnoses, *comorbidity* (the presence of other disease processes), functional ability to carry out activities of daily living, and abilities to implement a health treatment plan will suggest possible health care needs that the case manager will need to address. For example, the client with decreased functional abilities may need referral for help with household chores, and the client with diagnoses of cardiovascular disease and diabetes will require careful monitoring. Based on physiologic status, some clients may require skilled nursing care or specialized treatments such as intravenous infusions, oxygen administration, or physical therapy. Other biophysical factors that should be considered include medication use and the client's nutritional status. As noted earlier, population data regarding age composition or the incidence and prevalence of selected physical health conditions may indicate a need for the development of case management systems and services.

Psychological Considerations

Psychological factors may also influence individual clients' health care needs. A client with a psychiatric dis-order, for example, may require referral for continued therapy as well as social and emotional support. The presence of mental illness may also complicate the treatment plan for other conditions. For example, severely depressed clients may be unable to engage in the level of self-care required for managing their diabetes. In this instance, the case manager may arrange for frequent home health visits or transfer to an assisted living facility until the client is able to function effectively at home. Additional psychological factors that should be explored include fear and anxiety related to diagnoses, other stress experienced by clients, and clients' general coping abilities. In terms of population case management, a high incidence of suicide among disabled residents would be an indication of the need for case management programs.

Physical Environmental Considerations

Elements of the physical environmental dimension may also need to be addressed in the case management plan. For example, self-care at home may necessitate the use of assistive devices or equipment, and the case manager would arrange for the client to receive this equipment, or the home may require physical modification to accommodate the client's health status. For instance, clients with limited mobility may need to have a ramp installed or change sleeping arrangements to avoid climbing stairs. Other physical environmental dimension factors to be considered include the availability of running water, electricity, adequate heat or air conditioning, space for special equipment, and distance of the home to health care and other services. Environmental factors such as the presence of pollutants should also be considered. For example, a child who is being treated for lead poisoning will need environmental accommodations to prevent reexposure to lead.

Sociocultural Considerations

Sociocultural factors will also influence the types and extent of services to be included in the case management plan. Some factors to consider are the client's education level, support systems, economic status, occupation, transportation, and cultural beliefs and behaviors. For example, clients who live alone and have few social supports may require referrals for assistance with self-care or housekeeping, or institutional placement may be appropriate until the client can effectively engage in self-care. The case manager should also consider changes in family roles that may occur as a result of the client's condition and the effect these changes will have on the client and the family. Potential need for respite for family care givers should also be considered.

The client's economic status can profoundly influence the case management plan. Clients may need financial assistance to meet basic survival needs as well as help with health care needs. For example, a homeless client will need assistance with housing and possibly with food, clothing, and health care services. Occupation is

CULTURAL CONSIDERATIONS

Some cultural groups may exhibit distrust of health care providers. How might this distrust influence the case management situation? What actions could the nurse case manager take to minimize the influence of distrust on the client's ability and willingness to obtain health care services?

closely related to economic status and may also influence clients' health needs. The nurse will need to obtain information about the client's employment status and usual occupation. Is a return to work a relevant goal? If so, what must be accomplished for the client to be able to return to work? Will modifications be required in the work setting or in the tasks performed?

Transportation is another social factor that may influence the client's access to planned health services. Clients who are not able to get to provider agencies may be unable to avail themselves of services needed to meet identified goals. For example, the parent of a handicapped child may recognize the need for medical follow-up, but lack the means to get to the physician's office or specialty clinic. In this situation, the case management plan would incorporate transportation arrangements as well as links to health care providers.

Finally, language barriers may also influence the client's ability to follow through on referrals or to implement elements of the case management plan. The case manager should consider language when making referrals. Referrals should be made to providers who speak the client's primary language whenever possible. When this is not possible, the case manager may need to make arrangements for the services of an interpreter.

At the level of population case management, sociocultural factors will be particularly important in the design of case management programs to meet identified population health needs. Case management services will need to be culturally sensitive and may need to incorporate routine consideration of transportation issues or provision of health education services in multiple languages or for populations with low literacy levels.

Behavioral Considerations

Elements of the behavioral dimension that may affect case management include consumption patterns related to diet and substance abuse, rest and exercise, sexual activity, and other health-related behaviors. The nurse would assess special dietary needs that the client might have as well as the client's ability to meet those needs and willingness to do so. Clients with substance abuse problems may need referrals for treatment services in addition to services to meet other health care needs. If the substance abuse problem is not addressed, the client may be unable to follow through on other portions of the case management plan.

Rest and exercise behaviors may also indicate areas of service requirements. Does the client need a referral for an exercise program to lose weight or is there a need for physical therapy services to regain strength or range of motion? Or does the client have difficulty sleeping and need to arrange daily activities to accommodate rest periods? Similarly, the nurse would assess the effects of the client's condition on sexual function. If problems are noted, what services might be needed to deal with them? For example, a woman who has had a mastectomy might need the assistance of the Reach to Recovery program to deal with self-concept and body image issues. Finally, the nurse would assess the extent to which the client's condition poses special safety needs as well as the extent to which the client engages in routine safety measures such as seat belt use.

Health System Considerations

Information related to considerations discussed above helps the community health nurse identify the types of health care services that the client is likely to need. In the health system dimension, the nurse assesses the availability of those services in the client's community as well as influences related to the type and level of insurance coverage the client has. In addition, the nurse assesses the client's attitudes to health care services and providers. If there are needs for services that are not available locally, it may be necessary to transfer the client to a specialized facility elsewhere. This may necessitate arrangements for transportation, housing for the client or significant others, and admission to the new facility. Is home care an appropriate and cost-effective treatment option for this client? What service alternatives are covered by the client's insurance plan if he or she has one? Are there limitations on services to which the client is entitled, for instance a lifetime number of days in a skilled nursing facility? Other health system considerations include the need for and client's ability to make co-payments and whether or not preauthorization is required for certain services.

Client attitudes about the health care system and health care providers are another important consideration in assessing a case management situation. Clients may feel that they do not need or want any additional help or may prefer to receive care from a provider of an ethnic background similar to theirs. Clients may also resist certain types of services because of the emotional overtones attached to them. For example, elderly clients may refuse placement in a skilled nursing facility out of fear that they will never be able to return home. In some cultural groups, nursing home placement is viewed as abandonment of elderly parents and may be resisted by the family. By assessing these attitudes, the case manager will be able to plan for services that are acceptable to the client thereby facilitating plan implementation and goal accomplishment.

At the population level, the nurse case manager might assess the cluster of services available to meet the needs

assessment tips assessment tips assessment tips

ASSESSING THE CASE MANAGEMENT SITUATION

Biophysical Considerations

- How will the client's age influence the case management plan (e.g., service availability, eligibility, etc.)?
- What physical health problems or functional limitations affect the need for case management or the case management plan?
- Does the client's health status require specialized treatments or interventions? What is the client's level of understanding of health problems, recommended treatments, medications, and so on? What side effects of treatment must be addressed?

Psychological Considerations

- Does the client have any existing mental illness?
- Is the client confused? Does the client have the intellectual capacity needed to implement the management plan?

Physical Environmental Considerations

- Is the client's home environment adequate to meet needs? What modifications may be required in the home environment?
- Are there features in the external environment that will adversely affect the client's health (e.g., great distances to shopping or health care facilities, pollution, etc.)?

Sociocultural Considerations

- What are the client's income and education levels? How do they affect health status?
- What are the client's living arrangements? Does the client live alone? If so, is the client capable of self-care or will assistance be needed? Is the client responsible for the care of other family members? Is the client capable of providing the care needed?
- Is the client's support system adequate to meet the need for assistance? Is respite needed for family members who care for the client?

- Is the client employed? Is a return to work a relevant goal of care? What is/was the client's occupation? Does his or her occupation pose any health risks or give rise to any specific health needs?
- Does the client have access to transportation? Are there special transportation needs?

Behavioral Considerations

- Does the client have special dietary needs? Special needs for rest or exercise? Are these needs adequately met?
- Does the client abuse alcohol or other drugs? Does the client use tobacco or caffeine? Does the use of these substances have specific health implications for this client?
- Is the client sexually active? Does sexual activity pose any particular health risks for the client? Will the client's health status affect sexual activity?
- Does the client use routine safety measures (e.g., seat belts) or have any special safety needs? Are these adequately addressed?

Health System Considerations

- Does the client have a regular source of health care?
- Does the client seek health care services when needed?
- What types of health services does the client need? Are needed health services available and accessible to the client?
- Does the client have health insurance? What services does his or her insurance cover?
- What are the client's attitudes to health care services? Do these attitudes interfere with his or her ability to obtain needed care?

---

of specific populations. The nurse could also explore existing interactions between service organizations and the need and desire for closer coordination of services.

DIAGNOSTIC REASONING AND CASE MANAGEMENT

Once the client's need for and acceptance of case management have been established and factors influencing the client's health status identified, the case manager

uses the assessment data to diagnose specific client health care needs. The preliminary diagnosis may reflect the need for case management and the factors contributing to that need. For example, the community health nurse case manager may diagnose a "need for case management due to limited self-care abilities." Secondary diagnoses would address specific areas of focus in developing the case management plan. These areas may be related to the biophysical, psychological, physical environmental, sociocultural, behavioral, or health system factors influencing the client's health. For example, in the sociocultural dimension the nurse might diagnose a "need for housekeeping assistance due to shortness of breath on exertion" for the client with emphysema. Similarly, a "need for home modification due to limited mobility and potential for falls" might be diagnosed in the physical environmental dimension.

Nurse case managers may also make diagnoses related to population case management. For example, the nurse might diagnose "fragmentation and duplication of services for persons with HIV infection" in the community. Another potential diagnosis at the population level might be the "need for case management services for pregnant adolescents from low-income culturally diverse families."

DEVELOPING THE CASE MANAGEMENT PLAN

The case manager works with the client, family, payers, and potential providers to develop a case management plan that meets the client's identified health care needs in the most efficient and cost-effective manner possible. Developing the case management plan involves two basic activities: determining levels of prevention within the health care dimension and selecting resources. Two other special considerations that may be incorporated into plan development are clinical pathways and discharge planning. Links to resources that may assist with case management planning are provided on the companion Web site for this book.

Determining Levels of Prevention

Planning may involve arranging for services at any or all of the three levels of prevention as appropriate to the client's situation. For example, the case manager may arrange for well child and family planning services for the adolescent with a newborn. He or she may also refer the adolescent to a parenting class and a teen parent support group and arrange for enrollment in an education continuation program. All of these interventions would be aimed at primary prevention.

When secondary prevention services are needed, the case manager may devise a case management plan in keeping with a clinical pathway, also referred to as a *care map* or a *critical pathway*. As noted earlier, a clinical pathway is a typical sequence of medical and nursing interventions based on knowledge of best practices that should be performed in the care of an illness episode related to a particular diagnosis or procedure. Clinical pathways are usually developed for commonly encountered diagnoses and reflect the typical plan of care for that diagnosis. Components of clinical pathways include aspects of care, phases of care, provider processes, and expected outcomes of care. These components are explained in more detail at right.

HIGHLIGHTS

Components of Clinical Pathways

- Aspects of care including assessment and diagnostic activities, treatments, medications, dietary interventions, activity, client and family education, discharge planning, and outcome evaluation
- Phases of care or the timing and intervals for specific interventions
- Functions, processes, or interventions implemented by the care team such as documentation processes, communication, and so on
- Outcomes of care in terms of clinical outcomes related to client health status and managerial outcomes related to costs and quality of care

Source: Powell, S. K. (2000). *Case management: A practical guide to success in managed care* (2nd ed.). Philadelphia: Lippincott.

Clinical pathways are diagnosis-specific, not client-specific, and although the case manager may use a clinical path as a foundation for developing a case management plan, the final plan should be tailored to the needs of the individual client. Deviations from the clinical pathway are called variances, and should be justified on the basis of client-specific assessment information. Analysis of variances can provide evidence of the need for change in the clinical pathways or evaluative data for case management. When using clinical pathways, nurse case managers should inform clients of the potential for variance so they are not alarmed when care deviates from the expected pathway.

Most clinical pathways have been established to direct care for clients with specific medical diagnoses, addressing secondary prevention needs. A few agencies, however, have developed clinical paths for primary prevention activities with selected groups of clients. For example, one health department has developed a clinical path for prenatal care, specifying activities to be accomplished in each trimester and the expected outcomes of those activities. A clinical path at the tertiary level of prevention might detail a typical rehabilitation plan following myocardial infarction.

Even when the case management plan is not based on a clinical pathway, it may include interventions directed toward tertiary prevention. For example, the case manager may arrange for a client who has had a stroke to receive physical therapy services designed to assist the client to regain lost function.

Population case management may also take place at any or all of the three levels of prevention. The previous example of developing case management services for low-income adolescents who are pregnant is primary prevention. Similarly, the creation of case management services for individuals with AIDS would address both secondary and tertiary levels of prevention, while specific case management activities for this group might also entail primary prevention of social isolation and other problems related to their condition.

Discharge planning is a special application of the case management process and involves identifying follow-up needs and arranging for care after discharge from a hospital or other institutional setting (Bull, Hansen, & Gross, 2000). Discharge planning has been described as "preparation for the next phase of care" (Delong, 2000), and research has shown that it enhances client involvement in their own care and reduces the potential for readmission (Erwin, 1999). Indicators of the need for discharge planning are similar to those for case management in general, but studies suggest that, at least for older clients, functional dependence is the best predictor of readmission and a significant indicator of the need for discharge planning (Rosswurm & Lanham, 1998).

Selecting Resources

The second major aspect of developing the case management plan involves selecting the resources, providers, and services to meet clients' identified health needs. Selection decisions will be based on considerations of appropriateness, acceptability to the client, quality, and cost. Selection of resources may also involve accessing clients' personal resources. Health care services selected should be appropriate to the client's needs as well as to other aspects of the client situation. For example, it might be necessary to find a health care provider who speaks Spanish or who has office hours congruent with the client's work schedule. The appropriateness of the setting for care should also be considered. For example, while periodic home care might be appropriate for a client who is relatively self-sufficient or who has a supportive family, an assisted living situation might be more appropriate for another client.

The nurse case manager should also consider client preferences and the acceptability of specific resources to clients in developing the case management plan. For example, a client who has suffered a stroke may reject an otherwise obvious choice for a rehabilitation program because it is too far from family. Similarly, a client with a substance abuse problem may not find a residential treatment center acceptable because it would mean sending her children to distant family members for care.

The quality of services provided is another consideration in the selection of resources. The case manager should be conversant with the competence of providers to whom he or she refers clients, and the quality of care should be monitored once the referral is made. Client complaints should be investigated and action taken to ensure provision of high-quality services.

Cost is the fourth area of consideration in developing the case management plan. In many instances, the services available to a given client are constrained by economic considerations and what may or may not be covered by their insurance plan. The case manager has to be conversant with a wide variety of insurance plans and the services that they cover. In most instances, services should be provided in the least costly setting that will meet the client's needs. The vagaries of insurance coverage, however, sometimes mean that services will be reimbursed only if they take place in certain types of settings. For example, under some plans, intravenous infusions are not covered unless they are provided in an inpatient setting.

The nurse case manager should also be familiar with two other concepts related to reimbursement for services: coordination of benefits rules and extracontractual benefits. *Coordination of benefits (COB) rules* designate the responsibility of payers when a client is covered by more than one form of insurance (Powell, 2000). For example, when clients have both Medicare benefits and a supplemental insurance policy, Medicare first pays its share of the cost of services. Then the supplemental plan is billed for remaining costs. The case manager should be familiar with the succession of responsibility among insurance plans in order to develop an effective case management plan. When clients need services that are not covered under an existing plan, the community health nurse case manager may be able to negotiate *extracontractual benefits,* or reimbursement for uncovered services. This is usually only possible when no covered alternative is available and the nurse can demonstrate that the additional coverage will prevent a greater expense to the payer (St. Couer, 1996).

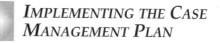

IMPLEMENTING THE CASE MANAGEMENT PLAN

Implementation of the case management plan involves communicating the plan, delegating, initiating referrals, and monitoring plan implementation.

Communicating the Plan

Clients and their significant others need to be informed of arrangements made for care and expectations of them in following through on the management plan. For example, clients may need to call to make a specific appointment with a provider even though care has been arranged by the case manager. Clients will also need to know about any payments required and the names of contact persons in agencies to which they have been referred. Additional information to be conveyed to clients relates to the expected duration and outcome of services.

The case manager also needs to communicate the case management plan to the providers who will be giving the necessary care. Client needs and expectations of the provider should be addressed as well as any previous plans and their effects, expectations for continued care, and any other information relevant to the client's situation.

Again, the case manager should be careful to obtain the consent of the client before providing such information. Finally, the payer should be informed of and approve the management plan. The nurse case manager should confirm and document that referral agencies and payers have received the information sent. He or she should also confirm that clients and family members understand the information provided.

Delegating

Delegation is the process of "transferring to a competent individual the authority to perform a selected nursing task in a selected situation" (Hansten, Washburn, & Kenyon, 1999b, p. 1). Delegation consists of four components referred to as the four "rights": the right task, right person, right communication, and right feedback (Hansten, Washburn, & Kenyon, 1999a). The tasks to be delegated must be within the scope of practice of the person or group to whom it is delegated. Similarly, the person or group must be competent and willing to assume the tasks. For example, the case manager would not delegate care of an older client to a daughter who is potentially abusive or to an elderly spouse who does not have the physical capabilities to provide the needed care. Similarly, in population case management, the nurse case manager would not delegate the development of a prenatal education program to a group that does not have that expertise.

Communication is a key element in delegation. The person or group to whom a task or tasks are being delegated must be informed of the expectations for their performance and any timelines involved in executing the task. Finally, the nurse case manager must monitor task performance and provide feedback to those to whom tasks are delegated. Recognition should be given for tasks well done and correction provided as necessary to improve performance. A summary of an article describing new graduates' perceptions of their ability to delegate is available on the companion Web site for this book. 🌐

Initiating Referrals

Referral is the process of directing a client to another source of information or assistance. It differs from delegation in that the nurse case manager relinquishes responsibility for the implementation of the portions of the plan of care for which the client is referred, although he or she retains overall responsibility for the quality of care provided (Bourguet, Gilchrist, McCord, & the NEON Research Group, 1998). Referrals to a variety of health care and related services may be part of case management for an individual client and his or her family. Four basic considerations enter into the decision to refer a client to a particular provider, agency, or service: the acceptability of the referral to the client, client eligibility for services, constraints operating in the situation, and community resources available.

Acceptability to the Client

The first consideration in making a referral is the acceptability of the referral to the client. Some clients may be unwilling to obtain help if they perceive it as "charity." In other cases, clients may have philosophies different from those of the referral resource. For example, a Southern Baptist client may be reluctant to accept assistance from an agency supported by the Roman Catholic Church. Barriers to acceptability of a specific referral may include fear of a strange agency or provider, prior negative experiences, lack of faith in the referral resource, failure to acknowledge a problem requiring referral, and concerns about costs. Finally, reaching out for assistance may be counter to the client's culture or frame of reference or following up on a referral may be preempted by client concerns with higher priorities.

Client Eligibility for Service

The second consideration in referral is the client's eligibility for the service provided. There are many determinants of eligibility for service. Sometimes, eligibility is based on financial needs, and clients may need to provide evidence of income and expenditures. In other instances, eligibility might be based on residence within a particular jurisdiction or membership in a particular group. For example, nonresidents are not usually eligible for state-supported medical assistance, or a particular agency may provide services only to members of a specific religious or ethnic group. Eligibility can also be based on age. As an example, senior citizens' groups usually do not provide services for anyone under the age of 55. Finally, eligibility is sometimes based on the existence of a particular condition. For instance, certain shelter services might be available only to abused women rather than to homeless people.

Situational Constraints

The presence of *situational constraints,* or factors in the client's situation that would prevent him or her from following through on a referral, is a third consideration. For example, does the client have transportation available to go to the appropriate place of care? If clients do not speak English, will they be able to find an interpreter to help them? The nurse making the referral should assess any situational constraints present and then take action to eliminate or minimize the effects of those constraints. The nurse case manager may also need to coordinate funding benefits among multiple agencies to prevent barriers to timely access to care (Ling, 1998).

Availability of Resources

Information related to each of the three previous referral considerations will be readily available if the nurse has thoroughly assessed each of the dimensions of health prior to developing the case management plan. Resource availability information, on the other hand, will be obtained through assessment of the community. The community health nurse case manager needs to be familiar with health care and other support services available in the community. Information on community resources can be obtained in a number of ways. Two major sources of information are the local health department and the yellow pages. Other resources are neighborhood information and referral centers, local government offices and chambers of commerce, and police and fire departments. The local library is also a source of information and may even have a directory of local resources.

It is not sufficient for the community health nurse to merely be aware of the existence of community resources. The nurse must know where these resources are located and understand the requirements for referral to each resource. The nurse should systematically collect information on the types of services a referral resource provides, criteria for eligibility for services, and whether any fee is involved. Information to be sought also includes indicators of the quality of services provided and the credentials and competencies of providers as noted earlier. The community health nurse case manager may want to establish a ***resource file*** or database to systematically organize and store information on area resources. Figure 12–1 ■ depicts a sample resource file entry. A copy of the resource file entry form is included on the companion Web site for this book.

The file could be organized according to categories of resources as in the following example:

- Developmental assessment
- Drug abuse
    - Diagnosis and treatment
    - Prevention
- Environmental services
    - Protection
    - Sanitation
- Family planning services
    - Contraception
    - Infertility
- Family services
    - Counseling
    - Family advocacy
    - Marital counseling
    - Parenting classes

Resource category: Transportation Funding source: Voluntary
Agency name: St. Martha's Catholic Church
Address: 3710 Montebank Rd, Otenada, Mississippi
Phone number: 817-3421 Business hours: Mon-Fri 8-4
Contact person: Mrs. Jefferson Title: receptionist / secretary
Source of referral: self or other
Eligibility: anyone without transportation - need not be members of church
Fee: none
Services: Provides transportation to church services as well as other services such as Dr.'s office, grocery shopping, etc. on periodic basis
Access: call to arrange transportation
Other comments: 1) Do not provide transportation on long-term basis, i.e., to work or school
2) depends upon availability of volunteer drivers
3) drivers trained to assist disabled riders

FIGURE 12–1 ■ *Sample Resource File Entry*

A particular agency with more than one type of service could be entered in several different categories or a cross-reference system could be used. The resource described in Figure 12–1 deals with transportation.

Information about the resource's funding source can be useful in tracking service availability. For example, if tax revenues have declined in the area, the community health nurse case manager may want to contact agencies funded by public money to determine whether services have been cut prior to making a specific referral. Also, it may be important to some clients to know that the services they receive from an agency are provided by tax dollars rather than "charity."

Of course, the resource file entry includes the referral resource's full name, address, and telephone number. The business hours notation may refer to when the agency is open or times when a particular service is offered. For example, the entry might read "Family planning: Monday, 9:00 A.M.–noon, Prenatal: Tuesday, 1:00–4:00 P.M."

It is helpful to have the name of a contact person in the agency as well. Referrals are facilitated when agency personnel are familiar with the person making the referral. Unfortunately, situations do occur where some agency employees are more inclined to accommodate professional colleagues than clients. When the case manager refers a client to an agency and gives that individual the name of a contact person who knows the nurse, the client who mentions that he or she was referred by the nurse may get a more prompt response than the client who does not have a specific person to contact. Having a specific contact person within the agency may also facilitate requests for services when the request is made by the nurse case manager rather than the client.

"Source of referral" in Figure 12–1 refers to the preferred originator of the referral. Some agencies accept referrals only from specific persons, usually physicians. If a professional referral is required, the nurse should specifically inquire about the acceptability of referrals from nurse practitioners, if they are available in the area. In the example in Figure 12–1, no specific referral source is required. Clients may request services on their own or be referred by anyone else.

As noted previously, information related to the eligibility of clients for service is very important. To make appropriate referrals, the nurse must know who is eligible for a particular service and who is not. This helps to minimize client frustration in being referred for services for which they do not qualify. The importance of a notation regarding fees is obvious. Clients need to know beforehand if they will be charged for services provided by the referral resource. The nurse should also be familiar with the types of insurance coverage accepted by the resource. For example, does the agency accept clients covered by Medicaid but not CHAMPUS? An additional notation might indicate whether or not the agency can help clients with financial arrangements for out-of-pocket expenses. The nurse should also know whether payment is expected at the time of services or if the client will receive a bill later.

Notation should also be made regarding the types of services provided by the resource. The entry regarding access refers to the means by which the client gains entry to the system. In the example in Figure 12–1, the client needs to call ahead for an appointment. Additional information under this entry would indicate any supporting documentation the client must provide to be eligible for services. Should he or she bring health insurance papers or just the policy number? Will the client need proof of residence, monthly expenditures, or medical expenses?

Finally, the nurse should obtain and store information regarding the competency of providers to whom referrals are made. Information about the credentials of providers, prior client complaints, malpractice actions, and so on can be recorded in the comments section as indicated in the third comment in Figure 12–1.

The type of information included in the sample resource file entry allows the community health nurse case manager to make appropriate referrals that do not waste clients' time and energy. It also allows the nurse to prepare clients for what they will encounter in following through on a referral. The file should be updated on a regular basis and as circumstances in various agencies change. Having a specific contact person in each agency may help to ensure that the nurse is notified of program changes. Experiences and reactions of clients following the use of a particular resource can also be used to update resource information and to evaluate the quality of service provided.

Monitoring Plan Implementation

Monitoring is another important aspect of implementing the case management plan. Once the plan is developed, the community health nurse case manager does not simply let the plan proceed to unfold on its own or close the case to case management services. Rather, the nurse case manager monitors the implementation of the plan and progress toward achievement of identified goals. Specific areas to be addressed at this stage include monitoring changes in the client's medical status (either positive or negative), social circumstances, and the quality of care provided; observing for changes in functional ability or mobility; and identifying evolving education needs. In addition, the nurse will assess the effectiveness of pain management if relevant and monitor changes in client or family satisfaction with services and their outcomes (Powell, 2000).

EVALUATING THE PROCESS AND OUTCOMES OF CASE MANAGEMENT

Evaluation is an integral component of the case management process. The community health nurse case manager focuses on three areas in evaluating case management: client outcomes, quality of care, and the case management process itself.

Evaluating Primary, Secondary, and Tertiary Intervention Outcomes

The community health nurse case manager evaluates client responses to health care services and the outcomes achieved. Did the client follow through on any referrals made? Has the client consistently performed the exercises recommended by the physical therapist? Outcome evaluation would focus on the degree of progress made toward identified goals. These goals may reflect primary, secondary, or tertiary prevention. Evaluation of primary prevention would assess whether or not health was promoted or specific problems were prevented. For example, the case management plan for a client with emphysema and hypertension might have included referral for influenza and pneumonia immunization. Evaluative questions would focus on whether the client received the recommended immunizations and remained disease free.

A secondary prevention goal might be control of the client's hypertension through education on correct medication dosage and administration. The client's blood pressure would be the criterion used to evaluate goal achievement in this case. Evaluation of tertiary prevention endeavors might focus on the client's ability to resume housekeeping chores and other functions after an exercise training program.

When desired client outcomes are not achieved, the community health nurse evaluates factors that may be affecting goal accomplishment. The case management plan would then be revised to modify or eliminate the effects of these factors. Difficulties in goal accomplishment may stem from an inappropriate case management plan, poor quality services, failures in plan implementation (on the part of providers or clients), or changes in the client situation. For example, the case management plan might include weekly physical therapy at a local outpatient facility. If the client's car breaks down and the client has no other source of transportation, the plan may not be implemented as designed and modifications will be needed.

Evaluating the Quality of Services

As noted earlier, the case manager is responsible for monitoring and evaluating the quality of services provided in implementing the case management plan. To obtain evaluative data in this area, the nurse might periodically visit providers to observe and discuss the quality of care given. For example, the nurse might ask an oncologist about the breadth of options usually presented to women with breast cancer. An oncologist who presents only one option to clients may not be the most appropriate referral for the case manager to make. The community health nurse case manager might also contact clients or family members to obtain their perceptions of the quality of services provided. The nurse should be particularly alert to situations in which clients discontinue services from one or more providers before goals are achieved. Exploration of the client's reasons for discontinuing services may indicate poor quality of care.

Quality of care should also be assessed in population case management. For example, the case manager might evaluate the interactions between agencies included in the system or the length of time clients had to wait for services from specific agencies. Evaluating the quality of care may involve the use of benchmarks. *Benchmarking* is a process of establishing comparative data between organizations. Clinical benchmarking reflects not only the best outcome actually achieved for a given group of clients or diagnosis, but should be based on the evidence of the best possible outcome (Ellis, 2000). Steps in the benchmarking process are presented below.

HIGHLIGHTS

Steps in the Benchmarking Process

- Identify the area of practice involved (e.g., control of blood pressure in hypertensive clients).
- Identify a patient-focused outcome (e.g., blood pressures consistently lower than 140/90).
- Identify factors and processes that affect the outcome (e.g., medication compliance).
- Identify benchmarks for the best practice for each factor (e.g., medication education provided on the initial visit and reinforced at each visit thereafter).
- Construct a scoring continuum for practice (e.g., medication education consistently provided on first visit, education delayed to subsequent visits, no education provided).
- Score current practice with comments on why scores were assigned (e.g., medication education delayed beyond first visit in 60% of cases).
- Compare results with the identified best practice.
- Share the results with others involved (e.g., physicians, nurse clinicians, etc.).
- Develop a plan of action for improving practice (e.g., identify and modify factors preventing medication education on initial visits).

Source: Ellis, J. (2000). Sharing the evidence: Clinical practice benchmarking to improve continuously the quality of care. *Journal of Advanced Nursing, 32*(1), 215–225.

Evaluating the Case Management Process

The third aspect of evaluation is the assessment of the case management process itself. Was the client really a candidate for case management services? Was the initial assessment accurate and complete enough to permit effective planning? Was the case management plan appropriate to the client's needs? Were the referrals appropriate? Could the case management process have been carried out more effectively, more efficiently, or in a more timely manner? The answers to these and similar

CRITICAL THINKING IN RESEARCH

Cost-effectiveness of case management services have usually looked at the costs of providing case management in comparison to the savings achieved in client care services. Cost-benefit analyses, on the other hand, weigh the cost of case management services against a variety of benefits that result from case management. If you were going to do such as study, what kind of benefits would you measure? How would you go about measuring them?

You can read a summary of a research article related to evaluation of case management services on the companion Web site for this book

questions will permit the community health nurse to revise the case management plan for a given client in a more effective way and will also enhance the nurse's overall case management ability.

Some case managers may be involved in one other aspect of evaluating case management, utilization review. *Utilization review* is a process of monitoring the necessity of care and the resources used and may involve preadmission review, concurrent review, retrospective review, or telephonics (Powell, 2000). In a preadmission review, the nurse case manager determines the appropriateness of the requested services before they are given. Areas for consideration include the need for the service and the appropriateness of the setting and level of services proposed. For example, the case manager may determine that a requested nursing home admission is not appropriate because the client can be effectively cared for at home for far less cost. Concurrent review takes place while services are being provided to determine client progress toward goals and the need to continue services. Telephonics is a form of concurrent review in which the information needed to determine the appropriateness of service continuation is obtained by telephone. In retrospective review, the case manager determines the need for and appropriateness of services after they have been provided with the intent of approving or denying reimbursement for those services. Utilization review is generally performed by case managers who have an identified role in reimbursement decisions and may or may not be required of community health nurse case managers.

Managerial aspects of the case management process should also be assessed, particularly with respect to population case management. Elements to be considered include the cost-effectiveness of care provided and the cost-effectiveness of case management services. Other considerations include client satisfaction with care and with the case management process. The elements of the case management process, including aspects of evaluation and utilization review are summarized in Table 12–2 ■.

Case management has been shown to be an effective nursing intervention used since the beginning of community health nursing practice. Community health nurses can improve their practice with more systematic use of the case management process with individuals as well as population groups.

■ **TABLE 12–2 Steps in the Case Management Process**

- Case selection
- Assessing the case management situation
    - Biophysical considerations
    - Psychological considerations
    - Physical environmental considerations
    - Sociocultural considerations
    - Behavioral considerations
    - Health system considerations
- Deriving nursing diagnoses to guide the case management plan
- Developing the case management plan
    - Determining the level of prevention
    - Selecting resources
- Implementing the case management plan
    - Communicating the plan
    - Delegating
    - Initiating referrals
    - Monitoring plan implementation
- Evaluating the process and outcomes of case management
    - Evaluating primary, secondary, and tertiary intervention outcomes
    - Evaluating the quality of care
    - Evaluating the case management process
    - Utilization review

APPLYING YOUR KNOWLEDGE IN PRACTICE

❧ CASE STUDY
Case Management in Action

Mrs. Davis is 67 years old. She was admitted to the hospital a week ago with a broken ankle. It is believed that she fractured her ankle stepping off a curb. Her bones are very fragile because of osteoporosis.

Mrs. Davis is retired and receives Social Security benefits. She lives with her son and 5-year-old grandson. Mrs. Davis's son is employed in heavy construction. Because of the recent rain, he has not been able to work consistently, and they have little savings. Mrs. Davis confides that she does not know how they will pay for the portion of the hospital bill that Medicare does not cover. Mrs. Davis usually takes care of her grandson when her son is working. She also does the housework, although her son does most of the heavy work around the house.

Mrs. Davis will be discharged later today. She has a follow-up appointment with the orthopedist in a week, but does not know how she will get there if her son is working that day. Mrs. Davis has been taught how to use a walker and will need to continue its use for several weeks.

- Is Mrs. Davis a candidate for case management? Why or why not?
- What are Mrs. Davis's health needs? How do biophysical, psychological, physical environmental, sociocultural, behavioral, and health system factors influence those needs?
- What desired outcomes would you establish for Mrs. Davis? Do these outcomes reflect primary, secondary, or tertiary prevention?
- How would you involve Mrs. Davis in developing the case management plan? Who else should be involved?
- What referrals would be appropriate for Mrs. Davis? What is the expected outcome of these referrals? How would you go about making the referrals?
- How would you evaluate the case management plan for Mrs. Davis? Be specific about the evaluative criteria you would use and how you would obtain the information to evaluate her care.

❧ TESTING YOUR UNDERSTANDING

- Describe at least five goals of case management. How do the goals of case management differ for clients and for health organizations? (p. 254)
- What are three types of negligence that may lead to legal action related to case management? How might they be avoided? (p. 255)
- What three types of criteria are used to determine the need for case management of individual clients or families? What criteria might suggest the need for population case management? (pp. 255–257)
- What types of considerations should be included in assessing a case management situation? Give examples of how factors in each area could affect the case management situation. (pp. 257–259)

- What are some of the factors that should be considered in selecting resources to meet clients' needs? (p. 261)
- What are the two major aspects of developing the case management plan? Give an example of each. (pp. 260–261)
- What four areas should be considered in implementing the case management plan? (pp. 261–264)
- What are three areas to be considered in evaluating case management? Is the focus on the client or the health care system? (pp. 264–266)

REFERENCES

Bedell, J. R., Cohen, N., & Sullivan, A. (2000). Case management: The current best practices and the next generation of innovation. *Community Mental Health Journal, 36*, 179–194.

Berry, V., Cranston, B., & Fox, T. (2000). Caremapping: What's in it for nurses? *Nursing Case Management, 5*, 63–72.

Blaha, C., Robinson, J. M., Pugh, L. C., Bryan, Y., & Havens, D. S. (2000). Longitudinal nursing case management for elderly heart failure patients: Notes from the field. *Nursing Case Management, 5*, 32–36.

Bourguet, C., Gilchrist, V., McCord, G., & the NEON Research Group. (1998). The consultation and referral process: A report from NEON. *The Journal of Family Practice, 46*(1), 47–53.

Bull, M. J., Hansen, H. E., & Gross, C. R. (2000). A professional-patient partnership model of discharge planning with elders hospitalized with heart failure. *Applied Nursing Research, 13*(1), 19–28.

Case Management Society of America. (1995). *Standards of practice for case management.* Little Rock, AR: Author.

Chan, S., Mackenzie, A., & Jacobs, P. (2000). Cost-effectiveness analysis of case management versus a routine community care organization for patients with chronic schizophrenia. *Archives of Psychiatric Nursing, XIV*(2), 98–104.

Davidson, J. U. (1999). Blending case management and quality outcomes management into the family nurse practitioner role. *Nursing Administration Quarterly, 24*(1), 66–74.

Delong, M. F. (2000). *The nurse as discharge planner.* Sunnyvale, CA: NurseWeek.

Ellis, J. (2000). Sharing the evidence: Clinical practice benchmarking to improve continuously the quality of care. *Journal of Advanced Nursing, 32*(1), 215–225.

Erwin, J. (1999). A simple plan: Discharge planning improves odds. *NurseWeek, 12*(13), 16.

Forkner, D. J. (1996). Clinical pathways: Benefits and liabilities. *Nursing Management, 27*(11), 35–38.

Fox, P. D., Etheredge, L., & Jones, S. B. (1998). Addressing the needs of chronically ill persons under Medicare. *Health Affairs, 17*, 144–151.

Gagnon, A. J., Schein, C., McVey, L., & Bergman, H. (1999). Randomized controlled trial of nurse case management of frail older people. *Journal of the American Geriatrics Society, 47*, 1118–1124.

Hansten, R. I., Washburn, M. J., & Kenyon, V. L. (1999a). Know what needs to be done: If I delegate all my tasks, what's left for me to do? In R. I. Hansten, M. J. Washburn, & V. L. Kenyon (Eds.), *Home care nursing delegation skills: A handbook for practice* (pp. 133–171). Gaithersburg, MD: Aspen.

Hansten, R. I., Washburn, M. J., & Kenyon, V. L. (1999b). The overall delegation process. In R. I. Hansten, M. J. Washburn, & V. L. Kenyon (Eds.), *Home care nursing delegation skills: A handbook for practice* (pp. 1–9). Gaithersburg, MD: Aspen.

Harris, L. E., Luft, F. C., Rudy, D. W., Kesterson, J. G., & Tierney, W. M. (1998). Effects of multidisciplinary case management in patients with chronic renal insufficiency. *American Journal of Medicine, 105*, 464–471.

Ling, C. (1998). *Case management basics.* Sunnyvale, CA: NurseWeek.

Michaels, C. (1997). Leading beyond traditional boundaries: A community nursing perspective. *Nursing Administration Quarterly, 22*(1), 30–37.

Nichols, D. J. (1996). Legal liabilities in case management. In D. L. Flarey & S. S. Blancett (Eds.), *Handbook of nursing case management: Health care delivery in a world of managed care* (pp. 424–442). Gaithersburg, MD: Aspen.

Powell, S. K. (2000). *Case management: A practical guide to success in managed care* (2nd ed.). Philadelphia: Lippincott.

Rosswurm, M. A., & Lanham, D. M. (1998). Discharge planning for elderly patients. *Journal of Gerontological Nursing, 24*(5), 14–21.

Schmidt, S. M., Guo, L., Scheer, S., Boydston, J., Pelino, C., & Berger, S. K. (1999). Epidemiologic determination of community-based nursing case management for stroke. *Journal of Nursing Administration, 29*(6), 40–47.

Schroeder, C. A., Trehearne, B., & Ward, D. (2000). Expanded role of nursing in ambulatory managed care, part II: Impact on outcomes of costs, quality, provider, and patient satisfaction. *Nursing Economics, 18*, 71–78.

Stanton, M. P., Walizer, E. M., Graham, J. I., & Keppel, L. (2000). Case management: A case study. *Nursing Case Management, 5*, 37–45.

St. Couer, M. (1996). *Case management practice guidelines.* St. Louis: Mosby.

Tahan, H. A. (1999). Clarifying case management: What is in a label? *Nursing Case Management, 4*, 268–278.

Taylor, P. (1999). Comprehensive nursing care management: An advanced practice model. *Nursing Case Management, 4*, 2–10.

Williams, D. B. (2000). Population care management: What's in it for your organization? *Nursing Case Management, 5*, 1.

CHANGE, LEADERSHIP, AND GROUP PROCESSES

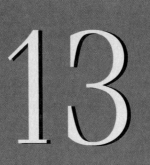

Chapter Objectives

After reading this chapter, you should be able to:

- Discuss the influence of driving forces and restraining forces in change.
- Describe four major considerations in planning for change.
- Identify three approaches to bringing about change.
- Describe the relationship of follower maturity to leadership style.
- Discuss the tasks involved in each of the five stages of group development.
- Describe two tasks in implementing the group process.
- Discuss two aspects of evaluation applicable to the change, leadership, and group processes.

KEY TERMS

cognitive dissonance 272
counterattitudinal behavior 272
disconfirmation 275
driving forces 271
empirical–rational approach 273
field theory 271
force field 271
moving 271
normative–reeducative approach 274
power–coercive approach 274
refreezing 271
restraining forces 271
unfreezing 271

Media Link

http://www.prenhall.com/clark

Additional interactive resources for this chapter can be found on the companion Web site. Click on Chapter 13 and "Begin" to select the activities for this chapter.

Reading about the accomplishments of early leaders in community health nursing, for example, Lillian Wald and her compatriots, one may wonder how these women came to exercise such influence. The answer lies in their knowledge and use of the change, leadership, and group processes. They knew how to use their leadership abilities to influence individuals and groups of people to achieve desired changes in society and in the health care system. Using these same processes, today's community health nurses can change health care and the health of those they serve.

The change, leadership, and group processes are interrelated. Community health nurses who seek to bring about change must exercise leadership, but leadership without systematic use of the change process may not achieve the desired outcome. Changes often result from the actions of a group of people rather than those of a single individual. Community health nurses exercise leadership skills to direct group activities that will accomplish desired changes. Having knowledge of these three interrelated processes is essential for effective community health nursing practice.

THE CHANGE PROCESS

Change as a process used by community health nurses involves a series of definite activities directed toward an identified goal. The change is planned and directed rather than spontaneous and unguided. Although we know that change does occur spontaneously and without direction, in this chapter change is explored as a planned process over which the community health nurse (and others) can exercise control. Conscious, deliberate, and intentional actions are designed to produce change.

THEORIES OF CHANGE

Community health nurses are involved in the change process at two levels, promoting behavior change in individual clients and families and promoting change in organizations or population groups. These levels of change are reflected in three types of theories related to change: personal change theories, organizational change theories, and community change theories (Thompson & Kinne, 1999). Community change theory will be addressed in Chapter 15. In this chapter, we will examine theories of personal change and organizational change theory.

Prochaska, Norcross, and DiClemente (1995) developed a stage theory of personal change in which an individual goes through five stages in accomplishing a change in behavior. These stages of change and their characteristics are presented in Table 13–1 ■. The client begins in the precontemplation stage in which there is no

■ **TABLE 13–1** **Stages of Personal Behavior Change and Associated Characteristics**

STAGE	CHARACTERISTICS
Precontemplation	No intention to change; possibility of change is not even considered
Contemplation	Development of an awareness of the need to change; change is considered; no commitment to change
Preparation	Intent to change is present; plans for making the change are developed and small preparatory changes may even be made (e.g., cutting down on the number of cigarettes a day prior to total smoking cessation)
Action	New behavior is implemented for at least six months
Maintenance	Activities to prevent relapse to previous behavior

intent to change and progresses through the period of contemplating change but taking no action, preparation for change, which may include small changes (Lawrence, 1999), to action in which the full change is implemented, to maintenance when the change becomes part of one's normal behavior. Although this model was developed for use in promoting personal behavior change in individuals, groups or organizations can also be assessed in terms of their readiness to engage in a desired change.

Interventions by the community health nurse as a change agent should be tailored to the stage at which the client is encountered. For example, action-oriented strategies are not particularly effective when clients are in the precontemplation or contemplation stages. In these stages, the nurse should focus on enhancing clients' awareness of the need for change. Similarly, in the contemplation stage, clients often focus on the most negative aspects of the proposed change and the nurse needs to assist them to develop a more balanced perspective by addressing both the positive and negative aspects of the change (Houlihan, 1999). A summary of a research study exploring the application of the stages of change model to dietary patterns among African Americans can be reviewed on the companion Web site for this book. 🌐

Kurt Lewin developed a set of microtheories that explain several aspects of change (Tiffany & Lutjens, 1998). The two most useful of these microtheories are field theory and the stages of change theory. Although these theories can be applied to change in individuals, they are most often applied to organizational change. Generally, three types of change occur in organizations, changes in structure (such as moving to a more or less centralized administrative structure or changes in lines of authority), changes in technology (methods and equipment used or ways of doing work), and changes in people (attitudes, expectations, behaviors, etc.) (Habel, 2000).

According to *field theory*, there are always two types of forces that affect the likelihood of change in any situation: driving forces and restraining forces (Lewin, 1951). These two types of forces work in opposition, and it is the relative strength of each that determines whether change will occur (Lewin, 1989b).

Force, in Lewin's theory, is a tendency to movement either toward change or away from change (Tiffany & Lutjens, 1998). *Driving forces* are those factors that favor or facilitate change. *Restraining forces,* on the other hand, impede change. For example, staff frustration with cumbersome charting procedures may be a driving force that motivates a change to computerized record keeping (a change in technology). In this situation, feelings of inadequacy regarding computer use and concern for depersonalization of clients may be restraining forces working against change. A field is the life space of the individual or group and a *force field* is the total of driving and restraining forces operating in a given situation.

Promoting change is a matter of changing the balance of the driving and restraining forces present in the force field (Colenso, 2000). Community health nurses can increase driving forces, decrease restraining forces, or do both to bring about change. It has been suggested, however, that weakening restraining forces may be a more effective approach (Skinner, 1994). Strengthening driving forces too much can result in precipitous and undirected change in an undesirable direction. When driving forces are stronger than restraining forces, change occurs.

⑥THINK ABOUT IT

What would you like to see changed in your nursing education program? What driving and restraining forces are operating in the situation? How might you influence these forces to promote change?

Lewin (1989a) also developed a three-stage theory of how change occurs, through unfreezing, moving, and refreezing. *Unfreezing* is the process of creating an awareness of the need to change and developing motivation for the change. *Moving* is the actual process of implementing or carrying out the planned change and involves "moving" to the next level of behavior (Lewin, 1989a). *Refreezing* is the process of internalizing the change so it becomes part of the normal routine. In the computerization example, refreezing occurs when the change to computerized charting has become internalized to the point that staff members wonder how they ever managed to chart the old way. Concepts of Lewin's field theory and stages of change are summarized at right.

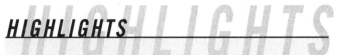

HIGHLIGHTS

Concepts of Lewin's Microtheories

Force: Tendency to movement toward or away from change

Driving forces: Forces promoting change

Restraining forces: Forces impeding change

Field: Life space of an individual or group

Force field: Total of driving and restraining forces operation in the situation

Unfreezing: Development of the awareness of the need for change

Moving: Carrying out the proposed change

Refreezing: Internalization of the change to become part of the normal routine

ASSESSMENT AND DIAGNOSIS IN THE CHANGE SITUATION

To bring about change, the community health nurse identifies a need for change and assesses the driving and restraining forces operating in the change situation and the stage of the client with respect to the change. The need for change may arise from factors in any of the six dimensions of health. For example, a new diagnosis of a chronic disease, a biophysical factor, may necessitate changes in diet or exercise levels. Similarly, a change in family structure with the birth of a first child is a sociocultural factor that may necessitate change in family roles. At the community level, widespread unemployment may necessitate changes in health care systems to provide access to care for those who have lost health insurance coverage.

Factors in each dimension may also serve as driving and restraining forces in the change situation. For example, the birth of a new baby (a sociocultural factor) may promote assumption of additional responsibilities by an adolescent sibling. At the same time, the egocentricity of the typical adolescent (a biophysical factor) may mitigate against this change. Similarly, changes in community leadership (another sociocultural factor) may be a driving force for change, while fear of encroachment on individual rights (a psychological factor) may be a restraining force.

The community health nurse also assesses where the client (individual, family, or population group) is with respect to the stages of change. Is the community even aware of the need for change? For example, does the community have an awareness of the extent of tobacco use among local high school students? If the community is aware, but maintains that preventing tobacco use is a parental function, community members may not be willing to change practices to prevent use. If, on the other

assessment tips assessment tips assessment tips

ASSESSING THE CHANGE SITUATION

- What factors in the biophysical, psychological, physical environmental, sociocultural, behavioral, or health system dimensions give rise to a need for change?
- What are the driving and restraining forces operating in the change situation?
- Where is the client in terms of the stages of change?
- What are the skills needed for the change? Does the client or organization have these skills?
- Who are the key people who will be involved in the change? Do their identified skills match those needed for the change?
- What are key people's typical responses to change? How versatile are they in their ability to adapt to change?

- What are the overall strengths and weaknesses of the organization with respect to the desired change?
- What developmental needs must be met for the change to occur?
- What are the potential weak links in the organization with respect to the desired change? What effects might these weak links have on implementation of the change?
- What other situational constraints may affect the desired change?

hand, the community perceives the need and its role in tobacco use prevention, changes may be made in local education programs to support nonuse.

A final aspect of assessing an organizational change situation is an analysis of the organization's capacity for making the change. This involves assessing the people involved in the change and the situation in which the change will occur (Bishop, 2001). The nurse would assess several areas related to the change situation. These include identifying the skills needed to implement the change, the key positions in the organization that will influence the change, and the degree to which the skills of the people occupying these key positions match the skills needed for the change. The change agent also assesses each individual's typical response to change and his or her versatility within the organization or adaptability to future changes. Information about specific individuals can then be analyzed to determine the strengths and weaknesses of the group as a whole with respect to the desired change. This information also leads to diagnoses of organizational and individual development needs as well as determination of the best people to play specific roles with respect to the change. Attention should also be given to potential "weak links" (e.g., what will happen to the change process if key individuals leave the organization?). Finally, the nurse assesses organizational constraints (e.g., budget) that may influence the change. Tips for assessing a change situation are presented above.

PLANNING FOR CHANGE

Change may occur with or without planning. In the absence of systematic planning, however, the change that occurs may not be desirable. As change agents, commu-

nity health nurses approach change through planned and goal-directed intervention.

Several general principles guide planning for change. If change is to be effective, the community health nurse and client both must participate in planning the change; however, not every person in an organization needs to be involved in planning for change (Freed, 1998). Another general principle is that participation in planning change reduces resistance to change. When people are expected to be resistant to the desired change, having them participate in planning the change engages them in *counterattitudinal behavior,* behavior not in keeping with their established attitudes and values. This counterattitudinal behavior results in *cognitive dissonance,* a state of psychological discomfort created by inconsistencies between one's attitudes and values and one's behavior. One way to decrease the resulting discomfort is to modify one's attitudes to be congruent with behavior. By planning a change not in keeping with one's present attitudes, one may begin to adjust those attitudes to reestablish consonance with behavior. In other words, participating in the planning of a change may result in decreased resistance to that change. For example, if your nursing program is planning a move to computerized course registration, students who may resist the change can be invited to help design the way in which online registration will occur. This may involve their testing of a proposed system and providing feedback on its ease of use. Actually using the system in the testing process will engage them in an unfamiliar and unwanted behavior, potentially decreasing their fear of the change and limiting the extent of their resistance.

Although participation in planning for change helps to decrease resistance to the change, it is highly unlikely that complete consensus will be achieved among those involved in the planning. Lack of consensus in planning leads to conflict that must be resolved. Conflict resolution is addressed later in this chapter in the discussion of the group process.

Another general principle is that change is not orderly; it usually causes confusion and, by its very nature, disturbs the usual routine of the organization. There is never a good time for change, and people will never be completely prepared for a change. There will always be some ambiguity in change. In addition, change almost always disenfranchises some individual or group within an organization, so change agents can expect some degree of unpopularity, no matter how beneficial the change in general. Finally, the major problem in planning and implementing change is not usually the development of a new behavior or process but the dismantling of prior ways of behaving (Freed, 1998). Principles of planning for change are summarized below. Working within the framework of these general principles, tasks to be accomplished in planning change include establishing goals and objectives, evaluating alternative approaches to change, delineating activities leading to change, and planning to evaluate the change.

Establishing Goals and Objectives

The first aspect of planning change is determining what change should accomplish. This entails setting both broad goals and specific objectives. Suppose a community health nurse wants to improve immunization levels among community residents. Increasing immunity in the population would be the broad goal, and immunizing 95% of children over 1 year of age against measles would be a specific outcome objective. In this instance, the goal and objective reflect primary prevention, and primary preventive measures would be indicated to achieve them.

Goals and objectives for change may also reflect secondary or tertiary prevention. At the secondary prevention level, for example, change in an obese client's dietary patterns would be desirable. In this instance, the goal would be a balanced diet for the client. Specific outcome objectives might include a decrease in caloric intake to 1,800 calories per day, inclusion of at least one iron-rich food in the diet daily, and adequate intake of vitamins and minerals. Similarly, a change to more effective coping strategies by an abusive parent would be the goal of tertiary preventive measures planned in an abusive family situation. A related outcome objective might be a decrease in the amount of alcohol consumed as a coping mechanism.

In developing outcome objectives for change, it is frequently wise to proceed incrementally, with achievement of a few objectives setting the stage for accomplishment of later changes. In this way, the nurse keeps the change at a manageable level so that clients do not become overwhelmed and resistant to the change.

Selecting an Approach to Change

Generally speaking, there are three approaches the community health nurse might take to bring about change: the empirical–rational approach, the normative–reeducative approach, and the power–coercive approach (Tiffany & Lutjens, 1998). Each is appropriate in some change situations. The choice of approach depends on the type of change to be achieved and the willingness and ability of those who must change.

The Empirical–Rational Approach

The *empirical–rational approach* to change assumes that people act reasonably and follow the promptings of rational self-interest when the need for change is revealed to them (Taccetta-Chapnick, 1996). In short, an awareness of a need for change results in change. Change is accomplished by providing information about the need for change and how to bring it about. The community health nurse as change agent informs those who need to implement the change of an unfavorable condition and a desirable course of action, and those individuals carry out the change.

This approach to change is effective in situations when it is clear where one's self-interest lies, when few restraining forces are operating, and when the change does not pose a threat to those who must implement it. For example, school officials made aware of hazards posed by damaged playground equipment will probably take steps either to repair or to remove the equipment. They can see the potential harm to the children and the possibility of lawsuits resulting from injuries, and they have no vested interest in retaining damaged equipment.

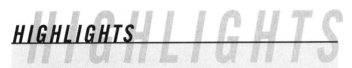

HIGHLIGHTS

General Principles of Planning for Change

- Participation in planning for change promotes acceptance and decreases resistance to change.
- Not everyone needs to be involved in planning the change.
- Complete consensus among the planning group is unlikely. Lack of consensus leads to conflict that must be resolved.
- Change is not orderly and creates tension and ambiguity.
- There is no really good time for change, nor are people ever completely prepared for change.
- Change almost always disenfranchises someone, so change agents are not always popular.
- Effective change relies less on the development of new behaviors or processes than on dismantling old ways of behaving.

The Normative–Reeducative Approach

Unfortunately, human behavior is not always rational and is often heavily influenced by attitudes, values, and emotions. For example, a mother may know that her child needs immunizations but hesitates because she does not like to see her child hurt by the injection. Rather than trying to increase the mother's awareness of the need for immunization, the community health nurse as change agent could employ a *normative–reeducative approach* to change, using educational strategies directed toward changing the mother's attitude. For example, the nurse might focus on how much greater the hurt would be if the child developed diphtheria, tetanus, or one of the other diseases preventable by immunization.

As another example, teenagers often see unrestrained drinking as evidence of adulthood. By using a normative–reeducative approach, the teens would be helped to see that refraining from drinking to excess is more characteristic of adult behavior than going on a Friday night binge. The approach to behavioral change in this instance focuses on their attitudes to drinking.

The normative–reeducative approach would be used in situations in which those who need to make changes have a vested interest in maintaining the current situation or in which there are emotional and attitudinal restraining forces at work, but where attitudes are open and amenable to change.

The Power–Coercive Approach

Some people, however, cannot be brought to change behavior by rational argument or attempts to change attitudes. In these situations, the *power–coercive approach* to change may be effective. This approach uses power to dispense reward and punishment to force change. As an example, children of parents who refuse to have them immunized are denied school entry unless there are religious or health reasons for nonimmunization. Using another example, empirical–rational strategies and normative–reeducative strategies have been somewhat effective in motivating people to use automobile seat belts. Others, however, do not use seat belts. For these individuals, laws mandating seat belt use are a power–coercive strategy to force a change in behavior.

Information obtained by the community health nurse in assessing the change situation indicates the driving and restraining forces that are operating. When restraining forces are related to misconceptions and lack of knowledge about the need for change, the change itself, or its consequences, the nurse would select the empirical–rational approach to bring about the desired change. When restraining forces include attitudes unfavorable to the desired change but amenable to modification, the normative–reeducative approach may be chosen. When the assessment indicates strongly rooted attitudes and values that impede change or strong resistance to change, the power–coercive approach may be used. This approach is also appropriate in situations where the need for change is immediate and there is no time for explanation or persuasion.

It should be remembered, however, that the power–coercive approach may result in temporary change and that those who are coerced may return to their previous behaviors as soon as coercion is removed. For these reasons, the power–coercive method is the least desirable of the three approaches to change. This approach generally is not used, except in situations in which clients' behaviors are clearly dangerous to themselves or others as in the case of a client threatening suicide, child abuse, failure to obtain necessary medical care for a minor, or someone with a communicable disease who refuses to refrain from infecting others.

The power–coercive approach may be warranted, however, in advocacy situations and other similar circumstances. For example, the community health nurse may find that the only way to motivate a landlord to comply with building safety codes is to threaten to report violations to the authorities. Similarly, health care providers who discriminate against certain types of clients may be motivated to change their behavior if threatened with the loss of their jobs.

Delineating Activities Leading to Change

The next step in planning change is to delineate specific activities required to accomplish the desired change. These activities would reflect process objectives for the change situation and may involve primary, secondary, or tertiary preventive measures. For instance, if an alteration is needed in an infant's diet to accommodate the slowed rate of growth normal at the end of the first year of life, dietary education for the mother would be a primary preventive measure directed toward this change. Similarly, providing clean syringes and needles for injection drug users might motivate them to stop sharing needles and prevent exposure to hepatitis C and HIV/AIDS.

Examples of secondary preventive strategies for change might include suggestions to minimize side effects of antituberculosis drugs to resolve the problem of noncompliance, or assisting teenage alcoholics to explore their reasons for drinking. Educating a parent on the role of bottle propping in recurrent middle ear infections in an infant might be a tertiary preventive measure designed to produce behavior changes in the parent that prevent a recurrence of otitis media in the child.

Planning to Evaluate Change

The last step in planning change is to plan to evaluate the effects of the change and the process used to achieve it. Consequently, the community health nurse needs to determine how the change will be evaluated, what data will be collected, and what data collection procedures will be used. In planning to evaluate change, criteria need to be developed that reflect the levels of prevention involved in the changes planned. If desired changes involve primary prevention, evaluative criteria will focus on the promotion of health and prevention of specific health problems. The emphasis in secondary prevention would be on criteria that reflect resolution of existing client problems. Evaluative criteria related to tertiary preventive measures would address prevention of complications or recurrence of problems. As an example, an objective for change at the level of primary prevention might be increased use of condoms among sexually active adolescents to prevent HIV infection. Evaluative criteria for the achievement of change would focus on the proportion of adolescents who use condoms consistently. Points to be considered in planning for change are summarized below.

HIGHLIGHTS

Considerations in Planning for Change

- Establish goals and specific expected outcomes for the change.
- Evaluate and select the appropriate approach to change based on the willingness of others to change, the type of restraining forces operating in the situation, and the immediacy of the need for change.
  - The empirical–rational approach focuses on awareness of the need for change.
  - The normative–reeducative approach focuses on attitudes toward the change.
  - The power–coercive approach uses power over rewards and punishment to enforce change.
- Delineate specific activities leading to the desired change.
- Plan to evaluate the change.

IMPLEMENTING CHANGE

Implementing the change involves employing strategies that will move the client (individual or group) through the stages of change. Strategies that promote unfreezing move clients through the first three stages of the personal change model (precontemplation, contemplation, and preparation).

Unfreezing may be approached somewhat differently in each of the three approaches to change discussed earlier. In the use of the empirical–rational strategy, the community health nurse as change agent may use a tactic known as disconfirmation to motivate others to change. *Disconfirmation* is an awareness that reality does not conform to the desired state of affairs. Creating disconfirmation involves presenting the client or target group with information to make them aware of differences between a desired state and reality. This awareness creates a feeling of discomfort with the current situation and fosters a willingness to change. For example, the commu-

nity health nurse might present figures on the number of adolescent pregnancies occurring in a specific school to make parents aware of a need for sex education. The desired state is an absence of teenage pregnancies, but, as the community health nurse makes clear, this is definitely not the reality of the situation.

A second tactic used in unfreezing is introducing guilt. This tactic might be used in the normative–reeducative approach to change. When people are made to feel guilty about a current situation, they may be more likely to reexamine attitudes and institute change. For instance, the community health nurse might point out what poor role models smokers are for their children and what the effects of secondhand smoke might be on children's health. Guilt over possible damage to their own children's health might motivate some smokers to quit.

Providing a climate of psychological safety is another tactic used in unfreezing in the normative–reeducative approach to change. Fear of a change and its effects is one of the major causes of failure to implement change (Butrie & Nowoholnik, 1998). Using the change to computerized charting as an example, the community health nurse might assure the group that they will receive detailed instruction and demonstration of the system and will have opportunities to practice and receive feedback before the new system is implemented. These activities lessen fears of making mistakes and decrease restraining forces working against the change. Attention to the emotional needs of those involved in a change can also help to create a climate of emotional safety (Nagaike, 1997).

Another important feature of unfreezing is dealing with resistance, some of which may have already been eliminated by creating a climate of psychological safety. Other steps, however, may be needed. Change, even when desired, produces stress. Stress creates discomfort, and people are often unwilling to experience even temporary discomfort in return for future gains. From this perspective, change is seen as "punishment" and constitutes a force restraining the desired change.

Resistance can be minimized by changing the person's perceptions of the change, that is, changing restraining forces to driving forces. The community health nurse can foster change by setting up the change situation such that the person(s) expected to change receives benefits that outweigh the "punishment" involved. This can sometimes involve a "trade." For example, a politician may be motivated to change his or her stance on an issue in return for election support from nurses. Similarly, a client who sees changing dietary patterns after a myocardial infarction as burdensome may be brought to see the advantages this will create in preventing another heart attack.

Functions of the community health nurse as change agent during the moving or action stage include introducing new information needed to bring about the change; modeling and/or encouraging performance of the new behavior; allowing ample time to practice the behavior; and providing a supportive climate and opportunities to voice feelings of fear, anxiety, frustration, and anger. Other functions include giving feedback on progress in implementing the change and acting as a motivator to maintain the momentum of the change.

Dividing the change into smaller segments and setting up effective communication channels can assist in the actual implementation of the change. The activities needed to implement the change may be delineated so that incremental change is possible. For example, if community health nurses are asked to convert all existing client records to a computerized charting system, they may feel overwhelmed. If, however, the change begins with newly opened records only, the change can be accomplished in manageable increments. As services to previously enrolled clients are terminated, there will be fewer and fewer records that have not been computerized.

Ongoing data collection is needed during the moving stage to monitor the change process. Providing avenues for those involved in the change to communicate problems experienced will smooth the implementation process. Communication permits evaluation of the implementation of change on an ongoing basis and allows modification of the planned change or the activities required to implement it, thus resulting in more effective change.

Functions of the change agent during the refreezing or maintenance stage of change include providing continuing motivation, directing the new behavior, and delegating greater responsibility for the change to others. Stages in implementing change and functions of the community health nurse as change agent are presented in Table 13–2 ■.

■ **TABLE 13–2** **Stages in Implementing Change and Functions of the Nurse as Change Agent**

STAGE	FUNCTION OF THE NURSE
Unfreezing (precontemplation, contemplation, preparation)	Create disconfirmation Introduce guilt Provide a climate of psychological safety
Moving (action)	Introduce new information required for change Encourage performance of new behavior Allow time to practice new behavior Provide supportive climate for change Provide opportunities to voice feelings about change Give feedback on progress of change Serve as an energizer Deal with resistance
Refreezing (maintenance)	Continue energizing activities Continue to direct new behavior Delegate greater responsibility for change to client or target group

EVALUATING CHANGE

Evaluating change involves assessing the change itself and the process used in achieving it. In evaluating change itself, the first question is whether the desired change was achieved. Has the individual client, family, or target group made the expected change in health-related behaviors? Are they now, for example, engaging in more effective communication patterns or eating a more appropriate diet? Is charting now done on the computer? Given the stage of change at which the client is encountered, it may be necessary to evaluate intermediate outcomes of change rather than ultimate outcomes (Gillis, 1995). For example, a community that was in the precontemplation stage of change may have moved to the preparation stage, but the ultimate objective of the change has not yet been achieved.

The second consideration in evaluating change is its effects. Even though the change has been achieved, it may not have accomplished the desired effect. For example, the client may have changed his or her dietary patterns and still not be losing weight, or more immunization clinics may have been established without appreciably raising community immunization levels.

In addition, change may have unanticipated effects that may or may not be desirable. For instance, the change to computerized charting may provide avenues for violation of client confidentiality because the computer increases access to client records, or the nurses may spend more time correcting computer errors than they spent in doing handwritten charting.

Another aspect of evaluating change is the assessment of the process used to achieve the change. Were the need for change and the driving and restraining forces accurately identified? Was the change well planned? Was the appropriate approach to change selected given the factors involved? Was resistance adequately addressed? What activities were involved in unfreezing, changing, and refreezing? Were these activities appropriate to the situation? Answers to these questions provide direction for action if the desired change has not yet been achieved and further attempts are warranted. They also assist the community health nurse to use the change process more effectively in the future. Components of the change process are summarized in Table 13–3 ■.

THE LEADERSHIP PROCESS

Initiating and directing change require leadership on the part of the nurse. The 1988 Institute of Medicine report, *The Future of Public Health,* noted a lack of leadership in public health. For this reason, community health nurses should prepare to provide leadership in the process of designing a health care system that will meet the health needs of the public. In this age of rising costs and diminishing resources,

■ **TABLE 13-3 Components of the Change Process**

Assessment	Assess the change situation in terms of:
	Factors giving rise to the need for change
	Forces driving change
	Forces restraining change
	Key skills needed for change and key
	positions involved
	Change response and versatility of
	those involved
	Match between skills needed and
	available
	Developmental needs of those involved
	in change
	Potential weak links in the organization
	Situational constraints affecting the
	change
Diagnosis	Diagnose the need for and capacity to change
Planning	Establish goals and objectives for change
	Evaluate approaches to change and select
	an appropriate one
	Delineate activities leading to change
	Plan evaluation of change
Implementation	Facilitate unfreezing/movement from pre-contemplation to preparation for change
	Facilitate movement/action toward the desired behavior
	Facilitate refreezing/maintenance of the desired behavior
Evaluation	Evaluate extent to which change has been accomplished
	Evaluate effects of the change
	Evaluate use of the change process

there is a particular need for leadership to ensure that health resources are adequate to meet those needs.

Leadership is defined as an intentional process in which one person attempts to influence the behavior of others to reach a specific goal (Pointer & Sanchez, 1997) or as a process of creating a bridge from what exists to what is desired (Koerner, 2000). Leadership in today's world is more than influencing the behavior of others; rather, it is the development of an environment that supports followers' creativity (Kerfoot, 1998). Creative leadership is characterized by a capacity to work effectively with others and to create negotiated partnerships, the ability to see new possibilities and relationships, fluency of words and ideas, and a capacity for moral courage and integrity (Koerner, 2000).

⑥THINK ABOUT IT

How might effective leadership after a natural disaster differ from effective leadership in your student nurses' organization?

LEADERSHIP MODELS

Over the years, a variety of theories have arisen to explain effective leadership. Early theories focused on personal traits of effective leaders and later ones on the leader's behavior. Motivational theories examined the factors that motivated followers and how leaders could influence those factors. Each of these types of theories failed to explain satisfactorily why some leaders were effective and some were not. More recently, contingency models and transformational models have been developed to explain effective leadership. Contingency models suggest that effective leadership is *contingent* on interactions among the leader, the followers, and the situation in which leadership occurs. In transformational models, the leader's role is to transform the situation into one in which followers will be empowered and motivated to act.

Situational leadership, developed by Hersey and Blanchard (Hersey, Blanchard, & Johnson, 2000), is a contingency theory of leadership in which effective leadership is a function of the interaction among the characteristics of the community health nurse as leader, the followers, and the task to be accomplished. In planning leadership, the community health nurse must select a style of leadership appropriate to all three of these components of the leadership situation.

One of four leadership styles that balance task-oriented and relationship-oriented behaviors by the leader may be appropriate to different leadership situations (Hersey, Blanchard, & Johnson, 2000). These four styles of leadership reflect a continuum of follower maturity and range from "telling," which is used with the least mature followers, to "selling" and "participating," used when moderate levels of follower maturity are evident, to "delegating," which is used with mature followers. Ideally, the nurse as leader will have developed the ability to use each of the four styles as needed in a given situation. These four styles will be discussed in more detail in the section on planning for leadership.

Situational leadership and the selection of a leadership style appropriate to a particular situation is a more traditional approach to leadership than transformational leadership. In transformational leadership, the focus of the leader is on assisting the group to create a vision in line with its purpose and values and creating the motivation to achieve it. Transformational leadership is characterized by a focus on planned action, promotion of risk taking, listening and providing feedback, leader trustworthiness, and concern for others (Taccetta-Chapnick, 1996). The transformational leader attempts to move followers to a level of maturity congruent with delegation and empowerment of the group to pursue their vision of organizational goals with minimal impetus from the leader.

ASSESSMENT AND DIAGNOSIS IN THE LEADERSHIP SITUATION

The community health nurse leader assesses the need for leadership and factors influencing the leadership situation as well as the identity of potential followers and their maturity relative to the tasks to be performed. The need for leadership and factors influencing the leadership situation might arise from any of the six dimensions of health. For example, a rising incidence of gonorrhea in the population (a biophysical factor) might require leadership to develop policies and programs that address the problem. Similarly, the nurse might see a need for leadership to address the problem of homelessness in the area (a sociocultural factor) or to provide access to care for uninsured populations (a health systems factor). Similarly, factors in each of the six dimensions may influence the ability to resolve problems requiring leadership. For example, a declining economy will affect the ability to provide jobs for homeless individuals. Similarly, high rates of mental illness among the homeless population may impede individuals' ability to hold a job. Assessment data related to these factors lead to diagnoses of the need for leadership.

Very often, a diagnosis of the need for leadership is also a diagnosis of a need for change. For example, in assessing a community's health needs, the community health nurse may note a high incidence of pedestrian fatalities at a particular intersection. Action is needed in the form of a traffic signal to permit safe pedestrian crossing; however, local residents have no idea how to go about arranging for installation of a traffic signal. In this instance, the nurse has identified both a problem that requires action and a need for leadership to bring about that action. The nursing diagnosis derived might be a "need for leadership in preventing traffic fatalities due to community members' lack of experience with group action."

The nurse also assesses and diagnoses potential followers with respect to their maturity in relation to the task to be accomplished. Maturity is a function of both

CRITICAL THINKING IN RESEARCH

Ellefsen (1998) conducted a study of the perceptions of community health nurses in Norway regarding the degree of influence they have in decision making. Nurse leaders and staff nurses in public health, home health, and nursing home settings participated in the study. The nurse leaders and nurses were perceived to have more influence on decision making in their respective practices than administrative leaders or political management. Differences were found among perceptions of decision making in the three settings. For example, the home nursing leader had less influence than the nurse leader in the nursing home, while staff nurses in home health had greater influence than those in the nursing home. Nurses in the public health setting perceived themselves to have the least influence among the three settings.

- What possible explanations might account for the differences in perceived influence among nurse leaders and staff nurses in the different settings?
- How might you conduct a study to see if your hypothesized explanations are correct?
- What kinds of tools might you use to measure influence in decision making? For what types of groups were these tools developed? Would they be appropriate for use with nurses and nurse leaders?

follower's expertise and motivation to act. Based on assessment data, the community health nurse should have an idea of both follower expertise and motivation regarding the action to be taken. An example of a possible diagnosis related to the traffic example is "adequate motivation for action, but lack of expertise in community organizing." A diagnosis related to city officials, another group of potential followers in the situation, might be "adequate follower expertise related to task, but poor motivation due to city budgetary constraints."

assessment tips assessment tips assessment tips

ASSESSING THE LEADERSHIP SITUATION

- What problems give rise to the need for leadership?
- What biophysical, psychological, physical environmental, sociocultural, behavioral, or health system factors influence the leadership situation?
- What is the task to be performed to resolve the problem(s)?
- Who are potential followers in the leadership situation?

- What is followers' level of expertise relative to the task(s) to be accomplished?
- What is followers' level of motivation regarding the task(s) to be accomplished? What factors influence followers' motivation?

PLANNING LEADERSHIP

Planning leadership involves two considerations: selecting an appropriate leadership style and preparing followers for action. Other aspects of planning, such as delineating specific activities, are based on the general principles of program planning that will be discussed in Chapter 15.

Selecting a Leadership Style

Based on the assessment of follower maturity the nurse may either engage in transformational leadership strategies to bring followers to the level of working independently to resolve the problem or select a leadership style appropriate to the situation. As noted earlier, one of four basic styles that differ in terms of follower maturity and their emphasis on task accomplishments and relationships can be selected. These styles are telling, selling or persuading, participating, and delegating.

Telling

For a situation in which task accomplishment is a priority and relationship concerns are less important, or followers have limited expertise or motivation, telling may be an appropriate leadership style. The nurse as leader tells the followers what to do and how to do it. For example, if the community health nurse encounters a client in cardiac arrest, he or she would direct one family member to call for emergency assistance and order another to assist with CPR. There is no time to explain why certain things must be done or to worry about offending family members. Immediate action is required.

Another situation may not be as urgent, but followers may lack the experience required to determine what needs to be done or how to do it. In this instance, a "telling" or directive approach is also appropriate. For example, when people first begin to use computers, one focuses on telling them the exact steps to take to accomplish a task rather than on the principles behind computer operations. As they become more familiar with the use of computers, one might then change the approach to explaining as well as telling followers what to do.

Selling

The second leadership style, selling, is used in situations in which both task accomplishment and interpersonal relationships are important. The leader works to persuade followers that a specific course of action should be taken. For example, the community health nurse might want to persuade school officials and parents that a school-based adolescent clinic is a good solution to health problems identified in this age group. The nurse as leader is not in a position to tell these people what to do, but must persuade them.

Participating

Participating is the third leadership style on the maturity continuum. A participative leadership style might be used by the community health nurse who is assisting parents of handicapped children to form a support group. In this instance, the nurse as leader would want to emphasize interpersonal relationships with less attention to the need to accomplish specific tasks. This leadership style is appropriate with a group of followers who are mature with respect to the group's goal, but need some guidance in reaching that goal. Leader and followers share in decision making, and the role of the leader is largely facilitative.

Delegating

The fourth leadership style is delegating. Followers are quite mature and can accomplish the group's goals with little or no direction from the leader. The nurse as a delegative leader places little emphasis on either task or relationship dimensions, but merely presents followers with a desired goal and leaves its accomplishment to them. For example, nursing faculty might delegate to the student organization the task of planning a graduation dinner, expecting students to take care of all the details with minimal input from the faculty. The four leadership styles discussed here are summarized in Table 13–4 ■.

■ **TABLE 13–4** Leadership Styles and Characteristics Features

STYLE	CHARACTERISTIC FEATURES
Telling	Emphasis on task accomplishment rather than interpersonal relationships
	Entails specific directions or orders given to followers without explanation
	Appropriate in emergency situations
	Appropriate when followers do not have expertise or motivation to act on their own
Selling	High emphasis on both task accomplishment and interpersonal relationships
	Entails persuasion of followers to take the desired course of action
	Appropriate when followers have expertise but not the motivation to act on their own
Participating	Emphasis on interpersonal relationships rather than task accomplishment
	Entails allowing and encouraging follower input into decisions on action to be taken
	Appropriate when followers have some expertise and are motivated to act but need some direction
	Appropriate when time is not a factor
Delegating	Low emphasis by leader on both task accomplishment and interpersonal relationships
	Entails informing followers of task to be done and leaving them to accomplish it
	Appropriate when followers are highly motivated and have the necessary expertise

⑥THINK ABOUT IT

Think of some effective leaders you have known. What made them effective? Would they have been equally effective in other kinds of situations? Why or why not?

Preparing Followers

The second aspect of planning leadership is preparing followers for action. This can involve either enhancing their abilities to accomplish the task involved or improving their motivation to act.

Enhancing Followers' Abilities

Enhancing followers' abilities to perform a desired action might involve teaching new skills or providing opportunities to practice previously learned ones. For example, if the action required of followers involves use of interpersonal skills, the leader may plan to review principles of group dynamics and interpersonal communication with followers. If the task involves use of computers, followers may need to develop skills or to broaden existing skills to encompass the desired action.

Improving Motivation

Because leadership is almost always directed to some type of action for change, improving followers' motivation to act may involve manipulation of the driving and restraining forces described earlier. The community health nurse may need to plan to reduce restraining forces, enhance driving forces, or both. These forces may reflect psychological factors influencing the leadership situation assessed earlier.

Different people may be motivated by different things. For example, some followers may act to get a traffic signal installed at a dangerous intersection out of fear of injury to themselves or their loved ones. Others may be influenced to act by altruistic motives or because they like the challenge presented by a tussle with city hall.

Knowledge of what motivates a specific individual permits the use of motivators that will reduce restraining forces and enhance driving forces, increasing the potential for accomplishing the desired action. For example, if action is needed to improve the quality of nursing care provided, some followers may be motivated by threats of job loss, whereas others will be better motivated by recognition of a job well done. The community health nurse who has thoroughly assessed the leadership situation will be able to plan rewards and sanctions that motivate specific followers to action.

 IMPLEMENTING THE LEADERSHIP PLAN

Two aspects of implementing a leadership plan are performance of designated activities by followers and performance of leadership functions by the leader. The first

aspect is a basic element of the nursing process and is not reiterated here. The second aspect of implementation is the performance of specific leadership functions by the nurse as leader. These functions include carrying out plans for follower preparation, coordinating and directing follower activity related to task accomplishment, and representing followers to outsiders.

Plans for preparing followers need to be executed. In this phase of implementation, the community health nurse provides whatever education is needed by followers to carry out the desired actions. The nurse also puts into operation planned rewards and sanctions designed to motivate followers.

In addition, the nurse coordinates group members' activities in planning and implementing the desired course of action. The amount of coordination required depends on the maturity of the group, their need for assistance, and

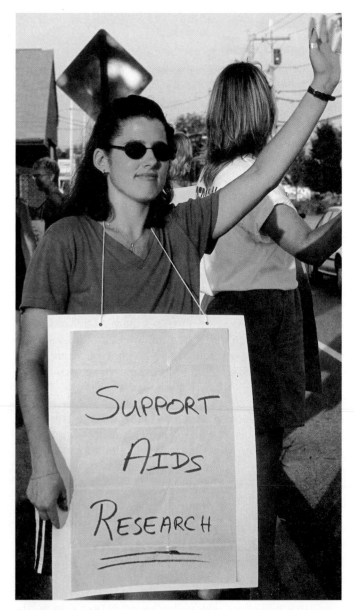

Community health nurses often assume active leadership roles in community action efforts.

■ **TABLE 13–5**   **Components of the Leadership Process**

Assessment	Assess the leadership situation in terms of:
	    Factors giving rise to the need for
	      leadership
	    Factors influencing the leadership
	      situation

Diagnosis	Diagnose the need for leadership Diagnose follower maturity
Planning	Select an appropriate leadership style Plan to prepare followers for action Delineate actions to be taken
Implementation	Enhance follower abilities Improve follower motivation Coordinate follower activities Represent group to outsiders
Evaluation	Evaluate actions accomplished Evaluate use of the leadership process

the leadership style employed. For example, if the task was appropriately delegated to a mature group of followers, there will be little need for extensive coordination by the nurse leader. If, on the other hand, the nurse selected the "telling" style of leadership, the leader might need to engage in quite a bit of coordination of follower activities.

Finally, the community health nurse leader serves as the group's spokesperson. He or she supports group decisions and defends those decisions to outsiders when necessary. For instance, if the task remains unaccomplished because of a lack of necessary materials, the nurse as leader may need to advocate for the resources needed for task accomplishment.

EVALUATING LEADERSHIP

As was true in the change process, evaluation in a leadership situation addresses the outcome of leadership as well as the process used. Was the desired action or change brought about? Was the leadership style selected appropriate to the task and to the level of follower maturity? Were followers adequately prepared for action? Components of leadership are summarized in Table 13–5 ■.

THE GROUP PROCESS

Change is often accomplished by group action or team work. This is particularly true of changes that occur in the health care delivery system. Many of the problems that affect population groups cannot be solved by the action of one health care provider, and cooperative activity by a group is required. Unfortunately, we have often been socialized to work independently, so teamwork is not a

skill easily learned by many of us. Teamwork has been defined as "a coordinated effort among several individuals who place the team's goals and interests above their own" (Hetherington, 1998, p. 30).

Community health nurses are often called on to initiate and direct group problem-solving activities; consequently, they must be conversant with the processes that govern the formation and operation of groups or work teams. Group process skills are needed by community health nurses who are members, as well as leaders, of groups.

Group action has a number of advantages over actions taken by individuals. The greater range of knowledge and expertise of group members provides a broader base from which to derive solutions to health problems. For example, if community health nurses are concerned about drug abuse among elementary school children, to address the problem they might form a group that includes school officials, police, child psychologists, and parents. Each member of the group has expertise that can contribute to solving the problem. Police personnel have knowledge of means by which drugs are circulated. School officials and parents can speak to factors in the school setting that contribute to drug traffic. The child psychologist can provide input into ways to motivate young people to refrain from using drugs. Working together, the group can generate a solution to the problem that is realistic and effective.

Another advantage to group activity is the increased efficiency realized by using each member's expertise and by eliminating duplication of effort. When people act cooperatively, those best suited to a particular function can perform that function. When one acts independently, one must carry out all the required functions despite one's level of expertise in those areas. In the drug abuse example cited earlier, school officials and teachers can work on curriculum aspects of a drug abuse prevention program while police concentrate on eliminating drug dealers from school grounds. Furthermore, group action also eliminates duplication of effort. For example, it is not cost effective for both the school system and the police department to develop independent drug education programs when drug education can be done more effectively and efficiently as a cooperative effort.

Finally, group action promotes communication among members of the group that may enhance problem resolution. Improved communication through group work can also lead to collaborative effort in other areas, which increases the resource network of each of the group's members.

 THINK ABOUT IT

What are some of the potential consequences when health-related groups fail to accomplish tasks of group development?

The role of the community health nurse in group action to solve problems frequently involves initiating the group and directing its activity. In other instances, community health nurses are asked to serve in groups formed by others. In either case, knowledge of the group process assists the nurse to make a greater contribution to the group effort.

Group development occurs in a series of stages: orientation, accommodation, negotiation, operation, and dissolution. These stages parallel the components of the nursing process. Specific tasks must be accomplished during each stage of group development for the group to function effectively. Each stage of group development with its related tasks is discussed in the context of the nursing process component to which it relates.

ASSESSMENT AND DIAGNOSIS IN THE GROUP SITUATION

Assessment and diagnosis in the nursing process are comparable to the orientation stage of group development, as depicted in Table 13–6 ▪. This stage is also sometimes referred to as the "forming stage," when group members come to know each other and assess their ability to function as a group (Drinka & Clark, 2000). Assessment in group work has two components: assessing the problem to be solved and assessing the group. The problem to be solved is assessed from an epidemiologic perspective, considering the biophysical, psychological, physical environmental, sociocultural, behavioral, and health care system factors that influence the problem and its solution.

Ideally, group members are selected because they have characteristics that enable them to contribute to the group. Unfortunately, that is not always the case, and the community health nurse working with a group needs to assess group members to identify their strengths and weaknesses. One potential barrier to effective group action is lack of knowledge of the abilities and characteristics of group members that could enhance or undermine group effort. Careful assessment of group members by the community health nurse can help to eliminate this barrier.

Factors in each of the six dimensions of health may also influence group members and their ability to function as a team. In the sociocultural dimension, for example, professional socialization often leads to territoriality, which interferes with effective teamwork. Professional socialization also creates unique professional languages, which may make communication difficult. Psychological dimension factors such as personal insecurity may make people in the group reluctant to try to work together or may lead to attempts to dominate the group. Similarly, if group members are separated by distance (a physical environmental factor), effective group work may be impeded.

Based on the assessment of group members, the community health nurse diagnoses group strengths and weaknesses. Diagnoses might also relate to group members' expertise and motivation relative to the problem to be solved. For example, the community health nurse

---

▪ **TABLE 13–6   Tasks of Group Development by Stage and Related Nursing Process Component**

NURSING PROCESS COMPONENT	STAGE OF GROUP DEVELOPMENT	GROUP DEVELOPMENT TASKS
Assessment and Diagnosis	Orientation (forming)	1. Selection of group members 2. Training for group participation 3. Identification of goals and purposes
Planning	Accommodation (norming)	1. Establishment of modes of decision making 2. Development of mechanisms for conflict resolution 3. Development of communication network 4. Development of climate conducive to group collaboration
	Negotiation (norming)	1. Negotiation of member roles 2. Development of methods of task assignment
Implementation	Operation (performing)	1. Assignment of specific tasks to accomplish group goals 2. Performance of actions to accomplish goals
Evaluation	Dissolution (leaving)	1. Planning of evaluative mechanisms for outcomes of action taken 2. Assignment of member roles and tasks in evaluation 3. Data collection 4. Analysis of evaluative findings 5. Possible group dissolution

CULTURAL CONSIDERATIONS

Some ethnic cultural groups, such as many Asians, are more attuned to work in groups than many Caucasian Americans. What features of their cultures promote effective group work? What features of the dominant culture in the United States inhibit effective work in teams?

might diagnose a "need for conflict resolution due to different perceptions of group goals by group members," or the nurse might derive a diagnosis of "effective group function due to successful accomplishment of tasks of group development." A third possible diagnosis might be a "need to educate members for group work due to inexperience with group dynamics." Assessment and orientation of group members should culminate in the establishment of group priorities and goals.

PLANNING THE GROUP PROCESS

There are two aspects to planning group work. One reflects the efforts of the group to resolve the problems in question. This aspect of planning uses the general planning principles discussed in Chapter 15. The second aspect involves planning the operation of the group itself and includes determining group modes of decision making, conflict resolution, communication, and role negotiation. These activities are carried out during the accommodation and negotiation stages of group formation, also referred to as the storming and norming stages (Drinka & Clark, 2000).

Selecting a Method of Decision Making

Group action requires group decisions, and decisions must be made after careful consideration by group members. To facilitate decision making, group members should agree on the method by which decisions will be made. Because most people are not familiar with group

processes or the deliberate need to select a decision-making strategy, the community health nurse may need to guide the group in this task.

Decisions can be made in one of six ways: by default, by the leader, by a subgroup, by majority vote, by consensus, or by unanimous consent. Decisions made by default result from a lack of response by the group. For example, if a class of senior nursing students, invited by faculty to plan a graduation reception, fails to respond, they have, in fact, decided not to have a reception.

The second method of decision making, in which decisions are made by the leader, is appropriate when a decision cannot wait on the slow-moving democratic process (e.g., when there is an emergency). The group may decide to give the group leader authority to make independent decisions in certain circumstances, but should decide in advance what those circumstances will be. In an effective group, this is not the method used for making most of the group's decisions.

In the third approach to group decision making, group decisions are made by a subgroup. This might involve "railroading," in which the subgroup uses its power and influence to force a decision on other group members. Conversely, the larger group may purposefully delegate the making of certain decisions to a subgroup. Many nursing organizations, for example, delegate authority to an executive board for decisions regarding everyday operation and make only major decisions as a total group.

Majority vote by group members, the fourth method of decision making, is already familiar to us. The fifth method involves consensus or agreement by all group members despite any reservations that individual members might have. Finally, decisions may be made by unanimous consent in which all group members agree without reservation. In both the consensus and unanimous consent methods, the group may take a relatively long time to reach a decision because of the need for all members to agree. For the purposes of true collaboration in a group, majority vote, consensus, and unanimous consent are the most appropriate methods for group decision making.

assessment tips *assessment tips* *assessment tips*

ASSESSING THE GROUP SITUATION

- What is the problem the group is expected to solve or task to be accomplished? What biophysical, psychological, physical environmental, sociocultural, behavioral, and health system factors are influencing the problem or task?

- What factors in the biophysical, psychological, physical environmental, sociocultural, behavioral, and health system dimensions affect members of the group?

- What is the capacity of the group to work together? What prior background do group members have in team or group work?

- What expertise do group members have relative to the task to be accomplished? To group roles?

- What organizational constraints may affect the work of the group?

Developing Mechanisms for Conflict Resolution

Breakdowns in the decision-making process are one source of conflict within the group. Other potential sources of conflict are unclear expectations, poor communication, differing values or attitudes, and competition for scarce resources (Habel, 2000). Lack of clear jurisdiction among group members and conflicts of interest may also be sources of conflict within the group (Umiker, 1998). Additional sources of conflict are interdependence when needs are not met and the existence of prior unresolved conflict between members or subgroups (Dove, 1998). Conflict is a normal component of group effort and is to be expected. In fact, many group behavior theorists include a conflict or "storming" stage in describing the development of groups over time (Drinka & Clark, 2000). If the group has developed mechanisms for conflict resolution before conflicts arise, conflict can often be a positive rather than a divisive experience for the group.

Recognition of conflict as a normal phenomenon is essential if the group is to plan ahead for conflict resolution. Again, many groups do not anticipate conflict, and when conflict occurs they are unprepared to deal with it. Strategies for resolving conflict constructively involve creating a climate conducive to discussion, identifying and eliminating sources of conflict, capitalizing on areas of agreement, and rationally considering alternative solutions to conflict. The community health nurse can explore these approaches to conflict resolution with members of the group and assist members to select the most appropriate approach.

Creating a climate in which disagreement is acceptable can minimize or resolve conflict. Conflict resolution requires that all parties be fully able to express their perspectives through open communication. Open communication cannot take place when there is pressure to conform and lack of acceptance of different opinions. Lack of communication hampers conflict resolution as well as contributing to conflict. As a group leader, the community health nurse may need to encourage group members to express thoughts and opinions that may not be congruent with those of other members. Through the use of interpersonal skills, the nurse can ensure that communications within the group are not accusatory, but deal with issues rather than personalities.

Recognizing the existence of conflict and identifying its sources and possible solutions are strategies for constructive use of conflict. A conflict that is ignored in the hope that it will resolve itself is likely to become worse. The community health nurse can encourage other group members to acknowledge that a conflict exists and help them explore the reasons for conflict. Again, the nurse should be alert to covert signs of conflict and bring them to the attention of the rest of the group. For example, a nurse working with a group trying to determine budget allocations among health care programs within the county may notice that representatives of programs for the elderly are maintaining a stony silence during the discussion. The nurse may comment on the fact that they have not participated in the discussion and ask why. In the ensuing discussion, it may be learned that these group members feel that too much money is being allocated to maternal–child health programs and that the elderly are being shortchanged. Once this conflict has been exposed, the group can begin work to resolve it.

Another strategy for resolving conflict involves identifying small areas of trust and agreement between group members that can be expanded. For example, although two group members may disagree on the "appropriate" approach to a problem, they can capitalize on their shared concern for clients' welfare. Finally, rational consideration of alternative solutions to a particular conflict using the group's decision-making process and the problem-solving process can result in conflict becoming a valuable learning experience in group problem solving. The community health nurse can assist the group to explore a variety of alternative solutions to a conflict and to select an approach that is agreeable to all members.

Developing Communication Strategies

Developing group communication strategies is another task in planning group operation. The importance of an effective communication network cannot be overemphasized. The group must develop a common language that facilitates communication, and members should refrain from using jargon familiar only to members of their own discipline. When it is necessary to use terminology unfamiliar to others, efforts should be made to translate it into the common language. The nurse in this situation can either play the part of the translator or ask other members for clarification. For example, some members of a group may use acronyms unfamiliar to others, such as HCFA. The nurse should then explain to the group that this stands for the Health Care Financing Administration. If the nurse does not recognize the acronym, he or she would ask for an explanation of its meaning.

The group should also agree on the form that communication will take. For example, communications may be verbal, written, or a combination of both, depending on the situation. Perhaps the group will decide that communication with sponsoring institutions should take the form of formal written memoranda, whereas communications between group members should be more informal verbal messages.

Consideration should also be given to the fact that communication takes place outside of regular group sessions. The content of these informal encounters between group members should not undermine group function or provide a forum for airing grievances or denigrating other members. The community health nurse who encounters unproductive communication outside of group meetings can bring relevant issues to the attention of the entire group so open discussion can take place and conflict can be avoided or resolved.

Establishing a climate in which group members feel respected and in which differences are accepted contributes to an effective communication network. This

ETHICAL AWARENESS

As a member of a client care team, you have obtained information that the client asks you not to share with other members of the team. The information you have received is pertinent to the team's decisions about the plan of care for the client. How would you resolve this dilemma?

means that all group members should be encouraged to participate and should receive positive reinforcement for their contribution whether or not others agree with it. In the beginning of the group's operation, the nurse group leader may need to ask reluctant group members for their ideas and opinions. As their participation is received positively, they will begin to volunteer remarks.

Negotiating Roles

Another task to be accomplished in forming an effective group is role negotiation. Professional roles tend to overlap, and role negotiation is crucial to effective group function. When two or more group members possess similar skills, the group must decide who will be responsible for exercising those skills. These decisions may be made as a general rule of thumb, so that one member always has responsibility for certain activities, or may change with the needs of the situation. For example, both teachers and nurses have educational skills. A group developing a health education program for the school system may decide that teachers will be responsible for general health education related to nutrition and hygiene, while the nurse will deal with more complex health topics such as substance abuse and sexually transmitted diseases.

One particular group role that must be negotiated is the role of leader. This position incorporates functions related to group administration, liaison with outside groups, teaching, and coordination of group effort. Additional team leadership roles may include providing information for group decision making, clarifying issues, refocusing the group's attention, and playing "devil's advocate" to promote exploration of alternative ideas (Breckon, 1998). The leadership role may be assigned to one member, may shift with the situation, or may reside with the group as a whole. In the last instance, no one member acts as the leader, and leadership functions are performed by the group as a unit. In many instances, community health nurses fulfill the leadership role within the group, particularly in groups composed largely of nonprofessionals. In other cases, the nurse may need to help the group identify who is best suited to lead the group, based on the needs of the situation.

IMPLEMENTING THE GROUP PROCESS

Implementation of the group process, sometimes called the "performing" stage of group development (Drinka &

Clark, 2000), involves actually assigning responsibilities for tasks required to achieve group goals and performing assigned tasks. Tasks are assigned on the basis of decisions made in the role negotiation phase of planning.

Planned group operating procedures are also executed during the implementation stage. Decisions are made using the method of decision making selected, and communication networks are established along lines determined by the group. If conflict arises during group operation, the group will employ the conflict resolution strategies selected during group formation.

EVALUATING THE GROUP PROCESS

Throughout the section on group process, we have alluded to stages of group development that coincide with the nursing process. The final stage of group development, the dissolution or "leaving" stage, is related to the evaluation component of the nursing process. Group tasks in this stage center around evaluation of both the outcome of group activity and the process used to plan and execute group action. Tasks of this stage actually begin during planning and prior to implementation of group actions. The group identifies outcome criteria and plans mechanisms for evaluating the effects of group effort in terms of those criteria. Group members' responsibilities in evaluation should be negotiated in the same manner as other group roles and assigned on the basis of competency. For example, if the group has implemented a school nutrition program, teachers may evaluate students' knowledge of nutrition, while the community health nurse evaluates indicators of nutritional status such as height, weight, and hematocrit.

In evaluating use of the group process, the effectiveness of group decision making, conflict resolution, communication, and role negotiation strategies may be addressed. Were roles allocated in a way that facilitated group goal achievement? Was communication between group members effective? Were conflicts within the group adequately resolved? Answers to these and similar questions can assist the group to work together more effectively in the future and can prepare group members to function effectively in other groups.

In some instances, the results of evaluation actually culminate in dissolution of the group. This may occur either because the group's purpose has been accomplished or because the group is not able to achieve its purpose. Tasks of the dissolution stage of group development, as well as tasks of other stages, are summarized in Table 13–6 in conjunction with the phases of the nursing process during which they occur. Table 13–7 ■ summarizes the components of the group process.

Community health nurses use the change, leadership, and group processes each day in their practice. All three of these processes can be used with individual clients, families, or population groups. Nurses using these processes may want additional sources of information

■ **TABLE 13–7 Components of the Group Process**

Assessment	Assess the problem to be addressed by the group Assess the members of the group in terms of factors influencing group function: 　Biophysical factors 　Psychological factors 　Physical environmental factors 　Sociocultural factors 　Behavioral factors 　Health system factors
Diagnosis	Diagnose group strengths and weaknesses, expertise, and motivation
Planning	Plan achievement of group goals Plan group operation in terms of: 　Methods for group decision making 　Mechanisms for conflict resolution 　Methods of communication 　Role negotiation
Implementation	Implement activities designed to reach the group goal Implement group operation procedures
Evaluation	Evaluate outcome of the group action Evaluate use of the group process

that will assist them in effectively incorporating these processes in practice. The companion Web site for this book contains links to several agencies and organizations that can provide additional resources. ⊕

APPLYING YOUR KNOWLEDGE IN PRACTICE

❧ CASE STUDY
Leading Community Change

In assessing the town of Clarkston, you, as a community health nurse, note that infant and maternal mortality rates are high. Part of the explanation lies in a lack of prenatal care for large numbers of pregnant women. The local health department prenatal clinic is always full, and clients may have to wait three months or longer for an initial appointment. Because many of the pregnant women in the community do not seek care until their pregnancies are fairly far advanced, they may deliver before they can be seen. Seven physicians with private practices in town provide obstetrical care, but their services are underutilized. This is primarily because most of the pregnant population come from low-income families and are on Medicaid, which these physicians do not want to accept. Because they are on the obstetrics staff of the local community hospital that accepts indigent clients, four of these physicians de-

liver many of the women who have not had prenatal care. Two physicians have been sued as a result of complications experienced by these indigent women.

- What changes or course of action might improve this situation?
- What would be the objective of your change? Be specific.
- What biophysical, psychological, physical environmental, sociocultural, behavioral, and health care system factors are acting as driving and restraining forces in this situation?
- As the leader in this change situation, who are your followers? How would you describe the maturity level of your followers?
- What leadership style would be appropriate in this situation? Why?

- How would you unfreeze this situation? What would you do to bring about the desired change? How would you promote refreezing?

- How would you evaluate the outcome of the change and your leadership as a change agent?

✜ TESTING YOUR UNDERSTANDING

- Describe the influence of driving and restraining forces in a change situation. Give examples of each type of force. (p. 271)
- What are the four major considerations in planning change? How might community health nurses be involved in each? (pp. 272–275)
- What three approaches may be used to bring about change? Describe situations in which each approach might be appropriate. (pp. 273–274)
- How does follower maturity relate to the selection of a style of leadership? What are the components of follower maturity? (pp. 278–279)

- What are the five stages of group development? What tasks need to be accomplished in each stage? (pp. 282–286)
- What are the two major tasks in implementing the group process? Give an example of the performance of each. (p. 285)
- What two aspects of evaluation are applicable to the change, leadership, and group processes? Give examples of evaluative criteria that you might use for each. (pp. 276, 281, 285)

REFERENCES

Bishop, C. H. Jr. (2001). *Making change happen one person at a time: Assessing change capacity within your organization.* New York: American Management Association.

Breckon, D. J. (1998). *Community health education: Settings, roles, and skills for the 21st century.* Gaithersburg, MD: Aspen.

Butrie, A. M., & Nowoholnik, H. (1998). Communicating and collaborating for change in the workplace. In D. J. Mason, & J. K. Leavitt (Eds.), *Policy and politics in nursing and health care* (3rd ed.) (pp. 289–293). Philadelphia: Saunders.

Colenso, M. (2000). *Kaizen strategies for successful organizational change.* Upper Saddle River, NJ: Prentice Hall.

Dove, M. A. (1998). Conflict: Process and resolution. *Nursing Management, 29*(4), 30–32.

Drinka, T. J. K., & Clark, P. G. (2000). *Health care teamwork: Interdisciplinary practice and teaching.* Westport, CT: Auburn House.

Ellefsen, B. (1998). Influence and leadership in community-based nursing in Norway. *Public Health Nursing, 15,* 348–354.

Freed, D. H. (1998). Don't shoot me: I'm only the change agent. *Health Care Supervisor, 17*(1), 56–61.

Gillis, A. (1995). Exploring nursing outcomes for health promotion. *Nursing Forum, 30*(2), 5–12.

Habel, M. (2000). *Developing your leadership potential.* Sunnyvale, CA: NurseWeek.

Hersey, P., Blanchard, K. H., & Johnson, D. E. (2000). *Management of organizational behavior: Leading human resources* (8th ed.). Upper Saddle River, NJ: Prentice Hall.

Hetherington, L. T. (1998). Becoming involved: The nurse leader's role in encouraging teamwork. *Nursing Administration Quarterly, 23*(1), 29–40.

Houlihan, G. D. (1999). The evaluation of the "stages of change" model for use in counseling clients undergoing predictive testing for Huntington's disease. *Journal of Advanced Nursing, 29,* 1137–1143.

Institute of Medicine. (1988). *The future of public health.* Washington, DC: National Academy Press.

Kerfoot, K. (1998). Leading change is leading creativity. *Nursing Economics, 12*(2), 98–99.

Koerner, J. G. (2000). Nightingale II: Nursing leaders re-membering community. *Nursing Administration Quarterly, 24*(2), 13–18.

Lawrence, T. (1999). A stage-based approach to behavior change. In E. R. Perkins, I. Simnett, & L. Wright (Eds.), *Evidence-based health promotion* (pp. 64–75). New York: John Wiley.

Lewin, K. (1951). *Field theory in social science: Selected theoretical papers.* New York: Harper & Row.

Lewin, K. (1989a). Changing as three steps: Unfreezing, moving, and freezing. In W. L. French, C. H. Bell, & R. A. Zawacki (Eds.), *Organizational development: Theory, practice and research* (p. 87). Homewood, IL: BPI Irwin.

Lewin, C. (1989b). The field approach: Culture and group life and quasi-stationary processes. In W. L. French, C. H. Bell, & R. A. Zawacki (Eds.), *Organizational development: Theory, practice and research* (pp. 85–86). Homewood, IL: BPI Irwin.

Nagaike, K. (1997). Understanding and managing change in health care organizations. *Nursing Administration Quarterly, 21*(2), 65–73.

Pointer, D. D., & Sanchez, J. P. (1997). Leadership in Public Health Practice. In F. D. Scutchfield & C. W. Keck (Eds.), *Principles of public health practice* (pp. 87–100). Albany, NY: Delmar.

Prochaska, J. O., Norcross, J. C., & DiClemente, C. C. (1995). *Changing for good.* New York: Avon.

Skinner, M. D. (1994). Getting to X. *Nursing Administration Quarterly, 14*(3), 58–63.

Taccetta-Chapnick, M. (1996). Transformational leadership. *Nursing Administration Quarterly, 21*(1), 60–66.

Thompson, B., & Kinne, S. (1999). Social change theory: Applications to community health. In N. Bracht (Ed.), *Health promotion at the community level* (2nd ed.) (pp. 29–46). Thousand Oaks, CA: Sage.

Tiffany, C. R., & Lutjens, L. R. J. (1998). *Planned change theories for nursing: Review, analysis, and implications.* Thousand Oaks, CA: Sage.

Umiker, W. (1998). Collaborative conflict resolution. In E. C. Hein (Ed.), *Contemporary leadership behavior: Selected readings* (5th ed.) (pp. 259–263). Philadelphia: Lippincott.

FAMILIES

The family is the basic social unit of American society. Defining family is difficult, however, because families can assume so many different forms. For the purposes of community health nursing, a *family* is a social system composed of "two or more persons who are joined by bonds of sharing and emotional closeness and who identify themselves as being part of the family" (Friedman, 1998, p. 9). Unlike those of other social systems, family relationships are characterized by intimacy, emotional intensity, and persistence over time (Fischer, 2000). This broad definition of family suggests that the principles of community health nursing applied to family clients must be flexible enough to meet the needs of many different family forms.

Types of Families

Families come in multiple sizes and configurations, each characterized by certain structural features and facing certain unique stresses. Among the family forms encountered by community health nurses in today's world are the traditional nuclear family, extended families, single-parent families, unmarried parents with children, single adults living alone, stepfamilies, binuclear families, cohabiting families, and gay and lesbian families. Each of these family types will be briefly discussed here.

NUCLEAR CONJUGAL FAMILIES

The *nuclear conjugal family,* or, more simply, the nuclear family, is composed of husband, wife, and children. Husband and wife are joined by marriage and their children are either biological offspring or adopted. The nuclear family is found in all ethnic and socioeconomic groups and is sanctioned by all religions. In the past, this type of family has been accepted as a social institution necessary to raise children properly. Today, the nuclear conjugal family is becoming less common in response to societal changes. In 1998, for example, 69% of U.S. households were considered family households and only 25% consisted of a married couple with children under 18 years of age. Slightly more than one fourth of U.S. families are *nuclear dyads,* married couples without children (U.S. Census Bureau, 1999). Nuclear dyads may result by choice, infertility, or movement of grown children out of the household. Approximately 5% to 10% of married women in the United States choose to remain childless (Friedman, 1998).

Another variant of the nuclear family is the *dual-earner family* which consists of two working parents with or without children. Dual-earner families exist primarily because of the need for increased income, and the number of such families increased 46% from 1974 to 1994. Challenges faced by these families include managing tasks related to housework and child care, managing the stress of two jobs, and maintaining family relationships (Friedman, 1998).

EXTENDED FAMILIES

The *extended family* consists of the family kin network such as grandparents, aunts, uncles, and cousins. Traditionally, extended families either shared household expenses and tasks or lived in close proximity and provided mutual support (Friedman, 1998). Like the nuclear family, the extended family has been affected by societal change. In the past, members of extended families often lived in close proximity to the nuclear family. But owing to increased mobility and the enticement of better jobs in other areas, families are more likely to live away from their extended kin network. Thus, the extended family is now more likely to be a long-distance unit with whom the nuclear family corresponds and visits. This phenomenon has limited the social, economic, and emotional support formerly available to members of a nuclear family from older and more experienced relatives.

As time passes and circumstances change, the nuclear family may take extended family members into the home. This typically occurs as a consequence of early marriage of children where the newlyweds must live with parents or when adult children return home following a divorce, an economic setback, or some other life crisis. Some adult children are remaining in the home due to economic constraints and older age at marriage. New living arrangements to incorporate extended family members into the nuclear family can also occur when aging parents can no longer live alone. The parent of a grown child may present adjustment problems for the nuclear family that has been separated from the parent for some time.

SINGLE-PARENT FAMILIES

The most common family unit to be encountered by community health nurses is the *single-parent family.* Single-parent families consist of an adult woman or man and children. Single-parent families result from divorce, out-of-wedlock pregnancies, absence or death of a spouse, or adoption by a single person. In 1998, 10% of U.S. households were single-parent families, and 27% of all family households were headed by a single parent. Most of these single-parent households (81%) were headed by women, although the number of single-parent families headed by men is increasing each year. The relative proportion of single-parent households varies among ethnic groups. For example, 23% of white families in the United States are single-parent families compared to 58% of African American families and 30% of Hispanic families (U.S. Census Bureau, 1999). Women as single parents out number men in each of the three groups.

Single-parent families are characterized by increasing poverty and role changes, role overload, and role conflict for the single parent. Research has indicated that children in single-parent families are generally worse off than their counterparts in two-parent families, particularly with respect to behavior problems (Friedman, 1998).

STEPFAMILIES

Stepfamilies are increasingly evident in American society. A *stepfamily* is composed of two adults, at least one of whom has remarried following divorce or death of a spouse. Stepfamilies can include children from either adult's previous marriage, as well as offspring from the new marriage. In 1988, 46% of marriages were remarriages for one or both parties, and 26% of married women in 1995 reported one or more previous spouses or cohabiting partners. The propensity for divorce and remarriage creates large numbers of new stepfamilies each year. Other terms used for stepfamilies include *blended, remarried,* or *reconstituted* families. The extended kin network of a step family can include stepgrandparents, stepaunts, stepuncles, and stepcousins, as well as an ex-spouse who is the biological parent of some of the children, but no longer a part of the household. The existence of stepfamilies may also contribute to the creation of a **binuclear family,** which exists when a child is a member of two nuclear households as a result of a joint-custody arrangement following the divorce of the child's parents (Friedman, 1998).

Stepfamilies face a number of unique challenges related to limited family loyalty, complexity of family interactions, preexisting parent–child coalitions, differences in the balance of power, multiple parental figures for children, and ambiguous family boundaries (Wright & Leahey, 2000). Complex relationships with extended kin networks and former spouses and unrealistic expectations of family relationships may further complicate life for members of stepfamilies (Friedman, 1998).

COHABITING FAMILIES

A *cohabiting family* consists of a man and a woman living together without being married. Individuals who choose cohabitation range in age from teens to retired elderly persons. The reasons cited for preferring this arrangement include the desire for a "trial marriage," the increased safety of living with another, and financial necessity. Cohabitation is becoming more prevalent in the United States. In 1995, for example, more than 41% of U.S. women reported cohabiting at some time in their lives and 7% were currently cohabiting. In 1998, there were 4.2 million cohabiting households in the United States, 1.5 million of which included children under 15 years of age (U.S. Census Bureau, 1999).

GAY AND LESBIAN FAMILIES

A *gay or lesbian family* is a form of cohabitation in which a couple of the same sex live together and share a sexual relationship. The homosexual family might include children and might resemble the traditional nuclear family in terms of the mutual support and sexual and economic interdependence of the couple involved. In addition to the usual stresses of family life, gay and lesbian families experience the added stresses created by a lack of societal and legal sanction and stigmatization that accompany known homosexuality.

COMMUNAL FAMILIES

A *communal family* is made up of several adults and children living together, usually because of a common religious or ideological bond or financial necessity. Communal families typically resemble traditional extended families in qualities of affection and interdependence, rituals, migration, and influence or control. Communal living can be more stressful than the typical nuclear family; this is because of crowding, more people and roles to deal with, and a general lack of privacy for couples and children to resolve differences. Communal families may exhibit monogamous or polygamous sexual relationships. Other family forms that are being seen with increasing regularity by community health nurses are foster families and skip-generation families.

Foster families consist of at least one adult and one or more foster children placed by the court system. Foster families may also include the adults' own biological or adopted children. Foster family composition may change frequently and exemplifies what has been called a *permeable family structure,* which encompasses many different kinship arrangements (Elkind, 1995). In 1996, nearly eight of every thousand U.S. children was in foster care (U.S. Census Bureau, 1999), and many of these children had been in several foster homes over time.

Skip-generation families are those in which grandparents are raising their grandchildren. Skip-generation families may occur because of working parents, drug use, or child abandonment. In 1998, more than 1.4 million children under 18 years of age were living with grandparents without the presence of either parent (U.S. Census Bureau, 1999). The family types presented here are summarized in Table 14–1 ■.

Community health nurses may record information regarding family composition and relationships among family members in the form of genograms or ecomaps. A *genogram* is a diagram of a family tree incorporating information regarding family members and their relationships over at least three generations. Information that may be included in a genogram includes dates of births, deaths, marriages, separations, and divorces; health status; ethnicity; occupation or unemployment; retirement; and significant family problems such as trouble with the law, family violence, or incest. Creation of a genogram is an excellent method of family engagement when the community health nurse first encounters the family (Wright & Leahey, 2000). A sample genogram is included in Figure 14–1 ■.

By convention, certain symbols have certain meanings in a genogram. For example, females are represented by circles and males by squares. Squares and circles marked with an "X" indicate deceased family members. A double circle or square indicates the *index person* or identified client. The lines connecting persons in the diagram indicate the character of relationships between them. Broader lines indicate stronger relationships, broken lines reflect distant or tenuous ones, and cross-hatched lines indicate conflictual relationships (Roth, 1996).

■ **TABLE 14–1** **Types of Families and Their Characteristic Features**

FAMILY TYPE	CHARACTERISTIC FEATURES
Nuclear conjugal family	Mother and father who are married with one or more biological or adopted children
Extended family	Kin network of the adult male and female of a nuclear family (e.g., grandparents, aunts, uncles, cousins)
Single-parent family	One adult male or female with biological or adopted children *most common*
Stepfamily	Reconstituted or blended family created by a second marriage in which one or both spouses have children from a previous marriage and possibly children of the new union
Binuclear family	A child (or children) who is part of two nuclear households as a result of divorce and joint custody
Cohabiting couple	A male and a female living together without marriage, with or without children
Gay or lesbian family	A cohabiting couple of the same sex, with or without children
Communal family	Multiple adults and children in one household who share household expenses and tasks and may share sexual relationships
Foster family	One or more adults and one or more court-designated foster children, with or without other biological or adopted children
Skip-generation family	One or both grandparents raising one or more grandchildren in the absence of the children's parents

An *ecomap* is a visual representation of relationships both within and outside of the family (Wright & Leahey, 2000). An ecomap can be used to depict the relationships of family members with each other and with outside forces such as health care providers, employers, and extended family members. The segment of the genogram including the household of interest may be contained within the larger central circle of the ecomap. Outside forces are represented by smaller circles on the periphery. Again, relationships are represented by the types of lines connecting the circles in the diagram. Figure 14–2 ■ presents a sample ecomap in which there are strong supportive relationships between the wife and the community health nurse and between the son and his teacher and conflictual relationships between the husband and his employer and between the family and the next door neighbor. There is also a tenuous relationship with the extended family.

Theoretical Approaches to Family Nursing

Many disciplines provide care and services to families and have developed theoretical models for dealing with families. Friedman (1998) grouped these theoretical approaches to family care as nursing models, social science models, and family therapy models. The application of selected nursing models to the care of families was addressed in Chapter 9. Family therapy models are not broad enough to address the aspects of family care by nurses, so we will focus our discussion on social science models as they are applied to holistic care of families by community health nurses. Three types of social science

models will be presented: systems models, developmental models, and structural–functional models. Other social science family models, such as transactional theory, stress theory, and family change theory, are useful in addressing selected family problems, but do not provide the broad scope of understanding required for community health nursing care of families.

SYSTEMS MODELS

Systems models conceive of families as open systems in which the whole of the system is more than the sum of its component parts or members, but also includes the interactions among them. The health of the family as a unit is influenced by interactions among members and between the family system and larger outside systems. The basic concepts of systems theory are derived from the work of biologist Ludwig von Bertalanffy and sociologist Talcott Parsons working independently to describe biological and social systems respectively (Friedman, 1998). Systems theory incorporates basic principles that can be applied to any kind of system from an automobile engine, to the human body, to families, to organizations, to communities, and so on (von Bertalanffy, 1973). A *system* is defined as "a complex of elements in interaction" with each other in which the interaction is ordered rather than random (von Bertalanffy, 1981). The "elements" that make up a system are also known as *subsystems*. Systems are hierarchical in nature, with some systems in turn constituting subsystems within more complex systems. For example, the cardiovascular system is a subsystem in the human body, a system that is itself a subsystem in the totality of an individual, who is a subsystem in a family system, and so on. In a family, the subsystems are the family members.

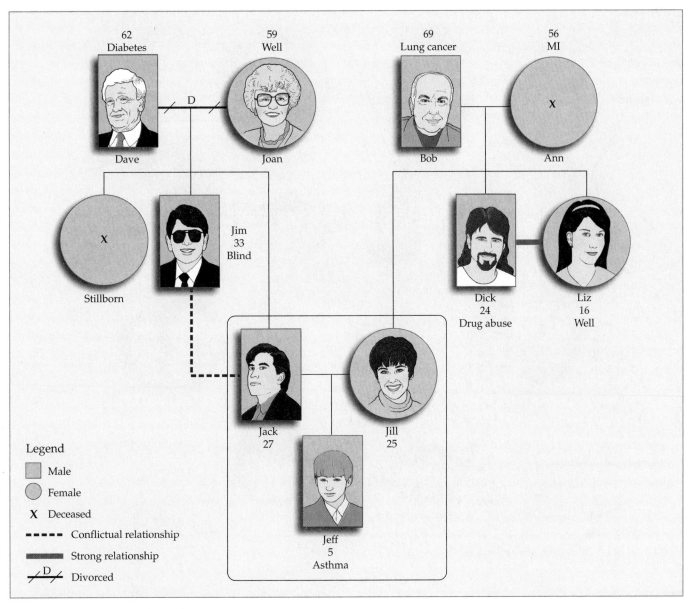

FIGURE 14-1 ■ *Sample Family Genogram*

Another concept of systems theory is the *suprasystem* or the context in which a given system functions. The next higher order system in the hierarchy is one aspect of the suprasystem for a lower order system. For example, the family is part of the suprasystem of an individual system, and the community is a suprasystem element for the family system. The concept of hierarchical systems is depicted in Figure 14–3 ■. The system of interest in any given situation is sometimes referred to as the *focal system* and other systems within the suprasystem as *interacting systems* (Friedman, 1998).

Any system is more than the sum of parts or subsystems of which it is made and also incorporates reciprocal interactions among its parts. This systems principle means that whatever affects one portion of a system will affect other portions because of their interdependence. The interrelationships between subsystems within the system, between subsystems and the suprasystem, and between the suprasystem and the system as a whole are important determinants of health and are one of the major foci in using a systems approach to community health nursing.

All systems have *boundaries* that define what is part of the system and what is not. For example, a community may have geographic boundaries such as city limits; whereas a family's boundaries are often (but not always) determined by blood and legal ties. The permeability of the system boundary determines whether one is dealing with an open or closed system. An *open system* is one that exchanges matter, energy, or information with the environment; a closed system does not. All of the systems of interest to community health nurses (individuals, families, and population groups) are open systems.

All systems also have two mutual goals: maintenance of a steady state and system growth and engage in three categories of processes designed to accomplish these goals. The first category of processes includes those

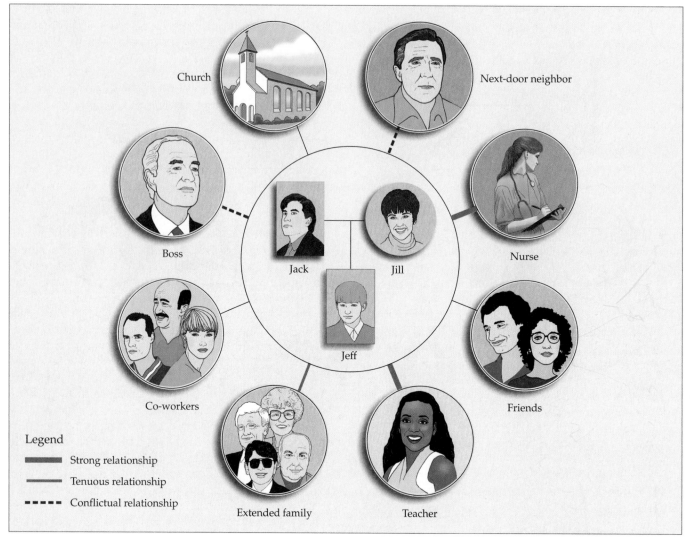

FIGURE 14–2 ■ *Sample Family Ecomap*

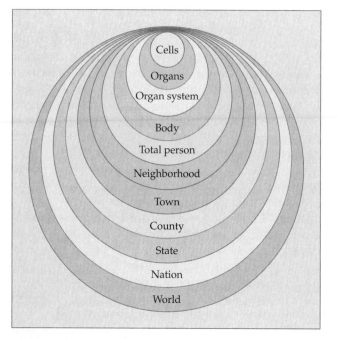

FIGURE 14–3 ■ *Hierarchical Systems*

needed to regulate exchanges with the environment. These processes are the input, throughput, and output processes. *Input* is the process whereby energy, matter, or information enter the system from outside the system's boundaries. *Throughput* is the process by which the material received into the system is transformed in some way, and *output* is what the system discharges back into the environment. In a family system, for example, input might include a report of a child's misbehavior in school. Throughput involves the processes by which the family acts on the report. The family might choose to ignore it, to criticize the child, or to explore and modify the child's reasons for misbehavior. Output would be the result of the processes used. If the family chooses to ignore the report, the behavior is likely to continue. If the family criticizes and punishes the child, the behavior may change, but the child's self-esteem may be damaged. If, on the other hand, the family attempts to explore the child's behavior and modify it, the behavior is likely to change, but the child's self-esteem will be left intact.

The second category, processes involved in system operation, includes those processes designed to limit expenditures of system energy, provide for organization, and prevent overload. Using these processes, a system may refuse to accept input. For example, the family may choose to suspend nonessential family tasks while one member is hospitalized. Internal processes, the third category of system processes, include subsystems change processes and adaptive processes. In subsystems change processes, a change in one subsystem results in changes in related subsystems. For example, when a new child is born into the family, relationships among family members will need to adapt to accommodate the new member. The teenage son or daughter, for instance, may need to assume more household responsibilities to free parents for care of the infant.

Adaptive processes, the second type of internal processes involve the systems concepts of entropy, negentropy, and feedback. *Entropy* is a state of system disorganization resulting from the demands of continual readjustment of subsystem interrelations. A certain level of entropy is necessary for the system to continue to function and to avoid stasis or cessation of activity. However, as entropy rises above optimal levels, the system's ability to work toward its goals decreases proportionately. For example, the number of family members' outside activities may increase beyond the capacity of the designated chauffeur to accommodate, and adjustments will need to be made to ensure effective family function.

Negentropy relates to an increase in order and organization, which allows energy to be used to meet system goals. Negentropy is necessary for maintenance of the steady state, but the system must periodically move away from this steady state in order for growth to occur. If, for example, the family refuses to adjust family roles to adapt to the increasing independence of adolescent members, family function and individual development are impeded.

Feedback is the process whereby the system output returns as input. Negative feedback tends to minimize changes in the system and contributes to maintenance of the steady state. Negative feedback, in essence, plays down any discrepancies between the desired state of affairs and things as they are. Using the school misbehavior as an example, if the outcome of family action is improved behavior, feedback from the school will not provoke further family action; the feedback indicates that the actual and desired behavior are congruent. Awareness of these discrepancies often results in system changes contributing to growth. In the example, positive feedback would indicate that the child's behavior still does not meet expectations, and the family system would probably take additional actions to improve his or her behavior.

DEVELOPMENTAL MODELS

Developmental models are based on the supposition that human beings and social units, such as families, develop in a logical fashion with predictable stages or milestones along the way. At each stage of development, the client is expected to accomplish specific tasks that provide a foundation for accomplishing the tasks of the next stage.

According to family developmental theory, families, like individuals, pass through predictable developmental or family life stages first described by Duvall (Duvall & Miller, 1990). There are differing expectations in each stage of family development. As the expectations change, so do interactions among family members. The term used for these stage expectations is *family developmental tasks.* The developmental tasks of each stage necessitate certain changes within the family in the roles of its members in order for the family to fulfill its functions.

Duvall divided the family life cycle into the eight stages presented in Table 14–2 ■. More recent family theorists such as Carter and McGoldrick (1999) have expanded the conceptualization of family stages as depicted in Table 14–2. In either model, each stage involves the accomplishment of specific tasks. At the same time that the family is engaged in accomplishing these tasks, family members are involved in accomplishing their own individual developmental tasks, which may parallel family tasks or conflict with them. The family must foster accomplishment of both family and individual tasks in order to function as an effective unit. Thus, there may be conflict or stress when the accomplishment of a family task is in direct opposition to task achievement by the individual. The family must develop healthy mechanisms for dealing with this type of conflict when it arises.

Families generally experience some stress as they pass from one stage to the next, since the transition usually involves one or more role changes. The family needs to negotiate these changes and respond by reevaluating roles and goals. For example, in Duvall's stage II, when the first child is born, the family enters a new stage that necessitates changes in the roles of both husband and wife and in their interactions with each other. Developmental tasks of each stage of family development are included in Table 14–2.

One of the criticisms of Duvall's developmental model is that it applies primarily to the traditional nuclear family. Carter and McGoldrick (1999) have identified developmental stages for divorced families and families resulting from remarriage. These stages are depicted in Table 14–3 ■. In applying developmental models, the focus of care is on identifying the family stage of development, assessing the degree to which the family has achieved the developmental tasks of that and previous stages, and engaging in action to promote accomplishment of developmental tasks.

⑥ THINK ABOUT IT

How would you intervene to help a family adjust to the stress of a young wife's return to work with three young children at home? How might your interventions differ if the stress was due to the children leaving home?

■ **TABLE 14–2** Duvall's and Carter and McGoldrick's Stages of Family Development with Associated Developmental Tasks

DUVALL'S STAGES OF FAMILY DEVELOPMENT	CARTER AND MCGOLDRICK'S STAGES OF FAMILY DEVELOPMENT

	Stage I: Single Young Adult
	Tasks: 1. Accept self-responsibility
	        2. Differentiate self from family of origin
	        3. Develop intimate peer relationships
	        4. Develop a career and financial independence

Stage I: Beginning Family
Tasks: 1. Establish a mutually satisfying marriage
        2. Develop new relationships with kin networks
        3. Engage in family planning
	Stage II: New Couple
	Tasks: 1. Achieve commitment to the new relationship
	        2. Form the marital relationship
	        3. Realign relationships with families and friends

Stage II: Early Childbearing Family
Tasks: 1. Establish a stable family unit
        2. Reconcile conflict in family and individual developmental tasks
        3. Facilitate accomplishment of members' developmental tasks
	Stage III: Family with Young Children
	Tasks: 1. Adjust the marriage to the presence of children
	        2. Distribute childrearing, household, and financial tasks
	        3. Develop new relationships with family members (parenting and grandparenting)

Stage III: Family with Preschool Children
Tasks: 1. Integrate second or third child
        2. Socialize children to familial and societal expectations and roles
        3. Begin separation from children	

Stage IV: Family with School-Age Children
Tasks: 1. Separate from children to a greater degree
        2. Foster education and socialization
        3. Maintain the stability of the marriage	

Stage V: Family with Teenage Children
Tasks: 1. Maintain the stability of the marriage
        2. Develop new communication channels
        3. Maintain family standards
	Stage IV: Family with Adolescents
	Tasks: 1. Adapt to growing independence of adolescent family members
	        2. Adjust to increasing frailty of own parents
	        3. Change parent–child relationships
	        4. Address marital and career issues

Stage VI: Launching Center Family
Tasks: 1. Promote independence of children
        2. Integrate spouses of children into the family
        3. Restore the marital relationship
        4. Develop outside interests
        5. Assist aging parents
	Stage V: Launching Children and Moving On
	Tasks: 1. Accept multiple entries and exits from family structure
	        2. Renegotiate the marital dyad
	        3. Adapt relationships to accommodate inlaws and grandchildren
	        4. Deal with disability and death of one's own parents

Stage VII: Family of Middle Years
Tasks: 1. Cultivate leisure activities
        2. Provide a healthful environment
        3. Sustain satisfying relationships with own parents and children
	Stage VI: Family in Later Life
	Tasks: 1. Accept the change in generational roles
	        2. Maintain function
	        3. Explore new roles
	        4. Assure support for middle and older generations
	        5. Deal with the death of others and one's own approaching death

Stage VIII: Family in Retirement and Old Age
Tasks: 1. Maintain satisfying living arrangements
        2. Adjust to decreased income
        3. Adjust to loss of spouse, relatives, and friends	

Sources: Carter, B., & McGoldrick, M. (1999). Overview: The expanded family life cycle: Individual, family and social perspectives. In B. Carter & M. McGoldrick (Eds.), *The expanded family life cycle: Individual, family and social perspectives* (3rd ed.) (pp. 1–26). Boston: Allyn & Bacon; and Duvall, E., & Miller, B. (1990). *Marriage and family development* (6th ed.). New York: Harper College.

■ **TABLE 14–3** **Developmental Stages of Divorced and Remarried Families**

DEVELOPMENTAL STAGES OF DIVORCED FAMILIES

Stage I: Decision to Divorce
Task:　Accepting the failure of the marriage

Stage II: Planning System Breakup
Tasks:　1. Addressing custody/property allocation issues
　　　　2. Dealing with extended family responses to the divorce

Stage III: Separation
Task:　Adjusting relationships among family members

Stage IV: Divorce
Task:　Overcoming hurt, anger, and other emotions precipitated by divorce

Stage V: Postdivorce
Tasks:　1. Functioning as a single-parent household or maintaining a noncustodial parental role and meeting financial responsibilities for former spouse and children
　　　　2. Maintaining relationships with kin networks
　　　　3. Rebuilding social networks

STAGES OF REMARRIAGE

Stage I: Entering a New Relationship
Task:　Making a commitment to the new relationship

Stage II: Conceptualizing and Planning the New System
Tasks:　1. Developing new relationships
　　　　2. Realigning prior relationships

Stage III: Remarriage and Reconstruction
Task:　Accepting a new model of the family

Sources: Carter, B., & McGoldrick, M. (1999). Overview: The expanded family life cycle: Individual, family and social perspectives. In B. Carter & M. McGoldrick (Eds.), *The expanded family life cycle: Individual, family and social perspectives* (3rd ed.) (pp. 1–26). Boston: Allyn & Bacon.

STRUCTURAL–FUNCTIONAL MODELS

A structural–functional approach to family nursing is based on the principle that all families possess structure designed to allow them to perform specific functions. The health of the family is dependent on performance of these necessary functions.

The two basic concepts of a structural–functional approach are structure and function. *Structure* is the pattern of organization of interdependent parts of a whole. Structural elements of a family include family members and family interaction patterns related to roles, values, communication patterns, and power structure (Friedman, 1998).

Structural elements affect families' abilities to perform functions that ensure continued survival and influence health. A *function* is one of a group of related actions that lead to accomplishment of specific goals, the goals of interest in family nursing being survival and health. Family functions fall into the five categories depicted in Table 14–4 ■. The affective function of the family reflects

---

■ **TABLE 14–4** **Family Functions and Related Goals**

FUNCTION	GOALS
Affective	Meet the emotional needs of family members
Socialization	Educate family members as contributing members of society Instill family attitudes and values in members
Reproductive	Ensure survival of family and society Regulate sexual activity Provide for sexual satisfaction
Economic	Provide financial resources sufficient to meet family needs
Provision of needs	Meet family member's needs for food, shelter, clothing, health care, etc.

---

its ability to meet the emotional and belonging needs of its members. The socialization function is designed to assist family members to become active contributors to the family and to the larger society and includes educating family members as well as transmitting attitudes and values. The reproductive function ensures continuity of the family and of society (Friedman, 1998). Another aspect of this function is control of sexual behavior and reproduction. The goal of the family's economic function is provision and appropriate allocation of family economic resources. This function is intimately tied to the provision of needs function, which reflects the family's ability to meet members' needs for food, shelter, health care, and so on. The relationship of structural and functional elements in families is presented in Table 14–5 ■.

Family structural elements may influence abilities to carry out required functions, thereby undermining family health. The community health nurse using a structural–functional approach to care first assesses how effectively the family performs expected functions and identifies any problems in functional areas. The nurse then identifies structural elements that are contributing to functional difficulties. Intervention using a structural–functional model is designed to improve functional performance. For example, ineffective communication patterns and fixed family roles are structural elements that may interfere with the family's ability to meet the affective needs of its members. In this case, nursing intervention would focus on improving family communication and redefining roles.

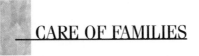

CARE OF FAMILIES

Community health nurses work with individual families and with families as an aggregate within the population. In doing so, they use the nursing process to assess family

■ **TABLE 14–5**   **Interrelationships Among Functional and Structural Elements in Families**

FUNCTIONAL ELEMENT	STRUCTURAL ELEMENTS
Affective function	*Role:* Who provides support, reassurance, encouragement? *Values:* How, when, and where is affection displayed? *Communication:* How are affective messages conveyed? By whom? *Power:* Do affective bonds confer power? Diminish power?
Socialization function	*Role:* Who socializes children? *Values:* How, when, and where are children socialized? *Communication:* How are standards communicated? Are accepted standards and behavior congruent? *Power:* Is socialization one-way or two-way? Is power maintained or diminished by socialization?
Reproductive function	*Role:* Who engages in reproductive functions? With whom? *Values:* When, where, and how are reproductive functions carried out? *Communication:* How is information about sexuality conveyed? How are sexual desires conveyed? By whom? Does reproductive activity also convey affection? *Power:* Is manipulation of the reproductive function used to confer power?
Economic function	*Role:* Who earns? Who spends? *Values:* How, when, and where are expenditures made? For what? *Communication:* How are economic needs communicated? To whom? *Power:* Who makes economic decisions? How?
Provision of necessities function	*Role:* Who provides what? *Values:* What should be provided? When? Where? How? To whom? *Communication:* How are needs communicated? To whom? *Power:* Who makes decisions about allocation of resources? How?

health, diagnose needs for care, and plan, implement, and evaluate care for families at both individual and societal levels.

 ## ASSESSING FAMILY HEALTH

Family health is an attribute of the family as a unit and encompasses more than the health status of individual family members (Soubhi & Potvin, 2000). Assessment of family health takes place with respect to individual families and the overall health of families within the population. The dimensions of health from the dimensions model provide an organizing perspective from which to assess family health at both levels. Areas of assessment address biophysical, psychological, physical environmental, sociocultural, behavioral, and health system considerations.

Biophysical Considerations

When the community health nurse first encounters a family, assessment begins by gathering data to identify the physical needs of family members. It is important to note that the physical status of each family member should be weighed as part of the family assessment. The physical health status of each member affects how the family functions and how members relate to each other.

For example, if a child has a chronic disease, the entire family must make adjustments to accommodate the youngster's special needs. The parents have to adjust their schedules to care for the child and ensure that the child is seen by appropriate health care providers. Siblings can assume household chores and provide some measure of care for their ill brother or sister. Other family members can assist with care and offer emotional support for the parents and children.

Knowledge of the sex, age, and race of family members, as well as information related to genetic inheritance, can guide the nurse in identifying problems and planning family care. For example, knowing that there are several young children in the home, the nurse may emphasize safety precautions when interacting with the family. An elderly family is more likely to have members with chronic, debilitating illnesses and may need closer scrutiny for evidence of these problems. The presence of older family members may contribute to *filial crises* in which they and their adult children are faced with acknowledging their mortality and accommodating role reversals. Multiple generations in the household may also result in the *sandwich generation* phenomenon in which younger adult members are caught between meeting the needs of their children and their aging parents (Richards, 1996). Or, a family's race may increase its members' risks for certain diseases such as sickle cell disease among African Americans and peoples of Eastern Mediterranean descent.

The community health nurse should also collect data regarding biophysical considerations at the aggregate level. For example, effective health care planning for families requires information about the proportion of elderly families and those with young children in the population and the number of families with disabled members or other individual health problems that may affect overall family health.

Psychological Considerations

The community health nurse assesses a variety of considerations in the psychological dimension of family health at both the level of the individual family and at the aggregate level. Areas for consideration include communication patterns, relationships and dynamics, emotional strengths, coping, child-rearing practices, family goals, and the presence or absence of emotional problems.

Communication Patterns

Communication patterns are an indicator of functioning in the psychological dimension. Both verbal and nonverbal modes of family communication should be considered, as should the listening ability of family members. How do members communicate values and ideas? When one family member talks, do others listen? Do they show anger or boredom while listening?

Mealtime is a good time to assess family interaction. It is here that the nurse can determine whether meals are a time of light conversation or heated argument, whether all family members eat together, and whether mealtimes contribute to family solidarity. It is also important to assess the content of communications. Are they superficial or does the family engage in values clarification discussions? The type of statements made or questions asked tell the nurse a great deal about family interactions. For example, "You are wrong about that" and "Tell me more about your feelings" indicate different attitudes about interactions among family members. The latter, open-ended response facilitates communication, whereas the previous accusatory statement impedes it.

The feeling tone expressed in communication is another indicator of the psychological environment. Family communications may contribute to interpersonal difficulties or facilitate cohesion and problem resolution. Sarcastic and resentful statements could block further communication between family members. For example, "When are you ever going to use your head?" does not facilitate communication. Other types of one-way communication include repeated complaints, manipulation through covert requests, insulting remarks, lack of validation, and inability to focus on one issue (Friedman, 1998).

The nurse should ascertain what areas of communication are taboo (off limits) for family members. Typical areas include feelings, sexual issues, and religion. For

Meals can be a time of family sharing.

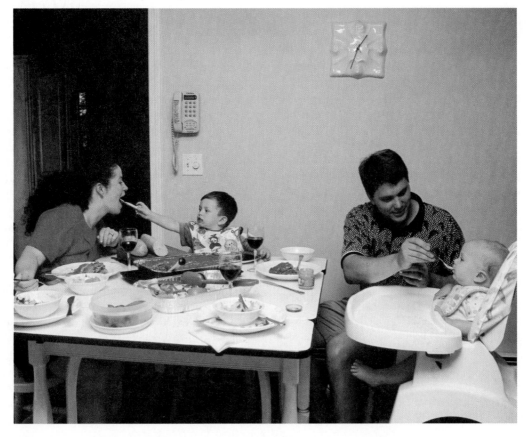

example, in some families, members are not expected to express feelings of anger. Another example would be an expectation that family members do not discuss family problems with outsiders. If certain topics are found to be taboo, the nurse may need to alter his or her approach to data gathering. For example, if one of the areas closed to discussion involves feelings, the nurse might try engaging in self-disclosure, thus acting as a role model. Another way to alter the approach is to gather data by examining areas related to the taboo issue. This may also help the nurse to identify the reason for resistance to communication about a specific area.

Communication patterns can influence the effectiveness of parenting, particularly in the area of discipline. Praise enhances the development of self-worth in the child, whereas negative or condescending communications

restrict the child's development. More about communications and child discipline can be found in Chapter 16.

The nurse should be aware of several dysfunctional communication patterns that may be employed within families. For instance, messages may be passed from one family member to another in a chainlike fashion that does not allow for reciprocal discussion, or communication may isolate a family member, as when the mother and children exclude the father from their discussions. Another problematic pattern is the wheel in which a central person directs what communication will be passed between family members. By way of comparison, a successful pattern of communication is the "switchboard" in which there is reciprocal communication among all family members. Figure 14–4 ■ illustrates these patterns of communication.

FIGURE 14–4 ■ *Family Communication Patterns*

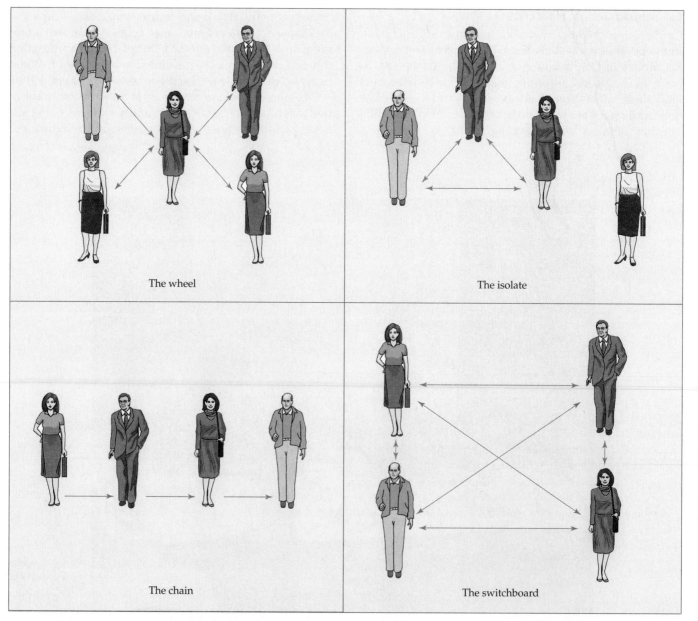

The wheel

The isolate

The chain

The switchboard

A final consideration is the degree of communication between the family and the suprasystem. Is the family open to new ideas and opinions from people outside the family? Are outsiders invited to participate in family discussions or are they expected to "mind their own business"?

Family Relationships and Family Dynamics

Family relationships and family dynamics are areas of concern in the community health nurse's assessment of the family's psychological environment. *Family relationships* are those bonds between family members that create identifiable patterns, such as subgroups and isolated members. *Family dynamics* describes the hierarchical patterns within the family. Power and leadership are the central focus for this area of assessment.

How does one assess relationships within the family? Initially, information regarding subgroups is compiled. For example, the nurse may notice that a mother–daughter subgroup has excluded the father from the decision-making process.

Communication within and between subgroups is then assessed in terms of both content (what is said) and process (who says it and how it is said). This is followed by identification of the relationship as supportive or close, demanding, maternal, and so on. Subgroups are described in terms of how they relate. For example, one may describe the sibling group as one that shares feelings and actions, or they may be described as alienated from each other.

Family dynamics are assessed by observing family leadership patterns. Who are the primary decision makers? Who controls conversations? Is there a leader in the family? What leadership style does the leader employ? (See Chapter 13 for a discussion of leadership styles.) Do family members respect the leader? Do they respect each other? Respect requires that children view parents as individuals as well as parents. Likewise, parents need to learn to respect their children as individuals.

Family Emotional Strengths

A family's emotional strengths become evident as the nurse observes interactions and communicates with family members over time. The nurse should look for evidence of family cohesion and the degree of sensitivity to others displayed by each family member. For example, the nurse might observe whether a mother anticipates her child's needs or whether there is a general feeling of warmth and caring. The nurse should also estimate the degree to which family members support and praise each other. The results of these observations help the nurse to estimate how well the family is meeting the emotional and psychological needs of its members.

Positive self-image on the part of a family member is the result of daily family interactions that bolster the individual's feelings of self-worth. A child who is criticized too often may develop a poor self-image. The nurse can assess the self-esteem of family members by observing nonverbal behavior as well as their communication patterns with others.

Coping Strategies

Identifying a family's coping strategies and defense mechanisms enables the nurse to assist families to deal realistically with stress and crisis. *Coping strategies* are behaviors that help a family to adapt to stress or change and are characterized by positive problem-solving methods that prevent or resolve crisis situations. Coping involves specific actions taken to manage demands on the family and to bring resources to bear on family problems. Research has identified several potential coping strategies that may be used by families (Astedt-Kurki, Hopia, & Vuori, 1999). These strategies include talking with family members, making positive comparisons with other families, expressing both positive and negative emotions, and having a positive attitude toward life. Other coping mechanisms demonstrated by families include having common rules and agreements, financial and emotional independence of adult members from each other, humor, and recognition of the limits of what the family or its individual members can achieve.

Defense mechanisms are tactics for avoiding recognition of problems. They may be used when the family cannot immediately determine how to solve a problem. Defense mechanisms are not considered problematic unless they interfere with coping and may actually be helpful in allowing time to organize resources before facing a problem. Examples of defense mechanisms include denial, rationalization, selective inattention, isolation, intellectualization, and projection. Characteristics of these defense mechanisms are summarized below.

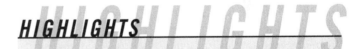

HIGHLIGHTS

Commonly Used Defense Mechanisms

Denial
Ignoring threat-provoking aspects of a situation or changing the meaning of the situation to make it less threatening

Rationalization
Giving a "good" or rational excuse, but not the real reason for responding to a situation with a particular behavior

Selective Inattention
Attending to only those aspects of the situation that do not cause distress or pain

Isolation
Separating emotion from content in a situation so one can deal objectively with otherwise threatening or emotionally overwhelming conditions

Intellectualization

Focusing on abstract, technical, or logical aspects of a threatening situation to insulate oneself from painful emotions generated

Projection

Attributing one's own motivation to other people

The use of coping strategies or defense mechanisms is seen most often when the family is faced with change. The community health nurse can assess how the family deals with change by observing behavior during life change events or by obtaining information on how the family has dealt with a major move, job change, or loss of a family member in the past. Working with a family in crisis is discussed more fully later in this chapter.

ⓖTHINK ABOUT IT

How does your family deal with stress? Are you more likely to employ defense mechanisms or coping strategies?

Child-Rearing and Discipline Practices

Another consideration in assessing the psychological dimension of family health is the child-rearing and discipline practices employed to socialize children. Such practices have the potential either for causing psychological problems among family members or for strengthening a sense of right and wrong in each child.

The nurse should determine the type of discipline used, who administers it, and the types of behavior that elicit disciplinary action. The nurse should also determine whether parents and other adults in the family support each other's decisions in matters of discipline. For example, if the child is punished by the mother, does the child attempt to avoid punishment by manipulating the father? If so, are the adults able to discuss and support a joint decision? Ultimately, parents need to teach self-discipline, so it is important to assess whether they provide adequate role models for children. For a more detailed discussion of discipline, see Chapter 16.

Family Goals

Family goals are an element of the psychological environment that may be difficult to assess because families often are not consciously aware of them. The nurse, however, can be aware of and observe for evidence of family goals; these include producing children and ensuring their survival, exchanging love and emotional support, and providing for economic survival or affluence.

Family goals are a function of family values and reflect a family's cultural background. Family goals also vary with a family's developmental stage, economic status, and the physical health of family members. Problems arise when there is disagreement on family goals. For example, the Gonzales family worked hard to send their son to college (a family goal). Before his sophomore year, the son refused to return to school, preferring instead to work as a plumber's apprentice.

Another element of the psychological dimension to be assessed in working with families is the presence or absence of mental or emotional illness among family members. Such illnesses not only affect the health status of individual family members, but can profoundly influence the health of the family unit (Wilson & Hobbs, 1999). Community health nurses working with these families should assess the impact of the illness on family function and should address the resulting health problems of both the individual and the family as a whole.

At the aggregate level, community health nurses can develop a picture of psychological dimension factors that have the potential for affecting the health of families within the population. The incidence and prevalence of family violence or suicide, for example, can suggest potential problems that may be faced by individual families as well as societal attitudes that may contribute to problems. Similarly, the extent of mental illness in the population may suggest psychological dimension factors impinging on family health.

Physical Environmental Considerations

The community health nurse's observational and interpretive skills are especially needed to assess the home environment. Within this setting, the family develops either functional or dysfunctional relationships. A chaotic, crowded, unsanitary, or unsafe home can contribute to physical and psychological health problems among family members.

To begin the assessment, it is important to describe the home and its condition. Information such as the address, whether the family owns or rents the home, whether the home is big enough for the family, the presence of safety hazards, and family plans for fire or other disasters are all relevant to the family's health status. Several potential hazards to be considered in assessing a family's physical environment are presented on page 305.

CULTURAL CONSIDERATIONS

What elements of culture influence psychological dimension factors in family health? How might these factors differ among an Anglo American family, an Asian American family, and a Hispanic American family? What similarities might you encounter among the three groups?

HIGHLIGHTS

Safety Considerations in the Family Environment

- Peeling paint (especially lead-based paint in older homes)
- Loose throw rugs, toys, or other safety hazards in walkways
- Broken furniture
- Broken stairs or stair railings (inside or outside the home)
- Broken porch floorboards or railings
- Hazardous materials within children's reach
- Plumbing that does not allow for sanitary disposal of human wastes
- Overcrowding
- Absence of fire alarms in the home
- Lack of a fire or other disaster plan
- Lack of a poison control plan (posted telephone numbers)
- Numerous house pets such as cats or dogs
- Close proximity to a heavily traveled highway
- Lack of a fenced-in yard for small children

ETHICAL AWARENESS

You are working with Mrs. Rhodes, who is pregnant with her third child. She has not yet told her husband that she is pregnant, because he beat her several times during each of her previous pregnancies. She is afraid that he will beat her again when he learns that she is pregnant. He doesn't believe that either of the other two children are his, even though Mrs. Rhodes says she has never been unfaithful to him. He tends to take his anger out on the older child, a 9-year-old boy, by yelling at him and telling him what a "piece of crap" he is. Mrs. Rhodes assures you that her husband has never physically abused either of the two children. Mrs. Rhodes tells you that she does not want to leave her husband because she still loves him and believes that he loves her. She does not want you to share the information she has given you with anyone, including the nurse midwife. What would you do in this situation?

Information about the neighborhood should also be obtained. Physical characteristics include the types of homes in the area, degree of industrialization, crime rate, and level of sanitation. Other important considerations include population density, common occupations of neighbors, availability of transportation, shopping facilities, health services, churches, schools, and recreational facilities. Each of these areas is assessed in relation to the specific needs of individual family members and of the family as a whole.

The community health nurse should note if there are any air, water, or noise pollution problems in the area that would increase the family's risks of disability and illness. It is important to determine what the sources of pollution are and the effects of pollution on the family.

After making this assessment, the community health nurse may want to question family members about perceptions of their environment. Does the family feel safe in this neighborhood? What are the hazards they perceive? Do they have an emergency plan if their safety should be jeopardized? Is the family aware of any existing pollutants in their neighborhood?

At the aggregate level, the community health nurse would obtain similar information about environmental conditions within the community. What is the proportion of unsafe housing in the community? What sources of pollution are present? What is the disaster potential in the community and how might a disaster affect resident families? The answers to these and other questions will give the community health nurse some idea of the environmental conditions that may be faced by families in general as well as those experienced by specific families.

Sociocultural Considerations

The sociocultural dimension of family health shares some of the influences of the psychological environment. For instance, relationships outside the family are the basis for a portion of personality development. Leadership ability of individual family members is developed in school and in cultural, social, and political organizations where family members have the opportunity to interact with others and to contribute to community endeavors. Family discussions of social, cultural, and political issues help to develop social awareness as children grow and encourage the children to become involved in community, county, state, and national politics or social movements. Areas for consideration in assessing the family's sociocultural dimension include family members' roles, religion, culture, social class and economic status, employment and occupational factors, and external resources.

Roles

One of the most interesting aspects of the sociocultural dimension is role enactment within families. *Roles* are socially expected behavior patterns that are determined by a person's position or status within a family. Each person in a family occupies several roles by virtue of his or her position. For example, the adult woman in a family typically has the roles of wife, mother, cook, and confidante. Roles can take two forms: formal and informal. *Formal roles* are expected sets of behaviors associated with family positions such as husband, wife, mother, father, and child. Examples of formal roles are those of breadwinner, homemaker, house repairman, chauffeur, child caretaker, financial manager, and cook. *Informal roles* are those expected behaviors not associated with a particular position. Informal roles influence the psychological dimension within the family by determining whether, how, and by whom emotional needs are met. Informal roles that may be present within any family group include the encourager, the harmonizer, the follower, the martyr, the scapegoat, the pioneer, the go-between, and the blamer. The nurse identifies the presence or absence of these and similar informal roles and examines their effects on family function and cohesiveness. Some informal family roles are described below.

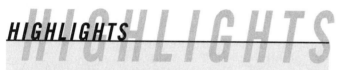

HIGHLIGHTS

Informal Family Roles

Encourager
Praises others and is able to draw others out and make them feel that their ideas are important

Harmonizer
Mediates differences by use of humor and smoothing over

Blocker
Tends to be negative to all ideas

Follower
Passively goes along with the group

Martyr
Wants nothing for self but sacrifices for the sake of others

Scapegoat
Identified problem member, serves as a safety valve, relieving family tensions

Pioneer
Moves the family into unknown territory and new experiences

Go-Between
Transmits and monitors communications among family members (often the mother)

Blamer
Fault finder and dictator

Next, the nurse may want to assess for evidence of role conflict. *Role conflict* occurs when the demands of a sin-

gle role are contradictory or when the demands attending several roles contradict or compete with each other. For example, a mother who works will experience role conflict when a business meeting she is expected to attend conflicts with her child's school play. Role conflict can also occur when one individual's definition of a role does not correspond with someone else's definition of the same role. For example, a husband may expect his wife to be responsible for all the cooking for the family, but the wife may work late and expect the husband to prepare an evening meal.

Role overload is another phenomenon that occurs in families when members assume multiple roles. *Role overload* occurs when an individual is confronted with too many role expectations at one time, even though these expectations do not contradict each other. For example, a mother with four children who returns to school and also has a part-time job may experience role overload in trying to meet the demands of housekeeping, cooking family meals, performing well on the job, and making straight As.

Flexibility of family roles and mutual respect for individuality are also considered in the assessment of the sociocultural dimension of family health. Family roles often change when a family member is absent, ill, or incapacitated and cannot fulfill his or her usual roles. It is important to assess the ability of family members to take on these unfilled roles and make the necessary role adjustments. When the ill or absent member is ready to resume roles, a readjustment may again be necessary. For example, when Frank had his heart attack, Beth had to go to work and assume the breadwinner role. Now Frank is recovered and can return to work. Beth likes her job and does not want to quit. Assistance in adjusting to changes in roles can alleviate conflict and stress in this and similar situations.

Role adjustments may also be required as the family progresses through its various developmental stages. For example, the parental role should be enacted differently with an adolescent child than with a preschooler. The nurse can assess the family's ability to adjust roles to the changing needs of its members and can also provide anticipatory guidance about adjustments that will be needed.

⑥THINK ABOUT IT

What formal and informal roles do you play in your family of origin? How have those roles changed over time?

Religion
The influence of religious beliefs and practices on the health of the family can be assessed by asking specific

questions about the importance of religion in family interactions and decision making and the role of religion for the family as a whole. For example, strong religious beliefs may prohibit the use of contraceptives, or health teaching may need to be modified in keeping with the family's religious convictions. Close affiliation with an organized church may also provide a source of emotional and/or material support for family members in time of need.

Culture

Family cultural information is an invaluable aid in building relationships and designing family interventions that will not conflict with cultural values. Does the family engage in cultural practices related to health? If so, are these practices helpful or harmful? What cultural factors will affect attempts to resolve family health problems? The nurse can compare the family's culture with that of the community in which they live and determine if there are differences present that may create problems for the family or the children of the family. Principles of cultural assessment, discussed in Chapter 6, are applicable to assessment of the social dimension of families.

Cultural factors may support or impede family abilities to adapt to changing environmental circumstances and may influence the health of individual members. For example, in one study, Korean immigrant women who worked were found to use two potential approaches to dealing with their role overload. Those who adhered to a traditional cultural expectation that the woman cares for home and children and attempted to work harder to do so experienced more depression than those women who abandoned the traditional role and negotiated with their husbands for help in these tasks (Um & Dancy, 1999).

Social Class and Economic Status

Social class delineations involve groupings of people based on financial status, race, occupation, education, lifestyle, and language. In America, the lower social class consists of people with less money, less education, and less access to resources such as health care.

The family's social class is important to the extent that it affects lifestyle, interactions with the external environment, and the structural and functional characteristics of the family. Economic status is closely tied to social class and education level. For instance, many single parents are members of lower socioeconomic groups, and most single-parent households are poor. The single female parent in many of these families either works outside the home or accepts welfare for economic support of her family. Often, the jobs available to such women are minimum-wage, menial jobs that allow some flexibility so they can care for their children. The single female parent often has no other adult to share in family decision making and must call on her children to carry out functions within the family that might have been her own if a male parent were present. The loss of Aid to Families with Dependent Children has forced many poor mothers to work, reducing their ability to provide reciprocal assistance with child care and other family supports previously available to them. This has been hypothesized to lead to the loss of support systems as providers of unreciprocated support attend to their own needs (Oliker, 2000).

The social class and economic status of a family can profoundly affect its health. Lack of financial resources can mean that the family does not have enough nutritious food, adequate shelter, or access to health care. The community health nurse can assess the family's social class and economic status and begin to make plans to assist the family through referral to community resources that will increase their access to food, better shelter, and health care.

Employment or Occupational Factors

Job-related factors that influence family health may present in three forms. First, the job might produce stress for the adult that results in illness. Second, the adult might be exposed to hazards that he or she brings home to other family members. Third, job-related problems and time constraints might interfere with family commitments.

Occupational or workplace stress can lead to a number of stress-related illnesses. Safety hazards within the work setting may cause injury and disability to the family breadwinner(s). The financial burden and stress of an occupation-related illness have led to divorce and the dissolution of families, among other problems. Similarly, job-related stress may lead to reduced energy for effective parenting and for maintaining the marital bond if one exists (Polatnick, 2000).

Sometimes, hazardous substances to which a working parent is exposed not only threaten the parent, but may also inadvertently be brought home to other family members. For example, nurses and other health care workers need to be aware that some infectious diseases may be transmitted to young children via clothing and shoes. Working with lead or other hazardous substances may also result in exposure of family members through contaminated clothing and other articles worn on the job (National Institute for Occupational Health and Safety, 2001).

Job-related family problems also might arise if a family member's work commitment conflicts with family commitments. Out of financial necessity, more parents are working, and they are working more hours than in the past. For example, in 1999, 72% of mothers with children under 18 years of age worked outside the home. Similarly, the average father now works approximately 50 hours a week and the average mother 41 hours per week, significantly reducing the time available for fulfilling parenting roles (Polatnick, 2000).

External Resources

To assist families in dealing with social environmental stressors, the community health nurse needs to identify external resources available to the family. External resources include those materials or sources of assistance available to the family from the community. The nurse's assessment of the family's external resources may suggest ways of dealing with identified health problems. Questions that elicit this information are those related to neighborhood sources of financial assistance, transportation, housing, health care, and education. The nurse should also investigate relational support systems such as kin networks, friends, and neighbors.

At the population level, the community health nurse should assess conditions that affect the social environment of families as well as the overall availability of social resources for families. What is the level of unemployment in the community? What is the availability of jobs, particularly for families with low education levels? What social and cultural attitudes prevalent in the population may affect family health and function? Similarly, the nurse would assess the resources available to families such as financial assistance, education for parenting, and so on.

Behavioral Considerations

The fifth area for consideration in family assessment using the dimensions model is family behavior. Areas of focus include family consumption patterns, rest and sleep patterns, exercise and leisure activities, and safety practices.

Family Consumption Patterns

A family's nutritional status can be assessed through physical assessment of each member and by observing the way in which the family selects, purchases, and prepares food. If any family members are nutritionally impaired, the nurse will need to determine the underlying causes. Is it lack of money to buy food? Does the person who prepares food lack information that would ensure good family nutrition? How is food prepared? Are cultural patterns evident in food selection, preparation, and consumption? For example, the excessive use of fried or high-fat foods sometimes seen among Latinos or families in the southern United States contributes to the increased incidence of atherosclerosis, heart disease, and stroke among members of these populations.

Other consumption patterns of interest to the nurse include the use of alcohol, drugs, medications, tobacco, and caffeine. Is the use of any of these substances causing a family member to be unable to carry out his or her role and functions within the family? Does the mother's smoking, for instance, aggravate her child's respiratory condition? Are prescription drugs being used as prescribed? Are any side effects evident from the use of prescription drugs? Are over-the-counter (OTC) products used appropriately? The answers to these and similar questions assist the nurse to identify problems arising from family consumption patterns. Similarly, aggregate-level data on consumption patterns, particularly those related to drugs and alcohol, can suggest problems that may be experienced by individual families.

Rest and Sleep

Family rest and sleep patterns may be a source of problems. For example, a new baby may sleep during the day and cry at night. This will adversely affect parents' rest and their subsequent performance the next day.

Another problem frequently encountered with respect to family sleep patterns is that of differing work schedules. If, for example, one parent works days and the other works nights, this situation may limit their opportunities to interact with each other and with their children. A parent's typical rest and sleep schedule may also require children to play at a neighbor's house during the day or find quiet pastimes at home.

Exercise and Leisure

Regular exercise is necessary for good health. The earlier children are included in such activities, the more likely they are to build lifetime habits of exercise. Exercise and leisure activities that include the entire family also promote cohesion. Assessment in this area includes consideration of the type and frequency of exercise engaged in by family members. At times, it is also helpful to plan leisure activities that are unique to certain members of the family. This allows for individuality among family members and promotes a balance between family togetherness and separateness that is needed for individual development. The nurse should explore whether there are exercise or leisure activities that include only the adults or only the children.

The nurse can also help the family to identify potential health risks involved in leisure activities. For example, are safety helmets worn by all family members on bike trips? What are the safety rules when the family goes swimming? Is a backyard pool covered when not in use to prevent a child from going in alone or falling in accidentally?

High costs and low income may limit the activities that families can do together, but should not eliminate them. The availability of low-cost recreational opportunities in the community is an area for assessment at the population level.

Household and Other Safety Practices

Safety practices such as use of seat belts, infant safety seats, cribs with safe spacing between rails and proper mattress width, proper disposal of hazardous substances, and safety education for children are important considerations in family assessment. Are these behavioral safety factors evident in the household? Who is the person most attentive to family safety issues? What family behaviors contribute to health risks for members? In assessing the behavioral dimension of family health, several safety practices should be considered; these considerations are presented on page 309.

HIGHLIGHTS

HIGHLIGHTS

Family Safety Assessment Considerations

- Consistent seat belt use
- Use of safety equipment such as eye and ear protection
- Use of infant safety seats
- Cribs with safe spacing between rails and proper mattress width
- Proper disposal of hazardous substances
- Safety education of children regarding not talking to or going with strangers, crossing the street safely, and using seat belts and safety equipment such as helmets, goggles, and ear protection
- Safe use of appliances and craft equipment such as saws, glues, and drills

Health System Considerations

Health system considerations in family assessment include the response of individual families to illness and their use of health services. At the aggregate level, assessment focuses on the availability and effectiveness of health services provided to families in the population.

Family Response to Illness

Assessing the biophysical, psychological, physical environmental, sociocultural, and behavioral dimension of health within families should give the nurse a general idea of family health and of the strategies family members use to remain healthy. But how do members deal with illness? Part of learning about this aspect of family life is determining who in the family decides when an ill family member should stay home from work or school and whether an ill member should receive health care. For example, in some families the mother decides who is ill and consults the father when she believes that the illness is severe enough to require the services of a health care provider. Family caregivers may themselves be in need of nursing intervention in order to function effectively in their caregiving role. Family care giving in chronic illness has been the subject of considerable research. A summary of one such study can be found on the companion Web site for this book.

In some families, home remedies or cultural health practices are used before consulting a health care provider. The community health nurse needs to assess if these practices are harmful to sick family members and whether to encourage the family to seek professional assistance. Chapter 6 provides more information on how the nurse can determine which cultural health practices may be harmful and how to help families choose other modes of care.

Use of Health Care Services

Accessibility, availability, and use of health care services by family members need to be assessed by the nurse. The community health nurse should explore how families deal with health problems. Family functions with respect to illness vary with the type of illness. For example, family functions in the case of acute illness include providing or obtaining health care, reassigning roles, and supporting the sick person. Additional functions in dealing with chronic illness include avoiding or coping with medical crises, preserving the family's quality of life, and arranging treatment modes and mechanisms. In the face of terminal illness, family functions also include dealing with shock and fear and minimizing pain and discomfort.

Do family members have a source of health care? Often, there may be providers available for mothers and children because of federal and state programs. Fathers and other young adult males, however, are often excluded from these programs. The nurse may be asked to help families find health care for excluded family members who become ill.

It is important to learn where family members go for health care and whether their choice provides any preventive health services or dental care. Many private medical doctors provide only sickness care, and families may need

Community health nurses should become familiar with services available to families in their areas.

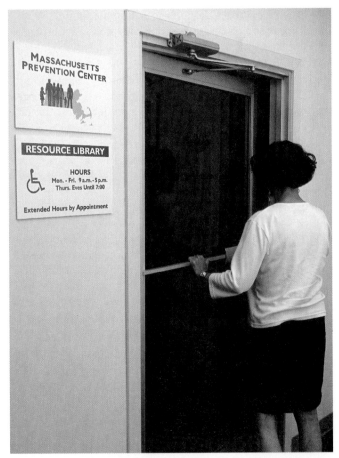

assessment tips assessment tips assessment tips

ASSESSING FAMILY HEALTH

Biophysical Considerations

- What is the age and gender composition of the family? How adequately have individual family members accomplished age-appropriate developmental tasks? Do individual family members' developmental stages create stress in the family?
- Do family members have any existing physical health conditions that are affecting the family? Is there a family history of genetic predisposition to disease?

Psychological Considerations

- What are the typical modes of communication in the family? How effective are family communication patterns? What areas are taboo in family communication?
- How cohesive is the family? Do family members exhibit close supportive relationships?
- How are decisions made in the family? By whom? Which family members have input into decisions? Who is responsible for carrying out family decisions?
- Who is the leader in the family? Does the leader use a leadership style appropriate to the age and abilities of other family members?
- Do family members express respect for each other?
- Is there evidence of violence within the family? What forms of discipline are used in the family? Is the discipline used appropriate?
- What emotional strengths does the family exhibit? How does the family deal with change? What coping strategies does the family use? How effective are these strategies? How well does the family deal with crisis?
- What are the family's goals? Do individual goals conflict or complement family goals? What values are reflected in the family's goals?

Physical Environmental Considerations

- Where does the family live? What is the physical condition of the home? Are there safety hazards in the home? Is plumbing adequate? Is the amount of space available adequate for the number of persons in the family? Does the family have an emergency plan?
- How safe is the neighborhood? Are there environmental hazards in the neighborhood?
- Does the family have access to necessary goods and services (e.g., grocery stores)?

Sociocultural Considerations

- What formal and informal roles are enacted by family members? How flexible and interchangeable are these roles? How congruent are family roles with those of the dominant culture? Is there evidence of role conflict? Role overload? How adequate were family role models? Are essential family roles being adequately performed? Are there expected changes in family roles? How will the family adapt to these changes?
- What cultural and religious factors influence family health status? What is the family's income? Is income sufficient to meet the family's needs?
- Are family members employed? What are the occupations of family members? Do occupational roles conflict with family roles?

Behavioral Considerations

- What are the food preferences and consumption patterns of the family? How are foods usually prepared? By whom?
- Do family members smoke, use alcohol, use other substances?
- What medications are used by family members? Is medication use appropriate? Are medications stored safely?
- Do family members get adequate rest and exercise?
- What kinds of leisure activities do family members engage in? Do leisure activities pose any health hazards?
- Do family members engage in appropriate safety precautions?
- Who in the family engages in sexual activity? Is there a need for contraceptives? What is the attitude of family members to sexual activity?

Health System Considerations

- How do family members deal with illness? Who makes health-related decisions in the family? Who carries out those decisions?
- What health-related behaviors do family members exhibit?
- What is the family's usual source of health care? Is the family's use of health care services appropriate? Does the family have health insurance? If so, are all family members covered? What services are covered?

CRITICAL THINKING IN RESEARCH

Medalie, Zyzanski, Langa, & Stange (1998) conducted a study of family physicians to determine the extent to which they actually provide a family focus to care. Their findings indicated that family physicians showed a high level of emphasis on families in one of two ways: use of a family history to focus care for individual clients or care for the family unit as a whole.

- What features of the physicians' practices do you think would differ based on their approach to inclusion of families in their practices? How might you go about testing your suppositions?
- What do you think the results of a similar study might be if you conducted it with different groups of nurses (e.g., nurses in neonatal intensive care units, oncology nurses, school nurses, etc.)? How might you go about conducting such a study?

information about where to go for preventive services such as immunizations, health teaching, and dental care.

Health care may be limited because of a lack of funds, language barriers, distance to health care facilities, transportation limitations, and many other problems. The nurse needs to determine these deterrents to access and find resources within the community to help families obtain health care.

Occasionally, even when families have health insurance, members are not able to take full advantage of this resource because they do not understand what services are covered (or not covered). The nurse can help them understand insurance benefits or refer families to resources in the community who can explain insurance benefits and how to use them.

At the aggregate level, the community health nurse should assess the availability of health services needed by families in the population. What illness-preventive and health-promotive services are available? Are they accessible to all families in the population or only to certain subgroups? What secondary and tertiary preventive services are available? How accessible are they to families in need of care? Tips for conducting an assessment of family health are presented on page 310. In addition, the companion Web site for this book provides an assessment tool that can be used by community health nurses to assess the health status of a specific family or families as an aggregate within the population.

DIAGNOSTIC REASONING AND CARE OF FAMILIES

The data obtained during family health assessment enable the nurse to make informed decisions about the health care needs of families. These needs are stated in the form of nursing diagnoses. The community health nurse may develop nursing diagnoses related to individual families or to families as a group within the larger population. For example, the nurse may diagnose "ineffective family coping due to changes in roles and relationships" in a newly constituted stepfamily. An example of an aggregate family nursing diagnosis might be "inadequate services for families experiencing chronic health problems in family members."

PLANNING AND IMPLEMENTING HEALTH CARE FOR FAMILIES

Based on nursing diagnoses derived from family health assessments, community health nurses plan nursing interventions to address identified needs. Again, these interventions may be directed toward improving the health of specific families or of all families within a population and may take place at the primary, secondary, and tertiary levels of prevention. Population level interventions will often involve the creation or expansion of an infrastructure that supports effective family function and provides services needed by families in the population (Meister, 1998). Links to resources for planning family care are provided on the companion Web site for this book.

Primary prevention for individual families may involve health promotion and protection or illness prevention. Teaching coping skills and modeling effective communication strategies with adolescents are two interventions that community health nurses might employ to prevent family crises. Similarly, the nurse may teach family members how to minimize lead exposure in residential areas with high levels of lead contamination in soil or water. At the aggregate level, primary preventive activities by community health nurses are more likely to be directed toward assuring the availability of health promotion and illness prevention services to families or toward environmental protection.

Secondary prevention activities with families may be aimed at assisting families to obtain needed care for existing health problems or helping families to deal with these problems. For example, the nurse might facilitate a family meeting to discuss role allocation in order to minimize role overload on a few family members. Similarly, the nurse might refer a family with a substance abusing member to community resources to help them deal with the problem.

THINK ABOUT IT

Why should community health nurses intervene to resolve families' socioeconomic problems as well as health problems?

Advocacy for secondary preventive services may be needed at the population level. The community health nurse may be actively involved in alerting health policy makers to the need for family services and in initiating plans for programs to meet those needs. For example, if the nurse's assessment indicates that most families in the population are dual-earner or single-parent families whose needs for child care services are not being met, he or she may initiate community efforts to provide additional child care resources.

With respect to tertiary prevention, community health nurses may assist families to cope with long-term health problems or to deal with the consequences of those problems. For example, a nurse might suggest home modifications that permit a disabled family member to be more functional within the family or help a family coping with Alzheimer's disease to locate respite care. Tertiary prevention activities at the aggregate level, on the other hand, might involve assisting the community to develop respite options for family care takers.

EVALUATING HEALTH CARE FOR FAMILIES

Evaluation begins as the nurse examines the adequacy of the assessment database and continues as he or she evaluates alternative approaches to meeting families' health care needs. Postintervention evaluation focuses on the achievement of objectives of family care and the processes and structures that promote accomplishment of these objectives.

Evaluation will occur at the level of individual families who receive care and at the population level. With respect to the care of individual families, the nurse would examine whether or not care has resulted in expected family outcomes. Is the family better able to cope with stress? Have communications between parents and adolescent children improved? The nurse would also assess the appropriateness of interventions employed and the quality of their implementation. Were the interventions appropriate to the family's cultural beliefs and practices? To family education level? Did the family experience frustration in following through on referrals because the nurse did not select appropriate resources or did not effectively prepare the family for acting on the referral?

At the aggregate level, evaluation will focus on outcomes and processes of care for groups of families rather than individual families. Is respite care readily available to families that need it? Is respite care provided in the most cost-effective manner? What are the effects of respite care on the level of stress experienced by families with disabled members? These and other questions can address outcome and process evaluation of programs designed to serve groups of families within the population.

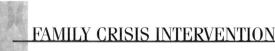

FAMILY CRISIS INTERVENTION

Family Stress

Stressful family life events and change are inevitable. Some families experience more stressful life events than do others and some are less able to cope with stress. Community health nurses can contribute much to families experiencing varying degrees of stress. In addition, community health nurses can offer anticipatory guidance based on an understanding of family development and stress theory that will assist families to prepare themselves for change and thus minimize stress.

Understanding stress theory enables the community health nurse to identify signs and symptoms of stress in families. It also helps the nurse to assist families experiencing stress whose methods of coping are inadequate to the situation. Stress theory is a scientific explanation for the physiologic and psychological effects of change on individuals or groups of people. Stress theory, in effect, states that any change, emotion, or activity that an individual or family experiences will cause stress. *Stress* is a nonspecific response to any demand that includes both physiologic and psychological components (Selye, 1978). This response is triggered by *stressors* or changes in the internal or external environment. When an individual or a family experiences stress, it may disrupt *homeostasis,* or balance. When this occurs, the individual or family attempts to adapt. *Adaptation* is a process of adjustment to change. Stress may be either positive or negative. Negative stress creates unpleasant effects and is called *distress.* If distress is extreme, the result may be disease in an individual or family dysfunction and disruption (Selye, 1978).

An example of family stress is the disruption of family homeostasis that occurs when a mother of four returns to work. This change has both positive and negative effects and necessitates other changes within the family. For example, the father may have to act as chauffeur for the children, cook occasional evening meals, or assist with other household chores. Another problem might be difficulty in obtaining adequate child care. The community health nurse can assess how the family is coping with the stress engendered by the mother's return to work and make suggestions to facilitate adaptation.

The experience of stress and successful adaptation to stressful events can be a growth-producing experience for the family. Families who learn together how to solve problems and adjust to stressors increase their resistance to the detrimental effects of future stress. Families who do not adapt well or ignore signs of distress are more likely to experience crisis.

Definition of Crisis

A family can view any situation as a crisis. What is a crisis for one family may not be a crisis for another.

Moreover, some families function and thrive on daily crises and would deteriorate if crisis situations were eliminated from their lives. Assessment and intervention, then, must be based on the family's perception of a crisis event.

A *crisis* occurs when a family faces a problem that is seemingly unsolvable. None of their methods of problem solving work. The problem becomes psychologically overwhelming, and anxiety and tension increase until the family becomes disorganized and unable to cope (Friedman, 1998). A crisis state is unlikely to be sustained for more than six weeks because it is difficult to endure the high stress and tension associated with crisis without breakdown or change. The result of a crisis can be either resolution, resulting in a healthier, more positive state of being, or loss of well-being and a higher potential for recurrent crisis. Temporary relief can be gained from the use of defense mechanisms, environmental action, or both. Resolution and more permanent relief and growth require appropriate coping mechanisms. During periods of crisis, families are more susceptible to change and are usually more open to help when it is offered. This receptivity affords the nurse the opportunity to produce change with very little intervention.

Types of Crises

There are two types of crises: maturational and situational. A *maturational crisis* is viewed as a "normal" transition point where old patterns of communication and old roles must be exchanged for new patterns and roles (Friedman, 1998). Every family experiences maturational crisis points, whether or not a crisis is actually experienced. Examples of transitional periods when maturational crises may occur are adolescence, marriage, parenthood, and one's first job. Such periods in life are usually predictable, so families can be prepared to use coping mechanisms that assist them through each transition period.

All the transitional periods experienced by families have in common a change in roles or the addition of new roles, and crises occur when a family is unable or unwilling to accept new roles. There may be a history of poor role modeling from parents that leaves children unprepared for new roles and unable to leave home successfully. There may be family members who are unable or unwilling to view one member in a new role. For example, it is sometimes difficult for parents to acknowledge that their teenage children need to make decisions for themselves.

A *situational crisis* can occur when the family experiences an event that is sudden, unexpected, and unpredictable. Such events threaten either biological, psychological, or social integrity leading to disorganization, tension, and severe anxiety. Examples include illness, accidents, death, and natural disasters.

Some crises may arise that contain elements of both situational and maturational crisis events. For example, a female may be going through the maturational transition of adolescence and encounter the situational crisis of an unwanted pregnancy. The multiplicity of crisis events further impairs the family's ability to cope.

Factors That Increase Susceptibility to Crisis

Why do some families go into crisis while others do not? Four categories of factors seem to play a part in determining whether or not a crisis will occur. These factors relate to (a) the stressor itself and the family's perceptions of the stressor, (b) other stressors impinging on the family, (c) family coping ability, and (d) the extent of family resources. Factors related to the stressor and how it is perceived by the family include the extent of the impact of the stressor on the family and the severity of that impact, the duration of the stressor and whether its onset was sudden or gradual, and the degree of perceived control the family has over the stressor. A stressor that is perceived as manageable is less likely to cause a crisis situation than one that is seen as uncontrollable. The cause and predictability of the stressor may also influence the occurrence of crisis. Stressors with unknown causes or unpredictable effects create greater anxiety and greater potential for crisis.

The family's perception of the stressor may be distorted by previous experience with crises that were not growth producing. For example, there are crisis-prone families who have a chronic inability to perceive or solve existing problems. Their inability to cope with problems results in an exaggerated response to new changes, and crises occur for them that would be averted by other families.

The extent of other concurrent stressors affecting the family may also be a determining factor in the development of a crisis. Multiple stressors may have additive effects that precipitate crises. As noted earlier, maturational and situational crises may occur simultaneously stretching family coping abilities beyond their limits. Existing family problems such as illness, unemployment, and marital strife, may make a seemingly minor stressor a precipitating factor in a crisis. Situational demands created by the stressor may also increase the potential for crisis. Unfortunately, situational demands created by the health care system may enhance the potential for crisis. For example, the illness of a child is a stressor; if taking the child to the clinic necessitates losing work time and money, this creates an additional burden for the family.

The family's coping mechanisms represent internal family resources important to crisis resolution. Among these resources are cohesion or closeness among family members, open communication, use of humor, control of the meaning of the problem, and role flexibility. The family's ability to cope lessens the impact of any crisis event. It is important to assess what degree of success has been achieved using these mechanisms in the past and whether the family is aware of the mechanisms used.

Situational support arises from external resources such as the extended family, community agencies, churches, neighbors, and friends of the family. The degree of security felt by family members in relationships with these support systems may be sufficient to avert crises.

Structure of a Crisis Event

In every crisis there are contributing factors that culminate in the crisis event. A hazardous incident or stressor of some sort triggers the sequence of events (Bomar & Cooper, 1996). Hazardous situations can arise from human biology as a result of aging, genetic factors, or illness; from the physical environmental, psychological, or sociocultural dimensions; as a result of behavior patterns such as drug or alcohol use; or from health care system problems such as lack of affordable medical care.

The hazardous situation is usually stressful and causes anxiety. The family experiences a reaction to the event characterized by depression or anger. Family members may use defense mechanisms, such as denial, to ease their discomfort before beginning to use coping mechanisms that help them deal constructively with the situation.

A precipitating event might occur that throws the family into acute anxiety and crisis. This event may be seemingly minor, but serves to tip the scales toward crisis. It overtakes coping mechanisms already stretched to the limits. For example, a father's unemployment is a hazardous event that makes the family vulnerable to crisis. Because of the mother's job and other supports, members are not yet in crisis. Then the car breaks down! This last event is perceived by the family as overwhelming and pushes members beyond their ability to cope. A crisis has occurred.

When coping mechanisms fail, the family resorts to different strategies. One person may laugh or cry a great deal; another might withdraw. Finally, the family is in full crisis, evidenced by inappropriate behavior and painful, stressful feelings. During this time they are unable to focus or concentrate and need clear, direct, precise direction. Figure 14–5 ■ depicts the structure of a crisis event.

ASSESSING THE CRISIS SITUATION

Interviewing during a crisis requires empathy, a calm demeanor, and a sensitivity to feeling tones that may not be readily apparent to others. Nondirective techniques are used. Inquiries and instructions need to be precise, concrete, and simple; a family in crisis is unable to focus and narrow the field to what must be done. Open-ended statements are used to encourage family members to speak spontaneously.

Human biological factors such as aging, genetic factors, and illness can contribute to the crisis. For example, an older couple has become unable to care for them-

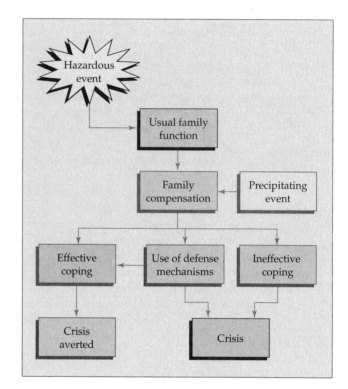

FIGURE 14–5 ■ *Structure of a Crisis Event*

selves adequately in their own home. None of their grown children has room to accommodate them and they are forced to move to an assisted living facility. This change in living arrangements may precipitate a crisis for the couple depending upon how they perceive the move. Finding the resources to pay for their care might also constitute a crisis either for the couple or for other family members.

As noted earlier, elements of the psychological dimension may also precipitate crises. For example, repeated episodes of depression leading to a family member's attempted suicide may result in a family crisis. Psychological factors also influence families' abilities to respond effectively to crises. The initial step in assessing a crisis situation is to review the events leading to the crisis. This gives family members a chance to discuss their perceptions of the event and affords the nurse an opportunity to assess perceptions, defense mechanisms, and coping strategies. A detailed history is not necessary. Just let them talk.

The nurse should determine if the family has ever experienced a similar event and how the family has reacted in the past. Past successful coping can be used to reassure members that they can cope with the current problem as well. Discussion of past events can be used to identify patterns that were not successful, and plans can be made to use alternative coping mechanisms. A major concern during a crisis is the potential for physical danger to family members. Individual family members must be assessed for suicidal or homicidal tendencies. If there are indications that a family member is contemplating

assessment tips assessment tips assessment tips

ASSESSING A CRISIS SITUATION

- What biophysical, psychological, physical environmental, sociocultural, behavioral, and health system factors are influencing the crisis situation? What is the hazardous situation facing the family? What was the precipitating factor in the crisis?

- What are the perceptions of family members regarding the crisis situation? What is the emotional response of family members to the crisis? Is there potential for harm to family members (e.g., homicide or suicide)?

- What defense mechanisms and coping strategies has the family employed? What effects have these strategies had?

- What internal and external sources of support are available to the family?

- What options for action are available to the family? What are the advantages and disadvantages of available options? To what extent are family members aware of available options?

violence to oneself or to others, immediate referral for psychiatric help is warranted. Assessment considerations related to suicide and homicide are discussed in more detail in Chapter 32.

When family members have had an opportunity to discuss the situation and are emotionally open to exploring solutions, an assessment can be made of external resources arising from the social environment. The nurse can determine if there are extended family members nearby, agencies that have been helpful for the family in the past, clergy, church members, or friends that the family want near them now.

Sometimes, sociocultural dimension factors such as unemployment, racial discrimination, and poverty can contribute to a crisis. For example, Mr. Lloyd's son needs surgery so he can walk. Arrangements were made but had to be canceled when Mr. Lloyd lost his job and his health insurance benefits. In this case, the community health nurse may want to determine whether an agency is available that can help the family to obtain the care their son needs.

Behavioral factors such as alcohol or drug use can constitute the hazardous event, be a precipitating event, or act as a defense mechanism for a family experiencing crisis. Alcohol and drug abuse can also impair a family's response to maturational and situational crises. The nurse must be alert to any evidence of alcohol or drug abuse and assist the family in seeking and obtaining assistance.

Assessment of health system considerations includes determining whether the family has insurance coverage for counseling, emergency care, or hospitalization should these be required to deal with the crisis. Counseling and medical services for potentially suicidal family members, accident victims, or members with drug and alcohol problems often must be sought for families that do not have any insurance or money. Identifying local, county, and state resources for families in need is an important responsibility for the community health nurse.

DIAGNOSTIC REASONING AND FAMILY CRISIS

Often, diagnostic reasoning and planning for crisis intervention occur at the same time. Working with families in crisis requires expertise in quickly determining family needs, knowledge of resources available that can be used spontaneously or with very little delay, and ability to teach problem solving. The primary diagnosis with a specific family experiencing crisis will relate to the existence of a crisis and the contributing factors involved. Using the example of the Lloyd family, the nurse might diagnose "family crisis due to father's unemployment and inability to pay for medical care necessitated by son's illness." Community health nurses may also derive nursing diagnoses related to family crisis at the population level. An example of such a diagnosis might be "lack of available crisis intervention services for low-income families."

INTERVENING IN A FAMILY CRISIS

Intervention in a crisis situation is guided by several general principles. First, the nurse should listen actively and with concern to family members' perceptions of and feelings about the event. Based on this assessment, the nurse can determine if immediate intervention is needed. Second, the nurse should encourage open expression of feelings and help the family gain an understanding of the crisis event. The nurse should also help the family accept reality and explore new ways of coping with problems presented by the crisis situation. The nurse may also need to link family members with a social network that can assist them to deal with the crisis. The community health nurse also engages in problem solving with the family and reinforces new coping strategies. Finally, the nurse needs to follow up with the family after the crisis has been resolved to engage in primary prevention for future crisis events. These principles are summarized below.

HIGHLIGHTS

General Principles of Crisis Intervention

- Listen actively.
- Encourage family members to verbalize their perceptions of the crisis situation and the emotions experienced.
- Encourage family acceptance of reality.
- Focus on development of effective coping skills.
- Develop social support systems to assist in crisis resolution.
- Assist the family in problem solving.
- Reinforce new, more effective coping strategies.
- Follow up to prevent future crises.

Crisis intervention focuses on secondary prevention and is directed toward helping members to discuss and define the problem and to express their feelings concerning the crisis situation. The nurse is an active listener and participates attentively, but the family must do the work. The emphasis is on bringing feelings out into the open. The nurse must be truthful, honest, and forthright, and should not give false reassurance about the situation.

It is important at this stage not to let the family's anxiety become contagious. If the nurse begins to experience anxiety, she or he should step back and attempt to regain perspective.

Exploration of coping mechanisms already used enables the nurse to help the family examine ways to cope. The nurse's involvement includes helping the family to explore other options for dealing with the situation. The pros and cons of each of these alternatives should be discussed with the family. At this stage, the nurse may need to be fairly directive in assisting family members to implement agreed-upon strategies for resolving the crisis. For example, if the family has decided to confront a substance abusing member with the need for treatment, the nurse may need to assign specific tasks to certain family members to implement the confrontation. She or he might have the wife obtain information on substance abuse treatment options under their insurance plan and assist the husband in determining how he will approach the problem with his substance abusing daughter. Following successful resolution of a crisis, the community health nurse should follow up with

the family to help them recognize their use of the problem-solving process, identify how the crisis might have been averted if possible, and engage in activities that will prevent future crises from occurring.

IMPLEMENTING PRIMARY PREVENTION TO AVERT CRISIS

Primary crisis prevention techniques are widely used by community health nurses because all families experience crises. Primary prevention includes providing anticipatory guidance related to common crises of family life and assisting families to develop effective coping strategies to combat the stress of situational crises.

It is impossible, and sometimes undesirable, to prevent a crisis situation from occurring; however, the nurse can assist the family to prepare for and cope with the event. For example, the birth of a child or change of employment may be a very desirable event. Such an event requires changes in lifestyle and family adaptation that might precipitate a crisis. The nurse can assist the family to explore areas in which change will be required, avenues for accomplishing these changes, and strategies for dealing with the anxiety related to change. Through primary prevention implemented via anticipatory guidance, a potential crisis may be averted even though the stressful event takes place.

EVALUATING CRISIS INTERVENTION

The evaluation process in crisis intervention is continuous as the nurse assesses the family's progress through the crisis event. More formal evaluation may also be conducted to review the entire process of intervention with the family. This includes systematic review of the crisis, the coping mechanisms used (old and new), and the result achieved. The emphasis is on reinforcing learning and strengthening the family for future crises.

Much of the work of community health nurses involves care of families in a variety of health care delivery settings. Family care should be based on the principles presented in this chapter and should contribute to the improvement of the overall health status of the population in which the family lives. Use of the nursing process in the context of community-focused care permits community health nurses to meet the health needs of family clients as well as those of the larger community.

APPLYING YOUR KNOWLEDGE IN PRACTICE

❧ CASE STUDY
A Family in Need

Alfinia Michaels is a 45-year-old single parent of two children, a boy of eight years and a girl of five. She has recently been diagnosed as having breast cancer and is scheduled to have a lumpectomy and reconstruction of her right breast in two weeks. Ms. Michaels is divorced and is responsible for the care of her 79-year-old father who has mild Alzheimer's disease. Her father is still capable of caring for himself during the day while she works, but cannot be left alone overnight and cannot care for the children. Ms. Michaels has one sister who lives approximately 150 miles away. She states that she and her sister have always been close. Ms. Michaels's former husband lives in the same community. He provides child support and health insurance for the children and takes them every other weekend. Ms. Michaels does not have health insurance because she works two part-time jobs, neither of which includes benefits. She tells the community health nurse she doesn't have any idea how she will pay for her surgery and the chemotherapy that will follow. She is worried about care of her father and her children during her hospitalization and afterwards.

- What biophysical, psychological, physical environmental, sociocultural, behavioral, and health system factors are influencing this situation?
- Is this a crisis situation? If so, what type of crisis would this be?
- What nursing interventions might the community health nurse employ with this family?
- How could the nurse evaluate the effectiveness of nursing intervention?

❧ TESTING YOUR UNDERSTANDING

- List at least five different types of families. What are the characteristic features of each type? (pp. 292–293)
- What are the basic components of family structure? What are the five major functions performed by families? Give some examples of how family structure might influence the ability to effectively perform family functions. (p. 299)
- What are the basic concepts of systems theory? How are these concepts applied to families? (pp. 294–297)
- How do Duvall's and Carter and McGoldrick's stages of family development differ? How are they similar? (pp. 297–299)
- Describe four considerations to be addressed in assessing family communication patterns. How might each influence family health? (pp. 301–303)
- What are the two central themes in assessing patterns of family dynamics? Give an example of the influence of each on family health status. (p. 303)
- How do formal family roles differ from informal roles? Give an example of each type of role. (pp. 305–306)
- Define stress, distress, homeostasis, and adaptation. Give an example of each. (p. 312)
- Give two examples of family stressors. (p. 312)
- How does a maturational crisis differ from a situational crisis? Give an example of each type of crisis. (p. 313)
- Describe the structure of a crisis event. Identify points at which nursing intervention could occur. (p. 314)
- Identify at least four principles of crisis intervention. How might the nurse employ each principle in working with families experiencing crises? (pp. 315–316)

REFERENCES

Astedt-Kurki, P., Hopia, H., & Vuori, A. (1999). Family health in everyday life: A qualitative study on well-being in families with children. *Journal of Advanced Nursing, 29,* 704–711.

Bomar, P., & Cooper, S. (1996). Family stress. In P. Bomar (Ed.), *Nurses and family health assessment: Concepts, assessment, and intervention* (2nd ed.) (pp. 121–138). Philadelphia: Saunders.

Carter, B., & McGoldrick, M. (1999). Overview: The expanded family life cycle: Individual, family, and social perspectives. In B. Carter & M. McGoldrick (Eds.), *The expanded family, life cycle: Individual, family and social perspectives* (3rd ed.) (pp. 1–26). Boston: Allyn & Bacon.

Duvall, E., & Miller, B. (1990). *Marriage and family development* (6th ed.). New York: Harper College.

Elkind, D. (1995). The family in the postmodern world. *National Forum, 75*(3), 24–28.

Fischer, L. (2000). Commentary. In B. D. Poland, L. W. Green, & I. Rootman (Eds.), *Settings for health promotion: Linking theory and practice* (pp. 67–76). Thousand Oaks, CA: Sage.

Friedman, M. M. (1998). *Family nursing: Research, theory, and practice* (4th ed.). Stamford, CT: Appleton & Lange.

Medalie, J. H., Zyzanski, S. J., Langa, D., & Stange, K. C. (1998). The family in family practice: Is it a reality? *Journal of Family Practice, 46,* 390–396.

Meister, S. B. (1998). Community infrastructures: Principles and strategies for improving child health services. In M. E. Broome, K. Knafl, K. Pridham, & S. Feetham (Eds.), *Children and families in health and illness* (pp. 268–279). Thousand Oaks, CA: Sage.

National Institute for Occupational Health and Safety. (2001). Occupational and take-home lead poisoning associated with restoring chemically stripped furniture — California, 1998. *Morbidity and Mortality Weekly Report, 50,* 246–248.

Oliker, S. (2000). Family care after welfare ends. *National Forum, 80*(3), 29–33.

Polatnick, M. R. (2000). Working parents. *National Forum, 80*(6), 38–41.

Richards, B. S. (1996). Gerontological family nursing. In S. M. H. Hanson & S. T. Boyd (Eds.), *Family health care nursing: Theory, practice, and research* (pp. 329–348). Philadelphia: Davis.

Roth, P. (1996). Family social support. In P. Bomar (Ed.), *Nurses and family health assessment: Concepts, assessment, and intervention* (2nd ed.) (pp. 107–120). Philadelphia: Saunders.

Selye, H. (1978). *The stress of life* (2nd ed.). New York: McGraw-Hill.

Soubhi, H., & Potvin, L. (2000). Homes and families as health promotion settings. In B. D. Poland, L. W. Green, & I. Rootman (Eds.), *Settings for health promotion: Linking theory and practice* (pp. 44–67). Thousand Oaks, CA: Sage.

Um, C. C., & Dancy, B. L. (1999). Relationship between coping strategies and depression among employed Korean immigrant wives. *Issues in Mental Health Nursing, 20,* 485–494.

U.S. Census Bureau. (1999). *Statistical abstract of the United States* (119th ed.). Washington, DC: Author.

von Bertalanffy, L. (1973). *General systems theory.* New York: George Braziller.

von Bertalanffy, L. (1981). *A systems view of man.* Boulder, CO: Westview.

Wilson, J. H., & Hobbs, H. (1999). The family educator. *Journal of Psychosocial Nursing and Mental Health Services, 37*(6), 22–27.

Wright, L. M., & Leahey, M. (2000). *Nurses and families: A guide to family assessment and intervention* (3rd ed.). Philadelphia: Davis.

CARE OF COMMUNITIES

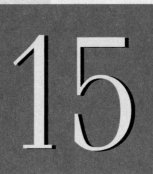

15

Chapter Objectives

After reading this chapter, you should be able to:

- Discuss the rationale for including community members in every phase of community assessment and health program planning.
- Describe at least three factors that influence the scope of a community or target group assessment.
- Describe factors in each of the six dimensions of health to be considered in assessing a target group or a community.
- Describe two levels of community nursing diagnoses related to the health status of a community or target group.
- Identify interventions at the primary, secondary, and tertiary levels of prevention that will influence the health of communities or target groups.
- Describe at least three considerations in planning screening programs for communities and target groups.
- Identify at least six tasks in planning health programs to meet the needs of communities or target groups.
- Describe three levels of acceptance of a health care program.
- Describe three types of considerations in evaluating a health care program.

Media Link

http://www.prenhall.com/clark

Additional interactive resources for this chapter can be found on the companion Web site. Click on Chapter 15 and "Begin" to select the activities for this chapter.

As noted several times in earlier chapters, the focus of community health nursing is on the health of population groups. In many instances, this focus entails providing care to whole communities or to target groups within communities. A *target group* is a subgroup within the community whose members exhibit particular health needs (such as victims of family violence) or are at particular risk for the development of problems (e.g., members of refugee groups).

In the past, interventions for such population groups frequently entailed health professionals' identification of problems and development and implementation of programs to solve them with minimal input from group members. More recently, health professionals have advocated the involvement of community members in all stages of intervention, from participation in identifying community needs and capabilities to the development, implementation, and evaluation of programs that enhance local capacity to meet those needs.

ORGANIZING FOR COMMUNITY INTERVENTION

The incorporation of community or target group members in health assessment and programming necessitates a certain level of community development or community organization. Achieving this level of development may be one of the first tasks of community health nurses and others working with population groups. Generally, there are four stages of nursing involvement with communities that facilitate community development (Moyer, Coristine, MacLean, & Mechthild, 1999). These stages are summarized below.

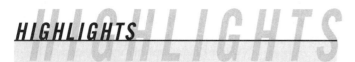

HIGHLIGHTS

Stages of Community Involvement

- *Identifying common ground:* Becoming acquainted with community organizations and their agendas, resources, and capabilities to identify the potential for collaborative action.
- *Establishing oneself as a community player:* Establishing one's presence in the community by engaging in cooperative activities that meet a common need but are not jointly planned.
- *Working on a common project:* Developing a joint initiative with other groups or agencies in the community.
- *Working on a multiagency, multisectoral project:* Collaborating in a joint community project that engages multiple partners from different sectors of the community.

Source: Moyer, A., Coristine, M., MacLean, L., & Mechthild, M. (1999). A model for building collective capacity in community-based programs: The elderly in need project. *Public Health Nursing, 4,* 247–256.

Once the nurse has begun the process of engaging with the community embodied in the stages of community involvement, he or she can begin to work on community development or community organization around health issues. The goal of community development is to develop community competence, which is characterized by four capabilities including abilities to (a) collaborate in needs identification, (b) agree on goals and priorities, (c) agree on means to achieve goals, and (d) collaborate in interventions required to accomplish group goals (Rissel & Bracht, 1999).

Community organization is defined as a planned process of community activation directed toward the use of available resources to accomplish community-identified goals consistent with community values. Community organization or community development occurs in stages similar to those of the nursing process that include assessment, design and initiation of an action plan, implementation, maintenance and consolidation, and dissemination and reassessment (Bracht, Kingsbury, & Rissel, 1999). These stages will be discussed in the context of the comparable stage of the nursing process later in this chapter.

Community development involves active participation by community members and is guided by several general principles. These principles include the following:

- Unless there is concerted effort to reach hidden groups within the community, only the more advantaged community members will participate.
- The extent of community participation will vary in different stages of community development.
- Complete community representation on steering committees is not necessary, and steering committee members may be selected on the basis of the expertise or perspective they bring to a particular project (Jewkes, 2000).

ASSESSING COMMUNITY HEALTH

In the past, a number of different approaches have been taken to assess the health needs of communities. These include an epidemiologic approach, which focused on trends in the incidence and prevalence of specific health conditions and risk factors, and a socioeconomic approach focused on social and economic features of a community and their effects on health. Another approach used is the behavioral approach, which emphasizes assessment of individual lifestyle behaviors and attitudes and the associated disease risks. More recently, however, emphasis has been placed on a community participation approach in which the community identifies for itself the health needs and issues to be addressed (Lawton, 1999). Participatory or *community-based research* is research in which community members are involved in all facets of the research process, from delineation of the research problem through data collection and analysis to use of findings (Israel, Schultz, Parker, & Becker, 1998).

⑥THINK ABOUT IT

What would be some of the advantages of involving community members in the assessment of community health needs? What challenges can you see to their inclusion as members of the assessment team?

In addition to the incorporation of community members in the community assessment process, there has been a concomitant shift away from a focus on needs or problems to a greater focus on community assets or capabilities (Sharpe, Greaney, Lee, & Royce, 2000). Traditional community assessments have focused on needs, problems, barriers, and community weaknesses and are "deficit based." Deficit-based needs assessments lead to fragmented approaches to community action and create the impression that only outside "experts" are capable of solving community health problems. Assets-based assessments, on the other hand, focus on the individual, organizational, and institutional resources available within the community and foster community capacity to deal with identified health needs (Ammerman & Parks, 1998). Community health nurses focusing on communities as clients should incorporate both the assets and deficits perspectives of community assessment, assisting the community to develop a complete picture of its health needs and the assets and resources available to meet those needs.

Community assessment is the process by which data are compiled regarding a community's health status and resources and from which nursing diagnoses are derived. An accurate assessment is the basis of any community health endeavor and is essential to planning any program designed to meet health-related needs. Community or target group assessment provides a *health index*, a summary of a population's health status, which serves as a basis for planning to meet health care needs. Without a clear picture of the health status of the community or target group, health care providers have no way of determining whether current programs meet health needs or how to plan programs that will.

Preparing to Assess the Health of a Community or Target Group

Community participation in needs and assets assessment is a form of community-based research in which community members are involved in all phases of the assessment (Israel et al., 1998). Selection of representative community members to participate in the assessment and

determination of their roles in the process are key features of community involvement. There needs to be a broad-based representation of different segments of the community that includes both members of community organizations who are familiar with the community and its needs and assets and grassroots community advocates who are not affiliated with any agency or organization. The inclusion of grassroots community members offsets the adherence to organizational agendas that may be displayed by members of specific agencies and provides a more comprehensive and balanced picture of the community (Kone, Sullivan, Senturia, Chrisman, Ciske, & Frieger, 2000).

Factors that facilitate collaborative effort between community members and the community health nurse researcher include joint development of operating procedures and joint determination of various aspects of the assessment. The role of the community health nurse in a participatory community assessment is generally one of education and facilitation. The nurse may need to educate community members regarding potential data sources and collection methods, data analysis, and data interpretation. The nurse may also serve as a coordinator for assessment team activities. A summary of an article describing a participatory community-based study is available on the companion Web site for this book.

The first step in preparing for a community assessment is to clarify the purpose and scope of the assessment. Other preparatory activities include determining the types of data to be collected, sources of data, and methods for data collection, organization, and analysis. The purpose for assessing a target group or community determines the types of data to be collected as well as the scope of the assessment. Community or group needs assessment may be conducted for a variety of reasons. For example, one may demonstrate the need for a specific kind of program to justify program funding, or fulfill a legal mandate to identify the health care needs of a community. Assessments may also be used as a basis for resource allocation decisions or to identify the needs of certain underserved segments of the population. Community members use the data derived from a community needs assessment to develop diagnoses and to plan, implement, and evaluate programs designed to promote health and resolve existing health problems through the use of available community resources.

The scope, or depth and complexity, of a community or target group assessment depends on a number of factors. First, if the purpose of the assessment is to determine the group's health status, the assessment needs to be much more extensive than if the purpose is to obtain additional data about a known problem. Second, the size of the population also affects the assessment. A small target group can be assessed in greater depth than a whole community for the same expenditure of money and effort. Third, the time available for the assessment may limit its scope. If information is required within a specified period, the assessment team may be limited in the depth of assessment possible. The degree of expertise of those conducting the assessment and the relationship between the cost and the perceived benefits of an in-depth assessment may be additional limiting factors. Finally, the political environment within the community may affect the comprehensiveness of any assessment. If policy makers or group members do not place a high priority on health, they are unlikely to support an extensive assessment of health needs.

When the scope of an assessment is limited, the assessment team needs to decide what categories of data are already available and what additional data are needed to accomplish the purpose of the assessment. In this chapter, the focus is on categories of data that would be collected in a comprehensive assessment of a community or a target group. In an assessment of lesser scope, the community health nurse and community members must determine what categories of data are essential to accomplish the purpose of the assessment and what information may safely be left out.

Usually, a variety of methods are used to collect the data. Both quantitative and qualitative approaches should be used to assess the health status and resources of communities or target groups. *Quantitative* approaches involve the collection of numbers of events. *Qualitative* approaches focus on examination of perceptions of health, attitudes, and health concerns as voiced by members of the population. For example, in obtaining information on the use of health care services by group members, quantitative methods would be used to gather data on the numbers of people who received care at various facilities; group members' perceptions of health care services and their reasons for using or not using them would be more easily obtained using qualitative methods of data collection.

Quantitative data may be obtained by reviewing statistics compiled by health care agencies and other sources at the local, state, and national levels. For example, the assessment team might obtain information on the racial composition of a community from published census figures or on the incidence of child abuse from records kept by child protection agencies or law enforcement officials. Newspaper reports are a source of quantitative data about injuries, crime, and residential fires. It has been noted that news stories often contain more detailed information about such incidents than official reports. The assessment team might also obtain quantitative data by conducting surveys and compiling figures on the frequency of certain responses. For example, community members might ask a sample of elderly persons how often they see a physician.

Quantitative data can also be obtained through observation. For example, one way the adequacy of protective services in a community could be assessed is to determine the location of fire stations. Assessment team members might drive through the community, note each fire station on a map, and then calculate the maximum distance from a fire station of any point in the community.

Surveys and observations can also provide qualitative data about a community or target group. Community or group members can be asked about their attitudes toward health and health care services or about their perceptions of community health needs. Qualitative data can also reflect community leadership and the readiness of a community for change. Because people's opinions and perceptions vary greatly, a diversity of community members should be approached for information. Such diversity is particularly evident in comparing opinions of residents in a community and those of health care providers in the area.

Community members might also interview members of the community and key informants. *Key informants* are people who, because of their position in the community, possess information and insights about the community. Key informants include both formal and informal community leaders. Examples of key informants include public officials, school and health care personnel, prominent businesspeople, and local clergy. Again, it is important not to restrict interviews to these sources, but also to interview typical residents of the community because of the possible differences in perceptions of the community's health needs.

Asset mapping is another means of collecting data about a community, particularly regarding its resources. *Asset maps* are geographic maps of the community indicating the location of specific community assets. A community assessment may involve the development of several asset maps, each related to a different type of community resources. For example, one asset map might indicate the location and types of educational resources available in the community, while another identifies agencies and organizations providing health care services. In addition to asset maps, community members engaged in community assessment may conduct capacity inventories that catalog the skills, expertise, and capabilities of individual community members and community organizations (Sharpe et al., 2000).

Different methods of data collection are appropriate to different types of information. Appropriate methods for gathering specific data needed to assess the health of communities or target groups are addressed later in this chapter.

Where does one find the information needed for a community or target group assessment? Before beginning an assessment, community members can usually identify several potential sources. Additional sources are usually uncovered during the course of the assessment, but the group needs an identified starting point for data collection.

A community or target group is assessed using data from many sources. Usually, the local chamber of commerce can supply information regarding community size, history, industry, and facilities for transportation, communication, and recreation. Information about many population characteristics such as age, sex, race and language, income and education levels, employment, and marital status can be obtained from the most recent census figures, as can some statistics related to housing. Similar information related to a particular target group may be less easy to find unless the group is one that is of interest to government officials or other agencies that gather statistics. For example, information about people with certain types of cancer might be available from a local cancer registry, while information about older persons could be obtained from the local office on aging.

Basic data from the most recent census may be found in public and university libraries. Updated data and information collected for special projects is also available online at the Census Bureau Web site (*http://www.census.gov*) and from the online version of *Statistical Abstract of the United States* (http://www.census.gov/statab).

Local school systems are good sources of information regarding the availability of education facilities and immunization levels. Various religious groups in the community can be identified in the yellow pages of the telephone directory; further information on religious affiliation can be sought from local houses of worship. Some local information in this area may also be available through an Internet search.

The yellow pages and the Internet may also list health care services and resources, transportation, and formal communication networks. In some communities, local agencies compile lists of referral resources for a variety of health-related services. A local Headstart program, for example, is required by federal standards to provide this type of information to parents of children enrolled.

Information about protective services can be obtained from the local government or police and fire departments. Statements of the adequacy of services can be validated in interviews with members of the community or target group or with insurance company representatives. The local health department can provide statistics related to births, deaths, and morbidity, as well as data on the availability and use of health resources and services. Information on water supply and waste disposal can also usually be obtained from health department sources.

Local government officials can provide information on the priority given to health care programs in the budget. Many industries provide some forms of health care services and would also have records of expenditures of this nature, as would insurance companies. Local voluntary and official health care agencies can also be sources of information on health care financing (see Chapter 22).

Area maps define the size of a community and the presence or absence of recreational facilities. Maps also show thoroughfares that link the community with other areas.

Other possible sources of organized data include the local hospital association, local chapters of professional and business organizations, and voluntary agencies, such as the American Diabetes Association. Key persons in the community, both official and unofficial, can provide information as well. Specific sources of information are addressed later in this chapter in relation to the categories

of data that constitute a community or target group assessment. General sources of qualitative and quantitative assessment data are listed in Table 15–1 ■.

For some types of information, however, no records are available. Such information must be obtained by the assessment team through personal observation and through contact with other members of the community or target group. Community attitudes toward health are one example of this type of data. Figures on the use of

■ **TABLE 15–1**   **Sources of Community Assessment Data**

TYPE OF DATA	SOURCE	EXAMPLE
Quantitative	Census figures	Age composition of population
		Racial composition of population
	Local agencies	Child abuse incidence figures from child protective services
		Diabetes admissions from hospitals
		Immunization levels from schools
	Community surveys	Frequency of health services use
		Common health problems
	Observation	Number and types of educational institutions
		Number and types of recreational opportunities
	Newspaper reports	Incidence of homicide
		Incidence of motor vehicle fatalities
	Telephone book	Number and types of health care providers
		Number and types of churches
Qualitative	Community surveys	Attitudes toward health
		Attitudes toward specific health issues
	Key informant interviews	Perceptions of community health needs
	Resident interviews	Perceptions of health needs
	Observation	Quality of housing
	Participant observation	Barriers to health care for handicapped individuals

health care services can provide a partial and indirect indication of attitudes, but nonuse may reflect the effects of cost or other barriers rather than a low priority given to health.

In addition to determining appropriate data collection methods, the nurse and community members preparing to conduct a community assessment explore methods for organizing and analyzing the data obtained. When modes of data organization and analysis are identified as much as possible prior to data collection, interpretation of the masses of information obtained becomes much easier.

Elements of a Community Assessment

Community health nurses and community members can use a dimensions of health perspective to guide the assessment of a community or target group. Biophysical, psychological, physical environmental, sociocultural, behavioral, and health system factors influencing community health are examined.

Biophysical Considerations

Human biological factors influencing community health reflect specific physical attributes of community members. The first of these attributes is age. Others reflect the genetic inheritance and physiologic function of community members.

The age composition of the population is an important indicator of probable health needs. Typically, there is an increased need for health services in areas with large numbers of the very young and the very old. Large numbers of women of childbearing age increase needs for prenatal and family planning services. Accident prevention is a major consideration in communities with large numbers of school-age and younger children. Information on the age composition of the population can be obtained from census figures for the census tracts that make up the community.

Another community factor related to age composition is the annual birth rate, which provides information on the growth of the younger segments of the population. The annual birth rate is calculated on the basis of the number of live births during the year in relation to the total population of the community. As is true of several of the other rates discussed in Chapter 10, the proportion of live births to the population is multiplied by 1,000 to give the rate of births per 1,000 persons. Birth statistics are usually compiled by official local and state health agencies and can be obtained from these sources.

Age-specific death rates also provide valuable information regarding the health status of the community (Rohrer, 1999). An age-specific death rate is the number of deaths in a particular age group compared with the population within that group. Because of the relatively small number of deaths in some age groups, the multiplier used in calculating age-specific death rates is 100,000. Excess deaths (deaths over the number that would be expected for that age group in the general

population) for any age group in the community would indicate the presence of health problems. Mortality statistics are available from official state and local health agencies.

The average age at death also provides an indication of overall community health. If people in the community typically die at a relatively young age, this suggests the existence of health problems that are contributing to these early deaths. Native Americans, for example, have shorter expected life spans than the rest of the population because of the high incidence of such health problems as chronic disease and alcoholism and high rates of homicide. Information on age at death may be compiled by local health agencies, but may also be obtained by a review of death certificates or examination of obituaries published in local newspapers.

Some typical community assessment data related to age composition are included in Table 15–2 ■. It is often helpful to include comparison data to identify trends over time. The community represented in Table 15–2, for example, has experienced a slight increase in the older adult population and a decline in the number of youngsters.

One feature of the genetic inheritance of the population is its distribution by gender. Many health problems such as obesity, hypertension, and various forms of cancer are more prevalent in one gender than in the other. Knowing the gender distribution in the community sharpens the index of suspicion with regard to these problems. Knowing the composition of the population with respect to gender assists the assessment team to identify health needs and plan programs to meet them. For example, the knowledge that women constitute 79% of a community's population might suggest the need for easily accessible detection programs for cancer of the cervix and breast.

The racial composition of a community is another important factor in assessment. Knowledge of the ethnicity and racial origin of the population helps to pinpoint health problems known to be prevalent in certain groups, such as sickle cell disease in African Americans and diabetes in some Native American tribes. Data on both the gender and racial composition of the community population are available in census figures as well as from state and local agencies. Sample assessment data reflecting a community's genetic inheritance are included in Table 15–3 ■.

Information about physiologic function in a community is derived from morbidity and mortality data as well as other health status indicators such as immunization levels. Mortality rates of concern to the community health nurse include the crude death rate, cause-specific death rates, and death rates among specific segments of the population, such as the elderly, minority groups, and the homeless.

The crude death rate reflects all deaths in the population regardless of age or cause of death and is calculated using the formula presented in Chapter 10. The crude

■ TABLE 15–2   Sample Community Assessment Data Related to Age

		1995 N	1995 Percent	1985 N	1985 Percent
Age Composition	Birth–1 year	5,827	6	6,380	7
	1–5 years	7,932	9	7,863	9
	6–12 years	9,347	10	8,476	10
	13–20 years	12,701	14	9,340	11
	21–30 years	10,838	12	11,795	13
	31–50 years	12,397	14	14,832	17
	51–65 years	10,492	11	9,508	11
	66–80 years	15,438	17	13,802	16
	Over 80 years	6,739	7	5,127	6

		1995	1985
Age-Specific Death Rate per 100,000 Population	Birth–1 year	27	35
	1–5 years	58	40
	6–12 years	110	80
	13–20 years	154	175
	21–30 years	75	77
	31–50 years	90	87
	51–65 years	169	185
	66–80 years	203	213
	Over 80 years	254	267

Average annual birth rate for last 10 years: 268 per 100,000 population

Average age at death: 72 years

death rate presents a picture of the overall health status of the community, but it does not suggest the presence of specific health problems that may be contributing to deaths.

Cause-specific death rates, on the other hand, provide information about a community's specific health problems. Cause-specific death rates are the number of deaths in the population attributable to specific conditions such as diabetes, heart disease, and suicide. They are calculated in proportion to the total population using a multiplier of 100,000. When death rates due to specific causes are higher than those of populations with a comparable age composition, health care programs may be needed to deal with these causes of death. Mortality statistics are

■ TABLE 15–3   Sample Community Assessment Data Related to Genetic Inheritance

Race/Ethnic Group	MALE N	MALE Percent	FEMALE N	FEMALE Percent	TOTAL N	TOTAL Percent
White non-Hispanic	19,003	56	33,511	58	52,514	57
Hispanic	6,787	20	8,667	15	15,454	17
Asian/Pacific Islander	3,733	11	8,089	14	11,822	13
African American	3,393	10	6,355	11	9,748	11
Native American	1,017	3	1,156	2	2,173	2
Total	33,933	100	57,778	100	91,711	100

compiled by state and local health departments. Information on mortality may also be available from other sources. For example, insurance companies or trauma centers might be able to provide information on motor vehicle fatalities, and homicide figures may be available from local law enforcement agencies.

The majority of health problems are nonfatal, and many existing health problems in the community are not brought to light by examining mortality statistics alone. For this reason, those conducting a community assessment must consider morbidity as well as mortality rates. Morbidity rates reflect the extent of illness present in the community. The two morbidity statistics of greatest significance in community assessment are prevalence and incidence rates. Prevalence rates indicate the *total* number of cases of a particular condition at any given time. Incidence rates indicate the number of *new* cases of the condition identified over a period. For example, eight new cases of tuberculosis may have been diagnosed in Buffalo County last month (incidence), but 39 people in the county are currently under treatment for active tuberculosis (prevalence).

Local and state health departments compile statistics on the incidence and prevalence of certain reportable health conditions. These conditions include many communicable diseases, but may also include other conditions for which special surveillance programs are in place. For example, in some areas information is compiled on newly diagnosed cases of hypertension. Another indicator of community morbidity is the *rate under treatment* or the number of people seeking assistance for specific health problems (Witkin & Altschuld, 1995). For example, the number of people being treated for depression says a great deal about the mental health of the population and may be obtained from local treatment facilities. For other conditions, the assessment team may need to seek other sources of data. Cancer registries may be a source of information about the incidence and prevalence of certain forms of cancer, and local health care facilities and providers may have figures related to the incidence of other conditions. For example, the local hospital may have data on the number of clients hospitalized for diabetes, myocardial infarction, and other conditions.

Immunization levels within the community also provide information on the physiologic function of community members. Information on immunization levels is usually extrapolated from immunization figures derived from school records. In areas where a large number of school-age children are not immunized, there are probably also large numbers of unimmunized younger children, and overall immunization levels in the general population are also likely to be low. School immunization records, however, are not always an accurate indicator of high immunization levels. Because immunization is required for school entry in most places, school-age children may be immunized, while younger children remain unimmunized. For additional data on immunization levels, the assessment team might want to examine

■ **TABLE 15–4** Sample Community Assessment Data Related to Physiologic Function

DATA ELEMENT	1995	1985
Mortality		
Cardiovascular death rate (per 100,000 population)	568 deaths	793 deaths
AIDS death rate (per 100,000 population)	207 deaths	150 deaths
Cancer death rate (per 100,000 population)	350 deaths	317 deaths
Morbidity		
Measles incidence (per 100,000 population)	35 cases	30 cases
Hypertension incidence (per 100,000 population)	2,130 cases	2,353 cases
Hypertension prevalence (per 100,000 population)	8,875 cases	8,038 cases
Immunization level among school-age children	92%	85%

the records of public immunization clinics as well as those of private physicians who provide immunization services.

Comparison figures on morbidity and mortality at state and national levels can be obtained from state health departments and from various federal publications, respectively. One publication that contains a great deal of information on morbidity and mortality statistics is the *Morbidity and Mortality Weekly Report* published by the Centers for Disease Control and Prevention (CDC). Such data is also available online at the CDC Web site (*http://cdc.gov*). National morbidity and mortality data can also be obtained from health and life insurance companies as well as specialty agencies concerned with specific health problems, such as the American Cancer Society and the American Heart Association. Sample data reflecting a community's physiologic status are presented in Table 15–4 ■. Again, comparison data indicate changes in community health problems over time.

Similar information would be obtained if the focus of the assessment is a target group within the population; however, the information gathered would be tailored to the group assessed. For example, assessment team members would assess the physical health conditions occurring in the target population and those to which they are particularly prone because of their condition. Similarly, team members would note any special considerations related to biophysical factors such as immunity (e.g., the need for communicable disease prophylaxis for persons with immunosuppression).

Psychological Considerations

The psychological environment within the community influences the health of community members by increasing or mediating their exposure to stress and affects the ability of the community to function effectively. In addition, elements of the psychological dimension may enhance or impede community action to resolve identified health problems. Some of the areas to be considered in assessing the psychological environment include the future prospects of the community, significant events in community history and the community's response to those events, communication networks existing within the community, and the adequacy of protective services. Other considerations in this area include evidence of psychological problems such as suicide and homicide rates and identifiable sources of stress within the community.

Learning about a community's prospects helps those conducting the community assessment to gain a clearer picture of the psychological climate within the community. If a community is growing and productive, for example, apathy regarding community problems is less likely than might be the case if the community is economically depressed and faltering. A community that is in decline or has multiple problems is also more likely to have multiple sources of stress that affect the health of its residents.

Similarly, information about a community's history can provide insight into previous and current health problems and how the community has dealt with them. Historical information may also provide some clue as to how the community will deal with subsequent problems and where community strengths lie. For example, historical information on the cohesive response of community members to a past crisis suggests a strength that will enable the community to face future crises.

The psychological environment created by relationships between subgroups within the community should also be explored. Harmonious relations between groups indicate a psychological climate that is conducive to cooperative community action to resolve identified problems. Tension and distrust between groups, on the other hand, may make resolution of community health problems more difficult. The assessment team should be alert to unrest and conflict between groups within the community and the implications of such psychological tensions for the health of the community and its members.

The adequacy of protective services provided by law enforcement, fire, and other emergency personnel can profoundly influence the psychological climate of an area. Adequate protective services help to create a psychological environment that enhances feelings of personal safety and security. Where these services are inadequate to meet residents' needs, stress and insecurity are created and can negatively influence the health of the population. Those assessing the health of a community would obtain information about the availability and quality of police and fire services, as well as information on the availability and adequacy of legal services, services for victims of abuse, and consumer protection services.

Communication is an important contributing factor in the psychological climate of a community, therefore, the adequacy of communication networks should also be explored. This includes the availability and accessibility of a telecommunication infrastructure in the community (Bingler, 2000). Communication in the community may be formal or informal. Formal channels include media such as radio, television, and newspapers, as well as the form that public announcements may take. Informal communications take place outside of these channels and may also influence the health of the community. For example, rumors about a particular religious or ethnic group may serve to exacerbate intergroup tension and strife. The degree of trust placed in official formal communications is another element of the psychological dimension that may enhance or detract from community health.

Other indicators of the psychological environment in a community include annual incidence rates for homicide and suicide. Rates for specific subgroups within the community should also be examined, for there is usually considerable variation among different racial and ethnic groups. For example, both suicide and homicide rates are frequently higher for minority group members than for the general population in most communities. Examination of these figures and their distribution in the population may help to identify factors contributing to poor psychological health in certain subgroups or in the population in general.

Finally, the assessment team would want to identify common sources of stress within the environment. Widespread unemployment, lack of available housing, and crowded living conditions are sources of stress in a community. These and other sources of stress serve to create a psychological environment that is not conducive to health.

Information on the psychological dimension of community health is obtained primarily through observation and through interviews with area residents. Again, it is important to get a broad representation of community membership among the people interviewed. Data about the psychological environment of a rural community with severe problems might include the following:

- Community population has declined by 15% in the last five years.
- Twenty-five percent of the town was destroyed in a tornado and flood seven years ago; only 20% of the buildings destroyed have been replaced.
- Ten percent of local businesses have gone bankrupt in the last three years.
- The only local newspaper closed two years ago.
- There are no radio or television stations in town.
- The volunteer fire department is able to respond to fire calls within an average of 15 minutes.
- Medical emergency calls receive a response within an average of 20 minutes.
- Suicide incidence is 50 per 100,000 population.

Again, similar types of information would be collected with respect to a target group with special attention to certain kinds of information. For example, the attitudes of the general population toward the target group may have a profound effect on their mental health. Similarly, members of some target groups (e.g., those with HIV infection) may have a high incidence of depression and suicide because of their condition.

Physical Environmental Considerations

Physical environmental factors affecting a community include its location, its type (e.g., rural, urban, or suburban) and size, topographical features, and climate. Other physical factors to be assessed include the type and adequacy of housing in the community and considerations related to water supply, nuisance factors, and potential for disaster.

The location, climate, and physical geography or topography of the community provide indications of some health problems likely to be identified in the course of the assessment. An area that is heavily wooded, for example, might increase the index of suspicion for problems such as Rocky Mountain spotted fever and Lyme disease. On the other hand, a dry, arid desert area would be more conducive to problems of heat exhaustion.

Size and population density, as well as the type of community, are other factors that influence the types of health problems encountered and resources available in the community. Certain health problems are more prevalent in urban areas than in rural ones and vice versa. Statistics indicate that suicide is more prevalent in urban communities, whereas one would expect a problem like rabies to occur more often in a rural area where wild animals are likely to be infected. Urban dwellers are less likely to encounter rabid animals because of regulations regarding vaccination of pets. Rural and urban areas also have unique strengths. For example, rural communities are often characterized by a tendency for neighbors to help each other, whereas urban areas generally have a greater variety of health care services within close proximity.

Housing is another important physical environmental factor. Inadequate, unsafe, or unsanitary housing conditions contribute to a variety of health problems including communicable diseases spread by poor sanitation, lead poisoning due to lead-based paint in older homes in poor repair, and unintentional injuries resulting from safety hazards. Overcrowding has been found to increase the incidence of a number of health concerns. Communicable diseases are spread more rapidly in crowded conditions, and the prevalence of stress-related conditions such as alcohol abuse, suicide, and other forms of violence increases with crowding as well.

The source of a community's water supply is another important physical environmental consideration. Are most residents supplied by local water systems or do they have independent wells? Those conducting the community assessment should investigate the *potability*, or *drinkability*, of the community's water. Is the community's water supply safe for drinking, or does it pose biological or chemical hazards to health? Moreover, the assessment team should explore the presence or absence of fluoride in the water supply as an indicator of dental health.

Disposal of wastes is another area of consideration in assessing the physical environment of a community. The assessment team should ascertain disposal methods for various types of materials. Of particular concern is the disposal of hazardous wastes. Do disposal methods ensure adequate safeguards for the health of the public, or is there potential for environmental pollution as a result of waste disposal? Concerns about hazardous waste disposal were addressed in Chapter 7.

Team members may also need to assess whether physical factors within the community contribute to accidental injuries. For example, particularly dangerous intersections may be the sites of frequent motor vehicle accidents, or large numbers of swimming pools in the area may contribute to the incidence of drownings.

Nuisance factors such as insects, noxious plants, and other substances may provide physical health hazards or prove offensive to the senses, thereby decreasing the quality of life in the community. Nearby dairy farms, for example, might provide insect breeding grounds that contribute to the incidence of insect-borne diseases, or there might be an airport that presents a noise hazard. Another consideration in terms of nuisances is the presence of various pollutants in the environment. The effects of pollution and the community health nurse's responsibility with regard to pollution were discussed in Chapter 7.

Finally, within the community's physical environment there may be the potential for either natural or manmade disasters. Is the community located on a major fault line and subject to earthquakes? Is a chemical manufacturing plant close by that presents a potential hazard? Assessment of the potential for disaster and the community health nurse's role in planning for disaster response are addressed in more detail in Chapter 27.

For the most part, the physical environmental characteristics of a community can be observed. For example, the nurse or other members of the community might drive through the community assessing its geographic features, nuisance factors, and the general adequacy of housing. Information about pollution, water supply, and waste disposal might be obtained from local government bureaus or the nearby public health agency. Data on population size and density are available from census figures or from local government agencies. This information, as well as information on the typical climate and geographic features, may also be available in local publications or from the chamber of commerce. Sample assessment data reflecting features of a rural community's physical environment include the following:

- Fifty percent of residential units contain lead-based paint.
- Annual temperature ranges from 33° to 109°F.

- Rabies incidence is 53 per 1,000 wild skunks and raccoons.
- Thirteen percent of local wells are contaminated with pesticides.
- Poor maintenance of local roads and wandering livestock pose safety hazards.
- Thirty percent of surrounding land is forested; 70% is used for dairy farming.
- A river running through town floods approximately every five years.

Assessment of a target group within the population would entail gathering similar data. Special attention should be given to any physical environmental needs engendered by membership in the target group. For example, if the target group is handicapped individuals in the community, the assessment team would examine handicapped access to public buildings, recreational facilities, and so on. Similarly, the group might pay special attention to the effects of air pollution on groups of people with chronic respiratory conditions.

Sociocultural Considerations

From the previous discussion it is clear that sociocultural and psychological dimensions are closely interrelated. Social and cultural factors influence the psychological dimension and have other effects on health as well. Considerations in assessing the sociocultural dimension include information about community government and leadership, language, income and education levels, employment levels and occupations, marital status and family composition, and religion. Other areas to be addressed include transportation and the availability of goods and services needed by residents.

A community's government and power structure are important considerations in terms of planning and implementing programs designed to solve community health problems and to make effective use of community resources. Who holds the purse strings? How are decisions made? Who are the decision makers in the community? Community members conducting the health assessment should identify formal and informal community leaders. In one isolated community, for example, no program was successful unless it first received approval from one elderly matriarch. It was she who controlled the community despite the presence of elected officials.

Information on the community's official leadership can be obtained from the mayor's office or from other local governmental agencies. Informal leaders may be more difficult to identify, but, if they do not already know this information, assessment team members can ask key informants in the community (e.g., school principals, clergy, and official leaders) who the informal leaders are. Other health care providers and business leaders might also provide information on informal leadership within the community.

Language is another important sociocultural factor affecting the health of community members. The nurse and others should assess the degree to which language presents a barrier to health education or to the provision of other health care services. Again, key informants in the community can provide information about languages spoken. Schoolteachers and principals, for example, are knowledgeable about languages spoken by their students. Those conducting the community assessment may also derive this information from personal observation in the community. For example, they may spend time observing stores where large segments of the population shop or check for newspapers and radio and television broadcasts in languages other than English.

Another aspect of language to be assessed is the use of colloquialisms by local residents. Are there unique ways in which community members express themselves? Unfortunately, much of this information is gleaned by trial and error on the part of the nurse; however, the nurse can ask key informants about the use of colloquialisms and about their meaning.

Closely related to language are the cultural affiliations of community members. Assessment team members need to identify the host of cultural factors within the community that affect its health status (see Chapter 6). Information on cultural groups in the community can be obtained from key informants and through observation.

The average income of community residents also has bearing on a community's health status. It has been noted, for example, that there is a strong relationship between the economic status of the population and certain critical indicators of health. Economic status influences the ability of residents to provide for basic necessities and to gain access to health care services. In addition, the income of residents influences the tax base of the community and the types of services the community is able to provide its citizens. For example, when many residents are unemployed or have low incomes, they have less money to spend. Businesses take in less money and community revenues from sales and other taxes are decreased. Consequently, the community is less able to provide essential services for its citizens.

Income is closely related to education level. People who have received a lesser education may have lower-paying jobs. They also tend to have less health-related knowledge, and, consequently, lower levels of health. Both income and education levels are indicators of a community's standard of living and, indirectly, of its health status. The prevalence of several acute and chronic conditions in the population (e.g., tuberculosis, pneumonia, and heart disease) tends to decline as income and education levels rise. Information on income and education levels can be obtained from census figures. This information may also be available from local government agencies or school districts.

In addition to determining the education level of the population, the community's education resources should be examined. This information enables the assessment team to make diagnoses regarding the adequacy of community resources for meeting identified health needs. The telephone directory is a good starting place for obtaining information on education facilities in the area. Assessment team members can then interview administrators of those facilities or review their brochures and other publications to determine the types of education programs offered. Local school personnel can also provide information on education opportunities in the community.

Because large numbers of people within a community are usually employed, it is important to assess the types of occupations and health hazards involved. Persons in some occupational groups are at higher risk for certain health problems than those in other groups. For example, histoplasmosis is a frequent occurrence among people who work with birds (e.g., poultry farmers), and black lung (pneumoconiosis) is prevalent among coal miners. Information about community businesses and industries is available from the local chamber of commerce. The numbers of people employed in specific occupations can be obtained from major employers in the area.

Questions should be asked about other health hazards presented by jobs in the community. Address the potential for exposure to hazardous substances (e.g., asbestos and chlorine gas), radiation, noise, or vibration, as well as the potential for injury due to falls or use of hazardous equipment. In addition to determining the potential for occupational injury or illness, the assessment team would obtain figures on the extent to which such conditions occur. This type of information may be obtained from the illness and accident records of major employers or may be available from the state occupational health agency.

In addition to information about employment, the level of unemployment in the community provides an indication of possible health problems. Unemployment contributes to stress and to decreased income levels that affect access to health care as well as other necessary goods and services. Unemployment figures can be obtained from state or local employment offices. Occupational data derived from a community assessment might include the following:

- Ten percent of the local workforce is unemployed.
- Seventy-five percent of working adults are employed in textile manufacture; 25% are in service occupations.
- Local health care workers are at increased risk of HIV exposure because of the high rate of HIV seropositivity in the community.
- There is a moderate to severe risk of chemical exposures in the manufacture of synthetic textiles.
- Fifteen percent of textile workers report significant hearing loss.

Religious affiliations within a community can either foster or impede health practices. The nurse and others conducting the community assessment should be aware of religious beliefs that may affect health or may influence the acceptability of health programs to community members. For example, some religious groups may be

averse to the idea of providing on-site health care services in high schools because of the fear that contraceptive services will be provided (see Chapter 6 for more information on the influence of religion on health). Similarly, local religious groups may provide significant community resources and should be included in assets assessment. Again, the telephone directory and Internet data can provide a picture of the religious groups represented in the community, and the membership rosters of specific houses of worship can provide information on the number of people affiliated with each religious group.

Marital status and family composition are social environmental factors that might influence the health of communities. Those conducting the community assessment determine the number of single-parent families and older persons living alone. Generally, married individuals have lower death and illness rates than those who are unmarried; therefore, information about marital status in the community can provide clues to overall health status. Information on marriage and family composition is available from census data for the community.

Accessibility of transportation is an important factor related to the use of health services and is, therefore, a necessary component of the community assessment. Transportation difficulties compound health problems where large numbers of people are poor or elderly, chronically ill or disabled, mothers with small children, and persons who are poorly motivated with respect to health. The assessment team can obtain information on the number of families with cars from community census data. Information on other forms of transportation can be gleaned from the telephone directory or Internet and by contacting bus and taxi companies to determine routes and fares.

In addition, the assessment team members would obtain data on the types and adequacy of goods and services available to community members, including recreational programs, local shopping facilities, prices for goods and services, and social service programs for community members. Much of this information can be obtained through participant observation. For example, the nurse might shop in local stores or look for recreational pursuits. Information about the number and types of stores and services is also available in the telephone directory and possibly on the Internet. Newspaper advertisements provide information on local prices. Finally, assessment team members can contact personnel at local social service agencies to obtain information about the services offered. Data related to a community's sociocultural environment might include the following information:

- Elected community officials represent the white segment of the population; all have been in office a minimum of 15 years.
- A large influx of Spanish-speaking migrant workers (5,000 to 6,000 people) occurs every spring.

- The average annual family income of year-round residents is $28,000; the average annual income for migrant families is $12,000.
- The average number of years of school completed by the resident population is 12; for migrant workers, the average is 3.
- Ninety percent of adult residents are married; 60% of the migrant population consists of males without families in the area.
- The town contains three elementary schools, one junior high school, and one high school.
- Ninety percent of the resident population is Protestant (major denominations: Methodist and Lutheran); 80% of the migrant population is Roman Catholic.
- Seventy-five percent of the residents and 25% of the migrant workers own cars; there is no public transportation available in town.

Assessment of a target group would include similar types of information as they affect the health of target group members. For example, the employment and economic status of refugee immigrants might differ significantly from those of the general population. Similarly, groups experiencing language barriers may have difficulty obtaining needed health care services.

Behavioral Considerations

Behavioral factors influence the health status of a community and its members. Areas to be addressed in this portion of the assessment include community consumption patterns, leisure pursuits, and other health-related behaviors.

Consumption patterns play a major part in the development of health or illness. In assessing consumption patterns in the community, the assessment team would examine dietary patterns and the use of potentially harmful substances.

ETHICAL AWARENESS

You have been working with a group of community residents to assess the health needs of the community. Part of the effort has involved focus group sessions with several ethnic minority groups in the community to elicit their perceptions of community health. Some of the comments made in the focus groups indicate dissatisfaction with the services of the major primary health care provider in the community. This provider is concerned about the effect these comments will have on his clientele and wants to have them eliminated from the assessment team's report. Other team members do not think this is appropriate. The provider is a member of the assessment team and has been one of the primary funders of the assessment. As leader of the assessment team, what would you do in this situation?

Information is needed on the general nutritional level of community members and on specific dietary patterns. For example, information would be sought on the prevalence of overweight individuals in the population or the incidence of anemia in school-age children. Another area for consideration is any ethnic nutritional patterns that might influence health either positively or negatively. For example, movement away from traditional tribal foods to typical American dietary practices has contributed to obesity and a variety of chronic diseases among many Native Americans. Information on dietary patterns may be obtained by interviews and surveys of community residents as well as by observation of foods purchased in grocery stores.

The use of harmful substances is another area to explore. Those conducting the assessment should determine the level of alcohol consumption within the community, both for the community at large and for specific target groups. The extent of both legal and illegal drug use may also merit investigation, including the types of substances abused and the typical sources of abused substances. Finally, the assessment team would determine the number of residents who smoke and whether that number is increasing or decreasing. Indirect indicators of use of alcohol, drugs, and tobacco include the extent of sales of these items in the community. This information can be obtained from interviews with personnel in stores that sell these items or from information about the related taxes collected. Information on substance abuse may be reflected in law enforcement agencies' records regarding arrests or accidents related to drugs and alcohol. Information can also be obtained on the number of admissions to drug and alcohol treatment facilities. Community self-help groups, such as a local chapter of Alcoholics Anonymous, may also provide information on the extent of substance abuse problems. Data reflecting a community's consumption patterns might include the following:

- Local diets are typically high in saturated fats due to frying foods; diets are also low in calcium, iron, and vitamin C.
- The incidence of moderate to severe anemia is 150 per 1,000 children.
- Annual per capita alcohol consumption is 3.64 gallons.
- Ten percent of the adult population smoke tobacco.
- The annual rate of arrests for illicit drug use is 15 per 1,000 population.
- The annual rate of arrests for driving under the influence of drugs or alcohol is 30 per 1,000 population.
- The annual death rate for motor vehicle accidents involving alcohol is 202 per 100,000 population.
- Thirty-five percent of all motor vehicle accidents in town are alcohol related.

Information about leisure activities prevalent in the community can also indicate the potential for certain kinds of health problems. For example, boating, water-skiing, and related recreational activities increase the risk of drowning and similar accidents. On the other hand, if watching television is the primary form of recreation, there may be increased potential for heart disease and other conditions associated with a sedentary lifestyle. The presence or absence of recreational opportunities in the community may also affect the psychological environment and the ability of community members to deal with stress effectively. Information on leisure-related exercise is usually obtained by means of interviews and surveys. To determine the extent of community interest in various forms of exercise, assessment team members might also contact groups that offer exercise-related classes or sell related equipment. In addition, they can observe for joggers or other exercise enthusiasts as they move about the community. Information on recreational opportunities can be obtained from the telephone directory and the Internet, from direct observation, and from events publicized in the newspaper or other means of communication employed in the community.

Members of the community conducting the health assessment should also examine the prevalence of other health-related behaviors by community members. For example, information would be obtained on the extent of seat belt use in passenger vehicles or the use of safety devices in certain occupational settings. The assessment team would also be interested in such behaviors as the extent of heterosexual and homosexual activity and use of condoms and other forms of protection against conception and sexually transmitted diseases. Two negative indicators of contraceptive use are the proportion of births that are illegitimate and the local abortion rate. In areas with a high prevalence of injection drug use, assessment team members would also try to obtain information on the extent of needle sharing and other practices that contribute to the spread of HIV/AIDS infection and hepatitis C. Much of this information is available only through observation and through interviews of key informants in the community.

The assessment team would collect similar information regarding behavioral considerations as they affect the health of members of a particular target group. Again, there might be specific information relevant to the target group that is not particularly relevant to the general population. For example, target group members may have specific dietary needs (e.g., a diabetic diet) that differ from those of the general population.

Health System Considerations

Health care system factors can profoundly affect the health of a community. Needs assessment in this dimension involves identifying existing services, assessing their level of performance, and identifying areas in which services are lacking. In assessing the community's well-being, community members would obtain information on the type of health services available to residents. What types of primary, secondary, and tertiary preventive services are available? How adequate are these services to meet the needs of the people? The assessment team would examine the availability and accessibility of specific types of services and how effectively they are used. For example, one might inquire as to the percentage of pregnant women who receive prenatal care and at what point in the pregnancy care usually begins. Team members might also investigate the availability of services provided by emergency medical personnel and by emergency rooms or trauma centers. Other questions relate to the availability and accessibility of certain types of health care providers. For example, there may be several physicians in town, but none of them provide prenatal services because of malpractice concerns.

Information on health care services available in the community may be obtained from the telephone directory, the Internet, word-of-mouth, and from personal observation. Referral services provided by professional organizations or agencies such as local senior citizens groups can also supply information on health care providers and facilities in the community. Health care institutions are also a source of information on services provided and fees involved.

Community members engaged in a community assessment would also determine to what extent available services are overused or underused. What factors contribute to overuse and to underuse? For example, emergency room services might be overused because many community members cannot afford a regular source of health care and seek care only in crisis situations. Conversely, the services of clinics and physicians might be underused because they are offered at inconvenient times or places or because people have no means of transportation to such services, or residents may simply not be aware of the need for or availability of certain services. Utilization figures can be obtained from health care facilities and providers in the community.

Another area for consideration is the financing of community health care. Questions to be addressed include who pays for health care services, adequacy of funding sources for meeting community health needs, priority given to health-related concerns in planning community budgetary allocations, extent of health insurance coverage among community members, and availability of funds to pay for care for the indigent (see Chapter 5). Information on health insurance may be available from insurance agencies or major health care facilities in the area. Health care facility records may also contain data on the percentage of the population without health insurance. Information about recipients of Medicaid and Medicare benefits is available from the agencies that administer these programs.

Financing of health care can also provide an indirect indication of prevailing community attitudes toward health. For example, adequate health care budgeting indicates that health is considered a public priority. Budgetary information can be solicited from public officials. Other considerations related to the health care system include community definitions of health and illness and the use of culturally prescribed health practices and practitioners. Community assessment data related to the health care system might include the following:

- Ten percent of the local government's budget is allocated to health services.
- Local insurance coverage is as follows:
  - Eligible for military health care services: 15%
  - Covered by Medicare/Medicaid: 30%
  - Covered by private insurance: 43%
  - Uninsured: 12%
- Only 3% of private health care providers accept Medicaid.
- Seventy percent of Medicaid-reimbursable services are provided in emergency departments.

- Civilian health care providers in town include:
  - Family practice physicians: 3
  - Internist: 1
  - Pediatricians: 2
  - Dermatologist: 1
  - Cardiologist: 1
  - Neurosurgeon: 1
  - Orthopedist: 1
  - Obstetrician/gynecologist: 1
  - Osteopath: 1
  - Advanced practice nurses: 5 (1 nurse midwife, 2 pediatric nurse practitioners, 2 family nurse practitioners)
- There is one hospital in town; its utilization rate is 85% of capacity.
- The local emergency medical service receives an average of 3,440 calls per month.

assessment tips assessment tips assessment tips

ASSESSING THE COMMUNITY OR TARGET GROUP

Biophysical Considerations

- What is the age composition of the population? What is the community's annual birth rate? What are the age-specific death rates in the community? What is the average age at death of community members?
- What is the racial and ethnic composition of the population? What is the relative proportion of men and women in the community? In specific age groups? What genetically determined illnesses, if any, are prevalent in the community?
- What are the cause-specific mortality rates for the community? What physiologic conditions are prevalent in the community? What is the extent of disability within the community? How does the community compare with state and national morbidity and mortality figures?
- What is the overall immunization level in the community?

Psychological Considerations

- What stressors are present in the community? How does the community deal with crises? What significant events have occurred in the history of the community? What was the community's response to those events? What are the community's prospects for the future?
- How cohesive is the community? Is there evidence of tension between groups in the community?

- How adequate are protective services in the community?
- What are the formal communication channels in the community? The informal channels?
- What are the prevalence rates for mental illnesses in the community? What is the community homicide rate? Suicide rate?
- What are the rates of crime in the community? What types of crimes are prevalent?

Physical Environmental Considerations

- What type of community is this (e.g., rural, urban)? Where is the community located? How large is the community? How densely populated? What topographical features could influence the health of community members? What is the local climate like?
- What is the quality of housing in the community? Is affordable housing available? Are dwellings in good repair?
- What is the community's source of water? Is the community water supply adequate to meet community needs? Is it safe for consumption? How does the community handle waste disposal?
- What plants and animals are common in the area?
- Is there evidence of environmental pollution that may affect health?
- Are there nuisance factors present in the community? If so, what are they? How do they affect health?

- Is there potential for disaster in the community? If so, what kind of disasters are likely? What is the extent of community disaster preparation?

Sociocultural Considerations

- How are community decisions made? Who makes them? Who holds power in the community? How is that power exercised? What is the community's governance structure? How effective is community governance? Who are the formal and informal leaders in the community?

- What cultural groups are represented in the community? What languages are spoken? What cultural beliefs and behaviors are prevalent in the community? What is the character of relationships between members of different cultural groups in the community?

- What religious affiliations are represented in the community? What effect do they have on community life and health?

- What is the education level of community members? What educational resources and facilities are present in the community?

- What is the income level and distribution within the community?

- What is the rate of unemployment in the community? Who are the major employers in the community? What kinds of occupations are represented within the community? What occupational health hazards are present in the community?

- How accessible is transportation in the community?

- What is the marital status of community members? What is the typical family structure in the community?

- How accessible are goods and services to community members?

Behavioral Considerations

- What are the usual food preferences and consumption patterns in the community? What is the nutritional level in the community? What percentage of the population is overweight? Underweight?

- What is the extent of drug abuse in the community? How easy is it to obtain drugs?

- What is the extent of alcohol and tobacco sales in the community? What is the prevalence of arrests related to alcohol and other drugs? What is the extent of smoking in the community? What is the rate of hospital admissions for health problems related to alcohol, drug, and tobacco use?

- What exercise and leisure opportunities are available to community members? To what extent are they utilized? Do leisure activities pose any health or safety hazards?

- What is the attitude of the community to sexual activity? To homosexuality? What is the prevalence of unsafe sexual practices in the community? What is the extent of contraceptive use in the community?

- To what extent do community members engage in safety practices (e.g., seat belt use)?

Health System Considerations

- What types of primary, secondary, and tertiary preventive services are available in the community? How accessible are these services to community members? Are the types of services available adequate to meet community health needs? Are available services culturally relevant to members of the population?

- To what extent are available health care services utilized? What barriers to service utilization exist in the community?

- Are there alternative health services available in the community? To what extent do members of the community use alternative health services? What is the level and quality of interaction between alternative and scientific health care systems in the community?

- How are health care services financed? What proportion of the population has health insurance? What level of priority is given to health care services in budgeting local funds? What are community attitudes toward health care services and providers?

Again, a target group assessment may focus on health system factors particularly relevant to the needs of the group. For example, the availability and adequacy of physical therapy services would be particularly relevant to a target group with physical disabilities. Tools for assessing communities and target groups from the perspective of biophysical, psychological, physical environmental, sociocultural, behavioral, and health system dimensions are available on the companion Web site for this book.

DIAGNOSTIC REASONING AND COMMUNITY HEALTH

The collection of data on factors influencing the health status of a community or a target group is the first step in identifying group resources and group health needs. To be of any value, the data must be interpreted and analyzed to derive nursing diagnoses. In other words, assessment data are used to identify health-related needs that are amenable to nursing action and the resources that will support action. Community or target group nursing diagnoses should reflect existing, emerging, and potential threats to health, as well as community and group strengths or competencies.

Diagnostic reasoning in the care of communities involves comparing community needs assessment data to identified standards to uncover community or group health problems and to identify assets. One type of standard that may be used in data analysis is the general health status of the state or the nation. For example, the community health nurse can compare data for the community or target group with data for the state or the nation as a whole. In doing so, the nurse might ask the following questions: How does this group stand in relation to the larger population on a variety of measures of health status? Is the local birth rate higher or lower than that of the state or the nation? How do death rates compare? For example, the southern region of Georgia has been labeled the "stroke belt" because the death rate for cerebrovascular accidents far exceeds that of the rest of the nation. Do morbidity rates for various illnesses exceed national and state rates? How do income and education levels compare?

Another standard with which to compare present data is found in the history of the community or target group. How do current rates compare with those of a year ago? Five years ago?

Members' perceptions of areas of need are a third type of standard with which to compare the data gathered. What health problems are mentioned in interviews with group members? What problems are perceived by other health care professionals and community or target group leaders? What are the expectations of the community or target group regarding these problems?

Diagnostic reasoning gives rise to statements of health needs or risk in the population. A second stage of community diagnosis involves a comparison of the health care needs identified and the resources available to meet those needs. This may be referred to as a diagnosis of "need–service match" or mismatch (Porter, 1987). Data for this level of nursing diagnosis would be found in the assessment of the health care system. If members of the assessment team found community health care resources inadequate to meet the needs posed by the increased risk of suicide in a vulnerable population, they would make a diagnosis of "need–service mismatch due to inadequate (or inaccessible) suicide prevention services."

The team might also make positive diagnoses related to the health status of a community or target group. For example, a preliminary diagnosis might indicate a vulnerable population group (e.g., children) at risk for certain health problems (such as communicable diseases). Examination of assessment data, however, might indicate that there are few problems with immunizable childhood diseases because of easy accessibility of immunization services and high immunization levels in the population. In this situation, the team's diagnosis might be a "need–service match due to accessibility and use of immunization services."

PLANNING HEALTH CARE FOR GROUPS AND COMMUNITIES

Whenever a diagnosis of need–service mismatch is made, planning to meet the unmet need is warranted, and the community health nurse should engage community members in planning health care delivery programs to meet the identified needs of the population. Systematic planning is essential to effective health care programming. Community health nurses, in particular, are aware of community health needs and of the kinds of programs that will be acceptable to members of target populations. The process used in planning health programs is similar to that used to plan care for other types of clients but is somewhat more involved. Considerations in planning at the group level include setting priorities, determining the level of prevention involved in meeting identified health needs, and developing health care programs to meet those needs. Sources of assistance in planning health care programs are available through links provided on the companion Web site for this book.

Setting Priorities

Once nursing diagnoses have been derived, they must be assigned priority for intervention. Community members must be able to set priorities that allow for the best use of available resources. Priority setting is even more important when the client is a community or a target group than in the care of individuals or families, because care of communities and target groups usually necessitates a greater expenditure of resources. This frequently means that only the highest-priority needs will be addressed because of limited resources available.

The criteria used to prioritize community or target group needs are essentially the same as those used in working with individuals and families: (a) severity of the threat to the community's health, (b) degree of the community's concern about the need, and (c) extent to which meeting one need depends on meeting other needs. It is likely that the priorities of the community or target group involve needs that are easily perceived. Community participation in the assessment process helps community members to become aware of less obvious needs that might have greater priority than the more obvious ones.

The process of assigning priority to the health needs identified in a community assessment involves the development of criteria for decision making, establishing standards for minimally acceptable levels of the criteria, and assigning weights to the criteria. For example, a high-priority problem will usually meet criteria of severity, significant community concern, and high cost to society. A standard for severity might be that a minimum of 20% of the population be affected by the problem; whereas significant community concern would be evident if 10% of community members surveyed mentioned a particular problem as needing attention. Possible standards for cost to society might be the number of days of lost school or work attendance or the actual monetary cost for medical treatment for the problem. Each of these three criteria (and others developed) would be given a weight reflecting its relative importance in decisions about priorities. For example, high societal cost might be given greater value than the level of community concern about a given problem. All of the problems identified in the community needs assessment would be evaluated in terms of the weighted criteria, and those with higher priority scores would be addressed first in efforts to resolve community health problems.

Determining the Level of Prevention

Programs for meeting the health needs of communities or target groups may be needed at any of the three levels of prevention. Primary prevention programs are designed to promote the health of the population and prevent specific illnesses. An exercise program for senior citizens is an example of a health promotion program aimed at a target group. Community education programs on water safety or prevention of accidents in the home are primary preventive measures for a community. Primary prevention involves education programs of any kind designed to promote the public's overall health. For example, parenting classes for expectant couples could help prevent child abuse, and sex education in the school system could minimize problems of adolescent pregnancy and sexually transmitted diseases. Immunization programs are another example of primary prevention for a community or target group.

Secondary prevention involves identifying and resolving existing health problems in members of the community or target group. Specific secondary interventions may focus on screening programs or control programs for community health problems.

Screening Programs

One major area of program planning related to secondary prevention for communities and target groups is the development of screening programs. *Screening* is the preliminary examination or testing of a person to determine whether or not he or she might have a particular condition and whether further diagnostic testing is indicated. Screening procedures are not diagnostic. Instead, they serve to indicate the possibility that a particular disease or condition is present. Positive screening test results are always an indication of the need for further diagnostic procedures. Screening is frequently used with large population groups because it is considerably less expensive than conducting a battery of diagnostic tests when the majority of people can be expected to have negative results. Screening procedures are available and recommended for breast and cervical cancer, testicular cancer, colorectal cancer, skin cancer, hypertension, and diabetes. Screening may also be done for several sexually transmitted diseases such as syphilis and gonorrhea and for the human immunodeficiency virus (HIV) that causes AIDS. Screening for tuberculosis is also available. Another form

of screening is the periodic health examination in which the person is examined for signs and symptoms of several common diseases.

Several factors need to be considered in decisions to implement large-scale screening programs. These factors can be divided into three groups: (a) considerations regarding the condition that is being screened, (b) considerations regarding the test itself, and (c) considerations related to the target group for the program. Any condition for which screening is warranted should have several characteristics. First, the condition should affect a sufficient number of people to make screening cost-effective. Second, the condition should have relatively serious consequences. For example, although it would be cost-effective to screen for the common cold because of the number of people affected, the effects of colds are usually minor and thus do not justify screening. The third consideration is the availability of an acceptable treatment. It is not realistic, generally speaking, to screen for a disease for which there is no treatment. (A significant exception to this criterion is screening for HIV infection. In this case, knowledge of being HIV-positive allows the infected individual to take precautions that can help limit the spread of the disease and minimize its effects.) Fourth, there should be a significant preclinical period between the time of exposure and the development of clinical symptoms to allow for treatment before the person becomes symptomatic. Finally, early diagnosis and treatment need to make a difference. If the outcome is the same whether the condition is treated early or late in its course, there is no point in screening. If, on the other hand, earlier treatment increases the chances of being cured, as is the case in breast cancer, then screening is appropriate.

The second group of factors influencing decisions for mass screening relates to the screening test itself. These factors are the sensitivity and specificity of the screening test as well as the cost, ease of administration, and acceptability of the procedure. *Sensitivity* refers to the ability of the test to identify accurately those persons with the disease (Valanis, 1999). A sensitive screening test would be able to detect the presence of a condition even when very little of the indicator that the test reacts to is present. For example, if a screening test relies on the presence of a particular substance in the blood, a sensitive test would give a positive result even when a small amount of that substance is present. The *specificity* of a screening test reflects the extent to which it excludes those who do not have the disease (Valanis, 1999). A positive result on a highly specific test would indicate the potential presence of only one condition, rather than two or three possible conditions.

Other considerations with respect to the screening test itself are cost, ease of administration, and acceptability. Screening tests should be relatively inexpensive compared with specific diagnostic tests. They should also be easy to administer to large groups of people and not require expensive or sophisticated equipment to conduct the test. Finally, the test should be acceptable to those who are intended to participate in the screening. This means that the test should not be overly painful, embarrassing, or anxiety provoking. The test should not have objectionable side effects. It would be unwarranted to screen people using a test whose potential side effects are worse than the symptoms of the disease in question.

Another consideration in deciding for or against mass screening projects is the population to be screened. The target group must be identifiable and accessible to screeners. If the target group for screening is not easily identifiable, screening programs may not reach those most in need. Adult women, for example, have been identified as being vulnerable to breast and cervical cancer, and this population can easily be screened for these conditions during the course of routine checkups. If the appropriate target group is less easily identified or unlikely to come forward (e.g., injection drug users or homosexuals), screening programs are less likely to be successful.

When conditions related to the illness, the screening test, and the target population are met, large-scale screening programs can prove worthwhile. When these conditions are not met, screening is unlikely to be effective in improving the health of communities. Disease, test, and target group considerations in planning large-scale screening programs are summarized below.

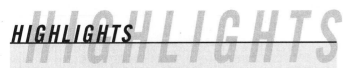

HIGHLIGHTS

Disease, Test, and Target Group Considerations in Screening

Disease Considerations

- The disease affects a sufficient number of people to make screening cost-effective.
- The disease is relatively serious.
- An effective treatment is available for the disease.
- The preclinical period is sufficient to allow treatment before symptoms occur.
- Early diagnosis and treatment make a difference in terms of outcome.

Test Considerations

- The screening test is sensitive enough to detect most cases of the disease.
- The screening test is specific enough to exclude most other causes of positive results.
- The screening test costs little, is easy to administer, and has minimal side effects.

Target Group Considerations

- The target group is identifiable.
- The target group is accessible.

Control Programs

Some of the same programs described as primary preventive measures may also be employed in secondary prevention designed to alleviate existing health problems. When a community or target group is already experiencing a high rate of sexually transmitted diseases (STDs), education on the transmission and prevention of STDs would be a secondary preventive measure. The intent of the program is to control an existing problem (high rate of STDs), rather than prevent a problem from occurring.

The kind of secondary prevention programs planned for a given community or target group varies with the types of problems identified in the assessment. For example, if child abuse is prevalent in the community, parenting classes for abusive parents would be an appropriate secondary preventive measure. Similarly, if there is a high rate of hypertension among group members, clinics could be established to screen for, diagnose, and treat this problem. In another community, a program to enforce seat belt legislation could be used as a secondary preventive measure for a high rate of motor vehicle accident fatalities.

Tertiary prevention programs for communities or target groups are designed to prevent complications of identified problems or prevent the recurrence of a problem. For example, if a community is experiencing an epidemic of measles, mass immunization programs to control the epidemic would be used as a secondary preventive measure. When the epidemic is under control, a program designed to maintain immunity levels among

CRITICAL THINKING IN RESEARCH

Healey (1998) conducted a study to determine the prevalence and characteristics of tobacco use in three counties in Pennsylvania. He examined the extent of cigarette use in children under 18 years of age and the age of onset of cigarette use as well as gender differences in cigarette use. He also noted the extent of continued cigarette use among children. Study findings were used to provide the impetus for two community initiatives to reduce the prevalence of tobacco use among children in the area.

- What other kinds of prevalence data might be used as a catalyst for community action?
- How might you go about obtaining similar data related to another health behavior (e.g., bicycle helmet or seat belt use)?
- Who would you involve in participatory community-based research related to your topic? Why would you include these people in your research team?
- To whom should your findings be disseminated? Why? How would you go about disseminating your fir[...] to these individuals or groups?

community members would be a tertiary preventive measure designed to thwart future epidemics.

Tertiary prevention is also designed to prevent consequences of existing problems. For example, when an earthquake occurs and safe water supplies are limited, programs to conserve or to purify water help to limit additional health effects of the earthquake that may arise from drinking contaminated water.

General Principles of Program Planning

Planning is a collaborative and systematic process used to attain a goal. Planning is collaborative in the sense that persons who will be affected by the planned program need to be involved in its planning. It is systematic in that change is consciously and deliberately brought about. Several general principles of program planning have been identified in the literature. Program planning should be population based. In other words, planned health programs should be appropriate to the population to be served and based on an understanding of the community's circumstances and the health problems experienced. Another principle is that members of the community, as well as health care professionals, should be actively involved in developing solutions to health problems.

In addition, programs should be based on epidemiologic and scientific data. Epidemiologic data suggest factors contributing to health problems that might be amenable to intervention. Research findings from the social sciences should also be used to plan programs that are acceptable to community residents.

Multiple approaches are often needed to address health problems arising from multiple causes. For this reason, planning should focus on both long-term and short-term outcomes that address the multiple contributing factors involved. Planning should also balance community needs and resources, and should make the best use of those resources to resolve identified health problems.

Planning should be based on a recognition of the interaction of multiple factors influencing health. This suggests that interventions encompassing the health care sector alone may not be comprehensive enough to resolve health care problems. For this reason, a wide variety of societal segments should be involved in health problem resolution. This means that intersectoral components of the community must work collaboratively rather than in isolation.

Broad community participation in health program planning has several advantages. Extensive participation promotes multiple points of view and may generate a wider array of potential solutions to community problems. Broad participation also leads to better refinement of programs and greater acceptance within the community. With multiple agencies and segments of society involved, there is also less chance for duplication of existing programs and more effective use of community resources.

⑥THINK ABOUT IT

Why have nurses not been very active or visible in health program planning efforts in the past? Are the reasons for nonparticipation by community members similar or different? What could be done to promote the involvement of both nurses and community members in program planning?

Finally, health care planning should be flexible enough to accommodate changes in community circumstances. This necessitates the development of broad strategies that can be implemented in a variety of ways. Flexibility may also require the interchangeability of some health care personnel within a plan, for example, using both physicians and nurse practitioners to provide primary care services to underserved populations. Principles of health program planning are summarized below.

HIGHLIGHTS

General Principles of Program Planning

- Planning must be population based and include broad community participation.
- The community must share responsibility for health problems and their solution.
- Planning should be based on epidemiologic and scientific data.
- Multiple interventions are needed to deal with the multiple causes of most community health problems.
- Planning should focus on both long-term and short-term change.
- Planning should balance needs and resources.
- Planning should be based on a recognition of the interactive nature of influences on health.
- Planning should be flexible.

The Planning Process

The process of planning health care programs for groups of people involves several discrete activities. These include selecting the planning group, developing planning competence, formulating a philosophy, establishing program goals, developing alternative solutions, evaluating alternatives and selecting a solution, and developing program objectives. Other planning activities are delineating the program theory or model, identifying resources, delineating actions required to accomplish objectives, evaluating the plan, and planning evaluation. These activities may or may not occur in the sequence in which they are presented here, but may occur simultaneously or in a slightly different order. What is important is that each one does occur at some point in the process.

Selecting the Planning Group

Those involved in planning should include key community or target group members expected to benefit from the program (Bracht et al., 1999). Potential beneficiaries of the program need to feel a sense of "ownership" of the program. For example, if the health need is one arising from adolescent sexuality (e.g., high incidence rates for STDs among teenagers), adolescents should be encouraged to provide input into planning a viable program to meet the need. They are the best judges of what will be acceptable to themselves and to their peers. A community or target group leader should also be identified to coordinate the planning process.

Other categories of persons to be included in the planning group depend, to a certain extent, on the type of problem to be solved; however, some general guidelines may prove helpful. It is wise to involve diverse segments of the community whenever possible to provide a widespread base of support for the resulting program. Individuals who have the authority to deal with the problem should certainly be included in the planning group. Those in a position to promote acceptance of the program such as media representatives, key community leaders, and influential citizens should also be invited to participate.

Another group that should be involved are those who are going to implement whatever program is planned. For example, if the program involves some type of educational campaign, local educators should be included in the planning process. Experts knowledgeable about the problem should also be included. These individuals can contribute to the group's understanding of the problem and provide knowledge of possible alternative solutions.

Both implementer and expert categories may involve health care professionals. The need to involve health care professionals in planning health care programs may seem obvious, but there are some additional, not so obvious, advantages to their inclusion in the planning group. In addition to providing technical input into the plan, health care professionals, especially community health nurses, have insights into local health care practices that affect problem resolution either positively or negatively. Furthermore, they can help legitimize the program and foster its acceptance in the community. Finally, health care professionals may be able to make the structural changes in the community's health care system that will be required for a successful program.

The last category of persons who should be involved in planning are individuals or groups who are likely to resist the program. This is one effective way of reducing opposition. Once these people have contributed to a plan that is acceptable to them, they are usually committed to the program and will work toward its acceptance by others.

Developing Planning Competence

Once the planning group is assembled, the first step in program planning is developing necessary planning competence. Few health care professionals or consumers have any educational background or experience in program planning. For this reason, the community health nurse may find it necessary to educate members of the planning group in regard to planning processes and activities. It may also be necessary to prevent the group from engaging in activities for which an adequate foundation has yet to be provided. In doing so, the community health nurse needs to exercise well-developed skills in leadership and group dynamics addressed in Chapter 13. Other tasks to be accomplished at this stage of planning include establishing the organizational structure of the group and clarifying the roles and responsibilities of planning group members.

Formulating a Philosophy

The next step, formulating a philosophy, is not often carried out as a conscious activity, but is an assumption on the part of group members. For example, there must be some type of commitment to adequate health care for prison inmates before a group would even consider planning a program to meet prisoners' needs. It is, however, important that the philosophies of various members of the planning group be compatible. Therefore, group members should be encouraged to verbalize their philosophies and to identify and deal with areas of conflict between philosophies. The development of a joint philosophy is sometimes referred to as "visioning" and is a process in which group members develop a collective view of what they hope to accomplish (Sharpe et al., 2000).

Establishing Program Goals

Goals flow from the group's philosophy and describe the overall intent of the group with respect to the problem to be solved. Again, goals must be developed by the group as a whole to ensure consistency. Goals are usually stated in general terms as a desired ultimate outcome. In the prison example, a possible goal might be "to provide adequate health care services for inmates." This goal, stated very generally, gives no indication of possible means of achieving the desired outcome. Objectives, on the other hand, are stated as specific expected outcomes that contribute in some way to realizing the goal. Objectives are discussed more thoroughly later in this chapter.

Developing Alternative Solutions

The next step in the program planning process is developing alternative solutions to the identified health need. Here, the planning group should be encouraged to exercise creativity in attempts to develop alternatives. A suggestion that appears absurd on first presentation may be found to be quite feasible on investigation. Inappropriate alternatives will eventually be eliminated during the next step of the planning process—evaluation of alternatives in terms of critical criteria for problem resolution.

Evaluating Alternatives and Selecting a Solution

One of the components in the planning stage of the nursing process is the development of critical criteria against which any solution to a particular problem must be weighed. Critical criteria for solutions are also required when the client is a community or target group rather than an individual or a family. Examples of critical criteria for solutions to community problems might be that such solutions fit within available budgetary resources or that they be acceptable to ethnic or religious groups within the community.

Potential solutions to community problems should always be evaluated in terms of cost, feasibility, acceptability, availability of necessary resources, efficiency, equity, political advantage, and identifiability of the target group. Generally speaking, an alternative that costs less will be viewed more favorably, other factors being equal, than one that costs more, or one alternative may be selected over another because its implementation is more feasible. For example, it is considerably easier to install a traffic light at an accident-prone intersection than to build a bridge to route one intersecting road over the other.

Potential solutions should also be evaluated in terms of their acceptability to policy makers, implementers, and the community. Policy makers are unlikely to approve an alternative that diminishes their power or authority, and implementers are certainly unlikely to accept a potential solution that requires them to work overtime or without pay if another alternative is available. Similarly, community members affected by the proposed program may find one alternative more acceptable than another for a variety of reasons.

Alternative solutions may also differ in terms of the resources needed to implement them. Generally speaking, an alternative that requires fewer resources or for which resources are already available is more likely to be endorsed than one that requires extensive or scarce resources. For example, a group seeking to improve the nutritional status of schoolchildren may select an alternative that makes use of existing facilities used to prepare meals for senior citizens rather than one that necessitates providing kitchen facilities in each school. Efficiency is a related criterion on which alternative solutions to a particular problem can be evaluated. An efficient alternative makes better use of available resources and is usually viewed more favorably in making planning decisions than an inefficient one. An asset-oriented assessment can provide a picture of the resources already available within the community or target group and can assist in assessing the relative resource needs of alternative solutions.

Questions of equity also arise in evaluating alternative solutions to a problem. Alternatives that unfairly discriminate against one segment of the population are usu-

ally rejected. For example, one alternative to the problem of dealing with teen pregnancy might be to provide contraceptive services in the larger high schools. If, however, these schools tend to serve the upper-middle-class segment of the community while lower-class students attend smaller schools, this alternative would discriminate against a segment of the community also needing service.

Political consequences also need to be considered in evaluating the alternative solutions to specific problems. For instance, an alternative plan that provides services to a highly vocal voting bloc might be viewed more favorably by politicians than one that serves a less politically involved minority group. Evaluation of alternatives may also involve forecasting regarding the effects of other possible events on the problem or its solution. For example, if a vaccine for HIV infection is likely to be available in the near future, the community may not want to put a lot of resources into a condom promotion program.

Finally, alternative solutions should be evaluated in terms of the identifiability of the target group. One potential solution for preventing the spread of AIDS might be to screen all prostitutes in the community for HIV infection. It is somewhat difficult, however, to identify this group of people, as prostitution is an illegal activity in most places. It might be easier to screen everyone who requests services for STDs because this group is sexually active and is also identifiable.

Consideration of possible sources of opposition also contributes to selection of the most appropriate alternative. If it is known that members of the community PTA would vigorously oppose a "sex fair" as a means of educating adolescents on sexual issues, another less threatening alternative would be more appropriate.

There are two basic types of opposition to proposed programs: rational and irrational. Rational opposition is based on sound reasoning and should be seriously considered, as it may prove beneficial to the planning effort. Rational opposition does pose problems to the extent that it lends support to irrational opposition and also tends to sway individuals who are undecided as to the merits of the planned program.

Irrational opposition can arise from several sources. It may result from a general attitude of conservatism in which only proven interventions are held to be acceptable. As a rule, conservatives usually discount innovative ideas as possible solutions and prefer to remain with more traditional approaches.

The second type of irrational opposition arises out of cultural patterns and social reactions to change in general. For example, agricultural change programs initiated by Peace Corps volunteers in India were considerably less successful than programs fostering small industries. The farmers were responding to centuries of culturally ingrained patterns of farming, whereas the small businessmen were engaged in pursuits that held no strong cultural connotations.

Opposition may also arise from perceptions that a particular course of action poses a threat to the power, prestige, or economic security of certain members in or outside of a group or community. For example, starting a clinic staffed by nurse practitioners to improve the accessibility of health care may be seen by local physicians as a threat to their economic security.

Another source of irrational opposition is usually unconscious in nature and results from feelings of overall vulnerability. This type of opposition is usually found in the same group of people, whatever the issue addressed. Because of their own personal insecurity, change of any type may be threatening to these individuals.

Additional sources of resistance to health care programs include reluctance to spend money on health care, legal obstacles across jurisdictions, and unreasoning self-reliance. Reluctance to spend money can often be overcome by accurate documentation of the costs of the problem and the cost-effectiveness of problem resolution. For example, a county sheriff's department got council approval for a nursing clinic in the county jail by documenting the decrease in the cost of health care for prisoners when a nurse was available.

Jurisdictional obstacles can be overcome by including in the planning body persons with authority and prestige in the problem area. Pride or unreasoning self-reliance can also be an obstacle to utilization of health programs. For this reason, any alternative selected must be acceptable to the group for which it is designed. One method of accomplishing this is including members of the target group in the planning body.

The community health nurse should assist the planning group to determine the relative weight to be given to each of these considerations in evaluating alternative solutions. Those considerations that are weighted most heavily become the critical criteria against which all potential solutions are evaluated. The remaining considerations are those that are nice if they can be met, but not absolutely necessary. For example, if there is an unlimited source of funding for dealing with certain types of problems, cost might not be a critical criterion for selecting a solution to the problem in question. Conversely, it may be that criteria of cost, feasibility, and acceptability are considered critical and others are viewed as less important. Once the criteria have been established, the group can proceed to evaluate all of the potential solutions generated and select the one(s) most appropriate to the situation.

Developing Program Objectives

Once alternative solutions have been evaluated in light of critical criteria and a solution selected, the process of planning a specific program based on that alternative begins. At this point, the planning group sets specific program objectives. Objectives are statements of specific outcomes expected to result from the program that contribute to the realization of the overall goal.

For objectives to be useful, they should meet several criteria. Perhaps the most essential of these is that the objective be clearly stated and measurable. A well-stated objective includes some means of measuring the outcome expected and evaluating the effectiveness of the effort. For example, if the overall goal is to improve children's nutritional status, one program objective might relate to hematocrit levels. It is not, however, sufficient to state that hematocrit levels will improve; the extent of improvement expected also needs to be specified. A measurable objective could be that "75% of school-age children in the community (or target group) will have hematocrit levels within normal limits." A more precise objective would include a definition of normal hematocrit levels: "75% of school-age children in Evanston will have hematocrit levels of 35% or greater." In this objective, a measure of the expected hematocrit level is specified as is a measure of the number of children expected to achieve it. This objective is measurable and precise.

Another criterion of good program objectives is the inclusion of a specific time frame within which the outcome is expected to occur. A time frame can easily be added to the previous objective to state that "a hematocrit reading of 35% or greater will be achieved in 75% of the school-age children in Evanston within six months of initiating a school-based food supplement program." As stated, this objective also meets several other criteria for program objectives. It is reasonable and practical to expect a significant increase in hematocrit levels after six months of an iron-rich diet. To expect it in two weeks would not be reasonable. It would also be unreasonable to expect that all of the children would achieve normal hematocrit levels as a result of the program. Seventy-five percent is reasonable.

The objective also meets the criterion of being within the competence of the planning group to accomplish. This would not be true, however, were the planners a group of electrical engineers. It is also legal, provided one has the permission of parents to provide nourishment to children in need of it and to obtain hematocrit levels. It fits the moral and value framework of the community and carries minimum unpleasant side effects. The latter would not be true, however, if the alternative chosen called for injectable iron preparations that are painful to administer. Finally, the objective, as stated, will probably be acceptable to those implementing the program, and it is hoped that it will fit within the budgetary limitations of the school system. Criteria for effective program outcome objectives are summarized on page 342.

Program planners usually develop two types of program objectives: outcome objectives and process objectives. The examples of objectives provided above are outcome objectives and specify the expected results of the program in terms of changes in clients' health status or behavior. Process objectives specify the means to achieve outcome objectives. A process objective related to the problem of childhood anemia, for example, might be "provision of 75% of the recommended dietary allowance for iron in a school meal program." The inclusion of iron-rich foods in a school meal program is the means by which normal hematocrit levels among school-age children are expected to be achieved. Process objectives are later broken down in the planning process into specific activities necessary for their achievement.

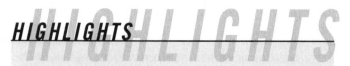

HIGHLIGHTS

Criteria for Effective Program Objectives

Measurability

The objective is measurable so as to determine whether it has been achieved.

Precision

The expected outcome is clear and precisely stated.

Time Specificity

The objective includes a statement of the time within which it is expected to be accomplished.

Reasonability or Practicability

The objective is practical and able to be met with a reasonable amount of effort.

Within Group Competencies

The objective is within the competence of the planning group to accomplish, given members' expertise and authority.

Legality

The objective is legal.

Congruence with Community Morals and Values

The objective is consistent with the values and morals of implementers and members of the community or target group.

Carries Minimal Side Effects

The objective has minimal side effects, and these effects are acceptable to program beneficiaries.

Fits Budgetary Limitations

The objective fits the community's budgetary limitations.

Delineating the Program Theory

A relatively new step that has been incorporated into health program planning is the development of a program theory or logic model. A *logic model* is a description of the connections between program events that lead to the accomplishment of the intended outcomes (Centers for Disease Control and Prevention [CDC], 1999). The

logic model links program activities to program outcomes and can be evaluated in terms of the accuracy of assumptions about those links. The model may be a schematic representation of the program such as that depicted in Figure 15–1 ■ or may be a series of if–then statements that describe the connections between program activities and expected outcomes (Goodman, 1998). For example, "if" iron-rich foods are provided in the school setting and "if" children eat them, "then" hematocrit levels should increase. Similarly, "if" hematocrit levels increase, "then" levels of anemia among school-age children will decrease.

Identifying Resources

Once objectives have been established, the planning group can proceed to identify resources needed to implement the program. Resources include personnel, money, materials, and time. To continue with the previous example of improving the nutritional status of children, if the alternative selected was an iron-rich school meal program, a variety of resources are required to institute such a program. Many of these resources may have been identified in the course of the asset-oriented community assessment. Personnel needed include people to develop menus incorporating iron-rich foods palatable to school-age children and people to purchase, prepare, and serve the food as well as to wash dishes. Funds to purchase food and the equipment with which to prepare and serve it are also needed. Material resources needed include the

FIGURE 15–1 ■ *Partial logic model for a school meal program*

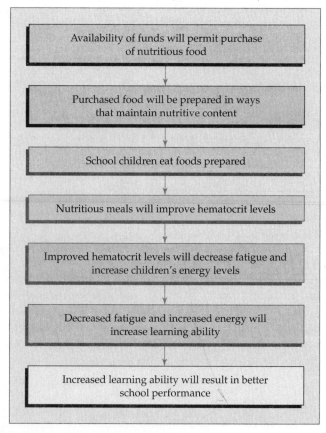

dishes, silverware, pots and pans, and cooking facilities. Other needs include the equipment and health care personnel who will check hematocrit levels.

Not only must the planning group decide what resources are required but they must also specify how these resources can be obtained. Will the PTA have a fund-raising drive? Will a grant proposal for federal assistance be submitted? The final consideration with respect to resources is that of time. The time needed to put the program into operation must be determined.

Delineating Actions to Accomplish Objectives

The next step in the planning process is delineating specific actions required to carry out the program. This is usually considered the "nitty-gritty" of planning, and many planning groups mistakenly jump immediately to this phase of activity. For planning to be effective, however, this step must be preceded by those discussed earlier.

In this phase of planning, the step-by-step details of the plan are developed. To a large extent, many of the major activities involved in carrying out the program have already been delineated in the development of the program theory. Using the example of the school meal program, some of the actions needed include presenting the problem and the proposed solution to the PTA, planning fund-raising projects, and purchasing equipment and supplies. In addition, the health department nutritionist would plan adequate menus. Advertisements for cooks and enlistment of parent volunteers to help prepare and serve food would be initiated, and so on, down to the last detail. Other areas that may need to be addressed include legal issues, development of program policies and procedures, ways of informing families of the program, and forms and recording procedures.

Evaluating the Plan

When the detailed plan has been constructed and specific activities delineated, the plan itself should be evaluated. Is the plan based on identified needs of the target group or is it unrelated to those needs? Is the plan flexible enough to adapt to changing circumstances in the foreseeable future? How efficient will the planned program be? Could program efficiency be improved by modification of the plan? Finally, how adequate is the plan? Have all constraints and contingencies been addressed? Answers to these and similar questions enable the planning group to evaluate the plan and to identify the need for any modifications before implementation. Again, the program theory or logic model can assist in evaluating the plan itself. Are the cause-and-effect relationships assumed in the model based on knowledge? Are the links clear and direct, or have some necessary activities been forgotten?

Planning Evaluation

The final component to be considered in program planning is planning evaluation of program effectiveness. This may seem a bit premature because the program has not even started; however, it is essential. Unless planning for program evaluation is incorporated at this stage, the data needed for evaluating program outcomes will not be available when the time arrives for actual evaluation.

Planning evaluation involves four considerations. The first of these is determining criteria on which the program should be evaluated. The second consideration is the types of data to be collected and the means used to collect the data. Determining the resources needed to carry out the evaluation is the third consideration in planning evaluation. Finally, the planning group should determine who will evaluate the program. All of these considerations are addressed in greater detail under the nursing process heading "Evaluating the Program." At this juncture it is sufficient to reemphasize the point that planning evaluation begins during program planning, not after the program has been implemented.

Effective health program planning involves all of the steps discussed up to now. When steps are ignored or bypassed, the program planned is likely to be less effective and its implementation may prove more difficult. These steps are summarized below.

HIGHLIGHTS

Steps in the Planning Process

- Selecting the planning group
- Developing planning competence
- Formulating a philosophy
- Establishing program goals
- Developing alternative solutions
- Evaluating alternatives and selecting a solution
- Developing program objectives
- Delineating the program theory
- Identifying resources
- Delineating action to accomplish objectives
- Evaluating the plan
- Planning evaluation

IMPLEMENTING THE PLAN

It is not enough for the planning group to plan for a health care program to meet identified health care needs. The group must also ensure that the plan is implemented as designed. The goal of implementation is to integrate program activities into community networks in such a way that the program is sustained as long as the need for it exists (Bracht et al., 1999). Implementing a health program involves several considerations. These include getting the plan accepted, performing the tasks involved in implementing the program, and using strategies that foster implementation of the program as planned.

Plan Acceptance

Acceptance of the planned program occurs at three levels. The first level is acceptance by community policy makers. If policy makers have been represented on the planning group, this level of acceptance should already have been achieved.

The second level of acceptance involves convincing those who are to carry out the plan to implement it for everyday operation. Again, if program implementers have been adequately represented in the planning effort, this level is already partially achieved. All that remains is for the implementers to convert the plan into an operational program.

Acceptance and participation in the planned program by members of the target group is the third level of acceptance. If, for example, the planned program involves providing contraceptive services to sexually active adolescents, the third level of acceptance involves adolescents' participation in the program. Acceptance at this third level may require marketing the program to the intended target population. *Marketing* is the design and use of methods to influence people's choices of actions to be taken (Fos & Fine, 2000), in this case adolescents' choice to obtain contraceptive services.

⑥THINK ABOUT IT

Should sex education be a required topic in public junior and senior high schools? How would you go about getting such a program accepted by the community?

Tasks of Implementation

Three basic tasks are involved in program implementation: activity delineation and sequencing, task allocation, and task performance. Necessary activities have been broadly outlined in plan development. Now they must be specified and subactivities identified. This involves identifying needed categories of action and the skills required for their performance. At this point, implementers would determine the appropriate sequencing of activities and might establish a time frame for their accomplishment.

Task allocation involves identifying the expertise of program implementers relative to the skills needed for effective implementation of the plan. Also at this point, responsibility is assigned for various activities delineated. Such assignments must be communicated to those involved, and they must be provided with whatever

Community clean-up projects promote efforts for a clean environment.

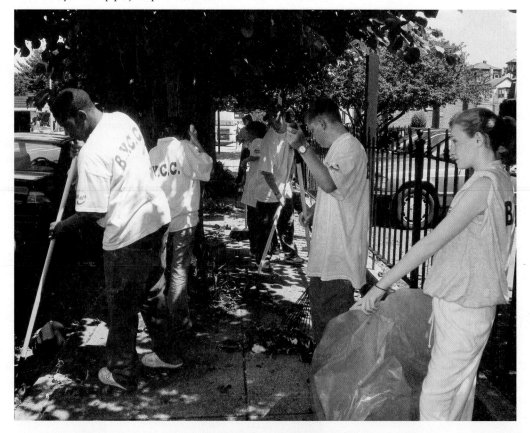

education or training is required for implementing the plan. Finally, the activities themselves are carried out and the planned program is put into operation.

Strategies for Implementation

Program implementation can be enhanced if several specific implementation strategies are employed. The first of these strategies is to assign responsibility for coordination of the total effort to one person. Identifying preparatory steps to each activity and listing them in sequence also fosters implementation of the program as planned.

Another strategy that enhances program implementation is periodic consultation with those implementing the program to address any difficulties that arise. Finally, the chances of implementing the program as planned are enhanced when everyone involved is clearly informed of expectations and the time frame for meeting expectations.

Using the school meal program as an example, implementing the plan might involve designating the school nurse as the program coordinator, staging a PTA bazaar to raise funds after delineating all of the activities involved in doing so, hiring and training personnel, and developing menus. Other implementation activities would include purchasing food, supplies, and equipment and preparing and serving the meals.

It is important that members of the planning group, or designated others, monitor implementation of the plan to determine any barriers to implementation or any changes needed in the plan itself. Monitoring should address at least five areas: the adequacy of funds budgeted to carry out the plan, the ability of personnel to address program needs, the adequacy of other program resources, the timing of actual activities versus the planned sequence of action, and the production of the planned output (Veney & Kaluzny, 1998). Again, using the school meal example, the planning group might note whether or not the funds budgeted for the program are sufficient to cover program costs and whether the nutritionist can develop menus that tempt children's appetites. Similarly, the group might note whether or not there are sufficient plates and tableware to meet the demand as well as the appropriateness of the planned activity sequence. Should purchasing processes be adapted to better fit the school's budget process? Finally, the group would monitor the number of meals being prepared and whether or not they are being eaten by the schoolchildren.

EVALUATING THE PROGRAM

Evaluating the effects of health care programs is an essential feature of community health nursing care of communities and target groups. Program evaluation is needed for many of the same reasons that a systematic process is used in program planning. Health care providers recognize the limitation of available resources and must be accountable to the community members who use the program and, particularly, to the community members who pay for the program. They must be able to justify the program's existence and continuation. This can be done only by documenting the effectiveness of programs in solving the problems at hand.

Evaluation of a particular program may be undertaken for a variety of reasons. Some of these include justifying program continuation or expansion, improving the quality of service provided, determining future courses of action, and determining the impact of the program. Other reasons for evaluation might be to call attention to the program, to assess personnel performance, or to assuage political expectations. Evaluation is frequently conducted because it is required by a funding agency.

Several general principles of program evaluation have been identified and are summarized below. First, program theory or the logic model as well as the outcomes of the program should be evaluated. Program evaluation measures also need to be tailored to the specific program and community that is being evaluated. This means that standardized evaluation measures should be used with caution and their use justified by the needs and purposes of the evaluation. The evaluation approaches used should be guided by the questions asked. As we will see later, the purpose for which the evaluation is being conducted strongly influences the approaches taken. Evaluation of health programs should take into account the multiple levels at which interventions may occur. For example, a program may address individual attitudes and behaviors while also addressing policy issues that impede or promote health care services, and program effects at each level should be evaluated. Community health problems arise from a complex interaction of social, cultural, economic, and other factors, and so, health programs should be evaluated in the context of the complex environment in which they function. Similarly, programs develop in stages, and evaluation should be appropriate to the stage of program development. Finally, the evaluation process should involve *stakeholders,* those concerned with the outcomes of the evaluation (e.g., program beneficiaries, staff, funders, etc.) in meaningful ways (Goodman, 1998).

HIGHLIGHTS

General Principles of Program Evaluation

- Program theory, as well as program outcomes, should be evaluated.
- Evaluation measures should be tailored to the program and community in which they are being used.
- The approach taken to evaluation should be guided by the questions asked.
- Multiple levels of program effects should be evaluated as appropriate.
- Health programs should be evaluated in the context of the complex factors that influence health.
- Programs should be evaluated in terms of their stage of development.
- The evaluation process should involve stakeholders in meaningful ways.

Considerations in Program Evaluation

Purpose Considerations

The purpose of the evaluation influences all other aspects of the process. For example, if the purpose of the evaluation is to justify continuing a program, the evaluation will focus on determining whether the program has a beneficial effect on the health of the population group for which it is designed. On the other hand, if the purpose is to decide whether programs are under- or overused, evaluation will focus on the number of persons served. In other words, the purpose of the evaluation influences the types of data collected and how they are used.

Evaluator Considerations

The second area for consideration is who should conduct the evaluation. A number of choices are possible. The program can be evaluated by those who implement it or who benefit from it. Evaluation by people who are involved in the program has some disadvantages in that there is a certain amount of bias on the part of those with a vested interest in retaining the program. The advantages of an inside evaluator are familiarity with the program and knowledge of sources of data that will be needed.

Another possibility is to employ someone from outside the program to conduct the evaluation. This person is likely to be relatively objective in his or her approach to evaluation, but faces the disadvantages of not being well acquainted with the program and, possibly, of being unable to identify appropriate sources of data. This alternative is also rather expensive.

A third possibility, and one that is in keeping with participatory research in community assessment, and community participation in program planning, is empower-

ment evaluation. *Empowerment evaluation* is defined as the "use of evaluation concepts and techniques to foster self-determination" among community members (Wallerstein, 1999). Empowerment evaluation assists communities to develop the skills to assess and improve their own quality of life. In empowerment evaluation, the community health nurse evaluator serves as an educator, advocate, and facilitator, and community members determine the focus and methods for the evaluation and participate in data collection and analysis and use of the findings.

Ethical Considerations

Ethical conflicts must be anticipated in program evaluation. Participation in the evaluation should be voluntary for staff and clients alike. This poses some problems in that staff members are sometimes unwilling to reveal information that reflects poorly on them or on the program that employs them. To circumvent this reluctance, the evaluator needs to have a variety of sources of data that provide an overall picture of the program and its effects.

Confidentiality is another issue. Persons who provide data need to be assured that their individual responses will not be identifiable. There is also the question of who will have access to the findings of the evaluation. Should findings be shared only with those involved in the program? With their supervisors? With funding agencies or regulatory bodies? The use to which findings can be put is also of concern. Can the evaluator publish the information? Will it be used to fire personnel?

Finally, the evaluation team must consider the risks and benefits accruing from the evaluation. Is there potential for harm to the participants, either clients or staff? Do the anticipated benefits of the evaluation outweigh any possible risks?

Type of Evaluation

The last major consideration in evaluating a health care program is the type of evaluation to be conducted. There are three basic types of evaluation: structure, outcome, and process evaluation, each of which can be broken down into subtypes or approaches.

STRUCTURE *Structure* reflects the delivery system characteristics of the program including its organization, the types of personnel employed, types of clients served, and so on (Aday, Begley, Lairson, & Slater, 1998). Evaluative questions related to program structure might include the following: Do program staff have the education and expertise to carry out the program and meet identified community needs? Are there barriers to access to services for some segments of the community? If so, what are they and how can they be overcome? Is the program reaching the population for which it was designed?

OUTCOME EVALUATION *Outcome evaluation* focuses on the consequences of the program for the health and welfare of the population, irrespective of how well organized or how efficient the program was. Outcome evaluation documents the effects of the program and justifies decisions to continue, modify, or eliminate it. The two subtypes of outcome evaluation are evaluation of *effect* and assessment of *impact*.

A program's effect is the degree to which specific outcome objectives were met. Using the previous example of the school lunch program, the effect of the program is evaluated when one determines whether 75% of the school-age children have a hematocrit level of 35% or greater within six months of the start of the program. If they do, the program can be considered effective. If not, the evaluator must determine to what degree the objective has been met and whether continuation of the program is warranted. For example, if the objective was achieved with 60% of the participating children, extending the program would probably be considered. If, on the other hand, only 20% of the children achieved normal hematocrit levels, alternative solutions to the problem may need to be considered.

The impact of a program is how well it serves to attain overall goals. If the goal was to improve the nutritional status of school-age children, for example, the achievement of improved hematocrit levels does contribute to goal achievement. If, however, the goal was to improve the children's learning ability through adequate nutrition, increasing hematocrit levels may or may not contribute to its achievement. In this case, one would need to know not only the hematocrit levels but also the amount of learning that has taken place to state that the program has had an impact on meeting the overall goal. One may find that hematocrit levels did indeed rise, but no improvement in learning ability occurred. In this instance, the program was effective in accomplishing its objective, but accomplishing the objective did not lead to achievement of the overall goal.

Health programs can have a number of outcomes. Often, the outcomes arise out of the program's stated objectives as in the examples above. Other outcomes may also be of interest. Usually, however, it is not feasible or even possible to examine all of a program's possible outcomes, so the evaluation team will need to decide which outcomes will be the focus of program evaluation. Several criteria have been suggested for making this decision. First, the outcomes studied should be valued by persons involved in the program, the recipients, the implementers, or the funders. Second, a multidimensional array of outcomes should be examined to provide information about the overall worth of the program. Outcomes should be selected for which objective and measurable data can be obtained. Fourth, the outcomes selected should be logically connected to the program and should be effects that can be attributed to the program rather than to other factors. Finally, both long-term and short-term outcomes of the program should be assessed whenever possible (Schalock, 1995).

For each outcome selected, the evaluation team will develop one or more outcome measures to assess that outcome. **Outcome measures** involve the assessment of one or more variables related to expected program results (Fos & Fine, 2000). Tests of children's hematocrit levels and tests of learning ability might be outcome measures selected to evaluate the school meal program.

PROCESS EVALUATION   The third type of evaluation is *process evaluation*. Here, one is concerned with the quality of interactions between program staff and recipients (Aday et al., 1998). Process evaluation examines program performance and may take the perspective of quality assurance or quality improvement. The focus in quality assurance is on making sure that the processes by which care is provided meet certain established standards. If the standard has been met, no action is warranted and program operation continues unmodified. Quality improvement, on the other hand, is designed to produce "a continuous stream of improvements in order to provide health care that meets or exceeds consumer expectations" (McLaughlin & Kaluzny, 1999). The philosophy behind quality improvement, also referred to as continuous quality improvement (CQI) or total quality management (TQM), is that clients' needs and expectations change over time and that an effective health care program is continually changing to better meet those needs. This can be achieved only if the processes of care are being continually examined and improved as needed. Quality improvement focuses on enhancing the processes of care to create more effective outcomes. General areas to be examined include the effectiveness of services in meeting client needs, the accessibility and acceptability of services to the client population, optimization of resource use, and needs for improvement in care processes. The types and aspects of program evaluation presented here are summarized below.

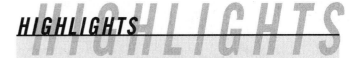

HIGHLIGHTS

Types and Aspects of Program Evaluation

Structure Evaluation
Evaluation of program delivery characteristics and their effects on program processes and outcomes

Outcome Evaluation
Effect: Evaluation of achievement of outcome objectives
Impact: Evaluation of the program's influence on meeting overall goals

Process Evaluation
Quality assurance: Evaluation of care processes based on identified standards
Quality improvement: Continuous improvement in care processes to better meet or exceed client expectations

In designing a program evaluation, the evaluation team needs to decide which types of evaluation are appropriate. A particular program can be evaluated with respect to any one aspect or a combination of several. The aspects selected depend on the purposes of the evaluation and the time and other resources available. Most health program evaluations will incorporate several aspects of evaluation.

The Evaluation Process

Like any other systematic process, evaluation takes place in a series of specific steps. Some of these steps, such as planning the evaluation, have already been completed as part of the total planning process. Other steps include collecting data, interpreting data, and using evaluative findings.

Planning Evaluation

Goals for the evaluation, evaluative criteria, types of data needed, and appropriate methods of data collection were established as part of the planning process. Evaluative criteria and type of evaluation are based on the purpose of the evaluation. If the intent of the evaluation is to determine the extent to which outcome objectives are met, evaluative criteria will be derived from those objectives. In the school meal program example, evaluative criteria related to outcome objectives would be hematocrit levels of children participating in the program. If the intent is to assess the efficiency of the program, evaluative criteria would include the amount of food wasted and the number of hours spent implementing the program.

Data needed to conduct the evaluation are determined and data collection procedures established. Planning evaluation also involves determining the necessary equipment and supplies. Items needed to evaluate accomplishment of the school meal program's outcome objectives would include parental consent forms for hematocrit testing, capillary tubes, lancets, and a microcentrifuge. Other equipment and supplies would be needed to evaluate other aspects of the program.

Collecting Data

The evaluative criteria chosen influence the types of data collected and the manner in which they are collected. For the hematocrit criterion, data include participating children's hematocrit levels, which need to be collected by testing blood samples at periodic intervals before and during the program. There needs to be a baseline level for each child before the program to determine whether hematocrit levels have increased, so data collection related to evaluation must begin before the program itself starts. Data collection related to food wasted might include review of purchase orders and periodic observation of the amount of food discarded at the end of the day.

Interpreting Data

The next step in the evaluation process is interpreting the data collected. In this step, data are compared with the evaluative criteria. In evaluating the achievement of the outcome objectives of the school meal program, the evaluation team would compare the children's hematocrit levels after starting the program with those obtained before the program. If an increase is noted in most children, the program has been somewhat effective. The team would also determine how many of the children had now achieved a normal hematocrit level. If 75% or more of the children now have normal levels, the program has met its objective.

In examining data related to the efficient use of supplies, the evaluation team would look at what percentage of food purchased is actually consumed and what percentage is wasted. If the criterion derived from process objectives specified that less than 5% of food and supplies purchased is wasted and the team finds that closer to 10% is actually wasted, the program processes are not operating as efficiently as planned.

Disseminating and Using Evaluative Findings

Effective use of evaluation findings requires that they be disseminated to those who need them (CDC, 1999). This includes those who will make decisions regarding the program as well as those who are contemplating similar programs.

Hopefully, the findings of the evaluation are used as a basis for decisions about the program. Basically, three decisions can be made based on evaluative findings: to continue, to modify, or to discontinue the program. If the evaluation team finds that the program's objectives are being achieved, they may recommend continuing the program. If the team finds that only a few children are participating in the program, they may recommend either stopping the program or taking steps to increase participation. For example, perhaps the menu needs to be changed to include nutritious foods that are more acceptable to the target group. Looking at program efficiency, if the assessment team finds that 10% of the food purchased is being wasted, various waste control practices may need to be instituted. The dissemination and use of evaluative findings and the other steps in program evaluation are summarized on page 349.

Factors in each of the six dimensions of health are considered by community health nurses in assessing the health needs of communities and other population groups. Planning to meet those needs then employs an organized and systematic process involving development of planning competence, developing goals and objectives based on program theory, and delineating resources and actions needed to accomplish goals and objectives. Implementation and evaluation of health care delivery programs are also systematic processes employed by community health nurses.

HIGHLIGHTS

Components of the Program Evaluation Process

- Planning evaluation
    - Setting evaluation goals
    - Developing evaluative criteria
    - Determining the data needed
    - Establishing data collection procedures
    - Determining resources needed
- Collecting data
- Interpreting data
- Disseminating evaluative findings
- Using evaluative findings to make decisions regarding:
    - Continuing the program
    - Modifying the program
    - Discontinuing the program

APPLYING YOUR KNOWLEDGE IN PRACTICE

✖ CASE STUDY
Caring for Copper City

You are the community health nurse assigned to Copper City, a small town in New Mexico, with a population of 3,000. You have just arrived in town and have been given the task of assisting community members to assess the health needs of the community and developing a plan to meet those needs. Your assessment committee consists of yourself, one of the local physicians, the elementary school principal, two teachers, pastors of two local churches, the owner of one of the local copper mines, and five community residents.

During the assessment, the assessment team obtains the following information: Copper City is a small town run by a city council and a mayor. Most of these officials are administrators of the local copper mines or owners of large chicken farms in the area. The town is in a largely rural area, and lies 50 miles from Tucumcari. The surrounding countryside is hot and arid.

The ethnic composition of the town is 80% Caucasian of European ancestry and 20% Latino, primarily of Mexican descent. Fifty percent of the town's population is under 8 years of age. There are very few elderly persons in the community, because Copper City is a relatively new town that grew up around copper mines discovered in the last 20 years. The birth rate is 30 per 1,000 population. Approximately 10% of all births are premature, and the neonatal death rate is 50 per 1,000 live births. Only about 10% of the women receive prenatal care during their pregnancies.

The major industries in the area are copper mines and chicken farms, which employ approximately 85% of the adult men and 50% of the women. The majority of the Latino population works on the chicken farms. The remaining 15% of the adult men and another 20% of the adult women are employed in offices and shops in the town. The unemployment level is 0.5%, far lower than that of the state and the nation.

The average annual family income is $8,000, and 75% of the population is below the poverty level. Nearly one third of those below the poverty level receive some form of aid such as Medicaid or Temporary Aid to Needy Families (TANF).

The predominant religion among the Caucasian population is Methodist, and among the Latino group it is Roman Catholic. There are two Methodist churches in town, one Catholic church, and a small Southern Baptist congregation.

Many of the Latino group subscribe to alternative health practices. They frequently seek health care from a local *yerbero* (herbalist). They may also drive to a nearby town to solicit the services of a *curandera* (faith healer). Close to one third of the Latino population speaks only Spanish.

The average education level for the community is tenth grade. For the Spanish-speaking group, however, it is only third grade. Education facilities in the town include a grade school and a high school. The high school also offers adult education classes at night. There is a Head Start program that enrolls 50 children, but no other child care facilities are available.

There is a high incidence of tuberculosis in the community, and anemia and pinworms are common problems among the preschool and school-age children. Several of the men have been disabled as a result of accidents in the mines.

The only transportation to Tucumcari is by car or by train, which comes through town morning and evening. About half of the families in town own cars.

There is one general practice physician and one dentist in the town. The nearest hospital is in Tucumcari, and the funeral home hearse is used as an ambulance for emergency transportation to the hospital. The driver and one attendant have had basic first aid training but have not been educated as emergency medical technicians. The county health department provides family planning, prenatal, well-child, and immunization services one day a week in the basement of the larger of the two Methodist churches. In addition to yourself, the staff consists of a physician, one licensed practical nurse, a master's-prepared family nurse practitioner, and a nutritionist. The well-child and immunization services are heavily used, and immunization levels in the community are high among both preschoolers and school-age youngsters.

- What are the biophysical, psychological, physical environmental, sociocultural, behavioral, and health system factors influencing the health of this community?
- What assets are present in this community that might assist with problem resolution?

- What community nursing diagnoses might you derive from the assessment team's data?
- What health problems are evident in the case study? Which do you think are the three most important problems for this community? Why have you given these problems priority over others? Do you think other members of the assessment team would prioritize them differently? Why or why not?
- Select one of the three top-priority problems and design a health program to resolve it. Be sure to address the following:
   Level of prevention involved
   Who should be involved in the planning group, why, and how you would obtain community participation in planning
   Additional information you would need, if any, and where you would obtain that information
   Goals and objectives for the program
   Resources needed to implement the program
- How would you gain acceptance of your program?
- How would you go about implementing the program?
- How would you conduct outcome and process evaluation of the program?

❧ TESTING YOUR UNDERSTANDING

- Why should community or target group members be incorporated into all phases of community assessment and program planning and evaluation? (pp. 320–321)
- What kinds of factors influence the scope of a community or target group assessment? Give an example of the influence of each factor. (pp. 321–322)
- What biophysical, psychological, physical environmental, sociocultural, behavioral, and health system factors should be addressed in a comprehensive community or target group assessment? (pp. 324–334)
- What are the two levels of nursing diagnoses related to the health status of a community or a target group? Give an example of a diagnosis at each level. (pp. 334–335)

- What are the three types of considerations in planning screening programs for communities or target groups? Give an example of how considerations in each category might influence the decision to institute a community screening program. (pp. 336–337)
- Identify at least six tasks in planning a health program to meet the needs of communities or target groups. What would be the role of the community health nurse with respect to each task? (pp. 338–343)
- What are the three levels of acceptance of a health care program? How might community health nurses influence acceptance at each level? (p. 344)
- What are three types of considerations in evaluating a health care program? How might each influence the program evaluation process? (p. 346)

REFERENCES

Aday, L. A., Begley, C. E., Lairson, D. R., & Slater, C. H. (1998). *Evaluating the healthcare system: Effectiveness, efficiency, and equity.* Chicago: Health Administration Press.

Ammerman, A., & Parks, C. (1998). Preparing students for more effective community interventions: Assets assessment. *Family & Community Health, 21*(1), 32–45.

Bingler, S. (2000). The school as the center of a healthy community. *Public Health Reports, 115,* 228–233.

Bracht, N., Kingsbury, L., & Rissel, C. (1999). A five-stage community organization model for health promotion: Empowerment and partnership strategies. In N. Bracht (Ed.), *Health promotion at the community level* (2nd ed.) (pp. 83–104). Thousand Oaks, CA: Sage.

Centers for Disease Control and Prevention. (1999). Framework for program evaluation in public health. *Morbidity and Mortality Weekly Report, 48*(RR-11), 1–40.

Fos, P. J., & Fine, D. J. (2000). *Designing health care for populations: Applied epidemiology in health care administration.* San Francisco: Jossey-Bass.

Goodman, R. M. (1998). Principles and tools for evaluating community-based prevention and health promotion programs. *Journal of Public Health Management Practice, 4*(2), 37–47.

Guimei, M. (2001). Community workers as extension of nursing personnel. *Journal of Nursing Scholarship, 33,* 13–14.

Healey, B. J. (1998). The use of prevalence data to unite the community in prevention programs. *Journal of Public Health Management Practice, 4*(6), 88–92.

Israel, B. A., Schultz, A. J., Parker, E. A., & Becker, A. B. (1998). Review of community-based research: Assessing partnership approaches to improve public health. *Annual Review of Public Health, 19,* 173–202.

Jewkes, R. (2000). Evaluating community development initiatives in health promotion. In M. Thorogood & Y. Coombes (Eds.), *Evaluating health promotion: Practice and methods* (pp. 129–139). New York: Oxford University Press.

Kone, A., Sullivan, M., Senturia, K., Chrisman, N. J., Ciske, S. J., & Frieger, J. W. (2000). Improving collaboration between researchers and communities. *Public Health Reports, 115,* 243–248.

Lawton, L. (1999). Approaches to needs assessment. In E. R. Perkins, I. Simnett, & L. Wright (Eds.), *Evidence-based health promotion* (pp. 325–332). New York: Wiley.

McLaughlin, C. P., & Kaluzny, A. D. (1999). Defining quality improvement: Past, present and future. In C. P. McLaughlin & A. D. Kaluzny (Eds.), *Continuous quality improvement in health care: Theory, implementation, and applications* (2nd ed.) (pp. 3–10). Gaithersburg, MD: Aspen.

Moyer, A., Coristine, M., MacLean, L., & Mechthild, M. (1999). A model for building collective capacity in community-based programs: The elderly in need project. *Public Health Nursing, 16,* 205–214.

Porter, E. J. (1987). Administrative diagnosis: Implications for the public's health. *Public Health Nursing, 4,* 247–256.

Rissel, C., & Bracht, N. (1999). Assessing community needs, resources, and readiness: Building on strengths. In N. Bracht (Ed.), *Health promotion at the community level* (2nd ed.) (pp. 59–71). Thousand Oaks, CA: Sage.

Rohrer, J. E. (1999). *Planning for community-oriented health systems* (2nd ed.). Washington, DC: American Public Health Association.

Roman, L. A., Lindsay, J. K., Moore, J. S., & Shoemaker, A. L. (1999). Community health workers: Examining the helper therapy principle. *Public Health Nursing, 16,* 87–95.

Schalock, R. L. (1995). *Outcome-based evaluation.* New York: Plenum Press.

Sharpe, P. A., Greaney, M. L., Lee, P. R., & Royce, S. W. (2000). Assets-oriented community assessment. *Public Health Reports, 115,* 205–211.

Valanis, B. (1999). *Epidemiology in health care* (3rd ed.). Stamford, CT: Appleton & Lange.

Veney, J. E., & Kaluzny, A. D. (1998). *Evaluation and decision making for health services* (3rd ed.). Chicago: Health Administration Press.

Wallerstein, N. (1999). Power between evaluator and community: Research relationships within New Mexico's healthier communities. *Social Science & Medicine, 49,* 39–53.

Witkin, B. R., & Altschuld, J. W. (1995). *Planning and conducting needs assessments: A practical guide.* Thousand Oaks, CA: Sage.

One of the most effective ways to improve the health status of a community is to maintain and enhance the health of its children. In 1998, children under 15 years of age constituted 21.5% of the U.S. population (U.S. Census Bureau, 1999). Children who receive effective health care services, particularly health-promotive and illness-preventive services, are less likely to develop a variety of acute and chronic health problems. When working with children with physical, mental, or emotional health problems, community health nurses also endeavor to promote the child's ability to reach his or her fullest potential.

Goals for primary prevention for children include promoting normal growth and development, developing positive parent–child relationships, preventing health problems, and developing strengths and resources. When children are ill or have a health problem, the community health nurse also works toward goals related to secondary and tertiary prevention. Goals of secondary prevention reflect efforts to accurately diagnose and treat health problems. Tertiary prevention goals in the care of children include restoring function and preventing problem recurrence, preventing complications, adapting to long-term effects of illness, and minimizing the effects of health problems on the child and family.

Achievement of primary, secondary, and tertiary prevention goals for children requires a societal infrastructure that includes certain core services without which children's health is imperiled. These core services include timely health- and illness-related care, nutritional support, safe and adequate housing, safe child care, and effective school health programs. Additional core services include health education systems, recreational opportunities, illness and injury prevention programs, family support systems, public accountability for access to care, and integrated health, education, and human services programs (Meister, 1998).

In addition to caring for individual children and their families in a variety of settings, community health nurses help to assure that these core health services are present in the communities they serve. In this chapter, we will examine community health nursing roles with respect to individual children and to children as an aggregate. Care of children in particular settings, such as the home and school are addressed in later chapters of this book.

⑥THINK ABOUT IT

Why are community health nurses better prepared than some other providers to promote health and prevent illness in children?

HEALTH PROBLEMS OF CONCERN IN THE CARE OF CHILDREN

In addition to general concerns for health promotion and illness prevention, several specific health problems are of concern to community health nurses caring for children. Some of these problems are infant mortality and low birth weight, congenital anomalies, HIV infection, unintentional injury, handicapping and chronic conditions, fetal drug and alcohol exposure, and child abuse.

The importance of community health efforts to improve the health of the nation's children is seen in the fact that more than 60 of the national health objectives for the year 2010 directly address the health needs of children and adolescents, and more than 40 additional objectives address those needs indirectly (U.S. Department of Health and Human Services [USDHHS], 2000). These objectives can be found on the Healthy People 2010 Web site through the link provided on the companion Web site for this book.   🌐

Infant Mortality

In 1970, infant mortality in the United States was 29.2 deaths per 1,000 live births (U.S. Census Bureau, 1999). By 1997, the rate of infant mortality had dropped to 7.2 per 1,000 births (National Center for Health Statistics, 1999). Despite these gains, U.S. infant mortality rates remain higher than those for most other developed nations. Infant mortality is even higher for some segments of the population. Nearly twice as many infants in minority groups die before they are a year old (Davis, Okuboye, & Ferguson, 2000), and infant mortality is 28% higher among women with less than a high school education than among those with higher educational attainment (USDHHS, 2000). Although current infant mortality rates are the lowest in history in this country, the rate of decline has slowed considerably in the last decade. Primary causes of death are congenital anomalies, low birth weight, respiratory distress syndrome, sudden infant death syndrome (SIDS), and effects of maternal complications during pregnancy (Regional Perinatal System, 2000).

Low Birth Weight

Low birth weight among those infants who survive also presents problems. *Low birth weight* is a weight less than 2,500 grams or 5 pounds at birth, and *very low birth weight* is a birth weight less than 1,500 grams or 3.3 pounds (USDHHS, 2000). In 1997, 7.5% of all babies born in the United States were of low birth weight (Forum on Child and Family Statistics, 1999). Again, figures are worse for certain segments of the population. For example, in 1997, 13% of African American babies were of low birth weight compared to 6.5% of white babies, and babies born to women with lower education levels are more likely to have lower birth weights (USDHHS, 2000).

Low birth weight is associated with younger and older maternal age, poor maternal weight gain, multiparity, and lack of prenatal care. Other factors associated with low birth weight include low income and maternal smoking and alcohol and drug use (Davis et al., 2000). Other contributing factors include vaginal infection and domestic violence (USDHHS, 2000).

Low-birth-weight infants are more likely to die in the first year of life than infants with normal birth weights. Effects of low birth weight include multiple developmental and neurological disabilities. Very-low-birth-weight babies are even more likely to exhibit many of these problems (USDHHS, 2000).

Congenital Anomalies

In 1997, infant mortality due to congenital anomalies was 1.6 per 1,000 live births (USDHHS, 2000). Congenital anomalies affect approximately 120,000 U.S. babies each year, and contribute to 20% of the infant mortality in the United States. Although many children with congenital anomalies die in utero or during infancy, modern medical technology has increased the number of children with anomalies who survive, with fewer than 7% dying in the first year of life (National Center on Birth Defects and Developmental Disabilities, 2001c). In recent years, there has been an increasing prevalence of several congenital abnormalities in newborns. These abnormalities include anomalies of the central nervous system (hydrocephalus, encephalocele); eye (congenital cataracts); cardiovascular system (ventricular and atrial septal defects, tetralogy of Fallot, pulmonary and aortic valvular stenosis, patent ductus arteriosus); gastrointestinal system (intestinal atresia, tracheoesophageal anomalies); genitourinary system (renal agenesis and hypoplasia); and musculoskeletal system (clubfoot), as well as cleft lip and palate and chromosomal abnormalities (Down syndrome, trisomy 13, trisomy 18).

HIV Infection and AIDS

Other areas of concern are HIV infection and the growing number of AIDS cases in children. As of June 1998, more than 8,000 cases of AIDS had been diagnosed in youngsters under 13 years of age. The vast majority of these cases are attributable to perinatal transmission from infected mothers. Vertical transmission—transmission of HIV infection from mother to baby—may occur in utero, during delivery, or, less commonly, via breastfeeding. In addition to newborn infection, vertical transmission of HIV infection is thought to be related to fetal demise and miscarriage. Therapy for HIV-infected mothers and cesarean section delivery have been shown to decrease the likelihood of perinatal transmission of disease by 87% (Regional Perinatal Programs of California, 1999). Treatment of both mothers and infants also appears to lengthen the time to onset of disease. For example, from 1986 to 1997, 48% of infected children progressed to symptomatic AIDS by three years of age; with treatment options, this figure dropped to 3% of children with symptoms by age three and a projected one third remaining symptom free at age 13. However, the question of these children's ability to transmit disease in adolescence remains (National AIDS Clearinghouse, 1998).

Despite these gains, HIV infection and AIDS in the pediatric population remain significant problems. In 1999, an estimated 620,000 children worldwide were newly infected with HIV, and 3.8 million of the world's children had died of AIDS since the beginning of the epidemic (United Nations, 1999).

Unintentional Injury

Unintentional injuries are a frequent occurrence among children, resulting in extensive morbidity as well as mortality. In fact, unintentional injuries are the leading causes of death in children (USDHHS, 1998b). Specific causes of injury mortality differ with age, with infants more likely to die of choking and toddlers and preschool children of burns, poison, and drownings. Motor vehicle accidents are a frequent cause of death for all children, contributing to approximately 500 child deaths per year (National Center for Injury Prevention and Control, 2000). Fires are another cause of significant mortality in children accounting for 2.1 deaths per 100,000 children in 1997 (USDHHS, 2000). In 1998, drowning caused more than 1,000 deaths among children under 15 years of age and was the second leading cause of injury-related death in this age group (National Center for Injury Prevention and Control, 2001a).

Unintentional injuries among children also result in significant morbidity. For example, in 1997, there were 460 nonfatal poisonings for every 100,000 children under the age of 4 in the United States (USDHHS, 2000). Injuries leading to restricted activity or medical intervention occurred at a rate of 27.6 injuries per 1,000 children under age 15 years in 1996, and accounted for a total of 16 million injuries in people from birth to age seventeen (U.S. Census Bureau, 1999).

Head trauma is a frequent result of injury occurring during sports and recreational activities. In 1997, 252 children were killed in bicycle crashes with motor vehicles. Virtually none of these children (only 3%) were wearing helmets at the time of the accident. An additional 374,000 children and adolescents were injured in bicycle-related incidents (National Center for Injury Prevention and Control, 2001b).

Many injuries are related to playground equipment and unsupervised play (National Center for Injury Prevention and Control, 1999). Each year more than 211,000 playground injuries occur, 36% of them severe injuries with 3% requiring hospitalization. Seventy percent of the injuries occur on public playgrounds, but 67% of fatalities occur on home play equipment (National Program for Playground Safety, 1999b). Approximately one fourth of playground injuries occur while children are playing without adult supervision. Others are the

CRITICAL THINKING IN RESEARCH

The U.S. federal government has ruled that all research receiving federal support include children if relevant to the study. Why is such a ruling appropriate? What ethical dilemmas might this policy pose? In what types of studies would inclusion of children as subjects not be appropriate?

---

result of unsafe playground conditions. In one study of children's playgrounds, 75% of playgrounds had appropriate surface materials under play equipment, but in 56% the depth of materials was insufficient to prevent serious injury. In addition, 25% of the playgrounds had equipment that was broken or was potentially hazardous (National Center for Injury Prevention and Control, 1999).

Firearms injuries are a serious concern in the health of children. In 1998, for example, 121 deaths occurred in children due to accidental firearms discharge. An additional 1,500 unintentional firearms injuries occur among children each year. Most of these injuries occur in the home and involve improperly stored weapons. In some studies, 75% to 80% of first- and second-grade children in homes with guns knew where the guns were located (National Safe Kids Campaign, 2001b).

Handicapping and Chronic Conditions

The health of children in the United States is also influenced by a variety of chronic or handicapping conditions. Chronic and handicapping conditions in children fall into several categories: sensory impairments; motor handicaps; mental retardation; pervasive developmental disorders; learning disabilities; speech and language disorders; emotional, behavioral, and conduct disorders; and chronic diseases. An estimated 8% of children encounter activity limitations due to chronic disease, and 12% of school-age children and adolescents have difficulty with one or more daily activities, most related to school performance (Forum on Child and Family Statistics, 1999).

Asthma is one of the most prevalent and disabling conditions among today's children. In 1998, an estimated 5 million children were affected (USDHHS, 1998b). Asthma prevalence increased by approximately 5% each year from 1980 to 1995 (National Center for Environmental Health, 2000), and both prevalence and mortality continue to increase each year. Approximately 12% of hospitalizations in children aged 1 to 9 years are due to asthma (McCormick, Kass, Elixhauser, Thompson, & Simpson, 2000), and the rate of hospitalization for asthma among children under five years of age in 1997 was 60.9 per 10,000 children, more than three times that for any other age group. Children in this age group also visit emergency departments for asthma at a rate of 150 per 10,000

children—twice as high as any other group. Although younger children have more frequent hospitalizations for asthma, children aged 5 to 14 years are at the greatest risk of death, with a 1998 mortality rate of 3.2 deaths per million children (USDHHS, 2000).

Pervasive developmental disorders include such conditions as mental retardation, cerebral palsy, autism, and learning disabilities. Mental retardation occurs at a rate of 131 per 10,000 children (USDHHS, 2000), and an estimated 12 of every 1,000 school-age children have some degree of retardation. In 1995–1996, special education services for this population cost approximately $3.3 billion, and it is estimated that the costs of caring for a mentally retarded child may be as high as 10 times those of caring for a normal child (National Center on Birth Defects and Developmental Disabilities, 2001f). Cerebral palsy develops in approximately 10,000 babies each year. Cerebral palsy is frequently accompanied by multiple physical disabilities and mental retardation. It is estimated that cerebral palsy may have a lifetime cost for care of $503,000 per child (National Center on Birth Defects and Developmental Disabilities, 2001d).

Although the prevalence of autism in the United States is not known, European and Asian figures suggest that as many as two in every 1,000 children may be affected. Autism and related disorders require extensive long-term care and special education services that cost about $8,000 per child per year in normal school settings and as much as $30,000 to $100,000 per year in specialized or residential settings (National Center on Birth Defects and Developmental Disabilities, 2001b).

Far more children are affected by learning disabilities, the next category of disabling condition. A *learning disability* is defined as being two or more years behind agemates in one academic area. In 1994–1995, 4.5% of children aged 6 to 14 years had a diagnosed learning disability, and slightly more than 6% had difficulty with school work (U.S. Census Bureau, 1999).

In 1998, malignant neoplasms were the fourth leading cause of death in children aged 1 to 4 years and the second leading cause among 5- to 14-year-olds (National Center for Health Statistics, 2000b). Many more children are surviving childhood cancers and need to learn to adjust to cancer as a chronic condition. Childhood risk factors for malignant neoplasms include environmental exposures to carcinogens, viral exposures (e.g., the Epstein–Barr virus that causes infectious mononucleosis), genetic characteristics, and other existing conditions such as some congenital anomalies, immunodeficiency states, and chromosomal anomalies.

Insulin-dependent diabetes mellitus (IDDM) occurs in approximately 123,000 children under age 20 years or 0.16% of the child population in the United States (National Diabetes Information Clearinghouse, 2001). Heart disease is another cause of mortality and chronic illness in children. From 1996 to 1998, the death rate for heart conditions was 16 per 100,000 children under one year of age, most often related to congenital heart defects.

Heart disease, however, still claims lives among older children with a mortality rate of 1.4 per 100,000 among children 1 to 4 years of age (National Center for Health Statistics, 2000b). Many more children are living with heart disease as a chronic condition. Hypertension, a risk factor for heart disease, may be associated with childhood obesity, but it is more likely due to an underlying medical condition such as coarctation of the aorta, renal artery stenosis, drug and toxin ingestion, and chronic pyelonephritis and glomerulonephritis (Kenney, 1997). Routine blood pressure measurements starting at 3 years of age are recommended to identify youngsters with hypertension.

Juvenile arthritis is a collection of syndromes that have in common chronic arthritis beginning in childhood. Although precise incidence and prevalence are unknown, worldwide approximately 1 in every 1,000 children is affected. Children most often display symptoms of arthritis between 1 and 4 years of age and between 10 and 13 years (Rheumatism and Arthritis Foundation of Tasmania, 2001). Arthritis in children can affect single or multiple joints, and virtually any joint may be involved. Early diagnosis and consistent care is required to prevent disability in children and exacerbation of disabling effects with age.

Approximately 2% to 4% of children experience at least one seizure sometime during their childhood (Seay & Janas, 1997). Most seizures experienced by children are a manifestation of underlying acute systemic or central nervous system diseases such as meningitis and encephalitis, metabolic disturbances such as hypoglycemia and hypocalcemia, or intoxications. Some children, however, experience recurrent seizures that constitute a seizure disorder or epilepsy. Most of these children obtain good seizure control with antiepileptic drug therapy, but the disease is still a frightening one for both parents and children.

The presence of these and other chronic illnesses in children creates special needs for community health nursing care. These illnesses may also necessitate creative approaches to general health promotion and illness prevention in these youngsters.

Attention Deficit Hyperactivity Disorder

Attention deficit hyperactivity disorder (ADHD) is characterized by poor attention span, impulsive behavior, and hyperactivity. Attention deficit with associated hyperactivity is frustrating for the children affected and for everyone who interacts with them. ADHD is estimated to affect as many as 3% to 5% of children, with boys twice as likely to be affected as girls (LeFever, Dawson, & Morrow, 1999). Many of these children have associated learning disabilities, and estimates of educational costs for children with ADHD in the United States range from $3.5 to $4 billion per year. Other effects of ADHD include impaired family life and social interac-

tions, low self-esteem, and increased prevalence of accidental injury and functional impairment. ADHD is also associated with delinquency, school dropout, and mental health problems in adulthood (National Center on Birth Defects and Developmental Disabilities, 2001g). Children with ADHD may also experience related problems such as disruptive behavior disorders, mood disorders, Tourette's syndrome, and anxiety disorders. In addition, they are more likely than other children to engage in risk behaviors such as smoking, impulsive behavior, substance abuse, and crime. Many of these comorbid conditions go undiagnosed and untreated (National Center on Birth Defects and Developmental Disabilities, 2001a).

A relatively large number of school-age children receive psychostimulants (e.g., Ritalin) as treatment for ADHD, yet only a small percentage of these children show improvement of problematic behaviors. In addition, the effects of these drugs on academic performance are unclear, suggesting potentially inaccurate diagnoses and overprescription (LeFever et al., 1999).

Fetal Alcohol and Drug Exposure

It is estimated that 1 in every 10 babies born in the United States has been exposed to tobacco, alcohol, or illicit drugs in utero. During 1996–1997, for example, 13% of pregnant adult women reported smoking during pregnancy, 14% reported alcohol use, 1% reported binge drinking, and 2% reported use of illicit drugs (USDHHS, 2000). Community health nurses are often involved in assisting either biological or foster parents to care for these children. *Fetal alcohol syndrome (FAS)* is a condition resulting from maternal alcohol consumption during pregnancy and is characterized by growth retardation, facial malformations, and central nervous system dysfunctions that may include mental retardation. Overall, estimated incidence rates for FAS in the United States range from 3 to 22 babies per 10,000 live births, contributing to 1,300 to 8,000 babies born with FAS each year (National Center on Birth Defects and Developmental Disabilities, 2001e). Incidence of FAS is even higher in some segments of the population. For example, FAS incidence rates for some Native American tribes are four times higher than for the general population (May, Brooke, Gossage, & Croxford, 2000). Societal costs for fetal alcohol syndrome are estimated to range from $75.6 million to $321 million per year (Egeland et al., 1998). Long-term effects of FAS include inability to hold down a job, impulsivity, social withdrawal, poor judgment, and mental retardation.

Even those infants exposed to moderate amounts of alcohol during pregnancy may have long-term effects. It is estimated that three to four times as many infants have fetal alcohol effects as have FAS (USDHHS, 2000). Approximately 1 in 29 pregnant women continues to drink throughout pregnancy, increasing the potential for fetal alcohol effects in their offspring (National Center on Birth Defects and Developmental Disabilities, 2001e).

Fetal drug exposure also has adverse effects on children. Use of cocaine during pregnancy, for example, increases the incidence of stillbirth, low birth weight, and congenital malformations. Use of cocaine also increases maternal risk of hepatitis B and HIV infection. Fetal drug exposure has also been shown to result in neurological abnormalities and developmental delays and increased risk of sudden infant death syndrome (SIDS). Similar fetal effects have been noted for tobacco and marijuana use (USDHHS, 2000).

Child Abuse

Child abuse is an area of serious concern to community health nurses. Increasing incidence of all forms of child abuse has been noted since 1980, and in 1997, 984,000 children experienced some form of maltreatment; more than 1,000 of these children died. The U.S. incidence rate for child fatalities due to maltreatment was 13.9 per 1,000 children under the age of 18 years. Most of the maltreatment (56%) involved neglect, while 25% involved physical abuse, 12.5% sexual abuse, and 6% emotional abuse (USDHHS, 2000). Child abuse is often linked to intimate partner abuse of the child's mother, with both forms of abuse occurring in approximately 50% of cases in several studies (National Center for Injury Prevention and Control, 2001c). Child abuse is addressed in detail in the section on family violence included in Chapter 32.

Evidence of all of the problems discussed above highlights the need for community health nursing services to children. Such services can help to prevent the occurrence of these and other problems affecting children and to minimize their effects on both the child and the child's family. Community health nurses can also be aware of the extent to which these problems occur within the population and work toward programs that prevent their occurrence or address their consequences among children and families affected.

ASSESSING CHILD HEALTH

Community health nurses care for individual children and their families and for children as an aggregate within the population. At either level, care begins with an assessment of health needs incorporating considerations in each of the six dimensions of health.

⑥THINK ABOUT IT

How does the information that you would collect in assessing a child differ from assessment information for an adult?

Biophysical Considerations

Human biological factors that may influence children's health include age and maturation levels, genetic inheritance, and physiologic function.

Age and Maturation

Areas to be assessed with respect to maturation and aging include growth and development. *Growth* is an increase in body size or change in the structure, function, and complexity of body cells until a point of maturity. Growth parameters considered in the nurse's assessment of the child include weight, height, and head and chest circumferences. With respect to height and weight, the nurse assesses the individual child in relation to normal values for the child's age and in comparison to the child's own previous growth pattern. Height and weight should be plotted on a graph at periodic intervals to establish the child's growth pattern. Plotting facilitates comparisons with age norms. Height and weight are also examined in relation to each other and to other growth parameters. Plotting a child's height in relation to his or her weight is demonstrated in Figure 16–1 ■. Marked deviations from normal values for the child's age, changes in previous growth patterns, and marked incongruence among growth parameters are indications of a need for further evaluation.

Head circumference is another indicator of growth that is usually measured and plotted on a graph until 1 to 2 years of age. Head circumference is measured at the largest diameter of the head, with the tape measure circling the forehead and the occipital bulge, as indicated in Figure 16–2 ■. Head circumference is always evaluated in conjunction with chest circumference measured at the nipple line, as indicated in Figure 16–2. The ratio between head and chest circumference changes dramatically in the first year of life. At birth, head circumference is

FIGURE 16–1 ■ *Plotting height in relation to weight*

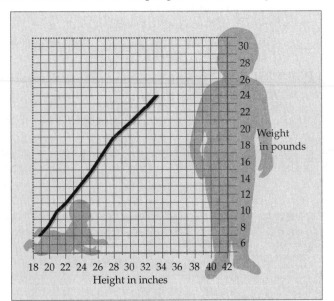

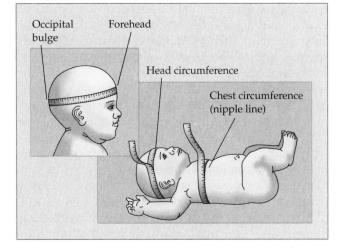

Occipital bulge
Forehead
Head circumference
Chest circumference (nipple line)

FIGURE 16–2 ■ *Measuring head circumference and chest circumference*

approximately three fourths of an inch greater than chest circumference. By 1 year of age, the two measurements are approximately equal. Beyond 1 year of age, chest circumference should exceed head circumference, and the difference in the two measurements will continue to increase with age until adult proportions are reached.

A marked departure from the expected ratio between head and chest circumference may indicate neurological, cardiovascular, or respiratory problems. For example, an overly large head might indicate hydrocephaly, whereas a small head may be related to microcephaly or poor bone growth of the skull. A large chest might be due to respiratory difficulties or cardiac enlargement. A small chest, on the other hand, could reflect malnutrition or other causes of poor bone growth.

The nurse assesses the child in terms of these growth parameters, noting deviations from age norms or changes in the child's own growth pattern. Such deviations or changes are examined to determine whether they indicate the presence of health problems. For example, deviation from age norms may be related to metabolic or hormonal disorders, poor feeding, overfeeding, neglect, or familial characteristics, to name a few underlying factors. Unexpected changes in the child's previous growth patterns may result from either physical or emotional causes. General guidelines for assessing growth patterns in individual children are presented in Table 16–1 ■.

At the population level, the community health nurse would determine the extent of growth retardation. In 1997, for example, 8% of low-income children under 5 years of age were below the fifth percentile of height for age. Slightly more African American and Asian children were growth retarded than other subgroups in the population (USDHHS, 2000). Widespread growth retardation may be an indication of poor nutrition, infectious diseases, chronic disease, or poor health care in the population.

Development is a process of patterned, orderly, and lifelong change in structure, thought, or behavior that

■ **TABLE 16–1**   **General Parameters for Assessing Growth in Children of Selected Ages**

AGE GROUP	ASSESSMENT PARAMETER
Neonate (birth–30 days)	Median weight of a full-term infant: 7 to 7¼ lbs. Loss of several ounces in first few days Return to birth weight by 10 to 14 days of age Median length at birth: 19¾ to 20 in.
Infant (1–12 months)	Doubles birth weight by 4 to 5 months of age Triples birth weight by 1 year of age Gains 10 in. in length by 1 year of age Head circumference increases by about 4¾ in. (12 cm) by 1 year of age
Toddler and preschool child (2–5 years)	Quadruples birth weight in the second year of life Gains 5 in. in height in the second year of life Gains 3 to 5 lbs. per year from age 2 to age 5 Grows 2 in. per year from age 2 to age 5 Head circumference increases by 1 in. in the second year
School-age child (6–12 years)	Gains 3 to 5 lbs. per year through age 10 Grows 1½ to 2½ in. per year through age 10 Boy: Gains 15 to 20 lbs. per year through age 12; grows 4½ to 5 in. per year through age 12 Girl: Gains 20 to 25 lbs. per year through age 12; grows 5 to 6 in. per year through age 12

occurs as a result of physical or emotional maturation. The community health nurse assesses the child's development in terms of *developmental milestones,* which are critical behaviors expected at specific ages. Developmental assessment may be approached in a number of ways. The most widely used tool for assessing the development of individual children from birth to age 6 is the Denver Developmental Screening Test (DDST). This test provides a gross measure of the child's fine motor and gross motor development, personal–social development, and language development. Although the test is easy to administer and can indicate problem areas related to the child's development, it is not a diagnostic tool and does not indicate the possible causes of developmental delays. The DDST is also useful as an aid in providing parents with anticipatory guidance regarding their child's behavior. (Test kits, score sheets, and directions for performing a DDST can be purchased from DDM, Inc., P.O. Box 6919, Denver, CO 80203-0911.)

An abnormal DDST should be repeated in two to three weeks. If results on the retest are similar, a more in-depth developmental assessment is warranted. In addition to

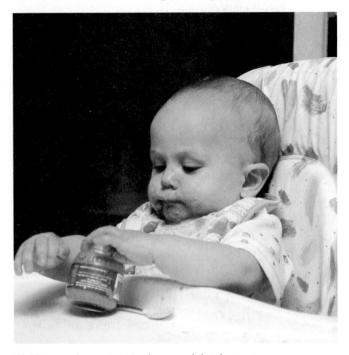

Children need opportunities for normal development.

retesting, the nurse would also explore factors that may be contributing to delayed development. For example, if the child is not given the opportunity to engage in certain activities, a developmental delay may occur. Mothers who will not let their children feed themselves because of the "mess" may be contributing to a delay in personal–social development on the part of the individual child. Similarly, if the child always gets what he or she wants by pointing, language development may be delayed. Other potential reasons for developmental delay include neurological deficits, mental retardation, and neglect.

The DDST is a useful tool for assessing the development of children from birth through age 6. The development of older children should also be assessed. A few assessment tools are available for use with older children, but these are less widely used and less well known than the DDST. For children over age 6, a general assessment in terms of accomplishment of specific milestones for their age is probably sufficient. Major developmental milestones for children of various ages are presented in Table 16–2 ■.

Community health nurses would also assess child development at the aggregate level. What is the extent of developmental delay or retardation in the population? What risk factors for retardation are present in the community? At what age do children in different segments of the population become sexually mature? The answers to these and similar questions will assist the nurse in planning health care programs appropriate to the needs of the child and adolescent population.

Genetic Inheritance

Genetic inheritance is another of the biophysical considerations in assessment of children's health. Two intrinsic

genetic factors that influence child health are gender and racial or ethnic background. Male and female children and children of different racial and ethnic groups tend to experience different types of health problems. For example, the nurse would want to direct more attention to a review of systems related to the urinary tract in school-age girls than boys because urinary tract infections occur more frequently in girls than in boys in this age group. Similarly, screening tests for sickle cell anemia should be routinely conducted on African American children and others at risk. Community health nurses should be familiar with the gender and ethnic composition of the child population in their communities.

Other information about genetic inheritance is obtained from the individual child's family history. Information obtained in the family history should include the age and health status of family members as well as any history of illnesses that may have a genetic component. If family members are deceased, the cause and age at time of death should be recorded, if known. The community health nurse should ask specifically about the presence of such conditions as cancer, heart disease, allergies, diabetes, kidney disease, hypertension, seizure disorders, emotional problems, and other chronic conditions in family members. Notations about conditions identified in the family history should include the family member or members affected. Notations should also be made of the absence of specific diseases within the family configuration. Family information can be described in a narrative format or diagrammed in a "genogram" as described in Chapter 14. At the population level, information regarding the prevalence of conditions with tendencies to genetic transmission will alert the community health nurse to the potential for these problems in children.

Physiologic Function

The third aspect of assessment in the biophysical dimension is physiologic function. Information on various aspects of an individual child's physiologic functioning can be obtained from the history of present and past health problems, review of systems, physical examination, results of routine screening tests, and review of the child's immunization status. The review of systems is tailored to the age of the child. For example, the nurse would not need to ask questions related to sexual activity when the client is an infant. Similarly, questions about urinary tract function for an infant would center around the number of wet diapers and any strong odor to the child's urine.

Physical examination of a child is also somewhat different from that of an adult. Differences are found in both the way the examination is conducted and in the findings. Most examiners adopt a head-to-toe approach when systematically examining an adult. This is not particularly appropriate with young children. With children, the nurse starts the examination with noninvasive techniques and leaves invasive procedures, such as the examination of

■ **TABLE 16–2** Developmental Characteristics of Individual Clients at Selected Ages

AGE		DEVELOPMENTAL CHARACTERISTIC
Birth–1 month	Neurophysical	Newborn reflexes intact, head lag present, follows objects to midline, responds to noise
	Psychosocial	Regards human face, quiets when picked up
1–2 months	Neurophysical	Follows objects 180°, holds head up in prone position, head erect and bobbing when supported in sitting position
	Psychosocial	Vocalizes other than crying, smiles responsively
2–4 months	Neurophysical	Newborn reflexes diminishing, sits well with support, rolls from side to side, grasps rattle
	Psychosocial	Laughs aloud, initiates smiling, enjoys play activity
4–6 months	Neurophysical	Reaches for and gets objects, puts objects in mouth, rolls over completely, supports own weight when standing, tooth eruption
	Psychosocial	Turns to voice, begins stranger anxiety, strong attachment to mother
6–9 months	Neurophysical	Sits alone, bounces, stands holding on, thumb–finger grasp
	Psychosocial	"Mama" or "dada," plays peek-a-boo and pattycake, imitates speech sounds
9–12 months	Neurophysical	Pulls to stand, creeps or crawls, walks holding on, sits from standing position, uses a cup with help
	Psychosocial	Gives toy on request, speaks two to three words, gives affection, indicates wants
12–18 months	Neurophysical	Scribbles, points to one or more body parts, uses a spoon, climbs and runs, plays ball, beginning bowel training
	Psychosocial	Likes to be read to, 10-word vocabulary
18–24 months	Neurophysical	Opens doors, turns on faucets, can throw or kick a ball, walks up and down stairs alone, daytime bowel and bladder control established
	Psychosocial	Parallel play, two- to three-word sentences, imitates household tasks
2–3 years	Neurophysical	Dresses with help, rides a tricycle, washes and dries hands
	Psychosocial	Separates easily from mother, uses pronouns, perceives danger, understands sharing and taking turns
3–5 years	Neurophysical	Dresses with decreasing supervision, hops on one foot, catches bounced ball, heel-to-toe walk
	Psychosocial	Gives whole name, recognizes three colors, draws person with more than six parts, tells a story, operates from rules
5–10 years	Neurophysical	Physical growth slows, motor coordination increases
	Psychosocial	Begins peer identification, forms friendships, learns more rules, begins sexual identification, increases use of language to convey ideas, begins to understand cause and effect
11–14 years	Neurophysical	Begins pubertal changes, gawkiness
	Psychosocial	Importance of peer group conformity, strong identification with sexmates, learning one's role in heterosexual relationships, begins to establish an identity, more abstract thought, negative attitude to family
15–18 years	Neurophysical	Completes pubertal changes and adolescent growth spurt, better able to handle the new "body"
	Psychosocial	Develops an independent identity, establishes relationships with members of the opposite sex, adopts an adult value set, moves away from family relationships.

ears and throat, until last. Similarly, different techniques may need to be adopted to examine the ears of a child or the abdomen of a ticklish child. The examination also takes place at a slower rate because of the need for extensive explanation and reassurance for the child.

There are also differences in what is considered normal and abnormal in the findings of a pediatric physical. For example, normal values for vital signs vary considerably in young children compared with those for adults. Also, some findings that would be considered definitely abnormal in an adult are perfectly normal in children of certain ages. One such finding is a positive Babinski reflex in an infant. This is an expected response, and a negative Babinski reflex at this age would be an abnormal finding. It is beyond the scope of this book to describe all of the differences in physical findings between children and adults. Community health nurses working with youngsters should, however, become familiar with these differences so they can accurately assess children's health status.

Assessing physiologic function also involves obtaining information about current and past conditions experienced by the child. Of particular concern are the types of conditions discussed at the beginning of this chapter. The nurse should ask about the presence of these conditions or any other diagnosed health problem. In addition, the nurse would also be alert to the signs and symptoms of a variety of problems that commonly occur in children. Some of these common problems are listed in Table 16–3 ■.

Information about the child's physiologic function may also be obtained by means of several routine screening tests performed at periodic intervals. The following are indications for the use of several routine screening measures (Newborn Screening Task Force, 1999; USDHHS, 1998a).

Age	Screening Test
Birth	Phenylketonuria (PKU), hypothyroidism, hearing, hemoglobinopathies, sickle cell, galactosemia, maple syrup urine disease, homocystinuria, biotidinase, congenital adrenal hyperplasia (requirements vary from state to state except for PKU and hypothyroidism)
1 month	Lead
1–2 months	Head circumference
3 months	Blood pressure (and periodically thereafter)
3–4 months	Vision (and periodically thereafter)
6 months	Hematocrit or hemoglobin
9 months	Tuberculin skin test (PPD)
11–18 years	Use of tobacco and alcohol (and periodically thereafter)
Periodically	Height and weight, dental

The nurse should also assess the child's immunization status. Has the child received immunizations appropriate to his or her age? Guidelines for childhood immunizations are summarized in Table 16–4 ■. For the very young infant, the nurse would also explore the mother's immune status, as immunity in the newborn is derived from transplacental transfer of maternal antibodies. If the mother has had chickenpox, for example, the child will probably have some protection against this disease. This is also true for diseases against which the mother has been immunized.

Similar information is gathered at the population level. What is the prevalence of conditions common in children? Do these conditions occur disproportionately in some segments of the population? What are the overall immunization levels in the community? Do immunization levels vary among subpopulations? If so, what fac-

■ **TABLE 16–3** Common Physical Health Problems in Children and Organ Systems Affected

ORGAN SYSTEM	COMMONLY ENCOUNTERED PROBLEMS
General	Anemia, communicable diseases, fever, failure to thrive, physical abuse
Cardiovascular system	Murmurs
Gastrointestinal system	Abdominal pain/appendicitis, colic, constipation, diarrhea, food allergy, spitting up, vomiting
Integumentary system	Abrasions, bruises, burns, diaper rash, eczema, impetigo, lice and scabies, monilial infection, other rashes, swollen lymph nodes
Musculoskeletal system	Congenital hip dysplasia (CHD), fractures, scoliosis, sprains and other muscle injuries
Neurological system	Headache, hearing loss, visual problems, speech problems, developmental delay
Respiratory system	Allergic rhinitis, asthma, bronchitis, bronchiolitis, croup, otitis media, pharyngitis, pneumonia, upper respiratory infection
Urinary system	Bedwetting, urinary tract infection

tors contribute to this variation? For example, in 1998, only 73% of African American children 19 to 35 months of age were completely up to date on immunizations compared to a national average of 82% for white children (California Department of Health Services, 2000). In 1999, overall immunization coverage was 99% for three doses of diphtheria–tetanus–pertussis (DTaP), 90% for three doses of polio, 96% for three doses of *Hemophilus influenzae* type b (Hib), 92% for one dose of measles–mumps–rubella (MMR), 88% for three doses of hepatitis B, and 59% for a single dose of varicella vaccine among U.S. children 19 to 35 months of age. Despite this high overall coverage, the extent of coverage in many ethnic populations was considerably less (National Immunization Program, 2000).

Psychological Considerations

There are large numbers of seriously emotionally disturbed children in the United States, many of whom go unrecognized and untreated (USDHHS, 2000). Children's mental health problems may manifest as emotional disorders characterized by internal feelings of anxiety or depression, or as behavioral disorders characterized by

■ **TABLE 16–4** Routine Pediatric Immunization Schedule

AGE	HBV	DTaP	Hib	IPV	PCV	MMR	Td	VARICELLA
Birth	#1*							
1 month	#2*							
2 months		#1	#1	#1	#1			
4 months		#2	#2	#2	#2			
6 months	#3*	#3	#3	#3*	#3			
12 months			#4*		#4*	#1*		#1*
15 months		#4*						
4–6 years		Booster		#4		Booster		
11–12 years, then every 10 years							Booster*	

HBV, hepatitis B virus; DTaP, diphtheria and tetanus toxoids and acellular pertussis; Hib, *Hemophilus influenzae* type b; IPV, inactivated polio vaccine; PCV, pneumococcal conjugate vaccine; MMR, measles–mumps–rubella; Td, tetanus and diphtheria toxoids, adult type
* Indicates earliest acceptable time of dose, doses may be given within a window of time beginning at the time indicated.
Sources: National Immunization Program. (2001). Recommended childhood immunization schedule—United States, 2001. *Morbidity and Mortality Weekly Report, 50,* 7–10.

disruptive behaviors. Community health nurses should routinely assess children for evidence of emotional problems and should explore factors in the psychological environment that may contribute to those problems. The child's psychological environment is a product of forces within and outside the child. Areas for consideration related to the psychological environment include the individual child's reactivity patterns, parental expectations and discipline, parental coping abilities and mental health status, parent–child interaction, and the child's self-image. The nurse should also consider the potential for child abuse within the family or child care environment.

Reactivity Patterns, Parental Expectations, and Discipline

Reactivity patterns are a set of typical responses to environmental stimuli displayed by a particular child. These patterns are part of the child's internal psychological environment. Reactivity patterns may persist throughout life and may influence the way others react to the child, thereby affecting the child's self-image and ability to interact meaningfully with others.

Knowledge of a child's reactivity patterns can suggest some potential problems that the child may encounter in his or her interactions with the outside world. Such knowledge also aids the nurse in designing interventions to assist families to adapt to their youngster's reactivity patterns or to aid children in adapting patterns to better fit the world around them.

Many of the difficulties in relationships between parents and children, and between the father and mother regarding their children, stem from unrealistic beliefs about things that children should and should not do. Community health nurses can help prevent such difficulties by assisting parents to develop realistic expectations of children's behavior. For example, it is unrealistic to expect a 3-year-old not to wet the bed occasionally. The community health nurse can explain to parents that the depth of a child's sleep at this age is such that urges to empty one's bladder are not sufficient to wake the child, and accidents occur. Similarly, the negativism of a 2-year-old is normal behavior, not evidence of deliberate disobedience. The nurse should explore with parents their expectations of children's behavior to determine whether these expectations are realistic in light of the child's age and developmental level, as well as his or her physical status.

Discipline is frequently an area of concern for parents and children alike. Many parents need assistance in knowing when and how to discipline children appropriately. The nurse should assess parental approaches to discipline and the appropriateness of disciplinary measures used. The nurse should also determine the extent to which parents adhere to the principles that should guide discipline. These principles and related assessment questions are presented in Table 16–5 ■.

Discipline can take any of several forms, and the community health nurse should ascertain the approach taken to discipline and the effectiveness of that approach. Verbal discipline is very effective with some children.

■ **TABLE 16–5** Principles of Effective Discipline and Related Assessment Questions

PRINCIPLE	ASSESSMENT QUESTIONS
1. Determine what is important.	Have parents determined what behaviors are never acceptable?
	Is there good rationale for this determination?
	Do parents say "No" automatically?
2. Be consistent.	Are parents consistent in what is considered unacceptable behavior?
	Do parents allow children to wear them down until they let unacceptable behavior pass?
	Do parents agree on what behavior is unacceptable, or can children manipulate parents?
	Have parents determined situations in which certain behaviors, otherwise allowed, are not acceptable?
	Have parents explained to children the reason for the difference in what is allowable at some times and not at others?
3. Never act in anger.	Do parents control their anger before disciplining children?
	Do parents use a "cooling off" period when needed?
	Have parents explained the reason for the cooling off period so children will learn appropriate ways of dealing with anger?
4. Allow time for compliance.	Do parents allow time for children to comply with directions, or do they expect instant obedience?
	Do parents respect children's need to complete a task in which they are engaged before complying with parental instructions?
5. Set limits ahead of time.	Do parents establish rules of behavior prior to disciplining certain behaviors on the part of the child?
	Do parents use knowledge of child growth and development to anticipate children's behavior?
	When children engage in unacceptable behavior that is not addressed in previously established rules, do parents give a warning before instituting punishment?
6. Be sure the child understands the rules.	Are parents clear on what behavior is expected of the child and what behavior is unacceptable?
7. Prevent rather than punish unacceptable behavior.	Do parents take steps to prevent unacceptable behavior before it occurs, rather than punishing it afterward?
	Do parents remove sources of temptation for young children?
	Do parents provide adequate supervision for children?
8. Be sure that discipline is warranted.	Do parents ascertain the facts of a situation before punishing children?
	Are parental expectations warranted given the developmental level of the child?
	Have rules been clearly established and made clear to the child?
	Do parents attempt to determine the reason for the child's behavior and explain what is wrong when the child's intentions were good?
9. Be sure that discipline is meaningful.	Do parents make sure that the child understands the reason for punishment?
	Do parents explain how the child can correct his or her behavior?
	What form of discipline do parents use?
	Is the form of discipline used effective in modifying the child's behavior?

When verbal discipline is used, the nurse should make sure that parents are focusing on the child's behavior and not the child. The idea should be conveyed that it is the *behavior* that is unacceptable, not the child. If physical punishment, such as spanking, is used, the nurse should ascertain that it is used appropriately and with caution.

Children should not be spanked with anything other than the hand and then only where no damage can occur (e.g., on the buttocks). The nurse should also be sure that parents refrain from using too much force even in spanking.

Removal of privileges is another effective means of discipline. When parents use this approach to discipline, the nurse should determine that the "punishment fits the crime" whenever possible and that the child is helped to see the connection between his or her behavior and the restriction imposed. For example, if a young child has purposefully broken another child's toy, he or she can be made to give up a similar toy for a certain period of time. Another effective method of discipline is time-out. Time-out effectively stops the behavior and affords the child an opportunity to contemplate its consequences. Whatever the form of discipline used, the nurse should ensure that it is employed in a way that leads to the accomplishment of its purposes.

Assessment considerations related to expectations and discipline at the population level might include cultural attitudes to children and child-rearing practices. How are children viewed in the society? Does that view differ among segments of the population? How do societal views of children influence expectations of children's behavior and forms of discipline used for unacceptable behavior?

Parental Coping and Mental Health

Another psychological dimension consideration in assessing the health of individual children or children as an aggregate is the level of parental coping skills and mental health. The ability of a child's parents to cope with the stresses and frustrations of parenthood and everyday life influences the child's psychological environment. Parents who are unable to cope with their own frustrations are likely to take some of their frustration out on the child. Even when this is not so, children are sensitive to the atmosphere around them and may feel insecure and uncertain in a situation in which parents are under obvious stress.

Community health nurses should assess coping strategies used by parents and the effectiveness of their use. In addition, community health nurses can identify ineffective parental coping mechanisms that may contribute to a psychological environment that is not conducive to the child's physical or emotional health. Parents can be asked what stressors they perceive in their lives and how they deal with stress.

In addition to parental coping skills, the presence of parental psychopathology can influence the health of children in the home. For example, parental depression may contribute to child neglect when one or both parents do not have the psychic energy to meet children's physical or emotional needs. Similarly, parental psychopathology (e.g., anxiety, affective, and substance abuse disorders) has been associated with emotional disorders among children. In assessing the population with respect to the effects of coping behaviors and psychopathology on child health, the community health nurse would determine the kind and extent of stressors to which parents in the community are subjected. Incidence and prevalence of substance abuse and mental health problems in the population can also give the nurse some idea of the level of coping strategies employed in the population and their relative effectiveness.

Parent–Child Interaction

The quality of interaction between parent and child is another important factor in the child's psychological environment. In assessing this area, the nurse would observe the pattern of interaction between parent and child in the nurse's presence. Do parents relate well to the child, or do they scream and yell over minor misbehavior? Do parents convey a sense of concern for the child and his or her welfare, or do they ignore the child unless the behavior impinges on the parents' level of comfort? Answers to these and similar questions provide the nurse with a picture of typical interactions between parent and child.

In the child with a chronic illness or disability, the quality of parent–child interactions may be profoundly influenced by the parents' response to the child's condition. These children tend to have higher incidence rates for emotional problems than do physically healthy children (Faux, 1998). The community health nurse can assess the parental response to the child's condition and identify any problem areas that may adversely affect the child's emotional status.

There is considerable evidence that parental responses to children with chronic or handicapping conditions may involve what has been called "chronic sorrow." Chronic sorrow appears to be triggered by periodic events that highlight the "disparity" between actual reality and idealized reality regarding one's child. Several authors have noted that the grief response to chronic illness or disability in one's child may not follow the time-bound grief response noted with bereavement or the death of a loved one. Instead the grief response seems to occur in two phases. The first phase is one of initial impact, denial, and grief. The second phase entails coping with the management of the condition and adaptation to a changed life, but is characterized by emotional turmoil, but at less severe levels than in the previous stage (Lowes & Lyne, 2000). Community health nurses can assess how well parents have adapted to the demands of their child's condition as well as the extent to which they experience chronic sorrow and its influence on interactions with the child. At the aggregate level, information about the prevalence of chronic and disabling conditions among children can alert the community health nurse regarding the potential for chronic sorrow among parents in the population.

Self-Image

Another area to be addressed in relation to the child's psychological environment is the child's self-image. The nurse can determine the individual child's self-perceptions by asking the child to "Tell me about yourself." A similar approach would be to ask the child to describe things that he or she does well. A child who has difficulty answering this question may not have a very strong self-image. For younger children who cannot easily articulate their feelings about themselves, nurses might watch for self-punishing behavior (e.g., slapping oneself or saying

"I'm dumb") or ask them to draw and explain pictures of themselves. The prevalence of emotional health problems among children such as depression, eating disorders, anxiety, and so on can provide the community health nurse with an aggregate picture of children's self-image in the population. Similarly, the nurse might look at media portrayals of children's activities. Are they all negative, or are there stories of positive contributions made by children in the news media?

Potential for Child Abuse

Child abuse is a major deterrent to psychological health among children. Inability to cope with life's stresses is one of the primary contributors to child abuse, a growing area of concern for community health nurses. The community health nurse should be alert to evidence of actual or potential child abuse. Although child abuse has both physical and psychological effects on children, it is factors in the psychological environment that place families at risk for the occurrence of abuse. Guidelines for child abuse assessment include considerations of parent characteristics and role expectations, child characteristics and behavior, and environmental stressors. Parental characteristics that increase the potential for child abuse include a history of abuse or parental abandonment when they themselves were children, feelings of hostility to or alienation from their own parents, and physical or emotional health problems experienced by the child's parents. Unrealistic parental expectations of the child, verbalizations of hostility or disappointment in the child, parental expectations that the child should always understand the parents' feelings, and a belief that the child does not love the parents enough are also parental indicators of potential for abuse.

Characteristics of the child may also signal potential for abuse. Such characteristics include prematurity, early separation from parents, developmental disability, obvious differences from siblings, difficulty concentrating, and inappropriate ways of expressing needs. The nurse should also be aware of environmental stressors such as financial pressures, social isolation, alcoholism or drug abuse, spousal abuse, and poor school performance that may indicate a potential for abuse.

Community health nurses should also be alert to signs of actual abuse or neglect. Some of these include evidence of obvious injury; torn, stained, or bloody underwear; an enlarged anal opening; signs of malnutrition and poor hygiene; and failure to thrive. Nurses should also be suspicious of stories that are inconsistent with injuries presented or with the child's stage of development and of inappropriate behavior on the part of adults in the situation (e.g., belligerence, being overly concerned, or refusing to allow diagnostic tests). Children may also display unusual behavior such as being excessively withdrawn or extremely passive. Abused children may cling to parents with unusual force or be remarkably detached from them. Whenever any form of child abuse is suspected, community health nurses are required by law to make a report to the local child protective service. The nurse makes an initial telephone report, followed by a detailed written report within a specified time period, which may vary from one jurisdiction to another.

The nurse should be alert to families at risk for child abuse and work to help them develop positive parenting skills as described in this chapter. The development of such skills may help to prevent abuse or to eliminate it in families where it already exists. The problem of child abuse and potential nursing interventions are addressed in more detail in Chapter 32.

Physical Environmental Considerations

Safety hazards are a major factor in the physical environment that influence the health of children of all ages. Safety concerns are related to the child's physical surroundings and the child's ability to gain access to dangerous substances. The nurse should assess both the presence of hazardous conditions in the environment and parents' and children's knowledge of safety-related behaviors.

The community health nurse also assesses the knowledge of and adherence to safety practices among parents and other caretakers. Areas for consideration relative to caretaker practices include the amount of supervision provided for the child and parental use of safety devices. Child safety practices in both the home and the child care environment should be considered if they are different.

Considerations in assessing child safety factors vary with the age of the child. Specific questions related to safety assessment for infants, toddlers and preschool children, and school-age children are presented in Table 16–6 ■. Community health nurses should assess parents' knowledge and use of safety practices in the home as well as the presence of safety hazards in the community. Are parents knowledgeable about safety concerns appropriate to their children's ages? Do they engage in appropriate safety practices in the home related to dangerous products and objects and potentially dangerous behaviors as indicated in Table 16–6?

Toys are another safety concern for children. Many toy-related injuries result from physical impact with or ingestion of the toy. The primary factors involved in toy-related injuries are selection of toys inappropriate to the child's age and improper use of the toy. The nurse should assess the safety and appropriateness of toys and the safety of any playground equipment in the home or day care environment. Some considerations include the ground surface on which equipment is placed and the state of repair of equipment. Energy-absorbing mats, wood chips, and sand under equipment reduce the likelihood of injuries due to falls. Concrete, asphalt, and packed earth, however, are very dangerous. The nurse should also determine whether equipment is properly anchored and free of obstructions. Equipment should also be in good repair and children should be supervised in its use.

■ **TABLE 16–6** Questions for Assessing Environmental Safety for Children of Selected Ages

AGE GROUP	ASSESSMENT QUESTIONS
Infant (birth–1 year)	Is the child left unattended on elevated surfaces? Is an approved car seat restraint used consistently? Do parents routinely fasten safety straps in high chairs, strollers, swings, and infant seats? Do parents use flame-retardant sleepwear? Does the infant have his or her own crib? Is plastic film that might suffocate the child left on or in the crib? Are there dangling drapery or other cords near the crib in which the child could strangle? Are slats on the crib sufficiently close together that the child cannot get his or her head stuck? Has nontoxic paint been used on crib surfaces? Are bumper pads used to prevent injury? Are soft pillows removed from the bed? Do mobiles or toys have sharp surfaces or small parts that can be swallowed? Are toys free of strings that could choke the child? Are siblings' toys with small parts kept out of the infant's reach? Do parents refrain from giving a bottle in bed or propping a bottle?

Toddler (2–3 years)	Are car seats used consistently?
	Is the child adequately supervised during waking hours?
	Do parents check the child periodically during naps?
	Has the environment been childproofed so that:
	    Electrical outlets are covered?
	    Sharp objects and poisonous substances are locked away, not just placed out of reach?
	    Medications and other hazardous substances are kept in appropriate containers?
	    Safety latches or locks are on cabinets used to store hazardous items?
	    Child-resistant containers are used correctly?
	    Dangling electrical cords have been eliminated?
	    Stairs are gated?
	    Bathroom doors are kept closed to prevent the child from falling in the toilet?
	Have parents inspected play equipment for hazards?
	Is the surface below playground equipment padded in some way?
	Are toys appropriate to the child's age and ability?
	Do parents leave the child unattended in the tub?
	If the family has a pool, is it adequately fenced?

Preschool child (3–6 years)	Has the home been childproofed as above?
	Are pot handles turned away from the edge of the stove?
	Are car seats or seat belts used consistently?
	Is play equipment safe?
	Are toys used appropriately, with adult supervision as needed?
	Is the child adequately supervised at all times?
	Has the child been given safety education regarding:
	    Talking to or going with strangers?
	    Crossing the street?
	    Fire safety?
	    Water safety?

School-age child (6–12 years)	Is play equipment safe?
	Are sports and play activities well supervised?
	Are sports activities age appropriate?
	Are seat belts used consistently?
	Has the child been given safety education regarding:
	    Sports?
	    Bicycling?
	    Water safety?
	    Opening the door to strangers or letting others know one is home alone?
	    Correct use of medications?
	Does the child know how to swim?
	Is a helmet used consistently for bike riding and other activities as appropriate?
	Are firearms kept in the home? If so, are they locked up? Is ammunition kept locked in a separate place from guns?

Other safety considerations include supervision of sports activities and seeing that such activities are appropriate to the age and development of the child. Elementary school children, for example, should not engage in contact sports such as football. Youngsters of this age should be taught safety rules for sports and bicycling, including the use of helmets and other protective equipment. Seat belt use and the ability to swim are other important areas for assessment.

Exposure to firearms is a major concern with children. The nurse should explore whether firearms are present in the home, or in the homes of friends, and how access to firearms is controlled. The nurse should also be aware of the prevalence of firearms in the population and the uses to which they are put. Guns should be kept away from all children, and youngsters in early adolescence should be taught gun safety. Even if guns are not present in their own homes, they may encounter guns in the homes of friends and need to be aware of the hazards.

Conditions in the larger environment also affect the health of children. Despite progress in recent years, many children still have elevated blood lead levels (BLLs). In 1998, for example, 7.6% of children in 19 states had BLLs greater than 10 μg/dL (National Center for Health Statistics, 2000a). Elevated BLLs in children are often associated with older low-income housing in urban areas. The community health nurse should also assess local housing policies as they relate to lead and other safety hazards. Research has indicated that jurisdictions with strong enforcement of housing policies have lower levels of lead poisoning in children than those with limited enforcement (Brown et al., 2001).

Air pollution also affects the health status of children. Air pollution has been shown to slow children's lung development by as much as 10%, with higher concentrations of pollutants causing greater impairment (Gauderman et al., 2000). Both indoor and outdoor air pollution also cause exacerbations of disease in children with asthma, and the nurse should be alert to the extent of pollution in the community and its effects on child health (Hricko, Preston, Witt, & Peters, 2001).

Sociocultural Considerations

Factors in children's sociocultural environments that contribute to health or illness should also be assessed. In younger children, the nurse might observe interactions with others in the environment, including the nurse. Parents can be asked about the child's interaction with siblings and with peers. The nurse should determine whether such interactions are normal for the child's age. For example, parallel play (play alongside of, rather than with, other children) is to be expected of toddlers; sharing and interactive play would not be expected to occur until preschool years. Competitive games and activities with rules are normal interactive behaviors for school-age children.

Older youngsters can also be asked about their friends and what kinds of things they do together. In addition, parents may offer their perspective on how the child interacts with agemates at school and in other settings.

Another area for assessment related to children's environment is culture and its effects on health. Cultural groups may have different child-rearing practices, and the nurse should become familiar with those of individual families as well as those found in the population at

Child-rearing practices may vary considerably from one cultural group to another.

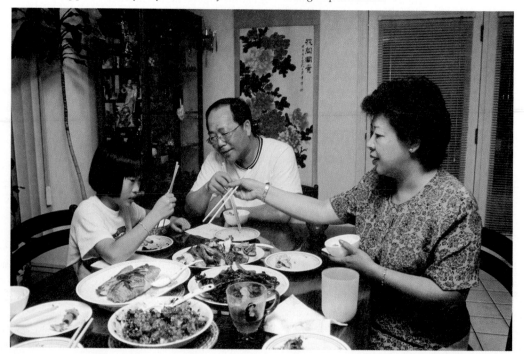

large. Other factors within the social environment may also influence children's health. For example, high levels of unemployment may mean a lack of available health care for children or, in some cases, lack of money for adequate nutrition, housing, and other necessities. In 1999, nearly one fifth of children under 18 years of age lived in families with incomes below poverty level (U.S. Census Bureau, 1999), and another 8% live in extreme poverty (Forum on Child and Family Statistics, 1999). For minority children, figures are even more alarming. For example, 35% to 41% of children in ethnic minority groups live at poverty level or below (Flores, Bauchner, Feinstein, & Nguyen, 1999). Low income is a significant factor in homelessness among children; families with children currently make up 40% of the homeless population in the United States (Better Homes Fund, 1999). Health concerns of the homeless are addressed in more detail in Chapter 20.

Other family considerations in assessing the health status of children include family composition and employment. In 1996, 68% of U.S. children lived with both parents, down from 77% in 1980. In addition, 76% lived with at least one full-time working parent, and 41% lived with single mothers who worked full time (Forum on Child and Family Statistics, 1999). More children are also living with grandparents. The number of children living with grandparents increased by 44% from 1980 to 1990, and in 1997, 4 million children in the United States lived with grandparents. Approximately 11% of American grandparents report raising a grandchild for six months to three years, and the percentage of grandparents raising grandchildren is even higher in inner-city areas (30% to 50%). In addition to the effects on children of not having their parents, these grandparents are particularly vulnerable to depression, social isolation, and poverty, and are more likely than grandparents without parenting responsibilities to have limitations in activities of daily living (Minkler & Fuller-Thomson, 1999).

Prejudice in the social environment may also affect children. For instance, they may be subjected to ridicule by other children at school because of their dress, physical appearance, family culture, or religion. Family religious affiliation may provide social support, but can also lead to potential health problems. For example, children

who receive exemption from immunization on the basis of religious beliefs are 22 times more likely to get measles and 6 times more likely to get pertussis than immunized children. When these children are in child care or elementary school settings, their risk increases 62-fold and 16-fold, respectively (California Department of Health Services, 2001). At the aggregate level, the community health nurse should be aware of the extent of such exemptions as well as other social conditions that affect child health in the population.

Behavioral Considerations

Behavioral factors can be important contributors to health or illness in children. Areas of primary concern include nutrition, rest and exercise, child care, school performance, and use of hazardous substances.

Nutrition

Childhood growth and appropriate development are facilitated by adequate nutrition. Both malnutrition and obesity contribute to childhood morbidity and mortality. In 1996, most U.S. children had poor nutritional status, with only 24% of 2 to 5 year olds and 6% of teenagers eating a balanced diet. In part, these findings are the result of poor family nutrition and eating habits, but an unsettling 4% of children under 18 years of age in the United States experienced moderate to severe hunger in 1997 (Forum on Child and Family Statistics, 1999).

The community health nurse should assess parental knowledge of children's nutritional needs as well as nutritional practices related to children. Nutritional status should be assessed in relation to the child's age and nutritional needs. Specific questions related to assessment for children of different ages are included in Table 16–7 ■. At the aggregate level, the community health nurse should explore the effects of economic conditions on the nutritional status of children in the population including the prevalence of diseases caused by nutritional deficits as well as the prevalence of overweight in children.

Rest and Exercise

Another area for consideration with respect to lifestyle factors and their influence on child health is the ratio of rest to exercise. With infants, the nurse would assess sleeping patterns and the length of periods of sleep and periods of wakefulness. One problem that may become evident at this point is the child whose schedule does not coincide with that of the rest of the family, so the nurse should be sure to ask when sleep periods occur. The nurse would also note whether the child appears to be sleeping more or less than would be expected at that age.

Activity level should also be assessed. Is the child normally active or listless and apathetic? Lethargy may be a sign of a variety of physical health problems including acute illness, hypothyroidism, and anemia. Hyperactivity should also be noted. Hyperactivity in young infants is a frequent consequence of drug exposure during pregnancy.

CULTURAL CONSIDERATIONS

Child-rearing practices can vary significantly from one cultural group to another. Differences in child-rearing practices can create problems when cultures interact with each other or when members of ethnic cultural groups interact with health care professionals. What are some examples of these types of cross-cultural difficulties involving ethnic groups in your area? How might they be addressed?

■ **TABLE 16–7** **Questions for Assessing the Nutritional Status of Children of Selected Ages**

AGE GROUP	ASSESSMENT QUESTIONS
Infant (birth–1 year)	Is the child breast- or bottlefed?
	If breastfed:
	How often does the child nurse?
	How long does the child nurse?
	Does mother alternate breasts?
	Is mother's nutritional intake adequate?
	Does the child seem satisfied?
	If bottlefed:
	How often does the baby eat?
	How much formula is consumed in 24 hours?
	What type of formula is used? Is it iron fortified?
	Do parents prepare formula correctly?
	Do parents use appropriate feeding techniques (e.g., not propping the bottle)?
	Does the infant tolerate the formula well?
	Is the infant gaining weight?
	At what point did parents introduce solids?
	How much solid food does the baby eat?
	Do parents use individual foods rather than less nutritious combination foods (like vegetable and beef combinations)?
	Is one new food introduced at a time? Over several days?
	Has the child started eating table food?
	Is the child weaned from the bottle by 1 year?
Toddler and preschool child (2–5 years)	What foods is the child eating?
	How much food is the child eating?
	Is the child's diet well balanced?
	Are finger foods and variety encouraged?
	Are nutritious snacks provided?
	Is the child given small portions initially and allowed to ask for more to enhance independence?
	Is the child's growth pattern normal for his or her age?
School-age child (6–12 years)	Is the child's diet well balanced?
	Is junk food avoided?
	Are snacks nutritious?
	How much does the child eat?
	Is the child overweight or underweight?
	Is the child's height within normal limits for his or her age?

Lack of exercise among children is a factor contributing to the increasing prevalence of childhood obesity. For many children, television and video games have largely replaced outdoor play. The community health nurse should assess the extent of regular exercise obtained as well as the type of activity performed. At the community level, the nurse would explore the extent of physical activity among children in schools and other settings.

Recreational activities may also pose health hazards, and potential for injury or other health effects should be assessed. Do children use appropriate safety equipment during sports activities? Are helmets consistently used for bicycling, skateboarding, roller blading, and skiing? Do hazardous substances used in children's or parents'

hobbies pose potential health hazards? These and other similar areas should be considered by the nurse in his or her assessment of child health.

Child Care

Child care is a factor in the health of a child that coincides with a family's dual wage-earner lifestyle or with a single-parent lifestyle when the parent works. In 1997, 48% of U.S. children were enrolled in preschool, many because of their parents' work schedules. Day care enrollment has both advantages and disadvantages. Children aged 12 to 23 months in day care are 2.3 times more likely than children cared for at home to have invasive *Streptococcus pneumoniae* infection. For those 24 to 59 months of age, the risk is 3.2 times greater than for stay-at-home peers. There is also a higher risk for episodes of acute otitis media among children in out-of-home day care (Centers for Disease Control and Prevention [CDC], 2000). Day care, on the other hand, has been found to contribute to enhanced intelligence, development, and school achievement and has been associated with long-term effects of employment, lower adolescent pregnancy rates, higher socioeconomic levels, and decreased criminality later in life. Day care has also been found to have positive effects on mothers' employment, education, and interaction with their children (Zoritch, Roberts, & Oakley, 1998). The nurse assessing factors influencing the individual child's health should ask the questions about child care arrangements suggested below.

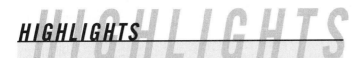
HIGHLIGHTS

Assessing Child Care Arrangements

- Who cares for the child?
- Where does child care take place?
- Are child caretakers qualified to care for children? Have background checks been done on child caretakers?
- Have parents requested references from private child caretakers other than family members?
- Is there more than one adult in the child care setting? Does the setting meet recommended adult-to-child ratios?
- Have parents inspected the child care premises for potential safety hazards?
- Do parents "drop in" to witness the quality of care provided to children in the child care setting and the extent of supervision of children's activities?
- Do parents investigate unusual stories reported by children?
- Have parents made contingency plans for care of the child when he or she is ill or when the child caretaker is unavailable?
- Are child care facilities licensed, if appropriate?

In assessing child health in the aggregate, the community health nurse would consider the availability and accessibility of child care to working parents. He or she would also determine the relative proportion of child care that takes place in licensed child care and home day care settings. Information about the relative preparedness of child care workers to care for children is another indicator of potential effects of child care on the health of children in the population.

School Performance

School performance is another lifestyle consideration for school-age children. The nurse obtains information on the individual child's response to the school environment and on performance in school. Children can be asked how they like school. Information on performance can be obtained from both children and parents. Areas of academic and interpersonal strengths and weaknesses should be identified, and the nurse should also try to gain some insight into family attitudes toward education because these will influence the child's performance. Do parents assist the child with learning tasks? What are parental expectations with regard to school performance? Are they too high or too low? What efforts, if any, are being made to assist the child with problems related to school performance? The child's ability to interact with peers and any school behavior problems should also be determined. In the overall population, the nurse should assess school performance on standardized tests, as well as evidence of school unrest or violence that may be found in local news media or in conversation with local police or school officials.

Exposure to Hazardous Substances

The effects of fetal drug and alcohol exposure were discussed earlier in this chapter. Unfortunately, infants are not the only members of the pediatric population exposed to drugs and alcohol, not to mention tobacco. Both passive and active exposure to tobacco occurs among children. Passive smoking has been linked to increased incidence of respiratory infections, otitis media, and asthma. Older children may actively experiment with tobacco or use alcohol and drugs. For instance, in 1998, 22% of twelfth graders and 16% of tenth graders reported daily smoking, and 9% of eighth graders had smoked cigarettes in the past 30 days. Similarly, 14% of eighth graders, 24% of tenth graders, and 32% of twelfth graders reported having had five or more alcoholic drinks at one time in the last two weeks. Illicit drug use was reported by 12%, 22%, and 26% of these age groups, respectively (Forum on Child and Family Statistics, 1999). Family substance use and abuse as well as the extent of use and abuse of tobacco, alcohol, and other drugs in the population should also be explored.

Health System Considerations

Assessment of the health system dimension includes consideration of attitudes toward health and health care, usual sources of health care, and use of health care services. Particular consideration should be given to the use of primary preventive services related to immunization and dental care.

Another area for consideration is how health care services for children are financed. In 1999, nearly 14% of U.S. children were uninsured, with more than 23% of poor children having no health insurance (U.S. Census Bureau, 2000). Homeless children are particularly unlikely to be insured. Unfortunately, a significant portion of uninsured children (40%) in 1998 were eligible for Medicaid, but were not enrolled (Selden, Banthin, & Cohen, 1998). Not surprisingly, as family incomes decline, the percentage of

ETHICAL AWARENESS

Geltman and Meyers (1998) conducted a study to determine whether or not pediatricians would change their decision to refer a child for child protective services if the referral was likely to lead to deportation of the family. Half of their sample said they would consider not abiding by mandatory child abuse reporting laws if the report would lead to deportation of the family. What would you do if faced with a suspected case of child abuse in a family illegally residing in the United States?

uninsured children increases. These figures indicate that those least able to afford out-of-pocket health care costs are those least likely to have health insurance coverage. The end result is lack of access to health care. In 1996, for example, more than 8% of children had no regular source of care, and nearly 13% received care in emergency departments limiting their access to primary prevention services (McCormick et al., 2000).

Because of the lack of access to health care, the concept of promoting a "medical home" for each child in the United States arose. A medical home is a regular source of health care that is characterized by access to preventive care, 24-hour availability of ambulatory and inpatient care, continuity, access to subspecialty referrals and

assessment tips assessment tips assessment tips

ASSESSING THE INDIVIDUAL CHILD'S HEALTH

Biophysical Considerations

- What is the child's age? Are the child's growth and developmental level commensurate with his or her age? Are there impediments to normal development?
- Is the child a boy or girl? Is the child's sex congruent with parental desires?
- Does the child have any existing physical health problems? Are there any problems with physiologic function (e.g., constipation, spitting up)? Does the child have a history of frequent illnesses?
- Has the child received age-appropriate screening tests? Are the child's immunizations up to date for his or her age?

Psychological Considerations

- Does the child exhibit evidence of psychological health problems?
- What is the attitude of family members toward the child? Are parental expectations of the child realistic? Is discipline appropriate to the child's age and abilities? Is there evidence of child abuse?
- What are the child's reactivity patterns? Do the child's reactivity patterns create conflict within the family?
- What is the quality of parent–child interaction? How adequate are parental coping skills? Do parents exhibit evidence of mental illness?
- How adequate is the child's self-concept?

Physical Environmental Considerations

- Are there safety hazards present in the home or child care environment? Is the home effectively child-proofed? Do parents use age-appropriate safety measures?
- Does the neighborhood present any health or safety hazards for the child?

Sociocultural Considerations

- Does the child interact effectively with others?
- What roles does the child play in the family? Are these roles age appropriate?
- What are the effects of family culture on the child's health?
- Are there factors in the family's social environment that may affect health (e.g., unemployment)? What is the family's economic level? Is family income adequate to meet the child's needs? Are parents employed outside the home?
- Are child care arrangements safe and appropriate to the child's age and developmental level?
- How is the child's school performance? Does the child receive educational support from parents?

Behavioral Considerations

- What are the child's usual diet, rest, and activity patterns? Are they age appropriate?
- Is there evidence of substance abuse in the family? Is the child exposed to tobacco smoke? Does the child use alcohol, tobacco, or other drugs?
- What recreational activities is the child involved in? Do these activities pose any health or safety hazards?
- Has the child received age-appropriate sex education? Is the child sexually active? If so, does the child engage in safe sexual practices? Has the child been subjected to female genital mutilation?

Health System Considerations

- Does the child have a regular source of health care? How does the family finance health care services?
- Do parents have adequate knowledge of basic illness care practices?

interaction between providers and school and community agencies as needed, and maintenance of a central health record for the child. The concept of a medical home is particularly crucial for children with special needs because of the potential for fragmentation of their care (Forsman, 1999).

The nurse should also explore parental knowledge of the care of minor illness in the home. Do parents know not to give aspirin to children? Does the caretaker know how to take a child's temperature? Are parents aware of when to take a child for medical care? What illness care practices are employed by the family? Are any of these practices potentially harmful? A tool that may be used by the community health nurse to assess the health needs of individual children is available on the companion Web site for this book.

Community health nurses assessing the health needs of children in the aggregate should consider the extent of uninsured children in the population as well as effort made to link children to medical homes. The nurse would also determine the type, adequacy, and availability of health care services for children, particularly those related to health promotion and illness prevention and those designed to meet special needs in the child population.

DIAGNOSTIC REASONING AND THE CARE OF CHILDREN

Based on the data gathered in the assessment of individual children or the overall child population, the community health nurse derives diagnoses or statements based on child health and health care needs. Both positive and problem-focused nursing diagnoses should be made from the data obtained. Diagnoses may reflect the need for primary, secondary, or tertiary preventive measures. For example, a positive community nursing diagnosis related to primary prevention is "high immunization levels due to high parental motivation and access to immunization services." On the other hand, a problem-focused nursing diagnosis related to immunizations is "lack of appropriate immunizations for age due to lack of transportation to immunization clinics." Another problem-focused nursing diagnosis related to primary prevention is "potential for child abuse due to unrealistic parental expectations, parental stress, and poor parental coping abilities."

Nursing diagnoses related to secondary prevention are necessarily problem focused because secondary prevention is warranted when actual health problems exist. Examples of nursing diagnoses for the individual child at this level include "need for medical evaluation and treatment due to possible otitis media" and "need for referral to child protective services due to probable child abuse." Diagnoses related to secondary prevention might also be made at the population level; an example might be "lack of services available in the community to meet the needs of children with developmental problems." Nursing

diagnoses at this level might also reflect physical environmental, psychological, sociocultural, or behavioral considerations affecting children's overall health status.

At the level of tertiary prevention, nursing diagnoses focus on the need to prevent complications of existing problems or to prevent the recurrence of problems. For example, the nurse might derive a nursing diagnosis of "need for education on proper infant feeding techniques due to practice of propping bottle" to prevent recurrent middle ear infections, or the nurse might diagnose a "need for emotional support due to imminent death" for a child with AIDS. The intent in this latter diagnosis is to direct nursing care to preventing family complications of a terminal illness. Community health nurses may also derive diagnoses related to the health needs of groups of children. An example of a diagnosis at this level might be "potential for measles epidemic among preschool children due to low immunization rates."

PLANNING HEALTH CARE FOR CHILDREN

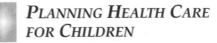

As in the care of any client, planning nursing care for children involves prioritizing needs, developing criteria for approaches to meeting those needs, evaluating alternatives, and selecting a course of action. Objectives for care must be developed and specific interventions related to needs for primary, secondary, and tertiary prevention planned.

Client participation in planning is desirable. Most often, this participation includes the child's parents or other caretakers; however, it is important for the nurse to remember that participation by the individual child in planning for his or her own care is also important. Children, as well as parents and other community members, may also be involved in planning health programs for groups of children.

Interventions selected should be appropriate to the problems identified as well as to the age and developmental level of children. For example, toys designed to enhance motor development should be challenging but not beyond the child's capability to use. If such strategies are not capable of implementation by the child, frustration will result. As another example, it may be appropriate to make a preadolescent responsible for soaking a sprained ankle periodically, but this would not be appropriate for a first-grader.

Nursing interventions for the health problems of children include primary, secondary, and tertiary preventive measures. In dealing with the well child, emphasis is placed on primary prevention—health promotion and prevention of illness. Initial intervention for the acutely ill child is geared to secondary prevention for the illness, with later attention to primary and tertiary prevention. For children with chronic conditions, the initial focus of care may be either secondary or tertiary prevention; however, primary prevention would not be neglected.

One general measure that cuts across all three levels of prevention is the provision of access to health care services for health-promotive, illness-preventive, restorative, and rehabilitative care. The community health nurse may be instrumental in referring children and their parents to appropriate sources of health care. The nurse may also need to refer families for financial assistance with health care needs. At the population level, the community health nurse may be actively involved in the design, implementation, and evaluation of programs to meet the health care needs of groups of children.

Primary Prevention

Primary preventive activities are designed to promote child health and to prevent illness. Major considerations in primary prevention include promoting growth and development, nutrition, safety, immunization, dental care, and support for parenting.

Promoting Growth and Development

To develop properly, children need an environment conducive to growth and development. Community health nurses can assist parents and communities in creating such environments. One of the ways in which this assistance may be provided is in the form of anticipatory guidance. *Anticipatory guidance* is the act of providing information to parents regarding behavioral expectations of children at a specific age before children reach that age.

Such information allows parents to engage in activities that promote development and to cope with some of the more negative aspects of that development. Anticipatory guidance can be provided to the parents of individual children or in parenting classes for groups of parents. For example, the community health nurse might warn parents with children about to turn 2 of the negative behavior typical of this age group. Parents need to know that this negativism is an attempt on the child's part to become autonomous and is normal behavior. They should be assisted to deal with this behavior in such a way that autonomy is fostered while the child's safety is ensured and discipline is maintained. The community health nurse can also reinforce the consistent use of the principles of discipline presented earlier.

Most parents are concerned about their children's development and ability to accomplish developmental milestones. Parents can be told when to expect children to perform various activities, but should also be informed that children develop at different rates. Toilet training is a common parental concern. Many parents attempt toilet training before their children are physically ready. The nurse can inform parents that toilet training is not appropriate until a child is walking. It is not until this time that sufficient sphincter muscle development has occurred to permit the child to control defecation. Parents can be encouraged to look for signs that children are ready to begin toilet training, such as squatting behaviors, hiding behind furniture, or pulling at their clothing when they feel the urge to defecate. Children may also demonstrate readiness by displaying curiosity about parents' eliminative behavior.

When a child has begun to demonstrate some of the signs of readiness for toilet training, parents should determine patterns of defecation and urination and should time trips to the bathroom to coincide with these patterns. If the child normally defecates after a meal, then meals should finish with a trip to the toilet. Children should not be left unattended in the bathroom and should not be encouraged to play during this time. Two to three minutes on a "potty seat" is sufficient. If the child is successful in defecating or urinating on the potty seat, he or she should be praised. Accidents, however, should be ignored. Parents should also be aware that early in the training process, children have very limited sphincter control. When children indicate a need to go to the bathroom, they mean "now!" Parents who tell the child to "wait" are inviting trouble, and accidents that occur in these situations are not the children's fault, but the parents'.

Teething is another developmental concern for parents. Children are frequently irritable when cutting their first teeth. Parents can be encouraged to provide safe teething objects for children. Teething objects that can be placed in the freezer are comforting. Parents can even place an ice cube inside a washcloth to make a cold, hard surface for children to teethe on. The nurse should discourage the use of commercial liquid teething preparations as these may irritate the gums.

Promoting growth and development in children with chronic illnesses or disabilities should also be a concern for the community health nurse. Parents may need to be encouraged to allow their youngster to engage in behaviors that facilitate development. For example, the nurse may need to remind parents of a blind child that the child can use other senses to compensate for lack of vision and that they should encourage the child to engage in activities appropriate to his or her age, rather than overprotect the child. Parents may also need to learn about specialized activities they can do to facilitate children's development. Information on these types of activities can be obtained from a variety of agencies and organizations that address the needs of children with specific conditions or special needs. Links to some of these agencies are provided on the companion Web site for this book. 🌐

Providing Adequate Nutrition

Childhood growth and appropriate development are facilitated by adequate nutrition. Here again, the primary function of the community health nurse is educating parents to provide adequate nutrition for their children. The nurse may also provide referrals to assistance programs or participate in the development of such programs as needed.

Much of the malnutrition found among children in this country is due to inadequate knowledge of nutrition on the part of parents. The community health nurse can help to alleviate such problems by educating parents on the nutritional needs of children at various ages. Parents should be told that children under 6 months of age should be maintained on breast milk or formula alone, because early introduction of solid foods contributes to food allergies and overweight in later life. The community health nurse may want to encourage prospective parents in decisions to breast-feed rather than bottle-feed their infants because of the number of advantages posed by breast-feeding. These advantages include facilitating maternal–child bonding, improved developmental outcomes, fewer infections, reduced allergy potential, convenience, faster return to a prepregnancy weight, and reduced fertility. This last holds true at the aggregate level, but not necessarily for the individual; therefore, breast-feeding should not be suggested as a mode of contraception. The nurse should also be alert to factors that may impede breast-feeding success: lack of peer and professional support for breast-feeding, the need to return to work and inability to effectively pump one's breasts, and commonly experienced problems such as sore nipples.

Some parents, for a variety of reasons, prefer to bottle-feed their infants and should be supported in this decision by the community health nurse. These parents may also need information prior to delivery to ensure that they use an appropriate and nutritious formula, prepare formula properly, adequately refrigerate formula and clean bottles and nipples, and provide nurturance during feeding using correct feeding techniques.

When solid foods are introduced, parents need to be aware that they should introduce new foods slowly to allow for identification of food allergies. They should give a new food for several days without introducing any other new substance to allow time for the development of allergic symptoms. Juices can be introduced between 4 and 5 months of age with the exception of orange juice, which may cause some allergies. Parents should be cautioned against using adult apple juice as it has not been pasteurized and may contain bacteria that can cause severe diarrhea in infants. Solid foods can be introduced at about 6 months of age (once the child is able to sit with support and has good head control), beginning with easily digestible cereals such as rice cereal (Hambidge & Krebs, 1997).

Once the baby has been able to tolerate several different types of cereal, parents can begin to introduce an array of vegetables, beginning with yellow vegetables and progressing to green. Vegetables should be introduced before fruits to avoid the development of a preference for the sweeter fruits and later resistance to eating vegetables. After the child is eating a variety of cereals and vegetables, fruits can be introduced, followed by meats. Again, parents should start with the more easily digested meats such as lamb.

Parents can either prepare pureed foods themselves or purchase commercially available baby foods. If using commercially processed foods, parents should be taught to evaluate food products for their nutritive value. Parents should be made aware that they should buy plain items rather than combinations of foods. For example, they should purchase vegetable and meat separately and mix them if desired, rather than buy the vegetable and meat combination. This is both more economical and more nutritious for the baby. Plain fruits should be purchased over the baby desserts as these merely add unneeded calories and expense.

Parents also need to understand the eating habits of children. The nurse should encourage parents to provide nutritious meals and snacks for youngsters of all ages and to avoid offering junk food. Parents should also avoid food fads such as the use of raw milk and other "natural" foods that may actually be harmful to children (examples of potentially harmful foods are raw eggs and unpasteurized honey).

Many children begin eating finger foods at 6 months of age (Hambidge & Krebs, 1997). Parents should see that children are carefully supervised to prevent choking on small pieces of food. Table foods may be started within a few months, and children may begin drinking from a cup at mealtime (retaining the bottle at nap- or bedtime). Parents can try any table food to see how a child responds. They should, however, be sure that their children are getting a well-balanced diet and that they are carefully supervised to prevent choking. If small vegetables such as peas and lima beans are provided, parents might want to mash them, as children have been known to put such small objects into any bodily orifice, including the ears, nose, and vagina.

Many parents become concerned about their toddler's apparent loss of appetite. Community health nurses need to reassure parents that this is a normal phenomenon resulting from the slower rate of growth that occurs at this age. Again, the primary concern should be the quality of what is eaten rather than the amount. Parents may want to arrange several small meals and nutritious snacks throughout the day rather than the usual three meals. Toddlers and preschoolers also react well to foods that can be eaten "on the go" because they are much more interested in playing than eating. Small portions and colorful meals also tempt a flagging appetite.

School-age children should receive well-balanced diets that provide them with sufficient energy to engage in all of their activities in and out of school. At this age, children tend to be very strongly influenced by what their peers are doing and eating, and parents may need to insist on nutritious foods without making the child feel too different from his or her peers.

Besides providing parents with information on nutritional needs and eating habits of children at various ages, the community health nurse may be called on to provide assistance in budgeting for adequate nutrition. In this area, the nurse can assist parents in the development of lower-cost menus that provide adequate nutrition. Nurses may also be involved in referring parents to sources of financial assistance with nutrition.

Special attention may be needed in meeting the nutritional needs of children with chronic conditions or disabilities. For example, the parents of a young child with diabetes may need to adapt family dietary patterns to accommodate the child's diabetic diet, or the parents of a child with a cleft lip and palate may need assistance in learning feeding techniques to prevent aspiration of food. Based on an assessment of parents' (and children's) knowledge of special dietary needs, the nurse may educate parents or help them develop the skills needed to meet the nutritional needs of their children.

Promoting Safety

Adequate supervision is the major primary preventive measure for promoting the safety of children of all ages. The community health nurse can educate parents regarding safety hazards and measures to keep children safe. Infants and young children should never be left unsupervised, even for short periods, unless they are sleeping soundly in a crib or are otherwise confined, as in a playpen. Even then, frequent checks by parents are indicated.

Children, even when securely restrained, can somehow manage to climb out of high chairs or strollers. Even small children can tip over swings and infant seats. For these reasons, as well, children should not be left unattended. Parents should also be taught not to leave infants alone on elevated surfaces from which they might fall. Care should also be taken that young children are not left unsupervised, even for a few minutes, in the bath.

Another primary preventive measure is instructing parents on the need for consistent use of safety devices such as seat belts and restraints in cars, strollers, high chairs, infant seats, and swings. Community health nurses may also need to be involved in advocacy programs to make safety equipment, such as car seats, available to children in low-income families or to promote legislation related to child safety practices. At present, for instance, no state completely protects child passengers in motor vehicles, since booster seats are not required in any state through age 8 (National Safe Kids Campaign, 2001a). Community health nurses can be actively involved in promoting appropriate use of child restraints in keeping with the principles presented below. Parents can also be encouraged to insist on the use of safety helmets for any child over 6 months of age in any form of wheeled conveyance. Helmets are particularly important for older children riding bicycles or skateboards or roller blading or skiing.

- Use restraints with labels indicating that they meet federal standards and were manufactured after January 1981.
- Do not use any restraint that has been involved in a crash.
- Position restraints in rear seats, on front-facing seats only, and never place them in front of an airbag.
- Make sure the seat belt is appropriate to the type of restraint.
- Do not use automatic or passive seat belts to secure restraints.
- Use a locking clip if the seat belt has a free-sliding buckle tongue. (It is wise to have a locking clip available for use in other vehicles as needed.)
- Use a top tether for the restraint if lap belts lock only on impact or with a sudden stop or if the top of the restraint can be moved more than an inch forward or 1 to 2 inches to the side.
- Route the seat belt according to instructions to secure the restraint.
- Tighten the seat belt around the restraint as much as possible, pressing the restraint tightly into the upholstery.
- Make sure the restraint harness is threaded correctly for the height of the child.
- Tighten the restraint harness so that no more than two fingers fit between the harness and the child's shoulder.
- Position the harness tie at the level of the child's armpit.
- Register the restraint on purchase to be notified in the event of a recall.

Source: Evenflo. (1997). *Safe passage.* Piqua, OH: Author.

The community health nurse should also instruct parents about age-appropriate toys and the need to examine toys frequently for sharp edges, damage, or other conditions that might present safety hazards. Parents can also be encouraged to establish rules for the appropriate use of toys and for toys that are not to be used without adult supervision. The National Safe Kids Campaign (2001e) has developed guidelines for the selection and use of toys that the community health nurse can pass on to parents to enable them to make their children's environment a little safer. These guidelines are presented below.

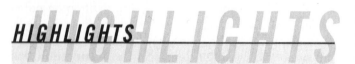

HIGHLIGHTS

Principles of Child Restraint Use

- Use rear-facing restraints for infants (5 to 20 lbs.), forward-facing seats for toddlers (20 to 40 lbs.), and booster seats for older children (30 to 60 lbs.).

HIGHLIGHTS

Guidelines for Toy Safety

- Select toys appropriate to the child's age, ability, and interest.
- Establish ground rules for playing with the toy.
- Select toys with clear instructions for parents and child on use of the toy.

- Select toys that are sturdily constructed.
- Avoid toys with small parts for young children.
- Avoid toys that propel or shoot objects.
- Avoid toys with sharp edges or points.
- Avoid toys with strings longer than seven inches.
- Avoid cap guns as caps can explode with little friction.
- Supervise use of toys with electrical heating elements (use recommended for children over 8 years of age only).
- Consider the environment in which toys are used.
- Inspect toys for damage, and repair or discard damaged toys.
- Teach toy safety and safe toy storage.
- Use proper safety equipment.
- Check the National Safe Kids Campaign Web site (*http://www.safekids.org*) for toy recall notices.

Source: National Safe Kids Campaign. (2001). *Toys: Protecting your family.* Retrieved April 14, 2001, from the World Wide Web, *http://www.safekids.org.*

Promoting school and playground safety are also important primary prevention activities for children. Each year, approximately 2.2 million children under 14 years of age experience school-related injuries, and 80% of school-age children will see a school nurse for an injury within two years (National Safe Kids Campaign, 2001d). Community health nurses can advocate for safe school conditions as well as for the presence of school nurses to address the injury and other needs of the school-age population. Similarly, community health nurses can assist communities to achieve the goals of the National Program for Playground Safety (1999a) which include:

- The design of age-appropriate playgrounds
- Installation of proper absorbent surfaces under all play equipment
- Proper supervision of children on playgrounds
- Proper maintenance of playground equipment

Community health nurses can also assist in providing safety education for children. Areas that should be addressed include watching for cars, crossing streets, talking to strangers, answering the phone or the door, playing with fire, and poisonous substances. Children should also be taught safety rules for sports and bike riding, water safety, and safety with firearms.

Childproofing the home is another area of primary prevention for the young child. This involves placing hazardous objects where children cannot access them and eliminating other safety hazards from the environment. Safety instruction for parents should be geared toward the age and developmental level of the child. Before the child begins creeping, parents need to think of covering electrical outlets and keeping small objects out of the

reach of young children. Stairways should be inaccessible, as should sharp objects and medications of all kinds. Because children learn at a surprisingly early age to climb to reach an objective, sharp objects and poisons should be kept in areas with sturdy locks or latches that the child cannot open, rather than placed out of reach.

As noted earlier, poisoning is a common occurrence in young children, and in the United States in 1998, 1.1 million unintentional poisonings and 69 deaths occurred in children under 5 years of age (National Safe Kids Campaign, 2001c). Parents should also be discouraged from putting toxic substances in unlabeled or usually innocuous containers. The child who sees liquid in a soda bottle may drink it, even if it tastes as bad as bleach or gasoline. Poison precautions suggested by the American Academy of Pediatrics (1997) are summarized on page 378. Special attention should be given to supervising the

Promoting safety (e.g., turning pot and pan handles away from reach) is essential for keeping children from danger.

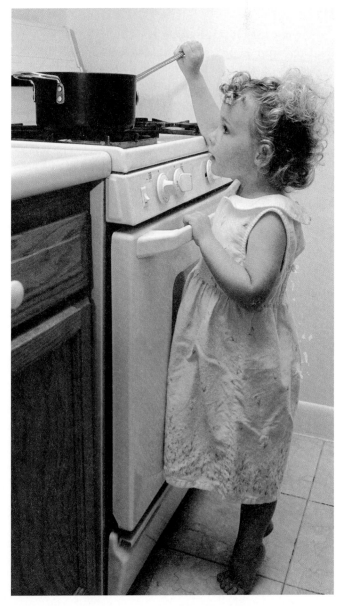

activities of young children when visiting friends or relatives whose homes may not be childproofed.

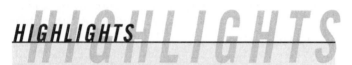

HIGHLIGHTS

Principles of Poison Prevention

- Keep all poisons locked away from children.
- Use safety latches on drawers and cabinets containing potentially harmful substances.
- Don't put poisons in other containers.
- Buy and keep all medications in childproof bottles.
- Discard leftover prescription medications.
- Don't store toothpaste and similar items in the same area as hazardous substances.
- Don't take medications in front of children or describe them as "candy."
- Check medication labels carefully at every administration.
- Buy the least toxic products available.
- Don't run an automobile or use kerosene heaters or wood- or coal-burning stoves in enclosed areas.
- Put the telephone number of the local poison control center in a prominent place by the telephone.
- Keep syrup of ipecac available, but use only on instructions from a health care provider or poison control center (dose: 1 month to 1 year—check with a poison control center; 1 to 10 years—1 Tbsp. followed by two glasses of water).

Source: American Academy of Pediatrics. (1997). *Protect your child from poison.* Elk Grove Village, IL: Author.

Dealing with firearms is an important safety consideration for school-age children. Parents should be encouraged to eliminate firearms or to make them inaccessible to children, never to leave a gun loaded, and to store ammunition apart from weapons. As noted earlier, preadolescent youngsters should be taught the principles of gun safety, and all children should be discouraged from pointing even toy guns at other people.

Immunization

Immunization is a particular concern of the community health nurse working with children and their families. Immunization not only protects the individual who is immunized, but maintaining high immunization levels in the community leads to smaller numbers of susceptible persons and less risk of exposure for those who are not immunized. Unless contraindicated, a child's immunizations should begin at 6 to 10 weeks of age. All infants should be immunized against diphtheria, tetanus, and pertussis (DTaP); polio (IPV); measles, mumps, and rubella (MMR); *Haemophilus influenzae* type b (Hib);

hepatitis B (HBV), and varicella (chickenpox). Pneumococcal conjugate vaccine (PCV) is also recommended for routine administration, but has not yet been adopted in many jurisdictions. Children at particular risk for pneumoccocal disease (e.g., those with sickle cell disease or other immunocompromising or chronic conditions; African American, Alaskan Native, Navajo and Apache children; and children in day care) should certainly be immunized (CDC, 2000). The routine schedule for these immunizations was presented in Table 16–4. Older children should also be immunized with DTaP, IPV, HBV, and MMR vaccines. A single dose of the recently approved chickenpox vaccine is recommended for unimmunized persons over age 11.

⑥THINK ABOUT IT

How can we assure that all children are adequately immunized?

Immunization is of particular concern for children with immunodeficiency problems. For example, live virus vaccines may be contraindicated for children with AIDS. Measles immunization may be considered in children with AIDS, as measles in individuals who have AIDS can be extremely serious, and the benefits of immunization outweigh its risks. Immunization for pneumococcal pneumonia and annual influenza immunization should be provided for children with chronic illnesses or disabilities, including those with AIDS.

In addition to referring individual children for immunizations and educating their parents about the need for immunizations and possible side effects, community health nurses may also need to educate providers regarding valid contraindications for immunization to avoid missed immunization opportunities. Similarly, community health nurses may be of assistance in achieving the 2010 objective to have 95% of U.S. children under the age of 6 included in population-based immunization registries. As of 2000, only 21% of children in this age group were included in local registries (National Immunization Program, 2001).

Dental Care

Dental health is another area of concern in primary prevention with children. From 1988 to 1994, 16% of children aged 2 to 4 years and 29% of those aged 6 to 8 years had untreated dental decay. Access to preventive dental care is particularly poor for children in low-income families. In 1996, for example, only 20% of children and adolescents in homes with incomes at or below 200% of poverty level received any preventive dental care (USDHHS, 2000).

Dental hygiene should begin as soon as the first tooth erupts. At this time parents can be encouraged to rub teeth briskly with a dry washcloth. Later, parents can begin to brush the child's teeth with a soft toothbrush. Older children can be taught to brush and floss their own teeth with adult supervision. Use of a fluoridated toothpaste should be encouraged in areas with unfluoridated water; parents can give fluoride-containing vitamins to infants in such areas. In addition to instructing parents of individual children regarding the need for preventive dental care, community health nurses can be actively involved in promoting fluoridation of community drinking water.

Community health nurses can instruct parents to wean infants from the bottle before a year of age to prevent bottle-mouth syndrome. The use of sugarless snacks and rinsing the mouth after eating—when brushing is not possible—can also be encouraged. Finally, community health nurses should encourage parents to obtain regular dental checkups for children and to get prompt attention for dental problems. Financial assistance may be needed for such services for low-income families. In such cases, the community health nurse should make a referral for Medicaid in those areas where dental care is covered or work to promote the availability of such services in the population.

Support for Parenting

Another major consideration in primary preventive activities for child health is support for parenting. As noted earlier, unrealistic parental expectations of children, excessive parental stress, and poor parental coping skills may contribute to child abuse. These conditions also create a psychological environment that is not conducive to health for either parents or children. Such conditions can be modified by community health nursing support in the parenting role. Parents can be assisted to develop realistic

expectations of child behavior through anticipatory guidance and help with skills related to communications and discipline. The community health nurse can also help parents to identify children's reactivity patterns and develop approaches to dealing with children that minimize some of the negative aspects of specific patterns.

In addition, community health nurses can engage in activities that minimize parental stress. This may involve referral for financial assistance, arrangement of respite care, assistance with finding work or adequate housing, or whatever is required to meet family needs. At the same time, the nurse can assist parents to identify coping strategies that work for them. Parents may also need assistance in problem-solving skills to decrease their own stress levels. Additional areas to be addressed in supporting parenting include counseling related to development, nutrition, physical activity, safety, violent behavior and firearms, STDs and HIV, family planning, and tobacco and drug use as appropriate to children's ages (USDHHS, 1998a).

Other Primary Preventive Activities

Additional primary preventive measures may be warranted for children with specific illnesses. For example, parents of children with AIDS and other immunosuppressive conditions should be taught to minimize exposure to opportunistic infections. Special intervention may also be warranted to create a healthy self-image in children with chronic conditions or disabilities. For example, the physically handicapped child can be helped to develop skills such as artistic ability that contribute to a positive self-image. Primary preventive interventions employed by community health nurses in caring for children are summarized in Table 16–8 ■.

■ TABLE 16–8   Primary Preventive Interventions in the Care of Individual Children

Promoting growth and development	Provide anticipatory guidance to parents. Assist with accomplishment of developmental tasks. Provide assistance with developmental concerns.
Promoting adequate nutrition	Educate parents regarding children's nutritional needs. Provide assistance in meeting nutritional needs.
Promoting safety	Encourage parents to provide adequate supervision of children. Educate parents regarding safety concerns appropriate to the child's age. Eliminate hazardous conditions from the environment. Assist parents to provide safety education appropriate to child's age and health status.
Immunization	Educate parents regarding the need for immunization and immunization schedules. Refer parents to immunization services. Educate parents about side effects of immunizations. Modify immunization practices or provide additional immunizations for children with special needs.
Dental care	Encourage adequate dental hygiene. Encourage regular dental checkups.
Support for parenting	Assist parents to develop realistic expectations of children. Take action to minimize parental stress. Assist parents to develop effective coping strategies and learn child care skills.

Secondary Prevention

Secondary prevention is geared toward resolution of health problems currently experienced by children. Activities are directed toward screening for conditions, care of minor illness, referral for diagnostic and treatment services, and dealing with illness and treatment regimens.

Additional Screening Procedures

Although many screening tests are routinely conducted as part of the assessment of a child's health status, assessment data may indicate a need for additional screening tests. As part of secondary prevention aimed at detecting existing health problems, the nurse can either conduct or make referrals for these additional tests. For example, lead screening may be indicated for children who live in areas with high lead levels in ambient air or who reside in areas with older housing where lead-based paint was used. Blood lead levels would also be obtained for children who exhibit signs of lead poisoning (see Chapter 7).

Other screening tests may be warranted by assessment data. Children who are at risk for HIV infection should be referred for screening. Children at risk include those born to mothers who are injection drug users or partners of injection drug users or of bisexual males. Children who exhibit signs of immunodeficiency or opportunistic infections associated with AIDS (see Chapter 28) should also be referred for screening. Similarly, screening for hepatitis B antibodies may be conducted for children who have been exposed to the disease.

Care of Minor Illness

Many of the health problems experienced by children can be treated by parents at home; however, many parents are quite inexperienced in dealing with minor childhood ailments. They may require help in determining when illness can be dealt with at home and when the assistance of health care professionals is required. The community health nurse can educate parents on the signs of illness in children, appropriate measures to be taken at home, and when to seek medical intervention. Common areas of concern that the nurse addresses are teething, fever, diarrhea and constipation, vomiting, and rashes. Parents should be acquainted with what is normal and what is abnormal, as well as what home remedies are appropriate and what might be harmful.

Besides providing such information, the community health nurse frequently is called on to assess a child's health status and recommend appropriate interventions or make a referral for medical assistance. Potential interventions for minor problems in children and indications for referral for medical assistance are addressed in Appendix A, Nursing Interventions for Common Health Problems in Children.

Referral

Community health nurses frequently encounter health problems in children that require further diagnostic evaluation and treatment. Unless the nurse is also a nurse practitioner, he or she will most probably refer the family to another source of diagnostic and treatment services. Referrals made should be appropriate to the condition suspected and to the circumstances of the situation. Considerations in making referrals and the referral process were addressed in Chapter 12.

In addition to making referrals for diagnosis and treatment services, the nurse may also educate parents and children about probable diagnostic and treatment procedures. For example, if the nurse suspects that a child may have hepatitis, he or she will explain the need for diagnostic blood tests to the parent (and to the child, if the child is old enough to understand) and will describe the typical treatment for hepatitis.

Referrals may be made for assistance with physical, psychological, or social health problems. In the case of child abuse, for example, the nurse might make a referral for evaluation and treatment of the physical effects of abuse on the child. At the same time, the nurse may refer both the perpetrator and the victim of abuse (or other family members) for psychological counseling. Finally, the nurse may refer for assistance those families whose social factors create stress and contribute to the potential for abusive behavior. At the population level, community health nurses may also be involved in advocacy for and development of secondary prevention programs to deal with health problems of children and adolescents.

Dealing with Illness and Treatment Regimens

When an illness requiring medical intervention has been diagnosed, the community health nurse may engage in several secondary preventive interventions related to the diagnosis and its treatment. These interventions include educating parents and children about the condition and its treatment. For example, parents of a child with a newly diagnosed case of diabetes may need information on diet, exercise, and the effects of infection on insulin needs, as well as instruction on how to give insulin. Parents of a child with otitis media may need directions on the use of the antibiotic prescribed. Parents and children should also be given information on the side effects of medications or treatments. For example, parents should be warned about the potential side effects of radiation therapy for cancer and educated on ways to minimize these consequences as much as possible.

Secondary prevention may also entail informing parents and children about what to expect regarding a chronic disease and its treatment. For example, they should be informed that diabetes or essential hypertension can usually be controlled with therapy but will not be cured, and that the child will probably need to take medication for the rest of his or her life. On the other hand, parents should be informed that symptoms of an ear infection should abate within a day or so of starting antibiotic therapy but that medication should be completed.

The community health nurse may also be responsible for monitoring the effect of treatment and the child's health status between visits to a physician or nurse practitioner. In addition, the nurse will observe the child for evidence of medication side effects or other adverse effects of therapy. For example, the nurse may observe a child with ADHD to determine whether medication results in diminished hyperactivity or whether the child exhibits any medication side effects.

Monitoring compliance with a treatment regimen is another secondary preventive measure in the care of children with acute and chronic conditions. The community health nurse periodically needs to assess the child's or family's compliance with medication or other treatments. If noncompliance occurs, the nurse needs to determine factors contributing to noncompliance and plan interventions that enhance compliance. For example, if parents have not been giving their child prescribed antiepileptics because they cannot afford them, the nurse may make a referral for financial assistance or help the family budget their income more effectively. If, on the other hand, parents stopped giving antibiotics prescribed for the child's otitis media because the child got better, the nurse will educate them on the need to finish the prescribed medication.

Secondary prevention for children with conditions like arthritis, cancer, or other illnesses that cause pain include interventions for pain control. Parents and children may need to be encouraged to use pain medications before pain becomes uncontrollable, or they may need suggestions for dealing with side effects related to pain medication.

Support for parenting is particularly needed by parents of children with chronic or terminal illnesses or disabilities. Parents may need assistance or referral in dealing with feelings of guilt and anxiety engendered by the child's condition. In addition, the community health nurse may provide assistance in developing new child care skills necessitated by the child's condition. Referral to groups of parents with children who have similar problems may provide parents with avenues of emotional, social, and material support.

Another area in which the community health nurse may be able to support parents of children with serious health problems is respite care. Parents need to be able to maintain their own lives and care for other children, in addition to meeting the needs of the ill child. The nurse may need to encourage parents to take some time for themselves. Frequently, this entails assisting parents to obtain respite care so they can be sure the child's needs are adequately being met while they are away. If respite care services are not available or are inaccessible to some segments of the population, the community health nurse can advocate for such services and help design and implement respite programs.

Parents and other family members also need to be encouraged to maintain a family life that is as normal as possible. The ill or disabled child should be incorporated into family activities whenever possible, and family members should be encouraged not to let the child's condition become the focus of family life. Family members should be assisted to discuss problems posed by the child's condition and to engage in active problem solving to resolve those concerns. Other avenues for providing support to parents of chronically ill or disabled children include giving information about the child's condition and its treatment, providing emotional support, focusing on positive aspects of the situation, encouraging use of existing support networks, and helping families to expand sources of support.

Families of terminally ill children need additional support in coming to terms with the eventuality of death. The nurse can determine the family's stage in the grief process and design interventions that help them successfully pass through these stages. Interventions suggested for assisting families to deal with perinatal deaths may also be useful in anticipating the death of a child. These include supporting the family's cultural and spiritual beliefs, providing continuity of care, providing time to deal with grief, and encouraging the expression of grief. Acknowledging the life of the child and recognizing and facilitating cultural and religious rituals are also suggested (Gardner, 1999). Referrals for counseling or for hospice services may also be helpful in working with families of terminally ill children.

⊚THINK ABOUT IT

Should dying children be told about their prognosis? Why or why not? Should some children be told and not others?

Tertiary Prevention

As is the case with secondary prevention, tertiary prevention is geared toward the particular health problems experienced by children. Generally, there are three aspects to tertiary prevention with children: preventing recurrence of problems, preventing further consequences, and, in the case of chronic illness or disability, promoting adjustment.

Preventing Problem Recurrence

Community health nurses may educate parents and children to prevent the recurrence of many health problems experienced by children. For example, the parent may need information on the relationship of bottle propping to otitis media to prevent subsequent infections. Similarly, education about the need to change diapers frequently, to wash the skin with each diaper change, and to refrain from using harsh soaps to wash diapers may help prevent continued diaper rash.

Preventing Consequences

Tertiary prevention related to preventing further consequences of health problems is most often employed with children with chronic conditions. For example, the child with diabetes requires attention to diet, exercise, and medication to control the diabetes and prevent physical consequences of the disease itself. At the same time, attention must be given to promoting the child's adjustment to the condition and normalizing his or her life as much as possible. Nursing interventions would be geared toward convincing the child to stick to his or her diet and promoting the child's social interactions with peers.

The nurse might also need to intervene to prevent or minimize the consequences of the child's condition for the rest of the family. For example, the nurse might need to point out to parents that in their concern for the child with a chronic heart condition, they are neglecting the needs of siblings. Tertiary prevention for an infant with AIDS may entail educating parents on the disposal of bodily fluids and excreta to prevent infection of other family members.

Tertiary prevention may entail a wide variety of activities on the part of the nurse, from education on how to deal with specific conditions to referral for assistance with major medical expenses. Nurses may also need to act as advocates for children with chronic conditions. The example that most readily comes to mind is the need for advocacy for children with AIDS who are still well enough to attend school.

Emotional support by the nurse is a very important part of tertiary prevention for children with chronic conditions. Parents' and children's feelings about the condition need to be acknowledged and addressed. The nurse can also reinforce positive activities on the part of parent or child. Again, this support may need to be extended as families go through the grieving process. Grieving will probably occur with most chronic illnesses, even those that are not terminal, and the nurse should be prepared to reassure families that their feelings of grief are normal and to support them through this process.

Promoting Adjustment

The community health nurse may also engage in activities that are designed to return the child and family to a relatively normal state of existence. For children with chronic illnesses or disabilities, this means restoring function as much as possible, preventing further loss of function, and assisting the child and his or her family to adapt lifestyles and behaviors to the presence of a chronic condition. The community health nurse might accomplish this by encouraging the family to discuss problems posed by the child's condition and to view the condition in the most positive light possible. The nurse should also encourage the family to normalize family life as much as possible. For example, if the Little League activities of a sibling have been curtailed because of an exacerbation of the child's illness, parents should make an attempt to reinstitute those activities as soon as the youngster's condition is stable, or the family can be encouraged to call on members of their support network to take the sibling to baseball practice and games.

IMPLEMENTING NURSING CARE FOR CHILDREN

Planned nursing interventions may be implemented by the nurse, by family members or others responsible for the child, or by the child. The nurse should be certain that the child or family members are motivated and capable of carrying out planned care activities. This might necessitate interventions by the nurse to improve motivation or to help the child or family members develop the skills needed to implement the plan. The processes involved in motivating and educating people to take action were addressed in Chapters 10, 11, and 13.

During the implementation phase of nursing intervention, the nurse should check frequently with the child and the family to determine that the plan is indeed being implemented. If it is not, the nurse would assess reasons for noncompliance and plan interventions to facilitate implementation. The nurse should also determine whether the family is experiencing any problems with implementation. Perhaps the nurse has arranged for physical therapy for a handicapped child, but visits by the therapist are interfering with the mother's work schedule. In this case, the nurse might explore the options for providing therapy in the school or in a day care setting instead of the home.

At the population level, implementation entails carrying out planned health care delivery programs and follows the guidelines for implementation discussed in Chapter 15.

EVALUATING NURSING CARE FOR CHILDREN

The effectiveness of nursing interventions for the individual child is assessed in the same manner that care of any specific client is evaluated. Has intervention fostered the child's growth and development? Is the child's nutrition adequate for normal needs? Is the child up to date on his or her immunizations? Are physical or psychological hazards present in the child's environment? Is the child receiving health care as needed? Have acute health care problems been resolved?

The community health nurse would also examine the extent to which care has contributed to the adjustment of the child and family to an existing chronic disease or disability. Are parents comfortable and adequately prepared to parent a child with special needs? Do they perform this role adequately? Have complications of the child's condition been prevented?

The community health nurse would identify criteria that provide the answers to these and similar questions. Data would then be collected relative to the criteria to determine whether nursing intervention has resulted in improved health status for the child and whether specific client care objectives have been met. If, for example, the child is anemic, the criteria used to evaluate nursing interventions related to this problem might include hemoglobin or hematocrit levels and the number and type of iron-rich foods in the child's diet. Evaluative data would be used to modify the plan of care or to determine the appropriateness of terminating services.

The community health nurse may also be involved in evaluating the effects of interventions at the aggregate level. This might entail evaluating the extent to which national objectives for children's health have been achieved. Evaluative data regarding the status of several of these objectives are summarized below.

Community health nursing services to young children are one of the most effective means of enhancing the health of the population. Community health nurses can educate parents and children on health-promoting behaviors and provide early intervention for existing health problems to minimize their effects on the health of individual children and on the population during childhood and as children age.

HEALTHY PEOPLE 2010

GOALS FOR THE POPULATION

Objective	Base	Target
1-9a Reduce pediatric hospitalizations for asthma (per 100,000 children)	23.0	17.3
6-9 Inclusion of children with disabilities in regular education programs	45%	60%
8-11 Eliminate elevated BLLs in children 1 to 5 years of age	4.4%	0
14-22 Achieve and maintain effective vaccination in children 19 to 35 months of age for universally recommended vaccines	43–93%	90%
15-20 Increase use of child restraints	92%	100%
15-33 Reduce maltreatment and maltreatment fatalities of children (per 1,000 children)	13.9	11.1
16-1c Reduce infant deaths (per 1,000 live births)	7.2	4.5
16-2 Reduce child death rates (per 100,000 children)		
a. 1–4 years	34.2	25
b. 5–9 years	17.6	14.3
16-10 Reduce		
a. low birth weight	7.6%	5%
b. very low birth weight	1.4%	0.9%
19-4 Reduce growth retardation in low-income children	8%	5%
21-2 Reduce untreated dental decay in young children	16%	9%
27-9 Reduce child tobacco exposure at home	27%	6%
28-4 Reduce blindness and visual impairment in children and adolescents (per 1,000 children)	25	20
28-12 Reduce otitis media in children and adolescents (visits per 1,000 children)	344.7	294

Source: U.S. Department of Health and Human Services. (2000). *Healthy people 2010* (Conference edition, in two volumes). Washington, DC: Author.

APPLYING YOUR KNOWLEDGE IN PRACTICE

CASE STUDY
Promoting Child Health

You have received a referral to visit Mrs. Kwon, a 24-year-old mother with a newborn baby. There is also another child in the family, Mandy, who is 3. Mrs. Kwon's pregnancy and delivery were uneventful, and mother and baby were discharged after two days in the hospital. When you make your home visit, Mrs. Kwon tells you that the baby is spitting up an ounce or so of formula after each feeding but had gained almost a pound at her two-week visit to the pediatrician yesterday. Otherwise, the baby is doing well.

When you first arrive in the home, Mandy is sitting with her back to you watching cartoons on television. The TV is rather loud and she does not seem to be aware that a visitor has arrived. While you are talking to Mrs. Kwon, Mandy turns around and sees you. She picks up her rag doll and comes to lean against her mother's knee with her thumb in her mouth. She seems to be rather pale compared with her mother's coloring.

Mandy pulls at her mother's sleeve to get her attention. When Mrs. Kwon continues to tell you about the baby spitting up, Mandy hits the infant with her doll.

Mrs. Kwon scolds her and then tells you that Mandy used to be a very good girl, but ever since they brought the new baby home, she has been throwing tantrums and sucking her thumb.

- What biophysical, psychological, sociocultural, behavioral, and health care system factors are influencing the health of these two children?
- What screening tests and immunizations should these two children have had?
- Based on the data presented above, what are your nursing diagnoses?
- How could you involve members of the family in planning to resolve the problems identified?
- What primary, secondary, and/or tertiary preventive measures might you employ with this family?
- What community resources for child health would be helpful to this family? How would you go about locating them?
- How would you go about evaluating the effectiveness of your nursing interventions?

TESTING YOUR UNDERSTANDING

- What are nine problems of concern to community health nurses working with children? (pp. 354–358)
- What is the difference between growth and development? How would you go about assessing each? (pp. 358–360)
- What are three safety considerations in assessing the physical environment of infants? Toddlers and preschool children? School-age children? (pp. 366–368)
- List at least five areas to be addressed in relation to children's psychological environment. Describe how factors in each of these areas might affect the child's health. (pp. 362–366)
- Identify at least three behavioral considerations in assessing the health status of a child. Give an exam-

ple of the influence of each on a child's health. (pp. 369–371)
- What are five primary preventive measures appropriate to all children? What modifications might be needed in these measures when caring for a child with a chronic or terminal illness or a disability? (pp. 374–379)
- What are four approaches to providing secondary preventive services to children with existing health problems? Give an example of the use of each. (pp. 380–381)
- What are the three considerations in tertiary preventive measures for children with existing health problems? Give an example of each consideration. (pp. 381–382)

REFERENCES

American Academy of Pediatrics. (1997). *Protect your child from poison*. Elk Grove Village, IL: Author.

Better Homes Fund. (1999). *America's homeless children*. Newton, MA: Author.

Brown, M. J., Gardner, J., Sargent, J. D., Swartz, K., Hu, H., & Timperi, R. (2001). The effectiveness of housing policies in reducing children's lead exposure. *American Journal of Public Health, 91,* 621–624.

California Department of Health Services. (2000, March). *African American immunization update*, p. 1.

California Department of Health Services. (2001, February 14). *Miniupdate*, 1.

Centers for Disease Control and Prevention. (2000). Preventing pneumococcal disease among infants and young children: Recommendations of the Advisory Committee on Immunization Practices (ACIP). *Morbidity and Mortality Weekly Report, 49*(RR-9), 1–33.

Davis, L., Okuboye, S., & Ferguson, S. L. (2000). Healthy people 2010: Examining a decade of maternal & infant health. *AWHONN Lifelines, 4*(3), 26–33.

Egeland, G. M., Perham-Hester, K. A., Gessner, B. D., Ingle, D., Berner, J. E., & Middaugh, J. P. (1998). Fetal alcohol syndrome in Alaska, 1977 through 1992: An administrative prevalence derived from multiple data sources. *American Journal of Public Health, 88,* 781–786.

Faux, S. A. (1998). Historical overview of responses of children and their families to chronic illness. In M. E. Broome, K. Knafl., K. Pridham, & S. Feetham (Eds.), *Children and families in health and illness* (pp. 179–195). Thousand Oaks, CA: Sage.

Flores, G., Bauchner, H., Feinstein, A. R., & Nguyen, U. D. T. (1999). The impact of ethnicity, family income, and parental education on children's health and use of health services. *American Journal of Public Health, 89,* 1066–1071.

Forsman, I. (1999). Children with special health-care needs: Access to care. *Journal of Pediatric Nursing, 14,* 336–338.

Forum on Child and Family Statistics. (1999). America's children: Key indicators of well-being, 1999. Retrieved August 31, 1999, from the World Wide Web, *http://www.childstats.gov.*

Gardner, J. M. (1999). Perinatal death: Uncovering the needs of midwives and nurses and exploring helpful interventions in the United States, England, and Japan. *Journal of Transcultural Nursing, 10,* 120–130.

Gauderman, W. J., McConnell, R., Gilliland, F., London, S., et al. (2000). Association between air pollution and lung function growth in Southern California children. *American Journal of Respiratory and Critical Care Medicine, 162*(4), 1–8.

Geltman, P. L., & Meyers, A. F. (1998). Immigration reporting laws: Ethical dilemmas in pediatric practice. *American Journal of Public Health, 88,* 967–968.

Hambidge, K. M., & Krebs, N. F. (1997). Nutrition and feeding. In G. B. Merenstein, D. W. Kaplan, & A. A. Rosenberg (Eds.), *Handbook of pediatrics* (18th ed.) (pp. 50–84). Stamford, CT: Appleton & Lange.

Hricko, A., Preston, K., Witt, H., & Peters, J. (2001). Air pollution and children's health. Retrieved January 4, 2001, from the World Wide Web, *http://www.usc.edu/schools/medicine.*

Kenney, K. (1997). Hypertension. In J. A. Fox (Ed.), *Primary health care of children* (pp. 452–454). St. Louis: Mosby-Year Book.

LeFever, G. B., Dawson, K. V., & Morrow, A. L. (1999). The extent of drug therapy for attention deficit-hyperactivity disorder among children in public schools. *American Journal of Public Health, 89,* 1359–1364.

Lowes, L., & Lyne, P. (2000). Chronic sorrow in parents of children with newly diagnosed diabetes: A review of the literature and discussion of the implications for nursing practice. *Journal of Advanced Nursing, 32*(1), 41–48.

May, P. A., Brooke, L., Gossage, J. P., Croxford, J., et al. (2000). Epidemiology of fetal alcohol syndrome in a South African community in the Western Cape Province. *American Journal of Public Health, 90,* 1905–1912.

McCormick, M. C., Kass, B., Elixhauser, A., Thompson, J., & Simpson, L. (2000). Annual report on access to and utilization of health care for children and youth in the United States—1999. *Pediatrics, 15,* 219–230.

Meister, S. B. (1998). Community infrastructures: Principles and strategies for improving child health services. In M. E. Broome, K. Knafl., K. Pridham, & S. Feetham (Eds.), *Children and families in health and illness* (pp. 280–294). Thousand Oaks, CA: Sage.

Minkler, M., & Fuller-Thomson, E. (1999). The health of grandparents raising grandchildren: Results of a national study. *American Journal of Public Health, 89,* 1384–1389.

National AIDS Clearinghouse. (1998, autumn). AIDS and pregnancy continue to pose treatment and prevention challenges. *HIVFrontline*, p. 7.

National Center for Environmental Health. (2000). Measuring childhood asthma before and after the 1997 redesign of the National Health Interview Survey—United States. *Morbidity and Mortality Weekly Report, 49,* 908–911.

National Center for Health Statistics. (1999). Mortality patterns—United States, 1997. *Morbidity and Mortality Weekly Report, 48,* 664–668.

National Center for Health Statistics. (2000a). Blood lead levels in young children—United States and selected states, 1996–1999. *Morbidity and Mortality Weekly Report, 49,* 1133–1137.

National Center for Health Statistics. (2000b). *Health, United States, 2000.* Washington, DC: Author.

National Center for Injury Prevention and Control. (1999). Playground safety—United States, 1998–1999. *Morbidity and Mortality Weekly Report, 48,* 329–332.

National Center for Injury Prevention and Control. (2000). Motor-vehicle occupant fatalities and restraint use among children aged 4–8 years—United States, 1994–1998. *Morbidity and Mortality Weekly Report, 49,* 135–137.

National Center for Injury Prevention and Control. (2001a). *Drowning prevention.* Retrieved April 21, 2001, from the World Wide Web, *http://www.cdc.gov/ncipc.*

National Center for Injury Prevention and Control. (2001b). *Preventing bicycle-related head injuries.* Retrieved April 21, 2001, from the World Wide Web, *http://www.cdc.gov/ncipc.*

National Center for Injury Prevention and Control. (2001c). *The co-occurrence of intimate partner violence against mothers and abuse of children.* Retrieved April 21, 2001, from the World Wide Web, *http://www.cdc.gov/ncipc.*

National Center for Birth Defects and Developmental Disabilities. (2001a). *ADHD long-term outcomes: Comorbidity, secondary conditions, and health risk behaviors.* Retrieved April 21, 2001, from the World Wide Web, *http://www.cdc.gov/ncbddd.*

National Center on Birth Defects and Developmental Disabilities. (2001b). *Autism among children.* Retrieved April 21, 2001, from the World Wide Web, *http://www.cdc.gov/ncbddd.*

National Center on Birth Defects and Developmental Disabilities. (2001c). *Birth defects and pediatric genetics.* Retrieved April 21, 2001, from the World Wide Web, *http://www.cdc.gov/ncbddd.*

National Center on Birth Defects and Developmental Disabilities. (2001d). *Cerebral palsy among children.* Retrieved April 21, 2001, from the World Wide Web, *http://www.cdc.gov/ncbddd.*

National Center on Birth Defects and Developmental Disabilities. (2001e). *Fetal alcohol syndrome.* Retrieved April 21, 2001, from the World Wide Web, *http://www.cdc.gov/ncbddd.*

National Center on Birth Defects and Developmental Disabilities. (2001f). *Mental retardation among children.* Retrieved April 21, 2001, from the World Wide Web, *http://www.cdc.gov/ncbddd.*

National Center on Birth Defects and Developmental Disabilities. (2001g). *Public health issues in ADHD: Individual, system, and cost burden of the disorder workshop.* Retrieved April 21, 2001, from the World Wide Web, *http://www.cdc.gov/ncbddd.*

National Diabetes Information Clearinghouse. (2001). *Diabetes statistics.* Retrieved April 22, 2001, from the World Wide Web, *http://www.diddk.nih.gov/health/diabetes.*

National Immunization Program. (2000). National, state, and urban area vaccination coverage levels among children aged 19–35 months—United States, 1999. *Morbidity and Mortality Weekly Report, 49,* 585–589.

National Immunization Program. (2001). Progress in development of immunization registries—United States, 2000. *Morbidity and Mortality Weekly Report, 50,* 3–6.

National Program for Playground Safety. (1999). *National action plan for the prevention of playground injuries.* Retrieved June 17, 1999, from the World Wide Web, *http://www.uni.edu/playground.*

National Program for Playground Safety. (1999b). *Statistics about playground related injuries.* Retrieved June 17, 1999, from the World Wide Web, *http://www.uni.edu/playground.*

National Safe Kids Campaign. (2001a). *Car.* Retrieved April 14, 2001, from the World Wide Web, *http://www.safekids.org.*

National Safe Kids Campaign. (2001b). *Firearms.* Retrieved April 14, 2001, from the World Wide Web, *http://www.safekids.org.*

National Safe Kids Campaign. (2001c). *Poison.* Retrieved April 14, 2001, from the World Wide Web, *http://www.safekids.org.*

National Safe Kids Campaign. (2001d). *School/Playground.* Retrieved April 14, 2001, from the World Wide Web, *http://www.safekids.org.*

National Safe Kids Campaign. (2001e). *Toys: Protecting your family.* Retrieved April 14, 2001, from the World Wide Web, *http://www.safekids.org.*

Newborn Screening Task Force. (1999). *Serving the family from birth to the medical home: Newborn screening: A blueprint for the future.* Washington, DC: Health Services and Resources Administration.

Regional Perinatal Programs of California. (1999, spring). HIV transmission: Mode of delivery and risk of vertical transmission. *Perinatal Care Matters,* pp. 2–3.

Regional Perinatal System. (2000). Infant mortality statistics released. *Crib Sheet, 12*(4), 3.

Rheumatism and Arthritis Foundation of Tasmania. (2001). *Who gets arthritis?* Retrieved April 22, 2001, from the World Wide Web, *http://www.tased.au/tasonline/raft.*

Seay, A. R., & Janas, J. (1997). Neurologic and muscular disorders. In G. B. Merenstein, D. W. Kaplan, & A. A. Rosenberg (Eds.), *Handbook of Pediatrics* (18th ed.) (pp. 631–658). Stamford, CT: Appleton & Lange.

Selden, T. M., Banthin, J. S., & Cohen, J. W. (1998). Medicaid's problem children: Eligible but not enrolled. *Health Affairs, 17,* 192–200.

United Nations. (1999). *Report on the global HIV/AIDS epidemic.* Retrieved August 24, 2000, from the World Wide Web, *http://www.unaids.org/epidemic_update.*

U.S. Census Bureau. (1999). *Statistical abstract of the United States, 1999* (119th ed.). Washington, DC: Author.

U.S. Census Bureau. (2000). *Health insurance coverage: 1999.* Retrieved November 17, 2000, from the World Wide Web, *http://www.census.gov.*

U.S. Department of Health and Human Services. (1998a). Clinical preventive services for normal-risk children. *Prevention Report, 13*(1), 10.

U.S. Department of Health and Human Services. (1998b). Task force on environmental health and safety risks to children. *Prevention Report, 13*(1), 3.

U.S. Department of Health and Human Services. (2000). *Healthy people 2010* (Conference edition, in two volumes). Washington, DC: Author.

Zoritch, B., Roberts, I., & Oakley, A. (1998). The health and welfare effects of day-care: A systematic review of randomized controlled trials. *Social Science and Medicine, 47,* 317–327.

WOMEN AS AGGREGATE

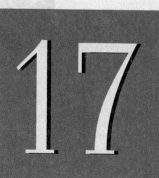

Chapter Objectives

After reading this chapter, you should be able to:

- Identify at least two factors in each of the dimensions of health as they relate to the health of women.
- Identify health problems common to women.
- Describe at least three unique considerations in assessing the health needs of the lesbian client.
- Identify concerns in primary prevention for women.
- Describe areas of secondary prevention activity with women.
- Describe two elements of secondary prevention of physical abuse of women.
- Describe at least two actions that the community health nurse can take to provide more sensitive and effective care to lesbian, bisexual, and transgender clients.

KEY TERMS

coming out 399
female genital mutilation (FGM) 391
homophobia 400
infertility 389
menarche 388
menopause 389
osteoporosis 390
perimenopause 388
postmenopause 389
premenopause 388
reparative therapy 403

Media Link

http://www.prenhall.com/clark

Additional interactive resources for this chapter can be found on the companion Web site. Click on Chapter 17 and "Begin" to select the activities for this chapter.

In 1998, there were nearly 110 million women over 15 years of age in the United States, roughly 52% of the adolescent and adult population (U.S. Census Bureau, 1999). Women have unique health care needs, not only because of their anatomy and reproductive functions, but also because of their vulnerability within society. Women live longer than men and experience more chronic health problems. Community health nursing services to women can greatly improve the health of the overall population.

The importance of improving the health of women in the United States is reflected in the national health objectives for the year 2010. Multiple objectives specifically target the health needs of women (U.S. Department of Health and Human Services [USDHHS], 2000). These objectives can be viewed by accessing the link to the Healthy People 2010 Web site provided on the companion Web site for this book. Selected objectives are included at the end of this chapter.

This chapter addresses care of adolescent, young adult, and middle adult women. The health needs of older women are the focus of Chapter 19.

ASSESSING WOMEN'S HEALTH

Care of female clients begins with an assessment of health status. Factors influencing health status are examined according to the six dimensions of health: the biophysical, psychological, physical environmental, sociocultural, behavioral, and health system dimensions. Community health nurses assess the health status of individual women as well as the status of women as an aggregate within the population.

Biophysical Considerations

Biophysical factors are of concern to the community health nurse assessing the female client. Specific areas for consideration include genetic inheritance, maturation and aging, and physiologic function.

Genetic Inheritance

Women are prone to a number of genetically related or genetically linked conditions. For example, cancers of the breast have been shown to occur more frequently among women whose mothers, sisters, aunts, or grandmothers have had similar cancers. Similarly, diseases of the thyroid gland seem to occur more frequently among women than men, as do diabetes, asthma, various forms of dermatitis, and hay fever–type allergies, all of which may involve genetic predisposition to disease.

Maturation and Aging

In general, physical maturation of females follows the developmental schedule for children presented in Chapter 16. Sexual maturation, however, follows a unique trajectory in women. Stages of sexual maturation are summarized at right.

Menarche, the first appearance of menstrual flow in the adolescent girl, usually occurs between 12 and 13 years of age. Menarche that occurs too early (age 8 or younger) is associated with precocious puberty, an anomaly of the endocrine system. Delayed menarche (after age 18) is also a signal that the endocrine system is not functioning properly. Either early or late onset of menses is cause for referral for medical evaluation. Menarche may appear earlier or later than average in some ethnic populations, and the nurse should be familiar with population parameters for the onset of menstruation.

The physical changes that occur just prior to and with menarche have the potential to create physical or psychological problems for the adolescent. Assessment of preadolescent girls should include the extent of sexual changes, knowledge of menstruation, and preparation for the event. If menarche has occurred, other considerations related to menstruation may include menstrual regularity, extent and duration of flow, and the experience of dysmenorrhea, or painful menstruation. The nurse would also inquire about signs and symptoms of premenstrual distress (premenstrual syndrome) such as depression, irritability, nervousness, tension, inability to concentrate, breast tenderness, bloating, edema, fatigue, headache, and food cravings. Symptoms of premenstrual distress may be severe and require medical referral or may be less severe and respond to dietary changes and exercise.

Premenopause is the period of a woman's life in which she is most likely to become pregnant. These child-bearing years generally last from menarche to age 40, when women enter the perimenopausal period (Goldsmith & Shelby, 1999). Areas for assessment in this stage include pregnancy rates, the proportion of unintended pregnancies in the population, the extent of prenatal care, and information on pregnancy outcomes for women and children. Consideration should also be given to the availability and use of contraceptive methods by women who do not desire to become pregnant.

Perimenopause is a transition period between premenopause and menopause, when the physical and hormonal changes that herald cessation of menstruation occur. Another term for this stage of sexual maturation is the *climacteric* (Holden & Miller, 1999). Perimenopause may last from two to eight years, but the average is four years. In 2000, an estimated 19 million women were in their perimenopausal years and experienced any of a number of discomforts associated with this period including hot flashes, night sweats, and sleep disturbances and insomnia. Additional effects of perimenopause may include painful intercourse, more frequent urinary tract infections, and stress incontinence and urinary urgency. Mood changes are typical of this period and may be more pronounced in women with a prior history of depression. Pregnancy may still be possible, and women who do not wish to become pregnant should use some form of contraceptive for 12 months after their last menstrual period (Goldsmith & Shelby, 1999). Hormone replacement therapy is often highly effective in addressing the discomforts of the perimenopausal period.

Menopause is the cessation of menstruation that occurs with advancing age. Menopause has occurred when the woman has been without menses for 12 months. The average age for menopause is 51 years (Lilly Center for Women's Health, 1998), but normal menopause can occur as early as age 40 (Holden & Miller, 1999). Some women experience menopause as a result of surgical interventions such as hysterectomy.

Postmenopause extends from menopause until death and may cover as much as one third of women's lives (Lilly Center for Women's Health, 1998). Because of the hormonal changes that occur with menopause, the postmenopausal period is a time of increased risk for a number of health problems. Several of these such as osteoporosis and heart disease are discussed in the section addressing physiologic function.

Other areas for consideration with respect to maturation and aging include the effects of aging in general on health status (which will be addressed in Chapter 19) and women's emotional maturation. Community health nurses would assess the effects of aging as well as emotional maturity among female clients. At the aggregate level, the nurse should assess the relative proportion of women at different ages and different stages of sexual maturation in the population. These data will provide a picture of the health care needs of women as a subsegment of the population.

Physiologic Function

Women's physiologic function is also assessed. Special considerations in assessing the female client include reproductive issues of pregnancy and infertility, the presence or absence of specific illnesses, and immunization levels.

REPRODUCTIVE ISSUES Pregnancy is one of the most prevalent problems related to human physiology in the adolescent girl. In 1997, a baby was born to 32.6 out of every 1,000 girls aged 15 to 17 years, and in 1996, 264,000

abortions were performed on girls 15 to 19 years of age (U.S. Census Bureau, 1999). Nearly half of all pregnancies among women 15 to 44 years of age in 1995 were unintended (USDHHS, 2000).

Pregnancy is more often associated with complications, prematurity, and fetal and maternal mortality among adolescents than among older women, but all women are at some risk of complications during pregnancy. In fact, in 1997 nearly one third of deliveries were associated with serious complications of pregnancy, occasionally resulting in death. The maternal mortality rate for 1997 in the United States was 8.4 deaths per 100,000 live births (U.S. Department of Health and Human Services, 2000).

Community health nurses would assess individual women for pregnancy and associated discomforts and complications. At the population level, nurses would assess pregnancy and birth rates as well as rates of maternal mortality and pregnancy complications.

The incidence of infertility among U.S. women is increasing. **Infertility** is the inability to conceive and have a child. In 1995, 13% of U.S. married couples had difficulty becoming pregnant (USDHHS, 2000). Causes of infertility among women include the occurrence of sexually transmitted diseases that damage fallopian tubes, environmental toxins affecting ova, and a tendency to postpone pregnancy until the late thirties or early forties. Women in the perimenopausal period may ovulate less frequently than younger women, thereby becoming less fertile than they would have been in their twenties.

Infertility can have serious consequences for the individual and the couple who are unable to conceive, including:

- Feelings of guilt, especially among women, who are usually the focus of the search for a cause
- Expense of diagnostic and other procedures
- Obsession with the inability to conceive
- Disapproval and pressure from family to adopt or try other methods to conceive
- In some cultures, perceptions of the female as less than a woman

The community health nurse can assess the individual woman's desire to have children and any attempts made to conceive. Data on the prevalence of infertility should also be obtained as well as information on probable causes of infertility in the population.

ILLNESS Assessment of physiologic function also includes the collection of data related to the presence or absence of physical illness. For the individual client, the nurse would obtain information about existing physical health problems, either acute or chronic. At the population level, the nurse would focus on the incidence and prevalence of diseases affecting women.

The leading causes of mortality in U.S. women in 1995 were (a) heart disease, (b) cancer, (c) stroke, (d) chronic pulmonary disease, (e) pneumonia and influenza, (f) diabetes,

(g) accidents, (h) Alzheimer's disease, (i) nephritis, and (j) septicemia. Other conditions affecting women may not cause death, but contribute to significant morbidity. Leading worldwide causes of physical morbidity in women include osteoarthritis, cerebrovascular disease, diabetes, and rheumatoid arthritis (Lilly Center for Women's Health, 1998). Several of these conditions and their effects on women's health will be briefly considered.

More than 500,000 deaths occur in U.S. women each year as a result of heart disease. Women are more likely than men to die within one year of myocardial infarction (MI) (44% and 27% respectively) and are more likely to have a second MI (31% versus 23% for men). Heart disease causes greater mortality among women than all of the next 16 causes of death combined (Lilly Center for Women's Health, 1998). In 1998, the rate for female heart disease mortality was 93.3 per 100,000 women. Although this is a significant decrease from the 1950 rate of 233.9 per 100,000 women (National Center for Health Statistics, 2000b), considerable work remains to be done in preventing heart disease in women.

Cancer is another significant cause of mortality and morbidity in women. In 1998, the U.S. mortality rate for women for all cancers was 105.5 per 100,000 women. For breast cancer, the rate was 18.8 per 100,000 which is a decrease from 23.3 in 1950. Lung cancer deaths, on the other hand, have increased sixfold since 1950 rising from 3.9 per 100,000 women to 27 per 100,000 (National Center for Health Statistics, 2000b). Mortality rates for thyroid cancer also rose by 35% from 1973 to 1994, while those for cervical cancer decreased by 40% in the same period (Lilly Center for Women's Health, 1998). In 2000, more than 182,000 new cases of breast cancer and 12,800 cases of cervical cancer were expected to be diagnosed, leading to 41,200 and 4,600 deaths respectively (Lawson, Henson, Bobo, & Kaeser, 2000).

Chronic pulmonary diseases, including asthma, are also major contributors to death and disability in women. In 1998, the age-adjusted mortality rate for chronic obstructive pulmonary diseases was 18.8 per 100,000 women, slightly more than twice the 1950 rate of 8.9 per 100,000 women (National Center for Health Statistics, 2000b). Asthma incidence in women increased 82% from 1982 to 1992, but increased by only 29% for men. Asthma mortality also increased by 59% from 1981 to 1995 (versus 34% for men) (Lilly Center for Women's Health, 1998). Women also account for 75% of all adult hospitalizations for asthma. The increased prevalence and severity of asthma in women may have a hormonal cause as some women with asthma get exacerbations of their disease just before and during their menstrual period, at menopause, or while on oral contraceptives or hormone replacement therapy. Hormonal changes in pregnancy affect asthma differentially, with approximately one third of women experiencing symptom relief, one third worsening symptoms, and one third no difference in symptoms. When asthma is exacerbated by pregnancy, it may

have consequences for both mother and fetus, including low birth weight, intrauterine growth retardation, preterm labor, toxemia, elevated blood pressure, hyperemesis, and vaginal hemorrhage (Holden & Miller, 1999).

Nationally, 5% of women have diabetes (National Women's Law Center, Focus/University of Pennsylvania, & The Lewin Group, 2000), and gestational diabetes mellitus (GDM) occurs in approximately 4% of all pregnancies in the United States. GDM incidence may be as high as 14% in some ethnic populations with high overall diabetes incidence (Regional Perinatal System, 2000). In addition to its direct effects on women's health and lifestyle, the presence of diabetes increases the risk of heart disease three- to sevenfold in women compared to a two- to threefold increase in men (Lilly Center for Women's Health, 1998).

Autoimmune diseases also cause greater morbidity and mortality in women than men. Autoimmune diseases include 24 different conditions such as lupus erythematosus, type 1 diabetes, rheumatoid arthritis, multiple sclerosis, and several other diseases that occur relatively rarely. Taken together, these diseases constitute a leading cause of death and the fourth leading cause of disability in women (Lilly Center for Women's Health, 1998; Walsh & Rau, 2000). Rheumatoid arthritis is the most common chronic condition in women and is expected to affect 36 million U.S. women by 2020 (Lilly Center for Women's Health, 1998). Approximately 23% of U.S. women over 40 years of age experience some activity limitation as a result of arthritis (National Women's Law Center et al., 2000).

Human immunodeficiency of virus (HIV) infection and acquired immune deficiency syndrome (AIDS) are specific forms of autoimmune disease not categorized with the 24 discussed above. Although initially a disease of gay men, the percentage of women with active cases of AIDS has tripled in the last decade (National Women's Law Center et al., 2000). Women accounted for 20% of new AIDS cases in 1998 compared to only 7% in 1985 (USDHHS, 1998b). In 1998, the age-adjusted female mortality rate for AIDS was 2.2 per 100,000 women, (down from 5.2 per 100,000 in 1995) (National Center for Health Statistics, 2000b), and the incidence rate for new cases was 8.8 per 100,000 women (USDHHS, 2000).

Another concern during the perimenopausal and postmenopausal years is osteoporosis. *Osteoporosis* is a common metabolic bone disease characterized by a loss of bone minerals that weakens bones so that fractures occur more easily. Women may experience loss of up to 50% of bone tissue over a lifetime. Approximately 25 million women (80%) have some degree of osteoporosis (Hughes, 1998), and 7 of 10 women have moderate to severe bone density reduction. Osteoporosis is the leading cause of fractures in adult women. Approximately 50% of women lose their independence following a fracture, and there is a 24% higher mortality rate in women who have had fractures. In 1996, there were 23 million U.S. women over age 50 years at risk for fracture due to osteoporosis, and in

1995 the direct medical costs to society for fractures in women over 45 years of age was $11 billion. This figure is expected to increase sixfold by 2020 (Lilly Center for Women's Health, 1998). Risk factors for osteoporosis include age, small thin body frame, menopause, poor calcium intake, being Caucasian or Asian, family history of osteoporosis, smoking, lack of weight-bearing exercise, and excessive alcohol intake (Hughes, 1998). Chemotherapy for breast cancer is another risk for osteoporosis for some women (*Excellence in Clinical Practice*, 2000).

Arthritis and osteoporosis are two of many conditions that contribute to disability in women. Approximately 4% of women in the U.S. receive Social Security disability payments (National Women's Law Center et al., 2000). In 1996, 16.5% of women experienced restricted activity days compared to 12.3% of men, and 6.9% of women experienced bed disability days compared to 4.9% of men (U.S. Census Bureau, 1999).

In addition to being aware of the incidence and prevalence of these conditions and their effects in the population, community health nurses should be alert to signs and symptoms of their presence in individual women clients. Nurses should also be aware of risk factors for these conditions exhibited by individual women and in the population. Risk factors for many of these conditions are addressed in Chapter 29.

One other physical condition that may affect some women in the population or a significant portion of the women in some segments of the population is female genital mutilation, also known as *female circumcision* or *infibulation*. **Female genital mutilation (FGM)** is the alteration of female genital tissue ostensibly to promote virginity, but in reality to maintain male dominance. It may take place anytime from birth to adolescence, and as many as 100 million women worldwide may have been victims of FGM (Brady, 1998).

A variety of religious groups practice FGM, including some Christian sects as well as some Muslim groups. It has been reported in Africa, the Middle East, Malaysia, and Indonesia. Although illegal in Canada, the United States, and most parts of Europe, community health nurses may encounter immigrant women from other parts of the world who have been subjected to FGM. Families in some cultural groups may take their daughters back to their countries of origin in order to have the procedure performed.

The community health nurse working with women who have experienced FGM may discover three levels of mutilation. The least severe is *sunna*, in which only the prepuce is removed. *Clitoridectomy* involves removal of the entire clitoris and parts of the labia minora. *Infibulation*, the most extensive form of FGM, involves removal of the clitoris, labia minora, and parts of the labia majora and stitching the sides of the area together to leave only a small opening for passage of urine and menstrual blood. The effects of FGM may include wound infection, HIV and hepatitis B virus (HBV) infection, pelvic inflammatory disease, hemorrhage, menstrual pain, painful urina-

tion, and urinary tract and vaginal infections. Long-term effects may include infertility and serious complications of childbirth including severe perineal tears, fistulas, postpartum hemorrhage, infection, and increased incidence of stillbirth. Some victims of FGM may view it as a source of pride and symbol of acceptance in their cultural group, but the consequent infertility may be psychologically devastating (Brady, 1998). Community health nurses should ask women clients about their exposure to FGM. Gynecologic and urologic referrals may be needed for these clients, as well as referrals to mental health professionals to help them deal with the psychological effects of this abusive practice. Community health nurses should also be aware of cultural groups within the population that engage in FGM and develop culturally sensitive ways of discouraging this practice.

IMMUNITY   The last aspect of physiologic function to be considered in the assessment of women's health is immunization levels. Women's immunization rates, like those for all adults are lower than recommended. In 1995, for example, only 43% of women aged 50 to 64 years received influenza vaccine, and only 22% had ever received pneumococcal vaccine. For tetanus, fewer than half of women in this age group were fully immunized (Singleton, Greby, Wooten, Walker, & Strikas, 2000). Community health nurses should assess the immunization status of individual women clients as well as immunization levels in the population as a whole.

Psychological Considerations

Factors in the psychological dimension can have a profound effect on women's health. Areas of particular concern to community health nurses assessing women's health are stress and coping abilities and the psychological implications of sexual identity.

Stress and Coping

The first area for consideration related to the psychological dimension and its effect on women's health is the extent of women's exposure to stress and their abilities to cope with that stress. It is well known that stress contributes to a variety of illnesses in both men and women. For example, stress plays a part in the development of tuberculosis and hypertension. Severe life events and the stress that accompanies them have also been shown to be related to breast cancer in women. In one study, stress was found to interact with women's personal psychological traits to affect health. Women in this study who were subjected to medium to high levels of stress who were less assertive, less hardy, and less able to express themselves had more physical symptoms than women who scored favorably in these areas (Kenney & Bhattacharjee, 2000). Women, in general, have been found to be less happy and to experience more stress than men. In fact, U.S. women as a group report an average of 3.5 days per month when their mental health was not perceived as good (National Women's Law Center et al., 2000).

Learned coping skills are an important facet of the psychological dimension of health that the nurse assesses. How does the individual woman client normally handle adversity? What factors in the environment strengthen her ability to cope? What coping strategies does she use and how effective are they? Is the client at risk for suicide or other health problems due to poor coping abilities? Women at all ages are less likely than men to commit suicide, but a significant number of women each year succumb to despair and end their lives. In 1998, the age-adjusted suicide mortality rate for women was 4.0 per 100,000 women, down from 6.8 per 100,000 women in 1970 (National Center for Health Statistics, 2000b). Although suicide mortality is only about one fourth that of men, women are twice as likely as men to experience depression, and approximately 11 million women experience depression each year (Lilly Center for Women's Health, 1998). Population estimates of depression in women as well as rates for attempted and completed suicide are important data for an aggregate assessment of women's health.

Sexuality

Elements of both the psychological and social dimensions affect issues of sexuality in women, but because of the implications of sexuality for women's mental health, they will be addressed under the psychological dimension. Many women are embarrassed to discuss issues of sexuality, and teenagers, in particular, may have a number of fears and misconceptions. In assessing adolescent girls, the community health nurse obtains information related to attitudes and anxieties about menstruation as well as knowledge of menstrual physiology and hygiene. Social factors such as family and cultural attitudes and knowledge and parental education level may affect family willingness or ability to assist the young girl with the physical, emotional, and practical issues posed by menarche.

The nurse cannot assume that older women do not have some of the same concerns regarding menstruation and sexuality as teenagers. Women may have questions about their sexuality, guilt about sexual activity or possible infertility, and difficulty in developing healthy sexual identities. As we will see later in this chapter, these concerns are frequently magnified for the lesbian client. Community health nurses should assess women's comfort with sexuality and their sexual identity and assist them to voice concerns in these areas.

Sexual activity by women, especially teenagers, may have a variety of psychological precursors. For example, the adolescent may think that if she is still a virgin at age 15, there is something wrong with her. Or, if she perceives her mother as asexual or "Madonna-like," she may rebel and seek sexual outlets totally unlike those of her mother. The nurse assesses clients' knowledge and attitudes about sexual identity and sexual activity.

Menopause, at the other end of the reproductive spectrum, also has psychological implications. In our society, menopausal women have not been held in high esteem.

ETHICAL AWARENESS

Approximately one in every 2,000 babies born each year in the United States have both male and female physical or hormonal characteristics. Genital reassignment surgery is performed on 100 to 200 of these babies each year (Sember, 2000). Since parents do not know what gender identity the child will adopt in later life, do you think they should wait until the child is old enough to participate in the decision to have surgery performed? Why or why not? If surgery is performed in infancy, should the child be informed? Why or why not? If yes, when should the child be informed?

Women have been barred from productive work on the basis of their menopausal symptoms. Society's lack of regard for the older woman adds to her emotional symptoms, thereby limiting her abilities to cope with physical and psychological changes occurring at this time.

One's sexual identity is constructed from societal and cultural definitions as well as self-perceptions. Traditionally, people tend to think of sexual identity as male or female, but in reality there are multiple possible ways in which women can think of themselves. A typology of female sexual identities is presented below. Women may experience considerable confusion and distress in the development of a sexual identity, particularly if the identity that seems right for them violates family or cultural norms. One's sexual identity may or may not coincide with one's sexual activity. For example, a woman who identifies herself as a lesbian may engage in sexual activity with women, or may engage in bisexual or heterosexual activity or be celibate (Gruskin, 1999). Community health nurses can explore sexual identity issues with women clients using non–value-laden terminology that does not suggest assumptions that the client has accepted a heterosexual identity.

HIGHLIGHTS

Typology of Sexual Identities Among Women

- *Heterosexual female:* A woman who has sex or primary emotional partnerships with members of the opposite gender
- *Lesbian female:* A woman who has sex or primary emotional partnerships with members of the same gender
- *Bisexual female:* A woman who has sex or primary emotional partnerships with members of the same and the opposite gender
- *Transsexual female:* A woman who desires to be a permanent member of the opposite gender (female to

male—FtM) or a man who has received genital reassignment surgery or hormone therapy to become a female (male to female—MtF)

- *Transvestite female:* A woman who dresses in male attire
- *Transgenderist female:* A woman who lives life in a part-time or full-time role as a member of the male gender
- *Androgynous female:* A biological female who adopts characteristics of both genders and neither
- *Intersex female (hermaphrodite):* A person who has physical and/or hormonal features of both genders

Sources: Sember, R. (2000). *Transgender health concerns.* In Gay and Lesbian Medical Association & Center for Lesbian, Gay, Bisexual, and Transgender Health (Eds.), *Lesbian, gay, bisexual, and transgender health: Findings and concerns* (pp. 32–43). New York: Author; and Solarz, A. L. (Ed.), (1999). *Lesbian health: Current assessment and directions for the future.* Washington, DC: National Academy Press.

Physical Environmental Considerations

Physical environmental factors also influence the health of women. They are exposed to physical environmental hazards both at home and in the work setting. In the home, environmental hazards include household chemicals used to clean, inhalants such as powders and sprays, and the potential for falls related to stools, stairs, and throw rugs. The effects of the workplace on women's health are covered later in this chapter during the discussion of the occupational component of the sociocultural dimension. Physical environmental dimension factors are particularly evident in rates for accidental injuries. Although women have far lower injury rates than men, significant morbidity and mortality are related to unintentional injuries in women. Another area for consideration is the reproductive effects of environmental pollutants, and the community health nurse should be alert to connections between environmental conditions and adverse pregnancy outcomes in the population.

Sociocultural Considerations

Many sociocultural dimension factors affect the health status of women. Among these are societal pressures regarding roles and relationships, occupational and economic issues, and violence and abuse.

Roles and Relationships

Women often define themselves in terms of relationships with others. Women's roles in these relationships are culturally defined by the society in which they live. Society even specifies how women should look, and women experience significant "pressure to be ornamental" (Crook, 1995). This often means that women engage in health risk behavior to attain the "perfect" image. This is exemplified in excessive dieting, cosmetic surgery, breast augmentation, and other attempts to alter one's appearance. Social expectations for thinness have also been correlated with increased smoking in women (Chesney & Nealey, 1996).

Many of women's relationships entail caregiving roles in which they have primary responsibility for the care of children, spouses, aging parents, and ill family members (Collins et al., 1999) that compound the stresses of daily life. In 1998, 22% of households with children under 18 years of age were headed by single women (U.S. Census Bureau, 1999). Overall, 9% of U.S. women care for sick or disabled family members, and two fifths of these women spend more than 20 hours per week in such care. For low-income women, the percentage of those who spend more than 20 hours a week in care of others is even higher, at 52%. These women are also half as likely as women with higher incomes to have paid help or respite care.

Women caregivers are often in poor health themselves. For example, one fourth of women caregivers in the United States describe themselves as in fair or poor health, and 54% have one or more chronic condition. More than half report symptoms of depression, and they are less likely than other women to receive health care for themselves (Collins et al., 1999).

Community health nurses should assess the effect of women clients' relationships on their health and the extent to which those relationships create additional stress. At the population level, nurses should also examine the proportion of women in the population who engage in family caregiver roles and the extent of support and respite services available to them.

Occupational and Economic Issues

Both occupational and economic issues can have direct and indirect effects on women's health. More than 13% of adult women in the United States live in poverty. Women earn less than three fourths of men's income, and the median annual income for all women is about $24,000 (National Women's Law Center et al., 2000). In 1997, more than twice as many women as men had annual incomes under $5,000 or between $5,000 and $10,000. (U.S. Census Bureau, 1999).

Lower income is frequently associated with higher incidence of disability, chronic disease, and generally poor health, and women's health status has been shown to decline as their income declines. For example, rates for diabetes and heart disease are twice as high for women with annual incomes less than $16,000 than for those with incomes over $35,000. One fourth of low-income women have disabilities severe enough to impair work or activities of daily living, three times the rate for women in higher income groups. Low-income women also experience twice the rate of anxiety and depression as higher-income women (Collins et al., 1999).

⑥THINK ABOUT IT

Why are women more likely than men to live in poverty? How does this state of affairs affect their health status?

Employment and occupation are sociocultural dimension factors that have profound effects on the health of many women. Many women in the paid labor force continue to work in traditional "women's jobs" such as nursing, teaching, the garment industry, and secretarial/clerical and service jobs. Although considered "women's work," these jobs are not without health risks. Physical risks arise from chemicals, radiation, infectious disease, noise, vibration, and repetitive movements.

As more women enter the world of "men's work" such as heavy industry, construction, mining, and factory work, they face a different set of physical hazards. Health risks arise from heavy lifting, use of dangerous machinery, and tools that were designed for larger men rather than smaller women. Minority women are at higher risk than white women for job-related injury because they often take jobs that others will not. Their economic need prevents them from saying no or quitting.

High-tech employment, once touted as safe, also entails health risks. The scrupulously clean area needed to produce a computer chip or to work with computers contains potential threats to human reproduction posed by radiofrequency or microwave radiation, video display terminal radiation, and arsine and chlorine gases. Working women today face essentially the same physical hazards as working men. They have the same risks for reproductive failure, respiratory ailments, skin disorders, and cancer. The health risks of the work setting are discussed in more detail in Chapter 24.

The psychological environment of the workplace can be as detrimental to women's health as its physical hazards. For example, studies have shown that it is not the female administrator who suffers the most from stress and depression, but women in the more traditional positions of secretary and clerk. It is postulated that stress is intensified by the lack of freedom to control one's work that secretaries and clerks experience. The "dead-end" quality of these jobs with little possibility of advancement may decrease incentive. In addition, the low salaries available for secretaries and clerks add stresses related to financial insecurity.

Another factor that contributes to stress among working women is role overload. In 1998, more than 71% of single women with families worked. Similarly, more than 6% of women held more than one job. Roughly one third of these women held two part-time jobs suggesting a lack of job-related health insurance. Another 50% held one full-time and one part-time job, and 2% held two full-time jobs. When asked about the reasons for holding several jobs, one third of all women indicated a need to meet regular household expenses. More than half (52%) of single women with families indicated the need to meet household expenses as a reason for multiple jobs (U.S. Census Bureau, 1999). In addition to the stress of holding more than one job, these women were faced with the responsibilities of parenting with less time to engage in parenting activities.

Social factors in the work environment also affect women's health. The world of work for women differs from that for men in several ways. First, more jobs are open to men than to women. In addition, those jobs that are open to women often provide unequal pay and levels of benefits compared with men in similar jobs. Finally, until a 1991 Supreme Court ruling, women were more often barred from work based on reproductive capacities than were men. Child bearing has also been blamed for women's late entry into the workforce and women's lack of training and education.

There are no uniform policies for paid medical or family leave for U.S. women despite federal mandates for such leaves, and only three states have provisions for medical or family leave beyond the federal mandate as well as paid disability leave (National Women's Law Center et al., 2000). Consequently, when a woman must have time off from work because of pregnancy or care of ill or disabled family members, she must often take it without pay.

Child care is another social environmental factor that creates problems for the working woman. Employer or community assistance with child care is practically nonexistent. Invariably, women must find quality child care on their own. If children are sick, it is usually the mother who stays home, often without pay, to care for them.

Disproportionate pay between traditional women's jobs and such "men's work" as road construction is a strong incentive for women to seek such jobs. Women who enter male-dominated jobs often feel pressure to prove they are equal to men in ability. They may not speak out against safety hazards because they do not want to appear weak or "unable to take it." Sexual harassment is another problem that may be encountered by women in the work setting. Although there are laws prohibiting such abuse, women may not complain because they need work so badly.

It is important to note that minority women must contend with a higher degree of discrimination and lack of job opportunity than white women. They are particularly subject to dead-end and hazardous jobs with low pay and few benefits. Minority women are also less likely to finish high school, more likely to become the head of a single-parent household, and more likely to have job-related illnesses than their white counterparts.

Social factors related to approaching retirement may affect the health status of the middle-aged woman. The woman who is nearing retirement needs to be aware of and plan for the financial shortfalls that are likely to occur with retirement. Leaving the workforce means living in poverty for many older people. Retirement assets are usually tied to lifetime income. Women who worked for low pay and poor benefits will have neither pensions nor full Social Security benefits. A divorced woman may draw Social Security from her ex-husband's account if they were married at least 10 years, but widows face declining incomes following the death of a spouse.

Community health nurses assess the individual woman's occupational and economic status and the effects of these factors on health. In addition, they obtain information about women's income levels, occupations, and other societal factors that may impinge on their ability to work or influence the economic and occupational effects on health for the population.

Violence and Abuse

Abuse of women is the product of many psychological and sociocultural dimension factors, and it fosters a psychological environment detrimental to women's health. Because it is primarily social and cultural conditions that allow abuse to continue, the issue is addressed here within the discussion of the sociocultural dimension. Psychological dimension factors contributing to abuse of women are also addressed. Psychological dependence on males and poor self-esteem on the part of both the victim and the abuser are some of the psychological causes resulting in abuse. Feelings of shame and worthlessness

may hamper the woman's ability to seek help while in an abusive situation. Societal attitudes toward abused women, colored by belief in some of the myths presented in Table 17–1 ■, often compound the problems of abuse for victims.

The community health nurse assesses clients for risk factors for and evidence of violence. Violence against women is a pervasive, underrecognized, and culturally condoned phenomenon in American society. Statistics indicate that 31% of women in the United States have been physically abused at some time in their lives, 3% (3 million women) in the last year (Collins et al., 1999). A significant subset of this abuse occurs during and after pregnancy. In one study, half of postpartum injury deaths were due to homicide compared to only 26% of injury deaths among nonpregnant women. This study confirmed prior findings on the incidence of homicide among postpartum women (Dietz, Rochat, Thompson, Berg, & Griffin, 1998). In 1998, the female rate of death from homicide was 3.2 per 100,000 women, a decrease

■ **TABLE 17–1 Myths and Truths About Abused Women**

MYTH	TRUTH
Battering occurs in a small percentage of the population.	An estimated 3 to 4 million women are beaten annually. Battering often goes unreported.
Violence among family members is a private matter, and it is a man's right to keep his woman in line.	Violence is not allowable in society. No one has the right to beat or rape a woman.
The abuse is not bad or the woman would leave. It is easy to leave an abusive situation.	Home is not unbearable all the time. Home offers comfort, memories, and shelter for the children. Many women are economically dependent on the abuser and have nowhere to go. The woman's culture or religion may prohibit separation or divorce. The legal system may also make it hard to leave an abusive situation. Women may fear the loss of their children or further abuse if they leave. Women endure abuse to keep the family together for the sake of the children.
Women tend to become helpless in abusive situations.	Abused women come to believe that they are worthless and that they have no one to turn to but the abuser. Health care workers perceive women as powerless and themselves as "rescuers."
Abused women are masochistic and enjoy being abused.	Abused women may feel that they deserve abuse, but they do not enjoy being abused.
Alcohol causes wife abuse.	Sober men do more damage than those who are drunk. Alcoholism is used as an excuse for abuse.
Battering is limited to minorities and the poor.	Abuse of women occurs in all socioeconomic and racial groups.
Women provoke men to beat or rape them.	Abusers and rapists lose control because of their own inadequacies, not because of the woman's behavior.
Batterers and abused women cannot change.	Batterers and abused women can be resocialized and can learn more effective ways to interact and relate to others.

CULTURAL CONSIDERATIONS

In some cultural groups, leaving a marriage for whatever reason is unacceptable to members of the culture as well as to individual women. What would you do if you encountered a woman from such a culture who was being physically or emotionally abused by her husband? Would your intervention be different if there were child abuse also taking place in the family? Why or why not?

from 4.5 per 100,000 women in 1980 (National Center for Health Statistics, 2000b).

Domestic violence such as spouse abuse is rarely a one-time event. By the time injuries are identifiable as inflicted by a batterer, a woman may have been abused for several years. If the woman does not ask for help or injuries are not discovered, battering usually increases in severity and frequency. Only four states have mandated assessment protocols, training, and screening for domestic violence and prohibit insurance companies from discriminating against victims of domestic violence (National Women's Law Center et al., 2000). Risk factors and prevention strategies for abuse of women are addressed in more detail in Chapter 32.

In assessing a potentially abused woman, the nurse needs to ask the client about depression, the possibility of suicide, and her risk of being killed by her partner. Another important consideration is the woman's willingness to leave the situation. Many women in such situations continue to hope that their partner will change or are fearful that the partner will hunt them down and further injure them if they try to leave. Another common fear is that the partner will attempt to win custody of the children if the woman leaves. Assessment at the aggregate level includes the prevalence of various forms of abuse of women as well as the presence of risk factors for abuse in the general population. Societal attitudes and responses to abuse are other important aspects of the assessment.

Behavioral Considerations

Behavioral dimension factors also affect the health of women clients. Areas of particular concern include consumption patterns, physical activity and exercise, sexual lifestyle, and attendant concerns with fertility control.

Consumption Patterns

The nurse assesses consumption patterns of the female client in the same terms as assessing any client. Specific areas for consideration include diet, smoking, and substance abuse. Dietary concerns may be particularly problematic among women, many of whom are obese or overweight or who engage in fad diets to attain or maintain a fashionably slim figure. Fad dieting is especially prevalent among adolescent females who also have high incidence rates for eating disorders such as bulimia and

anorexia nervosa. In addition to the influence of obesity and overweight on heart disease and other chronic health conditions, research indicates that overweight and obese pregnant women have a significantly greater risk for gestational diabetes mellitus, eclampsia, cesarean section, and delivery of a macrosomic child (a child with an abnormally large body) (Baeten, Bukusi, & Lambe, 2001).

Smoking is another consumption pattern that is problematic for women. Although the number of male smokers has declined rather dramatically in the last few years, the number of women who smoke has increased, leading to corresponding increases in lung cancer and heart disease among women. In addition to the increase in the number of female smokers, women are starting to smoke at younger ages and are less likely to stop smoking than men (Chesney & Nealey, 1996). The nurse assessing the individual female client obtains data about smoking, including the number of years the client has smoked and the number of cigarettes or other forms of tobacco smoked per day. Motivation to quit smoking should also be explored as part of the assessment. At the population level, the nurse would assess the extent of smoking among women in the aggregate.

Substance abuse among women is the third area of concern related to consumption patterns. Although women still tend to abuse alcohol and drugs less often than men, the incidence of such problems among females is increasing. Alcohol use is the 10th leading cause of morbidity among women worldwide (Lilly Center for Women's Health, 1998). In the United States, in 1998, 7% of adolescent girls and 21% of women 18 to 25 years of age reported binge drinking (National Center for Health Statistics, 2000b). Problems of drug and alcohol abuse are addressed in Chapter 31.

Sexual Lifestyle and Fertility Control

Assessment of women's sexual lifestyles may provide information related to potential health problems. For example, clients who are not sexually active and those who engage in exclusively homosexual activity have no need for contraceptive assistance, whereas the heterosexually active client who is not ready to have children may need such services. Information about the client's sexual activity may also suggest what form of contraception is most appropriate for those heterosexually active clients who do not wish to become pregnant. For example, the client with multiple sexual partners may prefer to use a barrier method of contraception rather than birth control pills to provide protection against sexually transmitted diseases as well as pregnancy.

Every woman from menarche to menopause has a right and responsibility to choose a method of fertility control that is effective, safe, and compatible with her lifestyle. The right to information on contraception and access to birth control agents is mandated by Title X of the Public Health Services Act and Titles V, XIV, and XX of the Social Security Act. The decision to use contraceptives reflects personal feelings about sexuality, self-concept, sense of autonomy and control, value system, relationship with the significant other, and the personal, social, and political power of women.

The ideal contraceptive method would be absolutely safe, 100% effective, easy to use, immediately reversible, free, and readily accessible to all. It would be acceptable to all religious and social groups, and its use would be independent of coitus. No single method available today meets all these criteria. In addition, there is no single method today that will meet the needs of an individual woman throughout her fertile years. The nurse should assess the need for contraception and biological and other factors that influence the need for contraceptive services. Information about various forms of contraception available to clients is presented in Table 17–2 ■.

Fertility control is particularly important for adolescents, for whom pregnancy poses greater disruption of life and potential for adverse physiological effects. Community health nurses can be especially effective in promoting contraception in this age group. In 1995, 19% of sexually active girls 15 to 19 years of age used no form of contraception (USDHHS, 2000). Community health nurses should assess the level of sexual activity among adolescent girls as well as the extent of contraceptive knowledge and use.

Another behavioral consideration related to female sexuality is the extent to which women engage in breast self-examination (BSE). All women beyond menarche should engage in monthly BSE, and community health nurses can educate women on the need and techniques for BSE. Community health nurses can also assess the degree to which BSE is emphasized in the local community by providers and lay groups. Cultural and ethnic groups may differ in their use of BSE. A summary of a research study describing differences in attitudes to and practice of BSE by African American and Caucasian nurses can be reviewed on the companion Web site for this book. ◉

Health System Considerations

Lack of attention to women's health needs, lack of illness prevention and health promotion resources, health insurance discrimination, and lack of support for the informal caregiver in the home are health care system issues that adversely affect women.

The medical system tends to focus on female reproductive problems, frequently to the exclusion of other health problems faced by women. Failure to recognize and deal with physical abuse is just one example of failure of the health care system to meet the needs of women. By and large, the health care system has only recently come to recognize the special health needs of the female client.

⑥THINK ABOUT IT

Do you think health care services provided for women are inferior to those provided to men? Why or why not?

Services provided by the health care system tend to focus on secondary and tertiary prevention of injury and disease. Few efforts are made to provide preventive health care, particularly for women. For example, in 1999 only 44% of female respondents to the National Health

Communities need health care facilities to deal with women's health problems.

■ **TABLE 17–2**   **Types of Contraception and Related Contraceptive Methods**

TYPE OF CONTRACEPTION	RELATED CONTRACEPTIVE METHODS
Abstinence	Abstinence from sexual intercourse
Barriers	Condom, diaphragm, cervical sponge, cervical cap
Fertility awareness	Basal body temperature, cervical mucous changes, position of cervix
Hormonal	Oral contraceptives, Norplant Progestasert (IUD), injections, postcoital contraception
Intrauterine device	Copper T, Progestasert, Paragard
Sterilization	Tubal ligation (female), vasectomy (male)

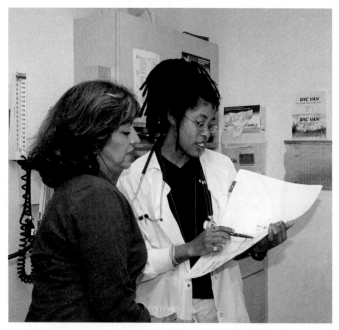

Interview Survey (NHIS) reported being counseled regarding hormone replacement therapy (Zhang, Tao, & Anderson, 1999). On a more personal level, those preventive health services that are available are not always offered at a time when busy working women can take advantage of them. Compounding this problem is the lack of provision for child care while women seek preventive health care services (Baird, 1998).

Another handicap for women is the cost of health care. Women pay almost 50% more for health care than do men (Baird, 1998). Women are also less likely than men to have employment-based health insurance, and they are more likely to work in part-time jobs or jobs that do not offer this benefit. Some insurance companies will not insure single women because of the likelihood of pregnancy and the more frequent occurrence of diagnosed disease among women than among men. Single women are also less likely to be able to pay the monthly insurance premiums. This situation is particularly hard on divorced and separated women with children who are already faced with financial difficulties. In a 1998 survey, 18% of women were either uninsured or had been uninsured for a portion of the previous year. Discontinuous insurance increases lack of access to care threefold due to the inability to develop a relationship with a consistent health care provider. Many of these women rely on emergency departments or hospital clinics for care, thereby increasing societal expenses for care (Collins et al., 1999).

Another problem for working women attributable to the health care system is the lack of support for the informal caregiver. Women may be forced to quit their jobs to care for a sick child or elderly family member but cannot expect the financial support that might be available for institution-based care of the loved one.

ⓖTHINK ABOUT IT

How can women influence the type of health care they receive?

The health care system has provided some services to deal with health problems posed by menopause. These have consisted primarily of hormone supplementation. Estrogen therapy, for example, reduces the occurrence of symptoms, reduces the rate of bone loss, and decreases cardiovascular risks, yet in 1997, only 27% of women were aware of the increased risk of osteoporosis after menopause (Lilly Center for Women's Health, 1998). Considerations in assessing health system influences on the health of women are summarized in Table 17–3 ■. A guide for assessing women's health is available on the companion Web site for this book.   ◉

■ **TABLE 17–3   Assessing Health System Influences on Women's Health**

HEALTH CONCERN	RELATED ASSESSMENT QUESTIONS
Need for secondary prevention screening	Have you ever had a Pap smear? When? What were the results?
	Have you ever had a mammogram? When? What were the results?
	When was your last eye examination? What were the results?
	Have you had an electrocardiogram? When? What were the results?
	Have you had a tuberculin skin test? When? What were the results?
	Have you had a breast examination? When? What were the results?
	Have you had recent blood tests? What were they for? What were the results?
Need for respite	Is there anyone who can relieve you so you can have a break from caring for your children (elderly parents)?
Access to health care	Do you have health insurance?
	If yes, do you know what services are covered?
	Where do you usually go for health care?
	How do you usually pay for health care?
	Are health care services provided at a time that is convenient for you?
	Do you have transportation to receive health care services?
	Are child care services needed and available while you seek health care?
	Are there any barriers that prevent you from getting the health care you need? If so, what are they?

ASSESSING LESBIAN, BISEXUAL, AND TRANSGENDER CLIENTS

Lesbians and bisexual and transgender women comprise a segment of the female population with whom the community health nurse will knowingly or unknowingly come in contact. According to various studies, an estimated 1.4% to 4.3% of U.S. women express these sexual identities. In one study of Massachusetts high school students, 3.4% of sexually active girls reported sexual activity only with other females, and 3% reported sexual activity with both males and females. Women in these subpopulations have many health needs in common with their heterosexual counterparts, but they also have unique needs that are not often known or acknowledged by health care providers.

The American Psychiatric Association recognizes that homosexuality is neither a choice nor a psychiatric disorder; it is a normal variant and an inherent part of a person's identity. Sexual orientation is not chosen; it is discovered. Being a lesbian means that a woman's primary affectional and sexual preferences are for other women. Lesbians exist in all cultures, races, religions, and classes. They cannot be identified by appearance, assumed role, or mannerisms. Lesbians are at high risk for misunderstanding and discrimination because they share the homosexual label with men, yet they have much in common with heterosexual women.

In examining lesbianism and other sexual orientations from a dimensions of health perspective, the goal is for the nurse to become better able to meet clients' needs by gaining greater understanding and insight into the similarities and differences between these subgroups and the heterosexual population. Using this knowledge, the nurse is then able to formulate a more sensitive and effective plan of care for the client.

Biophysical Considerations

There are no differences in the maturational or aging processes between lesbian, bisexual, and transgender women and heterosexual women. Sexual identity formation is a similar process of confusion, self-awareness, and acceptance, but leads to different outcomes in each group. Although it is sometimes assumed that the needs of lesbians are similar to those of gay men, their needs are actually quite different and differ as well from bisexual and transgender women. There have been no medical problems identified that are specifically attributable to being lesbian or bisexual, but there are some potential differences in risk factors that may put these women at higher risk for certain diseases.

From a gynecologic viewpoint, women who engage in sexual activity exclusively with other women seem to be at lower risk for some sexually transmitted diseases (STDs) than their heterosexual counterparts. Human papillomavirus (HPV), candidiasis, *Trichomonas vaginalis*, and bacterial vaginoses, however, are transmissible between women and occur even in lesbians who have not had sex with male partners (Silenzio & White, 2000a). Bisexual women, on the other hand, have the same risk of STDs as heterosexual women and may serve as a reservoir of disease for other women (Saunders, 1999). Complacency regarding risk for STDs should be discouraged, and lesbian and bisexual women should be as selective in their sexual partners as possible.

Although actual disease figures have not demonstrated an increased incidence of breast cancer among lesbian women (possibly because of underreporting in this largely hidden group), there is a higher prevalence of certain risk factors for breast cancer in this group (Meyer & Bowen, 2000). Nulliparity and late child bearing are both risk factors for breast cancer that are prevalent among lesbian women. Among lesbians over 40 years of age, approximately 3% develop breast cancer (Saunders, 1999).

Routine Pap smears are as important for the lesbian client as for heterosexual women. Studies have shown that lesbians have cervical dysplasia and carcinoma in situ. The incidence of these cervical disorders rises sharply in women who have had several sexual encounters with men, just as for their heterosexual counterparts. Approximately 11% of lesbians over 40 years of age develop cervical cancer (Saunders, 1999). Because lesbian women typically do not use contraceptive services (a common route to health care services for heterosexual women), they may miss opportunities for routine breast and cervical cancer screening. Similarly, lack of regular health care may minimize opportunities for routine blood pressure checks and cholesterol testing, placing lesbian women at higher risk for cardiovascular disease. Increased risk for heart disease may also lie in the fact that lesbian and bisexual women smoke more than their heterosexual sisters and tend to have a higher body mass index (Silenzio & White, 2000b).

Psychological Considerations

Psychological factors affecting lesbians are closely entwined with social factors. A woman who realizes that she has a same-sex orientation has three basic choices. She can live openly as a lesbian, thereby setting herself up for potential rejection by her family, loss of her job or professional reputation, and societal labeling and abuse. Second, she can deny her identity and put her energy into fulfilling the accepted female role. Third, she can live a lesbian life but maintain a heterosexual appearance.

The lesbian who does not live openly as a lesbian must deal, on a daily basis, with the fear that someone will discover who she really is. This involves the complex task of vigilance about how she looks and acts, where she is, who she is with, and what she says. This means that the lesbian must constantly monitor her responses and change pronouns to misrepresent the identity of her partners. She must hide from co-workers, family, or friends important life events such as a new relationship or the breakup of an old one. Although lesbian women grieve such losses, their grief is not sanctioned by society and is another source of hidden stress (Saunders, 1999). Recently, both lesbians and gays have also had to deal with increased fears of being "outed" by other, more militant homosexuals. *Outing* involves publicizing another's homosexuality without their consent (Gruskin, 1999).

An important emotional event lesbians experience is *coming out*. A lifelong process, **coming out** can be roughly defined as a woman's realization and admission to herself and to others of her same-sex orientation. Although the process of coming out usually occurs in the tumultuous years of the late teens and early twenties, it can happen at any phase in the lesbian's life. Coming out frequently encompasses critical aspects of awareness of same-sex feelings and attractions, initial lesbian encounters, participation in the lesbian subculture, labeling of self, and disclosure to significant others (Taylor, 1999). Stages of coming out have been delineated by several authors, but tend to fail to acknowledge that coming out may be more of a continuous process with no specific end point (Gruskin, 1999).

The coming out process may encompass contradictory feelings of excitement and relief at having found an inner answer to guilt, sadness, and anger about what the lesbian is losing or giving up. She must come to terms with any guilt she experiences for being different and for not fulfilling her role in the heterosexual lifestyle to which she has been socialized. She may also mourn the loss of her relationship with a husband or male lover, the fact that she may not fulfill parental expectations of a wedding and grandchildren, and that she will never be totally socially acceptable. Additionally, it has been found that many women go through the coming out process without the influence or support of the lesbian subculture, thereby adding isolation to the difficulty of the task. The coming out process may be even more difficult for lesbian women from minority cultures who already bear a certain amount of stigma due to membership in an ethnic minority group. These women may be marginalized by both the heterosexual ethnic community and the lesbian community since neither has a true picture of the difficulties they face (Solarz, 1999). Community health nurses should assess for feelings of guilt, isolation, or depression among lesbian, bisexual, and transgender women who have come or are coming to grips with their identities.

From a mental health perspective, although mental health is of concern among lesbians and bisexual women, they are no more likely to be diagnosed with psychiatric disorders than heterosexual women. Their level of social and psychological functioning is indistinguishable from that of their heterosexual counterparts. The community health nurse must be aware, however, of the medical and psychological implications of the emotional stresses that arise from the moral and social stigma attached by much of society to a lesbian, bisexual, or transgender identity. As a result of these stresses, lesbians and bisexual women may be at greater risk of mental distress, depression, substance abuse, and suicide (Meyer, Rothblum, & Bradford, 2000). Mental distress in transgender women may manifest in attempts at self-mutilation (Sember, 2000).

Some authors suggest that lesbian, bisexual, and transgender women may internalize negative social attitudes to their sexual identities, leading to greater risk of suicide. Whether or not this greater risk is an actual fact remains an area of controversy. One recent major study, the National Lesbian Health Care Survey, found no more depression in lesbians than in other women, but other studies have provided some evidence of risk (Meyer, Rothblum, & Bradford, 2000). There is some evidence, however, of greater risk of suicide in adolescent lesbians than in other adolescent girls. In one study, for example, 20.5% of lesbian high school students had made suicide attempts compared to 14.5% of heterosexual girls (Remafedi, French, Story, Resnick, & Blum, 1998). Another study reported similar findings (Faulkner & Cranston, 1999). The findings of these two studies support several prior studies indicating a greater risk for sui-

cide in young lesbians than in the general population (Meyer, Rothblum, & Bradford, 2000). This greater risk may be a result of dealing with the emotional turmoil of acknowledging a stigmatized sexual identity on top of the normal turmoil experienced in adolescence.

Sociocultural Considerations

Elements of the sociocultural dimension create problems that lesbian and bisexual women deal with on a daily basis. A woman cannot usually be a lesbian without experiencing social problems. The discrepancy between socially prescribed behaviors and sexual and affectional needs automatically sets up a conflict between the lesbian and her environment. Society tends to react to lesbianism as a personal identity rather than merely a sexual behavior. Thus, lesbians are identified in unidimensional terms. The routine conflict with the environment; homophobia; and religious, legal, familial, and economic constraints all combine to make life more difficult for the homosexual woman.

Homophobia, an irrational fear, hatred, or intolerance of homosexuals, encompasses a belief system that is believed to justify discrimination against gays and lesbians. Transgender females may be stigmatized by both the lesbian/bisexual group and by the heterosexual population (Meyer, Silenzio, Wolfe, & Dunn, 2000).

Homophobia is used to justify discrimination and abuse of homosexuals. As of 2000, only eight states had strong laws prohibiting employment discrimination based on sexual orientation (National Women's Law Center et al., 2000), and state and local laws supporting nondiscrimination are frequently overturned (Saunders, 1999). Homosexual activity is criminalized in 16 states (Meyer, Silenzio, et al., 2000), and lesbians are subjected to many forms of legal discrimination in employment, promotion, and so on (Gruskin, 1999). Lesbians are also discriminated against in terms of benefits usually granted to heterosexual marriage couples. For example, lesbians are not able to receive their partners' Social Security benefits on their deaths (White, Bradford, Silenzio, & Wolfe, 2000), nor can they file a joint tax return, claim family or bereavement leave, or inherit their partners' property (Gruskin, 1999; Solarz, 1999).

⑥THINK ABOUT IT

Should homosexual unions be legally recognized? Why or why not? What would the implications of this recognition be for the couple? For society?

In addition to legal sanctions, lesbian women risk the loss of social support due to rejection by family and friends. Loss of traditional sources of support have led to the creation of lesbian communities that offer a variety of health and social services as well as companionship and emotional support. In addition, many professional organizations have gay and lesbian interest groups and some local governments have developed special offices to address the needs of gay and lesbian populations (Sell & Wolfe, 2000). For example, the American Psychological Association (1999) has recently resolved to take a leadership role in promoting safe school environments to prevent discrimination and violence against gay and lesbian students.

Lesbian, bisexual, and transgender women are frequently subjected to verbal and physical violence. Approximately one half to one third of lesbians have reported being the object of a verbal hate crime, and 5% to 10% have been assaulted. Lesbian women, however, are no more likely than heterosexual women to have been sexually abused as children. It is estimated that only 13% to 14% of violent episodes are reported for fear of further stigmatization. In fact, 16% to 30% of lesbian, gay, bisexual, or transgender victims report victimization by police personnel (Dean & Bradford, 2000).

Lesbians may also experience violence, called *horizontal violence,* from their partners. An estimated 22% to 46% of women in same sex relationships report physical abuse by their partners, and 73% to 76% have suffered some form of abuse (Gruskin, 1999). These figures are similar to those reported by heterosexual women, and the potential for domestic violence in same-sex couples should not be ignored. Lesbian and bisexual women, as well as heterosexual women, should be assessed for evidence of abuse and the incidence and prevalence of domestic abuse in the community determined.

From a religious perspective, many Christian denominations advocate sexual activity only in the context of procreation. Most, especially fundamentalist denominations, consider homosexuality biologically unnatural, sinful, and condemned by the Bible, and religious traditions may cause a sense of shame in lesbians and bisexuals who adhere to more conservative religions (Gruskin, 1999). In a recent study, the majority of Americans still considered homosexuality to be immoral (Meyer, Silenzio, et al., 2000). Community health nurses should be sensitive to any feelings of guilt, abandonment, or anger or suicidal tendencies experienced by lesbian, bisexual, or transgender clients as a result of attitudes and values of the religious denominations to which they may belong. Coming out to family members may be particularly difficult in the context of a conservative religious background (Gruskin, 1999).

Many women realize and act on their same-sex preferences after they are married and have children; others choose to have children after coming out. It is estimated that there may be 1 to 5 million lesbians raising 6 to 14 million children. Research consistently indicates no negative outcomes for these children, in particular that children of lesbians are no more likely than other children to be gay or lesbian. In spite of these findings, courts may deny custody of children to a lesbian parent purely on the basis of her lesbianism (Scout, 2000).

Lesbian parents also face other potential legal difficulties related to their families. Some states prohibit adoption by gay or lesbian couples. Some lesbian women may choose artificial insemination in order to become pregnant. Because lesbians may be denied service by traditional sperm banks, they may enter into dubious agreements with known donors that may not be supported later in a court of law (Scout, 2000). Similarly, if the biological parent should die, the partner may have difficulty retaining custody of children unless guardianship has been legally specified (Gruskin, 1999). Community health nurses can explore with lesbian mothers the use and availability of legal safeguards.

Economically, lesbians usually earn lower wages than men or their heterosexual female counterparts despite higher educational levels (White, Bradford, Silenzio, & Wolfe, 2000). Those with children from a prior marriage have particularly little disposable income or time to engage in social activities. Also, because homosexuality is such a taboo subject, women in general are socialized to have a negative view of homosexuality. Although there are now several prominent public lesbian role models, many lesbians still have a very negative self-image.

For the majority of lesbians, disclosure of sexual preference in the work setting could lead to being passed over for promotion, subtle or overt harassment, or termination, particularly if they work with children or young women. As was mentioned under psychological factors, the ever-present fear of discovery adds immeasurable anxiety and tension to the inherent stress of work. Nevertheless, the economic and occupational achievements of lesbians are similar to those of their heterosexual counterparts.

Behavioral Considerations

Research suggests that lesbians have higher rates of smoking than heterosexual women, and young lesbians have been shown to smoke more than young gay males (Silenzio & White, 2000b). The lesbian subpopulation has been shown to have a higher rate of heavy smokers and fewer nonsmokers than among heterosexual women (Solarz, 1999).

Although lesbianism does not cause alcohol or substance abuse, there is a perception among researchers, clinicians, and lesbians themselves that such problems may be more prevalent and severe among lesbians than in the general population. In part, this is the result of earlier studies conducted on samples solicited in lesbian bars yielding biased samples. Among more recent studies, some researchers have found rates of alcohol and drug use comparable to those of heterosexual women and some have found higher rates (Silenzio, White, & Wolfe, 2000). There is some evidence, however, that younger lesbians have somewhat higher rates of tobacco, marijuana, and cocaine use than their heterosexual counterparts (Faulkner & Cranston, 1998; Silenzio, White, &

CRITICAL THINKING IN RESEARCH

James and Platzer (1999) presented several ethical considerations in conducting research with marginalized groups such as women with nonheterosexual orientations. These include issues of vulnerability, balancing researcher versus clinician roles, and the possibility of adding to negative stereotypes. Several of these issues are compounded when the researchers are members of the group studied. Marginalized groups may be vulnerable to bias and damage due to researchers' lack of familiarity with the culture and high levels of unmet needs. Confidentiality issues are particularly relevant when the group is characterized by social stigma. In addition, research with marginalized groups is frequently poorly funded limiting the availability of support counseling when participation in the research causes adverse psychological effects. Researchers who are themselves members of the marginalized group create a potential for bias and also face the ethical dilemma of possibly adding to negative stereotypes of the group if unfavorable findings are discovered (e.g., if research should indicate that children of lesbian parents have higher rates of attempted suicide than other children—which is *not* the case).

- To what extent do you think these ethical issues apply to research with women in general as well as to research with lesbians or bisexual or transgender women?
- What actions might researchers take to minimize potentially harmful effects of these ethical issues?
- How should researchers address the issue of maintaining the rigor of the research study in the face of identified clinical needs of subjects?

Wolfe, 2000). Bisexual women have been found, in some studies, to have higher rates of drug use, greater numbers of sexual partners, and more partners who have sex with prostitutes than strictly heterosexual women, suggesting that female bisexuality may be a marker for a variety of high-risk behaviors (Gonzales, Washienko, Krone, & Chapman, 1999).

Community health nurses can assist lesbian, bisexual, and transgender women clients by being alert to cues that would indicate patterns of substance abuse, by not assuming that the alcoholism is related to sexual preference, by respecting their reluctance to enter traditional treatment programs that are not designed to meet their needs, by being familiar with resources in the community to assist those women with substance abuse issues, and by involving their significant others in the treatment plan.

Some women who self-identify as lesbians may engage in high-risk sexual behaviors, for instance having unprotected sexual intercourse with injection drug users (Gruskin, 1999). It is estimated that 21% to 30% of self-identified lesbians continue to have male sexual partners, increasing their risk for STDs (Solarz, 1999).

Health System Considerations

Although women's health care concerns have, in general, tended to be ignored in the health care system, this propensity tends to be heightened when the woman is of color; a rape victim; addicted to drugs or alcohol; a lesbian, bisexual, or transgender female; or otherwise stigmatized. Three general types of barriers to health care for lesbian women have been identified: structural barriers, financial barriers, and personal and cultural barriers. Structural barriers relate to the availability and organization of health care services. For example, the short office visits mandated by managed care plans may limit the ability of lesbian and bisexual clients to develop the rapport with their providers required for optimal care. Similarly, lack of family insurance coverage may limit abilities for lesbian families to be cared for as a unit by providers who are familiar with the entire family. Finally, there is a systematic lack of recognition of the rights of partners in decision making, visiting, and so on (Solarz, 1999).

Financial barriers relate primarily to the lack of insurance coverage among lesbians. Because of their lack of legal status as a married couple, lesbian partners usually do not have access to spousal insurance benefits, and lesbian women are less likely than heterosexual women to be insured. Surveys of lesbians indicate that 12% to 27% of this population may be uninsured. In the National Lesbian Health Care Survey, 16% of lesbians indicated that they did not receive needed care because of costs (Solarz, 1999). Even for those with health insurance, many may not choose to seek care for fear of breach of confidentiality. This is particularly true of lesbians who are insured under an employer's self-insurance plan in which employers have access to employees' health records (White, Bradford, Silenzio, & Wolfe, 2000).

A variety of personal and cultural barriers also inhibit effective care for lesbian, bisexual, and transgender clients. Health care for women arises out of heterosexual assumptions and, as noted earlier, contraceptive needs are often a mode of entry for women into the health care system. Because they typically do not have contraceptive needs, lesbian clients may miss opportunities for preventive health and screening services readily available to other women (Ellerman, 1999). Lesbian and bisexual clients may also not seek care because of negative provider attitudes or fears of violation of confidentiality. For example, 40% of physicians in one study sometimes or often felt uncomfortable dealing with lesbian, gay, bisexual, or transgender clients, and many providers lack knowledge of the health needs of these populations. In some studies, 9% of lesbians reported that their partners were not allowed to accompany them to examinations and are not included in treatment discussions. Some gay and lesbian clients also reported rough or violent digital examinations after disclosure of their sexual orientation (White, Bradford, & Silenzio, 2000). In other studies, 6% of Canadian dentists were not willing to care for homosexual clients (McCarthy, Koval, & MacDonald, 1999), and beginning nursing students have been found less willing and less comfortable caring for sexual minorities than ethnic minorities. These findings were particularly prevalent among students from conservative religious backgrounds (Eliason, 1998). A few health care providers may even continue to advocate for reparative therapy. *Reparative therapy* is therapy designed to reverse a same sex orientation (Meyer, Silenzio, et al., 2000).

Counseling and preventive services often assume a heterosexual orientation, and intake forms and interview questions may make it difficult to alert providers to nonheterosexual orientations. Approximately 27% of lesbians in some studies have reported that their providers assumed that they were heterosexual, while 11% describe contraceptives being "forced" on them (Scout, 2000). Conversely, providers may fail to give counseling in areas where lesbian clients may be at higher risk (e.g., breast cancer risk factors) or to take these factors into account when making treatment decisions (Gruskin, 1999).

In order for effective care to occur, providers need to be aware of and knowledgeable regarding clients' sexual orientations, but the design of the health care system makes disclosure difficult and places the burden of disclosure on lesbian, bisexual, and transgender clients. Authors have described a two-phase decision process of disclosure of sexual orientation to health care providers. The first phase is the anticipatory phase in which the client assesses the risk of adverse effects of disclosure both imaginatively and cognitively. The second phase is the interactional phase in which the client begins preliminary disclosure, but closely monitors the provider's response and halts disclosure if it begins to seem dangerous (Taylor, 1999).

There are several suggestions that could be of value to community health nurses assessing lesbian, bisexual, and transgender clients. First, nurses need to examine their own attitudes toward sexuality and homosexuality. Although it is not necessary to sanction homosexual behavior, it is not ethical to discriminate against or deny the lesbian, bisexual, or transgender client supportive professional care that will assist in strengthening her self-esteem and realizing optimal wellness. As one observer has noted, "passing moral judgments is not a nursing function: such judgments can only impede the ability to give quality care" (Lawrence, 1975). If the nurse is unable to provide such care, the client should be referred to another provider.

Further suggestions are to refrain from recording a client's sexual preference on the record without her approval, to provide an atmosphere of openness and tolerance, and, most importantly, to involve the partner or designated other in the plan of care. Another problem arises when the practitioner automatically assumes the

client is heterosexual. Assessment questions can be less alienating if differently phrased. Nongender-type nouns such as *lover* and *partner* can be used. "Are you sexually active?" and "Do you use contraceptives?" are more appropriate than "When was the last time you had intercourse?" or "What kind of birth control are you using?" A question such as "Who would you like contacted in an emergency?" can also go a long way toward helping the lesbian, bisexual, or transgender client feel more comfortable. Other simple suggestions include providing nonheterosexually oriented publications and referral literature in waiting rooms, and developing educational literature that is culturally sensitive for these population groups. Tips for assessing the health of heterosexual and lesbian or transgender women are presented on page 404.

DIAGNOSTIC REASONING AND CARE OF WOMEN

Based on information obtained during assessment, community health nurses develop nursing diagnoses that direct further interventions. These diagnoses reflect both positive health states and potential or existing health problems and the factors contributing to them. Nursing diagnoses might relate to health problems experienced by an individual woman such as "role overload due to employment, single parenthood, and lack of a social support network." Or diagnoses may be made at the aggregate level regarding the health needs of groups of women. An example of a nursing diagnosis at this level might be a "need for adequate and inexpensive child care due to the number of single-parent working women and a lack of affordable child care."

PLANNING AND IMPLEMENTING HEALTH CARE FOR WOMEN

In planning to meet the identified health needs of female clients, community health nurses incorporate the general principles of planning discussed in Chapter 15. It is important to keep in mind the unique needs of female clients. Participation by clients in planning for health care is particularly important in view of the passive and dependent role expected of female clients by health care providers of the past. Women need to be encouraged to be active participants in health care decision making. Both community health nurses and their female clients may need additional resources in dealing with women's identified health care needs. Links to potential resources are provided on the companion Web site for this book.

Planning and implementing care for groups of women also need to be based on women's unique circumstances. Services should be offered at times when women, especially working women, can take advantage of them. Provision for transportation and child care services during

assessment tips assessment tips assessment tips

ASSESSING WOMEN'S HEALTH

Biophysical Considerations

- What is the woman's age? Has she experienced menarche? Menopause? Is she knowledgeable about these developmental stages and their physical and psychological effects? Is she experiencing any difficulties with menarche or menopause?
- Is the woman pregnant? Is she experiencing problems with the pregnancy? Fertility problems?
- Does the woman have any existing physical health problems or physical limitations?

Psychological Considerations

- What is the level of stress to which the woman is exposed? How effective are her coping strategies?
- Does the woman have a history of mental illness? Are there indications of current mental illness? Is she depressed or suicidal?
- What is the woman's attitude toward sexuality? Toward childbearing? Toward menopause? How does the woman define her sexual identity? What is her level of satisfaction with sexuality and her sexual orientation?
- Has the woman been subjected to female genital mutilation?

Physical Environmental Considerations

- Where does the woman live? Are there safety hazards in the woman's environment? Is the woman exposed to environmental health hazards?

Sociocultural Considerations

- What roles does the woman play? Is she satisfied with the roles she plays?
- Is the woman involved in an intimate relationship? Is the relationship satisfactory from her perspective?
- What is the extent of the woman's social support network? Is it adequate to her need for support?
- To whom has the lesbian, bisexual, or transgender client disclosed her sexual orientation? Has disclosure resulted in rejection or loss of significant relationships or social support?
- Does the woman have opportunities for social interaction with other adults?

- Is the woman responsible for the care of children or other family members? What effect does this responsibility have on her health? Is she supported in the caretaker role?
- Is the woman employed? If so, what is her occupation? Are there occupational health hazards present in her work setting? How does she balance work and home responsibilities? Have child care needs been adequately met?
- What is the woman's education level and income?
- Is the woman at risk for abuse? If so, what risk factors for abuse are present? Is there evidence of current abuse? What action has the woman attempted, if any? What barriers to action are present in the situation? What is the woman's attitude to abuse?

Behavioral Considerations

- What are the woman's usual food preferences and consumption patterns?
- What is the woman's sexual orientation? Is she comfortable with this orientation?
- Does the woman engage in unsafe sexual practices? If the woman is sexually active, is there a need for contraceptive services?
- Does the woman engage in monthly breast self-examination?
- Does the woman engage in appropriate safety practices (e.g., seat belt use)?

Health System Considerations

- What is the woman's usual source of health care? How does the woman finance health care? Does the woman receive routine screening measures? If the woman is pregnant, has she obtained prenatal care? Are there barriers to obtaining health care (e.g., language, lack of child care or transportation)?
- What is the reaction of health care providers to the lesbian, bisexual, or transgender client? Has the client encountered provider hostility or discrimination? Has she disclosed her sexual orientation to providers?

appointments might also need to be considered. Financing of such programs can be problematic, given the lower earning capacity of many women, and political activity to ensure program funding may need to be part of the planning process. Planning to meet the health needs of female clients may involve developing primary, secondary, or tertiary preventive interventions.

Primary Prevention

Four goals for women's wellness direct primary preventive interventions for women. These goals are as follows:

1. Maintaining balance, perspective, and priorities in life
2. Developing and maintaining healthy relationships

3. Developing and maintaining a healthy sense of self
4. Developing and maintaining a physically healthy body and preventing acute and chronic illness (Olshansky, 2000).

Primary preventive measures related to each of the goals will be briefly discussed.

Maintaining Balance, Perspective, and Priorities

Women may need assistance with a variety of conditions in their lives to help them achieve the first goal of wellness. For example, they may need referrals to existing social service programs to permit them to achieve economic balance. Similarly, they may need help in balancing multiple roles. Intervention in this area may be particularly important for single women with children who may be fulfilling both parental roles as well as the breadwinner role. Women caretakers may also need help in learning to balance personal needs with those of other family members or may need respite from continual demands on their time and energy.

For lesbian, bisexual, and transgender women, the aspects of life to be balanced may be even more complex, and community health nurses can assist them to find resources that help them to achieve the desired level of balance. For example, referrals may be needed to address legal problems of child custody or inclusion of partners in health-related decisions (e.g., drafting of a durable power of attorney).

There may also be a need to assist women to achieve balance in the work setting. The psychosocial environment of the work setting may need to be changed by means of several strategies. These strategies include educating and socializing women to expect wage equity and to believe that their work is as important as a man's; promoting legislation to prevent job discrimination; educating women about their rights; and encouraging women to challenge sexual harassment. Additional strategies include supporting women running for political office, influencing the legislative process, and promoting collective bargaining, mentoring, and networking among women. A final strategy is active participation in organizations working for changes to benefit women.

The community health nurse working in the occupational setting can provide primary preventive care for women by identifying and understanding stressors affecting women in the work setting, counseling regarding work options, encouraging women to report safety hazards (or the nurse can report them personally), encouraging organization of women in the work setting, fostering personal preventive measures such as the use of protective devices, and keeping a log of jobs and exposure to hazardous materials and health changes. Another major contribution can be made by community health nurses who have clients experiencing role proliferation. These nurses can assist clients to plan efficient use of time, to use outside help when possible, and to let go of minor household duties that can wait. Single parents particularly need help in this area.

Primary prevention for female clients also involves assistance in the development of coping skills and assertiveness. Interventions can be designed to improve women's self-esteem and to teach them how to cope with life stress in effective ways. These kinds of interventions may be particularly important for lesbian, bisexual, and transgender women who are subjected to multiple stressors.

Developing and Maintaining Healthy Relationships

Development of coping skills and self-esteem not only assists women in maintaining balance in their lives, but also assists in the development of healthy relationships. Another critical intervention in this area is prevention of domestic abuse. Community health nurses can assist in the development of societal conditions that prohibit abuse (e.g., strong sanctions for abusers, assistance for women at risk for abuse, etc.). Primary prevention of abuse is addressed in more detail in Chapter 32.

Developing and Maintaining a Sense of Self

Interventions in this area are important for all women, but may be particularly critical for lesbians, bisexual, and transgender women who are experiencing the coming out process or who are experiencing guilt over their sexual orientation. Abused women may also need to develop a strong sense of self to avoid blaming themselves for the abuse. Community health nurses can be active in the development of societal attitudes that value women and that promote economic and social status of women.

Young girls approaching menarche, women experiencing perimenopause and menopause, and infertile women may also be in particular need of interventions to assist them to develop or maintain strong self-images. Working women who are entering retirement or mothers who are experiencing the departure of children from the home may need help coming to grips with changes in their roles without feeling devalued or useless. Similarly, women who have decided to leave an abusive situation or obtain a divorce may need assistance in dealing with feelings of guilt, loss, and depression. Community health nurses can provide anticipatory guidance regarding all of these changes and assist women to work through them effectively without diminished self-esteem. In addition, nurses can provide assistance with the practical aspects of change (e.g., menstrual education, referral for hormone replacement therapy [HRT], financial assistance, etc.).

Developing a Physically Healthy Body and Preventing Illness

A number of primary preventive interventions center on promotion of physical health and prevention of illness. General measures for promoting health in women are similar to those for all clients and include adequate nutrition, rest and exercise, immunization, and abstinence from unhealthy behaviors such as tobacco, alcohol, and drug use. Attention should also be given to healthy behaviors such as the use of seat belts and other safety devices and use of preventive health services (including contraceptive services as needed). With respect to physical activity, women should also be educated regarding prevention of exercise-related musculoskeletal injury and encouraged to be realistic in goal setting and injury prevention (Gilchrist, Jones, Sleet, & Kimsey, 2000).

One of several health promotion strategies specific to women is provision of prenatal care. While some progress has been made in this area (only 1% of pregnant U.S. women in 1997 failed to receive any prenatal care at all), 17% of women delayed obtaining prenatal care beyond the first trimester of pregnancy (National Center for Health Statistics, 2000a). Reasons given for delaying receipt of care were lack of awareness of being pregnant, inability to afford care, and inability to get an appointment. Community health nurses can assist in early case finding of pregnant women and referral for services. In addition, they can advocate access to prenatal care services for all segments of the population.

For those women who do not wish to become pregnant, community health nurses can provide information about contraceptive options and make referrals for contraceptive services. At the aggregate level, community health nurses may need to advocate for the availability of such services, particularly for adolescents or low-income women.

Health promotion is also needed by women in the perimenopausal and postmenopausal years. These women should be educated regarding the need for hormone replacement and weight-bearing exercise to prevent osteoporosis and limit the risk of heart disease. There is also some preliminary evidence that HRT may be effective in preventing Alzheimer's disease in women (Goldsmith & Shelby, 1999). Education regarding calcium and vitamin D supplementation is also needed.

Communicable disease prevention entails such interventions as immunization and safe sex activities. Tetanus–diphtheria immunization is recommended at 10-year intervals for all adults including women (Briss et al., 1999), and women of child-bearing age who are not immune to rubella should receive one dose of measles, mumps, and rubella (MMR) vaccine. Similarly, women who do not have documented immunity to chickenpox should receive varicella vaccine. Other immunizations recommended, particularly for elderly women or those with chronic diseases, include annual influenza vaccination and one dose of pneumococcal vaccine (USDHHS, 1998a). Standing orders for nurses and pharmacists to give immunizations as needed and provision of immunizations in pharmacies, community centers, workplaces, churches, and so on can enhance the immunization status of women as well as other groups (McKibben et al., 2000; Postema & Breiman, 2000). Community health nurses may be involved in giving immunizations, making referrals to immunization sources, or assuring the availability of immunization services to women clients.

Education on barrier contraceptive methods should be given to sexually active women who are not in exclusive monogamous relationships for both partners. This is a need for all women, whether heterosexual, lesbian, bisexual, or transgender, who are at risk for STDs. Emphases in primary prevention interventions for women's health are summarized below.

HIGHLIGHTS

Primary Prevention Emphases in the Care of Women

Maintaining Balance, Perspective, and Priorities
- Maintaining economic balance
- Balancing multiple roles
- Balancing personal needs and care taking responsibilities
- Coming to grips with one's sexual orientation
- Balancing work and family responsibilities
- Balancing work and life stress
- Developing coping and assertiveness skills

Maintaining Healthy Relationships
- Preventing domestic violence

Maintaining a Sense of Self
- Developing and maintaining one's self-identity
- Anticipatory guidance for role changes

Maintaining Physical Health and Preventing Illness
- Obtaining adequate nutrition
- Obtaining adequate rest and exercise and preventing injury
- Immunization
- Abstaining from unhealthy behaviors (e.g., smoking, alcohol and drug use)
- Using safety precautions
- Obtaining prenatal care
- Preventing osteoporosis (with HRT, exercise, diet, etc.)
- Practicing safe sex

Secondary Prevention

Secondary prevention focuses on screening and diagnosis and treatment for existing health problems.

Screening

Routine screening procedures specifically recommended for women are summarized on page 407. Women should, of course, also be screened for other health problems that occur among both men and women, such as hypertension, diabetes, and skin cancers, and so on.

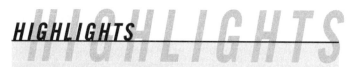

HIGHLIGHTS

Recommended Routine Screening Procedures for Women

- Blood pressure, height, weight, dental, alcohol use: periodically, age 18 to 75 years
- Papanicolaou test: every 1 to 3 years, age 18 to 75 years
- Cholesterol: every 5 years, age 45 to 65 years
- Mammogram: every 1 to 2 years, age 50 to 70 years
- Sigmoidoscopy: every 5 to 10 years age 50 to 75 years *or*
- Fecal occult blood: yearly, age 50 to 75 years
- Vision, hearing: periodically, age 65 to 75 years
- Gestational diabetes mellitus (GDM): first prenatal visit for women with risk factors (previous history of GDM, obesity, glycosuria, family history of diabetes, age over 25 years, prior poor obstetrical outcome, membership in a high-risk ethnic group, or medications that affect euglycemia) or at 24 to 28 weeks for all other pregnant women

Sources: Regional Perinatal System. (2000). Gestational diabetes mellitus: Screening and diagnosis. *Crib Sheet, 12*(4), 2; and U.S. Department of Health and Human Services. (1998). Clinical preventive services for normal-risk adults. *Prevention Report, 13*(1), 11.

Community health nurses can be particularly effective in educating women on the need and procedure for regular breast self-examination (BSE). The nurse can demonstrate the techniques involved in BSE and recommend that women examine their breasts monthly about one week after their menstrual period or, in the case of postmenopausal women, on the same day of each month. Nurses can also recommend periodic mammography and Pap smears for detection of breast and cervical cancers, respectively. Community health nurses may also refer clients to agencies that provide such services as well as educate them on the need for screening. Women of child-bearing age should also be screened for rubella immunity. Interventions at the population level may involve advocating for available screening and education services for women.

Women at risk for STDs should be screened periodically for gonorrhea, syphilis, and HIV infection. Women in high-risk groups include those with multiple sexual partners, injection drug users, and those who have sexual contact with drug users or bisexual men. Pregnant women in these high-risk groups should be particularly encouraged to undergo screening for STDs. This subject is discussed in more detail in Chapter 28.

Community health nurses may also be involved in case management for women whose screening tests are positive. These women may need assistance in accessing further diagnostic and treatment services (Lawson et al., 2000). At the aggregate level, community health nurses may need to be active in efforts to assure the availability and accessibility of screening, diagnostic, and treatment services for these women.

Diagnosing and Treating Existing Problems

Community health nurses refer female clients for medical or social assistance with any identified health problems. Problems unique to female clients for which secondary prevention may be required include infertility, fertility control, menopause, and physical abuse.

Treatment for infertility generally requires referral to a fertility specialist. The role of the community health nurse with respect to infertility focuses on case finding, referral, and support during a fertility workup. The nurse can also assist the client and her significant other in considering alternative options such as adoption, artificial insemination, and in vitro fertilization. The nurse may also refer couples to self-help groups for assistance in dealing with psychological problems of infertility.

Helping women who are having difficulty using a contraceptive method is another aspect of nursing care at the level of secondary prevention. Some women discover that they cannot use the method they have chosen and just stop using it. This can lead to unwanted pregnancy. The nurse can counsel, teach, and refer as needed to help each woman or couple find the best way to control fertility or to plan for children. Occasionally, secondary prevention in this area may entail presenting the client with options for dealing with the problem of an unintended pregnancy.

During perimenopause, referral to a physician or nurse practitioner for estrogen replacement therapy can take place if the client expresses discomfort related to hot flashes or has risk factors predisposing her to osteoporosis. If the client decides to be evaluated for estrogen replacement therapy, the nurse should describe what to expect during the initial visit. Generally, this visit entails a complete history and physical and several laboratory tests including a fasting blood glucose, complete blood count, blood lipids, liver function tests, and Pap smear. Some physicians also do an endometrial biopsy to determine the potential for endometrial cancer. This procedure is painful for the client and should be discussed by the nurse to alleviate fear and to assist the client to cope with the procedure.

Menopause may cause vaginal dryness and discomfort during sexual intercourse. The nurse can counsel women concerning longer foreplay and the use of vaginal lubricants to relieve the problem.

Some women also experience a decreased sexual desire. The community health nurse can help clients explore contributing factors in this experience such as depression, a feeling of being at the end of the reproductive years, and acceptance of a new phase of life. Self-help groups for women who are having similar problems are extremely beneficial during this stage of life. If there is no such group in the local community, the nurse might start one by inviting clients to meet and begin discussions.

Secondary prevention related to physical abuse of women has two dimensions. The first of these is dealing with the physical and psychological effects of physical abuse, and the second is dealing with the source of the problem itself. Recognizing the problem is a prerequisite to either dimension of treatment. Female clients should be asked in a caring and sensitive manner about any violence in their lives. Careful recording of the history and of information regarding old and new injuries is important in the diagnosis of abuse. Such a record may reveal a pattern the woman is unwilling or unable to admit to the nurse. If there is evidence of abuse, it is unethical for the nurse not to confirm this diagnosis with the client. Allowing the woman to describe what is happening to her through open-ended questions is therapeutic and can serve as the first step in stemming the cycle of abuse.

It is important that the nurse convey to the client that she does not deserve to be abused and that the nurse is concerned about her. These critical statements are needed to reveal to the client that someone cares and that she is not worthless, helpless, or deserving of abuse.

It is not easy for a community health nurse to intervene in an abusive relationship. Inherent in such situations are reasons to fear that intervention will not be successful, that the woman may become depressed and suicidal or resent the nurse for interfering in a private family matter, or that the male abuser may punish the woman or the nurse. Such fears have kept health care professionals from pursuing evidence and attempting to help women in abusive situations.

When the nurse is able to work through and conquer personal fear and is able to identify a client in an abusive relationship, the nurse should encourage the client to discuss the circumstances of her abuse. It is important that the client realize the danger inherent in her situation.

Once the diagnosis of abuse is made, the primary goal is to assist the woman to reestablish a feeling of control and to empower her to change the situation. Supportive counseling and reassurance are essential. The nurse should let the woman work out her problems at her own pace. Each woman has the capacity to change when she is ready. The nurse must realize that the victim will feel ambivalence in the relationship she has with her partner. The nurse should support realistic ideas for change and assist the client in altering unrealistic ideas. The nurse should help the client to clarify her beliefs about the situation. The nurse should also help to identify myths about abuse that the client may have internalized. For example, if the victim believes that she deserves the beatings, the nurse can assure the client that her partner is totally responsible for his or her own actions.

The nurse can help the client explore alternative plans for solutions to her problem. What are her personal supports? Is there anyone to whom she can go for help? The client may want to go home. If the client can do this without risk of suicide or homicide, the nurse should help her plan strategies for managing at home and provide her with resources for assistance or escape should the need arise. If necessary, however, the community health nurse can also help the woman to plan a quick getaway. The client needs to accumulate extra money, collect necessary documents like birth certificates and immunization records for children, pack a change of clothing, and carry a few emergency supplies. If the client has children, she should take them with her if she leaves or risk losing them to the abuser if he or she should claim that the client abandoned them.

It is important to remember that the nurse should avoid becoming another controller in the life of the client. The physically abused woman needs every opportunity to develop independence. Nurses tend to want to rescue victims to stop the violence. They cannot make decisions for the woman. Although nurses can provide information on shelters and other resources, they must allow the woman to make her own decisions.

Nurses should be familiar with the resources they recommend. Are they reliable? Will they assist the woman to become independent while providing a safe haven for her and her children? If the client is a lesbian, bisexual, or transgender woman, will her needs be effectively met in the shelter? Or will she be subjected to hostility and further abuse?

Community health nurses can also provide assistance in referrals for medical care for injuries and for counseling to deal with contributing factors and psychological effects of abuse. Such services may be needed for children as well as the woman. The woman should also be cautioned that her children may resist being removed from their home and other family members. If this should be the case, the community health nurse can help the client cope with grief and hostility on the part of the children. The client may also need help in dealing with her own grief over the loss of a significant relationship.

When adequate treatment facilities to meet the secondary prevention needs of women are not available, community health nurses can become actively involved in advocating for these services and in developing and implementing them. Community health nurses may also need to advocate for the availability of services for certain specific segments of the population, for example, low-income women or lesbian women.

Tertiary Prevention

As with all clients, tertiary prevention in the care of women focuses on rehabilitation and preventing the recurrence of health problems. Areas in which tertiary prevention are particularly warranted for the female client include pregnancy, abuse, and STDs. Tertiary prevention may also be needed to deal with some of the effects of menopause.

Tertiary prevention with respect to pregnancy involves the use of an effective contraceptive to prevent subsequent pregnancies. Again, the nurse may be involved in education, counseling, and referral for contraceptive services.

In the case of abuse, tertiary prevention necessitates the rebuilding of the woman's life and that of her family. This may involve developing new financial resources as well as ways of coping with problems. The woman needs to become self-sufficient. Again, referrals to a variety of agencies to help with employment skills and to provide counseling may be of assistance.

Women can also be helped to prevent recurrence of STDs or to cope with the life changes necessitated by a diagnosis of AIDS. Tertiary prevention related to STDs is discussed more fully in Chapter 28. Other tertiary prevention measures may be warranted for existing chronic health problems. Tertiary prevention for chronic physical and mental health conditions are addressed in Chapters 29 and 30.

EVALUATING HEALTH CARE FOR WOMEN

Health care provided to women should be evaluated using the evaluative process described in Chapter 15. Once more, it is important to evaluate both the quality of the care given and its outcomes. Because of the dependent role of many women, it is particularly important that they play an active role in evaluating the health care they are given. At the national level, the year 2010 objectives for the health of women can provide criteria for evaluating women's health care services. Evaluative information on selected national objectives related to women's health are presented below.

Women's health care needs are many and varied and are often poorly addressed by existing health care systems. Community health nurses may provide health care for women at all three levels of prevention: primary, secondary, and tertiary. Care may also be provided to individual women or to groups of women within the population, and often involves advocacy for services to meet women's needs.

HEALTHY PEOPLE 2010

GOALS FOR THE POPULATION

Objective	Base	Target
1-1 Increase the proportion of women with health insurance	87%	100%
2-9 Reduce the number of cases of osteoporosis	10%	8%
3-2 Reduce lung cancer deaths per 100,000 women	41.4	44.8
3-3 Reduce breast cancer deaths per 100,000 women	27.7	22.2
3-4 Reduce cervical cancer deaths per 100,000 women	3.0	2.0
9-1 Increase the proportion of pregnancies that are intended	51%	70%
9-3 Increase contraceptive use among those who do not desire pregnancy	93%	100%
9-10 Increase the proportion of sexually active adolescent girls who use effective barrier contraception	68%	75%
15-34 Reduce the rate of physical assault by intimate partners per 1,000 women	7.6	3.6
16-4 Reduce maternal deaths per 100,000 live births	8.4	3.3
16-5 Reduce pregnancy complications per 100 deliveries	32.1	20
22-1 Reduce the proportion of women with no leisure-time physical activity	43%	20%
24-1 Reduce asthma deaths per million women 35 to 64 years of age	23.5	9

Source: U.S. Department of Health and Human Services. (2000). *Healthy people 2010* (Conference edition, in two volumes). Washington, DC: Author.

APPLYING YOUR KNOWLEDGE IN PRACTICE

❧ CASE STUDY
Meeting a Woman's Health Needs

Susan is 25 years old, married, and the mother of two girls. She is pregnant for the third time. You have scheduled a home visit with her following a referral from the community clinic where she is receiving prenatal care. According to the referring agency, Susan does not always keep her appointments, and the baby is small for gestational age. The prenatal clinic requests that you teach nutrition and encourage her to keep her appointments.

When you arrive at the home, Susan is reluctant to allow you inside. She turns her face away and does not look at you as she answers your questions. Because you know that every woman has the potential for being a victim of physical abuse, you ask Susan if someone has hurt her. In a nonthreatening, caring, and sensitive manner you say, "I see many women in my practice who are in a relationship with a person who hits or abuses them. Did someone hurt you?" Susan begins to cry and says, "My husband hit me last night." She allows you to come in, and you observe that she has a black eye and a swollen jaw. Her two small children are thin and poorly clothed. The house, though neat, is sparsely furnished.

In speaking with Susan, you find out that her husband works in a local factory and has been denied a promotion and a raise in the last week. He seems to blame Susan for becoming pregnant again and causing more financial worries. Susan tells you that she has been missing appointments at the prenatal clinic because of her black eye and the lack of transportation when her husband is at work.

- What are the biophysical, psychological, sociocultural, behavioral, and health system factors operating in this situation?
- What are your nursing diagnoses in this situation?
- How would you address the two aspects of secondary prevention of physical abuse of women in this case?
- What other secondary preventive measures seem to be warranted in this situation?
- What primary and tertiary preventive interventions might be appropriate in working with Susan?
- How will you evaluate whether intervention has been successful?

❧ TESTING YOUR UNDERSTANDING

- What are the major human biophysical, psychological, sociocultural, behavioral, and health system factors that influence the health status of women? (pp. 388–398)
- What are some of the health problems common to women? Which of these problems also affect men's health status? How do these common problems differ between men and women? (pp. 389–391)
- What are some of the considerations that are unique in assessing the health needs of lesbian, bisexual, and transgender clients? (pp. 398–403)
- What are the major concerns in primary prevention for women? (pp. 404–406)

- Describe areas for consideration in secondary preventive activities in the care of women. Give examples of nursing interventions in each of these areas. (pp. 406–408)
- What are the two aspects of secondary prevention of physical abuse of women? (p. 408)
- What actions can community health nurses take to provide more sensitive and effective care to lesbian, bisexual, or transgender clients? (pp. 404–409)

REFERENCES

American Psychological Association. (1999). *Policy statements on lesbian, gay, and bisexual concerns: Resolution on lesbian, gay and bisexual youths in the schools*. Retrieved November 23, 1999, from the World Wide Web, *http://www.apa.org*.

Baeten, J. M., Bukusi, E. A., & Lambe, M. (2001). Pregnancy complications and outcomes among overweight and obese nulliparous women. *American Journal of Public Health, 91*, 436–440.

Baird, K. (1998). *Gender justice and the health care system*. New York: Garland.

Brady, M. (1998). Female genital mutilation. *Nursing98, 28*(9), 50–51.

Briss, P. A., Carande-Kulis, V. G., Bernier, R. R., Ndiaye, S. M., et al. (1999). Vaccine-preventable diseases: Improving vaccination coverage in children, adolescents, and adults. *Morbidity and Mortality Weekly Report, 48*(RR-8), 1–15.

Chesney, M. A., & Nealey, J. B. (1996). Smoking and cardiovascular disease risk in women: Issues for prevention and women's health. In P. M. Kato & T. Mann (Eds.), *Handbook of diversity issues in health psychology* (pp. 199–218). New York: Plenum Press.

Collins, K. S., Schoen, C., Joseph, S., Duchon, L., et al. (1999). *Health concerns across a woman's lifespan: The Commonwealth Fund 1998 survey of women's health*. New York: The Commonwealth Fund.

Crook, M. (1995). *My body: Women speak out about their health care*. New York: Plenum.

Dean, L., & Bradford, J. (2000). Violence and sexual assault. In Gay and Lesbian Medical Association & Center for Lesbian, Gay, Bisexual, and Transgender Health (Eds.), *Lesbian, gay, bisexual, and transgender health: Findings and concerns* (pp. 29–32). New York: Author.

Dietz, P, M., Rochat, R. W., Thompson, B. L., Berg, C. J., & Griffin, G. W. (1998). Differences in the risk of homicide and other fatal injuries between postpartum women and other women of childbearing age: Implications for prevention. *American Journal of Public Health, 88*, 641–643.

Eliason, M. J. (1998). Correlates of prejudice in nursing students. *Journal of Nursing Education, 37*(1), 27–29.

Ellerman, S. (1999). Opening up: Understanding the issues gay patients face. *NurseWeek, 12*(2), 10.

Excellence in Clinical Practice. (2000). Chemotherapy may cause bone loss in women. *1*(3), 4.

Faulkner, A. H., & Cranston, K. (1998). Correlates of same-sex sexual behavior in a random sample of Massachusetts high school students. *American Journal of Public Health, 88*, 262–266.

Gilchrist, J., Jones, B. H., Sleet, D. A., & Kimsey, C. D. (2000). Exercise-related injuries among women: Strategies for prevention from civilian and military studies. *Morbidity and Mortality Weekly Report, 49*(RR-2), 15–33.

Goldsmith, C., & Shelby, K. E. (1999). Perimenopause: Out of the shadows and into the light. *NurseWeek, 12*(11), 20–21

Gonzales, V., Washienko, K. M., Krone, M. R., Chapman, L. I., et al. (1999). Sexual and drug-use risk factors for HIV and STDs: A comparison of women with and without bisexual experiences. *American Journal of Public Health, 89*, 1841–1846.

Gruskin, E. P. (1999). *Treating lesbians and bisexual women: Challenges and strategies for health professionals*. Thousand Oaks, CA: Sage.

Holden, P., & Miller, C. L. (1999). Women and asthma, Part 2: Managing the disease. *NurseWeek, 15*(15), 16.

Hughes, T. (1998). *Osteoporosis prevention: What you need to know*. San Diego: Author.

James, T., & Platzer, H. (1999). Ethical considerations in qualitative research with vulnerable groups: Exploring lesbians' and gay mens' experiences with health care—A personal perspective. *Nursing Ethics, 6*(1), 73–81.

Kenney, J. W., & Bhattacharjee, A. (2000). Interactive model of women's stressors, personality traits, and health problems. *Journal of Advanced Nursing, 32*, 249–258.

Lawrence, J. (1975). Homosexuals, hospitalization, and the nurse. *Nursing Forum, 14*, 305–317.

Lawson, H. W., Henson, R., Bobo, J. K., & Kaeser, M. K. (2000). Implementing recommendations for the early detection of breast and cervical cancer among low-income women. *Morbidity and Mortality Weekly Report, 49*(RR-2), 37–55.

Lilly Center for Women's Health. (1998). *Women's health: Issues and trends*. Indianapolis, IN: Author.

McCarthy, G. M., Koval, J. J., & MacDonald, J. K. (1999). Factors associated with refusal to treat HIV-infected patients: The results of a national survey of dentists in Canada. *American Journal of Public Health, 89*, 541–545.

McKibben, L. J., Stange, P. V., & Sneller, V., Strikas, R. A., Rodewald, L. E., & Briss, P. A. (2000). Use of standing orders programs to increase adult vaccination rates: Recommendations of the Advisory Committee on Immunization Practices. *Morbidity and Mortality Weekly Report, 49*(RR-1), 21–26.

Meyer, I., & Bowen, D. (2000). Lesbian, gay and bisexual health concerns: Cancer. In Gay and Lesbian Medical Association & Center for Lesbian, Gay, Bisexual, and Transgender Health (Eds.), *Lesbian, gay, bisexual, and transgender health: Findings and concerns* (pp. 15–17). New York: Author.

Meyer, I., Rothblum, E., & Bradford, J. (2000), Mental health and mental disorders. In Gay and Lesbian Medical Association & Center for Lesbian, Gay, Bisexual, and Transgender Health (Eds.), *Lesbian, gay, bisexual, and transgender health: Findings and concerns* (pp. 21–26). New York: Author.

Meyer, I., Silenzio, V., Wolfe, D., & Dunn, P. (2000). Introduction/background. In Gay and Lesbian Medical Association & Center for Lesbian, Gay, Bisexual, and Transgender Health (Eds.), *Lesbian, gay, bisexual, and transgender health: Findings and concerns* (pp. 4–9). New York: Author.

National Center for Health Statistics. (2000a). Entry into prenatal care—United States, 1989–1997. *Morbidity and Mortality Weekly Report, 49*, 393–398.

National Center for Health Statistics. (2000b). *Health, United States, 2000*. Washington, DC: Author.

National Women's Law Center, Focus/University of Pennsylvania, & The Lewin Group. (2000). *Making the grade on women's health: A national and state by state report card*. Washington, DC: National Women's Law Center.

Olshansky, E. (2000). Goals for women's wellness. In E. Olshansky (Ed.), *Integrated women's health: Holistic approaches for comprehensive care* (pp. 69–80). Gaithersburg, MD: Aspen.

Postema, A. S., & Breiman, R. F. (2000). Adult immunizations programs in nontraditional settings: Quality standards and guidance for program evaluation. *Morbidity and Mortality Weekly Report, 49*(RR-1), 1–13.

Regional Perinatal System. (2000). Gestational diabetes mellitus: Screening and diagnosis. *Crib Sheet, 12*(4), 2.

Remafedi, F., French, S., Story, M., Resnick, M. D., & Blum, R. (1998). The relationship between suicide risk and sexual orientation: Results of a population based study. *American Journal of Public Health, 88*, 57–60.

Saunders, J. M. (1999). Health problems of lesbian women. *Nursing Clinics of North America, 34*, 381–391.

Scout. (2000). Family planning. In Gay and Lesbian Medical Association & Center for Lesbian, Gay, Bisexual, and Transgender Health (Eds.), *Lesbian, gay, bisexual, and transgender health: Findings and concerns* (pp. 17–18). New York: Author.

Sell, R., & Wolfe, D. (2000). Educational and community-based programs. In Gay and Lesbian Medical Association & Center for Lesbian, Gay, Bisexual, and Transgender Health (Eds.), *Lesbian, gay, bisexual, and transgender health: Findings and concerns* (pp. 13–15). New York: Author.

Sember, R. (2000). Transgender health concerns. In Gay and Lesbian Medical Association & Center for Lesbian, Gay, Bisexual, and Transgender Health (Eds.), *Lesbian, gay, bisexual, and transgender health: Findings and concerns* (pp. 32–43). New York: Author.

Silenzio, I., & White, J. (2000a). Sexually transmitted diseases. In Gay and Lesbian Medical Association & Center for Lesbian, Gay, Bisexual, and Transgender Health (Eds.), *Lesbian, gay, bisexual, and transgender health: Findings and concerns* (pp. 26–27). New York: Author.

Silenzio, I., & White, J. (2000b). Tobacco use. In Gay and Lesbian Medical Association & Center for Lesbian, Gay, Bisexual, and Transgender Health (Eds.), *Lesbian, gay, bisexual, and transgender health: Findings and concerns* (p. 29). New York: Author.

Silenzio, I. White, J., & Wolfe, D. (2000). Substance abuse. In Gay and Lesbian Medical Association & Center for Lesbian, Gay, Bisexual, and Transgender Health (Eds.), *Lesbian, gay, bisexual, and transgender health: Findings and concerns* (pp. 27–29). New York: Author.

Singleton, J. A., Greby, S. M., Wooten, K. G., Walker, F. J., & Strikas, R. (2000). Influenza, pneumococcal, and tetanus toxoid vaccination of adults—United States, 1993–1997.

In 1998, men constituted 48% of the U.S. population over 15 years of age (U.S. Census Bureau, 1999). A great deal of health-related literature has been written about specific problems that influence men's health status (e.g., cardiovascular disease, lung cancer, etc.). Very little, however, is written about the overall health needs of men. The health care of men has been fragmented, approached from an episodic perspective. Little effort has been made to provide comprehensive, holistic health services.

Lack of emphasis on holistic health for men is evident in previous versions of the national health objectives. Women, children, and the elderly are among the populations that have been specifically targeted in previous sets of objectives; men have not. Only in the most recent objectives is prostate cancer addressed (U.S. Department of Health and Human Services [USDHHS], 2000), despite the fact that the mortality rate for prostate cancer (33.8 per 100,000 men) was almost twice that of breast cancer in women (18.8 per 100,000) (National Center for Health Statistics, 2000). Many of the past and current objectives will benefit men. The lack of attention to the total health of men, however, is a justifiable concern of community health nurses. The focus of this chapter is on preparing community health nurses to provide holistic care to male clients.

In 1998, there were more than 102 million men over 15 years of age in the United States (U.S. Census Bureau, 1999). Clear differences exist between these men and their female counterparts in the epidemiology of certain health problems and health-related behaviors. These epidemiologic and behavioral differences are reflected in life expectancy, which in 1997 was 79.2 years for women and only 73.6 years for men (U.S. Census Bureau, 1999). The gap in life expectancy between men and women is an ironic reflection of the fact that our health care system—created by and still largely controlled by men—apparently does not serve men's health care needs well. Further evidence of this fact is noted in figures indicating that men have higher mortality than women for all 10 leading causes of death. In 1998, for example, men were three times more likely to die of AIDS, five times more likely to commit suicide, and almost twice as likely to die of heart disease as women (National Center for Health Statistics, 2000).

Just as women's health is not defined solely in terms of reproductive problems, men have unique health needs over and above those related to the male reproductive system. These needs are both biological and social and include the need to discuss health care concerns; the need to consider health risks posed by lifestyle and gender roles as well as by occupational, leisure, and interpersonal activities; the need for health education and information regarding their bodies and self-care; the need for comprehensive health assessment; the need for assistance with interpersonal relationships and parenting; and the need for health care services that take into account employment constraints in scheduling and location.

Men differ from women in their patterns of physical health disorders and health-related needs. These differences are attributable to (a) the physiologic differences between men and women (e.g., testicular cancer in men); (b) the differences in health-related habits and health-seeking behavior between men and women (e.g., men have fewer contacts with health care providers than women); (c) differences in social roles, stress, and coping; and (d) lifestyle differences between the sexes (e.g., men consume more alcohol and are more likely to resolve conflicts by resorting to violence) (Mann, 1996).

ⓖ THINK ABOUT IT

Why do you think men, rather than women, evolved as hunters and warriors?

ASSESSING MEN'S HEALTH

Community health nurses' assessment of men's health status occurs at the level of the individual client and at the population level. Such assessments can be framed in the context of the six dimensions of health to include biophysical, psychological, physical environmental, sociocultural, behavioral, and health system considerations.

Biophysical Considerations

Biophysical factors influencing men's health relate to elements of maturation and aging, genetic inheritance, and physiologic function.

Maturation and Aging

Maturation and aging play a significant role in many health risks and problems experienced by male clients. Certain physical disorders are associated with advanced age in men: cardiovascular disease, cerebrovascular disease, prostate cancer and hypertrophy, and hypertension. Other physical health concerns are more frequently associated with younger male clients: trauma, violence, and testicular cancer. In 1998, 10 million adolescent boys (age 15 to 19 years) constituted 10% of the male population in the United States. Another 14% of the population, or 14.1 million men were over 65 years of age (U.S. Census Bureau, 1999).

Physical sexual maturation in the male typically begins between ages 9.5 and 14 years and is completed between ages 14 and 18 years. Adolescent males are typically very concerned with sexual and physical development, often comparing themselves to other males and many times experiencing anxiety about the possibility that their development is delayed or inadequate. In some cases, this anxiety can be sufficient to cause social impairment or serious emotional distress, and the community health nurse should make a special effort to be supportive and accepting. The community health nurse can also assist adolescent male clients by offering information and reassurance about the normal patterns and variations in growth and development. In the majority of adolescent males, a degree of transient gynecomastia (enlargement of the breasts) occurs. This is variable in degree, but can be a source of significant concern to the adolescent; again, reassurance, explanation, and acceptance are of benefit.

During this period, adolescents become increasingly concerned with the values of peers and are increasingly focused on achieving acceptance from the peer group. They are prone to value peers over parents at this stage, and attitudes are more reflective of peers than family. Adolescent males often experience identity uncertainty, and may engage in a variety of behaviors that, although perhaps disconcerting to family or other adults, are necessary experiments in determining their self-concepts. Hormonal changes result in increased growth and libido, confronting adolescent males with the possibility of new (and perhaps anxiety-provoking) roles; these changes are also mirrored in the behavior of peers, on which the teenager tends to model his own behaviors and choices.

Adolescent males may feel embarrassed about the physical and emotional changes they experience. For example, they may have spontaneous and ill-timed erections or nocturnal emissions. Physical development and social circumstances, coupled with peer pressure and a desire to conform, may lead to varying degrees of sexual activity, presenting the risks of unwanted pregnancy and sexually transmitted diseases. It is not unusual for some of the adolescent male's sexual exploration to involve sexual contact with other males; approximately 50% of all males have had such contact at some point, and there is no correlation between such sexual activity and later sexual orientation (though the adolescent may again experience significant anxiety, guilt, or shame about this experimental behavior). Other adolescent males may begin to discover a same-sex orientation during these years and should be supported as well.

Over time, the adolescent male's preoccupation with sexual performance and activity as the major parameters of a relationship are increasingly replaced by romantic attributes and genuine caring; initially, these romantic views are often stereotypical and exaggerated, but this also changes as he progresses through early adulthood. Again, the nurse's role involves assessing the young male's development relative to existing norms; providing education about growth, development, sexuality, and related risks and safety precautions; and providing reassurance and guidance relative to the changes experienced.

Psychological maturity or the lack thereof is a significant contributing factor to trauma, substance abuse, and suicide. Certain health-related life experiences can also be viewed from a maturational perspective, particularly divorce (married males tend to live longer than divorced or never-married males) and retirement (which can result in a higher risk of isolation or depression), both of which are associated with poorer health and higher risk of suicide. Divorce is discussed more fully as a sociological fac-

tor later in this chapter. The health needs of older male clients, particularly those in retirement, are addressed in Chapter 19.

The nurse assesses the male client's maturational level by observing his behavior or interviewing him to elicit information about his concerns, interests, habits, and judgment. The nurse may also gather assessment data about a client's maturity level from indirect sources, such as reports from significant others and other health care professionals. At the aggregate level, the nurse would obtain information about the age composition of the male population.

Genetic Inheritance

Genetic factors play a significant role in the physical health of male clients and are an important area for nursing assessment relative to cardiovascular disease, hypertension, and cerebrovascular disease. Genetic factors also may play a role in testicular and prostatic cancer (and cancer generally), as well as in tendencies toward alcoholism and violence. Genetic factors may also influence a man's psychological health. They are, for example, suspected as a contributing factor in various mood disorders (which, in turn, often precipitate suicide among males).

The community health nurse assesses potential genetic contributions to a client's health status by obtaining a family history of the occurrence of physical and psychological disorders. It may be necessary to interview both the client and older family members and relatives to secure an accurate picture of genetically mediated health problems. At the population level, the nurse would obtain information on the prevalence of diseases with genetic components.

Physiologic Function

Men experience significant morbidity and mortality due to several physiologic conditions. Although considerable progress has been made in decreasing mortality related to heart disease, it remains the leading cause of death among U.S. men. Heart disease mortality declined 129% from 1950 to 1998, but in 1998 still accounted for an age-adjusted death rate of 166.9 deaths per 100,000 men. Most of these deaths result from myocardial infarction (MI), which contributed to a mortality rate of 196.7 per 100,000 white men in 1998 with similar rates among African American men and slightly lower rates among other ethnic minority groups (National Center for Chronic Disease Prevention and Health Promotion, 2001). More than one fourth (27%) of men who experience an MI die within one year, and 23% experience a second MI (Lilly Center for Women's Health, 1998).

Cancer also contributes to significant mortality among men. In 1998, the age-adjusted mortality rate for men for all neoplasms was 49.5 per 100,000 men. This represents an increase in mortality of 160% since 1950 (National Center for Health Statistics, 2000). In 1998, 184,500 new cases of prostate cancer were diagnosed in U.S. men, in addition to 91,400 cases of lung cancer, 64,600 cases of colorectal cancer, 39,500 cases of bladder cancer, and

24,300 cases of melanoma. Lung cancer deaths among men in that same year amounted to 93,100, with another 39,200 deaths due to prostate cancer, 27,900 deaths due to colorectal cancers, and 14,000 deaths due to pancreatic cancer. Despite the decrease in lung cancer deaths among men (4.2% from 1990 to 1994) and a rise in mortality among women, men still experience 39% more lung cancer deaths than women (Lilly Center for Women's Health, 1998). Similarly, men had a melanoma mortality rate more than twice that of women in 1997 (USDHHS, 2000). These figures serve to highlight the enormity of the problem of cancer among men.

As noted earlier, men also experience higher mortality rates from HIV/AIDS than women. In 1998, the HIV mortality rate was 7.2 per 100,000 men, more than three times that of women, but less than one third of the peak mortality in 1994, suggesting some effect of the new treatment options for AIDS and its opportunistic diseases. Chronic obstructive pulmonary disease (COPD) also accounts for significant mortality in men, with a rate of 25.9 per 100,000 men in 1998, again 43% higher than the rate for women (National Center for Health Statistics, 2000).

In addition to the burden of excess mortality, men also experience significant morbidity due to chronic diseases. For example, asthma incidence in men increased 29% from 1982 to 1992, and asthma mortality increased 34% in roughly the same period. Diabetes among men increases the risk for heart disease two- to threefold (Lilly Center for Women's Health, 1998). Men also experience a variety of activity limitations due to chronic conditions. In 1997, for example, 22% of men with arthritis had some activity limitation and 1.6% had difficulty performing personal care activities. Similarly, 31% of men 18 years of age and older experience limitations due to chronic back pain (USDHHS, 2000). Overall, in 1997, 13.1% of men experienced some form of activity limitation due to chronic disease (slightly less than women, at 13.4%) (National Center for Health Statistics, 2000).

Men also often achieve poorer control of chronic diseases than do women. For example, although men have lower rates of incidence for diabetes than women (2.6 per 100,000 men versus 3.7 per 100,000 women), they have higher mortality rates (87 versus 67 per 100,000 in 1997). Similarly, 28% of women with high blood pressure have their blood pressure under control compared to only 12% of men (USDHHS, 2000).

Men may also experience a variety of disorders involving the male reproductive system. The prostate gland, for example, is subject to infection (prostatitis), carcinoma, and nonmalignant hyperplasia (benign prostatic hyperplasia or BPH). The testes and surrounding structures also are prone to carcinomas and inflammatory diseases.

The symptoms of prostatitis, an inflammation of the prostate, typically include urinary flow restriction in association with fever, burning on urination, and perineal pain. The condition may also be accompanied by pyuria or hematuria. Prostatitis often accompanies cystitis. The condition may result as a consequence of sexually transmitted diseases and may develop into a chronic, recurring form. Because of this risk, it is especially important for the community health nurse to assess for the symptoms of this condition.

Benign prostatic hyperplasia commonly occurs in men over age 50, and approximately 40% of men over 70 years of age have some degree of BPH (Barry et al., 1997). Presenting signs and symptoms include urinary flow restriction (urinary frequency, hesitancy, terminal dribbling, bladder fullness or distention, or urinary incontinence). Nurses should assess male clients over the age of 50 for these symptoms and facilitate follow-up evaluation.

Epididymitis, or inflammation of the epididymis, is the most common form of intrascrotal inflammation. It usually presents as painful swelling within the scrotum and is frequently accompanied by urethritis. Complications include infertility, abscesses, and testicular atrophy. The condition may be idiopathic or result from sexually transmitted pathogens. Assessment by the community health nurse should include a review of the client's sexual habits for factors that would increase the risk of acquiring this infection (frequent sexual partners, failure to use condoms) in addition to assessing for the presence of signs or symptoms.

Impotence is another area of reproductive dysfunction experienced by a significant number of men. *Impotence* is a broad term for male sexual dysfunction and encompasses diminished sexual desire, inability to obtain or maintain an erection, premature ejaculation, absence of emission, or inability to achieve an orgasm. Impotence may arise from a variety of causes including male hormonal deficiencies, brain tumors, diseases of the spinal cord, diabetes, medication use (e.g., phenothiazines, imipramine, reserpine, fluoxetine [Prozac]), drug and alcohol use, surgical procedures (such as prostatectomy, rectosigmoid surgery, or aortic bypass), or stress. Whatever its cause, impotence, whether transient or long term, can be a devastating experience for the male client. Because men may be reluctant to volunteer information regarding sexual dysfunction to a nurse (especially a female nurse), the community health nurse needs to tactfully probe for evidence of problems in this area, assessing not only for the problem of impotence, but also for its effects on the client and his interaction with others.

Occurring primarily among men, inguinal hernia is relatively common. Usual symptoms include lower abdominal or groin pain on straining (when lifting and sometimes during bowel movements). Although typically manageable on a symptomatic level, inguinal hernias may require surgical repair. In some cases, herniation of the intestine through the inguinal canal(s) may lead to bowel obstruction and necrosis, a life-threatening situation. For this reason, the community health nurse working with a male client who is diagnosed with an inguinal hernia should carefully assess for the presence of persistent pain in the inguinal area, particularly if accompanied by persistent intestinal symptoms such as abdominal rigidity, pain, and cramping.

Another area to be addressed in assessing men's physiologic function is the presence of adverse effects related to accidental injury. Males at all ages have higher rates of unintentional injuries than females. This is particularly true for motor vehicle accidents. In 1997, for example, men were hospitalized nearly twice as often for nonfatal head injuries as women and nearly seven times more often for firearms injuries (USDHHS, 2000). Unintentional firearms mortality among men from 1993 to 1998 was eight times higher than among women (Gotsch, Annest, Mercy, & Ryan, 2001). As we will see later in this chapter, many of these differences arise from risk behaviors engaged in by men. Other factors that may contribute to accidental injuries and should be assessed by the community health nurse are sensory impairments. Both young and middle-aged men have higher incidence rates for visual and hearing impairments than women (U.S. Census Bureau, 1999). These impairments, if undetected and uncorrected, may contribute to a variety of physical and psychological health problems.

The last aspect of physiologic function to be considered in assessing the health status of men is immunization levels. Men, as well as women, should be immunized against tetanus and diphtheria (Td), influenza, and pneumococcal disease, and susceptible men should also receive varicella vaccine (USDHHS, 1998). Although men are more likely than women to have received Td vaccines in the last 10 years (59% versus 49% among persons 50 to 64 years of age), they are less likely to have received influenza vaccine in the past year or to ever have received pneumococcal vaccine (Singleton, Greby, Wooten, Walker, & Strikas, 2000).

Community health nurses should assess individual male clients for risk factors for physiologic dysfunction as well as signs and symptoms of existing disorders. In addition, when existing conditions are noted, the nurse should assess the degree of limitation posed by the problem. Because men are often reluctant to seek care for health problems, conditions tend to be more severe when help is sought. At the population level, community health nurses obtain information on the incidence and prevalence of acute and chronic conditions among men as well as the prevalence of risk factors for these conditions (e.g., the prevalence of smoking or overweight as risk factors for cardiovascular disease). In addition, they would assess immunization levels among the male population.

Psychological Considerations

Two related elements of the psychological dimension are of concern to community health nurses caring for men. These elements include socialization, stress, and coping abilities, as well as suicide as an outcome of ineffective coping.

Socialization, Stress, and Coping

Men, like women, have several basic psychological needs. These include the needs to know and be known to others,

to be mutually interdependent, to love and be loved, and to live meaningful lives. Society, however, has socialized both men and women to accept a stereotypical male role that makes it difficult to meet these needs. General dimensions of this stereotyped role include a need to actively differentiate oneself from women and refrain from behaviors ascribed to women (such as demonstrating affection or seeking help) and a need to see oneself as superior to others. Other dimensions include the need to be strong and self-reliant and to be more powerful than others, even if this means resorting to violence to demonstrate one's power.

Because of this stereotyped view of the masculine role, men experience social pressures to conform that sometimes conflict with health. Socialized to view the male role as strong or invulnerable, a man may have difficulty admitting health-related frailties to a community health nurse. Similarly, men who believe that taking physical risks is fundamental to their masculinity may experience more frequent health impairment from trauma. As seen from these examples, when societal messages about male roles are internalized by men, they become psychological factors influencing health-related behaviors.

⑥THINK ABOUT IT

In what ways were you socialized into gender roles? How closely do your internalized gender roles conform to those expected of society? What problems, if any, has gender created in your life?

Men may also have a stronger psychological need than women to see themselves as healthy and even invulnerable. Because men tend to value strength and endurance more than women, they are more likely to conceal or suppress pain and other perceived indicators of frailty. An example of this state of mind can be seen in the male post–myocardial infarction client who resumes shoveling snow against the recommendations of health care professionals and his family, and who continues it despite the return of the now-familiar angina. As a result of this need for strength in his self-image, the male client minimizes the importance of the problem. Consequently, when shoveling snow causes further angina, he may seek health care less readily and use it less effectively than would a female client in a similar situation.

Conversely, it should be noted that male values of strength and endurance do not always adversely affect a male client's health. Some men who value strength actually may be more motivated to exercise and maintain a higher level of general fitness and to seek preventive health care to preserve their sense of themselves as strong and invulnerable.

Another psychological barrier to men's health is the male client's conflicting response to feelings regarding a health problem. For example, a man who values strength may exercise regularly, but he may avoid having a swelling in his groin examined because he cannot cope effectively with the fear that the swelling may represent a threat to his sexuality. Despite widespread beliefs to the contrary, men may respond with surprising depth of emotion to perceived threats to health and self-sufficiency.

Men are exposed to different kinds of stress than women, and their ways of coping with stress differ. Much of the stress experienced by men may arise from their need to live up to societal expectations of masculine behavior. Men with nonextreme measures of trait masculinity have been shown to have better health, engage in more health-promoting behaviors, and have more extensive social support than those who exhibit extreme trait masculinity. Those with more extreme conceptions of masculinity are more likely to engage in risk behaviors and fewer health-promoting behaviors. They also tend to delay seeking treatment longer and exhibit more type A behavior than those with nonextreme trait masculinity. Extreme trait masculinity is also associated with depression and anxiety and with increased severity of myocardial infarction and poorer adjustment after infarction (Helgeson, 1995). Men may also experience more stress than women in similar situations due to cultural expectations and their own perceptions of their ability to cope with certain situations. For example, men may experience more stress when faced with a crying baby or serious illness in the family because they have been socialized to perceive themselves as unable to deal with these kinds of events (Copenhaver & Eisler, 1996).

Masculine expectations and socialization also lead to differences in approaches to coping between men and women. Men tend to be more oriented to action coping which may be reflected in independent and aggressive behavior or suicide (Helgeson, 1995).

Suicide

Although some sources report that females attempt suicide more frequently than males, males are much more likely to be successful in their suicide attempts. The age-adjusted death rate for suicide for men of all ages is four times that of females, and in 1998, suicide caused death in 17.2 per 100,000 men (National Center for Health Statistics, 2000).

It is important for community nurses to appreciate the often-concealed prevalence of suicide in a community. Suicide claims more lives annually than many of the diseases that health care professionals combat so effectively. Because suicide is such a frequent cause of mortality for males, it is important that the community health nurse directly address the issue with those male clients most at risk:

- Clients 15 to 24 years of age or older than 65 years
- Clients with chronic physical or mental disorders (particularly those that are progressively debilitating or that lead to deterioration in function)
- Clients who are depressed or who feel hopeless or helpless
- Clients with a recent history of significant loss (death of a family member, end of a marriage)
- Clients who are intoxicated
- Clients with a history of recent or remote suicides among peers or family members
- Clients with impaired muscle control

Clients who appear to be at risk for suicide should be directly but empathetically questioned about this possibility. For example, a nurse could state, "It would not be unusual for a person who's been through what you have to be thinking about suicide. Is that something you have considered?" Suicide assessment would further include distinguishing thoughts about suicide from actual intent and plans to initiate it, determining the client's access to lethal means of suicide (guns, heights, drugs), and the presence or absence of support persons who can ensure the client's safety. It is important that the community health nurse not allow his or her own denial of the reality of suicide to limit assessment of this important threat to a male client's well-being. At the aggregate level, community health nurses should be aware of the rates of attempted and completed suicide in subgroups within the male population. Nurses should ascertain the age and ethnic groups most affected as well as risk factors for suicide present in the population.

Physical Environmental Considerations

With the exception of the occupational environment, which is addressed in the discussion of the sociocultural dimension, the effects of the physical environment on men's health are much the same as they are on women's health. Pollution, overcrowding, and safety hazards adversely affect both. Men, however, may have increased exposure to environmental hazards due to occupational and leisure activity choices.

Sociocultural Considerations

Many influences on men's health arise from the sociocultural dimension. Some sociocultural dimension considerations in caring for men are violence and trauma, criminal justice issues, family interactions, and occupation and employment issues.

Violence and Trauma

Violence and trauma are often the effects of psychological and sociological factors. Men's socially reinforced aggressiveness and cultural role models that promote risk taking are frequently cited explanations for the significantly greater trauma-related morbidity and mortality rates among males. Figures for head injury and unintentional firearms injuries were presented earlier. Men also have twice the mortality related to motor vehicle accidents as women (21.7 per 100,000 men versus 10.4 per 100,000 women) (USDHHS, 2000).

Similarly, the death rate from homicide is more than three times higher for men than women. In 1998, homicides accounted for 11.3 deaths per 100,000 men. The rate of physical assault experienced by men is also higher than that for women (38.3 per 1,000 men versus 24.3 per 1,000 women in 1998) (USDHHS, 2000).

Although society tends to think of males as abusers rather than victims, the incidence of assault of men by intimate partners is relatively high, at 1.4 in every 1,000 men (USDHHS, 2000). Abused men typically experience the same negative societal and professional responses that female abuse victims might encounter (such as "blaming the victim" and disbelief). Additionally, many male victims either experience—or at least fear—accusations that they are homosexual. As a result, maintaining confidentiality is essential to the nursing care of the male victim of abuse.

Community health nurses should be alert to signs of abuse or assault among individual male clients. They should also obtain information on the prevalence of assault on male victims in the general population as well as risk factors for both violence and unintentional injury.

Men, as well as women, who have experienced trauma may suffer from an insidious and debilitating disorder that requires exceptional understanding and patience on the part of the nurse. *Posttraumatic stress disorder (PTSD)* is caused by exposure to traumatic events with which an individual is profoundly unable to cope. This disorder is characterized by disturbances in sleep (insomnia, nightmares), poor interpersonal relationships, modulation of emotions, vivid recollections of the traumatic episode, and periods of profound depression. Other reactions may include rage, homicidal impulses, and suicidal tendencies. Although this disorder can occur equally readily in men or women in the same circumstances (e.g., as a result of childhood sexual abuse), the much greater involvement in military combat by men and the resulting disproportionate exposure to the severe trauma of war (particularly the Vietnam War) have led to a significant number of American men with PTSD.

Community health nurses often encounter undiagnosed cases of PTSD, and they can be of tremendous value by case finding and by helping PTSD sufferers to seek or accept treatment. Community health nurses should assess clients who have experienced major psychological or physical trauma for the signs and symptoms of PTSD. These can occur at any time after the trauma, ranging from days to years later. Nurses should also assess for health issues frequently accompanying PTSD, including substance abuse, violence, and risk of suicide.

Criminal Justice Issues

Although men are not alone in their involvement with criminal justice issues, they comprise 89% of jail inmates and 94% of inmates of federal and state prisons. In 1997, there were 1.1 million men in prison, more than three and a half times the number of inmates in 1980 (U.S. Census Bureau, 1999). The prison system in general has been referred to as a "pocket of risk" (Polych & Sabo, 1995). Many inmates have been imprisoned for behaviors that put them at higher risk for health problems (e.g., substance abuse). The prison environment further enhances the risk of conditions like tuberculosis, hepatitis, and HIV infection. Not only are inmates themselves at increased risk of infection; the roughly 2 million annual admissions and discharges from jail and prison systems create a steady flow of infection into the system and back out into the general population. This risk to the general public is a concern for all community health nurses and nurses working with male clients should seek information regarding recent incarceration and be alert for signs of infection. Community health nurses may also be involved in follow-up activities with recently discharged inmates who have tuberculosis or HIV infection. In these cases, the community health nurse promotes continuity of care and continued therapy. Community health nurses may also be involved in care of men within the correctional system itself. This aspect of care is addressed in Chapter 26.

Family Interactions

By far, the largest proportion of men live within a family situation, which may create both positive and negative health effects. Marriage has been shown to have a protective health effect for men and less so for women; however, because of socialization to a stereotyped male role, men may have difficulty interacting within the family in ways that effectively meet the psychological needs discussed earlier. Differing role expectations between husband and wife may lead to marital conflicts and, in some cases, spouse or child abuse. Family violence and its effects on health are discussed in more detail in Chapter 32. It is, however, important for the community health nurse dealing with male clients to assess marital interactions and to engage in appropriate interventions.

Parenting is another aspect of family interaction that may prove problematic for men. Again, because of typical male socialization, many men have little or no child care experience. The increase in the number of working women has led to greater assumption of child care duties by men. The community health nurse should assess the male client's involvement in child care as well as the extent of his knowledge of effective parenting skills.

Divorce is another possible aspect of family interactions that can profoundly affect the health of the male client. Divorce is one of the most significant stressors a person can experience, and it frequently has a profound effect on physical and psychological health. Divorced men, in particular, have been shown to experience increased morbidity and mortality as compared with married men. Men may respond to divorce or its aftermath with intense anger, a profound sense of loss, or significant depression. Suicidal behavior occasionally occurs as the man reacts to the divorce as an assault against his self-image and self-worth, or homicidal behavior if he directs his anger toward his ex-spouse.

Divorce may also mean stressful battles for custody of any children born to the couple or part-time fatherhood if joint custody is the outcome. More and more divorced fathers have at least partial custody of their children. In 1998, 2.7 million U.S. households consisted of an adult male with children. This figure represents an increase of 59% from 1995 to 1998 (Barret & Robinson, 2000) and constituted 5% of all U.S. households (U.S. Census Bureau, 1999). Single parenthood may contribute to stress as well as economic deprivation. The community health nurse should assess the men in these families for needed assistance with parenting as well as for health effects of stress and reduced economic status.

Many men are single parents of young children.

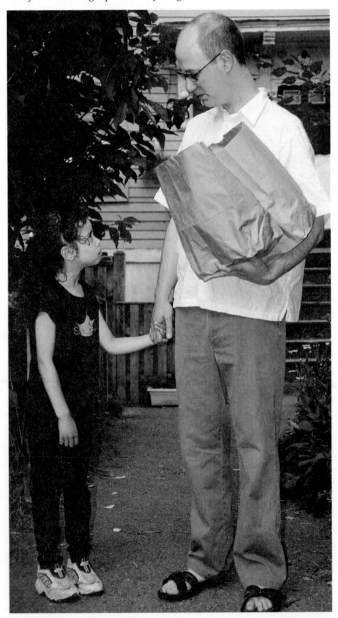

Assessment appropriate to the issue of divorce includes evaluating the client's style of coping with stress, for example, drinking alcohol as contrasted to talking with support persons. The nurse also assesses the client's access to support personnel as well as the client's psychological responses such as depression, suicidal behavior, and anger. Given the impact of divorce on physical health, it is also important to assess for stress-related physiological health problems such as exacerbation of hypertension, infectious illnesses, and cardiovascular disturbances. At the population level, the community health nurse would assess the extent of divorce and single male parenthood in the population.

One additional family consideration that may influence the health of men is caretaking responsibilities related to sick or disabled children or other family members. Approximately 4% of men in the United States have primary responsibility for the care of disabled family members (Collins, Schoen, Joseph, & Duchon, 1999). Although this is less than half the number of women caretakers, men may have more difficulties than women because they frequently have not been socialized to fulfill a caretaking role. Caregivers in general have been found to have poorer health status than noncaregivers and often experience stress and depression as well as chronic fatigue (Kelley, Buckwalter, & Maas, 1999; Teel & Press, 1999). In addition, caregivers have been shown to neglect their own health (Collins et al., 1999). This may be even more true of male caregivers since men in general tend to pay less attention to their own health needs than do women.

Occupation and Employment

Although the increase in the number of women in the American workforce has been significant, most hazardous occupations (such as mining and agriculture) are still performed by men. In 1997, 4 of every 100,000 workers, most of them male, died of injuries incurred on the job, and 3.8 million disabling injuries occurred in the work setting (U.S. Census Bureau, 1999). Men are exposed to a variety of workplace toxins that cause impaired fertility, chromosomal changes, fetal anomalies, miscarriage, and impaired sexual function (National Institute for Occupational Safety and Health, 1997). Other occupational hazards that men typically face more frequently than women include exposure to chemical agents, physical agents (temperature extremes, sunlight), mechanical agents (vibration, repetitive-use syndromes), and psychosocial agents (stress and burnout, role models of poor health habits such as smoking).

Particular psychological agents that are of concern in the work setting are stress and exposure to workplace violence. As noted earlier, men may adapt less well to stressful situations than women. Even more often than women, men may experience the stress of multiple jobs. In 1998, for example, nearly 6% of U.S. men held more than one job. In most instances (62%), this entailed one full-time and one part-time job; however, 4% of men with

CRITICAL THINKING IN RESEARCH

Neufeld & Harrison (1998) conducted a study of men caretakers of family members with impaired cognition. The study was based on equity theory which holds that relationships in which social support is nonreciprocal are usually terminated. The study examined men's perceptions of reciprocity in relationships in which the ability of the care recipient to reciprocate was minimal. Data were obtained in interviews with 22 male caregivers that occurred three to four times over an 18-month period and were confirmed in a focus group with seven of the caretakers. The authors found two types of caregiving relationships: those based on reciprocity over time and those based on obligation. Three types of reciprocity were identified: waived reciprocity, generalized reciprocity, and constructed reciprocity. Caregivers who waived reciprocity felt it was important in relationships, but impossible in the current situation. In generalized reciprocity, caregivers voiced expectations that their efforts would be returned to someone other than the caregiver (e.g., role modeling altruistic behaviors for children). In constructed reciprocity, the caregivers interpreted nonverbal cues from the recipient of care as indicating a response to care (e.g., looking more content, signs of interest).

More than half of the caretakers discussed caregiving in terms of obligation with no reciprocity. Caretakers also reported changes in reciprocal relationships with others as a result of their caregiving (e.g., loss of friends, inability to request help because they were unable to return it). Several men also reported lack of assistance or support from other family members.

- What are the implications of the findings of this study for practice?
- What additional research questions does this study suggest? How might you go about studying them? What data collection methods, other than interviews, might you employ?
- Do you think you would obtain similar findings if this study were conducted with women caregivers? Why or why not?

---

multiple jobs held two full-time positions. Like women, nearly one third of men in multiple jobs indicated a need to meet regular household expenses as the reason for dual employment. Another source of occupational stress is job-related travel. In 1997, 70% of men engaged in business travel compared to only 30% of women. Each trip covered an average of slightly more than three nights away from home (U.S. Census Bureau, 1999). For single male parents, such business trips pose the added burden of finding care for young children.

Workplace violence is also a source of occupational stress and potential injury. Men are more than twice as likely as women to be victims of workplace violence. From 1992 to 1996, men comprised 66% of victims of workplace violence (U.S. Census Bureau, 1999).

Assessment of occupational health pertaining to the male client would include determining the physical, chemical, and psychosocial hazards existing in the client's work environment. Whenever possible, community health nurses would collaborate with occupational health nurses in determining which risks would be most likely in a given work setting and in using those data to determine which health disorders or needs would be appropriate for further evaluation. For example, a nurse working with a male client who had been a coal miner for two decades would consult with occupational health nurses or other professionals to determine that "black lung" (pneumoconiosis) is a significant occupational hazard for miners. The community health nurse would then use this information to assess the client's respiratory function and activity tolerance. Additional assessment recommendations are presented in Chapter 24.

Men's economic status, although generally higher than that of women, can also affect their health. In 1997, nearly 29 million men (30%) over 15 years of age had annual incomes under $15,000. More than 500,000 single male–headed households (13.6%) had annual incomes below this level jeopardizing the health and welfare of children as well as men (U.S. Census Bureau, 1999). Low income has been consistently linked to poor health status and diminished access to health care services.

A final social environmental factor that may have a profound influence on the health of male clients is unemployment. Some authors make a distinction between the societal experience of unemployment and the individual experience of "joblessness." From this perspective, ***unemployment*** is the proportion of the workforce that is not employed at a specific point in time and is a statistical measure reflecting the general state of the economy. ***Joblessness,*** on the other hand, is the personalized experience of being out of work when one desires employment.

In 1998, 3.2 million men or 4.4% of the American male population over age 16 were without a job. Unemployment rates were highest among adolescent males (16.2%), but ranged from 2.8% to 8.1% of men in other age groups, with the next highest unemployment rate occurring in men 20 to 24 years of age. Approximately 52% of unemployment was due to job loss. Unemployment is an even more significant factor for single-men with children. In 1998, 14.5% of single male heads of households including children under 18 years of age were unemployed, more than three times the overall male unemployment rate (U.S. Census Bureau, 1999).

The effects of joblessness on health can be many and varied. At the societal level, increased cardiovascular and cerebrovascular mortality has been associated with increased unemployment levels as has cirrhosis mortality. Suicide and psychiatric hospitalization rates also increase in periods of marked unemployment. For the jobless individual, common health effects may include hypertension, cardiovascular disease, myocardial infarction, stroke, depression, aggression, psychosis, drug or alcohol abuse, and child abuse.

Community health nurses should assess male clients' employment status as well as unemployment levels in the population. They should also assess jobless males for signs of associated physical and emotional health problems. In addition, nurses can assess the strength of coping skills and support systems for helping male clients deal with joblessness. A further area for consideration is the potential for reentry into the workforce via job retraining and similar programs available in the community.

Behavioral Considerations

Behavioral factors of interest in assessing men's health include consumption patterns, leisure activities, and sexual behavior.

Consumption Patterns

In 1998, men were twice as likely as women to report binge drinking and use of cocaine. Men are also more likely to report regular marijuana use. The drug-related mortality rate among men is more than twice that of women at 8.3 per 100,000 men in 1997 compared to 3.6 per 100,000 women. Men are also more likely to be smokers, and in 1997, 27% of adult males smoked (USDHHS, 2000). Tobacco and alcohol use rates are even higher among adolescent males, with 35% of high school seniors reporting tobacco use, 9% reporting binge drinking, 26% reporting marijuana use, and 3% reporting cocaine use in 1999 (National Health Center for Health Statistics, 2000). Community health nurses should assess alcohol, tobacco, and other drug consumption by individual male clients as well as the prevalence of these behaviors in the population. Signs and symptoms of alcohol and drug use and abuse are presented below.

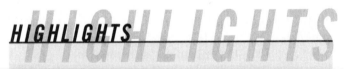

HIGHLIGHTS

Signs and Symptoms of Substance Use and Abuse

- Signs of intoxication (slurred speech, ataxia, unexplained behavioral changes)
- Alcohol odor to the client's breath
- Empty alcohol containers
- Unexplained sedation or hyperactivity
- Dilated or constricted pupils
- Increased vital signs
- Signs of withdrawal (increased vital signs, hallucinations, unexplained pain, irritability, diaphoresis, restlessness, delirium, seizures)

Diet is the final consumption pattern to be considered in assessing male clients. Although men are somewhat less likely than women to be obese, an average of 20% of U.S. men over 20 years of age were obese during the period of 1988 to 1994. Approximately one fourth of adolescent and adult men under age 65 eat two or more servings of fruit per day, while more than half consume three or more vegetables a day. Only one third of adult and adolescent men consume less than 30% of their calories as fat, and less than 5% consume less than 2,400 mg of sodium per day. Consumption of other nutrients by men remains similarly below recommendations (USDHHS, 2000). Community health nurses should assess individual male clients' dietary patterns for adequate balance and nutrient intake. Caloric intake should be assessed in light of size and activity level, and specific dietary deficiencies should be identified. Community health nurses should also assess general meal patterns and nutrient consumption at the population level, noting in particular the prevalence of obesity or specific nutritional deficiencies.

Leisure

Men and women increasingly share similar leisure patterns in American culture. Nevertheless, men still tend to be more active in competitive contact sports and, more often than women, to choose leisure activities involving some degree of physical risk (skydiving, white-water rafting, rock climbing). Participation in athletic sports is closely linked with images of masculinity and reinforces tendencies to aggressiveness and violence increasing the potential for injury. Expectations of masculinity may also lead men to downplay the severity of injuries, delay treatment, and take insufficient time for healing (White, Young, & McTeer, 1995). Men also tend to choose leisure activities associated with alcohol consumption. For these reasons, men experience relatively greater incidence of recreation-related trauma. Community health nurses should assess male clients' leisure pursuits relative to their risk of producing injury. They should also assess clients' understanding of the risks involved in leisure behaviors and knowledge and use of safety techniques or equipment to reduce health risks (e.g., eye shields and helmets during contact sports and bicycling).

ETHICAL AWARENESS

In their practice, community health nurses may uncover illegal activity. What would you do if you discovered that an adolescent in a family you are visiting is using illegal drugs? Would you report his activity? If so, to whom? If not, why not? Would your decision be any different if you had evidence that this person was supporting his or her drug habit by selling drugs to other youngsters? Why or why not?

Sexuality

Once separated by a double standard that encouraged sexual activity by men while discouraging it for women, male and female sexual behavior has grown to have more similarities than differences in many respects. Consequently, the psychosocial aspects of the sexually related health needs of men and women are very similar. For male clients, the differences often involve their physiology. For example, although cystitis is less common in men, males do develop prostatitis and urethritis. Community health nurses should assess male clients' sexual behaviors as they relate to health in a manner similar to that used for female clients, determining the client's knowledge and use of safe sexual practices, the presence or absence of symptoms of sexually transmitted diseases, and the presence of behaviors that may increase the risk of sexually related disorders. For example, 13% of sexually active adolescent males reported not using a condom at last sexual intercourse (USDHHS, 2000). The nurse should also address issues of sexual satisfaction and impotence. At the population level, nurses can obtain information on the incidence of sexually transmitted diseases and the prevalence of high-risk sexual behaviors among men.

Health System Considerations

Men tend to define health very differently from the way women define it, often viewing health as the ability to complete certain functions rather than as the presence or absence of specific symptoms. For example, a man who is obese, hypertensive, and diabetic may nonetheless feel in good health because he is able to perform what he considers to be necessary role functions at work and at home. Moreover, men tend to have fewer contacts with the health care system than do women, perhaps because of psychological and sociological factors such as a reluctance to see themselves as needing assistance. This is all the more surprising in that the majority of physicians are male, so male clients typically would have little difficulty obtaining services from someone of the same gender.

The U.S. health care system tends to focus on health from an illness perspective, with relatively little attention afforded to prevention. This state of affairs parallels the health-seeking behaviors of many male clients, who tend to focus on their health only when symptoms are significant enough to interfere with role function. Consequently, the relative lack of concern for prevention seen among many men is reinforced by the prevailing attitudes and operation of the health care system.

As is true of the population at large, men who are unemployed or employed in low-paying or part-time jobs typically lack health insurance and, therefore, experience a barrier to health care services. Men who are employed, however, may also find it difficult to obtain health care services because their work hours conflict with those of health care providers. Overall, a slightly higher percentage of men than women (17.6% versus 14.8%) were not covered by any form of health insurance in 1997 (U.S. Census Bureau, 1999).

Community nurses should assess male clients for self-images (e.g., invulnerability) that reduce the motivation to use health care services. Nurses should also assess men for other factors that serve as barriers or motivators related to obtaining health care services, such as work hours, value placed on health, ability to function in important roles despite health problems, and financial resources such as insurance.

ASSESSING GAY, BISEXUAL, AND TRANSGENDER MEN'S HEALTH

An estimated 2.8% to 9% of U.S. men are believed to be homosexual in their sexual orientation (Meyer, Silenzio, Wolfe, & Dunn, 2000). This figure includes both gay men (those who have a primary sexual or affectional orientation to members of the same sex) and bisexual men (those who may interact sexually with both men and women). Transgenderism is relatively rare, occurring in approximately one in 30,000 U.S. men. Rates of transgenderism are somewhat higher in countries like the Netherlands with policies that support genital reassignment surgery or so called "sex change operations" (Sember, 2000).

There is no general consensus on the use of the terms heterosexual, homosexual, and so on, primarily because the terms are defined differently by different groups. Homosexuality is culturally defined and what is considered homosexual in one culture may not be in another, even if it involves same-sex sexual activity (Murray, 2000). For example, 24% of African American men and 15% of Latino men who had sex with other men identified themselves as heterosexual (Scout & Robinson, 2000). Similar lack of clarity occurs in definitions of bisexuality. For instance, in one study, 82% of men who self-identified as gay also had sexual interactions with women, yet did not consider themselves bisexual (Taylor, 1999). Definitions may incorporate one or more of three dimensions: one's sexual identity orientation, sexual behavior, and/or sexual attraction (Sell, 2000). For the purposes of this book, self-identification as a gay, bisexual, or transgender individual will be used as the primary means of distinguishing membership in these groups. Readers should be aware, however, that different

CULTURAL CONSIDERATIONS

Homosexuality is defined differently in different cultures, and same-sex sexual activity may or may not be defined as homosexuality in a given culture. Explore some of the cultural groups in your area. How do they define homosexuality? When would a man consider himself to be gay or bisexual? When would a woman be considered a lesbian?

definitions have been used in some of the research that will be reported here. Where relevant, the term "men who have sex with men" (MSM) will be used since it encompasses both gay and bisexual men as well as some men who self-identify as heterosexual despite occasional same-sex sexual activity.

Gay and bisexual men are at increased risk of experiencing certain health problems when compared with heterosexuals, may have different health care needs, and may benefit from different approaches to nursing care. The Health Assessment Guide—Adult Man, available on the companion Web site for this book, can be modified to direct assessment of the homosexual client as well as the heterosexual male client.   ⊕

There exists a range of sexual orientations among individuals, with many being neither exclusively heterosexual nor exclusively homosexual. Research also suggests that most homosexually oriented persons do not differ in any psychological or social respect from their heterosexual peers. These views often conflict with those held by some people, and these conflicts may significantly affect the health behavior and status of gay, bisexual, and transgender men. Conflicts for these clients often arise out of myths related to homosexuality, some of which are presented below.

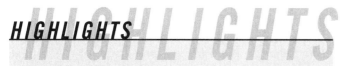

HIGHLIGHTS

Myths of Homosexuality

- Homosexuals are easily identified by their appearance.
- Homosexuality is due to disturbed parent–child relationships.
- Homosexuals do not marry.
- Homosexuals are antifamily.
- Homosexuals dislike children or are incapable of reproducing.
- Children of homosexuals are also likely to be homosexual.
- Homosexuals dislike members of the opposite sex.
- Homosexuality occurs because of parental dominance or abuse (dominant mother, aloof father).
- Homosexuality is contagious.
- Homosexuals will attempt to seduce "straight" males.
- Homosexuals sexually molest children.
- Gay men become fathers to identify with feminine roles and feelings.
- Bisexual individuals have relationships with males and females at the same time.
- Bisexual men are more masculine than gay men.

These myths lead to some of the discriminatory behaviors experienced by gay, bisexual, and transgender men.

For example, beliefs by some people that homosexuals are poor role models for young boys has led to prohibiting their functioning as adult leaders in the Boy Scouts of America. Other fears voiced are that homosexual leaders may sexually molest boys. Neither of these assertions has any basis in fact. The reality of homosexual existence and its implications for health are presented in the following discussion.

Biophysical Considerations

Gay and bisexual men experience significantly higher risks of selected physical health disorders. A major concern relative to the health of gay men is that of sexually transmitted diseases (STDs), particularly HIV infection and AIDS. Since 1981, 54% of all AIDS diagnoses occurred among men who have sex with men. In 1997, 4.7% of MSM tested for HIV infection had positive results compared to less than 1% of heterosexual men (National Center for HIV, STD, and TB Prevention, 1999). The relative proportion of AIDS due to homosexual behavior, however, has declined from 70% of new cases in 1987 (Polych & Sabo, 1995) to 38% of cases reported in 1999. This figure includes MSM who are also injection drug users (Scout & Robinson, 2000). Gay and bisexual men also experience higher rates of syphilis, gonorrhea, chlamydia, herpes, and genital warts (Silenzio & White, 2000a). Gay and bisexual men who have HIV infection are also at greater risk for serious complications of these diseases.

Gay, bisexual, and transgender clients experience a significantly greater risk of STDs because of the nature of their sexual practices and physiology. For example, anal-receptive intercourse readily traumatizes the highly vascularized intestinal mucosa, leading to increased susceptibility to entrance of infectious organisms. Among transgender men, sex work may be prevalent as a means of funding expensive genital reassignment surgeries (Sember, 2000). For these reasons, community health nurses need to assess carefully the safety of the sexual practices of these clients, their experience of symptoms suggesting STDs, and history of exposure to high-risk sexual partners. Nurses should also assess the prevalence of risk factors for STDs in the male homosexual population.

Oro-anal contact among gay, bisexual, and transgender men increases the potential for other infectious diseases. These include such diseases as *Salmonella* and *Shigella* infections, *Escherichia coli*, giardiasis, herpes simplex virus, and Epstein–Barr virus infections as well as hepatitis A, B, C, E, and G. Use of dental dams may serve to decrease transmission of these diseases. Other effects of receptive anal sex include trauma and allergic reactions to lubricants or latex condoms (Ungvarski & Grossman, 1999).

There is some evidence to suggest that gay, bisexual, and transgender men may also be at increased risk for certain forms of cancer. In part, this increased risk may relate to the effects of stress on the immune system, with clients who don't disclose their sexual orientation at even higher risk than other gay, bisexual, and transgender men.

Among gay and bisexual men with HIV infection, rates of Kaposi's sarcoma are thousands of times higher than in the general population. Incidence of Kaposi's sarcoma among gay and bisexual men has declined with the advent of more effective treatments for AIDS. The incidence of AIDS-related non-Hodgkin's lymphoma is also higher among MSM than among heterosexual groups. Gay and bisexual men also appear to be at increased risk for anal cancers, though not for cancers at other sites, than the heterosexual male population. This increased risk is thought to be due to the increased prevalence of human papillomavirus infection and smoking as risk factors among gay men. In addition, survival rates for gay men with cancer are lower than in the general population, probably due to HIV/AIDS co-morbidity and delay in disease detection and treatment (Meyer & Bowen, 2000).

Immunity is another consideration in the biophysical dimension. In addition to routine immunizations suggested for adults, gay, bisexual, and transgender men should also receive immunization for hepatitis A and B. Unfortunately, figures indicate low immunization rates for these diseases among the homosexual population (3%) (Silenzio, 2000). Community health nurses should assess immunity among individual clients as well as levels of immunity in the gay, bisexual, and transgender population at large.

Homosexual males are also vulnerable to other physiologic conditions found among their heterosexual counterparts. Due to discriminatory attitudes of some health care professionals and prior unpleasant experiences with the health care system, however, many homosexuals may not volunteer information about health problems or seek assistance. These barriers to care help to explain the lower cancer survival rates among this population. For this reason, community health nurses should carefully assess homosexual clients for evidence of physical illness.

Psychological Considerations

Psychologically, gay, bisexual, and transgender men may find themselves unable to access the usual support systems heterosexual men use to cope with health and social concerns. This may result in increased stress in some circumstances, though research suggests that most gay men adjust well to their circumstances and are no more uncomfortable in their circumstances than are their heterosexual male counterparts. One psychological factor is known to be a great concern for gay men: fear and anxiety related to encounters with homophobia and other potentially dangerous responses to their sexual orientation. As noted in Chapter 17, homophobia is an irrational fear of homosexuality that may manifest as discriminatory behavior, demeaning or derogatory comments and humor, or actual physical assaults.

Some gay men may feel compelled to conceal their sexual orientation from the heterosexual world to such an extent that they experience significant isolation; they cannot reveal their romantic joys or losses, share their longing for children, or display affection for another man (Taylor, 1999). This latter problem is more acute for gay men than for lesbians because people are more likely to perceive hugs, hand holding, or dancing between men as homosexual behavior (and, therefore, unacceptable) than if it were to occur between females. Some authors describe a trade-off between the stress, emotional inhibition, and internalized homophobia that may accompany nondisclosure and the risk of discrimination and violence that may result from disclosure. The effects of stress experienced by gay and bisexual men have been shown to be offset, however, by personal characteristics of hardiness and high self-esteem (Ungvarski & Grossman, 1999). Because of the importance of these psychological factors, community health nurses should assess coping skills and access to support systems, self-esteem, and preferences relative to privacy and confidentiality among gay, bisexual, and transgender male clients.

Another sensitive area for assessment with respect to the psychological environment is "coming out." As noted in Chapter 17, coming out is a process of acknowledging one's homosexuality to self and others. Some authors reserve the term *coming out* for one's personal acceptance of homosexuality, and use the term **disclosure** to describe the explicit revealing of one's sexual orientation to others.

The community health nurse explores with the gay male client where he is in the coming out process and how he feels about himself and his sexual identity. Because disclosure is frequently selective, confidentiality is a particularly important consideration, and the gay male client should be assured of the confidential nature of all information revealed. To maintain confidentiality, the nurse determines who else in the client's milieu is aware of his sexual identity.

Gay, bisexual, and transgender men may be at higher risk for mental distress and mental disorders, substance abuse, and suicide than the heterosexual population due to the stress of prejudice, discrimination, and risk of violence although evidence remains somewhat inconclusive for this group as a whole. There is some suggestion that men in this population may internalize negative societal attitudes to their sexual identities, resulting in difficulties in intimate relationships and the use of "emotion-focused" coping strategies such as high-risk sexual behaviors (Meyer, Rothblum, & Bradford, 2000).

It is unclear whether or not there is an increased risk for suicide or depression among gay and bisexual men as a group. Some research has indicated a higher lifetime prevalence of suicide ideation among MSM, but no greater prevalence of lifetime diagnosis of depression (Cochran & Mays, 2000). Other studies have found no relationships (Meyer, Rothblum, & Bradford, 2000). There is considerable evidence, however, that gay and bisexual youth may be at greater risk for suicide than heterosexual youth. In one study of high school students, for example, more than 28% of gay and bisexual males reported suicide attempts compared to 4.2% of heterosexual males (Remafedi, French, Story, Resnick, & Blum, 1998). In another similar study, high school students with exclusively same-sex sexual activity had eight times the incidence of four or more suicide attempts as heterosexual students (Faulkner & Cranston, 1998). Heightened risk for suicide may reflect increased perceptions of stigmatization in this age group. Being called *queer, gay,* or *faggot* have been reported by adolescents in general as the most upsetting form of sexual harassment experienced (Ungvarski & Grossman, 1999).

Transgender individuals have been found to experience a specific mental health problem called gender dysphoria which is believed to be endemic in the group. *Gender dysphoria* is a sense of incongruity between one's physical gender and one's self-perceptions (Sember, 2000). The American Psychiatric Association has retained the diagnosis of gender identity disorder in its *Diagnostic and Statistical Manual of Mental Disorders IV-TR*, but is moving to a consideration of pathology only in those individuals who exhibit significant levels of distress over their transgender identity (Meyer, Rothblum, & Bradford, 2000). These individuals may be at particular risk for suicide, auto-castration, or substance abuse. Psychological well-being seems to increase and gender dysphoria to disappear in most individuals who experience genital reassignment surgery (Sember, 2000). In the interim, however, community health nurses may need to be particularly alert to suicidal ideation in these individuals.

In addition to assessing individual gay, bisexual, and transgender clients for mental health problems, community health nurses should examine the prevalence of these conditions in the population. Nurses should also assess the availability of mental health services for those clients in need of them.

Sociocultural Considerations

Sociocultural dimension factors influencing the health of gay, bisexual, and transgender men are similar to those for lesbian women described in Chapter 17. Like homosexual women, gay, bisexual, and transgender men are subjected to discrimination and victimization in numerous aspects of their lives. For example, 20% to 24% of gay men experience violence or discrimination each year in New York City. There may be a greater difference in rates of childhood sexual abuse between homosexual and heterosexual men than between homosexual and heterosexual women. For example, in one study, 37% of gay men reported a history of sexual encounters with older stronger men, half of which involved force and 93% of which met criteria for sexual abuse. Similarly, gay men are disproportionately victimized by heterosexual men in prison settings. Most male-to-male sexual assaults involve unprotected anal intercourse with the attendant risks of trauma and STD (Dean & Bradford, 2000).

Family interaction is another element of the sociocultural dimension that affects the health of gay, bisexual, and transgender men. Disclosure of homosexuality to family members and their response, homosexual relationships, and homosexual parenting are the three primary aspects of family interaction to be assessed by the community health nurse.

Two different themes occur in families' responses to disclosure of a family member's homosexuality: loving acceptance or conventionality, which results in rejection of the homosexual family member. All families who come to know of homosexual members need to deal with feelings of grief, guilt, and fear for their child or sibling. Even before recognizing their sexual identities, gay, bisexual, or transgender men may have internalized homophobic attitudes based on parental comments heard in childhood. Such attitudes may contribute to self-hate and make disclosure to family members even more difficult (Owens, 1998).

For those families that are able to accept homosexuality in one of their members, acceptance appears to come about in stages similar to the stages of grief experienced with the loss of a loved one. The first stage is one of grief, followed by a period of denial during which parents may see their child's professed sexual identity as a "phase" that he or she will grow out of. This stage is followed successively by stages characterized by guilt and anger and, finally, acceptance (Barret & Robinson, 2000).

Parental response to the disclosure of homosexuality is strongly influenced by a variety of factors: the strength of traditional gender role conceptions, perceptions of the probable attitudes of significant others in the family's social network, and parental age and education level (younger and better educated parents tend to be more accepting). Affiliation with conservative religious ideologies and intolerance of other stigmatized groups are other factors that suggest a negative response to disclosure.

Gay males may face decisions about disclosure to wives as well as parents and siblings. Contrary to popular belief, many homosexual men are or have been married, and about half of these men have children. Some gay men do not become aware of their homosexuality until after marriage. Others marry in an attempt to deny or hide their sexual orientation. Responses of wives to the disclosure of homosexuality vary considerably and may include feelings of living with a "stranger," guilt, development of an asexual friendship or a semi-open relationship in which both husband and wife are free to take outside lovers, or a desire for divorce. Transgender identity changes can be particularly devastating to marital relationships as the spouse questions not only the husband's sexual identity, but her own as well (Sember, 2000). Community health nurses should assess the extent of clients' disclosure of their sexual identities and the effects of the responses received. Nurses should also assess the needs of family members for assistance in dealing with the disclosure.

Disclosure to family members is usually not a one-time event. As families grow and change, both the homosexual family member and others face decisions regarding disclosure to extended family members, to in-laws as siblings marry, and possibly to children and grandchildren (Barret & Robinson, 2000).

Parenting by gay, bisexual, and transgender men brings its own stresses, many of them similar to those experienced by lesbian parents. Gay or bisexual men may become fathers in a number of ways: in heterosexual relationships prior to coming out, as foster parents or through adoption, or in cooperation with a lesbian woman or surrogate mother. Gay fathers may be marginalized by both the heterosexual and homosexual communities, and partners may resent the intrusion of children into the relationship. Gay fathers may also be forced to be less open about their sexual identities than they might otherwise be in order to prevent court actions and potential loss of custody. This often means that they cannot openly live with a same-sex partner and may be denied the companionship and support afforded to heterosexual and even lesbian couples (Barret & Robinson, 2000).

Disclosure of one's sexual identity to children is another dilemma faced by gay, bisexual, and transgender men. Depending on when and how disclosure occurs, children may exhibit the same range of responses shown by other family members. Some guidelines for disclosure to children are provided below.

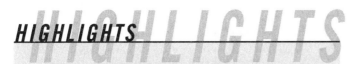

HIGHLIGHTS

Guidelines for Disclosure of Sexual Orientation to Children

- Come to grips with your own sexual identity before trying to explain it to children.
- Children are never too young to be told, but explanations must be couched in terms the child can understand.
- Disclose to children before they suspect or are informed by others.
- Plan the disclosure; do not let it occur in an impromptu fashion.
- Make the disclosure in a private setting where interruptions are unlikely.
- Inform the child in an objective and straightforward manner; do not "confess."
- Stress that your relationship with the child will not change.
- Be prepared for questions and respond to them honestly.

Source: Barret, R. L., & Robinson, B. E. (2000). *Gay fathers: Encouraging the hearts of gay dads and their families.* San Francisco: Jossey-Bass.

Gay men frequently establish long-term partnerships with same-sex partners. Gay couples' relationships are subjected to the same kinds of stress as heterosexual relationships, but this stress may be exacerbated by the absence of social support for the marital role. Therapists who work with gay and lesbian couples have identified several additional issues that threaten the stability of their relationships. These issues include differences in the stages of coming out between partners, differences with respect to extended family involvement, inequalities of power, and financial conflict and disparity in income (Barret & Robinson, 2000). With the exception of the stage of coming out, these same issues may also affect the stability of relationships among heterosexual couples.

The occupational risks and concerns experienced by gay men, another consideration in the social environment, relate primarily to avoiding discrimination and rejection in the workplace. No clearly established occupational health risks pertain to gay or bisexual lifestyles. It should, however, be noted that in occupational settings where masculine roles are stereotypical and exaggerated (e.g., construction), there may be an increased incidence of acting out of homophobic thinking, resulting in an increased risk of assault. Nursing assessment should focus on such potential safety risks and should consider the possibility that gay men who are unable to accept their sexual orientation may themselves enact exaggerated masculine roles and experience the related safety risks these behaviors may entail.

Behavioral Considerations

Among the many myths about the lifestyles of gay men are that they are very different from heterosexual men in nonsexual matters as well as sexual ones, that they have very different longings and romantic needs; and that they are highly promiscuous. In reality, the majority of gay men maintain lifestyles not significantly different from those of their heterosexual male counterparts. Some research, however, does indicate high-risk behaviors in some groups of gay and bisexual men. For example, bisexual men have been shown to be less likely to use condoms and engage in safe sexual practices than either gay or heterosexual men, and approximately one third of men who have sex with men do so without protection (Scout & Robinson, 2000). High-risk behaviors in general seem to increase with younger age. For example, in one study, same-sex sexually active adolescents were nine times more likely than heterosexually active adolescents to report daily alcohol use, four times more likely to be heavy drinkers, more likely to use marijuana, six times more likely to use cocaine, and five times more likely to use other illicit drugs (Faulkner & Cranston, 1998).

No clearly established difference has been shown in the consumption patterns of gay men in general, especially with respect to substance abuse. Prior findings related to the levels of alcohol abuse among homosexuals may be a function of sampling bias when subjects are recruited from gay bars. Research does suggest, however, that drug use among gay and bisexual men is associated with high-risk sexual behaviors. In addition, there is some evidence that use of several drugs may speed HIV replication or result in immunosuppression in individuals with HIV infection. Some drugs such as 3, 4-methylenedioxymethamphetamine (MDMA or *ecstasy*) may also interact with other medications such as viagra and ritonavir (a drug used to treat HIV infection) (Silenzio, White, & Wolfe, 2000). Research also suggests that gay men may have higher rates of tobacco use than the general population. In one study, for example, 41.5% of gay adults smoked compared to just under 29% of the general male population (Silenzio & White, 2000b). In another study, 48% of gay men reported smoking (Stall, Greenwood, Acree, Paul, & Coates, 1999).

In terms of nursing assessment and client behavior, an important area for assessment involves sexual behaviors. It is beneficial to stress the rationale for seeking this information, emphasizing that the community nurse's concern is based solely in the client's health risks and needs. Factors to evaluate include patterns of sexual activity, sexual exposure, and knowledge of sex-related risks and safety procedures. Bisexual men with female spouses may be even more concerned with privacy and confidentiality issues in order to maintain their concurrent heterosexual relationships; this may require significant amounts of reassurance and empathy from the nurse.

In spite of decreases in unsafe sexual practices among gay and bisexual men early in the course of the AIDS epidemic, there is growing evidence that some members of these groups are being less careful in their sexual practices. Minority men who have sex with men are contributing an increasing number of new cases of AIDS (52% in 1998 versus 31% in 1989) (National Center for HIV, STD, and TB Prevention, 2000). More gay and bisexual men are engaging in a practice called *barebacking*, which involves anal-receptive intercourse without the use of a condom. Much of the resumption of high-risk sexual behaviors by gay and bisexual men is related to the perceived effectiveness of current HIV therapy and the potential effectiveness of "morning after" treatment (Ungvarski & Grossman, 1999). In one study, 18% of gay and bisexual men were engaging in less safe sexual behaviors because of treatment advances (Scout & Robinson, 2000).

A high percentage of transgender men may engage in prostitution to pay for genital reassignment surgery. Because transgender prostitutes are stigmatized by both heterosexual and gay and lesbian prostitutes, they are often forced to take the least desirable customers who are least likely to agree to condom use. In addition, transgender individuals may resort to self-injecting hormones and engage in needle sharing, which increases their risk of HIV infection and hepatitis B (Sember, 2000).

Health System Considerations

Gay men may encounter homophobia among health care workers, and the perception of homophobia represents a significant barrier to health care. In a survey of members of the Gay and Lesbian Medical Association, 67% indicated seeing gay and lesbian clients receive substandard care based on their sexual orientation (White, Bradford, Silenzio, & Wolfe, 2000). Even when the health care provider, whether an individual or an institution, is devoid of homophobia, various circumstances may threaten the gay client and act as health barriers. For example, assessment questions about birth control practices, if answered truthfully, might have the effect of requiring that a client disclose his sexual identity. For the

client who fears loss of health care benefits (due to assumed higher risk of AIDS for all gay men), this is a situation to be avoided. Confidentiality issues may also prevent gay and bisexual men at risk for HIV infection from being tested (National Center for HIV, STD, and TB Prevention, 1999). Another problem in the current health care system is the lack of providers who are knowledgeable regarding the health care needs of gay, bisexual, and transgender clients. This lack is true among providers of mental health and other services as well. Inability to communicate effectively with gay, bisexual, and transgender clients may lead to inaccurate diagnoses and inappropriate treatment plans as well as impaired compliance with health-related recommendations (White, Bradford, & Silenzio, 2000). Some authors have identified the needs of providers who are caring for gay, bisexual, and transgender clients. These needs are summarized below.

HIGHLIGHTS

Provider Needs in the Care of Gay, Bisexual, and Transgender Clients

- Knowledge of high incidence conditions among gay, bisexual, and transgender clients
- Routine incorporation of harm reduction strategies in practice
- Awareness of the effects of societal homophobia and stigmatization on the health of gay, bisexual, and transgender clients
- Ability to create antihomophobic care environments
- Ability to assist gay, bisexual, and transgender clients to deal with stress
- Ability to distinguish between sexual identity and sexual behavior
- Ability to assist clients to decrease internalized homophobia
- Advocacy for health care policy to prohibit discrimination
- Research on the physical and mental health needs of gay, bisexual, and transgender clients
- Referral to and encouragement of the use of gay community support services
- Inclusion of significant others in treatment decisions
- Referral to other providers with greater expertise as needed

Source: Ungvarski, P. J., & Grossman, A. H. (1999). Health problems of gay and bisexual men. *Nursing Clinics of North America, 34,* 313–331.

Even when gay and bisexual men do receive treatment for existing health conditions, those treatments may create adverse effects. For example, there is some evidence that treatment of HIV infection with highly active anti-retroviral therapy (HAART), contributes to increased cholesterol levels, diabetes, and redistribution of body fat (lipodystrophy). Furthermore, saturation of some gay communities with less effective treatments early in the epidemic has led to the development of drug-resistant viruses. In fact, 16% of HIV-infected men in one study displayed resistance to one or more AIDS drugs. Perceptions of the availability of a "cure" for AIDS has also led to decreased funding of support services for those with the disease (Scout & Robinson, 2000).

⑥ THINK ABOUT IT

How might health care services be modified to better meet the needs of gay men?

The effects of the health care system on transgender men in the United States may be even more profound. Genital reassignment surgery is covered under national health insurance in the Netherlands, Great Britain, and Australia. In the United States, requests for coverage under Medicaid are addressed on an individual basis and are frequently not decided in favor of the client. The long-term effects of surgery have not been adequately studied although immediate responses to surgery have been almost uniformly favorable. Hormone therapy does, however, have some adverse side effects including a twentyfold increase in thromboembolism for men receiving estrogen, some reports of breast cancer, liver disease, increased risk for heart disease, increased blood pressure, sterility, mood changes, and a decreased sex drive, among others. For women receiving testosterone, side effects may include increased cholesterol and lipid levels, heart disease, mood changes, male pattern baldness, acne, and cessation of menses (Sember, 2000).

assessment tips assessment tips assessment tips

ASSESSING MEN'S HEALTH

Biophysical Considerations

- What is the man's age? Has he accomplished the developmental tasks relevant to his current and previous developmental stages? Has the man achieved sexual maturity?
- Does the man have any existing physical health problems? Is the man experiencing impotence or other sexual problems?

Psychological Considerations

- What is the extent of stress in the client's life? How has he been socialized to deal with stress? How effective are his coping strategies?
- Is the man depressed? Is he suicidal? Does the man have a history of mental illness? Does he exhibit current signs of mental illness? Signs of PTSD?

Physical Environmental Considerations

- Where does the man live? Is he exposed to safety or environmental health hazards?

Sociocultural Considerations

- How does the man deal with conflict? What is the quality of interpersonal interactions?
- Is the man a victim or perpetrator of family violence?
- What is the extent of the man's social support network?

- What effect do the man's education, occupation, and income have on his health?

Behavioral Considerations

- What are the man's typical behavior patterns? How do they affect health?
- Is the man sexually active? What is his sexual orientation? Is he comfortable with his sexual identity? Does he engage in unsafe sexual practices? Does he practice regular testicular self-examination?
- To what extent has the gay, bisexual, or transgender client disclosed his sexual identity? Is confidentiality a particularly important issue for him?

Health System Considerations

- How does the man define health? What is his attitude to health and health care? What is his usual source of health care? To what extent does he utilize health care services? Does he engage in preventive health care practices?
- How does the man finance health care?
- What is the reaction of health care providers to the gay, bisexual, or transgender client? How does this reaction influence attitudes toward and use of health care services?

DIAGNOSTIC REASONING IN THE CARE OF MEN

Community health nurses use data from their client and population assessments to identify health needs and determine appropriate nursing diagnoses. Nursing diagnoses for individual male clients may relate to educational deficits (e.g., "increased health risk due to lack of knowledge of testicular self-examination technique"), to barriers to health care utilization (e.g., "failure to cope with stress related to belief that men should not need help in coping"), to consequences of specific health problems (e.g., "pain due to overuse of strained ligaments," or "diminished self-esteem due to lost erectile function related to prostatectomy"). Nursing diagnoses may also relate to males as aggregates. For example, many young adult males living in poverty might suggest a diagnosis of "increased health risk related to socioeconomic pressures to participate in drug use and sales."

PLANNING AND IMPLEMENTING HEALTH CARE FOR MEN

Interventions to improve the health status of men in the population may occur at primary, secondary, or tertiary levels of prevention. The level of prevention chosen for community health nursing interventions depends on the status of health problems to be addressed.

Primary Prevention

Although it is difficult to generalize about male clients' attitudes toward health promotion activities, there are some commonly encountered patterns of health behavior among men. One such behavior is a tendency to view exercise as sufficient to compensate for unhealthy behaviors such as a high intake of fats in the diet. Men also tend to attribute greater significance to health changes they can sense than to those they cannot (e.g., they can sense pain but not elevated blood pressure). Because men tend to rate their health as very good or excellent more often than women, they may feel they do not need to be actively involved in health-promotion activities. They may also err in their health appraisal efforts, stemming from a tendency to believe that their past athletic or current work activities may provide for their present health needs ("When I was a teenager I would run all day." "I work hard all day in the fresh air. What could be healthier than that?")

One technique that can be used to promote positive behavioral change is *reframing,* which focuses on helping the client to see the same situation in a different light. A second technique for promoting change involves emphasizing alternate ways of coping with anxiety or fearfulness. Education, of course, is a crucial aspect of any primary prevention strategy. Education is perhaps most effective when teaching is initiated with school-age male youngsters, as this is the stage when lifelong health val-

ues and habits are forming. Health promotion by the client's family members is known to be a significant motivator and predictor of client compliance and outcomes, and involvement of family members in educational efforts and treatment planning is usually of significant benefit.

Primary prevention for health concerns specific to male clients focuses on increasing the client's use of health-promoting behaviors in the areas of cardiovascular and cerebrovascular disorders, hypertension, cancer, occupational disorders, substance abuse, violence and trauma, suicide, and PTSD.

⑥THINK ABOUT IT

What can nurses do to facilitate health-promoting behaviors among men?

Cardiovascular disorders involve education as a major primary prevention measure. Community health nurses provide education in home, school, or occupational settings, and emphasize knowledge of risk factors and preventive strategies. Nurses also emphasize methods to produce behavioral changes, recognizing that knowledge alone does not determine behavior. For example, most male clients *know* the importance of limiting fat-derived calories, but they fall short in being able to change their behavior because they lack understanding of their own behavioral dynamics (such as eating more when anxious).

Cerebrovascular disorders also involve education as a major preventive strategy. Community health nurses educate clients about the relationship between other health problems, such as hypertension and diabetes and cerebrovascular disease. They educate and motivate clients to maintain a weight and blood pressure appropriate to their age to control hypertension and minimize the risk of developing some forms of diabetes.

Hypertension can be minimized for many male clients by promoting a weight appropriate for the client's body build and by promoting regular exercise. A diet that excludes excessive sodium may have preventive value as well. For some clients, knowledge and use of stress management techniques such as stress compensators (relaxing walks, vacations) and relaxation techniques (progressive muscle relaxation, guided imagery) may assist in minimizing hypertensive changes. It is helpful to focus on the fact that the hypertensive client is typically asymptomatic, as this feature encourages denial and avoidance, which are common among male clients. Again, it is helpful to link efforts to control hypertension with the client's own values about health, such as invulnerability or physical activity. For example, the nurse could take advantage of the client's interest in sports by noting famous athletes with hypertension.

Primary prevention interventions for cancer include education regarding recognizing and limiting exposure to carcinogens in the workplace (such as chemicals and sunlight), around the home, or in the diet. The possibility of a link between stress and immune system function supports the promotion of effective stress management techniques. Lifestyle choices such as smoking and consuming large amounts of meat are believed to have a significant effect on an individual's risk of cancer. Ascribing healthy behaviors to masculine role images can increase cancer-preventive behaviors in male clients by tying such behaviors to male values such as strength and power. For example, a nurse could state, "Men do what makes them strong, not what makes them weak, and smoking weakens the body." It may also be helpful to reframe male clients' poor health habits as being the result of manipulation by advertisers (e.g., "I wonder whether eating all that meat might be because all your life the commercials have made eating meat seem like the right thing to do").

Primary prevention interventions for substance abuse focus on education at all age levels regarding the risks of substance abuse and on alternate means of coping with stress. Also important are efforts to assist males to redefine their social roles in healthier ways so that, for example, teenage males do not feel as compelled to drink or to behave as their peers might wish. In addition, community health nurses' activities that help reshape societal norms held by males, such as the anti-drinking publicity campaign undertaken by Mothers Against Drunk Driving, are also appropriate primary prevention measures.

Trauma and violence are complicated issues with many potential levels of nursing interventions. Primary interventions include educating male children on methods of coping with their feelings and countering social demands to take unnecessary risks or to participate in unhealthy behaviors. Teaching males nondestructive ways to express their feelings and initiating political activity on behalf of safety-related legislation (motorcycle helmet laws, enforcement of driving-under-the-influence statutes) are also appropriate as primary prevention interventions.

Important nursing interventions related to sexually abused male clients include educating key persons about the realities of male sexual abuse (schoolteachers, case managers, school nurses) and detecting families at risk. It is also important to facilitate referrals to treatment agencies specializing in sexual abuse of children or adults. Finally, although pairing male nurses with male clients for the purposes of providing care for issues involving male sexuality can be a very helpful strategy, this may not be the case with the child or adolescent male abuse victim, who may instead feel more secure working with a female nurse.

Primary prevention measures for suicide include helping a male client to avoid or cope with feelings of despair, hopelessness, or anger. Interventions that help a male avoid or cope with such feelings include role modeling, teaching disclosure of one's feelings, and prompting expression of a client's concerns through the use of empathy and acceptance. Also helpful are interventions designed to promote self-esteem and a positive self-image. Such interventions should begin with young males, prior even to school age. The community health nurse can promote the use of mental health resources that provide services to individuals or groups. Nurses can also educate families, children, workers, and other groups about the risk of suicide, factors that contribute to its occurrence, and appropriate ways to detect and respond to persons who are at increased risk of becoming suicidal. Males, especially those younger than 24 and over age 65, should be educated about their high degree of risk.

Posttraumatic stress disorder involves primary prevention of a more immediate sort—aiding the male victim to express his feelings about the traumatic experience in a supportive and accepting environment. By aiding the client to work through his feelings about the trauma rather than being overwhelmed by them, the community health nurse can prevent or minimize the severity of this disorder. Because PTSD is a complex psychological disorder, the community health nurse usually works in an adjunctive capacity with more expert or specialized providers within the mental health care system. Vietnam veterans with PTSD may benefit greatly from referral to peer-run "Vet Centers" and other support groups. A list of these is available from the Veterans Administration or local veterans organizations. Nurses should also understand that Vietnam vets with PTSD, and veterans in general, are distrustful of government-related providers. For this reason, a veteran may respond more favorably when the nurse relates to him as an individual rather than as an agent of a health care organization. A willingness to accept the veteran and a high level of trustworthiness are characteristics highly valued by Vietnam vets.

Primary prevention interventions for adolescents include aiding the adolescent to reevaluate images he holds regarding the male role, assisting the client to express his feelings through role modeling, teaching communication and social skills, conveying empathy and acceptance, and raising issues experienced by most male adolescents. Nurses can also intervene at the primary prevention level by promoting effective parent–child relationships via education about growth and development and communication skills, provided to both the client and his family.

Primary prevention measures for newly divorced men include referrals to peer support groups, encouragement of socialization and activities, and referral to mental health professionals when indicated (some mental health agencies sponsor special programs for newly divorced persons). It is also helpful for the community health nurse to provide support, assist the client to express his feelings, and guide him in coping with periods of crisis that may ensue.

For the gay or bisexual male client, providing education to increase the safety of sexual practices is an extremely important primary prevention measure. Community health nurses can perform a very valuable function by promoting safer sexual practices such as condom use and encouraging clients to reduce the number of sexual partners. These efforts are enhanced by conveying openness, showing acceptance of the client, and displaying an intent to address issues in a confidential and professional manner.

Immunization is another issue in health promotion with male clients. Adult men should receive immunization with tetanus and diphtheria toxoids every 10 years as well as varicella immunization if susceptible (Briss et al., 1999; USDHHS, 1998). Older men and those with chronic conditions should also receive influenza and pneumococcal vaccines. Hepatitis A and B immunizations are particularly important for gay, bisexual, and transgender men.

Secondary Prevention

Secondary prevention involves the earliest possible detection of health needs, using the assessment techniques described earlier in this chapter. It also encompasses the actual treatment of the health needs or disorders themselves. Secondary prevention roles for community health nurses working with male clients are appropriate for all disorders discussed in this chapter via special efforts to assess male clients in high-risk categories such as agricultural workers (trauma, skin cancer), teenagers (trauma, suicide, substance abuse), gay or bisexual males (AIDS), and those over age 50 (prostate cancer, cardiovascular disorders).

Community health nurses may also participate in health screening activities by providing or encouraging the client's use of such health measures as blood pressure screening and cardiovascular risk-assessment programs in public, educational, or occupational settings. Nurses can also facilitate the offering and use of screening examinations by other health care professionals within the community, such as rectal examinations and blood testing for prostate cancer and chest x-rays for lung cancer. Early detection of both prostate and testicular cancer is a very important area for secondary prevention by community health nurses.

One intervention that facilitates detection of testicular cancer is teaching the testicular self-examination (TSE) technique. Because testicular cancer occurs primarily in young men, the community health nurse can often educate and motivate clients efficiently (and minimize individual embarrassment in the process) by working with groups of males in school or work settings.

The TSE technique involves a gentle but thorough palpation of each testis, repeated monthly and akin to the procedure for breast self-examination. The male client should rotate each testis gently, moving his fingers so that all portions of the organ are palpated. He should feel uniform smoothness, without indentations, lumps, or

asymmetry within an individual testis. Abnormal findings, along with any other changes noted since the last TSE, should be promptly reported to the primary health care provider. It is helpful for the nurse to inform the client that it is normal for one testis to be larger than the other, and that the client may encounter other intrascrotal structures apart from the testes themselves, so that the client, for example, will not presume the epididymis is an abnormal finding. The ideal source of instruction for this technique would be direct guidance by a physician or nurse practitioner during a physical examination. Referrals to these providers are an appropriate form of secondary intervention.

Younger male clients may experience even more embarrassment about sexually related issues than their older counterparts, and significant attention to averting this embarrassment and anxiety is indicated. Humor may be a very helpful tool in that it is a common coping mechanism used by males in this age group for dealing with anxiety. Three-dimensional models, slides, and other teaching devices can be quite beneficial by giving the anxious male client something to focus on other than the (usually) opposite-sex nurse. Assignment of male nurses to this population may also reduce clients' hesitancy or embarrassment, as can creating an environment in which male clients can feel free to face and voice their fears about their own mortality.

The community health nurse is not usually directly involved in the detection and screening of prostate cancer. Detection is usually achieved by digital rectal examination or by ultrasound examination. In addition, blood screening for a prostate-specific antigen promises to be more effective than rectal screening alone at early identification of prostate cancer. Early detection of prostate cancer can also be aided by psychosocial nursing interventions. For example, education about the risk of this disorder among older males helps counter the denial experienced by many men (due to a need to perceive oneself as invulnerable, perhaps), and informing the client of the importance of annual digital rectal examinations increases health-promoting behavior. Many times, such teaching can be effectively enacted with male clients in work or social settings (e.g., a senior citizens' organization). It is important to stress the very positive prognosis that accompanies early detection to help motivate the client by compensating for the uncomfortable, but necessary, rectal examination.

Community health nurses do participate in the treatment of other illnesses experienced by male clients. In the case of ischemic and certain other cardiac disorders, for example, stress has been shown to impact negatively on treatment outcomes, in some cases leading to a threefold increase in mortality (e.g., in post–myocardial infarction clients). Treatment programs that identify high-stress clients during hospitalization, that track and reduce their stress levels after discharge, and that provide prompt assistance from nurses in the community when episodes of increased stress occur can result in significant reduction of the stress-related mortality experienced by post–myocardial infarction clients.

Prostatitis is another disorder with implications for secondary prevention by the community health nurse. Prostatitis is usually responsive to a regimen of antibiotics, and education about the nature of the disorder (particularly when sexually transmitted) and its treatment is the major area of nursing intervention. Because it is a personally intimate and uniquely male phenomenon, however, male clients are likely to exhibit embarrassment and avoidance. The nurse can manage this response pattern by being straightforward and matter-of-fact when discussing the issue and by noting that, although perhaps embarrassing, the disorder is not unlike having cystitis or other common infections. In effect, the nurse is using reframing. Interventions for prostatitis also apply to the rare case of epididymitis.

Benign prostatic hyperplasia (BPH) also involves the nurse at the secondary level of prevention. Here the nurse can educate the male client about his risk of developing this disorder, and by being straightforward and professional in demeanor, the nurse can reduce the client's embarrassment about assessment questions and examinations used to screen older male clients for this disorder. An important part of the detection process involves noting that rectal examination is essential for early detection of BPH as well as prostatic cancer. The nurse should instruct the client that, although this examination may not be pleasant, it serves a double purpose and is, therefore, doubly valuable. In terms of treatment, community health nurses may find themselves assisting the client with postoperative catheter care at home, and interventions to reduce embarrassment apply here as well.

Nurses can assist male clients with mild inguinal hernias to succeed in conservative treatment strategies and avert the need for surgery. One intervention involves education and encouragement to motivate the client's compliance with wearing supportive trusses, limiting exertion, and using proper body mechanics (to reduce straining and increased intra-abdominal pressure). Inguinal hernias involve both an intimate area of the body and an image of weakness rather than power. As a result, many men may delay treatment because of embarrassment or fear of surgery. Nurses can assist the client by helping him to overcome his embarrassment and reframing his interpretation of this disorder as a weakness. By being open and up front about this condition, the nurse can demonstrate that it does not require embarrassment, and in fact for many males is part of being a man. These interventions also promote compliance with conservative treatment approaches.

Tertiary Prevention

Tertiary prevention for male clients is directed at those disorders that influence the client in some ongoing manner or that have a likelihood of recurrence. The goals of tertiary prevention are to assist the client in coping with the continuing manifestations of his illness and to reduce the likelihood of future episodes of an illness. To this end, it is useful to group tertiary prevention measures into care directed toward those disorders that affect a male's sexual functioning or sexual identity or as they present a threat to notions about male strength. Tertiary prevention measures also would be directed at supporting a client's compliance with a long-term course of treatment.

One area for tertiary prevention measures by the community health nurse involves those disorders that affect the male client's sexual functioning or sexual identity, such as testicular and prostate cancers and any male reproductive system disorder. Male clients with testicular or prostate cancer may face significant emotional distress owing to the effect surgical treatment may have on their sexuality. Prostate cancer is treated by surgical removal of the gland in most instances. Although the prognosis is often excellent when discovered early, the surgery itself may result in impotence (though recent nerve-sparing surgical techniques have reduced this problem). Similarly, the treatment for testicular cancer is surgical removal of the affected testes followed by hormonal therapy. These treatments, along with their side effects (loss of fertility, emasculation), can have a profound impact on the client's self-image and psychosocial functioning.

An important area of tertiary prevention in this regard involves encouraging the male client to join support groups. Interaction with other men who have experienced the same problems can be very effective in facilitating the client's adjustment to a treatment that has so tangibly affected his sense of masculinity. On a one-to-one basis, the nurse can be accepting, supportive, and facilitative of the male client's expression of his feeling of loss.

Some disorders may affect the male client's sense of strength; this is particularly true of cardiovascular disorders. The heart is a symbol of masculine strength for some men. Consequently, cardiovascular disorders not only can leave residual symptoms and physiological impairment, but can also threaten a man's self-image. Men with cardiovascular disease often benefit from interventions that support their self-image as masculine and by discussing their feelings about their illness. As noted elsewhere, stress management training also can have a significant positive effect on the outcome of a male client who has cardiovascular disease. These interventions are essential to promote the client's adjustment and compliance with treatment.

Of course, community health nurses should also support and reinforce the male client's positive responses to cardiac rehabilitation efforts initiated in other treatment settings. Foremost among these would be weight control, limiting intake of saturated fats, maintaining regular exercise, compliance with follow-up examinations and medications, and control of other disorders that exacerbate cardiovascular disease (hypertension, diabetes).

In the case of some chronic disorders, especially those producing no overt symptoms, male clients tend to be lax about complying with long-term treatment recommendations. This is especially true for male clients with hypertension. Interventions that help the male client understand the importance of controlling this disorder and that build on his perceptions of masculinity are very helpful. Maintaining a regimen of antihypertensive medications may be especially difficult for male clients owing to side effects that interfere with what the client judges to be necessary masculine roles. Examples of such side effects could include impotence, dizziness, and decreased tolerance for physical activity. Nurses can assist the male client by teaching ways to compensate for these side effects, thereby helping him to maintain a sense of control over his own circumstances. In cases in which the side effects are not manageable and are affecting the client's masculinity (impotence), collaborating with the client's physician or assisting the client to discuss the problem with the physician can lead to acceptance of the treatment for hypertension.

Preventing recidivism, or rehospitalization, in instances of substance abuse is a major tertiary intervention in working with male clients. Interventions that decrease the likelihood of recidivism include encouragement of the client's use of therapeutic support groups (Alcoholics Anonymous) and education regarding factors that predispose the client to continued substance abuse (poor coping skills, co-dependent relationships, maintaining social contacts with abusers). It is also important for the community health nurse to consider the client's family and significant others when caring for the substance-

abusing male. Families and significant others can be either enablers of substance abuse or corrective forces leading to its elimination. Education of family and support persons as to those behaviors that produce improvement and those that permit further substance abuse is essential, and referrals to family treatment and support services are also of value. Links to resources that may be of assistance to community health nurses in planning health care for men are available on the companion Web site for this book. ◈

EVALUATING HEALTH CARE FOR MEN

As when working with other individual clients or aggregates, community health nursing plans and interventions are evaluated by determining the degree to which client goals have been met. It is also important to determine whether the interventions were efficient. Could the same results have been accomplished with less expense of time or other resources?

The community health nurse also needs to consider the client's reaction to nursing interventions. Is the client satisfied with the nurse's efforts and with the manner in which interventions were planned and implemented as well as with their results? The goal of evaluation is to ensure that client needs are met and to improve the nurse's abilities; inviting the critique of one's clients and colleagues is an excellent source of feedback.

HEALTHY PEOPLE 2010

GOALS FOR THE POPULATION

	Objective	Base	Target
2-3	Reduce the proportion of men with chronic joint symptoms who have difficulty in two or more personal care activities	1.6%	1.4%
2-11	Reduce activity limitation due to chronic back conditions (per 1,000 men)	31	25
3-1	Reduce cancer deaths (per 100,000 men)	258	158.7
3-2	Reduce lung cancer deaths (per 100,000 men)	81.6	44.8
3-7	Reduce prostate cancer deaths (per 100,000 men)	4.6	2.6
3-8	Reduce melanoma cancer deaths (per 100,000 men)	4.0	2.5
5-2	Prevent new cases of diabetes (per 1,000 men)	2.6	2.5
12-1	Reduce coronary heart disease deaths (per 100,000 men)	276	166
13-2	Reduce the number of AIDS cases among MSM	17,847	13,385
15-3	Reduce firearm related deaths (per 100,000 men)	21.4	4.9
15-32	Reduce homicides (per 100,000 men)	11.2	3.2
15-34	Reduce physical assault by intimate partners (per 1,000 men)	1.4	3.6

Source: U.S. Department of Health and Human Services. (2000). *Healthy people 2010* (Conference edition, in two volumes). Washington, DC: Author.

The effects of intervention at the aggregate level can be assessed in terms of the accomplishment of national health objectives. The current status of selected objectives related to men's health is presented on page 434. Information about objectives related to men's health is available on the Healthy People 2010 Web site, which may be accessed through links provided on the companion Web site for this book.

Men have a variety of health care needs that they may or may not acknowledge. Community health nurses can be actively involved in encouraging men to seek health care as needed. They may also provide direct services to male clients, particularly with respect to education for primary prevention.

APPLYING YOUR KNOWLEDGE IN PRACTICE

CASE STUDY
Caring for the Adolescent Male

You are a community health nurse working with a hypertensive, diabetic, middle-aged single mother for the past year. Her 17-year-old son has had hand surgery and has been added to your caseload for wound and cast care. On your next meeting with the mother, you discover that she is very upset about her son's behavior. He broke his hand when he punched a wall in a fit of anger, and the necessary care has hurt the family's very limited finances. The mother reports that she believes her son is drinking, and she is especially angry and upset about this because her ex-husband had deserted the family largely because of his own alcohol abuse. While the mother answers a phone call, you attempt to speak to the son. He seems wary but does concede he punches walls when angry. His view at present is that "It's no big deal—the cast will handle it." When asked about alcohol, he replies, "It's what we do . . . a little doesn't hurt anyone." When you begin to address the risks involved in this behav-

ior, he cuts you off by angrily retorting, "It's none of your damn business! Get lost and leave me alone!"

- What psychological and sociocultural dimension factors may be influencing the son's behavior? Are these typical or atypical of men in general? Of adolescent boys?
- What actual and potential health issues are raised by the lifestyle of the son and his past and present family situation?
- What primary interventions are indicated for the health risks present in the son?
- What secondary interventions are indicated for the health concerns affecting the son?
- How should the nurse respond to the client's denial and anger?
- How might the nurse's interventions be evaluated?

TESTING YOUR UNDERSTANDING

- What are the major considerations in assessing the biophysical, psychological, physical environmental, sociocultural, behavioral, and health system factors influencing men's health? (pp. 414–423)
- What are some of the factors that contribute to adverse health effects for gay, bisexual, and transgender men? (pp. 423–429)
- Identify at least four areas for primary prevention with male clients. How might the community health nurse be involved in each? (pp. 430–432)

- What are the major secondary prevention considerations for male clients. Give an example of at least one community health nursing intervention related to each consideration. (pp. 432–433)
- Identify areas of emphasis in tertiary prevention for male clients. How might the community health nurse be involved in each? In what kinds of situations might tertiary prevention be required? (pp. 433–434)

REFERENCES

Barret, R. L., & Robinson, B. E. (2000). *Gay fathers: Encouraging the hearts of gay dads and their families.* San Francisco: Jossey-Bass.

Barry, M. J., Fowler, F. J., Bin, L., Pitts, J. C., Harris, C. J., & Mulley, A. G. (1997). The natural history of patients with benign prostatic hyperplasia as diagnosed by North American urologists. *Journal of Urology, 157,* 10–15.

Briss, P. A., Carande-Kulis, V. G., Bernier, R. R., Ndiaye, S. M., et al. (1999). Vaccine-preventable diseases: Improving vaccination coverage in children, adolescents, and adults. *Morbidity and Mortality Weekly Report, 48*(RR-8), 1–15.

Cochran, S. D., & Mays, V. M. (2000). Lifetime prevalence of suicide symptoms and affective disorders among men reporting same-sex sexual partners: Results from NHANES III. *American Journal of Public Health, 90,* 573–578.

Collins, K. S., Schoen, C., Joseph, S., Duchon, L., et al. (1999). *Health concerns across a woman's lifespan: The Commonwealth Fund 1998 survey of women's health.* New York: The Commonwealth Fund.

Copenhaver, M. M., & Eisler, R. M. (1996). Masculine gender role stress: A perspective on men's health. In P. M. Kato & T. Mann (Eds.), *Handbook of diversity issues in health psychology* (pp. 219–235). New York: Plenum Press.

Dean, L., & Bradford, J. (2000). Violence and sexual assault. In Gay and Lesbian Medical Association & Center for Lesbian, Gay, Bisexual, and Transgender Health (Eds.), *Lesbian, gay, bisexual, and transgender health: Findings and concerns* (pp. 29–32). New York: Author.

Faulkner, A. H., & Cranston, K. (1998). Correlates of same-sex sexual behavior in a random sample of Massachusetts high school students. *American Journal of Public Health, 88,* 262–266.

Gotsch, K. E., Annest, J. L., Mercy, J. A., & Ryan, G. W. (2001). Surveillance for fatal and nonfatal firearm-related injuries—United States, 1993–1998. *Morbidity and Mortality Weekly Report, 50*(SS-2), 1–34.

Helgeson, V. S. (1995). Masculinity, men's roles, and coronary heart disease. In D. Sabo & D. F. Gordon (Eds.), *Men's health and illness: Gender, power, and the body* (pp. 68–104). Thousand Oaks, CA: Sage.

Kelley, L. S., Buckwalter, K. C., & Maas, M. L. (1999). Access to health care resources for family care givers of elderly persons with dementia. *Nursing Outlook, 47,* 8–14.

Lilly Center for Women's Health. (1998). *Women's health: Issues and trends.* Indianapolis, IN: Author.

Mann, T. (1996). Why do we need a health psychology of gender or sexual orientation? In P. M. Kato & T. Mann (Eds.), *Handbook of diversity issues in health psychology* (pp. 187–198). New York: Plenum Press.

Meyer, I., & Bowen, D. (2000). Lesbian, gay and bisexual health concerns: Cancer. In Gay and Lesbian Medical Association & Center for Lesbian, Gay, Bisexual, and Transgender Health (Eds.), *Lesbian, gay, bisexual, and transgender health: Findings and concerns* (pp. 15–17). New York: Author.

Meyer, I., Rothblum, E., & Bradford, J. (2000). Mental health and mental disorders. In Gay and Lesbian Medical Association & Center for Lesbian, Gay, Bisexual, and Transgender Health (Eds.), *Lesbian, gay, bisexual, and transgender health: Findings and concerns* (pp. 21–26). New York: Author.

Meyer, I., Silenzio, V., Wolfe, D., & Dunn, P. (2000). Introduction/background. In Gay and Lesbian Medical Association & Center for Lesbian, Gay, Bisexual, and Transgender Health (Eds.), *Lesbian, gay, bisexual, and transgender health: Findings and concerns* (pp. 4–9). New York: Author.

Murray, S. O. (2000). *Homosexualities.* Chicago: University of Chicago Press.

National Center for Chronic Disease Prevention and Health Promotion. (2001). Mortality from coronary heart disease and acute myocardial infarction—United States, 1998. *Morbidity and Mortality Weekly Report, 50,* 90–93.

National Center for Health Statistics. (2000). *Health, United States, 2000.* Washington, DC: Author.

National Center for HIV, STD, and TB Prevention. (2000). HIV/AIDS among racial/ethnic minority men who have sex with men—United States, 1989–1998. *Morbidity and Mortality Weekly Report, 49,* 4–11.

National Center for HIV, STD, and TB Prevention. (1999). Anonymous or confidential HIV counseling and voluntary testing in federally funded testing sites—United States, 1995–1997. *Morbidity and Mortality Weekly Report, 48,* 509–513.

National Institute for Occupational Health and Safety. (1997). *The effects of workplace hazards on male reproductive health.* Retrieved April 30, 2001, from the World Wide Web, http://www.cdc.gov/niosh/malerepro.

Neufeld, A., & Harrison, M. J. (1998). Men as caregivers: Reciprocal relationships or obligation? *Journal of Advanced Nursing, 28,* 959–968.

Owens, R. E. Jr. (1998). *Queer kids: The challenges and promise for lesbian, gay, and bisexual youth.* New York: Haworth.

Polych, C., & Sabo, D. (1995). Gender politics, pain, and illness: The AIDS epidemic in North American prisons. In D. Sabo & D. F. Gordon (Eds.), *Men's health and illness: Gender, power, and the body* (pp. 139–157). Thousand Oaks, CA: Sage.

Remafedi, F., French, S., Story, M., Resnick, M. D., & Blum, R. (1998). The relationship between suicide risk and sexual orientation: Results of a population based study. *American Journal of Public Health, 88,* 57–60.

Scout, & Robinson, K. (2000). HIV/AIDS. In Gay and Lesbian Medical Association & Center for Lesbian, Gay, Bisexual, and Transgender Health (Eds.), *Lesbian, gay, bisexual, and transgender health: Findings and concerns* (pp. 18–20). New York: Author.

Sell, R. (2000). Methodological challenges to studying lesbian, gay, bisexual, and transgender health. In Gay and Lesbian Medical Association & Center for Lesbian, Gay, Bisexual, and Transgender Health (Eds.), *Lesbian, gay, bisexual, and transgender health:*

Findings and concerns (pp. 43–47). New York: Author.

Sember, R. (2000). Transgender health concerns. In Gay and Lesbian Medical Association & Center for Lesbian, Gay, Bisexual, and Transgender Health (Eds.), *Lesbian, gay, bisexual, and transgender health: Findings and concerns* (pp. 32–43). New York: Author.

Silenzio, I. (2000). Immunization and infectious diseases. In Gay and Lesbian Medical Association & Center for Lesbian, Gay, Bisexual, and Transgender Health (Eds.), *Lesbian, gay, bisexual, and transgender health: Findings and concerns* (p. 21). New York: Author.

Silenzio, I., & White, J. (2000a). Sexually transmitted diseases. In Gay and Lesbian Medical Association & Center for Lesbian, Gay, Bisexual, and Transgender Health (Eds.), *Lesbian, gay, bisexual, and transgender health: Findings and concerns* (pp. 26–27). New York: Author.

Silenzio, I., & White, J. (2000b). Tobacco use. In Gay and Lesbian Medical Association & Center for Lesbian, Gay, Bisexual, and Transgender Health (Eds.), *Lesbian, gay, bisexual, and transgender health: Findings and concerns* (p. 29). New York: Author.

Silenzio, I. White, J., & Wolfe, D. (2000). Substance abuse. In Gay and Lesbian Medical Association & Center for Lesbian, Gay, Bisexual, and Transgender Health (Eds.), *Lesbian, gay, bisexual, and transgender health: Findings and concerns* (pp. 27–29). New York: Author.

Singleton, J. A., Greby, S. M., Wooten, K. G., Walker, F. J., & Strikas, R. (2000). Influenza, pneumococcal, and tetanus toxoid vaccination of adults—United States, 1993–1997. *Morbidity and Mortality Weekly Report, 49*(SS-9), 39–62.

Stall, R. D., Greenwood, G. L., Acree, M., Paul, J., & Coates, T. J. (1999). Cigarette smoking among gay and bisexual men. *American Journal of Public Health, 89,* 1875–1878.

Taylor, B. (1999). "Coming out" as a life transition: Homosexual identity formation and its implications for health care practice. *Journal of Advanced Nursing, 30,* 520–525.

Teel, C. S., & Press, A. N. (1999). Fatigue among elders in caregiving and noncaregiving roles. *Western Journal of Nursing Research, 21,* 498–520.

Ungvarski, P. J., & Grossman, A. H. (1999). Health problems of gay and bisexual men. *Nursing Clinics of North America, 34,* 313–331.

U.S. Census Bureau. (1999). *Statistical abstract of the United States, 1999* (119th ed.). Washington, DC: Author.

U.S. Department of Health and Human Services. (1998). Clinical preventive services for normal-risk adults. *Prevention Report, 13*(1), 11.

U.S. Department of Health and Human Services. (2000). *Healthy people 2010* (Conference edition, in two volumes). Washington, DC: Author.

White, J., Bradford, J., & Silenzio, V. (2000). Health communication. In Gay and Lesbian Medical Association & Center for Lesbian, Gay, Bisexual, and Transgender Health (Eds.), *Lesbian, gay, bisexual, and transgender health: Findings and concerns* (pp. 11–13). New York: Author.

White, J., Bradford, J., Silenzio, V., & Wolfe, D. (2000). Access to quality health services. In Gay and Lesbian Medical Association & Center for Lesbian, Gay, Bisexual, and

Transgender Health (Eds.), *Lesbian, gay, bisexual, and transgender health: Findings and concerns* (pp. 10–12). New York: Author.

White, P. G., Young, K., & McTeer, W. G. (1995). Sport, masculinity, and the injured body. In D. Sabo & D. F. Gordon (Eds.),

Men's health and illness: Gender, power, and the body (pp. 158–182). Thousand Oaks, CA: Sage.

By 2020, the elderly population throughout the world is expected to increase by 240%, and by that time it is anticipated that three fourths of deaths annually will be related to aging (International Council of Nurses [ICN], 1999). This same level of growth in the older population is occurring in the United States. In 1998, nearly 7% of the U.S. population was 65 to 74 years of age, while 4.4% were aged 75 to 84 years and another 1.5% were over 85 years of age. By 2050, people over 65 years of age are expected to comprise 20% of the U.S. population (nearly 9% aged 65 to 74 years, 7% 75 to 74 years of age, and another 4.6% over the age of 85 years) (U.S. Census Bureau, 1999). These figures amount to an unprecedented 400% increase in the proportion of people over 85 years of age (Tullman & Chang, 1999).

In part, the growth in the elderly as a percentage of the population is due to a lower birth rate and fewer young persons than in previous years. Another major contributing factor is increased longevity. Improvements in medical treatment and the use of advanced medical technologies to sustain life have resulted in a life expectancy of 73.6 years for U.S. men and 79.2 years for women. Projected life expectancy by 2010 is 74.1 years for men and 80.6 years for women (U.S. Census Bureau, 1999). Although life expectancy has increased, the quality of life for the elderly is often questionable. In working with older adults, individually or as an aggregate, community health nurses must be concerned with quality-of-life concerns as well as longevity.

This emphasis on quality of life can be seen in the focus of the national health objectives for 2010 addressing the health needs of the elderly. A major thread throughout these objectives is to reduce activity limitations that impair the quality of life for older persons (U.S. Department of Health and Human Services [USDHHS], 2000). These objectives can be viewed on the Healthy People 2010 Web site, which can be accessed through a link on the companion Web site for this book. A growing body of research has indicated that many consequences of the aging process are not inevitable, and efforts are needed to mitigate these consequences (Blackman, Kamimoto, & Smith, 1999).

Concern for the growing number of elderly in the population arises from the strain expected on the health care system of the aging of the "baby boomer" generation (those born between 1945 and 1955). In 1997, people over the age of 65 years accounted for 38% of hospital admissions with an average length of stay of 6.5 days compared to 5.5 days for younger people (Kovner & Harrington, 2000). The elderly also account for 30% of all health care expenditures in the United States (Zhan, Cloutterbuck, Keshian, & Lombardi, 1998). It is expected that by 2020 health care for the elderly will consume approximately 10% of the gross domestic product (GDP), more than twice that in 1995 (4.3%). Anticipated annual expenditures by 2020 will amount to $25,000 per elderly person, compared to only $9,200 in 1995 (Fuchs, 1999).

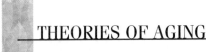

THEORIES OF AGING

Aging and circumventing aging are topics that fascinated humankind long before Ponce de Leon's search for the fountain of youth. Science cannot fully explain why aging occurs, but several theories have been advanced to explain the process. These theories tend to fall into four categories: stochastic, genetic, psychological, and sociological theories.

Stochastic Theories

Stochastic theories of aging are based on the assumption that the cumulative effects of environmental assaults eventually become incompatible with life. One of these theories, the *somatic mutation theory*, holds that prolonged exposure to background radiation of several types results in cell mutations that eventually lead to death (Ebersole & Hess, 1998).

The *error theory*, a second stochastic theory, is based on the belief that environmental changes interfere with cell function and protein synthesis, thus causing errors in reproduced cells. These errors multiply in a geometric progression until cells are no longer viable (Ebersole & Hess, 1998).

Genetic Theories

Genetic theories of aging are based on the assumption that aging is a part of the developmental process, with differences in that process genetically programmed from conception. *Neuroendocrine theory* holds that aging is the result of functional decrements in neurons and their hormones (Ebersole & Hess, 1998). In one version of this theory, for example, changes in the hypothalamic–pituitary system, over time, lead to changes in other body systems, possibly due to diminished responsiveness of neuroendocrine tissue to various signals.

Intrinsic mutagenesis theory holds that each person has a genetic constitution that regulates the replication of genetic materials. Over time, regulatory activity diminishes, creating mutations in cells that result in the effects of aging.

Immunologic theory holds that aging is an autoimmune process. As cells change with age, the body's immunological mechanisms perceive them as foreign bodies and destroy them. Finally, the *free radical theory* of aging is based on the belief that most physiologic changes of aging are due to damage caused by the action of free radicals, which are highly chemically reactive byproducts of metabolism. Generally speaking, these free radicals are rapidly destroyed by protective enzyme systems. Over time, however, it is believed that those radicals not destroyed accumulate to cause cell damage (Ebersole & Hess, 1998). Despite the stochastic and genetic theories of aging and related research, the physiologic processes involved in aging and the variability of aging among individuals remain unexplained.

Psychological Theories

A number of theories have also been advanced to explain the psychological aspects of aging. Jungian *psychoanalytic theory* regards aging as a time of developing self-awareness through reflective activity. Harry Stack Sullivan's *interpersonal theory* is developmental in nature. Maturity, in this theory, involves the development of satisfactory interpersonal relationships. The loss of these relationships over time is believed to result in a loss of interpersonal security and the consequent psychological aspects of aging.

In Abraham Maslow's *human needs theory*, physical aging and environmental changes contribute to difficulty in meeting basic human needs. These difficulties contribute, in turn, to the psychological effects sometimes seen with age. The greater the difficulty in meeting basic needs, the greater the impact of aging (Maslow, 1968). Maslow arranged these human needs in a hierarchy:

Survival needs	Oxygen, food, water, sleep, sexual activity
Safety and security needs	Protection from physical hazards, emotional security
Love and belonging needs	Affection from others, ability to feel and express affection for others, group identification, companionship
Esteem and recognition needs	Sense of self-worth, recognition of accomplishments by others
Self-actualization needs	Achievement of personal potential
Aesthetic needs	Order, harmony, and achievement of spiritual goals

Finally, in Erik Erickson's *theory of psychosocial development*, the degree of success experienced in accomplishing the developmental tasks in stages 1 through 7, as summarized below, influences the accomplishment of the tasks of the older adult in stage 8 (Erickson, 1963).

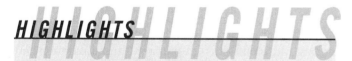

Erickson's Developmental Stages

Stage 1: Trust versus mistrust	Focuses on developing a sense of trust in oneself and others
Stage 2: Autonomy versus shame and doubt	Focuses on the ability to express oneself and cooperate with others
Stage 3: Initiative versus guilt	Focuses on purposeful behavior and the ability to evaluate one's own behavior
Stage 4: Industry versus inferiority	Focuses on developing belief in one's own abilities
Stage 5: Identity versus role confusion	Focuses on developing a clear sense of self and plans to actualize one's abilities
Stage 6: Intimacy versus isolation	Focuses on developing one's capacity for reciprocal love relationships
Stage 7: Generativity versus stagnation	Focuses on creativity and productivity and developing the capacity to care for others
Stage 8: Ego identity versus despair	Focuses on acceptance of one's life as worthwhile and unique

Sociological Theories

Sociological theories have also been advanced to explain the effects of aging. From the perspective of *disengagement theory*, the older person recognizes death as inevitable and so begins a process of withdrawal from society that permits the individual to enjoy old age and to prepare for death without causing social disruption when death occurs. The process may actually work in reverse, however, with society disengaging from and isolating older individuals as a result of *ageism*, which is prejudice or discrimination based on chronological age or appearance of age (Tullman & Chang, 1999).

Activity theory, on the other hand, posits continued engagement with society and the assumption of new roles and responsibilities by the older person. According to *continuity theory*, one's behavior becomes more predictable with age (Ebersole & Hess, 1998). For instance, the conservative person becomes more conservative and the adventurous person becomes more adventurous. Also, a change occurs in roles and relationships as the older adult becomes more concerned with introspection and self-reflection.

None of the theoretical perspectives presented completely explains the aging process and its effects, and,

CULTURAL CONSIDERATIONS

Ageism is primarily a product of the culture of Western industrialized nations. What other facets of culture do you think lead to ageism? What attitudes to the elderly are prevalent in other cultural groups? Why do you think these groups hold the attitudes to the elderly that they do?

■ **TABLE 19–1   Selected Theories of Aging**

PERSPECTIVE	THEORY	DESCRIPTION OF THEORY
Stochastic	Somatic mutation theory	Cumulative exposures to background radiation cause cell mutations incompatible with life.
	Error theory	Aging is the cumulative effects of errors in cell reproduction.
Genetic	Neuroendocrine theory	Aging is due to the effects of diminished response of neuroendocrine tissue to stimuli.
	Intrinsic mutagenesis theory	Genetic regulatory activity diminishes over time, resulting in cell mutations that eventually lead to cell death.
	Immunologic theory	Aging is an autoimmune process.
	Free radical theory	Aging is due to the accumulation of free radicals, by-products of cell metabolism, that interfere with cell function.
Psychological	Psychoanalytic theory	Aging leads to a focus on introspection and self-reflection.
	Interpersonal theory	The psychological effects of aging are due to the loss of satisfactory interpersonal relationships and consequent loss of interpersonal security.
	Human needs theory	Difficulty in meeting basic human needs results in the psychological effects of aging.
	Theory of psychosocial development	The degree of success achieved in developmental tasks in earlier stages affects one's response to aging.
Sociological	Disengagement theory	Recognizing death as inevitable, the older person begins to separate from society to provide for continuity of the social order.
	Activity theory	Interaction with society continues with assumption of new roles and responsibilities.
	Continuity theory	Previous personality traits become more pronounced with age and behavior becomes more predictable.

although nurses need a theory base for gerontologic nursing practice, it may be advisable to adopt more than one theory in working with older persons. Nurses must assess the individual needs of each client and select a theoretical perspective that best fits those needs. Theories of aging are summarized in Table 19–1 ■.

⑥THINK ABOUT IT

Which theory of aging do you think best explains the aging process? Why?

MYTHS AND REALITIES OF AGING

Aging is a normal human phenomenon. Although much research has been conducted recently on the aging process, aging itself remains a mystery surrounded by myths. Among the myths surrounding aging are beliefs that aging is a time of tranquility and that aging is syn-

onymous with senility. For many older adults, however, aging is a time of increased problems and decreased resources for dealing with those problems. Moreover, senility is not an inevitable consequence of aging. Many older persons retain their mental faculties well beyond the ninth decade of life.

Another myth is that old age is a time of reduced productivity. This is misleading. Many older adults remain productive throughout life. Societal factors, however, may limit opportunities for older adults to demonstrate their productivity. For example, many older adults are forced to retire at a specific age despite continued abilities to perform their jobs capably. Continued productivity among older persons is seen among those who do continue to work as well as among those who channel their energies into other areas after retirement. Retirees may continue to contribute to society through volunteer activities, artistic endeavors, or other pursuits.

⑥THINK ABOUT IT

In what ways, if any, does the saying "You can't teach an old dog new tricks" apply to the care of older clients?

Older persons are also thought by many to be resistant to change—again, a myth. Resistance to change tends to be a lifelong characteristic, not one developed with advancing age. Persons who have been relatively resistant to change throughout life will probably continue to resist change in their older years, whereas those who have welcomed change will probably continue to do so.

Finally, that aging is purely a matter of chronology, a uniform process that progresses at the same rate and with the same results for all, is a myth. The truth is that aging affects each individual differently, and the outcomes of aging may be very different from one individual to another. Myths of aging and related realities are summarized below.

- Older individuals are less productive then when they were young.
- Older people resist change.

- Aging is a uniform process.

- Many older individuals continue to be productive, although the manner of productivity may change.
- Older people are no more likely to resist change than younger people.
- Aging is a variable process.

The physical changes that occur, with variable speed and intensity, are additional realities of aging. These changes have the potential to cause health problems for older clients. Physical changes related to aging and their implications for health are summarized in Table 19–2 ■.

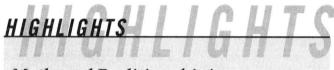

HIGHLIGHTS

Myths and Realities of Aging

Myth	Reality
• Aging is a time of tranquility.	• For many older clients, aging may be a time of increasing problems and diminishing resources.
• Senility is a universal experience with aging.	• Many older clients retain their mental faculties until death at advanced ages.

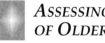

ASSESSING THE HEALTH OF OLDER CLIENTS

Effective nursing care for older clients requires an accurate assessment of the individual client's health status. At the aggregate level, it requires assessment of factors affecting the health status of the older population. Biophysical, psychological, physical environmental, sociocultural, behavioral, and health system factors may influence the health of older individuals and of the aged population. Consequently, the community health nurse

■ **TABLE 19–2 Common Physical Changes of Aging and Their Implications for Health**

SYSTEM AFFECTED	CHANGES NOTED	IMPLICATIONS FOR HEALTH
Integumentary system		
Skin	Decreased turgor, sclerosis, and loss of subcutaneous fat, leading to wrinkles	Lowered self-esteem
	Increased pigmentation, cherry angiomas	
	Cool to touch, dry	Itching, risk of injury, insomnia
	Decreased perspiration	Hyperthermia, heatstroke
Hair	Thins, decreased pigmentation	Lowered self-esteem
Nails	Thickened, ridges, decreased rate of growth	Difficulty trimming nails, potential for injury
Cardiovascular system	Less efficient pump action and lower cardiac reserves	Decreased physical ability, fatigue with exertion
	Thickening of vessel walls, replacement of muscle fiber with collagen	Elevated blood pressure, varicosities, venous stasis, pressure sores
	Pulse pressure up to 100	
	Arrhythmias and murmurs	
	Dilated abdominal aorta	
Respiratory system	Decreased elasticity of alveolar sacs, skeletal changes of chest	Decreased gas exchange, decreased physical ability
	Slower mucus transport, decreased cough strength, dysphagia	Increased potential for infection or aspiration
	Postnasal drip	

(continued)

■ **TABLE 19-2** Common Physical Changes of Aging and Their Implications for Health *(continued)*

SYSTEM AFFECTED	CHANGES NOTED	IMPLICATIONS FOR HEALTH
Gastrointestinal system	Wearing down of teeth	Difficulty chewing
	Decreased saliva production	Dry mouth, difficulty digesting starches
	Loss of taste buds	Decreased appetite, malnutrition
	Muscle atrophy of cheeks, tongue, etc.	Difficulty chewing, slower to eat
	Thinned esophageal wall	Feeling of fullness, heartburn after meals
	Decreased peristalsis	Constipation
	Decreased hydrochloric acid and stomach enzyme production	Pernicious anemia, frequent eructation
	Decreased lip size, sagging abdomen	Change in self-concept
	Atrophied gums	Poorly fitting dentures, difficulty chewing, potential for mouth ulcers, loss of remaining teeth
	Decreased bowel sounds	Potential for misdiagnosis
	Fissures in tongue	
	Increased or decreased liver size (2–3 cm below costal border)	Potential for misdiagnosis
Urinary system	Decreased number of nephrons and decreased ability to concentrate urine	Nocturia, increased potential for falls
Reproductive system		
Female	Atrophied ovaries, uterus	Ovarian cysts
	Atrophy of external genitalia, pendulous breasts, small flat nipple, decreased public hair	Lower self-esteem
	Scant vaginal secretions	Dyspareunia
	Vaginal mucosa thinned and friable	
Male	Decreased size of penis and testes, decreased pubic hair, pendulous scrotum	Lowered self-esteem
	Enlarged prostate	Difficulty urinating, incontinence
Musculoskeletal system	Decreased muscle size and tone	Decreased physical ability
	Decreased range of motion in joints, affecting gait, posture, balance, and flexibility	Increased risk of falls, decreased mobility
	Kyphosis	Lowered self-esteem
	Joint instability	Increased risk of falls, injury
	Straight thoracic spine	
	Breakdown of chondrocytes in joint cartilage	Osteoarthritis, joint pain, reduced abilities for activities of daily living
	Osteoporosis	Increased risk of fracture
Neurological system	Diminished hearing, vision, touch, and increased reaction time	Increased risk for injury, social isolation
	Diminished pupil size, peripheral vision, adaptation, accommodation	
	Diminished sense of smell, taste	Decreased appetite, malnutrition
	Decreased balance	Increased risk of injury
	Decreased pain sensation	Increased risk of injury
	Decreased ability to problem solve	Difficulty adjusting to new situations
	Diminished deep tendon reflexes	
	Decreased sphincter tone	Incontinence (fecal or urinary)
	Diminished short-term memory	Forgetfulness
Endocrine		
Thyroid	Irregular, fibrous changes	
Female	Decreased estrogen and progesterone production	Osteoporosis, menopause
Male	Decreased testosterone production	Fatigue, weight loss, decreased libido, impotence, lowered self-esteem, depression

explores factors in each of these six dimensions of health at both the individual and aggregate levels.

In addition to the routine aspects of any client assessment, there are some special considerations in assessing older clients. These considerations are summarized on page 445. Nurses need to differentiate normal effects of the aging process from evidence of pathology. Inaccurately attributing health problems to aging, by clients or health care providers, may lead to delays in obtaining needed care. Some of the common physical effects of the aging process that must be differentiated from organic disease are listed in Table 19–2. Additional physiologic effects of aging are reflected in changes in normal values for a variety of laboratory tests. For example, older clients may exhibit lower hematocrit and hemoglobin levels and higher blood glucose levels than younger people. Typical values for selected laboratory procedures are presented in Table 19–3 ■.

HIGHLIGHTS

General Considerations in Assessing Older Adults

- The normal effects of aging must be differentiated from pathology.

- Normal effects of aging are constantly being redefined.
- Normal laboratory values and other findings may differ between younger and older adults.
- Older clients may exhibit atypical signs and symptoms of illness.
- Older clients may exhibit a decreased tolerance for stress.
- Strengths that result from an older client's life experiences may provide a basis for health interventions.
- Loss is a persistent theme in the lives of older adults.
- Older clients usually exhibit multiple health problems that have complex interactions.
- Older clients may underreport symptoms of illness.
- Older clients may have multiple, nonspecific complaints that require explication.
- Older clients may have difficulty communicating their health needs.

■ **TABLE 19–3** **Changes in Normal Laboratory Values in Older Clients**

TEST	YOUNG ADULT NORMAL	OLDER ADULT NORMAL
Urine		
Specific gravity	1.003–1.030	1.016–1.022
Blood		
Hemoglobin	*Men:* 13–17 g/dL *Women:* 12–15 g/dL	10–17 g/dL
Leukocytes	4.0–10.0 x10³/mm³	*Men:* 4.25–14.0 x10³/mm³ Women: 3.1–12.0 x10³/mm³
Lymphocytes	26–36%	11–48%
Platelets	25,000–500,000	*Men:* 330,000–1,430,000 *Women:* 255,000–1,392,000
Serum albumin	3.3–5.0 g/dL	3.2–4.5 g/dL
Serum globulin	2.3–3.5 g/dL	*Men:* 3.1–3.4 g/dL *Women:* 2.8–3.4 g/dL
Glucose	60–110 mg/dL	*Men:* 52–135 mg/dL *Women:* 58–135 mg/dL
Protein	6.0–8.2 g/dL	6.0–7.8 g/dL
Sodium	136–145 mEq/L	*Men:* 134–147 mEq/L *Women:* 135–145 mEq/L
Potassium	3.5–5.5 mEq/L	*Men:* 3.5–5.6 mEq/L *Women:* 3.5–5.2 mEq/L
Blood urea nitrogen (BUN)	4–22 mg/dL	8–18 mg/dL
Creatinine	0.7–1.5 mg/dL	*Men:* 0.6–1.2 mg/dL *Women:* No change
Triglycerides	40–150 mg/100 mL	20–200 mg/100 mL
Cholesterol	120–220 mg/100 mL	*Men:* Decreases after age 50 *Women:* Increases from age 50–70, then decreases
Lactate dehydrogenase (LDH)	60–220 IU/L	71–207 IU/L
Serum glutamic transaminase (SGOT)	0–41 IU/L	8–33 IU/mL

Sources: Kennedy-Malone, L. Fletcher, K. R., & Plank, L. M. (2000). *Management guidelines for gerontological nurse practitioners.* Philadelphia: Davis; and Treseler, K. M. (1995). *Clinical laboratory and diagnostic tests: Significance and nursing implications* (3rd ed.). Norwalk, CT: Appleton & Lange.

In assessing older clients, community health nurses must also keep in mind that illnesses may present with atypical symptoms and that dysfunction in one organ system may exacerbate existing problems in another. Particular signs that should lead the community health nurse to suspect illness in elderly clients include cognitive changes or agitation, loss of bladder control, changes in dietary patterns, changes in activity or energy levels, and recurrent falls.

Because longevity may contribute to a variety of life experiences that increase resilience and coping abilities, the community health nurse should expect to find strengths as well as problems when assessing older clients. Longevity also means that most older clients have experienced a variety of losses (health, social roles, loved ones). Consequently, the nurse must consider the persistent theme of loss and the extent of the older client's ability to adjust to the losses experienced.

Considerations related to older clients' communication may also influence assessment of their health status. For example, older people tend to underreport symptoms of illness or may describe vague or nonspecific symptoms. Therefore, the community health nurse needs to be particularly thorough in the review of systems with an older client and will elicit specific information about symptomatology. In addition, the multiple concerns commonly voiced by older clients may make it difficult for the nurse to sort out relevant information and to complete a comprehensive assessment. Finally, older clients may have difficulty with the actual process of communication due to sensory or other neurologic deficits. In that case, the nurse may need to find alternate means of obtaining assessment data (e.g., a 20-question, yes–no approach or obtaining information from family members).

Biophysical Considerations

Biophysical factors that influence the health of older clients or populations include those related to maturation and aging and physiologic function.

Maturation and Aging

As noted earlier, aging affects the function of all body systems. Many of the changes brought about by the aging process are contributing factors in health problems frequently experienced by older persons, and community health nurses should assess the extent to which individual clients have experienced specific physiologic effects of aging.

Retirement and preparation for death are two other maturational issues that merit special attention. Retirement is an event avidly anticipated by many, but for some older clients retirement is a source of stress. Retirement has been found to result in changes in roles, relationships, self-esteem, use of time, and extent of social support (Rosenkoetter & Garris, 1998). For many older clients, these changes are positive, but for others they create problems that may influence health. Community health nurses should assess older clients' responses

to retirement and the presence of adverse effects on life and health. Nurses should also be aware of the extent of the retired population among the elderly in the community.

Preparing for death is a normal developmental task of the "old old" age group (people over age 85), but may be a significant issue for others with serious or terminal health conditions. In this area, the community health nurse considers the client's attitude toward death and acceptance of the inevitability of death, as well as the extent to which clients have put their affairs in order. Knowledge of the client's belief or nonbelief in an afterlife also enables the nurse to effectively assist clients with this task. Other issues that the nurse might explore with clients are provision of a durable power of attorney delegating to a significant other the power to make health-related decisions in the event of the client's incapacitation and the making of funeral arrangements. Care of terminally ill clients and their families will be addressed in more depth in the section on tertiary prevention.

Physiologic Function

In addition to assessing clients for commonly occurring age-related changes and their effects and developmental issues such as retirement and death, community health nurses should assess older clients for the presence of acute and chronic illnesses. At the aggregate level, nurses would obtain information on the incidence and prevalence of physical illnesses in the older population.

Although most older persons are in basically good health, 75% of those over 65 have one or more chronic conditions (Davis & Magilvy, 2000) that contribute to increased morbidity and mortality in this age group. In 1998, leading causes of death among persons over 65 years of age in the United States included: (a) heart disease, (b) cancer, (c) cerebrovascular disease, (d) chronic obstructive pulmonary disease (COPD), (e) pneumonia and influenza, (f) diabetes, (g) unintentional injury, (h) nephritis and related conditions, (i) Alzheimer's disease, and (j) septicemia. Worldwide health concerns among the elderly include confusion, immobility, sensory loss, nutrition, grief, depression, incontinence, mental illness, substance abuse, death and dying, and abuse (ICN, 1999).

Older persons in the United States have increased incidence and prevalence rates for a number of health conditions. For example, heart failure is the most frequent cause of hospitalization in older adults, and expenditures for hospitalization amount to $7.5 billion a year. Approximately one third to one half of readmissions for heart failure are preventable with adequate care (Blaha, Robinson, Pugh, Bryan, & Havens, 2000). Heart conditions affect far more U.S. men than women (394.8 per 100,000 men compared to 85.8 per 100,000 women in 1996). Women, on the other hand, have higher rates of hypertension (437 per 100,000 women) than men (271 per 100,000). Prevalence rates for arthritis are also high among persons over 65 years of age and increase with age (U.S. Census Bureau, 1999).

Cancer also affects the health of older clients. Older women, for example, have higher rates of breast cancer than younger ones, with half of all new cases diagnosed in women over 65 years of age (Fox, Stein, Sockloskie, & Ory, 2001). Similarly, prostate cancer, which occurs primarily in men over 50 years of age, is second only to lung cancer in male cancer mortality. More than 180,000 new diagnoses of prostate cancer and nearly 32,000 deaths were expected to occur in 2000 (National Center for Chronic Disease Prevention and Health Promotion, 2000). Community health nurses would assess individual clients for the existence of any of these diseases as well as for their effects on overall health. In addition, nurses would assess the incidence and prevalence of these conditions in the elderly population. Common health problems affecting the elderly are summarized below.

HIGHLIGHTS

Common Physical Health Problems Among Older Clients

Cardiovascular Problems
- Angina
- Atherosclerosis
- Congestive heart failure
- Hypertension
- Myocardial infarction

Gastrointestinal Problems
- Constipation
- Diverticulosis
- Fecal impaction
- Gallbladder disease
- Hemorrhoids
- Hiatal hernia

Hematopoietic Problems
- Anemia

Integumentary Problems
- Basal cell carcinoma
- Decubitus ulcers
- Herpes zoster infection
- Squamous cell carcinoma

Musculoskeletal Problems
- Arthritis
- Hip and other fractures
- Osteoporosis

Neurological Problems
- Alzheimer's disease
- Cerebrovascular accident
- Organic brain syndrome
- Parkinson's disease

Reproductive Problems—Female
- Breast cancer
- Cervical cancer
- Vaginitis

Reproductive Problems—Male
- Benign prostatic hyperplasia
- Impotence
- Prostatic cancer

Respiratory Problems
- Emphysema
- Influenza
- Pneumonia
- Tuberculosis

Urinary Problems
- Bladder cancer
- Incontinence
- Urinary tract infection

Assessment for the presence of acute and chronic conditions is best done using a systems approach. Nurses should keep in mind that, when assessing clients for signs of these conditions, symptomatology may differ markedly in younger and older persons. For example, older persons with pneumonia may not exhibit pain or fever, but only confusion and restlessness. Similarly, emphysema may present with weakness, weight loss, and loss of appetite.

Urinary incontinence is common among older adults. Incontinence may be either acute or chronic. Acute urinary incontinence is a short-term problem with a relatively sudden onset, whereas chronic incontinence is an ongoing problem. Causes of acute incontinence include urinary tract infections, fecal impaction or severe constipation, prostatic hypertrophy, and use of medications (e.g., diuretics, tranquilizers, sedatives). Chronic urinary incontinence may be categorized as stress incontinence, urge incontinence, overflow incontinence, or functional incontinence. *Stress incontinence* is involuntary loss of urine in response to pressure exerted on the bladder with coughing, laughing, and sneezing. *Urge incontinence* involves urine leakage accompanied by a sudden and severe urge to urinate. *Overflow incontinence* is involuntary loss of urine resulting from overdistension of the bladder and may be characterized by frequent or constant dribbling or manifestations of urge or stress incontinence. Finally, *functional incontinence* is incontinence due to organic problems existing outside the genitourinary system. Causes of functional incontinence may involve physiologic dysfunction such as neurological trauma or cognitive dysfunction as in organic brain syndrome. In addition to being distressing in itself, urinary incontinence is a risk factor for skin breakdown. Both incontinence and nocturia have been associated with fall-related injuries.

Reproductive system problems in older women include vaginitis with discharge or vaginal soreness and itching. Vaginal prolapse may also occur as evidenced by protrusion, low back pain, and pelvic pulling. Another problem that may occur as a result of scanty vaginal lubrication is dyspareunia, or painful intercourse.

Morbidity and mortality due to injuries and falls are also serious concerns among the elderly. In 1997, 17.2 of every 100 people over age 65 were injured (U.S. Census Bureau, 1999). From 1990 to 1997, an average 17 to 25 per 100,000 older people died as a result of motor vehicle accidents (Stevens et al., 1999). Many other injury deaths occurred as a result of falls. Approximately one third of all persons over 65 fall at least once in a given year, and half of these fall repeatedly (Resnick, 1999). Although only 10% of falls result in injury, falls are the leading cause of injury deaths in older age groups. Risk of mortality due to falls increases with age, and 70% of all fall deaths occur in people over 75 (National Center for Injury Prevention and Control, 2000a). Forty percent of falls among people in this age group result in hospitalizations (Resnick, 1999).

Older men are more likely than women to fall, and men are more likely to die as a result of a fall at all ages over 65 years. Women, on the other hand, are more likely to sustain a hip fracture as a result of a fall (Stevens et al., 1999). In 1996, 340,000 people over 65 years of age were hospitalized for hip fractures, 80% of them women. The incidence of hip fracture among women increased 23% from 1988 to 1996. Again, the risk of hip fracture increases with age, with women over 85 years of age at eight times the risk of women between 65 and 74 years of age (Stevens & Olson, 2000).

Only approximately one fourth of older persons who experience hip fractures will recover completely; another 50% will require the use of a cane, walker, or other assistive device. In addition to the suffering and disability experienced by individual clients, falls and resulting fractures contribute to extensive societal costs. Hip fractures cost more than $20 billion in the United States each year (Jech, 2000); by 2010 annual costs are expected to climb to more than $45 billion, reaching $240 billion per year by 2040 (National Center for Injury Prevention and Control, 2000b).

Risk factors for falls and fractures may be related to physical status, medication use, psychological or behavioral factors, or environmental conditions. Physical health factors include difficulties with gait or balance, muscle weakness, dementia, sensory impairments, osteoporosis, postmenopausal osteoporosis, osteoarthritis, illness, noc-

turia, and low body mass index. Medication use may contribute to postural hypotension, confusion, or other effects that enhance the risk of falling. Psychological and behavioral factors include fear of falling and lack of exercise. History of previous falls may make older clients hesitant to engage in physical activity, thereby diminishing muscle strength and increasing the potential for falling (Resnick, 1999). Environmental conditions include slippery surfaces, uneven floors, loose throw rugs and other objects that present trip hazards, poorly lighted hallways and staircases, and unstable furniture. Many of the factors in each of these categories can be eliminated or controlled, decreasing the potential for falls. Community health nurses should assess individual elderly clients for risks for injuries as well as for past injuries and their effects on health. They should also assess the prevalence of injury risk factors in the elderly population, the incidence of injuries in this group, and the aggregate effects of injury in terms of disability.

In addition to mortality and disease prevalence, disability is an area of concern in the elderly. More than one fourth of people aged 65 to 74 years in the United States have some functional limitations, rising to 43% in the 75- to 84-year-old age group and more than 60% of people over 85 years of age. More than one fourth of those over 85 years of age have limitations in activities of daily living (ADLs) and more than half experience limitations in instrumental activities of daily living. Furthermore, 18% of people over 70 years of age have visual impairments, 33% have hearing impairments, and nearly 9% experience both (Campbell, Crews, Moriarty, Zack, & Blackman, 1999). In 1994, 14 of every 1,000 people over 65 years of age used some form of assistive device, 99 per 1,000 people used hearing assistance, and 146.5 per 1,000 used a mobility device (cane, walker, etc.). In 1996, people over 65 years of age in the United States had an average of 12.6 days of bed disability per person (U.S. Census Bureau, 1999). All of these figures indicate the extent of disability among the elderly and the potential effects of disability on their quality of life.

Disabilities that can interfere with older clients' functional status are the last area for consideration in lifestyle assessment. *Functional status* is the ability to perform tasks and fulfill expected social roles. Assessment of functional status includes exploration of abilities at three levels of task complexity: basic, intermediate or instrumental, and advanced activities of daily living. *Basic activities of daily living (BADLs)* are personal care activities and include abilities to feed, bathe, and dress oneself, and toileting and transfer skills (getting in or out of a chair or bed). Intermediate or *instrumental activities of daily living (IADLs)* are tasks of moderate complexity, including household tasks such as shopping, laundry, cooking, and housekeeping, as well as abilities to take medications correctly, manage money, and use the telephone or public transportation. *Advanced activities of daily living (AADLs)* involve complex abilities to engage in voluntary social, occupational, or recreational activities.

Community health nurses should assess the degree of disability and functional limitation experienced by individual clients as well as the extent of disability present in the population. Potential questions for assessing functional status in terms of activities of daily living are presented below.

HIGHLIGHTS

Evaluating Activities of Daily Living

Basic Activities of Daily Living

Feeding
- Can the client feed him- or herself?
- Does the client have difficulty chewing?
- Does the client have difficulty swallowing?

Bathing
- Can the client get into or out of the bathtub or shower?
- Can the client manipulate soap and washcloth?
- Can the client wash his or her hair without assistance?
- Can the client effectively dry all body parts?

Dressing
- Can the client remember what articles of clothing should be put on first?
- Can the client dress him- or herself?
- Can the client bend and reach to put on shoes and stockings?
- Can the client manipulate buttons and zippers?
- Are modifications in clothing required to facilitate dressing (e.g., front-opening dresses)?
- Is arm and shoulder movement adequate to put on and remove sleeves?
- Can the client comb his or her hair?
- Can the client apply makeup if desired?

Toileting
- Is the client mobile enough to reach the bathroom?
- Is there urgency that may lead to incontinence?
- Can the client remove clothing in order to urinate or defecate?
- Can the client position him- or herself on or in front of the toilet?
- Can the client lift from a sitting position on the toilet?
- Is the client able to effectively clean him- or herself after urinating or defecating?
- Can the client replace clothing after urinating or defecating?

Transfer
- Is the client able to get from a lying to a sitting position unassisted?
- Is the client able to stand from a sitting position without support or assistance?
- Is the client able to sit or lie down without help?

Instrumental Activities of Daily Living

Shopping
- Is the client able to transport him- or herself to shopping facilities?
- Can the client navigate within a shopping facility?
- Can the client lift products from shelves?
- Can the client effectively handle money?
- Can the client carry purchases from store to car and from car to home?
- Is the client able to store purchases appropriately?

Laundry
- Can the client collect dirty clothes for washing?
- Is the client able to sort clothes to be washed from those to be dry cleaned?
- Can the client sort clothes by color?
- Can the client access laundry facilities?
- Can the client manipulate containers of soap, bleach, etc.?
- Can the client lift wet clothing from washer to dryer?
- Is the client able to hang or fold clean clothes as needed?
- Can the client put clean clothing in closets or drawers?

Cooking
- Is the client capable of planning well-balanced meals?
- Can the client safely operate kitchen utensils and appliances (e.g., stove, can opener, knives)?
- Can the client reach dishes, pots, and pans needed for cooking and serving food?
- Can the client clean vegetables and fruits, chop foods, etc.?
- Is the client able to carry prepared foods to the table?

Housekeeping
- Can the client identify the need for housecleaning chores (e.g., when the tub needs to be cleaned)?
- Is the client able to do light housekeeping (e.g., dusting, vacuuming, cleaning toilet)?
- Is the client able to do heavy chores (e.g., scrub floors, wash windows)
- Is the client able to do yard maintenance if needed?

Taking Medication
- Can the client remember to take medications as directed?
- Is the client able to open medication bottles?
- Can the client swallow oral medication, administer injections, etc., as needed?

(continued)

Managing Money
- Can the client effectively budget his or her income?
- Is the client able to write checks?
- Can the client balance a checking account?
- Can the client remember to pay bills when due and record payment?

Advanced Activities of Daily Living

Social Activity
- Does the client have a group of people with whom he or she can socialize?
- Is the client able to transport him- or herself to social events?
- Can the client see and hear well enough to interact socially with others?
- Does the client tire too easily to engage in social activities?
- Is social interaction impeded by fears of incontinence or embarrassment over financial difficulties?

Occupation
- Can the client carry out occupational responsibilities as needed?

Recreation
- Does the client have the physical strength and mobility to engage in desired recreational pursuits?
- Does the client have the financial resources to engage in desired recreational pursuits?
- Does the client have a group of people with whom to engage in recreation?
- Does the client have access to recreational activities (e.g., transportation)?

Some authors have suggested that assessments of functional abilities (e.g., abilities to perform ADLs and IADLs) are effective but alone may not be sufficient to accurately identify elders at risk for deterioration and rehospitalization. To increase the sensitivity of assessment, community health nurses can also assess physical performance tests such as the "chair stands" test, which is described below. Other measures of physical performance include tests of walking speed and standing balance (Bennett, 1999).

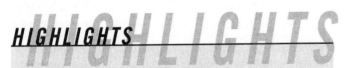

Conducting a "Chair Stands Test" of Physical Performance

Seat the client in a straight-back chair next to a wall. Ask the client to stand up from the chair with arms folded across his or her chest. If the client is able to do so, have him or her sit down and stand up again five times as

rapidly as possible. Score performance for five rise-and-sits only; if client cannot do five, score zero. Score the time from the initial sitting position to the final stand as follows: 4—less than 11.2 seconds, 3—11.2 to 13.6 seconds, 2—13.7 to 16.6 seconds, 1—greater than 16.6 seconds. Higher scores indicate greater lower body strength and endurance.

Source: Guralnik et al., cited in Bennett, J. A. (1999). Activities of daily living: Old fashioned or still useful? *Journal of Gerontological Nursing, 16*(5), 22–29. Reprinted with permission from Slack, Inc.

Another biophysical consideration affecting the health of older clients is infectious diseases. In 1996, the rate of infectious diseases among older people in the United States was 6.5 per 100 people, and 18% of those over 65 years of age developed influenza (U.S. Census Bureau, 1999). Influenza and pneumonia are particularly serious diseases in some older people. In 1996, for example, 90% of all deaths due to influenza occurred in people over 65 years of age (California Department of Health Services, 2000). In addition, tetanus appears to be more severe in older individuals with a greater risk of acute respiratory failure (Khajehdehi & Rezaian, 1998). All of these diseases are preventable with immunization, yet in the 1997 Behavioral Risk Factor Surveillance System (BRFSS) survey, a median of only 66% of people over 65 years of age in the reporting states had received influenza vaccine in the past year, and only 46% had ever received pneumonococcal vaccine (Janes et al., 1999). Similarly, in 1995, only 40% of older people reported having received a tetanus–diphtheria (Td) booster in the last 10 years (Singleton, Greby, Wooten, Walker, & Strikas, 2000). Reasons given for poor immunization rates included not knowing of the need for immunization, cost of or lack of access to immunization services, forgetting, concerns regarding potential vaccine effects, and failure of physicians to recommend vaccines or recommendations against vaccines by physicians (National Immunization Program, 1999). Community health nurses should assess older clients' immunization status as well as the presence of signs and symptoms of infectious diseases. In addition, they should assess immunization levels in this population and factors that impede effective immunization.

Psychological Considerations

Examination of factors in the psychological dimension includes assessing the individual client's psychological health status and related problems as well as the prevalence of such problems in the population. A psychological assessment involves considering the client's cognitive status, response to stress, affective status, and the potential for suicide.

Cognitive Assessment

In assessing the client's cognitive status, the nurse evaluates long- and short-term memory and orientation, powers of concentration and judgment, and ability to engage in mathematical calculations. Considerations in assessing cognitive status among older clients are presented below.

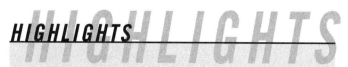

HIGHLIGHTS

Evaluating Cognitive Status

Attention Span

- Does the client focus on a single activity to completion?
- Does the client move from activity to activity without completing any?

Concentration

- Is the client able to answer questions without wandering from the topic?
- Does the client ignore irrelevant stimuli while focusing on a task?
- Is the client easily distracted from a subject or task by external stimuli?

Intelligence

- Does the client understand directions and explanations given in everyday language?
- Is the client able to perform basic mathematical calculations?

Judgment

- Does the client engage in action appropriate to the situation?
- Are client behaviors based on an awareness of environmental conditions and possible consequences of action?
- Are the client's plans and goals realistic?
- Can the client effectively budget income?
- Is the client safe driving a car?

Learning Ability

- Is the client able to retain instructions for a new activity?
- Can the client recall information provided?
- Is the client able to correctly demonstrate new skills?

Memory

- Is the client able to remember and describe recent events in some detail?
- Is the client able to describe events from the past in some detail?

Orientation

- Can the client identify him- or herself by name?
- Is the client aware of where he or she is?

- Does the client recognize the identity and function of those around them?
- Does the client know what day and time it is?
- Is the client able to separate past, present, and future?

Perception

- Are the client's responses appropriate to the situation?
- Does the client exhibit evidence of hallucinations or illusions?
- Are explanations of events consistent with the events themselves?
- Can the client reproduce simple figures?

Problem Solving

- Is the client able to recognize problems that need resolution?
- Can the client envision alternative solutions to a given problem?
- Can the client weigh alternative solutions and select one appropriate to the situation?
- Can the client describe activities needed to implement the solution?

Psychomotor Ability

- Does the client exhibit repetitive movements that interfere with function?

Reaction Time

- Does the client take an unusually long time to respond to questions or perform motor activities?
- Does the client respond to questions before the question is completed?

Social Intactness

- Are the client's interactions with others appropriate to the situation?
- Is the client able to describe behaviors appropriate and inappropriate to a given situation?

Loss of cognitive function is primarily due to dementia. *Dementia* is a loss of intellectual function in multiple domains including memory, problem solving ability, judgment, and others (Garand, Buckwalter, & Hall, 2000). Although more than 70 different conditions can cause dementia, 75% of dementia is the result of Alzheimer's disease. An estimated 5% to 10% of people over 65 years of age are affected by Alzheimer's disease, with the prevalence rising to 25% to 50% of people over age 85 (Boyd & Vernon, 1998). It is estimated that prevalence doubles for every five years of age beyond 65, and an additional 10% of older people may have milder forms of the disease that are not diagnosed (Hendrie, 1999). In 1997, there were an estimated 2.3 million people in the United States with Alzheimer's disease, and 68% of those were women. In the next 50 years, the prevalence of this conditions is expected to increase to 1 in every 45 older people (Brookmeyer, Gray, & Kawas, 1998). Worldwide prevalence is currently estimated at 20 million cases, but is expected to rise to 34 million by 2035, with approximately 2,000 new diagnoses each day between now and then (Haight, 2001).

Alzheimer's disease is a progressive disorder characterized by continuing decline in cognitive function, often accompanied by disruptive behavioral symptoms. Early stages are characterized by mild memory impairment, followed by geographic and temporal disorientation, difficulties with calculations and use of appliances, hesitancy in word finding, and decreased interest and initiative. Moderately severe disease involves short term-memory loss, difficulty with BADLs and IADLs, and behavior disturbances. In advanced disease, clients are chair-bound or bedfast, totally dependent, and have lost abilities to communicate and recognize others. They become mute and unresponsive, until, at last, they lose basic abilities such as swallowing (Boyd & Vernon, 1998).

Alzheimer's disease exacts a tremendous toll on the abilities of those it affects, the lives of their families, and society. Dementia accounts for 40% of functional dependence in the elderly (Aguero-Torres et al., 1998). Clients with Alzheimer's disease may exhibit pain from a variety of sources, including visceral, bone, and nerve pain and colic (Boyd & Vernon, 1998), and community health nurses should assess clients for nonverbal cues indicating pain. Nurses should also assess for disease effects in each of the three domains affected by Alzheimer's disease: behavior, cognition, and function. Assessment may be complicated, however, by the fact that many assessment measures depend on the cognitive abilities of the client. Community health nurses may need to rely on personal observation and information obtained from family members to get an accurate picture of the extent of disease effects.

Alzheimer's disease accounts for more than 7% of all deaths in the United States (Ewbank, 1999). Behavioral symptoms, which can occur at any time in the progression of the disease, are the leading cause of institutionalization (Garand et al., 2000). Financial costs are estimated at $58 billion per year, most of which is borne by the families of those affected. Family caregivers experience a variety of physical, emotional, and social problems as a result of their caregiving roles.

Response to Stress

There is considerable evidence that stress alters immune function. Age also causes declines in immune function and may increase susceptibility to illness. Research has suggested that depression causes greater immunologic impairment in older than in younger persons. In addition, the chronic stress of caregiving for family members with disabling conditions, particularly those with Alzheimer's disease, has been shown to adversely affect immune function. Declines in immune function have appeared to stabilize eventually, but do not return to prior levels immediately following the cessation of caregiving. There appears to be a dose-response phenomenon such that people exposed to greater stress have higher rates of respiratory diseases and those exposed to less stress have better response to immunizations (Robinson-Whelan, Kiecolt-Glaser, & Glaser, 2000).

Another source of stress is the presence and effects of chronic disability in one's life. Some authors have suggested that the degree of adverse response to disability may be a function of one's perceptions of control (Schulz, Heckhausen, & O'Brien, 2000). Chronic disease and disability affect control in multiple aspects of one's life, including functional abilities, occupation, and recreational pursuits. Community health nurses should assess the levels of stress experienced by individual clients, particularly elderly clients who are caring for disabled spouses or who experience disabilities themselves, as well as the health effects of stress.

Affective Assessment

Stress may contribute to affective changes in older clients. Considerations in the assessment of affective status include the presence of depression and saddened mood states. Depression and grief are commonly noted psychological problems among older adults. Information to be obtained in assessing clients for depression includes anniversary dates, recent changes in relationships, changes in physical health status or sleep patterns, fatigue, guilt, social isolation, alterations in mood or behavior, depressive symptoms such as depressed affect and apathy, history of depression, and recent losses or crises. Depression in the elderly may manifest in one of several forms: apathy, worry and agitation, somatization, or paranoia and resentment of others for failing to help. Assessment of depression is addressed in more depth in Chapter 30.

It is particularly important for the nurse working with older clients to distinguish depression from signs of delirium. Delirium usually has a rapid onset and is characterized by limited attention span and ability to concentrate, disorganized thinking, diminished consciousness, disorientation, increased or decreased psychomotor activity, or perceptual difficulties (e.g., hallucinations). Potential causes of delirium include adverse or toxic effects of medications, infection (e.g., urinary tract infection), electrolyte imbalance, small strokes, poor oxygenation, myocardial infarction, increased or decreased blood sugar levels, or hypotension. Delirium is usually reversible once the cause is eliminated, but may pose a medical emergency and requires prompt referral for treatment.

It is also important to keep in mind that sensory deficits may interfere with the assessment of psychological status and that such deficits must be compensated for to obtain an accurate assessment. To compensate for sensory deficits, the nurse should face the client, eliminate background noise, provide good lighting, speak clearly and slowly, and keep questions short.

The nurse should also try to reduce the client's anxiety, as this may interfere with obtaining an accurate picture of the client's abilities. The nurse can help to reduce anxiety by establishing rapport, explaining the purpose of the psychological evaluation, providing privacy, and limiting distractions. Other factors that may affect a psychological assessment include the client's use of medications, communication impairments, ethnic and cultural differences, and language barriers. Nurses may want to validate their findings regarding an older client's psychological status with family members to be sure that findings are consistent with typical behavior and not the product of the present situation.

Suicide Potential

Depression, in the extreme, may lead to suicide. Suicide rates are higher for older persons in the United States than for any other age group, and they increased 16% from 1990 to 1996 (Stevens et al., 1999). In 1998, the overall suicide mortality rate for persons over 65 years of age was 16.9 per 100,000 people. Suicide rates are nearly seven times higher for older men than for women in the same age group (National Center for Health Statistics, 2000). Community health nurses should assess older clients for suicide risk and obtain information on suicide rates in their local population. Assessment of suicide risk is addressed in more detail in Chapter 32.

Physical Environmental Considerations

Physical environmental concerns with older clients include the adequacy of housing, the existence of safety hazards in the home or community, the availability of necessary goods and services, and the effects of adverse weather conditions. The community health nurse assesses the adequacy of living conditions to meet clients' needs. For example, do living arrangements provide adequate space? Is there provision for privacy for the older person? Are living quarters adequately heated and ventilated? The nurse would also note whether there are adequate facilities for food storage and preparation.

A major concern in the assessment of the older client's physical environment is the presence of safety hazards. The community health nurse notes the presence of stairs, rugs, or other objects that might lead to falls and injuries. The nurse also assesses the adequacy of lighting and the presence or absence of tub rails and other safety features. Because of poor circulation, many older clients frequently feel cold and may use space heaters or kerosene stoves that present safety hazards. (See the Home Safety Inventory—Older Person, available on the companion Web site for this book.) 🔊

The neighborhood is another area of concern. Are fire and police services adequate to meet the needs of older clients? Is the neighborhood safe? Is transportation available if needed? Does the older person have access to shopping facilities and health care providers within a reasonable distance?

Both heat and cold have more profound effects on elderly persons than on younger ones due to changes in heat-regulating mechanisms that occur with aging. For example, 61% of heat-related deaths from 1979 to 1996 occurred in people over 55 years of age and half occurred in people over 65 (National Center for Environmental Health, 1999). Given recent energy prices, older persons on fixed incomes may have significantly more difficulty heating or cooling their homes than in the past. In areas of extreme temperatures, community health nurses should assess the extent of difficulty that older individuals may have in these areas as well as the availability of community support for subsidized energy services.

Sociocultural Considerations

Areas for consideration in assessing social and cultural factors influencing the health of older clients include social support, family roles and responsibilities, employment and economics, and potential for abuse.

Social Support

Nurses assess individual clients' social networks and the extent of available social support. A *social network* is the

Older adults may have poor nutritional intake.

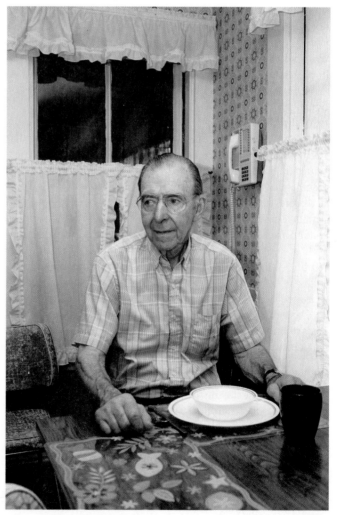

web of social relationships within which one interacts with other people and from which one receives social support. Social support includes emotional, instrumental, or financial assistance that the client receives from the social network.

In assessing the client's social network, the community health nurse identifies those persons with whom the client has frequent contact and whom the client feels able to call on for assistance. The nurse also explores with the client the types and adequacy of support available from members of the social network.

Family Roles and Responsibilities

Although 32% of the elderly in the United States live alone (Tullman & Chang, 1999), many others continue to live as part of family households. Family roles and responsibilities are other sociocultural dimension factors that may influence the health of older clients. As noted earlier, marriage has something of a health-protective effect, which is stronger for men than for women. Marital status has also been negatively associated with the potential for falls, possibly due to having the assistance of another person with daily activities (Resnick, 1999).

Marriage and other family roles may entail significant caretaking responsibilities for older clients. For example, 11% of U.S. grandparents have assumed primary responsibilities for the care of grandchildren for a minimum of six months, with most reporting this role over a longer period of time. Caretakers of grandchildren have been found to have higher rates of depression, poverty, and social isolation than noncaretakers. They also tend to have more difficulty with four out of five ADLs and have a 50% greater chance of ADL limitations than noncaretakers (Minkler & Fuller-Thomson, 1999).

As noted earlier, family caretakers bear most of the responsibility for care of disabled family members, particularly family members with Alzheimer's disease. Most often, such care becomes the responsibility of an elderly husband or wife, who may, themselves, experience significant disability due to chronic disease. It is estimated that more than 25 million family members provide $194 billion worth of care, and 80% of the care provided to functionally dependent and cognitively impaired individuals is uncompensated (Reinhard, Rosswurm, & Robinson, 2000).

Care of family members may be undertaken from a perspective of duty and obligation or on the basis of anticipated reciprocity. Caregivers frequently express difficulties in knowing what care to provide, how to provide it, and resources available to assist them. In some studies, as many as 59% of caregivers reported receiving no instruction in the care activities required of them, and it is possible that a significant portion of abuse of disabled elderly persons is a function of lack of knowledge rather than intent (Kelley, Buckwalter, & Maas, 1999). Informal caregivers also consistently exhibit diminished health status themselves and report such problems as increased fatigue, lack of energy, and

sleep problems (Teel & Press, 1999), as well as neglect of personal health needs.

The informal care network is jeopardized by a number of societal changes, the foremost among them being the increasing presence of women in the workforce, lower birth rates, and increase in mobility of family members (Hayes, 1999). Each of these changes decreases the availability of family members for assuming caretaking roles for older clients. In 1997, for example, 64% of those caring for frail elderly family members were employed, and 25% of these people provided personal care to elders. Approximately 10% of caregivers are forced to quit work, while another 11% take leaves of absence (usually unpaid). A further 7% reduced the number of hours worked. When caretaker responsibilities are heavy, as many as 30% of caretakers quit work (Lechner & Neal, 1999). While all of these strategies free up time for caretaking responsibilities, they also decrease the incomes of families that may already be constrained by the expenses entailed in chronic illness. Community health nurses should assess the burden of caregiving for older clients among family members, particularly when caretakers are themselves aged. Health and social effects of care giving should also be assessed. At the aggregate level, nurses should become aware of the extent of caretaker responsibilities among the older population as well as the availability of support programs for these caretakers.

Employment and Economic Factors

Economic and employment issues may also profoundly affect the health of older adults. In 1997, more than 4 million families in which the head of household was over 65 years of age had annual incomes under $10,000, and another 3.5 million had incomes of $15,000. Individual income in this age group may be even more reduced, with 495,000 men and more than five times as many women receiving annual incomes under $5,000. Overall, approximately 10% of the elderly in 1997 had incomes below poverty level, with figures even worse for minority elderly (26% of African American elderly and 24% of Hispanic elderly) (U.S. Census Bureau, 1999). Reduced income leads to decreased access to health care as well as reduced ability to provide for necessities such as nutrition and housing.

The elderly are more financially vulnerable than other segments of the population for several reasons. Many older clients are without health insurance, in spite of the Medicare program, and may not be able to afford the cost of health care for catastrophic or chronic conditions. In 1997, for example, approximately 1% of the population over 65 years of age had no health insurance coverage, and 11% of Medicare recipients reported delaying medical care because of cost (Janes et al., 1999). Older clients also tend to have fixed incomes that do not allow for increases in the cost of living, particularly increased housing costs. In addition, many older persons lack the financial assets to support long-term care if needed. Finally, the Social Security benefits received by many older clients are inadequate for meeting their needs but make them ineligible for many other forms of financial assistance. In one study, nearly 50% of minority women and 13% of white women with disabilities reported financial difficulties getting food (Klesges et al., 2001). Another effect of poverty among the elderly is a growing rate of homelessness in older age groups.

The community health nurse should assess the adequacy of the client's income for meeting basic needs as well as special needs arising from specific health conditions (e.g., the ability to pay for prescription medications). The nurse can also assess clients' abilities to budget their money and prioritize expenditures. At the aggregate level, the nurse should assess the extent of poverty and economic difficulties among the elderly population.

Another aspect of the sociocultural dimension to be addressed is occupation. Although many older clients will be retired, many more are continuing employment at later ages than was previously the case. For example, in 1997, 3.8 million older Americans (12% of those over age 65 years) were working or seeking work, and 34% of those 60 to 69 years of age were working. In recent surveys, a significant number of baby boomers planned to continue working into the retirement years. Nearly one fourth of those surveyed plan to continue work due to need rather than interest (Lewis, 1998). This aging of the workforce has implications for occupational injury incidence, which tends to increase with age. For example, nearly 7% of workers aged 55 to 64 years have some type of impairment that limits their ability to work safely. Vision and hearing impairments particularly increase the risk of injury (Zwerling et al., 1998). Community health nurses should assess the number of working elderly in the population as well as the occupational status of individual clients and any attendant health risks.

Abuse

The final social factors to be assessed in relation to the health of older clients are violence and evidence of or potential for abuse. Homicide, although not as frequent among the elderly as in other age groups, does occur. In 1998, for example, the homicide rate among those 65 years and over was 2.6 per 100,000 people (National Center for Health Statistics, 2000), with men twice as likely as women to be killed (Stevens et al., 1999).

Abuse of the elderly also occurs with some frequency. Estimates of the extent of abuse range from 820,000 to 1.8 million cases per year, or 4% to 10% of the U.S. population over the age of 65 years. Types of abuse perpetrated against the elderly include physical and sexual assault; physical, medical, or emotional neglect; financial or material exploitation; violation of personal rights; and abandonment. Potential causes of abuse include increasing socialization to violence in society, resentment by caregivers, family conflict, economic factors, ageism, and abrasive personality characteristics of the older person (Hogstel & Curry, 1999). Abuse of the elderly is addressed in greater detail in Chapter 32.

Behavioral Considerations

Considerations to be addressed in the behavioral dimension include diet; physical activity; personal habits, including medication use; and sexuality.

Diet

With respect to diet, the nurse should assess eating patterns and the adequacy of nutritional intake. Overall nutritional status, as well as intake of specific nutrients, is an important consideration. Both underweight and overweight increase mortality risks.

Although the prevalence of overweight decreases with age, many older clients have significant nutritional deficiencies. For example, only one third of those 65 years of age or older eat the recommended five or more fruits and vegetables a day (Kamimoto, Easton, Maurice, Hustin, & Macera, 1999). Similarly, only 28% of people over 60 years of age eat six or more servings of grains, and only 27% of women and 35% of men over 50 years of age consume the recommended amounts of calcium daily. Overconsumption of some nutrients is also a problem. For instance, from 1994 to 1996, only 34% of those over 60 obtained less than 30% of their calories as fat (USDHHS, 2000). The nurse should also evaluate compliance with specific dietary recommendations. Many clients need to restrict sodium intake or increase calcium. The older client with diabetes may or may not comply with a diabetic diet. Particular attention should be given to the amount of fluid and fiber in the diet.

Nurses should also explore with clients how foods are prepared and by whom. Many older clients have inadequate diets because they are not physically able to prepare some foods. Other problems impeding nutrition include lack of adequate cooking facilities, difficulties in chewing or swallowing, and poor dietary habits throughout life. In addition to assessing dietary intake, therefore, the nurse needs to identify factors contributing to poor nutritional status.

Physical Activity

The extent of physical activity among older persons is another lifestyle factor addressed in a comprehensive assessment. In the combined 1994 and 1996 Behavioral Risk Factor Surveillance System (BRFSS) surveys, the percentage of people who engaged in no leisure time physical activity ranged from 21% to 58% in various states, with a median of 35% for people aged 65 to 74 years. Among those 75 years of age or older, the prevalence of physical inactivity was even higher, ranging from 26% to 68% with a median of 46% (Kamimoto et al., 1999). Many older clients mistakenly believe that their need for exercise diminishes with age. Others may limit their physical activity due to hearing or visual impairment or other physical disabilities, lack of access to opportunities for exercise, or lack of support for participation in activity programs. Lack of exercise, however, has been associated with many of the physiologic changes experienced by the elderly as well as the development of specific health problems (Shin, 1999). Research has shown that moderate to high levels of recreational activity in the elderly are associated with decreased mortality and maintenance of functional status. Furthermore, exercise has actually resulted in improved coordination, gait, balance, and flexibility (Grove & Spier, 1999) and decreased potential for falls (Resnick, 1999). Again, the nurse should assess not only the extent of exercise but also factors that impede adequate exercise such as pain, fatigue, and weakness.

Personal Habits

One of the consequences of most chronic illnesses is the need for prolonged use of medication. Consequently, community health nurses assessing older clients with chronic illnesses need to assess medication use carefully. People over 65 years of age use 33% of all prescriptions filled in the United States, and as many as 25% of these prescriptions may be inappropriate (Whitelaw & Warden, 1999). A large majority of the noninstitutionalized elderly use an average of two to three prescription drugs daily in addition to a variety of over-the-counter medications. The number and the variety of drugs increase the potential for drug toxicity and drug interactions.

Nurses need to assess older clients to determine what medications they take, when and how these medications are taken, and the client's knowledge of side effects and signs of toxicity. Nurses should also explore with clients their use of nonprescription drugs and acquaint them with those that are contraindicated by their health status or because of other medications they are taking. Clients should also be assessed for signs of side effects or toxicity. Potential questions for assessing medication use in older clients are provided below left. Several drugs that pose health hazards for older clients are presented in Table 19–4 ■.

Nurses should determine the extent to which clients engage in other personal habits such as smoking, drinking, and caffeine consumption as well as the extent of motivation to change such habits. Nonsmoking and

HIGHLIGHTS

Evaluating Medication Use in Older Clients

- Is the client taking prescribed medications?
- Is the client taking over-the-counter (OTC) medications?
- Are any of the client's medications contraindicated by existing health conditions?
- Do OTC medications potentiate or counteract prescription medications?
- Do prescription medications potentiate or counteract each other?
- Does the client take prescription and OTC medications as directed (e.g., correct dose, route, time)?
- Does the client comply with other directions regarding medications (e.g., not taking with dairy products)?
- Is the client aware of potential food–drug interactions or drug–drug interactions?
- Are medications achieving the desired effects?
- Is the client experiencing any medication side effects?
- What is the client doing about medication side effects, if any?
- Is the client exhibiting symptoms of any adverse medication effects?

■ TABLE 19–4 Inappropriate Drugs for Older Clients

ANALGESICS/NSAIDS
Indomethacin (Indocin)
Pentazocine (Talwin)
Phenylbutazone (Butazolidin)
Propoxyphene (Darvon, Darvocet)

ANTIANXIETY AGENTS
Chlordiazepoxide (Librium)
Diazepam (Valium)
Flurazepam (Dalmane)
Meprobamate (Equanil, Miltown)
Pentobarbital (Nembutal)
Secobarbital (Seconal)

ANTIDEPRESSANTS
Amitriptyline (Elavil, Triavil, Etrafon)
Doxepin (Sinequan)
Imipramine (Tofranil)
Nortriptyline (Pamelor, Aventyl)

ANTIEMETICS
Trimethobenzamide (Tigan)

ANTIHYPERTENSIVES
Propranolol (Inderal)
Methyldopa (Aldomet, Amodopa, Dopamet)
Reserpine (Novoreserpine)

ANTISPASMODICS
Cyclobenzaprine (Flexeril)
Methocarbamol (Robaxin)
Carisprodol (Soma)
Orphenadrine (Banflex, Norflex, Neocyten)

HYPOGLYCEMICS
Chlorpropamide (Diabinese)

VASODILATORS
Dipyridamole (Persantine)

moderate alcohol intake are two factors found to be highly predictive of healthy aging. Despite the evidence that nonsmoking promotes health, 13% of people aged 65 to 74 years and nearly 7% of those over 75 years of age smoke (Kamimoto et al., 1999). In addition to the cardiac and respiratory effects of tobacco use, smoking has been found to increase the risk of hip fracture when falls occur. In fact, the risk for fracture among lean women who smoke is four to five times that of nonsmokers (Forsen et al., 1998).

Alcohol abuse is one more concern that may be identified in the elderly population. Both alcohol abuse and abuse of other drugs occur in two forms in the elderly population: prior abusers who are aging and older adults who seek escape from loneliness, depression, and social isolation. Because of metabolic changes, detoxification of alcohol, as well as other substances, is slowed, making the older person increasingly susceptible to the toxic effects of alcohol. Older individuals may also take a number of medications that interact with alcohol, thus increasing the dangers of abuse. Alcohol contributes to deleterious effects on a number of body systems that may already be impaired by age and chronic disease. For example, a definite dose-response relationship exists between the amount of alcohol ingested and blood pressure. For the client who is already hypertensive, alcohol abuse compounds the problem and impedes hypertension control.

Sexuality

The meeting of sexual needs is another important, but often overlooked, component of the assessment of social function. Older clients continue to have sexual needs. These may be fulfilled by a spouse if the couple is afforded the privacy necessary for sexual activity. For example, if older parents live with their children, their opportunities for sexual intimacy may be somewhat limited. The same may be true of older people in institutional settings. For clients who have no living spouse or whose spouse is unable to meet these needs, alternative methods of meeting sexual needs include masturbation and fantasizing.

Because most older people grew up in an era when sexuality was not a topic for discussion, they may find it difficult to talk about such needs with the nurse. Before addressing intimate issues, the nurse should first develop a rapport with the client. The nurse should also assure clients that sexual problems are not uncommon. For the older male client, the nurse should be aware that many of the medications taken for chronic illnesses, especially antihypertensives, may cause impotence.

Nurses should assess clients for problems with sexuality and identify any underlying factors. Nurses should also explore clients' satisfaction with their sex life. Another consideration in assessing this area is the potential for exposure to sexually transmitted diseases. Sexually transmitted diseases (STDs), including HIV infection, are a growing problem among older clients, and commu-

nity health nurses should assess for signs and symptoms of disease as well as risk factors for STD in individual clients and in the overall population of elderly persons. Nurses should also assess the environment of the older person to see whether it is conducive to sexual intimacy if this is desired. Finally, nurses should be aware of the potential for sexual abuse of older clients, particularly in institutional settings.

Health System Considerations

Health system dimension factors also influence the health of older clients. The advent of the Medicare program has improved elderly clients' access to health care services. Only 1% of the U.S. population over 65 years of age are not covered by any form of health insurance (U.S. Census Bureau, 1999), and, according to 1997 BRFSS data, 90% of people over 55 years of age have a regular source of health care. In spite of this level of coverage, however, only 75% to 80% of people in this age group had received a routine checkup in the past two years. Other preventive services were similarly lacking. For example, less than three fourths of older women had received a mammogram in the previous two years, and only 58% of women over 75 years of age had had a Papanicolaou smear. Similarly, only one fourth received testing for fecal occult blood. The percentage receiving blood pressure monitoring and cholesterol checks was somewhat higher at 95% and 85 to 88% of persons over 65 years of age, respectively (Janes et al., 1999). As noted earlier, immunization levels are not as high as desired among older persons, and some clients remain unimmunized on the recommendation of health care providers.

The health care system has other effects on the health of older clients as well. For example, provider emphasis on the risk of falls may increase fear of falling in older clients, encouraging them to reduce physical activity and putting themselves at greater risk of falls and injuries (Resnick, 1999). Similarly, the failure of the health care system to reimburse nursing services related to health promotion and education of both clients and caretakers can increase the potential for ill health (Kelley et al., 1999).

In assessing the influence of health care system factors on older clients' health, the community health nurse ascertains whether individual clients have a regular source of health care and the extent of health care utilization for both preventive and curative purposes. At the population level, nurses should determine the availability and adequacy of health care services to meet the needs of older clients. For both individual clients and the population, community health nurses would obtain information on mechanisms for financing health care and the extent of barriers to access health care services. Tips on assessing the health of older clients are presented on page 458. Health care system factors and other factors affecting the health of older clients can be assessed using the Health Assessment Guide for the Older Client available on the companion Web site for this book. ◈

assessment tips assessment tips assessment tips

ASSESSING OLDER CLIENTS' HEALTH

Biophysical Considerations

- What physiological effects of aging has the client experienced? How has the client responded to the effects of aging and decreased function?
- Does the client have any physical health problems or limitations? What effects do they have on the client's quality of life?
- What is the client's immunization status?

Psychological Considerations

- What causes stress for the client? How does the client cope with stress?
- What is the client's cognitive status? Usual mood? Is he or she depressed? Suicidal? Does the client have symptoms or a history of mental illness?
- Has the client recently lost spouse, friends, or relatives?

Physical Environmental Considerations

- How does the client's environment affect his or her health? Does the home environment pose health or safety hazards?
- Is the neighborhood safe? Are there shopping facilities accessible to the client?

Sociocultural Considerations

- What are the client's living arrangements? Are they adequate?
- What is the quality of the client's interactions with others? The extent of social support?
- Is the client at risk for or experiencing abuse? If so, what form does the abuse take?
- How do education, income, and occupational factors affect the client's health?
- Does the client have access to transportation?

Behavioral Considerations

- What are the client's typical consumption and health behavior patterns?
- What medications does the client take? Are they appropriate? Are they taken correctly?

Health System Considerations

- What is the client's usual source of health care? To what extent does the client utilize health care services when needed? Does the client receive routine screening and health promotion services?
- How does the client finance health care? Are health care services easily accessible to the client?

DIAGNOSTIC REASONING AND CARE OF OLDER CLIENTS

Based on the data derived from the in-depth assessment of older clients' health status, the community health nurse derives nursing diagnoses or statements of health care needs that require nursing action. Nursing diagnoses may be derived relative to each of the areas of assessment described above. For example, an individual client may have problems related to the normal aging process such as constipation and dry skin. There may also be nursing diagnoses related to existing chronic or communicable diseases. Similar types of diagnoses may reflect the prevalence of acute or chronic conditions in the elderly population.

In addition, the individual client may encounter factors in the physical environmental, psychological, or sociocultural dimensions that give rise to health needs. For example, a nursing diagnosis related to the physical environment of an individual client might be "safety hazard due to loose handrail on stairs." A comparable diagnosis at the aggregate level might be "unsafe housing conditions for elderly individuals due to buildings in poor repair." "Feelings of worthlessness since retire-

ment" and "social isolation due to death of family and friends" are sample nursing diagnoses for individual clients related to the psychological and sociocultural dimensions.

Behavioral factors may also give rise to nursing diagnoses. The diagnosis "shortness of breath due to emphysema and smoking" indicates the contribution of smoking, a lifestyle behavior, to a physiologic problem. The nurse may also derive nursing diagnoses reflecting health care system factors, for example, "lack of health promotion services available to older community residents."

PLANNING HEALTH CARE FOR OLDER CLIENTS

Community health nurses must be particularly mindful to involve clients and their families in the planning of care. Because older clients are particularly vulnerable to loss of independence, their involvement in planning their own health care is an important way to foster their sense of independence. Client involvement in planning is also likely to enhance compliance with the plan. Planning to meet the health care needs of older clients may take place at the primary, secondary, and tertiary levels of prevention. Links to resources that may be helpful to nurses planning care for older clients are provided on the companion Web site for this book.

Major emphases in planning health care for older clients should be on successful aging and promotion of self-care. As noted earlier, aging can result in loss of functional abilities, stamina, and so on, but these losses can be balanced to achieve successful aging. Balance focuses on three areas: selection, optimization, and compensation (Baltes & Baltes, 1998). Selection involves focusing on the more important aspects of life for the client. Perhaps older clients can no longer do everything they used to do, but they can be assisted to continue to do those things that are most important to them. Optimization relates to making the best possible use of available resources, either physical or material. For example, older persons can be assisted to budget limited financial resources to meet priority needs. Finally, compensation involves finding other means of accomplishing goals. For example, for the disabled client, this may include the use of assistive devices.

Enhancing self-care in older persons should be another major goal of nursing interventions. *Self-care* has been defined by the World Health Organization as activities undertaken by an individual or group to enhance health, prevent disease, limit illness, and restore health. Three types of self-care are appropriate to the elderly: adjustment to functional limitations, healthy lifestyle practices, and medical self-care (Konrad, 1998). Interventions to promote self-care will be included in the discussion of primary, secondary, and tertiary prevention with older clients.

Primary Prevention

As with other groups of clients, the most cost-effective means of providing health care to older clients involves primary prevention—preventing health problems before they occur. Areas of concern in planning health promotion for older clients include nutrition, hygiene, safety, immunization, rest and exercise, maintaining independence, and preparing for death.

Nutrition

Adequate nutrition is important for the older person to maintain health and prevent disease and further effects of existing chronic conditions. Nurses can assist older clients in choosing a diet that helps them attain and maintain health.

Adequate nutrition for health promotion frequently entails a reduction in caloric intake. Caloric needs decrease roughly 7.5% for each decade after 25 years of age. Recommended daily caloric intake for women aged 50 to 75 years is approximately 1,800 calories, whereas for women over 75, the recommendation is 1,600 calories. For men, approximately 2,400 calories per day are recommended from ages 50 to 75, dropping to 2,050 calories daily after age 75. Of course, specific caloric needs vary from person to person, and the nurse should assess the needs of each individual client.

Despite reduced caloric needs, older adults continue to require a balance of all other nutrients. Nutritional deficits are most frequently noted for calcium; iron; vitamins A, D, and C; and the B vitamins riboflavin and thiamine, as well as for dietary fiber. Community health nurses can promote the health of older clients by encouraging diets high in these nutrients as well as other essential nutrients.

Older adults need to remain part of family life.

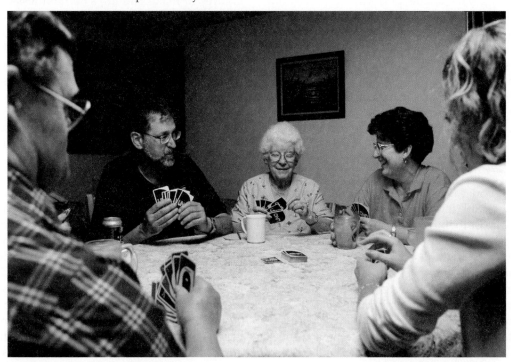

Older persons are frequent targets for food faddists promoting supplements. Unfortunately, dietary supplements are most often taken by those clients with relatively healthy diets who do not need them. Nurses can assist clients to obtain adequate nutrition by educating them regarding a well-balanced diet and can discourage expenditure of limited finances on dietary fads. Nurses can also educate clients as to the harmful nature of some food fads.

Other, more general interventions may also be needed to improve older clients' nutritional status by eliminating impediments to good nutrition. For example, social isolation may need to be addressed because people tend to eat better in company with others. Older clients can be referred to senior meal programs, or family members can be encouraged to drop by at mealtimes to eat with older clients who live alone. Interventions may also be required to deal with nausea, poorly fitting dentures, or other factors that may impede good nutrition. Community health nurses may also need to be active in the development and implementation of programs to meet the nutritional needs of the older population where these services do not already exist, or in increasing access to existing services for underserved segments of the population.

Hygiene

Promoting adequate hygiene is another aspect of health maintenance in the older adult. Skin care can be maintained by periodic bathing with mild soaps and the use of lotions to prevent drying and cracking of the skin. Clients should be discouraged from using water that is too hot and from using alcohol or powders that may further dry or irritate skin. Nails can be protected by a weekly manicure, including a massage with oil and shaping with an emery board. Dry and split nails can also be prevented by advising clients not to keep their hands in water or to wear protective gloves while performing household cleaning chores.

Adequate hygiene and hydration can protect the older client's remaining teeth and prevent dry mouth. Special toothpastes (such as Sensodyne) may be needed by clients who have sensitive gums. Toothbrushes should be firm enough to clean teeth, but not so hard as to injure gums. Clients should be encouraged to use a softer toothbrush on their own remaining teeth than they use on dentures. Clients may also need to be encouraged to seek preventive dental services, and community health nurses should work to assure the availability of such services to the older population.

Community health nurses can also educate older clients on the care of their hair and protection from sunburn. Hair should be brushed and combed daily, with a weekly shampoo and monthly conditioning. Care should be taken in the use of dyes or permanent solutions that may irritate fragile skin. Wearing a hat while outdoors will prevent sunburn due to thinning hair.

Wearing apparel may be another area for client education to promote health. Properly fitted clothing and shoes can prevent skin irritation and breakdown. Close-toed shoes and low heels are recommended for everyday wear. Shoes should always be worn with stockings, and socks should be changed daily. Older clients with functional limitations may need to be referred to home health services for assistance with hygiene. Homeless elderly, in particular, will have difficulty maintaining personal hygiene, and community health nurses may be involved in developing programs to meet their needs.

Safety

Three aspects of safety should be addressed when planning primary preventive measures for older clients: elimination of environmental hazards, home and neighborhood security, and prevention of elder abuse and neglect. Plans can be made to ensure the interior and exterior repair of the client's home. Community health nurses may need to be actively involved in assuring that building safety codes are met in residences that house older clients. Modifications can also be planned to accommodate special needs. For example, graduated ramps can replace steps to facilitate access by wheelchair or walker.

The community health nurse can also plan to educate older clients on home safety, and plans can be made to eliminate safety hazards in the home. All areas of the home, especially stairs, should be well lighted, and furniture should be placed so as to prevent falls. Because many elders experience nocturia, they may need to be encouraged to keep a nightlight burning to avoid disorientation or falls in the dark. Or the client can keep a flashlight close to the bed for nighttime use as needed.

Clients should be encouraged to keep electrical cords as short as possible and to tack them along baseboards to prevent tripping over them. If throw rugs must be used, they should be of the nonskid variety. Bathrooms can be equipped with tub rails or seats and handheld shower fixtures to make bathing safer and less arduous for the older person.

The use of space heaters and other portable heating devices should be discouraged because of the danger of burns and residential fires. Nurses should also encourage clients or their landlords to install smoke detection devices, as the elderly are particularly likely to be trapped by a fire and need sufficient warning to get out. To prevent burns, community health nurses can encourage clients to use electric blankets rather than hot water bottles in cold weather.

Older clients should also be warned about the potential for hypothermia. Persons over 60 years of age account for about half of deaths due to hypothermia each year. Clients with hypothyroidism and those using sedative–hypnotic drugs are particularly at risk for hypothermia and should be cautioned accordingly. Nurses should make sure that these and other elderly clients have an adequate caloric intake and that the homes of older persons are adequately heated. As noted earlier, hyperthermia is also an area of concern with older clients. Heatstroke can be prevented by limiting exertion in hot weather, increasing nonalcoholic fluid intake, taking cool baths, and using air conditioning. Although the use of fans will increase comfort, they are not particularly effective in reducing air temperatures and preventing heatstroke and exhaustion (National Center for Environmental Health, 1999). If clients do not have air conditioning, they can be encouraged to spend the hotter part of the day in areas that are air conditioned (e.g., an indoor mall, senior center). Again, community health nurses may need to take steps to ensure the availability of access to places where older clients can escape excessive temperatures.

Older clients should be educated regarding other health-promoting behaviors that minimize the risk of falls or their consequences. For example, weight-bearing forms of exercise (e.g., walking), maintaining body weight, and smoking cessation decrease the risk of fractures when falls do occur. Regular exercise programs, including Tai Chi training, can prevent falls from occurring by improving strength and balance. Other preventive measures for falls and fractures include review of medications that may cause physical limitations, dealing with postural hypotension, wearing sturdy shoes, increasing calcium intake, and eliminating safety hazards in the home.

Promoting home and neighborhood security is also of concern. Older clients should be cautioned to be careful about admitting strangers into the home and to refrain from walking alone in high-crime areas. Doors and windows should have secure locks, and cars should be locked even when kept in the garage.

In many neighborhoods, police and fire personnel can be notified of homes where older persons live. If this is the case, the nurse can encourage clients to provide such notification. Clients can also arrange for "disaster signals" to neighbors. For example, if neighbors do not see draperies opened by a certain time in the morning, they may decide to investigate.

Motor vehicles are a cause for concern in the safety of older adults. Although many older persons would like to retain their independence and continue to drive, they may not be able to do so safely because of a variety of sensory impairments. In this type of situation, the nurse can encourage older clients to find other ways of remaining mobile and maintaining their independence. Perhaps they can be encouraged to drive in the daytime, but not at night. Or the nurse might acquaint the older client with local bus routes and schedules. Many local organizations provide transportation at little or no cost to older people. Or the older adult can be encouraged to ride along with a younger friend.

Motor vehicles are also problematic when older people are pedestrians. In many areas, the bulk of pedestrian fatalities occur among elderly individuals. In areas where there are large numbers of elderly, nurses can campaign for traffic signals at heavily used crossings, strict enforcement of speed limits, and public awareness of the presence of older adults.

The last area of concern in promoting the safety of older clients is preventing abuse and neglect. Elder abuse and neglect frequently occur when those caring for elderly clients are unable to cope with the resulting stress. Providing support for these caretakers, teaching positive coping skills, and providing periodic respite care may help to prevent abuse. Assisting older clients to maintain their independence may also help prevent the development of a potentially abusive situation.

Immunization

Immunization of older adults is a special safety issue. Many adults in the United States, particularly older adults, have never been immunized for tetanus and are also unprotected against diphtheria. Current Immunization Practices Advisory Committee (ACIP) recommendations for adult immunization indicate a need for completion of the primary series of diphtheria and tetanus toxoids and boosters every 10 years. Annual immunization for influenza is recommended for all healthy adults over 65 years of age. Immunization against pneumococcal pneumonia is also recommended for older persons. Adults may also require immunization for hepatitis B, measles, mumps, rubella, and varicella if they do not have previously acquired immunity. Older clients may need to be referred to sources of inexpensive immunization. For example, many local health departments offer influenza and pneumococcal immunizations free or for a small charge. Community health nurses may also be involved in the development of immunization programs in places frequented by older clients (e.g., pharmacies, senior centers, etc.).

Rest and Exercise

Many people believe that the need for exercise decreases with age; however, older people need exercise as much as their younger counterparts. Community health nurses should encourage older clients to engage in moderate exercise on a regular basis. Encouraging clients to elevate the legs and refrain from crossing the legs will help to prevent venous stasis and skin breakdown.

Older clients also need adequate rest. Older people tend to sleep fewer hours at night than when they were younger. They continue to need rest, however, so daily activity patterns may need to be planned to accommodate an afternoon nap. Clients should also be encouraged to arrange activities to allow for rest periods throughout the day.

Maintaining Independence

Because of physical and economic limitations, it is sometimes difficult for older persons to maintain their independence. Decreased income and physical inability to care for oneself sometimes force older clients to give up their own residence and live with family members. Whatever the living arrangements of the older client, community health nurses should assist them to maintain the highest degree of independence possible. Some older clients may be able to continue to live alone if referred to supportive services such as homemaker aides, transportation services, and Meals-on-Wheels. When older persons are living with family members, the nurse can encourage family members to foster independence in the client. This may mean encouraging them to assign specific roles within the household to the older family member.

⑥THINK ABOUT IT

In fostering independence, what kinds of health risks do you think would be acceptable for an older client? Is there a point at which you would curtail some aspects of independence? If so, when and why?

Alzheimer's disease is one of the biggest threats to independence in the elderly. Although there is not yet any certainty, there is some evidence to suggest that use of nonsteroidal anti-inflammatory drugs (NSAIDs) or estrogen may delay the onset of Alzheimer's disease. Effects in research to date have been modest, but even modest gains may offset some of the tremendous societal burden expected of Alzheimer's disease in the next 50 years (Brookmeyer et al., 1998), and nurses may want to encourage clients at risk for Alzheimer's disease to discuss these options with their primary health care providers.

Life Resolution and Preparation for Death

As noted earlier, one of the developmental tasks to be accomplished by the older adult is preparation for death. This entails developing a personal set of goals and the ability to view one's life as having been meaningful and productive. Reminiscence is one way of accomplishing life resolution and achieving positive feelings about one's own life. The community health nurse must recognize and foster the older client's need to reminisce and should encourage other family members to do so as well. This is sometimes difficult given the nurse's busy schedule and the number of clients who need to be seen; however, nurses should be able to find some time during interactions with older clients to listen to these reminiscences and to help clients reflect on their lives. In spite of cognitive losses, reminiscence or "life review" has also been shown to be effective with some clients with Alzheimer's disease (Haight, 2001).

⑥THINK ABOUT IT

How would you help an older client work through the developmental task of preparing for death? Would your approach be different if the client had a terminal illness? Why or why not?

Preparation for death usually also entails a number of practical activities involved in getting one's affairs in order. Older clients may need to make decisions about funeral arrangements or the disposition of their belongings. Both nurses and family members should be encouraged to listen to clients in their reflections on such matters, rather than put them off with assurances that they "won't die for a long time yet." Nurses may also need to refer clients for legal assistance with wills, burial plans, and other financial arrangements. Many communities have low-cost legal aid services available to elderly clients. Community health nurses should keep in mind, however, the cultural differences in preparation for death that clients may exhibit (Mitty, 2001). For example, in many cultures, such decisions are believed to be the responsibility of children, and the dying client should not be bothered. In others, discussion of death is believed to hasten its occurrence, so clients are not willing to explore plans related to their deaths. Primary preventive interventions for older clients are summarized in Table 19–5 ■.

Secondary Prevention

Secondary preventive measures are undertaken when health problems have occurred and primary prevention is no longer possible. As noted earlier, older clients experience a variety of health problems related to the effects of aging. They are also subject to problems stemming from chronic and communicable diseases. Secondary prevention for communicable diseases and chronic conditions is addressed in detail in Chapters 28 and 29.

Skin Breakdown

Because of the fragility of older skin, skin breakdown is a common difficulty. The initial plan of care should be to prevent skin breakdown using the primary preventive strategies discussed earlier. Extremities should be inspected regularly for evidence of skin breakdown, and any breakdown noted should be cleansed properly and examined for signs of infection. Adequate dietary intake contributes to maintaining skin integrity and to healing when breakdown does occur. Care should also be taken to relieve pressure on bony prominences by frequent changes of position. When skin breakdown has already occurred, the nurse should make sure that the area is kept clean and dry. If healing does not occur, the client should be referred to his or her primary provider for evaluation.

Constipation

Constipation is another common problem in older clients. Again, the primary consideration is prevention through adequate fluid and fiber in the diet as well as adequate exercise. But when constipation does occur, the nurse can suggest the use of mild natural laxatives such as prune juice. Clients should be cautioned against the overuse of laxatives. Bulk products such as Metamucil or stool softeners should also be used with caution.

If necessary, the nurse or a family member can administer an enema. Nurses working with older clients

■ **TABLE 19-5** Primary Prevention Strategies for Older Clients

AREA OF CONCERN	PRIMARY PREVENTION STRATEGIES
Nutrition	Educate clients regarding nutritional needs.
	Promote caloric intake adequate to meet energy needs.
	Encourage well-balanced diet high in nutrient content (especially calcium, iron, vitamins A and C, riboflavin and thiamine, and fiber).
	Discourage participation in food fads.
	Maintain hydration.
Hygiene	Bathe periodically with mild soaps.
	Use lotion to prevent drying of skin.
	Keep hands out of water or wear gloves.
	Maintain oral hygiene with good toothbrush.
	Maintain hydration to prevent dry mouth.
	Brush and comb hair daily.
	Shampoo weekly with mild soap and condition monthly.
Safety	Wear hat to protect scalp from sunburn.
	Wear properly fitted clothes and shoes.
	Use electric blanket rather than hot water bottles.
	Provide adequate lighting, especially on stairs.
	Use a nightlight at night and keep a flashlight handy.
	Place furniture to prevent falls.
	Keep electrical cords short and tack along baseboards.
	Eliminate throw rugs if possible or use nonskid type.
	Install tub rails and other safety fixtures.
	Discourage use of space heaters, kerosene stoves, and similar devices.
	Install smoke alarms.
	Notify police and fire personnel of older person in home.
	Promote adequate and safe heating and ventilation of home.
	Provide door and window locks and keep car locked.
	Do not admit strangers to home.
	Ride with others or use public transportation rather than drive if senses are impaired.
	Use care in crossing streets.
	Promote family coping abilities and relieve stress to prevent abuse of older persons.
Immunization	Encourage adequate immunization for diphtheria and tetanus.
	Provide annual influenza immunization.
	Provide pneumonia vaccine.
Rest and exercise	Encourage moderate exercise on a regular basis.
	Arrange activities to accommodate rest periods as needed.
Maintaining independence	Provide support services that allow clients to live independently if possible.
	Encourage family members to foster independence.
	Encourage client participation in health care planning.
	Advocate for client independence as needed.
Life resolution and preparation for death	Encourage reminiscence.
	Assist client to discuss death with family members.
	Assist client to put affairs in order.

who are constipated should determine agency policy regarding whether an enema requires an order. If an order is required, the nurse can call to request the authorization. Care should be taken that the enema solution is not too hot and that the client is close to the toilet, as poor sphincter control occurring with age may result in the inability to hold the enema. Again, overuse of enemas is contraindicated. Fecal impaction that is unrelieved by enema should be referred to the primary care provider.

Urinary Incontinence

Urinary incontinence is a particularly distressing problem for some older adults. Incontinence may result in social withdrawal because of fear of embarrassing accidents in public. For clients with incontinence, not only are there the problems of hygiene and odor, but self-image is threatened by the inability to control one's bodily functions. Clients with stress incontinence should be referred for a urological consultation. Nursing interventions that may help urinary incontinence include encouraging clients to void frequently and teaching them Kegel pelvic floor exercises. Bladder training may also help to resolve the problem. Biofeedback techniques have been found to relieve both urinary and fecal incontinence in older adults. Environmental modifications that increase access to the toilet may also help, as can loose-fitting and easily removed clothing.

In some instances, incontinence becomes a chronic problem. For clients in this situation, the nurse needs to ensure that skin, clothing, and linens remain clean and dry, since urinary incontinence increases the risk of pressure sores. Sanitary pads, disposable underpants, or panty liners may prevent clothing and linens from becoming wet and may increase the client's confidence in going out in public. Frequent changes in such sanitary aids should be encouraged to prevent skin breakdown.

For bedridden clients, availability of a bedpan or urinal, or assistance to a bedside commode at frequent intervals, may reduce the frequency of linen changes. A bedside commode may also be of use to clients who are able to get up but have mobility limitations. The community health nurse may help arrange for the purchase or rental of these devices from durable medical equipment companies.

Sensory Loss

Planning to provide adequate lighting is particularly important in compensating for loss of visual acuity. If clients wear glasses, nurses should make sure that the degree of correction is appropriate and that glasses are kept clean. Nurses and clients should also take care that when glasses are removed they are placed in a safe but accessible location.

The use of large-print books, a magnifying glass, or books on tape can assist older clients to continue reading as a leisure activity. Taking medications may also be hampered by loss of visual acuity. When clients have difficulties reading medication labels, the nurse can color-code the labels. Colors used should be easily distinguishable, as there may be a loss of color discrimination with age, particularly with the colors blue, green, and violet.

The community health nurse can also suggest several measures that help to compensate for diminished hearing. Speaking clearly (not loudly) and at a lower pitch improves the older client's ability to hear. Properly functioning hearing aids also help some clients. Clients who are concerned about the unsightliness of old-fashioned hearing aids can be assured that there are many less noticeable devices available today. Speech should be slower, as many older persons have problems hearing rapid speech and have difficulty discriminating several specific sounds, among them s, z, t, f, g, and th. These auditory problems can be overcome by the use of multisensory input (e.g., using visual as well as auditory techniques in teaching older clients).

Eliminating background noise may also enhance the older person's ability to hear. Nurses working with older clients should always obtain feedback to be sure that clients have accurately heard and interpreted verbal messages. For clients living alone or others who must be able to use a telephone, the nurse can suggest voice enhancement devices that enable older people to hear better.

Because of older clients' diminished sense of touch, nurses should discourage clients from using hot water for bathing and from wearing open-toed shoes. Clients should be encouraged to check extremities periodically for injuries and to use extreme caution in working with sharp or other potentially harmful objects.

Decreased senses of smell and taste pose problems for older adults in that they may lead to diminished appetite. Older individuals can be encouraged to add additional spices and herbs to flavor foods; however, care should be taken that such condiments are not contraindicated (e.g., additional salt for the client with hypertension). Loss of the sense of smell is also problematic in that older clients may not be as easily able to tell when foodstuffs are spoiled or may not be able to smell smoke or a gas leak. Nurses may want to encourage clients using gas for cooking or heating to periodically check that pilot lights remain lit. They should also encourage the purchase of small amounts of perishable foods and rapid use before they spoil. Smoke detectors are also necessary devices in the homes of older clients.

Mobility Limitation

Related problems for older clients involve limitation of mobility and consequent impairment in the ability to carry out ADLs. Early diagnosis and treatment of diseases that cause mobility limitations have been shown to decrease the prevalence of upper and lower body limitations in spite of increased prevalence of the diseases that cause them (Freedman & Martin, 2000).

Nurses can explore options for assisting older clients with existing limitations to perform ADLs. Referral to a home care agency that has homemaker services may help with tasks such as housekeeping and grocery shopping. Home care agencies may also provide assistance with personal care services such as bathing and hair washing. There are also a number of mechanical devices that make it easier for older clients to care for themselves (e.g., special devices for clients with arthritis that make it easier to open jars or reach objects on shelves).

For clients who need outside assistance but do not have insurance coverage or cannot afford special services, volunteer services may be available through local churches or other social groups. Student workers are sometimes a good source of assistance with instrumental activities. Both high school and college students may be willing to provide services for small fees or for a room. The community health nurse can also explore service projects undertaken by sororities or fraternities at local colleges or universities that may provide assistance for older clients.

The nurse may refer clients who cannot cook for themselves to a Meals-on-Wheels program. For clients who are mobile, a referral for a lunch program at the local senior citizens center may be more appropriate. Such centers may also provide assistance with transportation to and from the center, for shopping, and for physician appointments.

Pain

The management of chronic pain is another common problem among older adults. In one study, almost half of older disabled women reported severe pain, and more than three fourths were using analgesics. However, nearly half of these women were using less than 20% of the maximum analgesic dose, while another 7% were using more than the maximum dose (Pahor et al., 1999). Undermedication may lead to failure to use medication because of perceptions that it "doesn't work." Undermedication may also be the result of fears of addiction. Community health nurses can help clients in pain distinguish between addiction and pseudoaddiction in which clients hoard pain medication out of fear of pain. These clients do not take pain medication indiscriminately as do those who are truly addicted, but reserve medication for pain (Todd, 1998).

As noted in Chapter 6, some forms of alternative therapies are being used for pain management. For example, acupuncture has been shown to be effective in treating some types of pain. Similarly, chiropractic techniques may be used for chronic back pain or headaches, and marijuana has been approved for treatment of intractable pain in terminally ill clients in some states. Community health nurses may make referrals to providers who practice alternative therapies, but should first assess the appropriateness of such referrals to clients' conditions.

Among clients with arthritis, 80% in some studies report significant pain. Clients experiencing pain are more likely than others to be depressed, and pain has been shown to worsen with depression due to a lack of serotonin and noradrenalin (Todd, 1998). In some studies, pain has not been shown to be associated with greater disability, but relationships between pain and depressive symptoms, sleep impairment, and diminished quality of life have been demonstrated (Ross & Crook, 1998). Community health nurses can assist clients in pain control by educating them regarding appropriate use of analgesics as well as other means of minimizing pain.

For clients with arthritis, pain may be controlled with the use of anti-inflammatory and analgesic agents such as aspirin or NSAIDs. When a mild analgesic is not effective, stronger medication may be prescribed by the pri-

mary care provider. Nurses should evaluate the appropriateness of any pain medication being taken by clients and should educate clients on the correct use of medications. They may also need to caution clients regarding overuse of some medications and discourage the use of medications that are contraindicated by the client's condition. For example, clients taking anticoagulants should not take aspirin for pain, because aspirin further increases clotting time and may lead to serious bleeding.

Clients with arthritis pain may do better if they do not attempt strenuous activity immediately after awakening when joints tend to be stiff and sore. Clients can be helped to plan activities for when their pain is at a minimum. Warm baths or soaks may also help to relieve pain. For other forms of pain, medication may again be used and the nurse should monitor its effectiveness. Nurses should also educate clients as to the adverse effects of specific pain medications and make sure that clients are familiar with the symptoms of adverse effects.

As noted earlier, clients with Alzheimer's disease may exhibit signs of various types of pain. Community health nurses should educate family members in the recognition of pain and use of appropriate control measures. For example, visceral pain demonstrated by moaning and restlessness may be addressed with acetaminophen for mild pain or narcotics for severe pain. Similarly, bone pain exhibited with signs of distress with movement can be relieved with NSAIDs. Tricyclic antidepressants, steroids, or anticonvulsants have been recommended for nerve pain that may be demonstrated by holding or rubbing painful areas. Finally, antispasmodics may be used for colic evidenced by abdominal guarding (Boyd & Vernon, 1998).

Pain management is also an area of concern in the care of clients with terminal illnesses such as cancer. Clients and family members should be encouraged to use or administer pain medication as needed without regard for potentially addicting effects. Studies of hospice clients have indicated that when pain medication is freely available, clients actually use less than when it is administered on a regulated schedule. Expense may be another impediment to effective pain control in clients with terminal illness as well as those with chronic diseases, and community health nurses may need to assist clients in finding resources to support the costs of pain medication, particularly since Medicare does not cover routine medication costs (although costs for pain medication for hospice clients is covered).

Confusion

Confusion is a problem encountered in some older clients. Confusion may be either a transient or a persistent condition. Transient confusion frequently occurs in new situations or in the dark. It may also occur when clients are moved away from familiar surroundings, as might occur following a move to a residential community or nursing home. In this case, confusion may be referred to as *relocation trauma*. Relocation trauma may even occur when the client is moved from one hallway or one bed to another.

Continuing confusion is most often associated with dementia, but is also a frequent side effect of many medications. Nurses should monitor orientation with respect to medication use. Other nursing interventions include improving sensory input, preventing malnutrition and dehydration, and preventing falls.

In working with confused older clients, the nurse and family members should plan for consistent intervention to reorient clients to their environment. Reality orientation interventions are based on the following general principles:

- Provide a calm environment without excessive stimulation.
- Establish and maintain a regular routine.
- Phrase questions and answers clearly and concisely.
- Speak directly to the client.
- Provide clear instructions or directions.
- Provide frequent reminders of date, time, and place.
- Refocus the client on reality and prevent rambling speech.
- Be firm but gentle.
- Be sincere.
- Be consistent.

Confusion is a symptom frequently encountered in clients with Alzheimer's disease. As noted earlier, there is some evidence to suggest that use of NSAIDs or estrogen may delay the onset of disease. In addition, acetylcholinesterase inhibitors may be used in the treatment of mild to moderate Alzheimer's disease. Approximately 30% of clients with Alzheimer's disease improve with these drugs; however, they do not stop or reverse the pathological progression of disease and may actually increase behavioral symptoms. They also have multiple cholinergic side effects (Garand et al., 2000). Until more effective medications are found, behavioral and environmental interventions seem to be most helpful in dealing with Alzheimer's disease.

Nurses working with families of clients with Alzheimer's need to provide a great deal of support. Families may need to consider nursing home placement and may need help in making arrangements. They may also need assistance in dealing with the guilt engendered by their inability to care for a family member, especially a spouse, at home.

For families who choose to care for the client with Alzheimer's at home, the nurse can help arrange home care or respite care. *Respite* is temporary relief from caregiving responsibilities that provides benefits for both client and caregiver. For the client, respite may result in increased opportunities for socialization, stimulation, and interaction with others; activities geared to their level of ability; time with trained caregivers; and a refreshed family caregiver. For caregivers, respite can lead to reduced stress, increased opportunity for socialization, vacation,

and time to oneself. In spite of these advantages, respite care services are often underused due to lack of awareness of their availability, cost, inflexibility, and guilt on the part of caretakers (Hayes, 1999).

Access to respite care appears to occur in three stages (Strang & Haughey, 1999). In the first stage, caregivers become aware of the need to get away from the caregiving situation. The second stage involves giving oneself permission to request assistance from others. Research has indicated that caregivers may be reluctant to request assistance because of their inability to reciprocate due to burdensome caretaking responsibilities (Neufeld & Harrison, 1998). In the third stage of access to respite care, caretakers need to have the social support resources available that make it possible for them to give up their caretaking responsibilities for short periods of time. Community health nurses can assist clients to identify sources of respite in their own social networks or refer them to formal respite care services if available. When such services are not available in the community, nurses can be active in advocating for their development as well as in planning and implementing such services.

Nurses can also encourage families of clients with Alzheimer's disease who wander to use an identification kit similar to that used for identifying lost children. Families can also create environments that permit wandering within safe parameters. Other interventions that may help families cope with clients with Alzheimer's disease include creation of a calm, consistent environment with minimal changes, provision of frequent rest periods with nocturnal restlessness, and encouraging reminiscence.

Depression

Depression is another area in which the nurse working with older clients may need to take action. Mild transient depression is a relatively normal phenomenon for most people. Depression may occur with the loss of familiar people and places or on anniversaries of those losses. It is normal, for example, for the older person to become somewhat depressed on the anniversary of a spouse's death or on the deceased person's birthday. In these instances, nurses can help clients to recognize their depression as a normal feeling. Encouraging them to discuss the loved one and to relive happy memories while acknowledging their feelings of sadness may help to alleviate the depression.

Severe depression, on the other hand, requires referral for counseling or other forms of therapy. Severe depression may be marked by continued inattention to personal hygiene, failure to take part in normal activities such as dressing or combing one's hair, and poor appetite. Depression may also be signaled by withdrawal from interaction with others. Again, the nurse should encourage the client to ventilate feelings regarding the cause of the depression, but should also refer the client for additional help as needed. The nurse should also clearly distinguish between clients who are depressed and those experiencing delirium. Evidence of delirium should prompt a referral for medical care.

Social Isolation

Social isolation is a relatively common problem among older adults, especially the "old elderly." Isolation may stem from a variety of circumstances mentioned earlier, including sensory deficits, communication difficulties, and loss of mobility.

Loss of family and friends is a significant contributor to social isolation in the elderly. As spouses and other family members or friends die, the social support system for the older person is reduced. In this instance, nurses can help older clients establish new social support systems by helping them get involved with other groups. Referral to an active senior citizens center may be appropriate. Many religious groups also have a variety of social activities for older persons. Special interest groups that incorporate people of all ages may provide an avenue for social interaction. For example, a local bridge club or garden club may be of interest to a particular client. The nurse can also encourage remaining family and friends to include the older person in their activities.

Loss of family and friends also leads to the problem of grief. Grief may also be engendered by anticipation of the client's own death, particularly when the client has a terminal illness. The nurse can assist clients to deal with grief by exploring with them their feelings about death. Acceptance of possible anger may be necessary as well.

If the client desires it, referral to a pastor or other source of spiritual counsel may be appropriate. Family and friends should be encouraged to talk with the client about the client's impending death, and the client should be allowed to make arrangements for disposition of personal property or plans for burial, if such planning is culturally acceptable to the client. As much as possible, dying clients should be allowed to continue in accustomed roles and should have control over decisions affecting their own life or death. If the client has a living will or durable power of attorney, the nurse should see that a copy of the document is placed in the client's record and that the document is adhered to by both family members and health care professionals.

Abuse and Neglect

Abuse or neglect of older persons is another problem for which nursing intervention may be required. Nurses should be alert to situations that have potential for abuse. Dependent elders who place a serious burden on caretakers or who were abusive parents themselves are at risk for abuse and neglect. Other situations in which potential for abuse is increased include reduced social status, other sources of stress for caregivers (e.g., unemployment or illness in other family members), and family dysfunction.

Resolving an abusive situation may require assisting caretakers to develop adequate mechanisms for coping with the frustrations of caring for an older adult. Persons in abusive situations can also be referred for counseling.

Respite care can help to reduce the burden of care of an older family member, and the nurse may need to help families arrange for such care. Removal of the older person and nursing home placement may reduce the potential for abuse. Finally, in situations in which abuse cannot be controlled, the nurse may arrange for placement of the older person in a temporary shelter while arrangements are made for other care. Abuse of older adults is discussed in more detail in Chapter 32.

Alcohol Abuse

Abuse of alcohol may warrant referral for a variety of services. Initially, the nurse may need to refer the client to a detoxification facility. Because of their diminished capacity to detoxify alcohol and other substances, older clients are at high risk for complications during detoxification and should be in a facility where adequate supervision is possible. Once detoxification has been accomplished, the client should be referred for ongoing counseling for his or her drinking problem. Referral to such groups as Alcoholics Anonymous may also be appropriate. Families with older alcoholic members may also need assistance in dealing with the problem, and referral to Al-Anon may help.

Older clients and their families should also be educated regarding the effects of alcohol and its potential for interaction with medication. Overuse of preparations containing alcohol should be discouraged as well.

Inadequate Financial Resources

Another common problem of older adults is inadequate financial resources. Many older people have reduced incomes that may not be sufficient to meet their needs. Nurses can refer clients to sources of financial assistance as appropriate. Clients who are receiving minimal Social Security benefits may be eligible for Supplemental Security Income (SSI). Referrals may also be made for food and other general assistance programs. Some utility companies provide reduced rates for older adults, which the client can inquire about. The nurse should become familiar with other local sources of financial assistance for older persons and make referrals to these agencies as appropriate.

The community health nurse may also be of assistance to older persons living on reduced incomes by helping them to prioritize expenditures and budget their income accordingly. The nurse may also provide information about lower-cost foods that provide adequate nutrition. Clients should be encouraged to buy staple goods in quantities that reduce prices. Perishable foods, however, should be purchased only in quantities that can be used before spoiling. The nurse may also encourage several older clients to buy items in bulk and split the costs to reduce expenditures for each individual.

Chronic Illness

As noted earlier, older persons experience a variety of chronic illnesses. Among these are arthritis, heart disease, hypertension, diabetes, and chronic lung conditions. Control of chronic disease in the elderly population requires four conditions (Wagner, 1999). First, there must be provisions for early identification and treatment of exacerbations of disease. Second, clients may need to make adjustments to their lifestyles to control chronic diseases and their consequences. Third, effective therapy must be initiated by providers and complied with by clients. Finally, clients must receive the support and resources necessary for them to adequately manage their conditions.

Secondary prevention for these conditions would include screening for specific diseases, diagnosis, treatment, and management. Community health nursing involvement in secondary prevention for these illnesses includes referral for medical services as needed, as well as supportive interventions during treatment and management. Community health nurses frequently educate clients regarding their conditions and the treatment recommended. Older persons may need instruction regarding their medications and possible side effects. In addition, the nurse monitors clients for treatment effects and for side effects and toxic effects of medications. They may also educate clients in other forms of symptom relief, for example, warm soaks for arthritic joints. Clients may also need emotional support in dealing with their disease and its effects. Additional secondary preventive measures for specific chronic diseases are addressed in Chapter 29.

Self-management of chronic disease is becoming an important issue given the rising cost of health care in the United States (Fries, Koop, Sokoloc, Beadle, & Wright, 1998). Self-management differs from self-care in that it involves implementation and appropriate modification of professional treatment recommendations for specific health problems (Stoller, 1999), while self-care is more general in nature. Goals for self-management include development of skills as well as understanding of disease; self-motivation and self-advocacy rather than dependency; attention to the influence of family, job, and other social factors; and development of skills in self-monitoring. Client self-management is facilitated by client information systems that promote education of and feedback to clients and family members; resources and programs to meet clients' information, behavior, and social needs; reorganized delivery systems to facilitate effective monitoring and follow-up with clients who are managing their own care; and decision support for providers who are not specialists in particular diseases (Wagner, 1999).

Nursing case management is often an effective vehicle for supporting self-management by clients since some may minimize the importance of symptoms of exacerbation of disease or fail to obtain care due to fears of hospitalization (Blaha, Robinson, Pugh, Bryan, & Havens, 2000). Unfortunately, this level of assistance is not often reimbursed under current health delivery systems. Medicare, in particular, needs to be refocused to support long-term management of chronic disease rather than episodic treatment of exacerbations (Whitelaw & Warden, 1999).

Communicable Diseases

Older clients are at higher risk than younger people for communicable diseases such as influenza and pneumo-

nia. Primary prevention of these diseases through immunization is desirable, but when this fails, the community health nurse may be involved in referring clients for medical care for these conditions as needed. Nurses also instruct clients in self-care during illness and monitor the effects of communicable conditions on health status. The nurse working with older clients with these diseases should be particularly alert to signs of complications, as these are more common in older individuals than in their younger counterparts. Controlling fever and maintaining hydration are two particularly important aspects of secondary prevention for communicable diseases in the elderly. Other aspects of secondary prevention in communicable diseases are addressed in Chapter 28.

Advocacy for Older Clients

Many times, nursing interventions for older clients involve advocacy. Advocacy may take place at the individual or aggregate level. At the individual level, the nurse may encourage family members to respect the client's need for privacy or allow the client to make his or her own health care decisions. Advocacy may also be needed in interactions with other health care providers. Advocacy may involve encouraging families to allow the client as much independence as possible. Intervention on behalf of the abused client is also a form of advocacy.

At the aggregate level, nurses can see that the needs of the older population are made known to public policy makers. They can become politically active to see that the needs of this group are being met by government agencies. They may also need to work with nongovernment agencies to ensure that the needs of older clients are met. For example, community health nurses might work with a coalition of religious groups to provide shelter for abused elders, or they might help a group of older adults establish some type of cooperative buying effort to decrease expenditures. There may also be a need to point out the needs of older persons to transportation authorities. Table 19–6 ■ summarizes secondary preventive activities that may benefit older clients.

■ **TABLE 19–6** Secondary Prevention for Common Problems in Older Clients

CLIENT PROBLEM	SECONDARY PREVENTION STRATEGIES
Skin breakdown	Inspect extremities regularly for lesions.
	Keep lesions clean and dry.
	Eliminate pressure by frequent changes of position.
	Refer for treatment as needed.
Constipation	Encourage fluid and fiber intake.
	Discourage ignoring urge to defecate.
	Encourage regular exercise.
	Encourage regular bowel habits.

CLIENT PROBLEM	SECONDARY PREVENTION STRATEGIES
Constipation (continued)	Use mild laxatives as needed, but discourage overuse.
	Administer enemas as needed; discourage overuse.
	Administer bulk products or stool softeners as indicated.
Urinary incontinence	Refer for urological consult.
	Encourage frequent voiding.
	Teach Kegel exercises.
	Assist with bladder training.
	Encourage use of sanitary pads, panty liners, etc., with frequent changes of such aids.
	Keep skin clean and dry; change clothing and bed linen as needed.
	Offer bedpan or urinal frequently or assist to bedside commode at frequent intervals.
Sensory loss	Provide adequate lighting.
	Keep eyeglasses clean and hearing aids functional.
	Eliminate safety hazards.
	Use large-print books or materials.
	Use multisensory approaches to communication and teaching.
	Avoid using colors that make discrimination difficult.
	Speak clearly and slowly, at a lower pitch.
	Eliminate background noise.
	Assist clients to obtain voice enhancers for phone.
	Use additional herbs and spices, but use with discretion.
	Purchase small amounts of perishable foods.
	Check pilot lights on gas appliances frequently.
	Encourage the use of smoke detectors.
Mobility limitation	Provide assistance with ambulation, transfer, etc.
	Assist clients to obtain equipment such as walkers and wheelchairs.
	Install ramps, tub rails, etc., as needed.
	Promote access to public facilities for older persons.
	Assist clients to find sources of transportation.
	Make referrals for assistance with personal care or instrumental activities.
Pain	Plan activities for times when pain is controlled.
	Encourage warm soaks.
	Encourage adequate rest and exercise to prevent mobility limitations.
	Encourage effective use of analgesics.

CLIENT PROBLEM	SECONDARY PREVENTION STRATEGIES
Confusion	Apply principles of reality orientation.
Depression	Accept feelings and reflect on their normality; encourage client to ventilate feelings.
	Refer for counseling as needed.
Social isolation	Compensate for sensory loss; enhance communication abilities.
	Improve mobility; provide access to transportation.
	Assist client to obtain adequate financial resources.
	Refer client to new support systems.
	Assist client to deal with grief over loss of loved ones.
Abuse or neglect	Assist caretakers to develop positive coping strategies.
	Assist families to obtain respite care or day care for older members.
	Refer families for counseling as needed.
	Arrange placement in temporary shelter.
	Assist families in making other arrangements for safe care of older clients.
Alcohol abuse	Identify problem drinking by older clients.
	Refer for therapy, Alcoholics Anonymous, or Al-Anon as appropriate.
	Observe for toxic effects of alcohol ingestion.
	Maintain hydration and nutrition.
Inadequate financial resources	Refer for financial assistance.
	Assist with budgeting and priority allocation.
	Educate for less expensive means of meeting needs.
	Function as an advocate as needed.

Tertiary Prevention

Tertiary preventive activities for older clients focus on preventing complications of existing conditions and preventing their recurrence. Tertiary prevention for the individual client depends on the problems experienced by the client. For example, tertiary prevention for an abused older client may include long-term counseling for family members, whereas prevention related to financial inadequacies may involve assistance with budgeting. Plans for tertiary prevention are often a component of discharge planning when older clients have been hospitalized. Unfortunately, research indicates that many clients who require referral for assistance on discharge do not receive it. In one study, for example, as many as 50% of hospitalized older clients experienced functional decline during hospitalization, yet only approximately half of those who were functionally dependent in one or more areas received referrals for home health services (Rosswurm & Lanham, 1998). Community health nurses can work closely with hospital discharge planners to ensure that clients are carefully assessed for functional limitations and that referrals for assistance are made accordingly.

In many instances, tertiary preventive measures are similar to those used for primary prevention. For example, primary and tertiary prevention for constipation both involve increasing fluid and fiber intake and exercise. Similarly, primary preventive measures to prevent skin breakdown can also be used to prevent a recurrence of the problem. Tertiary prevention measures used with older adults are presented in Table 19–7 ■.

■ **TABLE 19–7** Tertiary Prevention Strategies for Older Clients

CLIENT PROBLEM	TERTIARY PREVENTION STRATEGIES
Inadequate nutrition	Educate clients regarding nutritional needs.
	Promote caloric intake adequate to meet energy needs.
	Encourage well-balanced diet high in nutrient content (especially those with prior deficits).
	Discourage participation in food fads.
	Maintain hydration.
Skin breakdown	Bathe periodically with mild soaps.
	Use lotion to prevent drying of skin.
	Keep hands out of water or wear gloves.
	Elevate legs and refrain from crossing legs.
	Wear loose-fitting clothing and properly fitted shoes.
	Inspect extremities regularly for lesions.
	Relieve pressure on bony prominences by frequent change of position.
Constipation	Encourage fluid and fiber intake.
	Discourage ignoring urge to defecate.
	Encourage regular exercise.
	Encourage regular bowel habits.
	Use mild laxatives as needed, but discourage overuse.
	Administer enemas as needed; discourage overuse.
	Administer bulk products or stool softeners as indicated.
Sensory loss	Provide adequate lighting.
	Keep eyeglasses clean and hearing aids functional.
	Eliminate safety hazards.
	Use large-print books or materials.

CLIENT PROBLEM	TERTIARY PREVENTION STRATEGIES
Sensory loss (continued)	Use multisensory approaches to communication and teaching.
	Avoid using colors that make discrimination difficult.
	Speak clearly and slowly, at a lower pitch.
	Eliminate background noise.
	Assist clients to obtain voice enhancers for phone.
	Use additional herbs and spices, but use with discretion.
	Purchase small amounts of perishable foods.
	Check pilot lights on gas appliances frequently.
	Encourage the use of smoke detectors.
Confusion	Apply principles of reality orientation.
Abuse or neglect	Provide support for victim and caretakers.
	Assist families to obtain respite care or day care for older members.
	Refer families for counseling as needed.
	Monitor family situation closely.
	Assist families in making other arrangements for safe care of older clients as needed.
	Promote self-image of victim and abuser.
	Foster independence of victim and abuser.
Alcohol abuse	Provide support for abstinence.
	Refer to support group.
	Provide support to family in dealing with problem.
	Provide assistance in dealing with stress.
	Promote positive self-image.
Accidental injury	Eliminate safety hazards from environment.
	Encourage use of safety aids.
	Provide supervision for confused older person.
Social isolation	Assist client to build social support network.
	Refer to church or other groups for social activities.
	Provide means of transportation.

In planning health care to meet the needs of older clients, the nurse frequently makes referrals or obtains assistance for clients from outside agencies. In making referrals for older clients, the nurse should consider carefully the client's ability to follow through on the referral. The nurse should also explain carefully to the client what services may be provided by the referral agency and how to go about obtaining those services. In some instances, it may be necessary for the nurse to make arrangements for the client if the client is not able to do so. For example, some social service agencies make arrangements to visit a client's home if the client is unable to get to them.

Tertiary prevention is particularly warranted for clients with chronic diseases or terminal conditions. Community health nurses should intervene to promote adjustment to the presence of chronic illnesses. Chronic illness not only limits functional ability, which was addressed in terms of secondary prevention, but may also result in a variety of psychological consequences. It has been suggested that the psychological effects of chronic illness are the product of loss of control and diminished self-esteem. Chronic illness has been described as "undermining former self-images" (Helgeson & Mickelson, 2000). Chronic illness attacks self-esteem on a number of fronts by affecting many aspects of the definition of self, including body image, ability to care for oneself, social activity and relationships, physical capabilites, and vocational and recreational interests.

Approaches to dealing with the decline in self-image posed by chronic illness include social comparison, denial of impact, and finding meaning in the experience (Helgeson & Mickelson, 2000). In social comparison, clients compare their own state of health to that of someone else. Downward comparisons in which clients see themselves as better off than others promote favorable adjustment and result in fewer affective symptoms. Similarly, clients who deny the severity of the impact of disease in their lives (not the existence or the severity of the disease itself) tend not to let the condition interfere with major aspects of their lives, again promoting positive adjustment. For example, clients might rationalize that they can "still hike, just not as fast as before." Finally, clients who attempt to find some positive outcome from the experience of chronic disease (e.g., "making me more aware of the beauty of life") tend to adjust positively to the existence of chronic illness. On the other hand, clients who attempt to establish meaning in terms of a cause for the condition or approach the question of meaning as "Why me?" tend to have poorer adjustments to their illness. Community health nurses and family members can assist older clients with chronic diseases to engage in these strategies to promote optimal adjustment. Where adjustment is negative and clients exhibit depressive symptoms, nurses can initiate referrals for counseling or support groups.

Tertiary prevention is also important for clients with terminal illnesses as well as for their families. Interventions directed toward families can include encouraging them to expand their social support network, encouraging periodic solitude, maintaining their own health, and finding ways to nourish the spirit that fit with their con-

ceptions of spirituality (Furman, 2001). Pain control in terminal illness has already been discussed, but another intervention that may be warranted is referral for hospice services. Hospice services assist both the terminally ill client and family members to deal with the process of dying. The goals of hospice include establishing a relationship with clients and their families to assist them in living through the terminal illness and the death in the context of its meaning for them, releasing to the client and/or family the authority to determine the course of care, and providing a sustained presence during an experience of profound powerlessness (Boyd & Vernon, 1998). Hospice services can encompass help with home care, respite, volunteer support, counseling, and assistance with medications, comfort measures, physical therapy, and so on.

IMPLEMENTING CARE FOR OLDER CLIENTS

Nurse and client together implement the plan of care. Some activities of implementation may also be carried out by members of the client's family or by significant others. The extent of responsibility of each depends on the client's level of function and the ability of the client or others to carry out the actions required.

Frequently, implementing the plan of care involves educating the client (or significant others). Health education for older clients is based on the general principles of teaching and learning discussed in Chapter 11. There are also some unique considerations in implementing an education plan for the older adult.

Sensory losses need to be taken into consideration when teaching the older client. Strategies to circumvent hearing loss include using a lower-pitched voice; facing the client while speaking; employing nonverbal teaching techniques; using clear, concise terminology; and having the client use a hearing aid when possible. The effects of hearing loss can also be minimized by limiting background noise, reemphasizing important points, and supplementing verbal with written materials.

The use of glasses, a magnifying glass, and large print may help to minimize visual deficits. Learning can also be enhanced by visual materials using black lettering on white or yellow paper and providing adequate lighting and eliminating glare in the learning environment.

In implementing health education plans for the older client, the nurse may need to repeat material more frequently. Because of decreases in short-term memory, it may take longer for an older client to learn new material. Once material is learned, however, older clients retain it as well as younger ones. Multisensorial presentation, multiple repetitions, reinforcement of verbal content with written materials, and use of memory aids (e.g., a calendar for taking medications) may also assist learning in the older client.

Because response times are longer for older people than for their younger counterparts, lessons should proceed at a slower pace, and the nurse should allow increased time for responses on the part of the client. Self-paced instruction is helpful. Motivation to learn can be heightened by increasing client participation in the lesson and by setting easily attainable, progressive goals that enhance success and satisfaction. Irrelevant material can confuse clients and should be eliminated from the presentation.

Endurance may be somewhat limited in the older client, so teaching sessions should be kept short (10 to 15 minutes per session). Lessons should be scheduled at times of the day when the client is rested and comfortable. Health education for the older client should not be time limited, as the client may need more or less time to learn specific material. Again, learning should be broken down into small, progressive steps so that periodic success will continue to motivate the client. The teaching–learning process should also allow for rest periods as needed.

EVALUATING CARE FOR OLDER CLIENTS

The last aspect of care of older clients is evaluation. Evaluation should include an assessment of the current status of all identified health problems and the effectiveness of nursing interventions in resolving them. Evaluation should also consider the overall health status of the individual client and the quality of his or her life.

Some specific constraints need to be considered in evaluating the effectiveness of nursing interventions with the elderly. One of these is that the etiology of some problems may lie in other problems caused by aging itself and that these problems may not be capable of complete resolution. In this case, the nurse should evaluate the extent to which the effects of the problem on the client's life have been ameliorated. For example, it is not possible to eliminate arthritis pain. The nurse and client can, however, evaluate the extent to which interventions have limited the effects of pain on the client's ability to perform activities of daily living.

The second consideration is that the prognosis for one problem may be affected by the presence of other problems. For example, the existence of a terminal condition may make pain control increasingly difficult. In some cases, orientation and alertness might need to be sacrificed so as to control pain with the use of more powerful analgesics.

Evaluation must also take into account the possibility that one problem may diminish while another gets worse. Again, the example of pain control in terminal illness may lead to increasing confusion and disorientation that will entail other nursing interventions. Finally, the nurse and client must consider that deterioration in one area might lead to the development of additional problems that will need to be addressed. For example, decreased mobility leads to greater potential for constipation and skin breakdown. Therefore, while the status of individual problems needs to be assessed, there is a need to allow for a give-and-take or a realistic assessment of the ups and downs that may be involved in the care of the older person.

At the aggregate level, evaluation of the effects of care on the health of the elderly can be measured, in part, by the level of accomplishment of relevant national health objectives. The status of selected national objectives for the year 2010 related to the health of older clients is reflected on page 473.

Because older clients frequently have multiple health problems already, many people consider care for older individuals as incongruent with the population-focused health promotion emphasis of community health nursing. Primary, secondary, and tertiary prevention efforts by community health nurses, however, can decrease the burden of illness experienced by older clients themselves as well as by society.

HEALTHY PEOPLE 2010

GOALS FOR THE POPULATION

Objective		Base	Target
2-9	Reduce cases of osteoporosis in adults 50 years of age and older	10%	8%
2-10	Reduce hospitalization for vertebral fractures due to osteoporosis (per 10,000 persons over 65)	14.5	11.6
12-6	Reduce hospitalization for heart failure in:		
	a. Adults 65 to 74 years of age (per 1,000 people)	13.4	6.5
	b. Adults 75 to 84 years of age (per 1,000 people)	26.9	13.5
	c. Adults 85 years and older (per 1,000 people)	53.1	26.5
14-49	Increase immunization among those 65 years of age and older for:		
	a. Influenza	63%	90%
	b. Pneumococcal disease	43%	90%
21-4	Reduce the proportion of older adults who have lost all of their teeth	26%	20%
22-1	Reduce the proportion of adults with no leisure time physical activity as follows:		
	a. 65 to 74 years of age	51%	20%
	b. Over 75 years of age	65%	20%
24-10	Reduce activity limitation due to COPD in:		
	a. Men over 65 years of age	4.1%	1.5%
	b. Women over 65 years of age	3%	1.5%
27-1	Reduce tobacco use (older adults)	12%	12%

Source: U.S. Department of Health and Human Services. (2000). *Healthy people 2010* (Conference edition, in two volumes). Washington, DC: Author.

APPLYING YOUR KNOWLEDGE IN PRACTICE

✄ CASE STUDY
Caring for an Elderly Woman

Henrietta Walker is a 68-year-old African American woman who has been referred for community health nursing services following her discharge from the hospital. She was hospitalized after being found unconscious in her room by her 50-year-old daughter. A diagnosis of diabetes mellitus was made, and Mrs. Walker was placed on 15 units of NPH insulin daily. She and her daughter were instructed on injection technique and a diabetic diet at the hospital.

Mrs. Walker lives with her daughter and son-in-law and their three teenage boys (ages 18, 15, and 13). They live in a lower-class neighborhood, and the son-in-law works at the local textile plant. His income is barely enough for the family to live on. Mrs. Walker does not

know how she will pay her hospital bill. She has Medicare, Part A, and has a small Social Security income, but she does not have any supplemental health insurance.

Mrs. Walker's vision is failing, probably as a result of undiagnosed diabetes of long standing. She hears well but is 80 pounds overweight, so is unsteady on her feet. The family lives in a second-floor apartment, and there is no handrail on the stairs outside the apartment. Mrs. Walker tries to help out around the house because her daughter works. She says she does not want to be a burden to her daughter and her son-in-law. Mrs. Walker's husband died of a heart attack eight months ago, and that was when she came to live with her daughter. Mrs. Walker's daughter says that her mother's presence has caused some friction among the boys because the two younger ones now have to share a room.

- What are the biophysical, psychological, physical environmental, sociocultural, behavioral, and health system factors influencing Mrs. Walker's health?
- What nursing diagnoses can be derived from the information presented in the case study? Be sure to include the etiology of Mrs. Walker's problems where appropriate.
- How would you prioritize these diagnoses? Why?

- How would you go about incorporating client participation in planning interventions for Mrs. Walker's health problems?
- List at least three client care objectives that you would like to accomplish with Mrs. Walker.
- Describe some of the primary, secondary, and tertiary prevention strategies that would be appropriate in resolving Mrs. Walker's health problems. Why would they be appropriate?
- How would you evaluate your nursing intervention? What criteria would you use to evaluate care?

🐾 TESTING YOUR UNDERSTANDING

- What are some of the common myths related to aging? What is the reality related to each myth? (pp. 442–443)
- What are the four categories of theories of aging? What theories fit within each category? (pp. 440–442)
- What are some of the biophysical, psychological, physical environmental, sociocultural, behavioral, and health system factors that affect the health of older clients? (pp. 443–458)
- What are the major emphases in primary prevention in the care of older clients? Give examples of community health nursing interventions related to each. (pp. 459–462)

- Describe at least one secondary preventive measure for each of four common health problems encountered among older clients. (pp. 462–469)
- What considerations should influence the community health nurse's approach to health education with older clients? What nursing interventions might modify the influence of factors related to each consideration? (pp. 471–472)
- What four considerations unique to older adults influence the evaluation of nursing interventions in this population? (p. 472)

REFERENCES

Aguero-Torres, H., Fratiglioni, L., Guo, Z., Viitanen, M., von Strauss, E., & Winblad, B. (1998). Dementia is the major cause of functional dependence in the elderly: 3-year follow-up data from a population-based study. *American Journal of Public Health, 88,* 1452–1456.

Baltes, P. B., & Baltes, M. M. (1998). Savoir vivre in old age: How to master the shifting balance between gains and losses. *National Forum, 78*(2), 13–18.

Bennett, J. A. (1999). Activities of daily living: Old fashioned or still useful? *Journal of Gerontological Nursing, 16*(5), 22–29.

Blackman, D. K., Kamimoto, L. A., & Smith, S. M. (1999). Overview: Surveillance for selected public health indicators affecting older adults—United States. *Morbidity and Mortality Weekly Report, 48*(SS-8), 1–6.

Blaha, C., Robinson, J. M., Pugh, L. C., Bryan, Y., & Havens, D. (2000). Longitudinal nursing case management for elderly heart failure patients: Notes from the field. *Nursing Case Management, 5*(1), 32–36.

Boyd, C. O., & Vernon, G. M. (1998). Primary care of the older adult with end-stage Alzheimer's disease. *Nurse Practitioner, 23*(4), 63–83.

Brookmeyer, R., Gray, S., & Kawas, C. (1998). Projections of Alzheimer's disease in the United States and the public health impact of delaying disease onset. *American Journal of Public Health, 88,* 1337–1342.

California Department of Health Services. (2000, March). Flu and pneumonia immunization rates dangerously low for African American seniors. *African American Immunization Update,* 2.

Campbell, V. A., Crews, J. E., Moriarty, D. G., Zack, M. M., & Blackman, D. K. (1999). Surveillance for sensory impairment, activity limitation, and health-related quality of life among older adults—United States, 1993–1997. *Morbidity and Mortality Weekly Report, 48*(SS-8), 131–156.

Davis, R., & Magilvy, J. K. (2000). Quiet pride: The experience of chronic illness by rural older adults. *Journal of Nursing Scholarship, 32,* 385–390.

Ebersole, P., & Hess, P. (1998). *Toward healthy aging: Human needs and nursing response* (5th ed.). St. Louis: Mosby.

Erickson, E. (1963). *Childhood and society* (2nd ed.). New York: Norton.

Ewbank, D. C. (1999). Deaths attributable to Alzheimer's disease in the United States. *American Journal of Public Health, 89,* 90–92.

Forsen, L., Bjartveit, K., Bjornald, A., Edna, T., Meyer, H. E., & Schei, B. (1998). Ex-smokers and the risk of hip fracture. *American Journal of Public Health, 88,* 1481–1483.

Fox, S. A., Stein, J. A., Sockloskie, R. J., & Ory, M. G. (2001). Target mailed materials and the Medicare beneficiary: Increasing mammogram screening among the elderly. *American Journal of Public Health, 91,* 55–61.

Freedman, V. A., & Martin, L. G. (2000). Contribution of chronic conditions to aggregate changes in old-age functioning. *American Journal of Public Health, 90,* 1755–1760.

Fries, J. F., Koop, C. E., Sokoloc, J., Beadle, C. E., & Wright, D. (1998). Beyond health promotion: Reducing need and demand for medical care. *Health Affairs, 17*, 70–84.

Fuchs, V. (1999). Health care for the elderly: How much? Who will pay for it? *Health Affairs, 18*(1), 11–21.

Furman, J. (2001). Living with dying: How to help the family caregiver. *Nursing 2001, 31*(4), 31–41.

Garand, L., Buckwalter, K. C., & Hall, G. R. (2000). The biological basis of behavioral symptoms in dementia. *Issues in Mental Health Nursing, 21*, 91–107.

Grove, N. C., & Spier, B. E. (1999). Motivating the well elderly to exercise. *Journal of Community Health Nursing, 16*, 179–189.

Guralnik, J.M., Simonsick, E.M., Ferrucci, L., Glynn, et al. (1994). A short physical battery assessing lower extremity function: Association with self-reported disability and prediction of mortality and nursing home admission. *Journal of Gerontology: Medical Sciences, 49*(2), M85–M94.

Haight, B. K. (2001). Life reviews: Helping Alzheimer's patients reclaim a fading past. *Reflections on Nursing Leadership, 27*(1), 20–22.

Hayes, J. M. (1999). Respite for caregivers: A community-based model in a rural setting. *Journal of Gerontological Nursing, 16*(1), 22–26.

Helgeson, V. S., & Mickelson, K. (2000). Coping with chronic illness among the elderly: Maintaining self-esteem. In S. B. Manuck, R. Jennings, B. S. Rabin, & A. Baum (Eds.), *Behavior, health, and aging* (pp. 153–178). Mahwah, NJ: Lawrence Erlbaum.

Hendrie, H. C. (1999). Alzheimer's disease: A review of cross-cultural studies. In R. Mayeux & Y. Cristen (Eds.), *Epidemiology of Alzheimer's disease: From gene to prevention* (pp. 87–101). New York: Springer.

Hogstel, M., & Curry, L. C. (1999). Elder abuse revisited. *Journal of Gerontological Nursing, 16*(7), 10–18.

International Council of Nurses. (1999). ICN on healthy ageing: A public health and nursing challenge. *Journal of Advanced Nursing, 30*, 280–286.

Janes, G. R., Blackman, D. K., Bolen, J. C., Kamimoto, L. A., et al. (1999). Surveillance for use of preventive health-care services by older adults, 1995–1997. *Morbidity and Mortality Weekly Report, 48*(SS-8), 51–88.

Jech, A. O. (2000). A health crisis for the elderly: Taking a tumble. *NurseWeek, 13*(13), 20–21.

Kamimoto, L. A., Easton, A. N., Maurice, E., Hustin, C. G., & Macera, C. A. (1999). Surveillance for five health risks among older adults—United States, 1993–1997. *Morbidity and Mortality Weekly Report, 48*(SS-8), 89–124.

Kelley, L. S., Buckwalter, K. C., & Maas, M. L. (1999). Access to health care resources for family care givers of elderly persons with dementia. *Nursing Outlook, 41*(1), 47–14.

Kennedy-Malone, L., Fletcher, K. R., & Plank, L. M. (2000). *Management guidelines for gerontological nurse practitioners.* Philadelphia: Davis.

Khajehdehi, P., & Rezaian, G. (1998). Tetanus in the elderly: Is it different from that in younger age groups? *Gerontology, 44*, 172–175.

Klesges, L. M., Pahor, M., Shorr, R. I., Wan, J. Y., et al. (2001). Financial difficulty in acquiring food among elderly disabled women: Results from the Women's Health and Aging Study. *American Journal of Public Health, 91*, 68–75.

Konrad, T. R. (1998). The patterns of self-care among older adults in western industrialized societies. In M. G. Ory & G. H. DeFriese (Eds.), *Self-care in later life: Research, program, and policy issues* (pp. 1–23). New York: Springer.

Kovner, C. T., & Harrington, C. (2000). Nursing counts: Fast facts. *American Journal of Nursing, 100*(5), 33.

Lechner, V. M., & Neal, M. B. (1999). The mix of public and private programs in the United States: Implications for employed caregivers. In V. M. Lechner & M. B. Neal (Eds.), *Working and caring for the elderly: International perspectives* (pp. 120–139). Ann Arbor, MI: Braun-Brumfeld.

Lewis, R. (1998). Boomers may spend their retirement—working. *AARP Bulletin, 39*(7), 7.

Maslow, A. (1968). *Toward a psychology of being* (2nd ed.). New York: Van Nostrand Reinhold.

Minkler, M., & Fuller-Thomson, E. (1999). The health of grandparents raising grandchildren: Results of a national study. *American Journal of Public Health, 89*, 1384–1389.

Mitty, E. L. (2001). Ethnicity and end-of-life decision-making. *Reflections in Nursing Leadership, 27*(1), 28–31.

National Center for Chronic Disease Prevention and Health Promotion. (2000). Prostate cancer: Can we reduce deaths and preserve quality of life? Retrieved April 30, 2001, from the World Wide Web, *http://www.cdc. gov/cancer/prostate.*

National Center for Environmental Health. (1999). Heat-related illnesses and deaths—Missouri, 1998, and United States, 1979–1996. *Morbidity and Mortality Weekly Report, 48*, 469–473.

National Center for Health Statistics. (2000). *Health, United States, 2000.* Washington, DC: Author.

National Center for Injury Prevention and Control. (2000a). The costs of fall injuries among older adults. Retrieved April 30, 2001, from the World Wide Web, *http://www. cdc.gov/ncipc.*

National Center for Injury Prevention and Control. (2000b). Falls and hip fractures among older adults. Retrieved April 30, 2001, from the World Wide Web, *http://www. cdc.gov/ncipc.*

National Immunization Program. (1999). Reasons reported by Medicare beneficiaries for not receiving influenza and pneumococcal vaccinations—United States, 1996. *Morbidity and Mortality Weekly Report, 48*, 886–890.

Neufeld, A., & Harrison, M. J. (1998). Men as caregivers: Reciprocal relationships or obligation? *Journal of Advanced Nursing, 28*, 959–968.

Pahor, M., Guralnik, J. M., Wan, J. Y., Ferrucci, L., et al. (1999). Lower body osteoarticular pain and dose of analgesic medications in older disabled women: The Women's Health and Aging Study. *American Journal of Public Health, 89*, 930–934.

Reinhard, S. C., Rosswurm, M. A., & Robinson, K. M. (2000). Policy recommendations for family caregiver support. *Journal of Gerontological Nursing, 17*(1), 47–49.

Resnick, B. (1999). Falls in a community of older adults. *Clinical Nursing Research, 8*, 251–256.

Robinson-Whelan, S., Kiecolt-Glaser, J. K., & Glaser, R. (2000). Effects of chronic stress on immune function and health in the elderly. In S. B. Manuck, R. Jennings, B. S. Rabin, & A. Baum (Eds.), *Behavior, health, and aging* (pp. 69–82). Mahwah, NJ: Lawrence Erlbaum.

Rosenkoetter, M. M., & Garris, J. M. (1998). Psychological changes following retirement. *Journal of Advanced Nursing, 27*, 966–976.

Ross, M. M., & Crook, J. (1998). Elderly recipients of home nursing services: Pain, disability and functional competence. *Journal of Advanced Nursing, 27*, 1117–1126.

Rosswurm, M. A., & Lanham, D. M. (1998). Discharge planning for elderly patients. *Journal of Gerontological Nursing, 24*(5), 14–21.

Schulz, R., Heckhausen, J., & O'Brien, A. (2000). Negative affect and the disablement process in late life: A life-span control theory approach. In S. B. Manuck, R. Jennings, B. S. Rabin, & A. Baum (Eds.), *Behavior, health, and aging* (pp. 119–133). Mahwah, NJ: Lawrence Erlbaum.

Shin, Y. (1999). The effects of a walking exercise program on physical function and emotional state of elderly Korean women. *Public Health Nursing, 16*, 146–154.

Singleton, J. S., Greby, S. M., Wooten, K. G., Walker, F. J., & Strikas, R. (2000). Influenza, pneumococcal, and tetanus toxoid vaccination of adults—United States, 1993–1997. *Morbidity and Mortality Weekly Report, 49*(SS-9), 39–62.

Stevens, J. A., Hasbrouck, L. M., Durant, T. M., Dellinger, A. M., et al. (1999). Surveillance for injuries and violence among older adults. *Morbidity and Mortality Weekly Report, 48*(SS-8), 27–50.

Stevens, J. A., & Olson, S. (2000). Reducing falls and resulting hip fractures among older women. *Morbidity and Mortality Weekly Report, 49*(RR-2), 3–12.

Stoller, E. P. (1999). Dynamics and processes of self-care in old age. In M. G. Ory & G. H. DeFriese (Eds.), *Self-care in later life: Research, program, and policy issues* (pp. 24–61). New York: Springer.

Strang, V. R., & Haughey, M. (1999). Respite—A coping strategy for family caregivers. *Western Journal of Nursing Research, 21*, 450–471.

Teel, C. S., & Press, A. N. (1999). Fatigue among elders in caregiving and noncaregiving roles. *Western Journal of Nursing Research, 21*, 498–520.

Todd, C. (1998). Pain in the Elderly, Part 1: Assessing a complex population. *NurseWeek, 11*(3), 12–13.

Treseler, K. M. (1995). *Clinical laboratory and diagnostic tests: Significance and nursing implications* (3rd ed.). Norwalk, CT: Appleton & Lange.

Tullman, D. F., & Chang, B. L. (1999). Nursing care of the elderly as a vulnerable population. *Nursing Clinics of North America, 34*, 333–344.

U.S. Census Bureau. (1999). *Statistical abstract of the United States, 1999* (119th ed.). Washington, DC: Author.

U.S. Department of Health and Human Services. (2000). *Healthy people 2010* (Conference edition, in two volumes). Washington, DC: Author.

Wagner, E. H. (1999). Care of older people with chronic illness. In E. Calkins, C. Boult, E. H. Wagner, & J. T. Pacala (Eds.), *New ways to care for older people: Building systems based on evidence* (pp. 39–64). New York: Springer.

Whitelaw, N. A., & Warden, G. L. (1999). Reexamining the delivery system as part of Medicare reform. *Health Affairs, 18*(1), 132–143.

Zhan, L., Cloutterbuck, J., Keshian, J., & Lombardi, L. (1998). Promoting health: Perspectives from ethnic elderly women. *Journal of Community Health Nursing, 15*(1), 31–44.

Zwerling, C., Sprince, N. L., Davis, C. S., Whitten, P. S., Wallance, R. R., & Heeringa, S. G. (1998). Occupational injuries among older workers with disabilities: A prospective cohort study of the Health and Retirement Survey, 1992–1994. *American Journal of Public Health, 88,* 1691–1695.

HOMELESS CLIENTS AS AGGREGATE

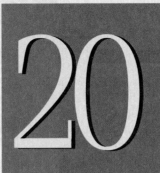

Chapter Objectives

After reading this chapter, you should be able to:

- Describe factors that contribute to homelessness.
- Identify biophysical, psychological, physical environmental, sociocultural, behavioral, and health system factors that influence the health of homeless clients.
- Describe approaches to primary prevention of homelessness.
- Identify major areas of emphasis in primary prevention of health problems in homeless clients.
- Identify areas in which secondary preventive interventions may be required in the care of homeless individuals.
- Identify strategies for tertiary prevention of homelessness at the aggregate level.
- Describe considerations in implementing care for homeless individuals.
- Identify the primary focus of evaluation for care of homeless clients.

Media Link

http://www.prenhall.com/clark

Additional interactive resources for this chapter can be found on the companion Web site. Click on Chapter 20 and "Begin" to select the activities for this chapter.

Who are the people that make up the growing homeless population? Contrary to popular belief, the typical homeless person is not the "skid row bum," a perpetually drunk male vagrant inhabiting a rundown district of a large city. Today, homeless people include families, single women with children, and the elderly, as well as single men. Most are poor, but some are not. Many have little education, but some are well educated. Many are mentally ill, but, again, many are not. Members of ethnic minority groups are overrepresented among the homeless population in the United States, but they are not the only ones who are homeless.

Community health nurses may encounter homeless clients in a variety of ways. For example, when going to visit another client at home, the nurse may be approached by homeless individuals asking for work, shelter, or food. Or the nurse may provide health care services for the homeless in shelters or in clinics. Or the nurse may meet homeless persons when following up contacts of persons with a communicable disease. In addition, community health nurses may participate in task forces mounted by local governments or religious groups to address the problems of homelessness. Wherever they encounter homeless clients, community health nurses must be prepared to assist them to deal with a variety of health and social needs.

DEFINING HOMELESSNESS

Homelessness can be defined in various ways. For the most part, the definition used is that included in the McKinney Homeless Assistance Act of 1987 in which a *homeless individual* is one who (1) lacks a fixed, regular, and adequate nighttime residence, and who (2) has a nighttime residence that is a shelter, an institution, or a place not intended as sleeping accommodations (Wojtusik & White, 1998). Although technically accurate, this definition ignores an estimated 7.5 million people who are "precariously or marginally housed," those who are forced to live with friends or family because of a lack of other housing alternatives. Not being homeless means one has adequate affordable shelter that includes basic services (e.g., access to water, adequate refuse removal) (Glasser & Bridgman, 1999).

THE PROCESS OF HOMELESSNESS AND ITS RESOLUTION

Homelessness is a process of disconnection from social systems that normally provide support in times of need or crisis (Walker, 1998). Conversely, its resolution involves a progressive reconnection.

Causes of homelessness can be conceptualized at two levels: the causes of increasing homelessness in the population and factors that cause a specific individual to become homeless (Phelan & Link, 1999). The first level of causes are structural causes, defects in the structure of society that create populations at risk for homelessness. At the second level, personal characteristics of a given person (or family) determine one's vulnerability to the effects of structural causes (Wright, Rubin, & Devine, 1998). For example, high unemployment levels and low wage scales are some of the structural causes that contribute to homelessness. Poor education or substance

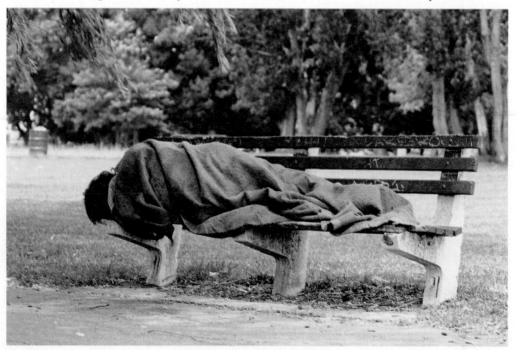

Due to overcrowding in shelters, many homeless individuals have no other choice but to sleep outside.

abuse, on the other hand, may make an individual less employable, thereby increasing his or her risk of consequent homelessness.

Some authors have identified four categories of factors that contribute to homelessness. Two of these, poverty and loss of affordable housing, are structural causes. The other two, behavioral disorders and impoverished social networks, are personal characteristics that may precipitate specific individuals or families into a state of homelessness. Only a small percentage of these individuals, however, are chronically or repeatedly homeless. For the majority of homeless, particularly homeless families, homelessness is a stage, not a permanent state of affairs, but one that requires intensive intervention nonetheless (Shinn et al., 1998).

Although the needs of the homeless population are not specifically addressed by the national health objectives for the year 2010 (U.S. Department of Health and Human Services [USDHHS], 2000), the majority of objectives targeted to low-income individuals also address the needs of homeless individuals. These objectives may be viewed by accessing the Healthy People 2010 Web site through the link available on the companion Web site for this book. ⬟

THE MAGNITUDE OF HOMELESSNESS

There are no exact figures on the number of homeless persons in the United States, and estimates encompass roughly 3% of the total U.S. population (Shinn et al., 1998). Homeless individuals can be found in almost any major city, in affluent suburbs, and in rural areas.

Who are the homeless? The homeless are by no means a homogeneous group. Recent literature speaks to the difference in composition between the homeless population of today and that of several years ago. In the past, most homeless individuals were men over the age of 45. Today, however, only slightly more than half of homeless individuals are single men. Recent figures indicate that approximately 14% of the homeless are single women, and one quarter are children under 18 years of age. Just over half of the homeless population is people aged 31 to 50 years. A large percentage (58%) of the U.S. homeless population are African American, 29% are Caucasian, and approximately 10% are Hispanic (Strehlow & Amos-Jones, 1999). It is estimated that more than 1 million children are homeless (Better Homes Fund, 1999), and growing numbers of adolescents are also included in the homeless population, although their exact numbers are difficult to determine (Ringwalt, Greene, Robertson, & McPheeters, 1998).

Many more families are becoming a part of the homeless population, which in the past was composed primarily of single individuals. It is estimated that families with children constitute as much as 40% of the homeless pop-

ulation nationwide (Better Homes Fund, 1999). Most of these homeless families are headed by single women and include preschool and school-age children (Strehlow & Amos-Jones, 1999).

Obtaining an accurate estimate of the numbers of homeless persons and identifying the factors that contribute to homelessness are difficult tasks. Many segments of the homeless population are hidden, and the factors that contribute to homelessness in one segment of the population may differ for other segments. Visit the companion Web site for this book to read a summary of an article discussing difficulties in identifying factors that contribute to homelessness. ⬟

HIGHLIGHTS

Two Homeless Women

Angela

Angela is an attractive woman in her late 30s. She and her 6-year-old daughter are staying temporarily at a shelter for homeless women with children. She has a college education and had her own business in New York. She has been divorced for a year, but her ex-husband still beat her regularly, so she decided to take her daughter and move to California. She sold her business and left without letting her ex-husband know what she was doing.

When Angela arrived in California, she used the money from her business to buy inventory and rent a place to begin again. She used the little money left over to pay the rent on a small apartment. After living in the apartment for a week, she discovered that the building housed an illegal drug lab run by the building's owner and that most of the other tenants were substance abusers. She decided that this was not an appropriate environment for her child, so she left. She was afraid to ask the landlord for her money back for fear that he would think she was going to the police. She had no other funds, so she and her daughter were homeless.

Angela was very close to her parents, but her father had recently had heart surgery and her parents could barely afford their mortgage payments. Angela did not think she could ask them for help. Fortunately, Angela knew that there were usually shelters available for homeless women with children, so she contacted the health department and was referred to the shelter.

Nancy

Nancy is also staying in the shelter. Nancy is in her early 30s and is tall, gaunt, and emaciated. She describes living for a year in a Volkswagen with her boyfriend and her 7-year-old son.

Nancy and her boyfriend were drug abusers and occasionally gave drugs to her son when he began to "snivel about being hungry." Nancy and her boyfriend worked odd jobs, but used the bulk of their income to support their drug habit.

Nancy's son was enrolled in public school but was frequently absent, and his school performance was poor. When school personnel began to investigate his absences, his circumstances were discovered, and he was placed in a foster home. Nancy voluntarily entered a drug detoxification center, but had no place to go when she was discharged. The social worker at the center made arrangements for Nancy to stay at the women's shelter. Nancy is currently trying to regain custody of her son.

ASSESSING THE HEALTH OF HOMELESS CLIENTS

The first step in the care of homeless clients is assessing their health status and the factors that influence their health. The community health nurse examines factors in the client's situation that contribute to homelessness as well as the health effects of their homeless state.

Biophysical Considerations

Biophysical factors, in conjunction with factors in other dimensions, may lead to homelessness. Conversely, homelessness has serious consequences for biophysical health that vary with age and prior health status.

The health effects of homelessness are exacerbated for both the young and the elderly. Homeless children are twice as likely as other children to to be in fair or poor health and four times as likely as children in families with annual incomes over $35,000. They also have a higher incidence of asthma and other respiratory conditions (Better Homes Fund, 1999). Although recent studies have not found homeless children to have significantly delayed development compared to housed poor children, older children in both groups show poorer development than children in higher-income families, suggesting cumulative developmental effects of poverty (Coll, Buckner, Brooks, Weinreb, & Bassuk, 1998).

Homeless mothers are more likely to be pregnant or have recently experienced childbirth than housed poor women (Shinn et al., 1998), and are more likely to experience adverse pregnancy outcomes such as low birth weight. They also tend to have higher rates of acute and chronic diseases than housed women, with 39% experiencing hospitalization, 22% subject to asthma, and 20% affected by anemia (Better Homes Fund, 1999).

Environmental conditions, including crowded shelters, place all homeless persons at increased risk for infectious diseases, particularly tuberculosis (O'Brien & Simone, 1999). In fact, in 1997, 6.5% of all new cases of tuberculosis in the United States occurred among homeless persons. This is an increase from 5.7% of cases in 1995 and

occurred in spite of an overall decline in tuberculosis incidence (Marks, Taylor, Burrows, Qayad, & Miller, 2000).

Mortality rates among homeless persons in one study were four times those of the general population of the area. In this and other studies, the homeless population had higher mortality rates from accidents and violence than the general population, and injury, heart and liver disease, poisoning, and ill-defined causes contributed to more than three fourths of deaths (Barrow, Herman, Cordova, & Struening, 1999).

The elderly are at particular risk of health problems stemming from homelessness. All of the usual problems of the elderly discussed in Chapter 19 are intensified by homelessness. The homeless elderly are particularly susceptible to the effects of communicable diseases, exposure, burns, and trauma due to alcoholic, physical, or mental impairment or assault. The elderly homeless population is also more likely than younger groups to experience chronic disability due to physical, mental, or emotional impairment.

Homeless persons experience a variety of acute and chronic health problems. In one study, for example, nearly half of the homeless persons studied reported their health as fair or poor. In addition to problems such as tuberculosis and asthma, the most commonly identified health problems included dental problems, vision problems, skin problems and problems with the feet, arthritis, hypertension, injury and trauma, hearing problems, heart disease, and gynecologic problems (Wojtusik & White, 1998).

Chronic health problems are compounded by the homeless person's difficulty in following a prescribed treatment regimen. For example, exposure to cold exacerbates the effects of chronic respiratory diseases, and an unstable diet places the diabetic at higher risk. In addition, because insulin syringes are highly valued by injection drug users, the homeless person with diabetes faces the risk of being attacked for the syringes in his or her possession. The homeless person with diabetes also might be tempted to sell the syringes.

Community health nurses working with homeless individuals or groups of homeless persons would be particularly alert for these commonly encountered health problems. In addition, they would assess individual clients for the presence of any other chronic or communicable diseases, as well as for high prevalence rates for these conditions in the homeless population.

Psychological Considerations

Psychological factors can lead to homelessness when people are unable to cope with the demands of daily life and have limited support systems. Estimates of the extent of psychiatric illness in the homeless population vary, but best estimates suggest that one third of the homeless population experiences severe mental illness. Approximately half of this group have dual diagnoses of mental illness and substance abuse, and half have physical co-morbidities as well (Shern et al., 2000). Homeless clients with psychiatric illness are often noncompliant with therapeutic recommendations, exhibit more symptoms, and have higher rates of hospitalization for mental illness than housed persons with mental health problems (Caton et al., 2000). Mentally ill homeless persons are also likely to display depression, detached affect, and slow responses that put them at risk for victimization on the streets (Walker, 1998).

Some homeless persons without preexisting mental illness exhibit psychological problems as a result of their homelessness. In general, though, nonpsychotic homeless adults have been found to be no more likely to exhibit depression or substance abuse than the general population (Caton et al., 2000). This does not seem to be true among homeless children, however, and approximately 20% of homeless children 3 to 5 years of age exhibit distress and emotional problems, with 12% exhibiting clinical symptoms and 16% displaying behavior problems. Among homeless children aged 6 to 17 years, one third have major mental disorders (compared to 19% of children in general), 47% exhibit anxiety and withdrawal (versus 18% of other children), and 36% display delinquent or aggressive behaviors (compared to 17% of children in general) (Better Homes Fund, 1999).

Psychological and physical abuse are contributing factors in the homelessness of many women with children. National figures indicate that 63% of homeless mothers have been abused by a male partner. Similarly, 8% of homeless children have been physically abused, and another 8% have been sexually abused (Better Homes Fund, 1999). Abuse is also a significant factor in homelessness among adolescents. In one study, 47% of homeless adolescents reported sexual abuse in their home situations and approximately one third left home because of sexual abuse by parents (Rew, Taylor-Seehafer, Thomas, & Yockey, 2001). Victims of abuse experience a variety of psychological effects, including posttraumatic stress disorder (PTSD), depression, somatic complaints, and suicidal ideation. The strain of homelessness compounds these effects.

Childhood abuse may lead to foster home placement. Foster placement in childhood is one of the most signifi-

CRITICAL THINKING IN RESEARCH

In research conducted with homeless persons, it is often difficult to know whether health problems such as mental illnesses, physical handicaps, or substance abuse should be considered contributing factors for homelessness or effects of homelessness.

- How might you design a study that could differentiate the reciprocal relationships among these conditions?
- What type of study design would you employ? Why?
- Where might you recruit your subjects? Why?

cant predictors of homelessness in adulthood (Zlotnick, Kronstadt, & Klee, 1998). There has been a 50% increase in foster placements since 1982, with more placement occurring among homeless than housed children. In fact, approximately 12% of homeless children are placed in foster homes compared to only 1% of the general child population. These rises in placement increase the risk of adult homelessness for these children, creating an intergenerational cycle of homelessness (Better Homes Fund, 1999).

Physical Environmental Considerations

Physical environmental factors also contribute to the effects of homelessness on health. Exposure to cold, even in the mildest climates, can lead to hypothermia. This is particularly true when people are lying on concrete or are clothed in wet garments. Overcrowding and poor sanitary conditions in shelters contribute to the spread of communicable diseases among a population that is already debilitated by exposure and poor nutritional status.

Unsafe physical environments also present health hazards for young children. In addition to the potential for physical injury, the restrictions placed by parents on children's activities in unsafe surroundings may result in developmental delays.

Sociocultural Considerations

Sociocultural dimension factors play a major role in the development of homelessness and in its effects on the health of homeless individuals and families. Changes in family structure and support, widespread unemployment, poverty, and urban redevelopment are some of the societal conditions that contribute to homelessness.

In some cases, homelessness may occur as a result of a breakdown in family ties. Mobility within the population has led to the breakup of extended family systems. This, in turn, results in a restricted social support network for families facing psychological and/or economic crises. High unemployment rates in some areas have led large numbers of individuals and families to move to other parts of the country in search of work. Others have fled countries plagued by poverty and violence. Many of these people arrive in a new locale to find the job market closed and a lack of available low-cost housing. Without an established social support network, they have no recourse but to live in cars, on the street, or in "welfare hotels."

Increases in poverty and consequent homelessness in the United States are, in part, the result of declining family income. In 1997, more than 10% of U.S. families had incomes below the poverty level, and 14% of family incomes were below 125% of poverty level (U.S. Census Bureau, 1999). The increases are the result of several social environmental factors, including changes in government assistance programs, diminished wages, and increased taxes.

⑥THINK ABOUT IT

What factors in your local community contribute to homelessness? What contributions might community health nurses make to modify these factors?

Changes in government programs to assist the poor have contributed to increased poverty and homelessness in two ways. First, the level of assistance provided has not kept pace with the rate of inflation. Consequently, individuals and families receiving aid fall deeper into poverty. Second, budgetary cutbacks have actually reduced benefits in some instances and stiffened eligibility requirements so that fewer of the working poor are eligible for aid. At the same time, taxes paid by the poor have increased. A further problem with the current system of public assistance is a need for persons to rid themselves of most of their resources to be eligible for help. In 1997, for example, only 38% of households with incomes below the federal poverty level received food stamp assistance, 21% received housing subsidies, and 47% received Medicaid benefits (U.S. Census Bureau, 1999).

In 1996, the Personal Responsibility and Work Reconciliation Act replaced the Aid to Families with Dependent Children (AFDC) program with the Temporary Aid to Needy Families (TANF) program placing lifetime limits on receipt of benefits and requiring recipients to be employed within two years of receiving benefits. The change also divorced Medicaid benefits from cash assistance programs. The intent of the legislation was to move recipients off the welfare rolls and to obtain gainful employment for them. Unfortunately, although many TANF recipients are finding employment, it is usually in low-paying jobs without benefits or sick leave, making it difficult for homeless women with children to provide adequately for their children. The federal legislation did not mandate support for child care for working mothers, and although some states provide this assistance, many do not, making it even more difficult for low-income women to adequately care for dependent children (Chavkin, 1999).

Unemployment is another major social factor contributing to homelessness. Although many people remain employed, there has been a shift in the job market from relatively well-paid manufacturing jobs to lower-paid employment in service industries (e.g., janitorial work). This phenomenon is referred to as ***structural unemployment*** or ***deindustrialization*** because it arises from changes in the nation's economic and occupational structure, such as the shifts from heavy to light industry and from manufacturing to service occupations (Snow & Anderson, 1993). The emergence of high-technology occupations requires new sets of skills that many displaced workers do not have. Such changes in the structure of the job market have resulted in a situation in which 6.2 million people were unemployed in 1998 (U.S. Census Bureau, 1999).

The percentage of homeless people who are jobless varies from group to group. Many homeless individuals work at low-paying jobs that do not provide sufficient income to meet basic survival needs. It is estimated that in 45 states, an individual would need to earn twice the

Thrift stores help poor and homeless clients to stretch strapped resources, but still may not meet all their needs.

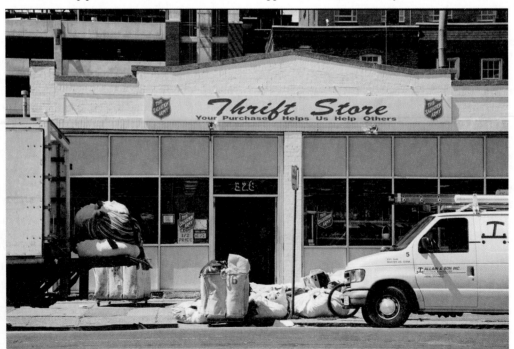

minimum wage to be able to afford rent for a two-bedroom apartment (Strehlow & Amos-Jones, 1999).

Finding employment is difficult for most homeless individuals. Those with mental illness find it hard to maintain a job, if they can get one, because of their instability. Homeless single women with children, who account for almost half of homeless families, have problems of child care while they work.

Even those homeless persons with employable skills in areas where jobs are available may have difficulty negotiating the employment process. Lack of transportation may make it difficult to go to an interview or to get to work when a job is found. In addition, job application and interviews take time, which may prevent the individual from securing food or shelter for the night when these are obtained only after long waits in line in competition with many other homeless persons. Moreover, the homeless person may also find that he or she is penalized for working by reduction or even loss of assistance benefits and publicly financed health care coverage. Homeless individuals who cannot find regular work may engage in day labor or "shadow work." Shadow work may involve selling junk, personal possessions, or plasma; begging or panhandling; scavenging for food, salable goods, or money; and theft (Glasser & Bridgman, 1999).

Loss of affordable housing for low-income individuals and families is a major contributing factor in homelessness. Eviction is a common precipitating cause and may result from inability to pay rent or mortgage. Furthermore, the redevelopment of urban areas with a consequent loss of many low-cost housing units also fosters homelessness. This process, called *gentrification,* occurs when low-income housing is displaced by higher-income space use such as luxury apartments, condominiums, or office buildings (Glasser & Bridgman, 1999). From 1973 to 1993, for example, 2.2 million low-rent housing units disappeared from the market while the number of low-income renters increased by 4.7 million. Similarly, 1 million single-room-occupancy units (SROs) were demolished from 1970 to 1980 and have not been replaced. Many of these units did not meet building safety codes and were condemned (Strehlow & Amos-Jones, 1999). Other units have been destroyed by arson (Walker, 1998).

ETHICAL AWARENESS

You are visiting a formerly homeless client, a single mother with three children under eight years of age. She has been in subsidized housing for only three months. She is now working, and you discover that she is making about $50 more than the maximum that allows her to qualify for her housing subsidy. You know that there is a long list of people who are waiting to obtain subsidized housing, many of whom are in worse straits than this mother. Will you report her increased income to the housing authorities?

The cost of housing in relation to income is another factor contributing to homelessness among the poor. The amount of family income spent on housing has steadily increased over the last few years, and families experiencing "worst case housing" are at higher risk for homelessness than other families. *Worst case housing* occurs when families with incomes below 50% of poverty level pay 50% or more of their income for housing (Better Homes Fund, 1999). In 1997, the median percentage of income spent on housing by families with incomes below poverty level was nearly 55% (U.S. Census Bureau, 1999).

Other social factors that contribute to homelessness in certain populations are divorce or separation and flight from abuse. Many women and their children are forced from their homes by abusive partners/fathers; another sizable group of homeless individuals are teenage runaways fleeing abusive home situations.

The effects of homelessness on health status are compounded by social factors such as lack of transportation and residency requirements for public assistance programs. Lack of transportation limits the ability of the homeless to secure housing, employment, and health

Single-room-occupancy hotels (SROs) provide low-cost shelter in many inner-city neighborhoods.

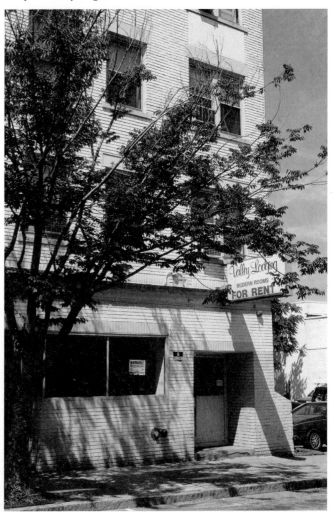

CULTURAL CONSIDERATIONS

Homelessness is much less prevalent among some cultural groups than others (e.g., Muslims). Why do you think this might be the case? What other cultural groups do you think might exhibit similar protective factors for homelessness? How would you go about determining whether or not your assumption is correct?

care, among other things. Other contributing factors include lack of knowledge about entitlements, inability to produce required documentation, complexity of application forms, and frequent changes in eligibility requirements from place to place and over time.

Crime is another effect of homelessness. Homeless men are twice as likely to report arrest as a comparable group of nonhomeless. They are also more likely to report multiple arrests. Often, the arrests of the homeless are for theft of items sold to purchase food or shelter. Other reasons for arrest include violation of vagrancy laws, the stigma of just being homeless, and the substitution of incarceration for needed treatment for mental illness. The extent of criminalization of homelessness is reflected in 23,600 arrests for vagrancy in 1997 (U.S. Census Bureau, 1999). The homeless are also at risk for robbery and assault. This is particularly true of homeless women, those with mental illness, and the elderly, who are less able to protect themselves and their belongings than homeless adult men.

Provision of shelter for the homeless may create problems in and of itself. The number of shelter beds available is often unequal to the needs of the population, especially in areas with large numbers of homeless. Competition for beds often results in intimidation of women and older persons in an attempt to force them to give way to stronger and more dominant males. Unless shelters are segregated by age or sex, or special shelters provided for homeless women, families, and the elderly, these groups may be prevented from making use of available shelter resources.

Shelters are also frequently governed by rigid rules and schedules that may not meet the needs of the homeless. For example, if meals are offered only at certain times, shelter residents may need to choose between food and searching for employment or meeting other needs.

Behavioral Considerations

Substance abuse is a behavioral factor that may contribute to homelessness when the abuser is unable, because of his or her addiction, to meet, or even care about, needs for shelter. Substance abuse may also lead to expenditure of money for alcohol or drugs that could be used for shelter. On the other hand, homelessness may lead to use and abuse of alcohol and drugs as a form of escape. It has been suggested that substance abuse may be a risk factor for homelessness in women, but not in

men, since homeless women have been found to have twice the lifetime rate of diagnosis for substance abuse as nonhomeless women (Caton et al., 2000).

Prostitution is a lifestyle that may arise as a result of homelessness in an effort to earn enough money for food and shelter. Prostitution is particularly prevalent among adolescent runaways who find no other way to earn enough money to support themselves.

Prostitution and injection drug abuse among some members of the homeless population place this group at risk for communicable diseases such as AIDS and hepatitis B. AIDS in and of itself may be a contributing factor in homelessness when persons with AIDS lose their jobs and their ability to provide shelter for themselves or their families. In many instances, avenues of assistance such as shelters and nursing homes that might otherwise assist terminally ill people may be closed to people with AIDS because of fear of the disease.

Homelessness also influences behavioral factors related to nutrition and rest, further compounding the health problems of this population. Inadequate nutrition among the homeless is a lifestyle factor leading to ill health. Even those homeless persons housed in shelters rarely have access to kitchen facilities. Some shelters do provide meals, but they are rarely adequate to meet the nutritional needs of those served. This is particularly true in the case of homeless children, who frequently exhibit anemia or serious growth failure, and who go hungry twice as often as housed children (Better Homes Fund, 1999). Homeless persons may also obtain foods from soup kitchens, fast-food restaurants, or trash cans and tend to have diets high in fat and low in vitamins and minerals (Alley, Macnee, Aurora, Alley, & Hollifield, 1998). The homeless often have difficulty meeting special dietary needs posed by chronic illness and pregnancy.

Homeless individuals may also have difficulty obtaining adequate rest. Because of increased crime and victimization at night, many homeless individuals may attempt to sleep in the daytime when they are less vulnerable to attack. This further limits their ability to obtain many services that are offered only during the day (Strehlow & Amos-Jones, 1999). The inability to rest frequently places homeless individuals at greater risk for a variety of health problems and worsens existing health conditions. For example, the inability to lie down to rest may lead to venous stasis and contribute to leg and foot ulcers. These adverse effects on circulation are made worse if the homeless individual smokes. Smoking also intensifies the effects of respiratory infections contracted from others in crowded shelters. In one study, smoking was reported by 71% of women using a clinic for homeless persons (Alley et al., 1998).

Health System Considerations

Deinstitutionalization of the mentally ill has been described as a major health care system factor in the growing number of homeless people. *Deinstitutionalization* is the process of discharging large numbers of mentally ill persons from mental institutions in an attempt to enable them to live in the least restrictive environment possible. This move was prompted by recognition of the appalling conditions prevalent in many institutions for the mentally ill. Although the intent of deinstitutionalization was laudable, the results were not. Unfortunately, there was no concurrent move to provide the community services needed for the mentally ill to live in noninstitutional settings, and many mental health providers prefer to work with the "worried well" rather than the severely disturbed clients who often become homeless (Walker, 1998). Many deinstitutionalized persons were virtually left to fend for themselves. Without the social or personal resources to provide adequate care for themselves, many of the deinstitutionalized became part of the homeless population.

ⓑTHINK ABOUT IT

Are there elements of the local health care delivery system that would make it difficult for homeless people to get health care?

A related social phenomenon is *noninstitutionalization* of the mentally ill. This refers to a lack of hospitalization of persons with mental problems who are in need of care. Often, particularly in urban areas, people with mental illness are not hospitalized until they have deteriorated to the point where they are a danger to themselves or others. Such tolerance of deviant behavior prevents mentally ill individuals from obtaining help when they need it and when they could most easily benefit from it.

Health care system factors also contribute to homelessness when overwhelming medical bills cause an individual or family to be unable to continue to afford paying rent or making mortgage payments. The effect of medical expenses on one's ability to provide shelter is particularly noticeable in the case of clients with catastrophic illness. These clients are already at risk for a variety of health problems, and homelessness further complicates their needs.

More often than causing homelessness, however, health care system factors make it more difficult for homeless individuals to obtain health care and to prevent or resolve health problems. Financial costs are one barrier to health care for the homeless. In 1999, nearly one third of the U.S. poor had no health insurance, and many of these people are part of the homeless population (U.S. Census Bureau, 2000). An estimated 20% of homeless children lack a regular source of health care (Better Homes Fund, 1999). Even for those who do have health insurance, recent increases in cost sharing (e.g., higher co-payments) may prevent homeless individuals, as well as

other medically vulnerable populations, from obtaining health care (Broyles, McAuley, & Baird-Holmes, 1999).

Cost is not the only barrier to health care access. Other problems include lack of transportation, long waits for service (which may mean missing a meal at the soup kitchen or being unable to obtain shelter for the night), fragmentation of services due to lack of case management, and billing practices that result in attaching the wages of those who make next to nothing. Lack of child care for other children may also prevent homeless parents from obtaining care for themselves or their children. Provider barriers include insensitivity to the needs and circumstances of the homeless and unwillingness to provide care to those with no means of payment. In one study, for example, 22% of homeless subjects indicated disrespect by health care staff as a barrier to obtaining care (Wojtusik & White, 1999).

Personal barriers posed by homeless persons themselves include priority placed on survival over health needs, denial of illness, fears of loss of personal control, lack of money, and embarrassment over personal appearance and hygiene. Homeless individuals and families may also lack the expertise or the energy to complete the processes involved in registration or application for services.

Lack of preventive care is a common problem among this population. Few pregnant homeless women receive prenatal care. These women and their offspring are at higher risk for complications of pregnancy than is the general population. Homeless women are also less likely to receive preventive services.

Preventive care is also lacking for young children. Homeless youngsters use emergency room services as a regular source of health care two to three times more frequently than the general pediatric population, suggesting a focus on crisis care rather than prevention. National figures indicate that 10% of homeless newborns do not receive preventive services and approximately one third lack immunizations. Overall, 70% of homeless children in shelters are not up to date on required immunizations (Better Homes Fund, 1999).

ⓑTHINK ABOUT IT

Why are some health care providers reluctant to care for homeless clients? What strategies can you suggest to minimize their reluctance to deal with this vulnerable population?

Compliance with treatment recommendations may also be difficult. Homeless clients may be unable to afford prescribed medications or may not have a watch to time doses correctly. They may not have access to water to

assessment tips assessment tips assessment tips

ASSESSING THE HOMELESS POPULATION

Biophysical Considerations

- What is the age composition of the homeless population? The ethnic and gender composition?
- What developmental effects has homelessness had? What acute and chronic health problems are prevalent? What is the prevalence of pregnancy?
- What is the immunization status of the homeless population (particularly children)?

Psychological Considerations

- What is the extent of mental illness in the homeless population? What is the extent of depression, anxiety, and suicide?
- What stresses are experienced by this population? How does the homeless population cope with stress?
- What are individual and group responses to being homeless? To seeking help?

Physical Environmental Considerations

- What are the effects of climatic conditions on the homeless population?
- Where do homeless individuals in the community seek shelter? How adequate are shelter facilities? What hygiene facilities are available to homeless persons?
- Do environmental conditions pose other health hazards for homeless individuals (e.g., flooding under bridges used for shelter)?

Sociocultural Considerations

- What is the community attitude to homelessness? To homeless individuals?
- What is the extent of family support available to the homeless individual? What is the extent of community support available for the homeless population?
- To what extent does family violence contribute to homelessness in the community?
- What effects do education, economic, and employment factors have on homelessness in the community? What proportion of the eligible homeless population are receiving financial assistance?
- What child care resources are available to homeless women with children?
- What education programs are available for homeless children?

- What transportation resources are available to the homeless population?
- What is the availability of low-cost housing in the community? What is the availability of shelter for homeless persons? For individuals with special needs?
- What proportion of the homeless population consists of families? What proportion of homeless families are headed by women?
- What is the extent of crime victimization among homeless individuals?

Behavioral Considerations

- What food resources are available in the community for homeless individuals? What nutritional deficits do homeless individuals exhibit? What is the nutritional value of food available to homeless individuals and families?
- What is the extent of drug and alcohol abuse in the homeless population?
- What is the prevalence of smoking in the homeless population?
- Are there facilities available in the community for homeless individuals to rest during the day? What health effects does lack of rest have on the homeless individual?
- What is the extent of prescription medication use among the homeless population? Do homeless individuals have access to resources to help with medication expenses?
- What is the extent of prostitution and unsafe sexual activity in the population?

Health System Considerations

- What health care services are available to homeless persons in the community? To what extent are these services integrated with other services needed by the homeless population? What is the availability of mental health services for homeless individuals? Drug and alcohol treatment services? To what extent are preventive health services available to and utilized by the homeless population?
- Where do homeless persons usually obtain health care? What are the attitudes of health care providers toward homeless individuals?
- How is health care for homeless persons financed?

take oral medications, and syringes for insulin may be lost or stolen. Other difficulties include retaining potency in medications exposed to frequent temperature changes and obtaining prescription refills.

Mental health services for the homeless population are also lacking. Some observers have noted a mismatch between traditional community mental health services and the needs of the homeless population. Comprehensive services are seldom offered at one location, and mental health services seldom address the social factors contributing to homelessness. Assessment of the health status of homeless clients can be guided by the assessment tips provided on page 486. A tool for assessing health needs in this population is available on the companion Web site for this book.

DIAGNOSTIC REASONING AND CARE OF HOMELESS CLIENTS

Based on the assessment of the health status of homeless clients and factors contributing to that status, nursing diagnoses may be derived at any of several levels. At the individual client level, the community health nurse may make diagnoses related to the existence of homelessness. As discussed before, the diagnostic statement includes underlying factors if identifiable, for example, "homelessness due to inability to pay for shelter" or "homelessness due to mental illness and inability to care for self."

Other kinds of diagnoses made at the individual or family level might relate to specific health problems resulting from or intensified by homelessness. As an example, the nurse might make a diagnosis of "stasis ulcers due to excessive walking and standing and inability to lie down at night" or "malnutrition due to inability to afford food and lack of access to cooking facilities."

Nursing diagnoses may also be made at the group or community level. For example, the community health nurse may diagnose a significant problem of homelessness in the community. Such diagnoses might be stated as an "increase in the homeless population due to recent closure of major community employer" or an "increase in the number of homeless families due to unemployment and reductions in public assistance programs." Diagnoses may also be made at the aggregate level relative to specific problems engendered by homelessness, for example, "increased prevalence of tuberculosis due to malnutrition and crowding in shelters for the homeless" or "increased incidence of anemia among homeless children due to poor nutrition."

PLANNING HEALTH CARE FOR HOMELESS CLIENTS

Planning done to meet the needs of homeless clients should focus on long-term as well as short-term solutions to problems. Planning should also reflect the factors contributing to the needs of the homeless in a particular locale. For example, if most of the homelessness in one community is due to unemployment, long-term interventions would most likely be directed toward improving employment opportunities in the area or increasing the employability of those involved. If, on the other hand, a significant portion of homelessness in the area is due to mental illness and inability to care for self, attention

would be given to providing supportive services for the mentally ill.

Planning should address the underlying factors contributing to homelessness as well as its health consequences. For example, providing shelter on a nightly basis may decrease the risk of exposure to cold for homeless persons but does nothing to relieve homelessness. In planning to meet the health needs of homeless clients, community health nurses may work independently or in conjunction with other health care and social service providers. When planning to address factors contributing to homelessness, however, the community health nurse frequently is part of a group of government officials and concerned citizens who have assumed responsibility for dealing with the overall problem of homelessness.

Efforts to alleviate homelessness and its consequences may take place at the primary, secondary, or tertiary level of prevention. Community health nurses may be involved in activities at any or all three levels. Whatever the level of prevention undertaken, nurses working with the homeless may be in need of assistance in resolving the problems engendered by homelessness. Links to resources to assist community health nurses working with homeless clients are provided on the companion Web site for this book.

As is true in caring for any client, planning care for a homeless client begins with giving priority to the client's health needs. In many instances, for example, the first priority would be obtaining shelter, a secondary preventive measure. Other health needs could then be addressed in terms of their priority. For each of the health care needs identified for the homeless client, the community health nurse would develop specific outcome objectives and design interventions at the primary, secondary, or tertiary level of prevention. Planning efforts should be a joint function of the community health nurse and the homeless client, who best knows his or her situation and the kinds of interventions that are likely to be successful in that situation.

Primary Prevention

Primary prevention may be directed at either preventing homelessness or preventing its health consequences. Primary prevention can occur at the individual or family level or at community levels. Community health nurses can help prevent individuals and families from becoming homeless by assisting them to eliminate factors that may contribute to homelessness. For example, if a family is threatened with eviction because of a parent's unemployment, the nurse can assist family members to obtain emergency rent funds from local social service agencies. The nurse can also encourage the family to apply for ongoing financial aid programs or assist the parent to find work.

As noted earlier, some people become homeless because of underlying psychiatric illness and an inability to deal with the requirements for maintaining shelter. Severely disturbed people may just wander away from home and take up residence on the streets. Homelessness in this group can be prevented by referrals for psychiatric therapy and counseling. A case management approach to the transition from hospital to home has been found to be helpful in preventing recurrent homelessness among the mentally ill (Susser et al., 1997). Nurses may also provide support services to families caring for mentally ill members to prevent these persons from becoming part of the homeless population. Placement in a sheltered home might also be an approach to preventing homelessness in the mentally disturbed person when family members either cannot or do not wish to care for the client. In addition, the community health nurse can monitor the effectiveness of therapy and watch for signs of increasing agitation or disorientation that may precede wandering. The nurse can also assist the disturbed person by giving concrete direction in such tasks as paying one's rent.

Runaway children and teenagers are another segment of the homeless population for whom homelessness could have been prevented through primary preventive interventions. Efforts of community health nurses to promote effective communication in families and to enhance parenting skills may prevent young people from feeling a need to run away. Similarly, efforts to prevent or deal with child abuse may prevent runaways.

Primary prevention at the community level to reduce the incidence of poverty and homelessness requires major changes in societal structure and thinking. Some suggested avenues for intervention include federal support for low-cost housing, increases in the minimum wage, and access to supportive services for the mentally and physically disabled to allow them to function effectively in society. Another suggestion aimed at reducing the incidence of poverty in families with children to prevent their homelessness is to provide child care assistance and paid parental occupational leaves as needed.

Creating employment opportunities and programs to train people with employable skills is another possible primary preventive measure for both poverty and homelessness. Current public job training programs, however, have been criticized for their failure to facilitate job placement for those who complete the programs. Job training programs directed specifically toward the local job market have been suggested as more appropriate approaches to unemployment. A living wage, child care, and transportation to and from work are other essential considerations if welfare-to-work programs are going to be effective (Chavkin, 1999). Another societal intervention could be to provide a guaranteed annual income to all citizens. Such an approach is exemplified in part by social insurance programs such as Social Security and unemployment insurance that are not restricted to the poor but available to all eligible participants. Other social programs that may help to prevent homelessness include legal assistance to prevent evictions as well as increased housing subsidies (Caton et al., 2000). Changes in housing codes and tax laws to prevent loss of welfare benefits or allowing tax credits in shared housing situations may

also be helpful. There is also a need for "discharge planning" for housing assistance for people displaced by building condemnation or renovation or release from prisons and other institutions.

Community health nursing involvement in such activities occurs primarily through advocacy and political action. As advocates, community health nurses can make policy makers aware of the needs of the homeless and can contribute in efforts to plan programs that prevent homelessness. Nurses can also engage in political activities such as those described in Chapter 4 to influence policies that help to eliminate these conditions.

Primary prevention may also be undertaken with respect to specific health problems experienced by homeless persons. Here, community health nurses may work with individuals, families, or groups of people. For example, community health nurses working with homeless substance abusers might advocate a program providing clean syringes to injection drug users. Failing that, the nurse might provide a simple bleach solution for injection equipment to minimize the risk of bloodborne diseases such as hepatitis and AIDS. Similarly, nurses may provide assistance to families with budgeting and meal planning to provide nutritious meals on limited incomes.

Community-based avenues for preventing homelessness among the mentally ill include providing access to services within the community that enable these persons to care for themselves adequately without institutionalization. Efforts may also be needed to ensure hospitalization for those persons who cannot be adequately maintained in the community. Treatment for substance abuse and secure places for convalescence after hospital discharge might also serve to prevent homelessness in this subgroup.

Also at the group level, nurses may engage in primary prevention for specific problems by encouraging community groups to provide shelters for homeless individuals. Nurses may also provide basic health care for the homeless, focusing particularly on primary preventive measures such as influenza vaccine and routine immunizations for children. For example, immunization services may be provided in nontraditional settings such as soup kitchens, shelters, and so on (Postema & Breiman, 2000). Adequate ventilation, reduced crowding, and use of ultraviolet lights in shelters may also help to prevent the spread of communicable disease.

Another area for primary prevention of the health consequences of homelessness is adequate nutrition. Community health nurses can advocate for food programs for the needy, including the homeless. They can also serve as consultants to existing food programs to ensure that meals are nutritionally adequate to meet the needs of the population served. Community health nursing activities in this area may also include attempts to arrange diets for homeless clients with special needs (e.g., assisting a diabetic client to select foods from those prepared in a shelter that approximate a diabetic diet as closely as possible).

Community health nurses can also work with other concerned citizens to initiate programs to provide adequate clothing and shoes for homeless clients. Efforts may also be needed to arrange for the homeless to bathe and wash their clothing. In some cities, day shelters that do not provide sleeping accommodations often provide homeless individuals an opportunity to shower and wash their clothing. These shelters may also provide a clean change of clothing on a periodic basis.

Another aggregate approach to preventing specific health problems among the homeless is providing universal access to health care through national health insurance or similar programs at the state level. Nurses can promote such programs through political activity and advocacy and may also be involved in implementing them by providing direct services to the homeless.

Secondary Prevention

Secondary prevention is designed to alleviate existing homelessness and its health effects. At the individual level, secondary interventions may include referral for financial assistance via "means-tested income transfers." *Means-tested income transfers* involve the distribution of cash or noncash assistance to individuals and families on the basis of income. As noted earlier, such programs frequently serve only the poorest of the poor and may necessitate loss of all resources before eligibility can be confirmed. Community health nurses may need to function as advocates to assist clients through the bureaucratic process frequently involved. This is particularly true for elderly clients and those with mental health problems. At the community level, nurses can advocate a review of eligibility criteria for means-tested income transfer programs so that a greater proportion of the homeless population is served.

Shelter is an immediate need for homeless individuals. The community health nurse can assist the homeless client to locate temporary shelter. This may be accomplished by means of referrals to existing shelters. If the nurse is not aware of homeless shelters provided in the community, he or she can contact a local YMCA or YWCA, a Salvation Army service center, or local churches for information on shelter availability. When organized shelter facilities are not available, the nurse may try contacting local houses of worship to see if members of religious congregations can provide shelter for a homeless person on a short-term basis. In making a referral for emergency shelter, the community health nurse would consider the needs of the particular client. Ideally, for example, the elderly and women and children would be referred to shelters where they are protected from victimization. Similarly, homeless persons with chronic health problems should be referred to shelters where health services are available and their conditions can be monitored on an ongoing basis.

At the aggregate level, community health nurses can work with government officials and other concerned citizens to develop shelter programs for homeless individuals or families. Avenues that might be pursued include school gymnasiums, churches, and public buildings. Many cities have used these and other buildings as temporary nighttime shelters for the homeless during cold weather. Plans might also be developed for more adequate shelters that provide other services as well as a place to sleep. In designing a shelter program, the community health nurse and other concerned individuals would employ the principles of program planning presented in Chapter 15.

For homeless persons with significant mental health problems, it may be necessary to create specialized shelters called *safe havens,* which are secure, stable places of residence that place few demands on those receiving help. Many mentally ill homeless individuals are not able to deal with the behavioral restrictions and other policies imposed by many typical homeless shelters. They need a place with limited restrictions that offers the same bed each night, a place to stay during the day, and a place to store their belongings. Because of the special needs of this segment of the homeless population, safe havens do not limit the length of stay for those served. Safe havens then become a stage in clients' progressive movement toward permanent housing in which they can learn to trust and relearn skills needed to maintain a permanent residence while unlearning the distrust required for survival on the streets. Homeless persons with mental illness also require services tailored to meet their needs. Although this population has been characterized as generally noncompliant with treatment recommendations, pilot projects that involve outreach; available, but not mandatory, group therapy; and case management services have been shown to be effective in assuring housing stability in this population (Rosenheck et al., 1998; Shern et al., 2000). In addition, provision of integrated services to this population has demonstrated reduced hospitalization costs by $5,900 per person per year (Walker, 1998).

Shelters are an emergency resource, not a solution to the problem of homelessness. Community health nurses should help homeless clients find ways to meet long-term shelter needs. For individual clients, this may mean referrals for employment assistance or other services to eliminate factors that resulted in homelessness. At the community level, nurses can participate in planning long-term solutions to the problems of homelessness. Unfortunately, such planning has not often been the focus of community attempts to deal with the problem. Community health nurses can advocate and participate in planning efforts to provide low-cost housing, employment assistance, job training, and other services needed to resolve community problems of homelessness. Initiating these planning activities may require political activity on the part of the community health nurse.

Planning for long-term resolution of the problem of homelessness for runaways involves a different set of strategies. The community health nurse can explore with the youngster his or her reasons for running away from home. Nursing interventions are then directed toward modifying factors that led the child to run away. For example, if the child was abused, the nurse can institute measures to prevent further abuse if the youngster returns to the home, or foster home placement can be arranged. If problems stem from poor family communication, the nurse can make a referral for family counseling or other therapeutic services. The nurse can also serve as a liaison between the child and his or her family, negotiating for changes that make the child's return possible.

Particular care should be taken to involve the child in planning interventions to resolve his or her situation. A child returned to his or her family unwillingly will probably run away again. In addition, such actions on the part of the community health nurse may also destroy any faith the child may have had in health care providers as a source of assistance.

At the aggregate level, community health nurses should alert community policy makers to the need for coordinated services for the homeless offered in a single location to meet the health and social needs of homeless clients (Rosenbaum & Zuvekas, 2000). They should also make sure that planning groups in which they participate plan services to address the needs of the homeless for housing, food, clothing, employment, child care services for working parents, and adequate preventive and therapeutic health care services. Planning should also include avenues for outreach and follow-up services, particularly for the homeless who may be lost to service. Such comprehensive programs require changes in health care and social systems that may necessitate legislation and public policy formation that can be guided by nursing input.

Community health nurses can also provide curative services for a variety of health problems experienced by the homeless. For example, they may make referrals for food supplement programs or provide treatment for skin conditions or parasitic infestations. They will also be actively involved in educating clients for self-care. Homeless clients may have difficulty with simple aspects of treatment regimens. For example, if the homeless client does not have access to a clock or watch, it may be difficult to take medications as directed. Nurses can suggest the use of medications that can be taken in conjunction with set activities, such as on arising or at bedtime.

The special needs of homeless children and older persons require particular attention. One suggestion is age-segregated shelters or services specifically designed for older persons and families with children to prevent their victimization by other subgroups within the homeless population. Special attention also needs to be given to meeting the nutritional needs of these vulnerable groups as well as those of pregnant women.

Tertiary Prevention

Tertiary prevention may be aimed at preventing a recurrence of poverty and homelessness for individuals, families, or groups of people affected. Conversely, the emphasis may be placed on preventing the recurrence of health problems that result from conditions of poverty and homelessness.

Community health nursing involvement in tertiary prevention may entail political activity to ensure the provision of services to relieve poverty and homelessness on a long-term basis. This means involvement by nurses in efforts to raise minimum wages or to design programs to educate the homeless for employment in today's society. Advocacy and political activity may also be needed to ensure the adequacy of community services for the mentally ill to allow them to care for themselves or to support their families as caregivers.

At the individual or family level, community health nurses may be involved in referral for employment assistance or for educational programs that allow homeless clients to eliminate the underlying factors involved in their homelessness. Moreover, nurses might assist clients to budget their incomes more effectively or engage in cooperative buying efforts to limit family expenses. Community health nurses may also be actively involved in monitoring the status of mentally ill clients in the home and in assisting families of these clients to obtain respite care and other supportive services needed to prevent the mentally ill client from returning to a state of homelessness. In such cases, nurses also monitor medication use and encourage clients to receive counseling and other rehabilitative services.

IMPLEMENTING CARE FOR HOMELESS CLIENTS

Acceptance of clients and their circumstances is an essential function of community health nurses working with the homeless. Dirty bodies and unwashed clothing are most likely the result of inadequate opportunities for hygiene rather than an indication that the client does not value cleanliness.

Another area in which understanding and acceptance may be required is failure to keep appointments. In the absence of timepieces and calendars, which may not be available to the homeless client, keeping appointments for health care and other services may be difficult. One suggestion is to provide clients with a photocopy of a date book on which they can keep track of days until their next appointment. Providing services on a walk-in basis is another way in which clients can be seen when the need arises, rather than at the convenience of the health care facility.

EVALUATING CARE FOR HOMELESS CLIENTS

Evaluating the effects of nursing interventions with homeless clients can take place at two levels: the individual level and the population level. At the individual level, evaluation of the effectiveness of interventions reflects the client care objectives developed by the nurse and client in planning care. For example, if an objective for a homeless family was to provide them with an income sufficient to meet survival needs, the nurse and family would determine whether this objective has been achieved. Does the family now have sufficient income to provide adequate housing, appropriate nutrition, and other needs? If the objective was to find employment for the mother or father, has this been accomplished?

Evaluation of aggregate-level interventions must also be undertaken. For example, nurses and other concerned individuals will want to determine whether shelter programs are sufficient to meet the needs of the homeless population. Evaluation of tertiary prevention programs focuses on the extent to which interventions prevent people from returning to poverty and again becoming homeless. Are job training programs effective in increasing the income of participants above the poverty level? Criticism of current welfare programs seems to indicate that such programs do not effectively relieve the problems of the poor and homeless. If current programs are not effectively alleviating the problem, other solutions must be sought; community health nurses must be actively involved in developing those solutions.

⑥THINK ABOUT IT

What agencies or organizations in your area are successful in assisting homeless people to obtain permanent housing? What factors contribute to these organizations' success?

The Working Group on Homeless Health Outcomes (1996) of the Bureau of Primary Health Care suggested that evaluation of programs for the homeless address both systems-level and client-level outcomes. Systems-level outcomes to be considered include ease of access to programs; the comprehensiveness of services offered; continuity of care, including appropriate referrals, follow-up, and case management; the degree to which an integrated set of services is provided; cost-effectiveness; focus on prevention; and client involvement in the design and implementation of services. Client-level outcomes include client involvement in and commitment to treatment, improved health status, improved functional status, effective disease self-management, improved quality of life, client choice of providers, and client satisfaction. These areas and related evaluative questions are summarized at right.

An additional focus for evaluation is the achievement of those national health objectives that relate to low-income individuals and families. The current status of some of these objectives is presented on page 492.

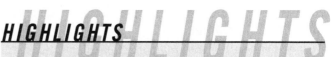

HIGHLIGHTS

Evaluating Services for Homeless Clients

Systems-Level Outcomes

Access to Care
- Are services provided in a location that is accessible to homeless individuals?
- Are services provided at times that do not interfere with the ability of homeless individuals to meet other needs?

Comprehensiveness of Services
- Do services address the wide spectrum of needs experienced by the homeless population?
- Can the agency provide or arrange for the full array of services needed?

Continuity of Care
- Do services provide for long-term involvement with clients rather than episodic assistance?
- Do services include an effective referral network?
- Is there provision made to follow up on the effectiveness of services provided to clients?
- Are case management services available to promote continuity of service?

Systems Integration
- Do homeless clients experience the service system as seamless?
- Are there gaps and overlaps between services provided?
- Are there multiple ways for clients to gain entry to the full range of services provided?

Cost-effectiveness
- Do services make efficient use of available resources?
- Do services result in cost savings to society in the form of reduced emergency room visits or hospitalizations, etc.?

Prevention Focus
- Are preventive services available?
- Are preventive services appropriate to clients in terms of age, gender, etc.?
- Are preventive services effectively utilized by the homeless population?

Client Involvement
- Are clients active participants in their own treatment planning?
- Are clients involved in the planning and implementation of services provided?
- Do clients function as role models, peer advocates, and outreach workers?

(continued)

Client-Level Outcomes

Involvement in Treatment

- Are clients committed to the treatment plan?
- Are clients compliant with treatment plans?
- Do clients continue to request services as long as they are needed?

Improved Health Status

- Have specific client health problems been resolved or ameliorated?
- Do clients perceive their own health status as improved?

Improved Level of Function

- Are clients better able to function emotionally and socially?
- Has the client's level of physical function improved?

Disease Self-Management

- Are clients able to effectively engage in self-care?
- Can clients minimize the effects of disease on everyday life?

Improved Quality of Life

- Do clients describe improvement in their quality of life?

Client Choice

- Do clients have choices among relevant treatment options or social service plans?
- Are these choices perceived by clients?

Client Satisfaction

- Have services provided met clients' expectations and addressed perceived needs?
- Do clients express satisfaction with services provided?

Source: Working Group on Homeless Health Outcomes, Bureau of Primary Health Care. (1996). *Meeting proceedings.* Rockville, MD: Health Resources and Services Administration.

Homelessness is a growing problem in the United States, and community health nurses may encounter homeless individuals and families in a variety of settings. Community health nurses can provide direct health care services to homeless clients. Nurses may also be actively involved in identifying and planning to deal with factors that contribute to homelessness.

HEALTHY PEOPLE 2010

GOALS FOR THE POPULATION

	Objective	Base*	Target
1-1	Increase the proportion of persons with health insurance	70% (74%)	100%
1-4	Increase the proportion of people with a source of health care	78% (81%)	96%
1-6	Reduce the proportion of families with difficulty or delay in obtaining health care	17% (17%)	7%
9-1	Increase the proportion of intended pregnancies	39% (47%)	70%
14-24	Increase receipt of all immunizations among children	70% (72%)	80%
19-4	Reduce growth retardation in low-income children	8%	5%
19-13	Reduce anemia in low-income pregnant women	29%	20%
19-18	Increase food security and reduce hunger	69%	94%
26-30	Reduce binge drinking	15% (15%)	6%
27-1	Reduce tobacco use by adults	34% (31%)	12%

*Baseline figures are for the poor, with figures for the near poor in parentheses.

Source: U.S. Department of Health and Human Services. (2000). *Healthy people 2010* (Conference edition, in two volumes). Washington, DC: Author.

APPLYING YOUR KNOWLEDGE IN PRACTICE

❧ CASE STUDY
A Homeless Family

Crystal is a 16-year-old girl with a 3-month-old baby boy. She has been referred for community health nursing services by her teacher at a special program for adolescents with children. In this program, the girls attend school while child care services are provided for the children. During the day, the girls participate in the care of their infants and learn about child care as well as the usual high school subject material. Crystal has been referred because she has not been coming to school and her teacher is concerned. The school does not have a home address or phone number for Crystal, but the teacher gives you the phone number of Crystal's grandmother. After several attempts, you finally contact the grandmother, who agrees to give Crystal a message to get in touch with you. The grandmother says that Crystal does not live with her and that she sees her only occasionally.

The following week you receive a call from Crystal. She is reluctant to give you an address, but agrees to come to the health department with the baby. When she arrives, she tells you that she has not been going to school because the baby was ill and cannot return to the child care center without a doctor's note that the baby is well. Crystal says she cannot afford to see a doctor. She has no health insurance and no money for health care. She began the application process for Medicaid but never followed through because it was "too much hassle." She lives with her mother and stepfather in a camper shell at a construction site where her stepfather is temporarily employed. She refuses to give you the location of this construction site, saying that they will probably move to a new site soon. Crystal says her parents provide her with food and formula for the baby, who appears clean and well nourished. The baby has not begun his immunizations, again because of lack of funds for health services.

Crystal says she is in good health but has not had a postpartum checkup. Although not currently sexually active, she has a steady boyfriend and is contemplating sexual intimacy with him. She asks about various types of contraceptives.

The father of her baby is no longer in the area and is not aware that Crystal had a baby. Crystal's own father is also removed from the picture and Crystal does not know where he is. When asked about her grandmother, Crystal says that they do not get along well and that her grandmother hardly speaks to her since she got pregnant.

Crystal is anxious to complete high school and enroll in a program to become a beautician. She tried recently to get a part-time job in a fast-food restaurant, but was told they wanted someone with experience. She socializes somewhat with the girls at school and goes with several of them to take their babies to the park and similar outings.

- What health problems are evident in this situation? What are the biophysical, psychological, physical environmental, sociocultural, behavioral, and health system factors influencing these problems?
- What primary prevention measures would you undertake with Crystal and her son?
- What secondary prevention measures would be warranted to deal with existing health problems? Describe specific actions that you would take to resolve these problems.
- What could be done in terms of tertiary prevention to prevent further consequences or recurrence of health problems in this situation?
- How would you evaluate the effectiveness of your interventions with Crystal? Describe the specific evaluative criteria you would use and how you would obtain the evaluative data needed.

❧ TESTING YOUR UNDERSTANDING

- What are some of the biophysical, psychological, physical environmental, sociocultural, behavioral, and health system considerations that contribute to homelessness or affect the health of homeless people? (pp. 480–487)

- Describe at least three approaches to primary prevention of homelessness. How might community health nurses be involved in each approach? (pp. 487–488)

- What are the major areas of emphasis in primary prevention of health problems among homeless clients? (pp. 488–489)
- What are three areas in which secondary preventive activities may be appropriate in the care of homeless clients? What kinds of secondary preventive measures might a community health nurse employ in these areas? (pp. 489–490)
- Identify at least two strategies for tertiary prevention of homelessness at the aggregate level. How might community health nurses be involved in implementing these strategies? (p. 490)
- What is the primary focus in evaluating care for homeless clients? Is this focus the same for evaluating care for individuals and families and care for groups of homeless people? (pp. 490–492)

REFERENCES

Alley, N., Macnee, C., Aurora, S., Alley, A., & Hollifield, M. (1998). Health promotion lifestyles of women experiencing crises. *Journal of Community Health Nursing, 15*(2), 91–99.

Barrow, S. M., Herman, D. B., Cordova, P., & Struening, E. L. (1999). Mortality among homeless shelter residents in New York City. *American Journal of Public Health, 89,* 529–534.

Better Homes Fund. (1999). *America's homeless children: New outcasts.* Newton, MA: Author.

Broyles, R. W., McAuley, W. J., & Baird-Holmes, D. (1999). The medically vulnerable: Their health risks, health status, and use of physician care. *Journal of Health Care for the Poor and Underserved, 10,* 186–200.

Caton, C. L. M., Hasin, D., Shrout, P. E., Opler, L. A., et al. (2000). Risk factors for homelessness among indigent urban adults with no history of psychotic illness: A case-control study. *American Journal of Public Health, 90,* 258–263.

Chavkin, W. (1999). What's a mother to do? Welfare, work, and family. *American Journal of Public Health, 89,* 477–478.

Coll, F. G., Buckner, J. C., Brooks, M. G., Weinreb, L. F., & Bassuk, E. (1998). The developmental status and adaptive behavior of homeless and low-income housed infants and toddlers. *American Journal of Public Health, 88,* 1371–1374.

Glasser, I., & Bridgman, R. (1999). *Braving the street: The anthropology of homelessness.* New York: Berghahn.

Marks, S. M., Taylor, Z., Burrows, N. R., Qayad, M. G., & Miller, B. (2000). Hospitalization of homeless persons with tuberculosis in the United States. *American Journal of Public Health, 90,* 435–438.

O'Brien, R. J., & Simone, R. S. (1999). Tuberculosis elimination revisited: Obstacles, opportunities, and a renewed commitment. *Mor-bidity and Mortality Weekly Report, 48*(RR-9), 1–13.

Phelan, J. C., & Link, B. G. (1999). Who are the "homeless"? Reconsidering the stability and composition of the homeless population. *American Journal of Public Health, 89,* 1334–1338.

Postema, A. S., & Breiman, R. F. (2000). Adult immunization programs in nontraditional settings: Quality standards and guidance for program evaluation. *Morbidity and Mortality Weekly Report, 49*(RR-1), 1–13.

Rew, L., Taylor-Seehafer, M., Thomas, N. Y., & Yockey, R. D. (2001). Correlates of resilience in homeless adolescents. *Journal of Nursing Scholarship, 33,* 33–40.

Ringwalt, C. L., Greene, J. M., Robertson, M., & McPheeters, M. (1998). The prevalence of homelessness among adolescents in the United States. *American Journal of Public Health, 88,* 1325–1329.

Rosenbaum, S., & Zuvekas, A. (2000). Health care use by homeless persons: Implications for public policy. *Health Services Research, 34,* 1303–1304.

Rosenheck, R., Morrissey, J., Lam, J., Calloway, M., et al. (1998). Service system integration, access to services, and housing outcomes in a program for homeless persons with severe mental illness. *American Journal of Public Health, 88,* 1610–1615.

Shern, D. L., Tsemberis, S., Anthony, W., Lovell, A. M., et al. (2000). Serving street-dwelling individuals with psychiatric disabilities: Outcomes of a psychiatric rehabilitation clinical trial. *American Journal of Public Health, 90,* 1873–1878.

Shinn, M., Weitzman, B. C., Stojanovic, D., Knickman, J. R., et al. (1998). Predictors of homelessness among families in New York City: From shelter request to housing stability. *American Journal of Public Health, 88,* 1651–1657.

Snow, D. A., & Anderson, L. (1993). *Down on their luck: A study of homeless street people.* Berkeley, CA: University of California Press.

Strehlow, A. J., & Amos-Jones, T. (1999). The homeless as a vulnerable population. *Nursing Clinics of North America, 34,* 261–274.

Susser, E., Valencia, E., Conover, S., Felix, A., Tsai, W., & Wyatt, R. J. (1997). Preventing recurrent homelessness among mentally ill men: A "critical time" intervention after discharge from a shelter. *American Journal of Public Health, 87,* 256–262.

U.S. Census Bureau. (1999). *Statistical abstract of the United States, 1999* (119th ed.). Washington, DC: Author.

U.S. Census Bureau. (2000). *Health insurance coverage: 1999.* Retrieved November 17, 2000, from the World Wide Web, *http://www.census.gov/hhes/hlthins.*

U.S. Department of Health and Human Services. (2000). *Healthy people 2010* (Conference edition, in two volumes). Washington, DC: Author.

Walker, C. (1998). Homeless people and mental health: A nursing concern. *American Journal of Nursing, 98*(11), 26–32.

Wojtusik, L., & White, M. C. (1998). Health status, needs, and health care barriers among the homeless. *Journal of Health Care for the Poor and Underserved, 9,* 140–152.

Working Group on Homeless Health Outcomes, Bureau of Primary Health Care. (1996). *Meeting proceedings.* Rockville, MD: Health Resources and Services Administration.

Wright, J. D., Rubin, B. A., & Devine, J. A. (1998). *Beside the golden door: Policy, politics, and the homeless.* New York: Aldine de Gruyter.

Zlotnick, C., Kronstadt, D., & Klee, L. (1998). Foster care children and family homelessness. *American Journal of Public Health, 88,* 1368–1370.

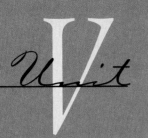

CARE OF POPULATIONS IN SPECIALIZED SETTINGS

ADMISSION

Her eyes would blur
so she couldn't see
to fill the syringes.
Often as not
she'd skip the dose
and damn the diabetes.

She'd get groggy
so she'd lose her balance
*   and fall—*
bound to break a hip one day
land in the hospital
die of complications.

The most complicated things
are simple
in the beginning.

I offer a house call
to check her sugar
and fill the syringes
a week at a time

I offer to enter
once every week
an uncharted world
not my own.

Enter, do for, exit
*   Simple!*
Enter, look around, listen
*   do for, exit*

Enter, wonder
Enter, ask

Enter deeper
Enter.

Reprinted with permission from V. Masson (1999),
Rehab at the Florida Avenue Grill. *Washington,*
DC: Sage Femme Press.

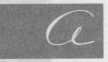

dmission reflects the intimacy of care provided in the home setting, one of many settings in which community health nurses practice.

CARE OF CLIENTS IN THE HOME SETTING

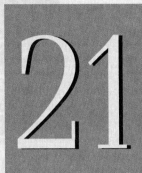

Chapter Objectives

After reading this chapter, you should be able to:

- Describe the advantages of a home visit as a means of providing nursing care.
- Identify characteristics of successful home visiting programs.
- Identify challenges encountered by community health nurses making home visits.
- Describe the relationship between home health nursing and community health nursing.
- Identify types of home health agencies and their distinguishing features.
- Describe major considerations in planning a home visit.
- Identify tasks involved in implementing a home visit.
- Identify potential distractions during a home visit.
- Discuss the need for both long-term and short-term evaluative criteria for the effectiveness of a home visit.

Media Link

http://www.prenhall.com/clark

Additional interactive resources for this chapter can be found on the companion Web site. Click on Chapter 21 and "Begin" to select the activities for this chapter.

Historical photographs of community health nurses often show them caring for clients in their homes. Indeed, home care was the initial focus of community health nursing. The home was where most clients were to be found and where community health nurses had to go to reach them. Today, the home is only one setting where community health nurses care for their clients. Despite the broadening of community health nursing over the years to encompass many other places and settings, the home visit remains a strategic tool for health care delivery. A home visit by a nurse is different from a social visit that might be made by friends or relatives. A *home visit*, as conceptualized in community health nursing, is a formal call by a nurse on a client at the client's residence to provide nursing care.

In spite of the continued use of home visiting as a nursing intervention, this approach to nursing is not always used as effectively as it might be because of several misperceptions about the effectiveness of home visits. Visit the companion Web site for this book to review a summary of an article that presents and refutes several of these misperceptions.

In 1996, more than 94,000 nurses were employed in non–hospital-based health care agencies in the United States. As of 1998, there were more than 10,000 U.S. home care agencies providing nursing home visits to more than 1.8 million people (Kovner & Harrington, 1998; National Center for Health Statistics, 2000). Public health nurses, those employed by official government health agencies, may also make home visits. In addition, community health nurses are employed in a variety of other home visitation programs. For example, in 1996 more than 59,000 clients received hospice services, many of them in their homes (National Center for Health Statistics, 2000). While the focus of home visits may vary among these agencies, the process of planning and conducting a home visit is essentially the same.

ADVANTAGES OF HOME VISITS

Why do community health nurses make home visits? It would seem to be more cost-effective for clients to come to the nurse. More clients might be seen in a given period if the nurse did not have to consider travel time or time wasted being lost in unfamiliar areas. What is there about a home visit that outweighs these obvious disadvantages?

The advantages of home visits can be viewed in terms of six major aspects: convenience, access, information, relationship, cost, and outcomes. With respect to convenience, many clients would prefer to be seen in their homes rather than clinics or other health care settings. Home visits permit health care services to be integrated into the client's usual routine. Moreover, during a home visit, clients are not subjected to the need to find transportation or to the long waits for service that frequently occur in other settings.

The access aspect of home visiting has two elements. First, clients who are immobile or lack transportation and cannot reach other care settings have access to care that might otherwise be unavailable to them. Similarly, community health nurses may gain access to clients who would not present themselves, for whatever reasons, for services provided in other settings. Second, home visits provide community health nurses with opportunities to identify other clients in need of services (Merrill, Turner, McLaughlin, & Milner, 1999).

In the information aspect, the nurse making a home visit has opportunities to obtain a variety of information that is less easily obtained in other settings. The nurse gets a complete picture of the client, whether individual or family, and of his or her environment. The nurse can see firsthand the effects of physical environmental, psychological, and sociocultural environmental factors on a client's health status. A home visit provides the nurse with information about possible resources and hazards that can influence a client's health. The interaction of family members during the visit might suggest the extent of a client's support network and the ability of family members to provide care. Similarly, detecting potential health hazards in a home, such as loose throw rugs in the home of an older client, can provide the stimulus for health education to promote physical safety.

In the home, the nurse can better assess the client's ability to perform activities of daily living (ADLs). Finally, frequent contact in the client's home may permit the nurse to identify minor health changes for which clients would not seek help. The nurse may then act to prevent major problems.

Because the community health nurse has a more complete picture of a client as a result of a home visit, the nurse has a better understanding of the client's needs and can better design interventions. Finally, during a home visit, the nurse is better able to monitor and evaluate the effects of interventions. For example, the client may tell the nurse in the clinic that he or she is adhering to a low-sodium diet as planned. If the nurse visits at home, however, and finds the client munching potato chips, it is readily apparent that dietary instruction has not been as effective as desired.

The relationship aspect of home visiting has the advantage of the client exercising autonomy and control. In the client's home the nurse is a guest; the client controls the situation. Effective community health nurses build on this aspect of control to foster clients' sense of empowerment. The nurse also acts as an enabler, assisting clients to find resources to take action on their own, and as an enhancer, helping clients build on personal strengths. These actions by the nurse lead to a collaborative atmosphere in which the client is fully involved in planning interventions, which in turn enhances the probability of successful implementation (Lasker, 1997).

Another advantage to the relationship aspect of a home visit is the privacy and sense of intimacy created. Clients often feel freer to raise sensitive issues in the privacy of

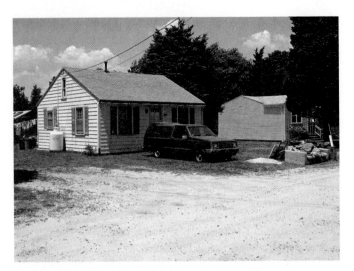
Community health nurses make visits to a variety of homes.

their own homes than in more alien health care settings (Cody, 1999). Thus, the community health nurse may gain more private insights into the client's situation.

The last element of the relationship aspect that frequently operates during a home visit is the continuity of the relationship itself. Often, community health nurses make several visits to an individual or family. This continuity intensifies the effects of the information dimension and other aspects of the relationship dimension, particularly intimacy. Continuity in the relationship may also permit services to others in the client's environment. For example, the nurse may provide education and referrals to enhance the health status of family caregivers (Chen, 1999; Neal, 1999b). On occasion, however, the long-term nature of many home visiting relationships may contribute to challenges that are addressed later.

The cost aspect of home visiting is one reason this mode of delivering health care services has experienced a resurgence (Goodwin, 1999). A RAND Corporation study of one home visitation program, for example, found no cost savings in visits to married women of higher income, but found significant cost reductions over the life of children of low-income unmarried women visited during pregnancy and for up to two years after delivery (Hellinghausen, 1998). Another study estimated cost savings of more than $18,000 per infant for a home visiting program after early discharge of low-birth-weight babies. These savings were realized through the elimination of lengthy hospital stays typical of these babies. Similarly, the cost of an effective child health clinic visit resulting from a home visitation program was estimated at $523 compared to an estimated cost of $2,900 for the usual fragmented approach to care (Kearney, York, & Deatrick, 2000).

The final aspect of a home visit that contributes to its value is client outcomes. Evidence suggests that clients recover equally well after hospitalization with home visitation at a significant cost savings (Penque, Petersen, Arom, Ratner, & Halm, 1999), and that well-designed

CRITICAL THINKING IN RESEARCH

Gagnon et al. (1999) conducted a study of the effects of nurse case management (including home visits) to frail elderly clients after discharge from a hospital emergency department. The focus of the visits was on health maintenance and promotion in clients over 70 years of age. In a comparison of experimental and control group subjects, they found no significant differences in quality of life, satisfaction with care, functional status, hospital admission, or length of hospital stay. Subjects in the experimental group who were visited by nurse case managers were more likely than those in the control group to use emergency department services. Some possible explanations for these findings suggested by the authors included an insufficient number of participants to show significant differences between groups, threats to internal validity (e.g., some control group subjects may have received community health nursing services), ineffective criteria for subject selection, and a weak intervention.

- How might you go about ruling out these possible explanations for the findings?
- What other possible explanations might account for the negative findings of the study?
- Would you expect the results to be similar or different if the subjects were younger or if the intervention had focused on disease management instead of health promotion and maintenance? Why or why not?

home visiting programs targeted to high-risk children and their families produce a number of positive health-related outcomes (Eckenrode et al., 2000; Kitzman, Olds, Henderson, & Hanks, 1997; Olds et al., 1997; Olds, Henderson, Cole, et al., 1998). In fact, a review of several studies of the effects of home visitation programs found decreases in rates of unintentional injury in children and decreased rates of child abuse in some studies. Other studies, however, found increased rates of abuse, possibly due to increased observation of families as a result of home visits (Roberts, Kramer, & Suissa, 1996). Studies of home health care visits also indicate positive effects. In one study, for example, 51% of clients were discharged from services because their needs had been met, and 46% were discharged with improvement in their condition (Lee & Mills, 2000).

CHALLENGES OF HOME VISITING

Despite the many advantages of home visits, this mode of health care delivery is not without challenges. Some of these challenges arise out of the diversity of clients and the multiplicity of their problems. Clients differ in age, ethnic background, culture, health status, and attitudes toward health and health providers. They do not usually experience isolated problems, but are faced with multiple problems that impinge on their health. The diversity of clients and the problems encountered in home visiting require the community health nurse to have a broad knowledge base to understand and deal with the variety of factors that may influence clients' health. The multiplicity of problems coupled with the diversity of clientele creates a variety of service demands that can seem overwhelming and lead to a great deal of stress for the visiting nurse.

Maintaining Balance

Other challenges in home visiting derive from the community health nurse's need to maintain balance in his or her interactions with clients. Areas in which a delicate balance is required are depicted in Figure 21–1 ■, and include a balance between intimacy and professional distance, assisting and devaluing clients, dependence and independence, altruism and realism, creativity and inadequacy, risk and safety, cost containment and quality, and, in some cases, health restoration and health promotion services.

As noted earlier, home visits create a sense of intimacy between nurse and client that is not found in other health care settings. This intimacy, while advantageous in some respects, can make it difficult for nurses to maintain an appropriate professional distance in order to be most therapeutic (Neal, 1999b). Although the home visit is not a social visit, a certain amount of socialization is necessary to establish rapport with clients. Nurses making home visits may disclose more about themselves than they would in other settings. Such self-disclosure can help establish rapport and a collaborative relationship with clients and help to equalize the balance of power between nurse and client (Cody, 1999), but the nurse must be careful to determine what level of self-disclosure is appropriate to the situation. In addition, the nurse will sometimes have to make difficult decisions: Should hospitality or gifts be accepted? The client's offering them may have cultural overtones and refusal to accept may damage the nurse–client relationship. Often, the nurse may feel that the client cannot afford to give what is being offered. In each situation, the nurse must judge the potential effects of accepting or rejecting hospitality and gifts. When refusal to accept small gifts might be interpreted by the client as rejection, the nurse should gracefully accept. If more expensive gifts are offered, the nurse

FIGURE 21–1 ■ *Maintaining balance in home visiting*

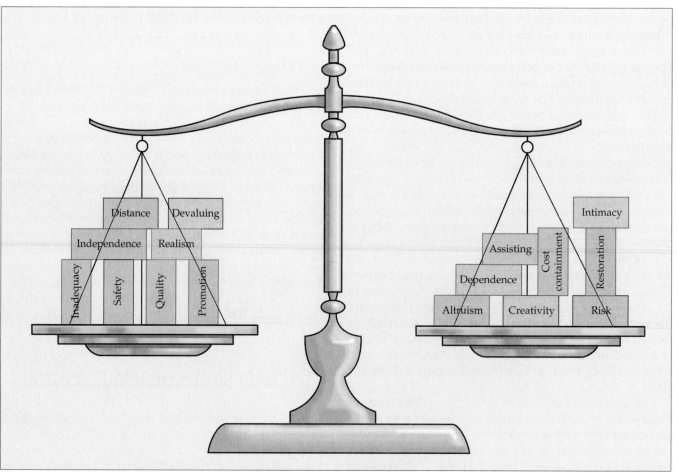

should decline tactfully. He or she might also indicate willingness to accept something of minimal monetary value. For example, the nurse might say, "I couldn't possibly accept that lovely vase, but I would love to have some of your delicious cookies" or anything else that seems appropriate. Such a response indicates acceptance of the client's offer while not accepting an expensive item.

Another challenge arises out of the need to assist clients without conveying that clients are inadequate, that is, without devaluing them. Too often, when people are required to accept the help of others, they begin to perceive themselves as inadequate. This is where a collaborative relationship can be very beneficial. In a collaborative relationship, nurse and client work together to resolve problems and the input of both is valued. Within this relationship, the nurse should convey a sense of self-efficacy that prevents clients from feeling inadequate to meet difficulties on their own.

The balance between assisting and devaluing clients affects self-determination. Clients have the right to determine for themselves whether they are going to comply with health providers' suggestions. Because of the relationship engendered in the home visit situation, nurses may feel tempted to trade on the relationship to subtly coerce clients into actions that are "in their best interest." In a truly collaborative relationship, however, client and nurse together determine goals and the actions to achieve them. The nurse must always keep in mind that veto power lies with the client.

Another area in which balance is required is the level of dependence or independence of client function. The goal of a home visit is to promote client and family self-sufficiency; however, many clients may not reach this level until well into a series of home visits (Neal, 1999b). Again, a collaborative relationship conveys the expectation that clients will do what they can, with assistance from the nurse as needed.

Because of the sometimes overwhelming nature of clients' problems, community health nurses making

home visits must also maintain a balance between altruism and realism. The nurse cannot resolve all of the client's problems and must focus on those problems that are amenable to nursing intervention. Nurses must also recognize that they will not be completely successful with all clients. The nurse, therefore, must learn to be satisfied with incremental progress rather than the dramatic improvements in clients' health status that may be seen in other health care settings. Having a realistic sense of what can be accomplished, given the resources available to client and nurse, will diminish the stress of insurmountable client problems.

Balance is also required between creativity and inadequacy. In the home situation, community health nurses frequently have to deal with a lack of materials and resources that would be taken for granted in other settings. Community health nurses have thus learned to exercise their creativity and "make do" with whatever resources are available. For example, the nurse might suggest to a mother with limited income that she use simple homemade toys to stimulate an infant's development, or the nurse might arrange for support services from friends and neighbors to assist a client on a short-term basis. The nurse, however, must recognize when "making do" is no longer feasible but, rather, is contributing to inadequate care. In this situation, the nurse must seek other avenues to obtain the resources necessary to provide adequate client care. For example, the amount of assistance needed may tax the resources of the client's friends and family, and professional care must be sought.

The need for balance in the area of risk and safety affects both nurse and client. The nurse must decide what level of risk is acceptable without unduly jeopardizing the safety of the client or the nurse's own safety. The nurse may need to weigh the relative risks of changing a potentially hazardous environment versus the disruption to the client's life that will result from the change. For example, a visiting nurse may have to help a family decide the best alternative for caring for an older family member no longer capable of self-care. Should the older person live with family members, seek a companion, or be placed in a nursing home?

The risk–safety balance issue affects the nurse as well. Nurses need to be aware of and minimize potential risks to their own safety in making home visits. Basic safety precautions frequently prevent risk situations. Table 21–1 ■ lists several suggestions for risk reduction in this area. On occasion, the nurse may need to balance client safety against his or her own safety. In this case, the decision of the nurse will be based, of necessity, on the factors operating in the particular situation and the relative risk to self and client.

Cost containment and quality must also be balanced. As noted earlier, one of the advantages of home visits is their cost-effectiveness. Providing care in the home is not inexpensive, however, and agencies that engage in home visiting need to be reimbursed for their services. At present, reimbursement is based too often on provision of

CULTURAL CONSIDERATIONS

You are visiting the home of an elderly German American woman to check her blood sugar. Her home is quite rundown and in need of several repairs. You notice that several of the window screens have holes and there are numerous flies in the home. Your client offers you a piece of coffee cake that a neighbor had brought her. Several of what appear, at first glance, to be raisins in the coffee cake are actually dead flies. Because of your client's diabetes and consequent retinopathy, she cannot see the flies. You know that among many German Americans hospitality is very important and that your client will be insulted if you decline the offer. What will you do?

■ **TABLE 21–1 Personal Safety Considerations in Home Visiting**

Appearance
- Wear a name tag and a uniform or other apparel that identifies you as a nurse.
- Do not carry a purse or wear expensive jewelry.
- Leave any valuables at home or lock them in the trunk of the car.

Transportation
- Keep your car in good repair and with a full tank of gas.
- Carry emergency supplies such as a flashlight and blanket.
- Always lock your car and carry keys in hand when leaving the client's home.
- Park near the client's home with your car in view of the home whenever possible.
- Avoid the use of public transportation if possible.
- Get complete and accurate directions to the home.

The Situation
- Call ahead to alert the client that you will be coming.
- Ask clients to secure pets before your visit.
- Walk directly to the client's home, without detours to local shops or other places.
- Keep one arm free while walking to the client's home.
- Avoid isolated areas, especially late in the day or at night.
- Knock before entering the client's home, even if the door is open.
- Make joint visits in dangerous neighborhoods or situations or employ an escort service if needed.
- Listen to the client's messages regarding potential safety hazards.
- Make home visits at times when illicit activity (such as drug transactions) is less likely to occur or when potentially dangerous family members will not be present.
- Carry a whistle that is easily accessible.
- Become familiar with personal defense techniques.
- Leave any situation that appears to hold a risk of personal danger.
- Stay alert and observe your surroundings.

ETHICAL AWARENESS

Although it is quite rare, community health nurses making home visits occasionally encounter situations that are unsafe and in which they must balance their own safety with that of their clients. Imagine that you are making a home visit to an elderly homebound woman who is being followed for hypertension. The woman's son was recently arrested for producing and selling methamphetamines after his mother reported his activities to the police. About 10 minutes after you arrive, the son comes out of the bedroom with a shotgun. He is obviously intoxicated. He tells you that he is going to shoot one of you. If you leave, he will shoot his mother. If you stay, he will shoot you. He tells you the choice is yours. What will you do?

technical care services rather than on clients' health needs. Frequently, nurses are not reimbursed for services such as health education. Until reimbursement policies are changed, community health nurses need to continue to provide these services within the context of reimbursable services while continuing to maintain productivity levels that ensure the fiscal viability of the parent agency.

The ability to meet client and family needs effectively must also be considered in balancing cost containment and quality. Sometimes the question is one of "cost containment for whom?" For example, it may cost society less to provide care in the home, but it may cost the family more. Family costs may include higher out-of-pocket costs for items not covered in the home setting by health insurance or lost wages if a family member needs to stay home to provide care.

The final balance that needs to be achieved in many home visit situations is related to the cost containment versus quality issue. Because health-promotive services are frequently not reimbursable in many home visit programs (particularly home health programs), nurses may need to maintain a balance between the provision of illness-related health restoration care and health-promotive care, the true focus of community health nursing. Again, community health nurses may need to incorporate these kinds of services into the provision of reimbursable acute care services. Community health nurses must also be able to provide needed services to family members and caretakers that generate revenue.

Effective community health nurses are able to maintain balance in each of the areas addressed here. In maintaining that balance, nurses provide effective holistic care and yet maintain their own integrity and sanity.

Other challenges may arise in home visiting. The first may arise in getting clients' permission to visit in the first place. Because of increases in violent crime, families may be reluctant to admit strangers into their homes. In addition, clients are often unaware of referrals to community health nurses or may perceive them as unwarranted or intrusive. Moreover, being identified as being in need of home visits may be interpreted by some families as "evidence of poor performance." In Great Britain, where home visiting is a routine health care service available to all families, this perception of labeling does not occur. In the United States, however, a home visit may be seen as evidence of inadequacy (Kearney et al., 2000). Because of this, community health nurses may be faced with the challenge of building rapport in an initial contact to permit a therapeutic interaction among nurse, client, and family. This task may be particularly difficult when clients do not have the option of refusing services, as in the case of suspected or confirmed child abuse.

Another challenge in home visiting is the ambiguity of the client situation. Visiting nurses repeatedly refer to the need to shift gears or move from a preconceived agenda to address more pressing needs identified in the family. Frequently, the nurse needs to accomplish this shift within relatively restrictive service parameters of a given agency. Finally, community health nurses may be challenged by the need to avoid client abandonment when services continue to be needed but funding sources have been exhausted. Avoiding abandonment may require very creative problem solving by nurse and client to ensure receipt of needed services. Finally, program attrition is another challenge that may limit the effect of home visit programs with an estimated 50% to 60% attrition from some programs (Navaie-Waliser et al., 2000).

CHARACTERISTICS OF SUCCESSFUL HOME VISITING PROGRAMS

Research has indicated that successful home visiting programs share several characteristics. One such characteristic is focusing on a broad spectrum of goals rather than a single area. Single-focus programs have a tendency to produce modest, short-term effects rather than lasting gains in health status. Similarly, programs that use professional staff as home visitors are more effective than those that use paraprofessionals or laypersons. Indeed, nurses have been shown to be one of the most effective groups to make home visits because of their broad knowledge base and ability to link clients with other aspects of the health care system (Olds, Henderson, Kitzman, et al., 1998). Nurses have also been shown to contribute to lower attrition rates in home visitation programs (Korfmacher, O'Brien, Hiatt, & Olds, 1999). More research is needed, however, to identify the appropriate mix of staff in most home visiting programs.

Effective programs also differ from less effective ones in terms of the intensity and duration of services (Kearney et al., 2000). Generally speaking, a single home visit does not accomplish much, but gains in health status can be seen with a series of visits. Finally, home visit programs are more successful when they are targeted to high-risk populations with multiple needs. These characteristics of successful home visiting programs give rise to the principles summarized below.

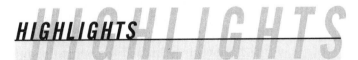

HIGHLIGHTS

Principles for Home Visiting Programs
- Participation in home visiting programs should be voluntary and client–visitor relationships should be collaborative.
- Home visiting programs should foster client progress toward personal goals in addition to program goals.
- Home visiting programs should address multiple goals and should encompass long-term as well as short-term gains in health status.
- Home visiting programs should permit flexibility in the intensity and duration of services provided.
- Home visiting programs should be sensitive to the diversity of clients and needs served.
- Home visiting programs require a well-educated staff.
- Expected outcomes of home visiting programs should be realistic.
- Evaluation of home visiting programs should focus on client outcomes, cost-effectiveness, and processes used in intervention.

PURPOSES OF HOME VISITING PROGRAMS

An array of health-related agencies conduct home visits, either as the major component of service or in addition to other services. Each agency has its own goals for the home visit program, but generally the purposes of visits can be grouped into four categories: case finding and referral; health promotion and illness prevention; care of the sick, which includes health restoration and maintenance; and care of the dying. Any given agency may incorporate several purposes within a home visiting program, but will usually emphasize one purpose over the others.

Case Finding and Referral

Some agencies engage in home visiting primarily to identify clients in need of additional services. These clients are then referred to appropriate sources of services to meet those needs. In this type of program, a minimum number of visits are usually required. In fact, the nurse frequently makes only a single visit to identify and deal with clients' needs. In other cases, the nurse might return to the home to follow up on referrals made.

Health Promotion and Illness Prevention

Health promotion and illness prevention are the primary focus of many visits made by community health nurses, particularly those employed by official public health agencies. For example, in many jurisdictions, community health nurses routinely make home visits to new mothers. Community health nurses working in special projects that focus on prenatal and child health also emphasize health promotion and illness prevention in their visits. For instance, special prenatal health projects frequently employ home visits as well as regular clinic appointments as a means of promoting maternal and child health. Similarly, home visiting programs to foster child development focus on health promotion and prevention of health problems.

In 1991, the U.S. Advisory Board on Child Abuse and Neglect recommended universal home visiting for families with young children to reduce the incidence of child mal-treatment (Roberts et al., 1996). Several studies, however, have indicated that home visits are more effective for some groups of clients than for others. Because of the potential costs of universal programs, programs targeted to specific at-risk individuals and families may be more cost-effective (Gomby, 2000). For example, in one study, women with greater social support needs and more healthy behaviors tended to stay in home visitation programs longer than those who had fewer needs and fewer healthy behaviors (Navaie-Waliser et al., 2000). In another study, home visits during pregnancy and infancy reduced the incidence of child abuse, but not in families with a high frequency of domestic violence (Eckenrode et al., 2000). The results of these studies reinforce the concept of targeted home visitation programs for health promotion and illness prevention.

Care of the Sick

Specific "home health" agencies are primarily geared to meeting the needs of the sick in their homes. *Home health care,* in this context, refers to the delivery of services in the home for purposes of restoring or maintaining the health of clients. The great majority of clients who receive home health services are elderly persons (69% of care recipients in 1998) who have a variety of chronic illnesses. Common diagnoses among clients who receive home health services include circulatory problems (24%), musculoskeletal problems (8%), respiratory problems (8%), central nervous system disease and sensory problems (8%), diabetes (6%), fracture (4%), neoplasms (4%), and decubitus ulcers (1%) (National Center for Health Statistics, 2000). The presence of multiple nursing diagnoses and difficulties with functional abilities are other indicators of the need for home health services (Lee & Mills, 2000; Rosswurm & Lanham, 1998). Indicators of potential needs for home health care services are summarized in Table 21–2 ■.

Care of the Dying

Specialized home visiting services are provided to people with terminal illness by hospice agencies. In addition to home visits by nurses, hospices also provide a variety of other services including visits by volunteers, caretaker respite, physical therapy, medications, durable medical equipment, counseling, and other spiritual care for clients and families. In 1996, hospice care was provided to more than 59,000 clients in the United States. Again, the majority of these clients (79%) were over 65 years of age, but just over one fifth were younger. Most terminally ill clients (58%) were admitted to hospice care with diagnoses of various kinds of neoplasms (National Center for Health Statistics, 2000).

Nurses employed by home health care agencies may also care for dying clients and their families. Family members, as well as dying clients, need information and support from

■ **TABLE 21–2 Clients Who Might Benefit From a Home Visit**

Indication	Type of Client
Physical needs and conditions	Pregnant clients
	Ill, disabled, or frail elderly clients living alone or with others whose health is impaired
	Clients with physical or emotional problems that make it difficult to carry out activities of daily living
	Clients discharged from hospitals or nursing homes with continuing health needs
	Clients who need special procedures that family members cannot perform or need help in performing
	Clients who require periodic monitoring of chronic conditions
	Terminally ill clients and their families
	Clients with certain communicable diseases (e.g., HIV/AIDS, hepatitis, tuberculosis) that require care over time
	Clients who need rehabilitation services
	Clients who are recovering from work-related injuries
	Postpartum clients who experienced perinatal difficulties
Emotional needs	Clients with chronic mental health conditions
	Clients who are anxious about their condition or their ability for self-care
	Families undergoing crises
	Clients who have experienced the death of a child
	Clients who are at risk for suicide or who have experienced a recent suicide in the family
Family role changes	Adolescent parents
	First-time parents and their newborns
	Caretakers who need assistance or reassurance
	Caretakers who miss work frequently to provide care to family members
	Families with multiply handicapped children
	Families in which caretakers are experiencing stress
Health education needs	Clients who have significant knowledge deficits regarding health promotion, an existing condition, or its treatment
Psychosocial needs	Clients who live in unsafe physical environments
	Children who are experiencing difficulty in school
	Clients who have no regular source of health care

Indication	Type of Client
Other needs	Clients who are noncompliant with health recommendations
	Clients who need periodic review of medications
	Clients who are at risk for abuse or who have experienced abuse
	Children with a history of fetal drug exposure
	Children with attention deficit disorder or developmental delay

nurses, and research has indicated that bereaved family members who received home visits during their loved one's illness showed less depression than those who were not visited (McCorkle, Robinson, Nuamah, Lev, & Benoliel, 1998).

Several aspects of the care of dying clients and their families were presented in Chapter 19. One additional aspect of care that should be addressed in the context of home health care is the use of advance directives. Several different kinds of advance directives exist and are summarized below. Nurses providing home services to dying clients should be familiar with the types of advance directives that have legal status in their states as well as with agency policies regarding the use of advance directives. Nurses should also be knowledgeable about the contents of advance directives, how they should be written, who should witness them, what instructions should be included, and, in the case of health care proxy or durable power of attorney documents, who can serve as the proxy agent (Madden-Bare, 1997).

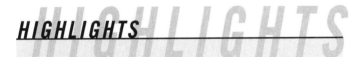

HIGHLIGHTS

Types of Advance Directives

Living will: A document delineating a client's specific wishes regarding use of extraordinary measures to prolong life

Do not resuscitate consent: A document granting the physician permission to write a "do not resuscitate" order

Health care proxy or durable power of attorney: A document designating a specific other person to make health care decisions in the event of incapacitation

HOME HEALTH AND COMMUNITY HEALTH NURSING

A number of authors distinguish between home health nursing and community health nursing. The distinction arose from the early split between personal health care services and public health services when official health agencies began to emphasize population-based screening and health promotion services. Authors who make this distinction base it on the fact that home health nursing is primarily illness focused and that it deals with individuals rather than population groups. Other authors, however, point out that home health nurses do deal with aggregate needs. From this perspective, home health nurses identify populations at risk and in need of home health services and define the role of home health nursing in meeting the needs of individual clients and the larger community. The community focus in home health comes in the planning of systems of care based on an assessment of community needs, characteristics, and resources.

Still other authors suggest that illness is both an individual or family problem and a community experience. This was the perspective of early community health nurses who provided personal health services in clients' homes and simultaneously campaigned to improve social conditions. These nurses and their supporters believed that the conditions of the sick in their homes influenced the health of society in general.

Although today home health nurses work primarily with ill individuals, they continue to employ the knowledge of environmental, social, and personal health factors. That knowledge is a combination of public health science and nursing practice and is the hallmark of community health nursing. It would seem, then, that the distinction between community health nursing and home health nursing is an artificial one and that home health is actually a subspecialty within community health nursing in which the primary but not sole focus is health restoration. Effective home health nurses who provide holistic nursing care employ principles of community health nursing within the segment of the population that is ill. This perspective is supported by the *Scope and Standards of Home Health Nursing Practice* (American Nurses Association, 1999), which states:

> Home health nursing is a specialized area of nursing practice with its roots firmly placed in community health nursing. By definition, community health nursing practice includes nursing care directed toward individuals, families and groups with the predominant responsibility for care being to the population as a whole. The health care needs of the client determine the appropriate augmentation of home health nursing skills with community health nursing practice (p. 3).

Home health nursing is characterized by holism, care management, resource coordination, collaboration, and both autonomous and interdependent practice. Interdependent practice involves collaboration with members of other health care disciplines, both professional (e.g., physicians, physical therapists) and nonprofessional (e.g., home health aides), as well as the client and family members.

Home health nurses, like other community health nurses, also practice autonomously and are responsible for the achievement of designated outcomes of care. Research has indicated that home health nurses pass through a series of stages in the development of autonomous practice (Neal, 1999a). In the first stage, the nurse is hesitant, dependent, uncomfortable with independent decisions; has difficulty negotiating with others; and asks multiple questions. The second stage is one of moderate dependence in which the nurse asks fewer questions, assists others with answers, displays developing confidence in decision making and receives validation for clinical decisions, is more resourceful and innovative, and displays beginning negotiation skills. The expert home health nurse functions autonomously and is confident, self-assured, and comfortable with his or her role; is adaptable, creative, and innovative; is autonomous and self-directed in decision making; coordinates care by others; and uses intuition in expert problem solving.

Types of Home Health Agencies

Home health agencies providing health restoration home visit services can be classified into several types including public or governmental, voluntary charitable, proprietary, institution-based, and hospice agencies (Rice & Smiley, 1996; Schulmerich, 1996). *Governmental agencies* are publicly funded units of government, usually health departments, that provide home health services. Governmental agencies are funded by tax revenues and occasionally by third-party payment. This type of agency frequently operates in areas where there are few other providers of home health services (e.g., the rural southeastern United States) or where financially strapped local governments have attempted to generate revenue by providing reimbursable home health services. Some policy makers suggest that this last activity is an inappropriate focus for official health agencies. Others, however, contend that in underserved areas or areas where private sector services are economically unstable, official health agencies provide a reliable source of care.

Voluntary home health agencies provide home health services on a nonprofit basis. These services are usually funded by charitable donations, fund raising, third-party payment, and some private payment. Visiting nurses' associations are examples of agencies in this category. Both voluntary and governmental agencies tend to care for large numbers of indigent clients with no other source of care, and many voluntary agencies have been forced to reduce the number or types of clients eligible for services because of the drain on limited resources posed by this clientele.

Proprietary agencies are independent home health agencies owned by individuals or corporations that operate on a for-profit basis. Their funding sources include third-party insurance payers and private fee-for-service payments. *Institution-based agencies* provide home health services under the auspices of a larger health organization, usually a hospital or health maintenance organization. Their funding often comes from a combination of proprietary and voluntary payment sources. Finally,

hospice agencies provide home services to the unique population of terminally ill clients. Hospice agencies may be independent voluntary agencies or affiliated with a larger proprietary agency or institution.

Any or all of the home care agencies described here may qualify as Medicare-certified agencies and may provide services under the Medicaid program as well. *Medicare-certified agencies* are home health agencies that have been approved by the federal Health Care Financing Administration (HCFA) to provide specific home health services directly reimbursable under Medicare, the federal insurance plan for the elderly and disabled. In 1996, Medicare paid for home health care for nearly 80% of persons over 65 years of age who received home health services. As noted earlier, older clients comprise the bulk of home health care recipients, which means that Medicare is supporting approximately 40% of the home health care received in the United States (Levit et al., 1998). Medicaid was the source of 7% of reimbursement for home care for older clients (U.S. Census Bureau, 1999).

Agencies that wish to be designated Medicare-certified agencies must comply with federal, state, and local standards for home health agencies and be licensed by the appropriate state or local body. In addition, clients who receive services reimbursed under Medicare must meet certain eligibility requirements in addition to being eligible for Social Security benefits (Green, 1998; Parness & Weinberg, 1997a). These requirements include certification of the need for care and a care plan developed by the client's physician. Periodically, this plan of care must be reviewed and updated with recertification of need for services. In addition, eligible clients must be homebound and need at least one of the following services: intermittent skilled nursing care; physical, speech, or occupational therapy; skilled observation and assessment; or case management and evaluation. Medicaid home care eligibility criteria vary from state to state and usually require clients to "spend down" their assets to become financially eligible for care. Other funding sources for home health care services include workers' compensation, private payment, and free care, which is required of most agencies receiving federal funds (Parness & Weinberg, 1997b). Types of home care agencies are summarized below.

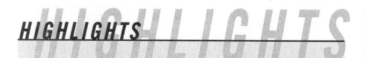

Types of Home Health Care Agencies

Governmental agencies: Governmental bodies that provide home health care services (e.g., local health departments)

Voluntary agencies: Nonprofit agencies that provide home health care services (e.g., Visiting Nurse Associations)

Proprietary agencies: Agencies that provide home health care services on a for-profit basis

Institution-based agencies: Home health care agencies that are part of a larger institution such as a hospital or managed care organization (e.g., Kaiser Home Care)

Hospice agencies: Specialized agencies that provide home health and in-patient services to terminally ill clients.

Medicare-certified agencies: Any of the above that meet the Medicare Conditions of Participation to receive Medicare reimbursement for home health care services.

Costs for Medicare-supported home health care have escalated continuously since the benefit was introduced. From 1987 to 1995, home health reimbursements by Medicare increased tenfold while Medicaid reimbursement for home care services increased fourfold (Kenney, Rajan, & Socia, 1998). In order to contain escalating costs, Congress passed the Balanced Budget Act in 1997, which changed the Medicare home health benefit structure to a prospective payment system to be implemented by the end of 2000 (Flaherty, 1998; Schroeder, 2000). This legislation also reduced Medicare home health payments by 31% initially with subsequent reductions of 2% and 15% prior to the implementation of the Interim Payment System (IPS), a prospective payment system similar to diagnosis-related groups (DRGs) for hospital care reimbursement. The IPS also placed a per-client cap on reimbursement based on the agency's past cost and utilization figures (Peters & McKeon, 1998). Agencies that provide services beyond the cap will not be reimbursed for them.

⑥THINK ABOUT IT

What are the implications of different types of home health agencies for the practice of community health nursing at the aggregate level?

Licensing of Home Health Agencies

Licensure of home health agencies is state or locally controlled depending on where the agency is located. In California, for example, licensing is a state regulatory function. Some areas require a certificate of need prior to licensing a home health agency. A *certificate of need* is a statement providing evidence of the need for home health services in that area that are not being met by existing agencies. The trend appears to be toward increasing regulation of licensure for home health agencies; thus, the reader is encouraged to seek out licensing requirements for agencies in his or her own area.

In addition to state licensure, home health agencies may become eligible for reimbursement for services

under Medicare by complying with the Medicare Conditions of Participation (COPs). Home health care agencies may also choose to be accredited by the Joint Commission on Accreditation of Healthcare Organizations (JCAHO) or the Community Health Accreditation Program (CHAP). Accreditation involves meeting more rigorous standards for quality of care and performance than the minimum standards set by state and federal governments (Green, 1998).

STANDARDS FOR HOME HEALTH NURSING

Individual home health nurses, as well as agencies, should meet established standards. The standards for home health nursing have been established by the American Nurses Association (ANA) (1999) and reflect standards for care of individual clients and standards of performance. The standards of care relate to assessment, diagnosis, outcome identification, planning, implementation, and evaluation; in other words, the use of the nursing process in the care of clients. Standards of practice relate to quality of care, performance appraisal, education, collegiality, ethics, collaboration, research, and resource utilization (Peters & McKeon, 1998). Each of the standards are accompanied by designated measurement criteria. The standards for home health nursing practice are summarized below.

HIGHLIGHTS

Standards of Home Health Nursing Practice
Standards of Care

Assessment: The home health nurse collects client health data.

Diagnosis: The home health nurse analyzes the assessment data in determining diagnoses.

Outcome identification: The home health nurses identifies expected outcomes to the client and the client's environment.

Planning: The home health nurse develops a plan of care that prescribes intervention to attain expected outcomes.

Implementation: The home health nurse implements the interventions identified in the plan of care.

Evaluation: The home health nurse evaluates the client's progress toward attainment of outcomes.

Standards of Professional Performance

Quality of care: The home health nurse systematically evaluates the quality and effectiveness of nursing practice.

Performance appraisal: The home health nurse evaluates his or her own nursing practice in relation to professional practice standards, scientific evidence, and relevant statutes and regulations.

Education: The home health nurse acquires and maintains current knowledge and competency in nursing practice.

Collegiality: The home health nurse interacts with and contributes to the professional development of peers and other health care practitioners as colleagues.

Ethics: The home health nurse's decisions and actions on behalf of clients are determined in an ethical manner.

Collaboration: The home health nurse collaborates with the client, family, and other health care practitioners in providing client care.

Research: The home health nurse uses research findings in practice.

Resource utilization: The home health nurse assists the client or family in becoming informed consumers about the risks, benefits, and cost of planning and delivering client care.

Reprinted with permission from American Nurses Association, *Scope and Standards of Home Health Nursing Practice,* © 1999 American Nurses Publishing, American Nurses Foundation/American Nurses Association, Washington, DC.

THE HOME VISIT PROCESS

Although home visits have some distinct advantages over care provided in other settings, to be effective, home visits must be focused, purposeful events. Like any other nursing intervention, the home visit should be a planned event with specified goals and objectives. The nursing process provides a framework for systematically organizing the home visit to make it an effective nursing intervention.

Initiating the Home Visit

Home visits by community health nurses are initiated for a variety of reasons. Many times, the nurse receives a request for a visit from another health care provider or agency. Reasons for such requests include health care needs related to specific health problems or needs for health-promotive services. For example, many hospital obstetrics units refer all first-time mothers for home visits by community health nurses to provide assistance in parenting and to promote a successful postpartum course and adjustment to parenthood. Similarly, a physician might request a home visit to educate a hypertensive client about prescribed medications.

Home visits might also be initiated by clients themselves. For example, a mother concerned about her child's recurrent nightmares may call and request a home visit by a community health nurse. Friends and family might also initiate a home visit. A neighbor might inform the nurse that he or she thinks the children next door are

being abused, or a mother may request a home visit to help her daughter deal with the loss of a child. Finally, the community health nurse may initiate a home visit. The nurse might note that a child seen in the well-child clinic is developmentally delayed and decide to visit the home to see if environmental factors are contributing to the delayed development.

CONDUCTING A PRELIMINARY HEALTH ASSESSMENT

Before the home visit the nurse conducts a preliminary assessment to review existing information about the client and his or her situation. Previously acquired client data should be reviewed and factors influencing client health status defined. If the client is already known to the nurse or the agency, a certain amount of data is available in agency records, notes from previous visits, and other material. Such data can be used by the nurse to refresh his or her memory regarding the client's health status.

If the client is new to an agency, data available will most probably be limited to that received with the request for services. In such a case, the nurse needs to look for general cues that suggest client strengths and potential problems. For example, if the home visit is requested for follow up on a newborn and his adolescent mother, the nurse knows that infant feeding, sleep patterns, maternal knowledge of child care, bonding, involution, maternal coping abilities, and family planning are areas that may need to be addressed with this family. Similarly, if the referral is for an elderly woman with uncontrolled hypertension, the nurse will identify areas related to diet, medication, safety, and exercise for investigation during the visit.

All aspects of the client's life should be reviewed to detect strengths, existing problems, and potential problems that may need to be addressed during the visit. Using the dimensions of health as a framework, the nurse reviews available information on biophysical, psychological, physical environmental, sociocultural, behavioral, and health system factors that influence the client's health status. By assessing client factors in each of these areas, the nurse enters the client's residence better prepared to deal with the wide variety of client needs likely to be encountered.

Biophysical Considerations

In the biophysical dimension, the nurse would consider the effects of age and client developmental level on health status. For example, if the family includes adolescent children, the nurse might focus on sexuality issues, while home safety might be more relevant to a family with small children. The nurse would also obtain information on existing physical health problems and the presence of disability in clients as well as immunization status and other physiologic factors that influence health.

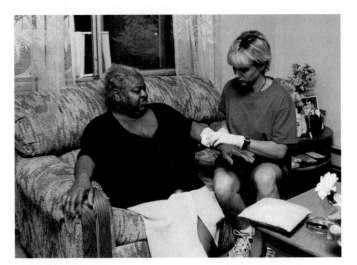

Community health nurses assess clients' physical health status.

Psychological Considerations

Considerations related to psychological factors include evidence of family stress and coping. Nurses making home visits may often find themselves called upon to provide emotional support to individual clients or families in crisis, particularly until other services (e.g., counseling) can be obtained (Cody, 1999). The client with a terminal illness and his or her family are particularly in need of emotional support by the nurse.

Physical Environmental Considerations

In the physical environmental dimension, the nurse obtains information about the home environment with particular attention to home safety needs based on the client's age and health status. Two home safety assessment tools, available on the companion Web site for this book, may be of help to the nurse in this aspect of the assessment.

Other environmental safety conditions may relate to the client's condition or to therapeutic regimens to be implemented in the home. Continuous chemotherapy infusions, for example, are successfully administered in homes, but they present unique safety hazards. For example, some agents are extremely toxic to skin tissue. Needles and other equipment used to administer these agents also present contamination and injury hazards.

Infection control is another safety issue related to provision of health care in the physical environment of the home. Infection control in the home has a dual focus: protecting the client and family and protecting the nurse. The nurse should adhere to the agency's standards of practice, incorporate universal precautions for preventing the spread of disease, and educate clients and family members in infection control measures.

Community health nurses change dressings for infected wounds, change intravenous sites, provide central line care, transfuse clients, and work with clients diagnosed with many communicable diseases. Continuous assessment of the environment for established infec-

tion control standards and outcome criteria is a necessary function of the community health nurse in the home setting. In the preliminary assessment, the community health nurse alerts him- or herself to the potential for problems related to infection control within the client's home environment.

Infection control procedures in the home are similar to those employed in other health care settings, but may require more creativity on the part of the nurse working in the client's home. For example, one community health nurse made an early morning visit to change an indwelling urinary catheter in a remote rural area 60 miles from the health department. Because the nurse knew he would be visiting the client before going to the public health center, he put the necessary supplies in his car the day before. Unfortunately, the temperature dropped during the night, and when the nurse went to inflate the bulb to keep the new catheter in place, the fluid was frozen in the syringe. The nurse did not have another catheterization set and could not return to the health center to get one, so he used the warmth of his sterile-gloved hand to thaw the syringe while maintaining a sterile field and keeping the catheter in place in the client's urethra.

The primary infection control measure in any setting is adequate handwashing before and after giving any direct care to clients. Hands should be thoroughly washed with soap and running water. Again, this may require some creativity on the part of nurses or family members in homes without running water. For example, the nurse may wet his or her hands, apply soap, and lather thoroughly, then ask a family member to pour clean water over the hands to rinse them. The nurse can also make a habit of carrying paper towels on home visits to avoid using towels that were used previously. The nurse may also identify a need to instruct family members in the importance of handwashing in the care of the client and as a general measure for preventing the spread of disease.

Infection control in the home, as in other settings, involves the use of sterile precautions in any invasive procedures, appropriate disposal of bodily secretions and excretions, and isolation precautions as warranted by the client's condition. Nurses working in the home with clients who have bloodborne diseases such as AIDS and hepatitis should use universal blood and body fluid precautions. These precautions apply to any body fluids, including blood, semen, vaginal secretions, cerebrospinal fluid, synovial fluid, pleural fluid, peritoneal fluid, pericardial fluid, and amniotic fluid, and feces, nasal secretions, sputum, sweat, urine, or vomitus that contains visible blood. Identification of the possible need for universal precautions during the preliminary assessment allows the community health nurse to plan effectively to promote personal safety and that of the client and family. Universal precautions to be taken by the nurse to prevent the spread of bloodborne disease are summarized on page 510.

Universal Precautions for Preventing the Spread of Bloodborne Diseases

- Use appropriate barrier precautions (e.g., gloves) to prevent skin and mucous membrane exposure when contact with human blood or other body fluids is anticipated.
- Wash hands and other skin surfaces immediately after contamination with blood or other body fluids.
- Take precautions to prevent injuries stemming from needles and other sharp instruments during or after procedures, when disposing of used equipment, or when cleaning used equipment.
- Do not recap, bend, or break used needles; place them in a puncture-proof container for disposal.
- Keep mouthpieces, resuscitation bags, or other ventilation devices at hand when the need for resuscitation is predictable.
- Refrain from direct care of clients and from handling client care equipment when you have exudative skin lesions or weeping dermatitis.
- Implement these precautions with all clients, not just those known to be infected with bloodborne diseases.

Source: Centers for Disease Control. (1988). Recommendations for prevention of HIV transmission in health care settings. *Morbidity and Mortality Weekly Report, 36*(Suppl. 2), 35–185.

Care should also be taken in the disposal of secretions and excretions of clients with other conditions. For example, sputum from clients with active tuberculosis should be handled with care, and the feces of chronic typhoid carriers should be disposed of in a municipal sewer system.

Sociocultural Considerations

Sociocultural dimension factors to be considered include the client's or family's economic status, interactions with the outside world, and occupational or employment considerations. The nurse would also obtain information on cultural or religious factors that influence the client's health as well as the extent of the client's social support system. Client–family interactions are another feature of the sociocultural dimension that may influence the client's health. The nurse would also be alert to information about family caretaker responsibilities and how these might affect the health of both the client and the caretaker.

Cultural factors should also be considered. For example, the client's cultural food preferences or modes of preparation should be considered in planning to meet nutritional needs. Similarly, child-rearing practices may affect the plan of care for a young child. For instance, in some cultural groups even very young children may make independent decisions about taking medications or adhering to other elements of a treatment plan. If this is the case, the nurse will need to work with both parent and child to assure compliance.

Behavioral Considerations

Behavioral dimension considerations would include information about consumption patterns and nutritional needs of the client based on age or health status. Information regarding substance use or abuse would also be relevant to the planning of effective nursing interventions.

Health System Considerations

The effects of the health system on the client are also an area to be addressed in the preliminary assessment. What is the source of payment for home health services? Does the client have access to other health promotion and health restoration services? Are these services effectively utilized by the client? Tips for the assessment of the individual client in the home setting are provided on page 511.

The reduction in Medicare reimbursement and the shift to prospective payment initiated by the Balanced Budget Act of 1997 has caused approximately 10% of Medicare certified home health agencies to go out of business and others to refuse care to Medicare clients (Flaherty, 1998; Schroeder, 2000). These changes have also resulted in fewer and shorter visits to clients and inability of some clients to obtain services at all.

The movement to managed care has also affected the provision of home health services and the availability of services to clients. Managed care organizations (MCOs) that do not include home health agencies within their organizational structure may contract with existing home health agencies and refer clients to these agencies. Although contract agencies are assured a steady stream of clients, MCOs usually pay discounted rates and authorize fewer visits per client than in prior health care delivery systems. This results in decreased revenue for these agencies. For agencies that do not have major contracts with MCOs, client referral has diminished significantly in areas of the country with high levels of managed care penetration (Peters & McKeon, 1998). Both of these effects of managed care have decreased the economic viability of some home care agencies, forcing many to close and again limiting client access to home care services in some areas. Community health nurses should be alert to these effects on the health of the population in need of home health care.

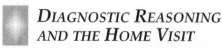

DIAGNOSTIC REASONING AND THE HOME VISIT

Based on the data available in the preliminary assessment, the nurse makes nursing diagnoses related to health conditions to be addressed during the home visit.

assessment tips assessment tips assessment tips

ASSESSING THE HOME VISIT SITUATION

Biophysical Considerations
- What are the ages of persons in the home? Do the age and developmental level of persons in the home give rise to specific health needs?
- Do any persons in the home have existing physical health problems?
- Does anyone in the home have difficulty in performing activities of daily living?
- Do persons in the home exhibit other physiologic states that necessitate health care (e.g., pregnancy)?

Psychological Considerations
- What is the emotional status of persons living in the home? How effective are coping strategies used by persons living in the home? Is there a need for respite for family caregivers?
- Is there a history of mental illness in anyone living in the home?
- Do persons in the home interact effectively with one another? What effects do interpersonal interactions have on health? What is the potential for domestic violence in the home?

Physical Environmental Considerations
- Where is the home located? Is the neighborhood safe? Are there environmental conditions in the neighborhood that adversely affect health?
- Are there safety hazards in the home? Does the home environment accommodate the age-related safety needs of persons living there?
- Is the home in good repair? Does it have the usual amenities (e.g., running water, heat, electricity, refrigeration, cooking facilities)?
- Is the home equipped to meet special needs of persons living there (e.g., safe administration of oxygen, mobility aids)?

- Does the home situation pose an infection risk for persons living there?

Sociocultural Considerations
- What are the education and economic levels of persons living in the home. How do they affect health status?
- What is the extent of social support available to those living in the home? Do they make use of available social support?
- Are persons living in the home employed? How does employment affect health status and health care needs?
- Are there religious or cultural practices in the home that influence health?
- Is there sufficient provision for personal privacy in the home?

Behavioral Considerations
- Does anyone living in the home have special dietary needs? Are those needs being met?
- Does anyone living in the home smoke? What are the potential health effects of smoking on persons living in the home?
- Is there evidence of substance abuse in the home?
- Do any of those living in the home use medications on a regular basis? If so, are they used and stored appropriately?

Health System Considerations
- Is health care utilization by persons living in the home appropriate?
- Are there barriers to access to health care services for persons living in the home?
- How are home care services reimbursed?

These diagnoses may be positive diagnoses, health-promotive diagnoses, or problem-focused nursing diagnoses.

The diagnostic reasoning process is used to derive nursing diagnoses. The nurse examines available data and then develops diagnostic hypotheses that seem to explain the data. Hypothesis evaluation takes place when the nurse actually makes the home visit and obtains additional data to confirm or disconfirm the diagnostic hypotheses. The diagnostic hypotheses generated from the preliminary assessment, however, give the nurse some direction for planning nursing interventions to be performed during the home visit.

Positive nursing diagnoses reflect client strengths evidenced in the preliminary assessment. For example, available data may indicate "effective coping with the demands imposed by a handicapped child due to a strong family support system." This diagnosis suggests that the nurse will reinforce family support as a factor contributing to effective coping.

Problem-focused nursing diagnoses may reflect actual problems for which there is evidence in the preliminary assessment data or potential problems. For example, an existing problem of "ineffective contraceptive use due to inadequate knowledge of contraceptive methods" may have been documented on a previous home visit. Unless there is also an indication that this problem has been resolved, the nurse will probably address it during the subsequent home visit. Preliminary assessment data may suggest potential problems as well. For example, the request for services might indicate that the client's husband is in the Navy and is due to leave on extended sea duty. This information would suggest a nursing diagnosis of "potential for ineffective coping due to loss of spousal assistance."

Nursing diagnoses might also reflect the need for health promotive services. For example, there will soon be a "need for routine immunizations" for a newborn child. Similarly, the mother has a "need for postpartum follow-up due to recent delivery."

Planning the Home Visit

Based on the preliminary assessment, the community health nurse makes plans for a home visit to address the health needs most likely to be present in the situation. Tasks to be accomplished in planning the visit include reviewing previous interventions, prioritizing client needs, developing goals and objectives for care, and considering client acceptance and timing. Other tasks of this stage include delineating activities needed to meet client needs, obtaining needed materials, and planning evaluation.

Reviewing Previous Interventions

The first step in planning is to review any previous interventions related to client health needs and the efficacy of those interventions. This information allows the nurse to eliminate interventions that have been unsuccessful in the past and to identify interventions that have worked.

Prioritizing Client Needs

The next task is to give priority to identified client needs. Client care needs may be prioritized on the basis of their potential to threaten the client's health, the degree to which they concern the client, or their ease of solution. It is often impossible to address all of the client's health problems in a single visit, so the nurse must decide which needs require immediate attention. For example, if the wife has been admitted to an alcohol treatment center and there is no one to care for the children while the father works, provision of child care and dealing with the children's feelings about the mother's absence may be the only things that can be accomplished on the initial visit. Other problems, such as poor nutritional habits and need for immunizations for the toddler, can be deferred until a later visit.

Developing Goals and Objectives

After determining which client needs will be addressed in the forthcoming visit, the nurse develops goals and objectives related to each area of need. Goals are generally stated expectations, whereas objectives are more specific. In the previous example, the nurse's goal might be to enable the family to function adequately in the mother's absence. In this instance, an outcome objective might be that adequate child care will be obtained so the father can return to work.

The health care needs that will be addressed during a home visit may reflect the primary, secondary, and tertiary level of prevention. When health care needs occur in the realm of primary prevention, goals and outcome objectives reflect positive health states or absence of specific health problems as expected outcomes of care. For example, a goal for primary prevention might be "development of effective parenting skills." A related outcome objective might be that the client "will display effective communication skills in relating to children."

Goals and objectives related to needs for secondary prevention focus on alleviation of specific problems. For example, a goal for a hypertensive client might be "effective control of elevated blood pressure" and the related outcome objective might be a blood pressure that is "consistently below 140/90." Similarly, goals and objectives for tertiary prevention reflect client achievement of a prior level of function or prevention of recurrence of a health problem.

Considering Acceptance and Timing

In planning a home visit, the nurse should consider the client's readiness to accept intervention as well as the timing of the visit and introduction of intervention. The nurse may find, for example, that a relatively minor problem with which the client is preoccupied must be addressed before the client is willing to deal with other health needs.

Timing is another important consideration in planning an effective home visit. If the visit interferes with other activities important to the client, the client may not be as open to the visit as would otherwise be the case. Other activities that compete with a home visit for the client's attention might be the visit of a friend, an upcoming doctor's appointment, getting the children ready for an outing, or even something as mundane as a favorite soap opera. Prescheduling or rescheduling home visits can make the visit a more effective intervention if something else is interfering.

Timing also relates to the degree of rapport established between client and nurse. Clients need time to develop trust in the nurse before intimate issues can be addressed. For example, a pregnant adolescent may feel too uncomfortable and threatened by the nurse during early visits to admit to prior drug use and ask about its effects on the baby. The nurse should judge the appropriateness of the timing in bringing up intimate issues for discussion and wait, if possible, until rapport is established with the client.

Delineating Nursing Activities

The next aspect of planning the home visit is the planning of specific nursing activities for each nursing diagnosis to be addressed. Planned interventions should be based on evidence of their effectiveness and may incorporate practice guidelines, agency procedures and protocols, or elements of clinical pathways. The federal Agency for Healthcare Research and Quality (AHRQ) (formerly the Agency for Health Care Policy and Research [AHCPR]) has developed practice guidelines for several problems relevant to home health nursing. Current guidelines include those related to pressure ulcer prevention and treatment and cardiac rehabilitation. Prior guidelines include those for acute pain management, urinary incontinence, cataracts, depression, sickle cell disease, early HIV infection, benign prostatic hypertrophy, cancer pain management, unstable angina, heart failure, otitis media with effusion, quality mammography, acute low back pain, poststroke rehabilitation, smoking cessation, and early Alzheimer's disease (Agency for Healthcare Research and Quality, 2001). Because of recent developments in treatment, these prior guidelines are no longer considered current, but may be of interest to home health nurses anyway. Current and prior guidelines may be accessed through the AHRQ Web page available through a link from the companion Web page for this book.

Agency procedures and protocols and clinical pathways may also be used as guides for planning nursing interventions during a home visit. Clinical pathways were addressed in detail in Chapter 12. Clinical pathways may differ from agency to agency and should be tailored to the goals and resources of the particular agency (Peters & McKeon, 1998). Components of clinical pathways are summarized below.

HIGHLIGHTS

Characteristic Elements of Clinical Pathways

Scope: The extent of the client episode to which the pathway is applicable (e.g., only home care services, or a continuum of care from hospital to home care)

Condition: The health problem or condition to which the pathway applies (e.g., pregnancy or congestive heart failure)

Activity categories: Activities required in the care of typical clients with the specific condition, may be more or less detailed, but ideally reflects activities for which reimbursement is sought

Outcomes: Expected outcomes of care for the client and family

Format: The way in which activities are organized and presented in the pathway (e.g., in a linear form, by treatment day or visit, by discipline)

Documentation: Use of the pathway itself to document interventions, in which case the pathway becomes part of the client's permanent record.

Adapted with permission from Peters, D. A., & McKeon, T. (1998). *Transforming home care: Quality, cost, and data management.* Gaithersburg, MD: Aspen.

The activities planned reflect the nurse's assessment of health care needs and the factors influencing them. In the previous example, referral to a Head Start program may provide assistance with child care, but only if the children involved are of the right ages. If the youngsters are of school age, the appropriate nursing intervention might be to help the father explore the possibility of an after-school program, if one is available, or have the children go home with the parents of a friend until the father can pick them up after work.

Nursing activities can focus on both health promotion and resolution of health-related problems. For example, the community health nurse might provide the parents of a toddler with anticipatory guidance regarding toilet training or assist parents to discuss sexuality with their preteen daughter. Other positive interventions might focus on providing adequate nutrition for a young child or promoting a healthy pregnancy for the pregnant female.

Specific interventions employed by the nurse include referral, education, and technical procedures. For example, the nurse might refer a family to social services for financial assistance, teach a mother about appropriate nutrition for the family, or check a hypertensive client's blood pressure. The actions selected should be geared to achieving the goals and objectives established while taking into account the constraints and supports in the individual client situation.

Obtaining Necessary Materials

One aspect of planning the home visit that does not apply to many of the other processes discussed in this unit is obtaining materials and supplies that may be needed to implement planned interventions. Because the nurse is going to be in the client's home, one cannot assume that necessary supplies will be available there. If the nurse plans to engage in nutrition education, he or she might want to leave a selection of pamphlets with the client to reinforce teaching. If planned activities involve weighing a premature infant, the nurse will want to take along a scale.

Equipment and supplies may also be needed for other procedures such as dressing changes, catheterizations, injections, and blood pressure checks. Because the nurse frequently does a physical assessment of one or more clients, additional equipment such as a stethoscope, percussion hammer, tongue blade, flashlight, and otophthalmoscope will need to be obtained prior to setting out for the visit.

Planning Evaluation

As with every other process employed by community health nurses, the planning phase of the home visit process concludes with plans for evaluation. The nurse determines criteria to be used to evaluate the effectiveness of the home visit. Criteria for evaluating client outcomes are derived from the outcome objectives developed for the visit. Because the outcome of nursing interventions undertaken during a home visit may not be immediately apparent, the nurse needs to develop both long-term and short-term evaluative criteria. Short-term criteria are likely to be based on client response to interventions. If, for example, the nurse makes a referral for immunizations, the mother cannot follow through on the referral and receive immunizations on the spot. The nurse, however, can evaluate the mother's response to the referral. Does the mother seem interested? Does she indicate that she will follow through on the referral? On subsequent visits, the nurse would employ long-term outcome criteria to evaluate the effects of interventions. In this instance, criteria would include whether the client had her child immunized.

Outcome evaluation addresses the level of prevention of nursing interventions. Evaluative criteria for primary preventive measures, for example, reflect health promotion or the absence of specific health problems. For example, criteria for interventions to foster immunity to childhood diseases would include whether immunizations were obtained and the presence or absence of immunizable diseases such as measles. If the client develops measles, primary prevention of this disease obviously was not effective.

Evaluation of secondary preventive measures focuses on the degree to which an existing problem has been resolved. For example, a client's hypertension may have been uncontrolled because of poor medication compliance. Evaluative criteria in this instance would include the degree of compliance achieved and the client's blood pressure measurements. Criteria to evaluate tertiary preventive measures reflect the degree to which a client has regained a prior level of health or prevented recurrent health problems. For example, have passive range-of-motion exercises helped a client recovering from a broken arm to regain strength and mobility? Or has parenting education by the nurse prevented further episodes of child abuse in an abusive family?

The nurse also develops criteria to evaluate implementation of the planned home visit. These criteria are derived from process objectives developed for the visit. For example, was the nurse adequately prepared to address the health care needs encountered during the visit? Were the appropriate supplies available for implementing planned interventions?

IMPLEMENTING THE PLANNED VISIT

The next step in the home visit process is conducting the visit itself. Several tasks are involved in implementing the planned visit. These include validating the health needs and diagnoses identified in the preliminary assessment, identifying additional needs, modifying the intervention plan as needed, performing nursing interventions, and dealing with distractions.

Validating Assessment and Diagnoses
The first task in implementing the home visit is to validate the accuracy of the preliminary assessment. Problems identified from the available data may or may not

exist when the nurse actually enters the home. For example, the nurse may find that the family's poor diet is not the result of lack of knowledge about nutrition, but stems from a lack of money to purchase nutritious foods, or the nurse may find that what appeared to nurses on the postpartum unit to be poor maternal–infant bonding was not actually the case. Similarly, the nurse may discover that expected strengths or positive nursing diagnoses do not accurately reflect the client's actual health status. For example, a mother who appeared to be coping effectively with her child's handicap may really have been exhibiting denial of the condition.

Identifying Additional Needs
During the visit, the nurse collects additional data related to biophysical, psychological, physical environmental, sociocultural, behavioral, and health system factors to identify additional health care needs. For example, when the nurse arrives to visit a new mother and her infant son, the nurse may find that the client's father has recently had a heart attack and been taken to the hospital. The client may be much more in need of assistance in finding child care for her new baby so she can spend time at the hospital than in discussing immunization and postpartum concerns. Or the nurse may find that, in addition to having a new baby, the client's husband is out of work and the 12-year-old has been skipping school.

Modifying the Plan of Care
Based on what the nurse finds in the course of the home visit, the initial plan of care may need to be modified. The nurse shares with the client the initial goals established for addressing health needs identified in the preliminary assessment, as well as additional problems identified, and together they set or revise goals. In doing this, the nurse might find a need to restructure priorities based on new data and client input. For instance, if the 2-year-old has cut her arm and is bleeding profusely when the nurse arrives, this problem takes precedence over the nurse's plan to discuss with the mother the potential for sibling rivalry. In other words, the nurse can either implement interventions as planned or modify the plan as the client situation dictates.

Performing Nursing Interventions
Once the plan of care has been modified as needed, the nurse performs whatever nursing interventions are warranted by the client situation. As noted earlier, these activities may include primary, secondary, and tertiary preventive measures. For example, the nurse working with a new mother might discuss parenting skills as a means of preventing child abuse (primary prevention), give the mother suggestions for dealing with the infant's spitting up (secondary prevention), and discuss options for contraception to prevent a subsequent pregnancy (tertiary prevention).

Any or all of the three levels can be emphasized depending on the situation encountered. For example, if the mother is inexperienced and concerned about child care skills in feeding, bathing, and parenting, the emphasis would be on primary prevention. Conversely, if the nurse arrives to find a baby screaming with gas pains, emphasis is placed on making the infant more comfortable and relieving the mother's anxiety. Once this has been accomplished, the nurse can focus on suggestions to prevent a recurrence of the problem.

Dealing with Distractions

One important consideration in implementing a home visit is dealing with distractions. Distractions are generally of three types: environmental, behavioral, and nurse initiated. Environmental distractions arise from both the physical and social environments and may include background noise, crowded surroundings, and interruptions by other family members or outsiders. The occurrence of such distractions during the home visit can give the nurse a clear picture of the client's environment and the way in which the client and family interact among themselves and with others. For example, if mother and child are continually yelling at one another during the visit, this suggests the existence of family communication problems. On the other hand, positive interactions between a mother and her young child provide evidence of effective parenting skills.

Despite the information that can be gleaned from these distractions, their negative effects on the interaction between client and nurse need to be minimized. Requesting that the television be turned off during the visit or moving the client to a more private area can minimize some distractions. Or the nurse may ask an intrusive younger child to draw a picture to allow parent and nurse to talk with fewer interruptions. If there are too many distractions that cannot be eliminated or overcome, the nurse can ask the client if there is a better time for the visit, when fewer interruptions will occur, and reschedule the visit for a later date. For example, subsequent visits might be planned to coincide with the toddler's nap.

Behavioral distractions consist of behaviors employed by the client to distract the nurse from the purpose of the visit. Again, the use of such distractions can be a cue for the nurse that certain topics are uncomfortable for the client or that the client does not quite trust the nurse or may feel guilty about something. The nurse can benefit from the distraction by exploring the reasons for the client's behaviors and working to establish trust with the client.

The last category of distractions originate with the nurse. These distractions create barriers to relationships with clients. Fears, role preoccupation, and personal reactions to different lifestyles can distract the nurse from the purpose of the home visit. Nurses may fear bodily harm, rejection by the client, or the lack of control that is implicit in a home visit. In today's violent society, fear of bodily harm is understandable and nurses making home visits should employ the personal safety precautions discussed earlier in this chapter.

Community health nurses may also create distractions by being so preoccupied with their original purpose that they fail to see the need to modify the planned home visit. No planned intervention is so important that it cannot be postponed if more important needs intervene. Nurses who continue to pursue predetermined goals in the light of other client needs reduce their credibility with clients and create barriers to effective intervention. For example, the nurse who insists on talking about infant feeding when the client just had an argument with her husband and fears he will leave her is not meeting the client's needs.

Finally, community health nurses may be put off by the contrast between their own lifestyle and that of the clients they are visiting. In dealing with feelings engendered by such differences, it is helpful to understand that one's own attitudes are the product of one's upbringing and that clients derive their attitudes in the same way. In dealing with lifestyle differences, the nurse must be aware of personal feelings and their impact on nursing effectiveness. The nurse must also determine what aspects of the client's lifestyle may be detrimental to health and focus on those, while accepting other differences in attitude or behavior as hallmarks of the client's uniqueness. Being thoroughly informed about cultural and ethnic differences also minimizes negative reactions by the nurse to such differences. Some of these differences are discussed in Chapter 6.

⑥THINK ABOUT IT

What kind of home visit distractions might arise from your own personal behavior? What could you do to prevent this kind of distraction?

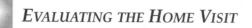

EVALUATING THE HOME VISIT

Before concluding the visit, the nurse evaluates the effectiveness of interventions in terms of their appropriateness to the situation and client response. This evaluation is conducted using criteria established in planning the visit. It may not be possible, at this point, to determine the eventual outcome of nursing care. The nurse can, however, examine the client's initial response to interventions. Was the mother interested in obtaining contraceptives? Is it likely that she will follow through on a referral to the immunization clinic? Did the client voice an intention to reduce salt intake? Could the client accurately demonstrate the correct technique for breast self-examination?

Evaluating the ultimate outcome of interventions may occur at subsequent visits. For example, on the next visit, the nurse might determine whether the mother obtained contraceptives. If she called but was not able to get an appointment, the nurse would determine the reason. Based on information obtained, there may be a need for advocacy on the part of the nurse. If the client did not seek contraceptive services, the nurse should determine the reason for her behavior. Was the client distracted by crises that occurred in the meantime, but plans to call for an appointment next week? Did she not have transportation to the clinic? Or maybe she does not really want contraceptives. If the client lacks transportation, the nurse might help her explore ways of getting transportation. If the client does not really want contraceptives, the nurse can either explore why or accept the client's wishes.

As noted earlier, evaluation of nursing interventions during a home visit should reflect the level of prevention involved. The nurse examines both short-term and long-term effects of interventions at the primary, secondary, and tertiary levels of prevention, as appropriate. For example, if the home visit focused on secondary prevention, evaluation will also be focused at this level. If several levels were addressed during the visit, evaluation will focus on the effects of interventions at each level.

The nurse also evaluates his or her use of the home visit process. Was the preliminary assessment adequate? Was information available that the nurse neglected to review, resulting in unexpected problems during the visit itself? For example, did the nurse ask about the husband's reaction to the new baby when the record indicates the client is not married? Did the nurse miss cues to additional problems during the visit? Was the nurse able to plan interventions consistent with client needs, attitudes, and desires? Was the nurse able to deal effectively with distractions? If not, why not? Answers to these and similar questions allow the nurse to improve his or her use of the home visit process in subsequent client encounters.

Evaluation of home visiting services must be undertaken at the aggregate level as well. Efforts to promote such evaluation include outcomes-based quality improvement and the use of the Outcomes Assessment Information Set. *Outcomes-based quality improvement (OBQI)* is the measurement of home health outcomes and the use of resulting data to improve systems of care (Crisler, 1998). A 1993 study by the Health Care Financing Administration (HCFA) indicated that quality management efforts in home health were driven by the needs of regulatory and reimbursement bodies rather than client care needs, that massive amounts of data were collected but seldom used for program improvement, and that multiple difficulties were encountered in collecting relevant data. These findings led to a focus on measurement of outcomes of care and the development of a standardized uniform data set for assessing client health status and care outcomes, the *Outcomes Assessment and Information Set (OASIS)* (Peters & McKeon, 1998).

OASIS is a standard set of assessment and evaluation items used to identify client needs and to track and docu-

ment the effectiveness of home care interventions. OASIS is intended to promote continuity of care and consistency across care givers and disciplines as well as to help determine the plan of care and document the effects of intervention (Carr, 1998). The current version of OASIS contains 10 client identification items and 79 items assessing the client's health and functional status. Data are intended to be collected at the initiation of services and every 60 days until discharge from Medicare-certified home care agencies, with a final entry at discharge from service (Peters & McKeon, 1998). The Balanced Budget Act of 1997 mandated the use of OASIS for Medicare-certified home health care agencies, with initial data obtained within 48 hours of initiating services (Schroeder, 2000).

It has been recommended that OASIS items be integrated into existing agency documentation formats to prevent duplication of effort and data. It has also been suggested that OASIS data be used to generate three kinds of reports: outcome reports, case mix reports, and patient tally reports. Outcome reports address the percentage of clients that achieve specific identified outcomes in a given period of time (e.g., the percentage of clients whose mobility improves). Outcome reports can be compared with those of other agencies as well as with prior time periods in a given agency to determine areas needing improvement. Case mix reports provide information on average values related to clients' health status at initiation of services (e.g., the number of clients with difficulties in multiple ADLs) and can be used to determine potential resource use and the types and number of staff required to address identified needs. The patient tally report combines client-specific outcome data with case mix data to identify areas in need of quality improvement (Peters & McKeon, 1998). For example, a particular client may show no improvement in pain control, a finding that might lead agency staff to examine this client's record in more detail to identify factors that are impeding pain control and to develop more effective modes of intervention in this area.

Home health agencies may also choose to use the Health Plan Employer Data and Information Set as a means of evaluating care given to clients as a whole. The *Health Plan Employer Data and Information Set (HEDIS)* is another data set developed to rate managed care organizations and to provide prospective purchasers (usually employers) with information needed to select a health care plan. HEDIS collects data and creates a "score card that measures eight dimensions of the organization: effectiveness of care, access/availability of care, satisfaction with care, health plan stability, use of services, cost, consumer choice, and specific health plan descriptive information. Home health organizations can use HEDIS score card information as a marketing tool if they compare favorably with other home care agencies, or they can use HEDIS information to make informed decisions about the feasibility of contracting to provide home care services to specific managed care organizations (Peters & McKeon, 1998).

DOCUMENTATION AND REIMBURSEMENT

Documentation is the last stage of the home visit. It is particularly important in home health care precisely because care is given in that setting. In the home, there are frequently no witnesses other than the nurse, the client, and possibly family members. In the event of an adverse effect of care, without adequate documentation, it may be the nurse's word against that of the client or family member. Accurate documentation is also required for reimbursement and for research to support the effectiveness of home care. Finally, when services are provided by a multidisciplinary team, good documentation facilitates coordination and continuity of care.

In documenting the home visit, the nurse must accurately record the client's health status, the nursing interventions employed, and the effectiveness of interventions. The nurse documents validation of diagnoses made in the preliminary assessment, as well as additional needs identified, by recording both subjective and objective data obtained during the visit. Goals and objectives established for addressing client health needs are also recorded. In addition, the nurse documents actions taken, client response to those actions, and the outcome of interventions if known. Also included in documentation are future plans and recommendations for subsequent home visits. As noted earlier, clinical pathways and OASIS may both be used for documentation purposes.

Reimbursement for services provided under Medicare is made by a fiscal intermediary. A *fiscal intermediary* is an agency designated by HCFA to act as a reimbursing agent and deal directly with home health care agencies. For example, in certain portions of Southern California, the Blue Cross–Blue Shield Insurance Company acts as a fiscal intermediary for home health agencies. In other parts of the country, private insurance carriers such as Aetna Life and Casualty and Traveler's Insurance Company serve as intermediaries. Home health agencies are reviewed periodically by representatives of the fiscal intermediary for adherence to Medicare guidelines related to services, documentation, and billing practices.

Fiscal intermediaries for Medicare reimbursement monitor agency documentation via periodic audits of nursing notes submitted with billing forms and on-site review visits. If inconsistencies or inappropriate statements are found, it is possible for reimbursement for all Medicare services to be denied, even those unrelated to the audited notes.

Medicare is not the only source of reimbursement for home health care services, and in some instances is not even the first source of reimbursement sought. It is important for home health nurses to be aware of the order in which reimbursement occurs. As a general rule, workers' compensation or no-fault insurance is the first payer for services where relevant, followed by commercial insurance, Medicare, Medicaid, private fee-for-

service payment, and, finally, free care (Parness & Weinberg, 1997b). Home health nurses should also be conversant with the types of services that are reimbursable.

TERMINATING HOME HEALTH SERVICES

The community health nurse may terminate home visiting services to a particular client when the goals and objectives established for care have been accomplished, when the duration of services surpasses allowable limits, when clients refuse continued services, or when a client dies. Other possible reasons for terminating services include safety concerns for the client or nurse, noncompliance with the treatment plan, needs that go beyond the capability of the agency to meet them, institutionalization, and repeated failure to find the client at home (Hogue, 1998; Sobolewski, 1997). In many of these instances, however, services should not be terminated until reasonable efforts have been made (e.g., to promote compliance or locate the client).

Obviously, it is less stressful for the nurse to terminate services to clients who no longer require them. Even then, the intimacy of the nurse–client relationship developed over a series of encounters may make it difficult for both nurse and client to "let go." In the case of agency moratoria on additional visits, clients with yet unmet needs may feel abandoned unless the nurse has made careful preparation for termination. Client refusal of services may be perceived by the nurse as a personal rejection, and the nurse will need to work through feelings of frustration and come to an acceptance of the client's decision without loss of self-esteem. Even in the case of a client's death, the nurse may find it difficult to terminate relationships developed with the client's family.

True abandonment of clients is grounds for legal action. Clients who claim abandonment, however, must be able to prove that the provider unilaterally terminated the relationship without reasonable notice when the client required further care to prevent harm. Repeated failure of the client to be home for scheduled visits can be construed as termination of the provider–client relationship by the client rather than the provider. The precise number of missed visits that constitutes termination of the relationship should be determined on the basis of consistent agency policy. In the face of repeated failures to keep appointments, the agency must notify the client of the possible consequences of this behavior and that he or she is perceived as having terminated the relationship. In the case of exhaustion of payment limits, clients can be offered the option of continuing services on a fee-for-service basis. If the client declines services on this basis, he or she is again perceived as terminating the relationship and cannot make a claim of abandonment against the agency (Hogue, 1998). Needless to say, all of these activities by the nurse and the client's response must be accurately documented to prevent a claim of abandonment. In such cases, the legal responsibility for care of the client has been met; the nurse will need to determine whether or not moral and ethical responsibilities have been met prior to deciding to terminate services to a client.

Effective termination actually begins with the initial home visit. The nurse should recognize and make clients aware that the relationship is necessarily time limited. It may be helpful at the outset of the relationship to specify a predetermined period during which services will be provided. The period designated may be mandated by agency policy or by mutually determined estimates of the time needed to accomplish established goals and objectives. As time passes, the nurse may need to remind the client that the time for termination is drawing near. When the time for termination actually arrives, the nurse and client can review goal accomplishment and the nurse can provide clients with continuing needs or surviving family members of deceased clients with referrals for sources of continued assistance. Some resources that may help community health nurses in making home visits are provided on the companion Web site for this book.

⑥THINK ABOUT IT

Under what circumstances should a home health agency discontinue services to a client? Is an agency ever justified in terminating services because the client cannot pay for them? Is an agency justified in refusing to begin services for clients who have no source of payment?

Home visits, as a form of nursing intervention, have been used by community health nurses since the early days of their practice, and home visits remain a viable alternative to other health care delivery settings. The nursing process provides a context for structuring home visits to provide health care to individuals and their families. The components of the home visit process are summarized in Table 21–3 ■.

■ TABLE 21–3 Elements of the Home Visit Process

Preliminary assessment	Review available client data to determine health care needs related to biophysical, psychological, physical environmental, sociocultural, behavioral, and health system dimensions.
Diagnosis	Develop diagnostic hypotheses based on preliminary assessment.
Planning	Review previous interventions and their effects. Prioritize client needs and identify those to be addressed during the visit. Develop goals and objectives for visit and identify levels of prevention involved. Consider client acceptance and timing of visit. Specify activities needed to accomplish goals and objectives. Obtain needed supplies and equipment. Plan for evaluation of the home visit.
Implementation	Validate preliminary assessment and nursing diagnostic hypotheses. Identify other client needs. Modify plan of care as needed. Carry out nursing interventions. Deal with distractions.
Evaluation	Evaluate client response to interventions. Evaluate long-term and short-term outcomes of intervention. Evaluate the quality of implementation in the home visit. Evaluate outcomes and quality of care at the aggregate as well as individual level.
Documentation	Document client assessment and health needs identified. Document interventions. Document client response to interventions. Document outcome of interventions. Document future plan of care. Document client health status at discharge.

APPLYING YOUR KNOWLEDGE IN PRACTICE

CASE STUDY
The Home Visit

You are a community health nurse working for the Hastings City Health Department. Your supervisor took the following request for nursing services by phone and passed it on to you because the address is part of your district. You know that this address is in an older residential area with a large Hispanic population.

Hastings City Health Department
Request for Nursing Services
Source of Request: *La Paloma Hospital Maternity Unit*
Date of Request: *7-12-02*
Client: *Maria Flores* Date of Birth: *10-21-82*
Address: *8359 Marlboro Way, Marquette, AR 36019*
Head of Household: *Juan Flores (client's father)*
Reason for Referral: *Delivered 5 lb. 7 oz. baby boy on 7-5-02. Gestational age 32 weeks. Baby remains in NICU with RDS. Prognosis good. Client had no prenatal care. Lives with parents and 2 younger sisters (ages 8 and 13). Both parents work, but family income insufficient to pay hospital bill. Family does not have insurance. Immigration status unknown. Request home assessment prior to anticipated discharge 8-1-02.*

- Based on the information you have, what health care needs related to the biophysical, psychological, physical environmental, sociocultural, behavioral, and health system dimensions would you identify in your preliminary assessment? List your diagnostic hypotheses.
- What nursing interventions would you plan for the health needs you are likely to encounter in a visit to this client? Identify your planned interventions as primary, secondary, or tertiary prevention measures.
- What supplies and materials might you need on this home visit?
- How would you go about validating your preliminary assessment and diagnostic hypotheses?
- What additional assessment data would you want to obtain during your visit?
- What evaluative criteria would you use to conduct outcome and process evaluation of care provided to this client and her family?
- On what basis would you make the determination to terminate services to Maria?

TESTING YOUR UNDERSTANDING

- What is the relationship between community health nursing and home health nursing? (pp. 505–506)
- Describe at least three advantages of home visits as a means of providing nursing care. (pp. 498–499)
- What are some of the challenges faced by community health nurses making home visits? (pp. 499–503)
- What are some of the characteristics of effective home visiting programs? (p. 503)
- Identify the major purposes of home visiting programs. How might programs differ with respect to purpose? (pp. 503–505)
- What are some of the types of home health agencies? In what ways do they differ? (pp. 506–507)
- Identify the major emphases in planning for a home visit. Give an example of each. (pp. 512–514)
- What are the major tasks in implementing a home visit? Give an example of the performance of each task. (pp. 514–515)
- What are some of the distractions that occur during a home visit? Give an example of each and describe actions by the nurse that might eliminate the distraction. (p. 515)
- Why is there a need for both long-term and short-term criteria for evaluating the effectiveness of a home visit? Give examples of the use of both types of criteria. (pp. 515–516)

In 1998, there were more than 58 million children 5 to 19 years of age in the United States (U.S. Census Bureau, 1999). These children spend seven to nine hours a day in school five days a week for an average of eight months, or between 22% and 27% of their waking hours (Miller & Spicer, 1998). Youth have been described as being at risk for "social morbidities" such as pregnancy, substance abuse, and so on, and health promotion efforts in schools can help to modify that risk (Parcel, Kelder, & Basen-Engquist, 2000).

Educational institutions have been identified as one of six categories of resources for healthy communities (Bingler, 2000), and the relationship between education and health is a reciprocal one. Health factors influence one's ability to learn. Education affects one's ability to engage in healthful behaviors. This reciprocal relationship makes the school setting an ideal place to provide health care.

Most school nurses are community health nurses practicing in a specialized setting. Given their community health preparation, school nurses retain their concern for the health of the community and apply the principles of community health nursing to the needs of the overall community as well as to the needs of the school population. This may be difficult at first, given the sometimes overwhelming nature of the needs of individual students (Raphael, 1998), but most school nurses eventually begin to see the patterns among the individual needs and identify population-based issues that require intervention (Merrill, Turner, McLaughlin, & Milner, 1999).

Community health nurses working in school settings have a threefold concern for the health of schoolchildren. First, the health of schoolchildren influences the health status of the community at large. Second, health-promotion and illness-prevention efforts directed at youngsters will improve their health status as adults. Finally, healthy children learn better and can take greater advantage of the educational opportunities provided to them.

The importance of the school health program as an avenue for improving the health of the population is evident in the number of national health objectives for the year 2010 that reflect health measures in schools (U.S. Department of Health and Human Services, 2000). These objectives can be reviewed on the Healthy People 2010 Web site accessed through the link from the companion Web site for this book. 🌐

HISTORICAL PERSPECTIVES

School nursing is one of several traditional roles for community health nurses. It originated with compulsory school attendance and a concern for the number of children being excluded from school because of communicable diseases (Allensworth, Lawson, Nicholson, & Wyche, 1997). Initial health activities in schools consisted of cursory physical inspections by physicians in New York City. Children who were found to have communicable diseases or parasitic infestations such as head lice were sent home. Because they

received no treatment for their conditions, these children were excluded from school for extended periods of time and continued to serve as reservoirs of infection for friends and family members still in school. In response to this problem, Lillian Wald assigned nurses from the Henry Street Settlement to four New York City schools in a pilot project in school nursing in 1902. During that first year, the number of school exclusions declined 90%. Because of the success of the project, the New York City Board of Health hired additional nurses to continue this type of work (Kronenfeld, 2000). By 1911, more than 100 cities had employed school nurses who conducted routine medical inspections, treated and educated students regarding minor illnesses on the spot, and made home visits to those students with more serious illnesses (Allensworth et al., 1997).

The potential of schools as avenues for promoting health and dealing with social ills was recognized considerably earlier than the advent of specific health-related services in the school setting. For example, Benjamin Franklin advocated physical exercise as part of the school curriculum and the report of the Massachusetts Sanitary Commission emphasized the importance of health education and the place of schools in providing it. In 1870, smallpox vaccination was required for school entry as a means of increasing immunization levels in the population, and in 1899 Connecticut made vision screening of schoolchildren mandatory.

In 1915, schoolchildren were enlisted as "modern health crusaders" by the National Tuberculosis Association to sell Christmas seals. This program also encouraged personal health behaviors by requiring participating children to keep a daily diary of 11 "health chores" (e.g., brushing one's teeth). Health education in schools arose from the temperance movement, which viewed schools as a vehicle for inculcating values antithetical to the use of alcohol, tobacco, and narcotics. These early attempts at promoting health education led to legislation mandating health education in schools in many states, and in 1928 the recommended health curriculum in the Sixth Yearbook of the Department of Superintendents of the National Education Association included topics such as mental, home, and sex hygiene; bodily functions as a basis for good health habits; causes of disease; nutrition; and posture (Allensworth et al., 1997).

Early school nursing focused on preventing the spread of communicable disease and treating ailments related to compulsory school attendance. By the 1930s, however, the focus had shifted to preventive and promotive activities including case finding, integration of health concepts into school curricula, and maintenance of a healthful school environment. Treatment of any health problems by the nurse was strongly discouraged to prevent infringement on the private medical sector.

School health nurses, dissatisfied with such a minimal role, continued to provide clandestine diagnostic services and treatment of minor ailments in addition to engaging in classroom teaching related to health. More recently, school nurses have begun to return to activities related to the diagnosis and treatment of health problems. Several factors account for current changes in the school nurse role. Among these are the number of families of school-age children in which both parents work. In these families, neither parent may have time to deal with routine health problems of their children. Other factors include the interest of school nurses in expanding their role, the failure of government programs (e.g., the Early and Periodic Screening, Diagnosis, and Treatment Program [EPSDT]) to resolve the health problems of school-age children, enrollment of handicapped youngsters in regular school programs, and consumer demands for alternative sites for providing health care to children. One other major factor is that approximately 40% of school-age children in the United States have no regular source of health care except for care rendered in emergency rooms (Sharma, 1999). For these children, in particular, the school nurse may be the only source of health care.

THE SCHOOL HEALTH PROGRAM

Health care is provided in schools for a number of reasons: the school environment itself may create hazards from which students must be protected; children need to be healthy to learn effectively; maintaining the health of children today produces healthier adults in years to come; and finally, there is a need to protect and enhance the health of the overall community. The national health objectives reflect these points.

The overall goal of a school health program is to enhance the educational process by removing health-related barriers to learning. More specific objectives of a school health program include decreasing morbidity and absenteeism, identifying and providing early treatment for existing health problems, managing special health needs, and promoting employee health and wellness. Additional objectives include serving a liaison function between the school, home, and community; contributing to staff development; serving as a resource to administrators on health and safety issues in schools; and assuring quality of and accountability for health services (Newton, Adams, & Marcontel, 1997).

These goals traditionally have been achieved through the three basic components of a school health program: health services, health instruction, and a healthy environment. More recently, other aspects of school life have also been considered integral features of a comprehensive school health program. According to the Committee on Comprehensive School Health Programs in Grades K–12 of the Institute of Medicine, a *comprehensive school health program* is defined as "an integrated set of planned, sequential school-affiliated strategies, activities, and services designed to promote the optimal physical, emotional, social, and educational development of students" (Allensworth et al., 1997, p. 60). Components of this comprehensive program include the traditional elements of health services, health education,

and a healthy environment, as well as physical education activities, nutrition services; staff health promotion; counseling, psychological, and social services; and parent and community involvement as identified by the Office of Disease Prevention and Health Promotion (1997). Components of a comprehensive school health program are depicted in Figure 23–1 ■.

The health services component of a school health program should provide a wide variety of health care services. Broadly categorized, these services include assessment and screening, case finding, counseling, health promotion and illness prevention, case management, remedial or rehabilitation services, specific nursing procedures, and emergency care. Examples of activities in each of these categories are presented in Table 23–1 ■.

The focus of the health education component of the school health program is educating students for health awareness and healthful behavior. Health education in the school setting focuses on both cognitive and affective learning. *Cognitive learning* involves acquisition of facts and information related to health and healthy behavior. *Affective learning,* on the other hand, refers to developing attitudes toward health and health behaviors that foster a healthy lifestyle. In the past, content areas for school-based health education included topics such as community health, consumer health, environmental health, family life, growth and development, nutrition, personal health, disease prevention and control, safety and accident prevention, and substance use and abuse. More recently, the health education curriculum has focused on the seven *National Health Education Standards* designed to promote health literacy. The components of health literacy are presented below.

HIGHLIGHTS

Components of Health Literacy

- Comprehension of health promotion and disease prevention information
- The ability to access health information and health promoting products and services
- The ability to engage in behaviors that promote health and reduce risk
- Analysis of the influence of culture, media, technology, and other social factors on health
- Use of interpersonal communication to enhance health
- The ability to set goals and make decisions regarding health
- The ability to advocate for personal, family, and community health

Source: Breckon, D. J. (1998). *Community health education: Settings, roles, and skills for the 21st century.* Gaithersburg, MD: Aspen.

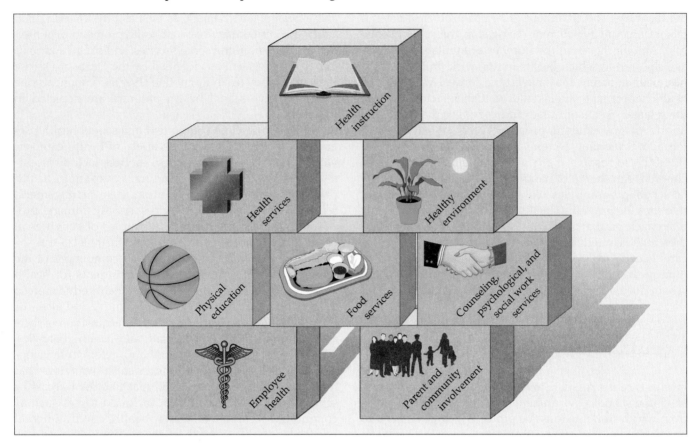

FIGURE 23–1 ■ *Components of the school health program*

The environmental component of the school health program includes activities directed toward improving the physical, psychological, and social environments of the school and the surrounding community. In the area of physical education, the emphasis is on promoting physical activity among school-age children, as well as developing attitudes to exercise and fitness that will continue throughout life. Positive attitudes and good food habits are also a focus of the nutrition component of the school health program in addition to provision of healthful diets while children are at school. Counseling and social work services are provided to assist students and their families to deal with changes and problem areas in their environments that may contribute to poor health and poor school performance.

The employee health component provides similar types of services for school employees in addition to assistance with physical health problems. U.S. schools employ 2.5 million teachers and 2 million other staff members. Services to school employees serve several purposes, among them the reduction in illness and absenteeism, enhancement of interest in health issues and willingness to address them with students, and the potential for role modeling healthy behaviors (Allegrante, 1998).

The final component of the school health program is directed toward fostering partnerships among school, family, and community that enhance the health of the overall community.

EDUCATIONAL PREPARATION FOR SCHOOL HEALTH NURSING

Depending on the requirements of the particular jurisdiction, nurses working in school settings may have varying levels of education (Felton & Keil, 1998). In some parts of the country, for example, the Southeast, a person designated as a "school nurse" may not even be a registered nurse. Because of the autonomy of nursing practice in the school setting and the complexity of health problems addressed, ideally the school nurse should be prepared at least at the baccalaureate level. This level of educational preparation guarantees that the nurse has the community health nursing background to deal effectively with the health needs of the school population.

In some states, employment as a school nurse requires advanced preparation beyond a baccalaureate degree in nursing. In California, for example, school nurses must complete a state-approved *school nurse credential program.* This is a nondegree program offered in an institution of higher learning that meets state requirements for educating school nurses.

■ TABLE 23–1 Sample Activities Related to School Health Service Categories

School Health Service Category	Related Activities
Assessment and screening	Preschool entry assessments Transfer student health assessments Special appraisals for high-risk students or students referred by other school personnel Routine screening Home visiting for comprehensive assessment Monitoring chronic conditions and treatment effects
Case finding	Identification of communicable diseases Identification of chronic diseases Referral for diagnostic and treatment services Immunization surveillance Surveillance for selected health events
Counseling	Counseling to decrease health risks Counseling regarding existing health problems Anticipatory counseling for students, parents, staff
Health promotion/illness prevention	Exclusion of students with communicable diseases Immunization of unimmunized students, staff Health teaching in and outside of classrooms Health promotion activities for students/staff (e.g., smoking cessation, weight control)
Case management	Liaison with community services Referral to outside services as needed Follow-up on referrals Fostering parental involvement Arranging transportation
Remedial/rehabilitative services	Speech therapy Physical therapy Behavior modification
Nursing procedures	Development of student care plans Administration of medications Specialized nursing procedures Teaching procedures to other staff
Emergency care	Development of emergency protocols First aid services Postemergency assessment

Other school nurses may be prepared at the master's level in nursing. These nurses frequently function as nurse practitioners, promoting health and diagnosing and treating minor illnesses (Brindis et al., 1998). Some, however, have advanced preparation in community health nursing and are involved in program planning rather than primary care of minor illnesses.

Curricular content for nurses with specific preparation for school nursing also varies widely, but there is some agreement on core curricular strands that should be included. These areas include content on the definition and actualization of the nursing role in school settings, the legal and educational parameters of special educa-

tion, health education principles and techniques, physical assessment skills specific to school nursing (e.g., audiometry and neuromaturational assessment) as well as general assessment skills, and content on the educational system (SEP, 1998).

There are only approximately 30,000 school nurses in the United States to care for children at the elementary, middle, and high school levels. Only a portion of these nurses have educational preparation specific to school nursing. Many schools have little or no nursing presence. In 83% of California schools, for example, administrative staff provide first aid services and dispense medications (Hopkins, 2000). Given the complexity of the school nurse role and the expansion of that role in many areas to addressing the health needs of families and communities, there is clearly a need for educational preparation of more school nurses.

STANDARDS FOR SCHOOL HEALTH NURSING

Like other areas of nursing practice, school nursing should be practiced in accordance with a set of minimum care standards. The first national *Standards for School Nursing Practice* were published in 1983 by the American Nurses Association, the National Association of School Nurses, and the National Association of State School Nurse Consultants. In 1993, these standards were updated in the document *School Nursing Practice—Roles and Standards* (Proctor, Lordis, & Zaiger, 1993). The current standards for school health nursing were revised in 1999 by the National Association of School Nurses and are summarized below. The standards for school nursing practice, like the standards for nursing practice in other specialty areas, reflect the use of the nursing process.

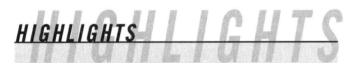

HIGHLIGHTS

Standards of Professional School Nursing Practice

Standards of Care

Assessment: The school nurse collects client data.

Diagnosis: The school nurse analyzes the assessment data in determining nursing diagnoses.

Outcome identification: The school nurse identifies expected outcomes individualized to the client.

Planning: The school nurse develops a plan of care/ action that specifies interventions to attain expected outcomes.

Implementation: The school nurse implements the interventions identified in the plan of care/action.

Standards of Professional Performance

Quality of care: The school nurse systematically evaluates the quality and effectiveness of school nursing practice.

Performance appraisal: The school nurse evaluates one's own nursing practice in relation to professional practice standards and relevant statutes, regulations, and policies.

Education: The school nurse acquires and maintains current knowledge and competency in school nursing practice.

Collegiality: The school nurse interacts with and contributes to the professional development of peers and school personnel as colleagues.

Ethics: The school nurse's decisions and actions on behalf of clients are determined in an ethical manner.

Collaboration: The school nurse collaborates with the student, family, school staff, community, and other providers in providing student care.

Research: The school nurse promotes use of research findings in school nursing practice.

Resource utilization: The school nurse considers factors related to safety, effectiveness, and cost when planning and delivering care.

Permission granted for reprint from the National Association of School Nurses, Inc. Castle Rock, Colorado

THE SCHOOL HEALTH TEAM

Health problems identified in individual children or in the community served by the school are frequently beyond the capabilities of the community health nurse acting independently. To meet the needs of the school population and the community, the school health nurse often needs to participate as a member of a team.

Because identified health problems may be the consequence of factors beyond the control of health care professionals, the school health team often consists of a variety of individuals, not all of whom have a health or medical background. The team acts to design a school health program that meets the health needs of students and of the larger community.

The school health team should use the strategies discussed in Chapter 13 to create an effective team that can address the health needs of the population. One of the critical features of group development for the school health team is negotiating member roles. Group members should clarify for themselves the roles that each will play, so that infringement on anyone's professional territory is avoided.

Specific members of the team will vary with the identified needs of the population, but some of those who may be involved, in addition to the nurse, are parents, teachers, administrators, counselors, psychologists, social workers, physicians and dentists, a health coordinator, food service personnel, janitorial and secretarial staffs, public health officials and other public officials, and students. Additional team members in some school settings include nurse practitioners; physical, occupational, and respiratory therapists; and speech pathologists.

Parents, of course, have the primary responsibility for the health of their children. With respect to the school health program, parents have a responsibility to reinforce health teaching at home and to follow up on referrals for assistance with health problems identified in their children. They should also provide input into the planning and evaluation of the school health program. Parents may also provide volunteer services for first aid or "sick room duty" when there is not a nurse employed full time.

Teachers also have a variety of responsibilities for the health of their students. Among these are the need to motivate students in the development of good health habits, to encourage student responsibility for health, and to observe them for signs of health problems. Teachers have a responsibility to model healthy behavior and to provide health instruction. Other responsibilities include assisting with screening efforts and measures to control the spread of disease and helping to identify factors in the physical, psychological, and social environments that are detrimental to the health status of students and coworkers. In addition, teachers may counsel students with health problems and may make referrals for assistance as appropriate.

School administrators include principals, district superintendents, and school board members. Administrators are responsible for the implementation of the school health program and should provide both material and nonmaterial support. They also function as liaisons between the school and the larger community. In collaboration with other team members, administrators participate in planning and evaluating the school health program. Other administrative responsibilities include hiring and evaluating health service employees and fostering collegial relationships among school health team members. Finally, administrators have the ultimate responsibility for the creation of a healthy and safe environment.

Some schools employ counselors, psychologists, or social workers or contract for their services as consultants. Counselors may provide emotional counseling or assistance to students in career decisions. Psychologists may also be involved in counseling for emotional problems. In addition, they may conduct psychological testing on selected youngsters to identify emotional problems or learning disabilities, or they may be called on to administer tests of school readiness to all incoming children. Social workers may likewise counsel students regarding problems and may provide referrals for students and families to assist with socioeconomic problems. When the services of these specialists are not available in a particular school setting, many of these functions may be assumed by the school nurse, if he or she is educationally prepared to carry them out, or the nurse might make a referral to an outside source of assistance.

Physicians and dentists usually are not employed by a school system, but they may provide services on a contract or referral basis. Under a contractual arrangement, physicians and dentists may spend a certain amount of time in the school assessing health and dental needs or making treatment recommendations. In other instances, students may be referred to their own physicians or dentists for follow-up treatment of identified health problems. Physical, occupational, or respiratory therapists may be employed in some school systems that provide comprehensive health services or may serve as outside

consultants in the care of individual children. School systems may also have similar kinds of interactions with speech pathologists.

The school nurse may function as the school's health coordinator, or the school health team may include a health coordinator who is not a nurse. The health coordinator may be a parent, teacher, or other person with some health-related preparation. Responsibilities of the health coordinator include serving as a liaison with families and with the community, arranging in-service education for staff, facilitating team relationships, and coordinating the health instruction program. Other areas of responsibility include planning for speakers on health topics, arranging health-related learning experiences such as field trips or health fairs, and reviewing materials for use in health education.

In schools where meals are provided, food service personnel are responsible for preparing and serving nutritious meals. They may also be responsible for planning menus, depending on their background and knowledge of the nutritional needs of school-age children.

The janitorial staff is usually responsible for maintenance of the physical environment. Remediation of physical health hazards usually comes under their jurisdiction as well. They also ensure the cleanliness of kitchen and sanitary facilities to prevent the transmission of disease.

Clerical personnel are responsible for maintaining student records and for processing family notification of screening test results and recommendations. They may also be responsible for notifying families in the case of student injury or illness.

Public health officials are not employed by the school, but still form part of the school health team in that they are responsible for inspection of school sanitation, cooking facilities, and immunization status. They also act to establish local health policy related to schools and other institutions and to safeguard the health of the overall community. Other public officials may also be involved in planning a school health program to meet the needs of the school's population. Fire or police personnel might be involved, for example, in designing safety education programs for children and their parents.

In older age groups, students within the school may also be part of the school health team. Student responsibilities include helping to maintain a healthful and safe environment and providing input regarding student health needs and planning to meet those needs. Older students should also be involved in evaluating the effectiveness of the school health program.

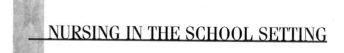

NURSING IN THE SCHOOL SETTING

Community health nurses working in school settings apply the nursing process to the care of individual students and their families, to the school population, and to the larger community.

ASSESSING HEALTH IN THE SCHOOL SETTING

Use of the nursing process in the school setting begins with assessing the health needs of the school population and identifying the factors influencing those needs. Areas for consideration include the biophysical, psychological, physical environmental, sociocultural, behavioral, and health system dimensions of health.

Biophysical Considerations

Areas for consideration related to the biophysical dimension include maturation and aging as they affect health and health behaviors, genetic inheritance, and physiologic function.

Maturation and Aging

School nurses work with students in preschool, elementary school, junior high and high school, and college and university settings. Consequently, the age of the client population influences the types of health problems that may be present. For example, prevention of childhood communicable diseases would receive greater emphasis in the preschool population, and sexuality issues and substance abuse would be of greater concern with adolescent populations. For college students, substance abuse and sexuality issues are also pertinent, as are stress-related problems stemming from academic pressures and being away from home.

Client maturation also influences the content and process of the health instruction component of the school health program. Basic hygiene conveyed via cartoon films is appropriate to the preschool or early elementary-age child; a frank discussion of sexuality and sexually transmitted diseases is appropriate with older groups of school children.

Genetic Inheritance

Aspects of genetic inheritance of particular interest to the school nurse are the gender and racial composition of the population. A predominance of females in an elementary school increases the frequency with which the nurse will encounter students with symptoms of urinary tract infection as these are common in girls of that age. In adolescent girls, on the other hand, there is increased risk of unwanted pregnancy. Boys of all ages tend to have more sports-related injuries with which the nurse must deal (Miller & Spicer, 1998).

Racial composition of the school population also influences the types of health problems encountered. For example, in schools with large African American populations, sickle cell screening might be included as a routine part of the school health program. The nurse must also be alert to the prevalence of other diseases that exhibit genetic predispositions, such as thalassemia and diabetes.

Physiologic Function

An important aspect of the human biological component of the assessment is the physiologic function of the school population. School nurses may encounter students or staff with self-limiting health problems or chronic conditions that affect their abilities to function effectively in the school setting.

Examples of self-limiting conditions include communicable diseases such as the common cold, influenza, and chickenpox and injuries such as a fractured arm or leg. Diabetes, seizure disorders, and minor visual or hearing problems are examples of chronic conditions that may have health and educational implications. Many of these conditions can be controlled if properly diagnosed and treated and do not necessarily interfere with the child's ability to function in school. Other chronic and handicapping conditions do interfere with school function. Examples are blindness, deafness, mental retardation, attention deficit hyperactivity disorder (ADHD), and long-term effects of fetal drug exposure. Conditions related to environmental or psychological stress may or may not affect physiologic function, although they may affect the child's ability to function effectively in the school situation.

The kinds of physical health problems seen by school nurses among students and staff are many and varied. Acute and chronic conditions commonly encountered in the school setting are listed in Table 23–2 ■.

The majority of health conditions seen in most school populations are acute respiratory illnesses. Ten percent of school-age children, however, have some type of chronic condition, and 2% of schoolchildren exhibit severe physical or developmental disabilities (Felton & Keil, 1998). The Individuals with Disabilities Education Act and section 504 of the Rehabilitation Act of 1973 mandated "mainstreaming" of children with disabilities (Hopkins, 2000). *Mainstreaming* is the process of placing children with disabilities and chronic illnesses in regular school settings rather than in specialized educational programs. The presence of these and other children with chronic health conditions in schools has increased the level of responsibility of school nurses and has increased the potential for medical emergencies in the school setting (Allen, Ball, & Helfer, 1998). School nurses need to be conversant not only with care of minor illness and injury, but with complex care of children with special needs.

⑥ THINK ABOUT IT

Are students with handicapping conditions better off in regular or specialized classrooms? Why?

Immunity is another important consideration related to physiologic function in the school population. The community health nurse working in the school setting monitors the immunization status of students and school

■ **TABLE 23–2**   **Acute and Chronic Physical Health Problems Encountered in the School Setting**

Organ System Affected	Conditions Encountered
Cardiovascular system	Heart murmurs, hypertension
Central nervous system	Mental retardation, blindness, deafness, attention deficit hyperactivity disorder, learning disability, seizure disorder, meningitis, cerebral palsy
Endocrine system	Diabetes mellitus, thyroid disorders
Gastrointestinal system	Encopresis, hepatitis, diarrhea, dental caries, constipation, peptic and duodenal ulcer
Genitourinary/ reproductive system	Sexually transmitted diseases, urinary tract infection, enuresis, dysmenorrhea, pregnancy
Hematopoietic system	Anemia, hemophilia, leukemia, sickle cell disease, lead poisoning
Immunologic system	AIDS and related opportunistic infections
Integumentary system	Acne, eczema, impetigo, lice, scabies, dermatitis, tinea corporis
Musculoskeletal system	Arthritis, sprains, fractures, scoliosis, Legg–Calvé–Perthes disease
Respiratory system	Upper and lower respiratory infections, strep throat, influenza, asthma, hay fever, pertussis, diphtheria, pneumonia
Other diseases	Measles, mumps, rubella, scarlet fever, chickenpox, infectious mononucleosis, otitis media, otitis externa, conjunctivitis, Lyme disease, cancer, hepatitis

employees. For example, maintenance personnel are at risk for tetanus because of the potential for dirty injuries, and their immunization status should be monitored. For female teachers and other school personnel of childbearing age, the risk of rubella during pregnancy is increased by working with children, and they should also be adequately immunized.

A final health problem frequently encountered in the school population that may have a physiologic basis is learning disability. Learning disabilities were discussed in Chapter 16.

Psychological Considerations

The psychological environment of the school can either foster good health or undermine it. Aspects of the psychological dimension to be assessed include the organization of the school day, the nature of relationships among students and school staff members, discipline and grading practices, and parent–school relationships.

Organization of the School Day

The nurse determines whether the organization of the school day is conducive to health. Assessment areas to be addressed include the extent to which periods of strenuous physical activity are alternated with periods of quiet study and the extent of opportunities for developing a variety of psychomotor as well as academic skills. The nurse also assesses whether mealtimes are arranged so that students have the energy reserves to handle the tasks of the school day. For younger children, this usually means providing a snack time. Another area for assessment is the scheduling of time for toileting activities. The nurse should determine whether children are given time to go to the lavatory or permitted to go when necessary to prevent chronic constipation or urinary tract infection. There should also be opportunities for children to obtain drinks of water. Such opportunities should increase in frequency with hot weather.

Peer Relations

The relationships of a student with his or her peers can create a psychological environment that is either conducive or detrimental to mental and physical health. The community health nurse can assess the extent to which students who have difficulties with peer relationships are encouraged to participate in group activities. Is there adequate adult supervision of student activities to moderate unhealthy peer relationships? If school personnel see that particular children are unable to participate or are even victimized, do they act to stop such behaviors? Are opportunities provided within the school setting and the curriculum for values clarification and learning about healthy interpersonal interactions?

Teacher–Student Relationships

Teacher–student relationships also affect the psychological climate of the school. The nurse assesses the quality of student–teacher relationships within the school in general and also between specific teachers and their students. Ideally, teachers are people who listen, reward appropriate behavior, maximize student assets, allow personal expression, and foster responsibility. Teachers who foster good student relationships tend to be enthusiastic and have a way of making learning fun. They exhibit a sincere concern for students and respect, accept, and trust them. They get to know their students well, encourage participation and curiosity, foster healthy competition, and encourage students to perform to their best potential. They also refrain from harsh or sarcastic comments, and they discipline students appropriately.

Unfortunately, not all teachers fit this picture. In assessing teacher–student relationships, the nurse identifies any tendencies on the part of teachers to use undue punishment or to make demands that students are incapable of meeting. Inconsistent demands or conflicting expectations on the part of a teacher can also create stress in students and lead to physical and mental health problems. Nurses might note that certain children are singled out for punishment by a particular teacher and may need to function as advocates. School nurses should also be alert to the potential for emotional, physical, or sexual abuse of students by teachers (and, on occasion, of teachers by students).

Teacher–Teacher Relationships

The relationships among teachers in a school and between teachers and other school personnel also influence the psychological environment of students. The nurse should assess the extent to which healthy teacher relationships—those that are supportive, encourage creativity and freedom, and foster cooperation—exist within the school. Effective relationships among teachers foster sharing and self-confidence, recognize achievements, and provide guidance for teacher development. In schools where teacher–teacher relationships are strained, students may get caught in the middle between teachers, or student morale may be undermined by the stress created by strife among teachers. For example, if the basketball coach and a particular high school English teacher do not get along well, the coach may demand that basketball players cut English class for an extra practice before a championship game, and the English teacher may threaten to fail any player that cuts class. In this instance, the students cannot win. If they cut class, they may fail English. Conversely, if they miss the practice, they may be dropped from the team.

Discipline

In discussing the characteristics of supportive teachers, the issue of discipline was alluded to. In addition to looking at disciplinary measures employed by individual teachers, school nurses should assess the school's philosophy regarding discipline. Discipline should be used for inappropriate behavior and should not be unduly harsh. It is estimated that 1 to 2 million instances of corporal punishment occur in U.S. schools each year, and the American Academy of Pediatrics (2000) has called for efforts to prohibit corporal punishments in all states. The nurse determines whether rules of behavior are clearly communicated to students and whether expectations are realistic. The nurse should also assess whether discipline, when warranted, is administered fairly and in a manner that does not diminish the student's self-respect.

A particular need in today's society is to prevent violence in and around the school setting. Violence within the school environment can be addressed by explicit codes of conduct that are clearly communicated to students and consistently and uniformly enforced. Weapons should be strictly banned from school campuses and the

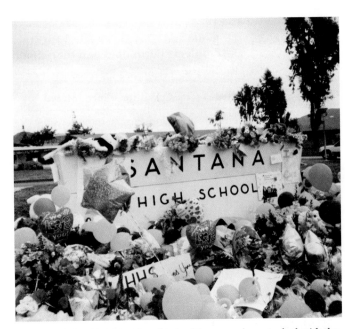

Community health nurses in school settings may have to deal with the aftermath of school violence.

ban stringently enforced. Despite such bans, however, Youth Risk Behavior Surveillance data for 1999 indicated that more than 70 incidents of weapons carrying occurred per 100 students. These incidents involved slightly more than 17% of students nationwide (Kann et al., 2000). Peer counseling and off-campus counseling sites to address interpersonal problems have been effective means of reducing violence. The community health nurse in the school setting can assess the level of violence on campus as well as the effectiveness of steps taken to prevent violence. The nurse can also examine the inclusion of conflict resolution strategies and content on interpersonal relations in the school's health education curriculum.

Grading

School and teacher grading policies should be clearly understood and should be fairly implemented. Particular grading practices are usually the province of the individual teacher, but the community health nurse can assess whether grading standards are consistent and grades are communicated to students privately to avoid humiliation. If graded work is displayed, the nurse can examine the extent to which student work is exhibited in a way that all students are made to feel good about some of their abilities. This is particularly important in elementary grades when children incorporate perceptions of their school performance into either positive or negative self-images.

Parent–School Relationships

Another area for assessment is the quality of relationships between school personnel and parents, which can have a strong influence on the psychological climate of the school setting. When this relationship is cooperative, students do not receive conflicting messages about what is expected of them. On the other hand, when relationships between parents and school personnel are adversarial, students may again be caught in the middle of a power struggle, or students may attempt to exploit the situation by manipulating both parents and teachers to their own advantage. Other areas that the nurse might explore in assessing the psychological environment are the quality of students' school performance and absenteeism and dropout rates.

⑥THINK ABOUT IT

How can school nurses motivate parent participation in school health activities?

Physical Environmental Considerations

The nurse assesses both the internal and external physical environment of the school. The external environment includes the area surrounding the school. Assessment considerations here include traffic patterns, water hazards, use of pesticides, and rodent control in the area. Other environmental concerns include the proximity of hazardous waste dumps or nuclear power plants, industrial hazards, and the presence of various forms of pollution. (See Chapter 7 for a discussion of environmental health issues.)

Several aspects of the school's internal environment, such as fire hazards and sanitation, are the responsibility of official agencies like the fire department and health department; however, there are other aspects of the physical environment that are rarely adequately assessed. The school health nurse needs to be alert to other hazards to physical safety that may be present in the school setting. Examples of these hazards are toxic art supplies, scientific equipment in laboratories, kitchen appliances in home economics classrooms, and chemical substances used either in chemistry labs or by maintenance and janitorial staffs. Animals in classrooms may also present safety hazards in terms of the potential for scratches and bites or disease transmission. Other conditions that may jeopardize safety include asbestos used in building materials, inadequate maintenance of fire hoses and extinguishers, and inoperable communications systems in the event of an emergency.

Other areas of concern are the safety of industrial arts classrooms, the gymnasium, and play areas. As noted in Chapter 16, the safety of outdoor play equipment should be inspected on a regular basis and repairs made as needed. A similar need exists for periodic assessment of sports equipment and practices. Other hazards associated with play areas include broken glass and other refuse on the playground. Hard surfaces below play equipment increase the potential for injuries stemming from falls.

Other assessment considerations with respect to the school's internal physical environment include noise levels within and outside of classrooms and adequacy of lighting, ventilation, heating, and cooling. Food sanitation should also be assessed. If hot meals are provided at school, cooking facilities should be inspected regularly. Such inspections are usually the official responsibility of the local health department, but the community health nurse should also assess these facilities periodically. If students bring their lunches, the potential for food poisoning from spoiled foods should be appraised.

Assessing sanitary facilities in the school is another area for consideration. Here, the nurse would examine the adequacy of toilet facilities for the size of the school population. The nurse would also periodically inspect sanitary facilities to make sure they are in good working order and do not pose hazards for the transmission of communicable diseases. Again, this area is usually the responsibility of health department personnel, but official inspections may occur only at lengthy intervals and the nurse should be aware of hazards that might arise in the interim.

Another area of concern with respect to sanitation is the use and cleaning of shower facilities. The nurse should assess that showers are adequately cleaned to prevent transmission of communicable conditions such as tinea pedis (athlete's foot).

Physical facilities for preventing the spread of disease by infected children should also be assessed. Are there places within the school where youngsters with infectious conditions can be isolated? All too often, these children are merely kept in the nurse's office until a parent can come for them. This presents opportunities for exposure of all those who visit the nurse while the child is there.

Special consideration should be given to the physical environment as it relates to handicapped children. Many physical barriers may exist, particularly in older schools, that limit the ability of handicapped youngsters to benefit from the education setting. Areas of concern include the presence of ramps, easily opened doors and windows, nonslip flooring, elevators, and curb modifications to eliminate the need to step up. Another consideration is access to toileting facilities by handicapped children. Are toilets accessible to wheelchairs? Are sinks placed so that a wheelchair can be maneuvered beneath them? Placement and height of mirrors, drinking fountains, and telephones is also of concern. Other considerations with respect to the environment of handicapped children are the adequacy of storage for wheelchairs and other special equipment, wheelchair space in classrooms and auditoriums, modification of laboratory and library carrels for wheelchair use, and adequacy of evacuation plans for the handicapped in case of emergency. The intent is to create a school that is barrier free so that all students, staff, and community members who may use the premises after school hours have access to facilities and equipment.

Sociocultural Considerations

The sociocultural dimension also plays a part in influencing the health status of members of the school community. The nurse needs to assess the community's attitudes toward education because these attitudes determine, in large part, the degree of support given to the schools and to health care within the schools. Community attitudes also affect the allocation of funds for both school and health programs.

The extent of crime in the school neighborhood is another aspect of the social environment to be assessed. Is violence a problem for children going to and from school? Is drug dealing going on in the area, and will youngsters be pressured to experiment with drugs?

A social factor that influences health in the school setting is the prevalence of families in which both parents work. Unfortunately, children are often sent to school when they are ill because there is no one at home to care for them. The nurse should assess the number of students who come to school ill and explore with parents their reasons for sending sick children to school. It may be a lack of awareness on the part of parents of the signs and symptoms of illness or an absence of other options available to parents.

The nurse should also assess before- and after-school care of children whose parents work. Many so-called "latchkey" children stay at home alone before and after school until parents return from work. Community health nurses can assess the availability of programs for children who are not mature enough to stay home alone and make referrals to these programs if they do not already exist within the school. In addition, nurses can assist parents to determine children's readiness to stay home alone and help to educate both parents and children on conditions that promote the safety of latchkey children (Kalthoff, 1998). The companion Web site for the book contains an assessment tool that may be of assistance to school nurses and parents in this regard. (See material related to Chapter 16.)

The social environment within the school is also influential. What is the socioeconomic status of students? Of school personnel? What is the racial or ethnic composition of the school population? Are racial tensions present? Do religious beliefs influence the health of the school population? For example, if there are large numbers of children whose parents object to immunization on religious grounds, the nurse needs to be particularly alert to signs of outbreaks of childhood diseases such as measles, rubella, and diphtheria.

Another area for consideration is the cultural backgrounds of students and school personnel. Are they similar? Do cultural practices influence students' health? Do differences in cultural practices create tension among students or between students and staff? Cultural factors may also lead to inappropriate diagnoses of ADHD for behavior considered perfectly normal in the child's culture or child abuse in the face of cultural health practices such as dermabrasion or cupping. (See Chapter 6 for a

CULTURAL CONSIDERATIONS

A large percentage of the children in your school are Mexican American or Mexican whose families have come to the United States for work. Most of the families are here legally, but some are not. Several teachers have referred some of these children to you because of frequent absences (often of three days to a week) that are interfering with their achievement in school. When you contact the families to determine the reasons for children's absences, you discover that the families are making frequent trips to Mexico for a variety of family events and celebrations. What will you do about this situation?

discussion of these practices.) In addition, parents from other cultural groups, particularly immigrants, may not be accustomed to the school routine and may include children in late night family activities leaving them too tired to perform effectively in school (Merrill et al., 1999). Children whose primary language is not English may also have difficulties in school, and the nurse should work to achieve culturally appropriate education for these children. Similarly, children of migrant families of whatever cultural or ethnic background may have their education disrupted by frequent moves.

Homelessness is another sociocultural dimension factor that can have a profound effect on the health of school-age children. Homeless children are more likely than their housed peers to be behind in their classes, need remediation, or repeat a grade (Better Homes Fund, 1999). As a result of the McKinney Homeless Assistance Act, homeless children are guaranteed access to free and public education. Under this act, homeless children may be eligible for other services that must be provided by schools receiving assistance funds. These services may include clothing, a place to bathe and change clothes, free or reduced-cost meals, school supplies, tutorial assistance, and access to medical care. The problems of homelessness and its effects on children's health were addressed in Chapter 20.

Homelessness is often the result of divorce or violence within families. Children may be homeless because their mothers are fleeing an abusive situation. In such circumstances and in disputes over child custody, the school system needs to be alert to the potential for abduction of schoolchildren by the other parent. Similarly, abduction and mistreatment by strangers is an area of concern, and the school nurse should assess school policies designed to prevent such occurrences for their adequacy and the extent to which they are enforced.

Behavioral Considerations

Enrollment in school is itself a lifestyle factor that influences health. School attendance increases one's risk of exposure to a variety of communicable diseases. Children generally experience an increase in the number of acute illnesses during the first few years of school whether this occurs at the day care/preschool level or with admission to elementary school.

The rigidity of the school day may also affect the health status of students. Attempts to postpone defecation or urination until prescribed times may lead to chronic constipation or to urinary tract infections. Likewise, inability to get a drink of water except at specific times may lead to dehydration, particularly in hot weather. The nurse should assess the effects of these aspects of regimentation on the health of students.

Nutrition is another behavioral dimension factor that should be assessed in the school population. The adequacy of lunches brought from home should be examined, as should evidence of poor nutrition of meals eaten at home. For example, the nurse would assess children for evidence of anemia or poor growth and development. In schools without a dietary consultant, the nurse should appraise the nutritional quality of school lunch and/or breakfast programs. Too often, food for such programs is purchased with an eye toward economy rather than nutritional value. School nurses may also encounter students who exhibit eating disorders and can assist with referrals for diagnostic and treatment services for these children.

Recreational activities should also be explored. The need to examine recreational and sports equipment for safety hazards has already been touched on, but the nurse should also be aware of the types of recreational and competitive activities engaged in by students. Is there ample opportunity for physical activity? Is it adequately supervised? Are sports and recreational programs appropriate to children's ages and developmental levels? For example, contact sports are not appropriate for children in lower elementary grades because of increased risk of injury. Another question is whether recreational activities are suited to children's interests. Are various opportunities available, or must all children engage in the same activity, whether they choose to or not? Is a gender bias evident in recreational opportunities provided? For example, is soccer restricted to boys while girls are expected to play hopscotch or jump rope? Attention should also be given to the recreational needs of teachers. Are teachers given a break from classroom and playground duties?

The physical education curriculum of the school will also influence students' exercise behaviors. Many schools do not include the exposure to physical education activities required to meet the national health objectives. Research has indicated that features of the school environment such as physical improvements and supervision influence physical activity by students before and after school and at lunch. For example, the presence of permanent grounds improvements such as installation of basketball and tennis courts and football and soccer goals increase the extent of physical activity by students. Similarly, adequate adult supervision also increases physical activity (Sallis et al., 2001). The school nurse should assess the extent to which the school physical education curriculum and the physical and social environments of the school promote physical activity.

Rest is another component of the behavioral dimension that is assessed. Nurses and teachers should note whether children appear to be getting sufficient sleep at night. The nurse should also examine the adequacy of rest periods provided for younger children. Are these periods appropriately incorporated into the school day? Are there adequate facilities for rest periods (i.e., cots or mats)? Facilities for rest periods are also an important consideration for handicapped children or those with chronic illnesses who may tire easily.

Other lifestyle behaviors should also be assessed, particularly among older students. The extent of tobacco use or use of alcohol or other drugs by students or staff should be explored as should the extent of sexual activity among preadolescent and adolescent students. Approximately half of all adolescents aged 15 to 19 years are sexually active (Kann et al., 2000), and the nurse should assess the extent of sexual activity in the school population. The nurse must also be alert to signs of pregnancy and sexually transmitted diseases as well as being aware of the potential for sexual assault in the school population. Similar assessments are needed with respect to substance use and abuse. In spite of the fact that 99% of school health education programs address problems of alcohol and drug use (Grunbaum et al., 2000), and that schools nationwide have policies prohibiting the use of tobacco, alcohol, and other drugs, use of these substances among preadolescents and adolescents remains high. In fact, in 1999, nearly 33% of students reported current cigarette use, 81% reported use of alcohol at some time in their lives, and 47% and 9.5% of students reported marijuana and cocaine use respectively (Kann et al., 2000). The nurse should assess the extent of substance use and abuse in the school population, ease of access to these substances in the community, and the adequacy and enforcement of school policies regarding their use. The nurse should also be alert to signs of substance use and abuse in individual students and school personnel.

Sexual activity by and with students may also be an area for community health nursing intervention. Community

ETHICAL AWARENESS

One of the teaching staff comes to see you to discuss a drinking problem that she has. Her drinking occurs primarily on weekends when she and her husband like to party. So far, her drinking has not affected her ability to interact effectively with the children in her third grade class. However, she has had a number of absences on Mondays after a weekend of heavy drinking. She asks you for a referral to an alcohol treatment facility and asks that you not tell the principal about her drinking problem. What will you do?

health nurses may be actively involved in sex education in school settings or in the identification and reporting of sexual abuse of children. Date rape and adolescent pregnancy may be other areas that prompt education and intervention by the community health nurse.

Health System Considerations

The health of the school population is influenced at both the individual and community levels. At the individual level, the community health nurse assesses the usual source of health care for individual children and their families. Do children have a regular source of health care? Do they make use of health-promotive and illness-preventive services as well as curative services? Or is health care for children crisis oriented, focusing only on the treatment of acute conditions? Do children have unmet health needs because their families cannot afford care?

At the community level, the nurse assesses the availability of health care services to meet the needs of the school-age population. Are health-promotive and illness-preventive services easily accessible in the community? Are services available for youngsters with special health needs (e.g., handicapped children)? Are specific pediatric or adolescent services available? Is there access to contraceptive services or treatment of sexually transmitted diseases for the adolescent population? Is community attention to possible child abuse adequate?

The nurse also assesses the relationship between the school and the health care community. Are private physicians conversant with regulations for excluding children with communicable conditions from school? Do physicians and other health care providers work cooperatively with school personnel to meet the health care needs of individual youngsters? Do health care providers in the community offer services within the school on either a paid or a voluntary basis?

Another consideration is the organizational structure for delivering health services in the school setting. New models of health care delivery in the schools include school-based and school-linked health centers or clinics and their natural extension, family health centers located in or near schools. The goal of these new models is to provide extended medical and mental health services at present, with the ultimate goal, in some models, of comprehensive ambulatory health care and social services (Dryfoos, 1999). A *school-based health center (SBHC)* is a program of integrated health and social services provided in a school setting and designed to ensure access to necessary services. A *school-linked health center (SLHC)* is a cooperative effort of health and social services personnel to provide coordinated education, health, and social services to a target population of students and their families. Services are usually provided at sites near involved schools.

Both SBHCs and SLHCs are efforts to provide accessible services to children who attend school. Family health centers extend these services to family members as well. Because of their centrality to community life, school-based clinics have been found to be a viable means of health care

CRITICAL THINKING IN RESEARCH

Critics of school-based health centers have indicated that evaluations of these programs to date have not assessed the long-term outcomes of these services in terms of health behaviors and health status measures. Other concerns include fears that health clinics may detract from, rather than enhance, the educational function of schools, duplicate services, or increase competition for resources with existing health services (Barnett, Nieburh, & Baldwin, 1998). Select one of these issues and design a study that would address the concern voiced.

- What variables would your study measure? How might you measure them?
- What potential exists for bias in your findings? How might you control for bias?
- What findings do you think might result from your study? What are the potential implications of your findings for school nursing practice?

delivery. From 1980 to 1994, the number of SBHCs and SLHCs increased fourfold, from 150 to 600 (Barnett et al., 1998). By 1998, the number of school-based clinics had increased to more than 1,000 (Sharma, 1999). In addition to providing direct health care services to students and school staff, clinic personnel may be involved in health fairs; crisis intervention teams; classroom, parent, and teacher education; student health clubs; and other health promotion activities. School-based clinics have been associated with more visits to health providers and fewer emergency department visits. No effects have been noted on sexual activity or contraceptive use, and other effects are difficult to assess because of the high turnover among students who use clinic services (Dryfoos, 1999). Programs such as SBHCs and SLHCs may already exist in a particular system, or the community health nurse can assess the potential for their successful development.

THINK ABOUT IT

What are the advantages and disadvantages of school-based health centers (SBHCs) compared to school-linked health centers (SLHCs)?

Another innovative program involves links between school nursing services and those provided by managed care organizations (MCOs) in areas of high managed care penetration or in schools that enroll large numbers of children who are involved in Medicaid managed care programs. In these programs, school nurses carry out many of the routine screening and health-promotion

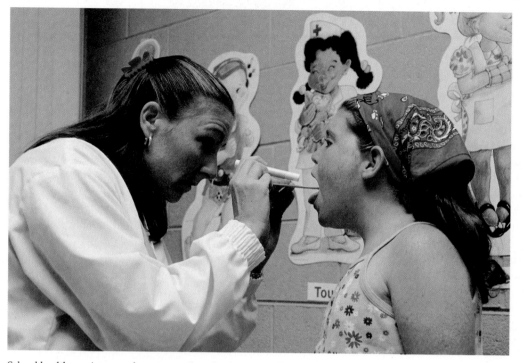

School health services may be some students' only source of health care.

activities among enrolled clients. For example, they can increase the percentage of tuberculin skin tests that are read by preventing parents from having to make a second trip to a provider's office for reading. School nurses also participate in multidisciplinary review of complex cases to prevent unwarranted referrals and increased costs for the MCO. MCO familiarity with the capabilities and value of school nurses has created a powerful ally for school nurses when school budget cuts are considered (Tarras, Nader, Swiger, & Fontanesi, 1998).

In spite of these recent growths in the presence of school-based clinics and other models for health care in schools, many schoolchildren remain without access to health care services in school or outside. In California, for example, only 7% of public schools have a full-time nurse, and 18% of schools have no nurse available at all, yet 94% of these schools have children with asthma and 45% have children who require daily blood glucose monitoring, conditions that argue for the consistent presence of a nurse (Hopkins, 1999).

Tips for assessing factors influencing the health of school populations are provided on the following page. A complete guideline for conducting a population-based health assessment in the school setting is available on the companion Web site for this book.

 ## DIAGNOSTIC REASONING AND CARE OF CLIENTS IN THE SCHOOL SETTING

The second aspect of the use of the nursing process in the school setting is deriving nursing diagnoses from assessment data. Diagnoses can be derived at two levels, in relation to individual students and in relation to the school population. Examples of diagnoses related to a population group are "safety hazard due to placement of play equipment on asphalt surface" and "need for drug abuse education due to high prevalence of drug abuse in the surrounding community." Diagnoses related to an individual student are "inability to participate in vigorous physical exercise due to exercise-induced asthma" and "need for referral to child protective services due to suspected physical abuse by father."

Each of the sample diagnoses provided above contains a statement of the probable underlying cause of the problem. Such a statement provides direction for efforts to resolve the problem. For example, one approach to the playground safety hazard might be to relocate play equipment in a sandy area. With the individual examples, measures might be taken to provide less strenuous forms of exercise for the asthmatic child or to make a referral for child protective services in the abuse situation.

PLANNING TO MEET HEALTH NEEDS IN THE SCHOOL SETTING

Planning to meet health needs identified in the school setting takes place at two levels: the macrolevel, at which the general approach to providing health services in the school is planned, and the microlevel, at which plans are made to meet specific health needs of members of the school population. The community health nurse working in the school setting participates in planning efforts at both levels.

assessment tips assessment tips assessment tips

ASSESSING HEALTH IN THE SCHOOL SETTING

Biophysical Considerations

- What is the age composition of the school population (staff and students)? Do any of the students exhibit developmental delays? Are there specific developmental issues related to the age of the student population (e.g., sexual development)?
- What is the relative proportion of males and females in the school population? What is the racial/ethnic composition of the school population?
- What chronic or communicable conditions are prevalent in the school population? What are the immunization levels in the school population?

Psychological Considerations

- Does the psychological environment of the school promote health?

Physical Environmental Considerations

- Are there health hazards present in the school or the surrounding neighborhood?
- Are food sanitation practices adequate to prevent communicable diseases, vermin infestation, etc.?
- Are school facilities adequate and in good repair? Are there adequate facilities for handicapped students or staff?

Sociocultural Considerations

- What are the community attitudes toward education? Toward the school? To what extent does the community support the school program?
- What sociocultural factors in the community affect the health of the school population?

Behavioral Considerations

- What health-related behaviors affect the health of the school population?
- What recreational opportunities are available to the school population? Do recreational activities pose health hazards? Are appropriate safety equipment and devices used (e.g., in sports)?
- Do any members of the school population use prescription medications on a regular basis? Are medications used, stored, and dispensed as directed?

Health System Considerations

- What health services are offered in the school setting? How are school health care services funded? Is funding adequate to meet health needs?
- How accessible are needed health services in the community? To what extent does the school population use available health services?

Macrolevel Planning

Health services are provided in keeping with an overall health services plan. The plan should specify the population to be served and the services to be provided. Typical categories of services include assessment of health status, problem management services, acute care services, and other preventive services such as immunizations and safety education. An additional component of the health services plan is specification of the personnel involved and of the resources needed to implement the program.

The health services plan should also address the nature of records to be kept. Categories to be addressed include clinical records related to the health of particular children or staff members, administrative records, and evaluative records. Planning for program evaluation should also be included in the plan. Finally, the plan should specify budgetary considerations related to salaries, facilities, and other expenses. Specific elements of the plan in each of these areas are listed in Table 23–3 ■. Initial development of a health services plan in the school setting would entail use of the program planning process described in Chapter 15.

Microlevel Planning

The school health program includes planning for activity at all three levels of prevention: primary, secondary, and tertiary.

Primary Prevention

Primary prevention in the school setting involves many of the same planning considerations as those used with children in general. Areas of emphasis in planning primary preventive measures in the school setting are immunization, safety, exclusion from school, health education, diet and nutrition, and exercise. Other concerns in primary prevention include developing a strong self-image, positive coping skills, and good interpersonal skills in students.

IMMUNIZATION Young children are at particular risk for a variety of communicable diseases for which immunization is possible. Immunizations against measles, mumps, rubella, diphtheria, pertussis, tetanus, and polio are required for school entry. Immunizations are also available for diseases caused by *Hemophilus influenzae* B, hepatitis B, varicella, and influenza. These diseases are discussed in more detail in Chapter 28.

The school nurse may be involved in referring individuals who are not immunized for appropriate services or may provide immunizations in the school setting. In addition to providing for routine immunizations, school nurses may also suggest other immunizations in the event of exposure to certain diseases, such as hepatitis.

■ TABLE 23–3 Elements of the School Health Plan and Related Considerations

Health Plan Element	Related Considerations
Population served	Ages and grades of students involved Extent of service to be given to staff
Services provided	Assessment/screening services First aid Acute care services Problem management services Immunizations Safety education Health education Counseling services
Personnel	Categories of health personnel Qualifications of health personnel Functions and responsibilities Staff development needs
Resources	Facilities Equipment Supplies/postage Health records Telephone
Record system	Clinical records for individuals seen Administrative records Immunization records Absenteeism records Program evaluation records
Program evaluation	Focus of evaluation Data collection procedures Data analysis procedures
Budgetary considerations	Salaries Facility construction and maintenance Equipment and supply costs Record-keeping costs Staff development costs

SAFETY Part of the school nurse's responsibility is to identify safety hazards and report them to those responsible for eliminating them. Safety education may also be the responsibility of the school nurse. In addition, the nurse might collaborate with others within and outside the school setting to reduce safety hazards in the surrounding area. Moreover, the nurse and other school personnel might become involved in cooperative efforts with local police to reduce drug traffic in the neighborhood.

There are generally three aspects of injury prevention in school settings, all of which may involve participation by school nurses. The first is educating students and staff regarding safe behaviors. The second lies in the develop-

ment of school policies related to adult supervision, aggressive behavior, and so on. Finally, community health nurses may be involved in planning to modify environmental factors that pose injury hazards (Allen et al., 1998).

EXCLUSION FROM SCHOOL One of the earliest responsibilities of the school nurse was to determine when children should be excluded from school because they had communicable illnesses. Children were also excluded from school as part of an effort to stop the spread of scabies, lice, and other parasites among a highly susceptible population. This responsibility still requires the school nurse to be knowledgeable of the signs and symptoms of communicable disease and infestation and to be aware of state and local regulations regarding school exclusion. Several conditions that usually warrant exclusion and guidelines for readmission are listed in Table 23–4 ■.

The responsibility of the nurse does not stop with excluding the affected child from school. The nurse should also educate parents and children regarding the need to stay home from school when they are ill and about care during illness. The nurse may also make referrals for medical care as needed. In addition, the nurse follows up on children excluded from school to make sure that they are receiving appropriate care and that they are able to return to school when there is no longer any danger of exposure to others.

HEALTH EDUCATION Health education in the school setting provides a foundation for healthy behaviors in adulthood. Most states and school districts require some form of health education at the elementary and junior and senior high school level. At the elementary level, health education is most likely to be incorporated into the total curriculum. Separate health courses are more likely at the junior and senior high level (Grunbaum et al., 2000).

⑥THINK ABOUT IT

Should health education be provided in the school setting by nurses or by teachers? Why?

The principles of health education discussed in Chapter 11 are particularly relevant to community health nursing in the school setting. The nurse may either serve as a resource for teachers on health content, provide health education classes, or both. The school nurse is also involved in the development of the health education curriculum. Activities involved in curriculum development in which the nurse may engage include the assessment of needs and resources, review of health curricula from other school systems, development of goals and objectives, and

■ **TABLE 23–4**   **Conditions Typically Warranting Exclusion from School and Guidelines for Readmission**

Condition	Readmission Guidelines
Bacterial conjunctivitis	After acute symptoms subside
Chickenpox	5 days after eruption of the first vesicles or after lesions are dried
Diphtheria	Until negative cultures of nose and throat are obtained at least 24 hours after discontinuing antibiotics
Hepatitis A	One week after onset of jaundice
Impetigo (staphylococcal)	24 hours after treatment is initiated
Influenza	After acute symptoms subside
Measles	4 days after onset of the rash
Meningococcal meningitis	24 hours after chemotherapy is initiated or when the child is sufficiently recovered
Mononucleosis, infectious	After acute symptoms subside Delay resumption of strenuous physical activity until spleen is nonpalpable
Mumps	9 days after onset of swelling
Pediculosis	24 hours after application of an effective pediculocide
Pneumonia, pneumococcal and *Mycoplasma*	48 hours after initiation of antibiotics or when child is sufficiently recovered
Pertussis	After 5 days of antibiotic therapy or when child is sufficiently recovered
Respiratory disease (viral) and upper respiratory infection	After acute symptoms subside
Rubella	7 days after onset of the rash
Scabies	24 hours after treatment
Streptococcus (strep throat, scarlet fever, impetigo)	24 hours after treatment is initiated or when child is sufficiently recovered
Tinea corporis	Excluded only from gym, swimming pool, or other activities where exposure of other individuals may occur; activities resume after treatment is completed

design of specific learning activities. In addition, the nurse may be involved in preparing teachers to participate in the health education program. Finally, the nurse participates in the implementation and evaluation of the program.

School nurses may also be involved in the provision of health education to school staff. For example, in spite of the fact that much first aid care is provided by school staff in the absence of a school health nurse, as few as one third of teachers are estimated to have received formal training in first aid or cardiopulmonary resuscitation (CPR) (Nguyen, 1998). School staff may also require education to enable them to promote their own health.

FOOD AND NUTRITION   Nutrition is another important aspect of health promotion with the school population. As noted earlier, when this function is not performed by a dietitian or nutritionist, school nurses assess the nutritional status of children and monitor the nutritional value of school lunches. When nutritional offerings are inadequate, the nurse works with school administrators and food service personnel to improve the nutritional quality of meals served. The nurse may also educate children and their parents regarding nutrition and good dietary habits.

EXERCISE AND PHYSICAL ACTIVITY   Exercise and physical activity are another important area for primary prevention in the school setting. The school health program must be designed to assure physical activity while students are in school and to promote continued activity throughout life. The Centers for Disease Control and Prevention (1997) has developed the following recommendations for promoting physical activity among young people:

- Policies should be established that promote enjoyable physical activity throughout life.
- Schools should provide physical and social environments that encourage physical activity.
- Schools should implement physical education curricula that promote enjoyable participation in physical activity and enable students to develop the skills and self-confidence to continue to be physically active.
- Schools should implement health education curricula that assist students to adopt physically active lifestyles.
- Schools should provide extracurricular programs that emphasize physical activities congruent with students' needs and interests.
- Parents and guardians should become actively involved in instruction and extracurricular activities related to physical activity.
- School personnel should be effectively trained to promote physical activity among students.
- Health services personnel should assess student activity patterns and counsel students regarding the need for physical activity.
- Communities should provide a range of sports and recreational opportunities for physical activity that are developmentally appropriate.

- Schools and communities should regularly evaluate physical activity instruction, facilities, and programs.

Community health nurses working in school settings can be actively involved in planning to implement these recommendations in their schools.

SELF-IMAGE   Sound mental health is promoted by a strong self-image developed throughout childhood. Health promotion in the school setting should focus on the development of a healthy self-image as well as a healthy physical self. School nurses can foster self-image development by serving as role models in their dealings with children. They can also suggest to teachers learning activities that enhance development of a positive self-image.

On occasion, school nurses may need to function as advocates for children who do not have a strong self-image or for those who may be emotionally (or physically) abused by family members, peers, or even teachers. As noted earlier, the nurse should be aware of disciplinary measures used in the school and be alert to forms of discipline or unfair exercise of authority that are harmful to a child's self-image. When such circumstances are identified, the nurse might discuss his or her observations with teachers or other personnel involved and suggest other avenues for achieving the goals of disciplinary action. When corrective actions do not result from these interventions, the nurse may need to bring the problem to the attention of the appropriate authorities such as the school principal or members of the school board.

Occasionally, this requires filing a report of child abuse. In addition to reporting the situation, however, the nurse has a responsibility to provide counseling or referral for assistance to those involved and to serve as a support person for both victim and abuser. In such cases, referrals may also be needed to address socioeconomic problems that may be contributing to the situation.

COPING SKILLS   Another aspect of primary prevention that should be fostered in schools is the development of coping skills. Students and personnel can be assisted to develop active problem-solving strategies that promote their abilities to cope with adverse circumstances. School health nurses can serve as role models in this respect and can also provide counseling that assists students and their families or staff to engage in positive problem solving. Nurses can also reinforce evidence of positive coping by making others aware of their abilities to cope. In addition, the nurse can present information on stress, and can offer strategies for dealing with stress that enhance the development of sound coping skills.

INTERPERSONAL SKILLS   The ability to interact effectively with others is essential to civilized society. Such abilities are not innate and must be learned. Education for effective interpersonal skills is another aspect of primary prevention with the school population. Again, the nurse can serve as a role model for effective interpersonal skills and can

educate students, parents, and staff regarding interpersonal interactions and the development of communication skills. The nurse can also provide information on group dynamics and communication skills that can enhance interpersonal skills within groups. For example, the nurse might promote role play in a class to which a handicapped child will soon be admitted or help youngsters learn how to express anger at a teacher in an appropriate manner. Aspects of primary prevention in the school setting and related community health nursing responsibilities are summarized in Table 23–5 ■.

Secondary Prevention

Secondary prevention deals with existing problems that require intervention. Generally speaking, secondary prevention involves screening for existing health conditions, referral, counseling, and treatment.

SCREENING   Screening is a major facet of most school health programs and an important responsibility of the school nurse. The goals of screening programs within the school setting include the obvious goal of detecting disease as well as identifying children with special needs that require adjustment of the education program, promoting the importance of primary preventive measures, and evaluating the effectiveness of current measures.

Screening can be used to detect health conditions that are amenable to treatment and that can be resolved with appropriate therapy. For example, vision screening is used to identify children with visual problems, the majority of whom can benefit from corrective lenses. Screening may also help to identify children with particular needs that necessitate adjustments in the education program. For example, developmental screening may help to identify youngsters with learning disabilities who will benefit from special education programs.

A screening program also provides an opportunity to stress the importance of primary prevention. Dental screening, for example, provides an excellent opportunity to educate students on the need for good dental hygiene. Finally, screening efforts provide one measure of the effectiveness of current preventive efforts. For example, hematocrit screening can provide evidence of one aspect of the efficacy of a school lunch program or nutrition education program in promoting good nutrition.

Screening is a cost-effective approach to the identification of health problems. Typical costs of a screening program include those of the screening procedure itself and of retesting those with positive results; time spent by the nurse in referral; costs of diagnostic and treatment services; special education costs; and costs of corrective maintenance (e.g., for hearing aids or replacing eyeglasses). These costs tend to be far less than the costs incurred when diagnoses are made later, after problems become more pronounced.

Screening programs typically undertaken in the school setting include screening of vision and hearing, dental screening, height and weight measurements, and screening

■ **TABLE 23–5** **Areas of Emphasis in Primary Prevention in the School Setting and Related Community Health Nursing Responsibilities**

Area of Emphasis	Community Heath Nursing Responsibilities
Immunization	Refer for immunization services as needed. Provide routine immunizations. Suggest additional immunizations as warranted by circumstances (e.g., an epidemic of hepatitis A).
Safety	Report safety hazards to appropriate authorities. Provide safety education. Collaborate in the development of school policies that promote safety. Collaborate with others to eliminate safety hazards in the community.
School exclusion	Determine need for exclusion from school. Explain need for exclusion to parents. Refer child for treatment of condition if needed. Educate children and parents on preventing the spread of communicable diseases. Follow up on children excluded from school to ensure appropriate care.
Health education	Participate in designing health education curricula. Provide consultation to teachers on health education topics. Provide in-service for teachers related to health education. Teach health education in the classroom. Arrange for other health education experiences (e.g., field trips or guest speakers). Arrange or provide health education for staff and/or families.
Food and nutrition	Provide consultation on menu planning. Educate children and families regarding nutrition.
Self-image	Provide a role model for teachers and others in positive interactions with children. Provide consultation to teachers on activities to enhance children's self-esteem. Function as an advocate for children who have poor self-esteem.
Coping skills	Provide a role model for students and staff for effective problem-solving skills. Provide counseling regarding problem-solving skills. Reinforce use of appropriate coping skills. Educate students and staff on stress and coping.
Interpersonal skills	Provide a role model for students and staff for effective interpersonal skills. Educate students, staff, and parents on group dynamics and communication skills.

for scoliosis. Other screening tests may also be employed depending on the needs of the population served by the school. For example, tuberculosis, lead, sickle cell, and diabetes screening may be conducted in communities with high prevalences of these conditions.

The community health nurse in the school setting may perform a variety of roles with respect to screening programs. The nurse might arrange for the screening to be done or might conduct the screening tests, or the nurse might train volunteers to perform certain screening procedures. Moreover, the nurse is responsible for informing students and parents of the results of screening tests and for interpreting those results (Caldwell et al., 1997). The nurse may also need to make referrals for follow-up diagnostic or treatment services. In addition, the nurse follows up on these referrals to make sure that students are receiving appropriate health care services.

REFERRAL School health nurses make a number of referrals. In addition to referrals for following up on positive screening test results, the nurse may make referrals for a variety of other services. For example, the nurse might refer children who are not immunized to the local health department for immunizations, or a referral for counseling might be needed for a child with behavior problems. School personnel may also be referred for health problems that require medical attention. In making these and other referrals, the school nurse uses the principles of referral discussed in Chapter 12.

COUNSELING Another important role for the school nurse in secondary prevention is that of counseling. As noted in Chapter 8, counseling involves assisting clients to make informed health decisions. Nurses may counsel individual students regarding personal problems, or they may assist students, families, and staff to engage in problem solving.

TREATMENT   School nurses may also be involved in the actual treatment of existing health conditions. Treatment can involve emergency care in the event of illness or injury. School nurse practitioners might even engage in medical management of minor illnesses such as antibiotic treatment of otitis media.

Nurses may also be involved in providing specific treatments designed to minimize the effects of acute and chronic conditions. For example, the nurse may need to dispense prescribed medications or engage in specific technical procedures. The need for expertise in the use of medical technology in the school setting has increased dramatically and derives from the inclusion of children with congenital anomalies, chronic illnesses, conditions related to perinatal factors (e.g., prematurity or meconium aspiration), genetic diseases such as sickle cell disease and Tay–Sachs, the long-term effects of injuries and infections, and developmental delays (Caldwell et al., 1997). The school nurse may also be involved in assisting students and staff with chronic illnesses such as diabetes or asthma to effectively manage their conditions.

School nurses may assist with physical therapy or perform procedures such as tracheosomy suction or catheterization. They may also be involved in programs for bowel or bladder training. Community health nurses working with handicapped children in the school setting may also find it necessary to educate other school personnel in procedures required and deal with the fears experienced by school staff regarding the child's condition.

Caring for children with special health needs in the school setting entails the development of an Individualized Health Care Plan (IHCP). Components of the IHCP include a health history, identification of special care needs (e.g., required procedures), an overview of the child's basic health status, and information about medications including who dispenses them, timing, dosages, routes of administration, and so on. Additional elements of the plan include special dietary or nutritional needs, transportation needs, requirements for specialized equipment, identification of possible problems and strategies to solve them, and a plan for emergency action and transportation. Finally, the IHCP should indicate review by the nurse, physician, parent, and school administrator and be incorporated in an easily retrievable location in the student's record (Caldwell, Janz, et al., 1997).

In addition to planning care for students with special needs, the community health nurse monitors the therapeutic effects and side effects of medications and other treatments. Emphases in secondary prevention in the school setting and related community health nursing responsibilities are summarized in Table 23–6 ■.

Tertiary Prevention

Tertiary prevention is undertaken to prevent the recurrence of a problem or to minimize the effects of an exist-

■ **TABLE 23–6   Areas of Emphasis in Secondary Prevention in the School Setting and Related Community Health Nursing Responsibilities**

Area of Emphasis	Related Community Health Nursing Responsibilities
Screening	Conduct screening tests or arrange for screening by others.
	Train volunteers in screening procedures.
	Interpret screening test results.
	Notify parents of screening test results.
	Make referrals for further tests or treatments as needed.
	Follow up on referrals to determine outcomes and to ensure appropriate care for identified conditions.
Referral	Refer children and families for health care and other services as needed.
	Refer other school personnel for needed services.
Counseling	Assist students, staff, or families to make informed health decisions.
	Counsel students, staff, or families regarding personal problems.
	Assist students, staff, or families to engage in problem solving.
Treatment	Provide first aid for illness or injury.
	Dispense medications prescribed for acute or chronic illnesses.
	Develop the IHCP for care of children with special health needs.
	Perform special treatments or procedures warranted by identified conditions.
	Teach others to perform special treatments or procedures.
	Monitor therapeutic effects and side effects of medications and other treatments.

ing one. To a large extent, tertiary preventive measures depend on the problems experienced by the student or staff member. Generally speaking, however, there are four aspects of tertiary prevention with which the school nurse is concerned: preventing the recurrence of acute problems, preventing complications, fostering adjustment to chronic illness and handicapping conditions, and dealing with learning disabilities.

ACUTE CONDITIONS   Preventing the recurrence of acute health problems depends on adequate treatment for existing problems and eliminating conditions that might lead to recurrence. For example, the school nurse might need to educate parents and children regarding the need to complete the course of therapy for otitis media, or education might be needed related to toileting hygiene (e.g., wiping from front to back) to prevent a recurrent urinary tract infection. The nurse might also engage in efforts to help an abusive parent or unduly harsh teacher find other ways to vent frustrations, or might make a referral to help alleviate financial difficulties that are taxing coping abilities.

PREVENTING COMPLICATIONS   Tertiary prevention is also directed toward preventing complications of either acute or chronic health problems. For example, the school nurse might encourage parents of a child with strep throat to complete a course of antibiotics to prevent cardiac and urinary complications. Similarly, the nurse might suggest a cushion and frequent changes of position to prevent pressure sores in a student confined to a wheelchair.

CHRONIC ILLNESS AND HANDICAPPING CONDITIONS   Tertiary prevention for children with chronic or handicapping conditions involves assisting them to adjust to their condition and preventing complications. Specific measures depend on the condition involved. For example, special arrangements for physical education might be needed to prevent recurrent attacks of exercise-induced asthma, and special attention to diet might be required for the diabetic child or staff member.

Major considerations in dealing with children with chronic illness in the school setting involve money, transportation and facilities, and equipment. Additional considerations include nutrition and psychological well-being. The school nurse may need to refer students and parents to sources of financial assistance as a way to deal with the long-term care requirements of chronic and handicapping conditions.

Transportation and facility considerations in the school setting include issues of physical access to facilities discussed earlier in this chapter. Another area for consideration is that of transportation to and from school and for field trips. The nurse identifies barriers to access in the school setting and serves as an advocate for the removal of those barriers. Likewise, the nurse attempts to arrange transportation and other circumstances so that students with chronic or handicapping conditions can participate in as many regular school activities, including field trips, as possible. Advocacy in this area might also be needed with parents of handicapped children who may have a tendency to overprotect them.

There may also be a need for special equipment to be used either at home or at school. The school nurse makes referrals to obtain such equipment or sees that necessary equipment is provided by the school itself.

Nutrition may be particularly problematic for schoolchildren with chronic diseases or handicapping conditions. Youngsters with diabetes, for example, may need assistance in adapting a school lunch program to a diabetic diet. Severely handicapped children may need assistance with eating or may need to be fed. The school nurse assesses the special nutritional needs of children with these and similar conditions and then assists the child, family, and other school personnel to meet those needs.

The final consideration with children who have chronic illnesses or handicapping conditions is that of psycholog-

ical well-being. These children should be helped to adjust to their conditions and to participate as normally as possible in the school routine. Parents, teachers, and other children may need to be discouraged from undermining the child's independence by "doing for" them. Values clarification exercises can help other children to understand the problems of the handicapped or chronically ill child rather than to make fun of them or pity them.

Psychological health may be particularly fragile among those children with AIDS. There is a need to provide emotional support for these children as they deal with a stigmatized illness that may cause others to withdraw from them in fear. Again, the community health nurse in the school setting may need to function as an advocate to prevent social isolation of these and other children with chronic or handicapping conditions. Other concerns about the child with AIDS are the need to protect the child from infection and the use of universal precautions when dealing with blood and body fluids; both of these concerns may heighten the child's sense of isolation and alienation. There is also a need to deal with the child's knowledge of his or her own mortality. Thus, the nurse may want to refer the child and family members for counseling. The nurse might also need to help other children, parents, and school personnel deal with their feelings of fear and grief related to AIDS and death.

LEARNING DISABILITY   Because there does not seem to be any form of primary or secondary prevention available for learning disability, the focus in working with learning-disabled children is on minimizing the effects of their disability.

Some of the interventions that may be planned to assist learning-disabled children are learning by activity;

ETHICAL AWARENESS

Lila, one of the students in your school is a third grader with a serious congenital heart defect that is not amenable to surgical repair. Lila voluntarily restricts her activities when she becomes fatigued or activities cause her to become dizzy. She is a bright, happy child, well liked by the other children, and is always involved in school activities that do not require too much physical exertion. Lila and her parents both know that her prognosis is poor and that she is "living on borrowed time." They have asked the child's physician to issue a "do not resuscitate" (DNR) order, which has been done and included in the child's school health record. One day while you are eating lunch, Lila's best friend runs to you to tell you that Lila has fallen down on the playground and the other children "can't wake her up." When you get to the playground area you find that Lila is not breathing and has no pulse. Will you abide by the DNR order in this situation?

involving multiple senses in learning activities; repetition; providing direction in small steps; and giving directions without irrelevant detail. Teaching at the appropriate level, a level that creates a challenge but does not lead to frustration, may also be helpful. Other useful strategies include avoiding drastic changes in activities, limiting distractions, and creating a climate in which success is ensured and reinforced as often as possible.

The nurse is involved in development of Individualized Education Plans (IEPs) that allow children with learning disabilities, as well as those with other chronic or handicapping conditions, to learn as easily as possible. Again, attention must be given to the psychological effects of being tagged *learning disabled*. The nurse may need to function as an advocate with parents, teachers, and other children to avoid the application of labels that undermine the child's self-esteem. The nurse can also function as a role model in providing positive reinforcement for the child's strengths and for his or her accomplishments, however small. Considerations related to tertiary prevention in the school setting and related community health nursing responsibilities are summarized in Table 23–7 ■.

In planning primary, secondary, or tertiary preventive measures in the school setting, the community health nurse may need information or assistance from outside sources. Links to sources of assistance for specific health problems among children or sources of information on school nursing are provided on the companion Web site for this book.

IMPLEMENTING HEALTH CARE IN THE SCHOOL SETTING

Implementing health care for individuals or groups in the school setting frequently involves collaboration between the nurse and other members of the school health team. At the individual level, for example, the community health nurse may need to contact the private physician of a child with a chronic illness with information about adverse effects of medications or to request a change in the medical treatment plan based on changes in the child's condition. The nurse also needs to solicit the cooperation of parents in following through on a referral for medical services, testing, counseling, or other services needed by their child.

Implementing care for groups within the school setting also requires collaboration between the nurse and others. For example, the nurse may invite local police personnel to participate in a drug education program to be presented in the school, or the nurse might work with teachers, media specialists, food service personnel, and others to implement an educational program on basic nutrition for elementary schoolchildren. Parental permission may be required in certain school-based health programs. For example, parents need to grant permission for screening procedures such as hematocrit testing. The nurse may also need to recruit parent or community

■ **TABLE 23–7**   **Areas of Emphasis in Tertiary Prevention in the School Setting and Related Community Health Nursing Responsibilies**

Area of Emphasis	Related Community Health Nursing Responsibilities
Preventing recurrence of acute conditions	Eliminate risk factors for the condition.
	Teach students, staff, or parents how to prevent recurrence of problems.
	Make referrals that can assist in eliminating risk factors.
Preventing complications of and promoting adjustment to chronic and handicapping conditions	Assist parents with finding sources of financial aid to deal with chronic and handicapping conditions.
	Facilitate meeting special nutritional needs.
	Assist with meeting special needs for transportation and facilities.
	Provide for special equipment needs.
	Promote psychological well-being.
	Assist students, families, and staff to deal with the eventuality of death in terminal illnesses.
	Refer for counseling as needed.
	Function as an advocate as needed.
Preventing adverse effects of learning disabilities	Provide consultation for teachers in dealing with children's learning disabilities.
	Participate in the design of IEPs for children with disabilities.
	Function as an advocate for the learning-disabled child as needed.
	Serve as a role model in positively reinforcing the child's accomplishments.

volunteers to assist with screening programs or with other health-related programs such as a health fair.

EVALUATING HEALTH CARE IN THE SCHOOL SETTING

Evaluating the effectiveness of care in the school setting focuses on the outcomes of that care. Evaluation can occur at two levels, the individual child or the total school health program. Evaluative criteria for the care of the individual child reflect the effects of nursing care on the youngster's health status. For example, if a child is no longer abused by his parent, or no longer has recurrent ear infections, or is now able to interact effectively with peers, the interventions of the nurse have probably been effective.

Evaluation of the overall school health program focuses on indicators of the health status of the total population. For instance, absentee rates might indicate how effective the program has been in preventing disease. Student screening test results may also provide information on the effectiveness of primary preventive efforts.

Changes in the prevalence of certain health problems within the school population may also indicate the efficacy of secondary preventive measures. For example, if alcohol abuse has been a problem among the student population, a declining prevalence of alcohol abuse would indicate that secondary measures are having an effect. Similarly, a decline in the teenage pregnancy rate would indicate that a sex education program is effective.

The processes used in evaluating the school health program are those discussed in Chapter 15. The school nurse collaborates with other members of the school health team in designing and implementing an evaluation of the program. Moreover, the nurse may also be involved in data collection related to the evaluation and in interpreting those data. Finally, the nurse should be actively involved in decisions made on the basis of evaluative data.

At the national level, national objectives for the year 2010 related to school health can provide additional evaluative criteria. Information on the current status of some of these objectives is presented below.

Community health nursing in schools provides an opportunity for promoting health and preventing illness in children and their families. Community health nurses working in school settings at all levels can also assist students and staff with existing health problems, as well as designing school health programs that promote the health of the general public.

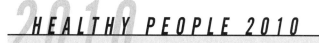

HEALTHY PEOPLE 2010

GOALS FOR THE POPULATION

	Objective	Base	Target
7-2	Increase the proportion of middle, junior, and senior high schools that provide comprehensive school health education related to:		
	b. Unintentional injury	66%	90%
	c. Violence	58%	80%
	d. Suicide	58%	80%
	e. Tobacco use and addiction	86%	95%
	f. Alcohol and other drug use	90%	95%
	g. Unintended pregnancy, HIV/AIDS, and STD	65%	90%
	h. Unhealthy dietary patterns	84%	95%
	i. Inadequate physical activity	78%	90%
	j. Environmental health	60%	80%
7-3	Increase the proportion of college students who receive information on six priority health risks	6%	25%
7-4	Increase the proportion of elementary, middle, junior high, and senior high schools that have a nurse-to-student ratio of at least 1:750	28%	50%
6-9	Increase the proportion of children and youth who spend at least 80% of their time in regular education programs	45%	60%
22-8	Increase the proportion of schools that require daily physical education for all students		
	a. Middle and junior high	17%	25%
	b. Senior high	2%	5%
22-9	Increase the proportion of adolescents who participate in daily school physical education	27%	50%
22-10	Increase the proportion of adolescents who spend at least 50% of time in physical education classes being physically active	32%	50%
27-11	Increase smoke-free and tobacco-free environments in schools (including all school facilities, property, vehicles, and events)	37%	100%

Source: U.S. Department of Health and Human Services. (2000). *Healthy people 2010* (Conference edition, in two volumes). Washington, DC: Author.

APPLYING YOUR KNOWLEDGE IN PRACTICE

❦ CASE STUDY
Nursing in the School Setting

Brandon is a third grader in the school where you work as a school nurse. He comes to see you because he "has a stomachache." This is his third visit to your office in as many days. Each day, you have seen him for a similar complaint but have found no physical evidence of illness. According to his teacher, his appetite has been good at lunch, although his lunches are large and not particularly nutritious. Brandon says he is not constipated and has not had any diarrhea or vomiting. His abdominal pain usually disappears after lying down in your office for about 20 minutes.

When you talk to the teacher, she tells you that lately the other children have been making fun of Brandon because he always comes in last in running games and can't run very fast during PE. Brandon is about 35 pounds overweight for his height and becomes short of breath with strenuous physical exercise. Brandon has two younger brothers who are both slender and have no difficulties with physical activity.

The teacher also mentions that Brandon has been talking during class and disturbing the other children.

She has tried to take him aside and explain why he should not talk in class, but he continues. His grades are not the best in the world (they're not the worst either), but he has been discouraged lately because he is having trouble mastering long division.

- What biophysical, psychological, sociocultural, behavioral, and health system factors are operating in this situation?
- What nursing diagnoses would you derive from the information provided above? How would you prioritize Brandon's problems? Why?
- Who else should be involved in developing a plan of care for Brandon?
- Write at least two outcome objectives for Brandon's care.
- What primary, secondary, and tertiary prevention measures would be appropriate in this case?
- How would you evaluate the effectiveness of your interventions with Brandon? Be specific.

❦ TESTING YOUR UNDERSTANDING

- What are three goals of a school health program? (p. 537)
- What are the basic components of a school health program? (pp. 537–538)
- What biophysical, psychological, physical environmental, sociocultural, behavioral, and health system factors may influence the health of the school population? (pp. 542–549)
- What are the major areas of emphasis in primary prevention in the school setting? Describe at least

two nursing activities related to each area. (pp. 550–553)
- What are the facets of secondary prevention in the school setting? Identify at least two community health nursing responsibilities related to each approach. (pp. 553–555)
- What are the major areas of emphasis in tertiary prevention in the school setting? How might the community health nurse be involved in each of these areas? (pp. 555–557)

REFERENCES

Allegrante, J. P. (1998). School-site health promotion for faculty and staff: A key component of the coordinated school health program. *Journal of School Health, 68,* 190–195.

Allen, K., Ball, J., & Helfer, B. (1998). Preventing and managing childhood emergencies in schools. *Journal of School Nursing, 14*(1), 20–24.

Allensworth, D., Lawson, E., Nicholson, L., & Wyche, J. (Eds.). (1997). *Schools and health: Our nation's investment.* Washington, DC: National Academy Press.

American Academy of Pediatrics. (2000). Corporal punishment in schools. *Pediatrics, 106,* 343.

Barnett, S., Niebuhr, V., & Baldwin, C. (1998). Principles for developing interdisciplinary school-based primary care centers. *Journal of School Health, 68,* 99–105.

Better Homes Fund. (1999). *America's homeless children: New outcasts.* Newton, MA: Author.

Bingler, S. (2000). The school as the center of a healthy community. *Public Health Reports, 115,* 228–233.

Brindis, C. D., Sanghvi, R., Melinkovich, P., Kaplan, D. W., Ahlstrand, K. R., & Phibbs, S. L. (1998). Redesigning a school health workforce for a new health care environment: Training school nurses as nurse practitioners. *Journal of School Health, 68,* 179–183.

Caldwell, T. H., Janz, J. R., Alcouloumre, D. S., Porter, S., et al. (1997). Entrance and planning process for students with special health care needs. In S. Porter, M. Haynie, T. Bierle, T. H. Caldwell, & J. S. Palfrey (Eds.), *Children and youth assisted by medical technology in educational settings: Guidelines for care* (2nd ed.) (pp. 41–62). Baltimore: Paul H. Brookes.

Caldwell, T. H., Sirvis, B. P., Still, J., Still, M., et al. (1997). Students who require medical technology in school. In S. Porter, M. Haynie, T. Bierle, T. H. Caldwell, & J. S. Palfrey (Eds.), *Children and youth assisted by medical technology in educational settings: Guidelines for care* (2nd ed.) (pp. 3–18). Baltimore: Paul H. Brookes.

Office of Disease Prevention and Health Promotion. (1997). *A comprehensive school health program.* Atlanta, GA: Author.

Centers for Disease Control and Prevention (1997). Guidelines for school and community programs to promote lifelong physical activity among young people. *Morbidity and Mortality Weekly Report, 46*(RR-6), 1–36.

Dryfoos, J. G. (1999). School-based health and social service centers. In T. P. Gullotta, R. L. Hampton, G. R. Adams, B. A. Ryan, & R. P. Weissberg (Eds.), *Children's health care: Issues for the year 2000 and beyond* (pp. 137–167). Thousand Oaks, CA: Sage.

Felton, J. S., & Keil, C. P. (1998). School nursing: A study of perceptions and visions. *Journal of School Nursing, 14*(3), 5–13.

Grunbaum, J. A., Kann, L., Williams, B. I., Collins, J. L., et al. (2000). Surveillance for characteristics of health education among secondary schools—School health education profiles, 1998. *Morbidity and Mortality Weekly Report, 49*(SS-8), 1–41.

Hopkins, M. E. (2000). More than just bandaids: School nurses tackle new challenges and an expanding role. *NurseWeek, 13*(13), 27.

Kalthoff, C. (1998). *Latchkey kids: Alternative needs for care . . . An assessment tool for parents.* San Diego, CA: Author.

Kann, L., Kinchen, S. A., Williams, B. I., Ross, J. G., et al. (2000). Youth Risk Behavior Surveillance—United States, 1999. *Morbidity and Mortality Weekly Report, 49*(SS-5), 1–94.

Kronenfeld, J. J. (2000). *Schools and the health of children: Protecting our future.* Thousand Oaks, CA: Sage.

Merrill, J., Turner, L. C., McLaughlin, J., Milner, G. (1999). Following in Wald's footsteps: Bringing health to the people. *Journal of the New York State Nurses Association, 30*(1), 5–8.

Miller, T. R., & Spicer, R. S. (1998). How safe are our schools? *American Journal of Public Health, 88,* 413–418.

National Association of School Nurses. (1999). *Standards of professional school nursing practice.* Scarborough, ME: Author.

Newton, J., Adams, R., & Marcontel, M. (1997). *The new school handbook: A ready reference for school nurses and educators* (3rd ed.). Paramus, NJ: Prentice Hall.

Nguyen, L. H. (1998). First aid training: The hidden dimension of injury control for school-based injuries. *American Journal of Public Health, 88,* 1557.

Office of Disease Prevention and Health Promotion. (1997). *A comprehensive school health program.* Atlanta, GA: Author.

Parcel, G. S., Kelder, S. H., & Basen-Engquist, K. (2000). The school as a setting for health promotion. In B. D. Poland, L. W. Green, & I. Rootman (Eds.), *Settings for health promotion: Linking theory and practice* (pp. 86–120). Thousand Oaks: Sage.

Proctor, S., Lordis, S., & Zaiger, D. (1993). *School nursing practice—Roles and standards.* Scarborough, ME: National Association of School Nurses.

Raphael, D. (1998). Emerging concepts of health and health promotion. *Journal of School Health, 68,* 297–300.

Sallis, J. F., Conway, T. L., Prochaska, J. J., McKenzie, T. L., Marshall, S. J., & Brown, M. (2001). The association of school environments with youth physical activity. *American Journal of Public Health, 91,* 618–620.

SEP. (1998). Education for practice: Identifying a "critical mass" of specialty content for school nursing. *Journal of School Nursing, 14*(3), 2, 4.

Sharma, S. (1999). Back to class: School-based clinics help keep uninsured kids healthy. *NurseWeek, 12*(10), 15.

Tarras, H., Nader. P., Swiger, H., & Fontanesi, J. (1998). The School Health Innovative Programs: Integrating school health and managed care in San Diego. *Journal of School Health, 68,* 22–25.

U.S. Census Bureau. (1999). *Statistical abstract of the United States, 1999* (119th ed.). Washington DC: Author.

U.S. Department of Health and Human Services. (2000). *Healthy people 2010* (Conference edition, in two volumes). Washington, DC: Author.

CARE OF CLIENTS IN WORK SETTINGS

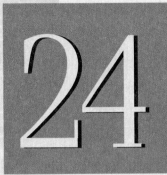

Chapter Objectives

After reading this chapter, you should be able to:

- Describe advantages in providing health care in work settings.
- Identify types of health and safety hazards encountered in work settings.
- Identify biophysical, psychological, physical environmental, sociocultural, behavioral, and health system factors that influence health in work settings.
- Describe spheres of social influence on the health of employees.
- Describe types of health care programs in work settings.
- Describe areas of emphasis in primary prevention in work settings.
- Describe major considerations in secondary prevention in work settings.
- Describe emphases in tertiary prevention in work settings.

Media Link

http://www.prenhall.com/clark

Additional interactive resources for this chapter can be found on the companion Web site. Click on Chapter 24 and "Begin" to select the activities for this chapter.

561

Because nearly two thirds of the U.S. population, or 137.6 million Americans, are employed, the work setting is an important place for promoting the health of the general population (U.S. Census Bureau, 1999). Although the work environment contributes to a wide variety of health problems, it also provides opportunities to influence a major segment of the population regarding personal health behaviors.

Over the years, employers have come to appreciate that healthy employees are more productive and that it is in the employer's interest to promote and maintain employee health. Moreover, the escalating cost of health insurance makes health promotion increasingly cost-effective. One way that some companies have chosen to decrease health-related costs is to provide on-site health care for employees.

⑥THINK ABOUT IT

Daykin (1999) has suggested that occupational health research should focus on unpaid as well as paid occupations as they relate to health issues. Areas suggested for research include unpaid housework and family caretaking. Another relatively neglected area of research is the health effects of sex work; research efforts in this realm have tended to focus on risk for sexually transmitted diseases, but have ignored other possible health effects (Scambler & Scambler, 1999). Do you think these occupational pursuits should be considered work and should be included in the research agenda for occupational health research? Why or why not?

The importance of health care in the occupational setting can be seen in the national health objectives for the year 2010. In fact, one entire section of the objectives deals with health and safety in occupational settings (U.S. Department of Health and Human Services [USDHHS], 2000b). These objectives can be reviewed on the Healthy People 2010 Web site, which can be reached through a link provided on the companion Web site for this book. ⬤

ADVANTAGES OF PROVIDING HEALTH CARE IN WORK SETTINGS

From a community health nursing perspective, there are a number of advantages to providing health care in work settings. They include the substantial amount of time that

people spend in this setting and the fact that this time is spent on a regular basis. In addition, when employees are present, they are essentially a "captive audience," subject to powerful pressures from peers and employers to engage in healthy behaviors. For example, nonsmoking peers may object to smoking in their work or recreation areas, or employers may provide financial or nonfinancial incentives for healthy behavior. Another advantage is that the workforce frequently consists of people who may be at risk for a variety of health problems or who may be motivated to maintain their health to ensure their continued ability to work. Because health care personnel are frequently in the setting and mechanisms are in place for communicating health messages, health promotion in work settings is efficient and cost-effective. More and more companies are acknowledging the advantages of providing health care in the occupational setting.

Failure to address occupational health issues leads to a variety of consequences and costs for businesses themselves, as well as for society as a whole. Employers currently pay 30% of U.S. health care expenditures, and are expected to be bearing half of the cost of care when health care expenditures reach the anticipated 14% of the gross domestic product (Reardon, 1998). In addition to the visible costs of dealing with health problems, health issues present other visible and hidden costs in the work environment. Visible costs include those related to sickness, absenteeism, and employee turnover. Hidden costs may include low productivity, poor-quality work, poor customer service, accidents, and legal claims arising from illness and injuries due to the work environment. Other potential hidden costs include difficult working relationships among employees, low employee morale, lack of innovation, and poor decision making, which can affect the future of the company (Williams & Cooper, 1999).

THE OCCUPATIONAL HEALTH TEAM

Community health nurses working in occupational health settings may be part of an occupational health team. In some small companies, the nurse is the only health care professional employed by the company. In such instances, other health care professionals interact with the nurse on a consultant basis. For example, the community health nurse might collaborate with an employee's primary health care provider to plan for the employee's return to work after an illness or injury. In other instances, the company may contract with outside providers for consultation services related to employee health needs.

Other companies have a well-developed occupational health team present within the facility. In addition to the community health nurse, such teams may include other nurses, physicians, safety engineers, industrial hygienists, counselors, ancillary nursing personnel (e.g., licensed practical nurses), toxicologists, emergency medical technicians, physicians' assistants, epidemiologists, laboratory and x-ray technicians, safety coordinators, and nurse practitioners. The functions and roles of most of these individuals are already familiar to the reader. A few, however, may be unfamiliar. A safety engineer, for example, is responsible for monitoring the safety of the physical environment in the work setting, and an industrial hygienist has similar responsibilities for identifying and controlling physical, biological, and chemical hazards in the work setting. Toxicologists may be involved in research on the toxic effects of chemical exposures in the work setting, as well as in contributing to plans for the control and treatment of such exposures.

OCCUPATIONAL HEALTH NURSING

Not all nurses who practice in occupational settings are community health nurses. The community health nurse, however, is uniquely prepared to meet the health needs of the working population because of his or her knowledge of community health principles. Occupational health nursing is not a new role for the community health nurse. Nurses may have been employed in work settings as early as 1888 and certainly by 1895 when the Vermont Marble company employed Ada M. Stewart (Parrish & Alfred, 1995). In 1943, a U.S. Public Health Service study recommended one nurse for every 300 employees to provide health services and advocacy in factories (Anglin, 1990). Since that time, the role of the occupational health nurse has been expanded along with other nursing roles. Several years ago, the U.S. Department of Labor defined *occupational health nursing* as "giving nursing service under general medical direction to ill or injured employees or other persons who become ill or suffer an accident on the premises of a factory or other establishment" (Hughes, 1979).

This definition did not, however, fully describe today's community health nursing role in work settings. It concentrates on the treatment aspects of care and the nurse's dependent functions and does not acknowledge the promotional and preventive aspects that are paramount in this practice setting. In the 1999 *Standards of Occupational and Environmental Health Nursing*, the American Association of Occupational Health Nurses (AAOHN) defined occupational health nursing as "the specialty practice that provides for and delivers health care services to workers and worker populations. The practice focuses on promotion, protection, and restoration of workers' health within the context of a safe and healthy work environment."

Educational Preparation for Occupational Health Nursing

Several types of nursing personnel may be found in occupational settings including registered nurses prepared in associate degree and diploma programs in nursing as well as in baccalaureate degree programs; licensed practical nurses; and nurses prepared at the master's level. Because of the need to apply principles of community health nursing, nurses who engage in the full scope of the occupational health nurse's role should be prepared at least at the baccalaureate level in nursing. Advanced preparation in occupational health nursing may result in certification by AAOHN. Nurses working in occupational settings might also hold master's degrees in nursing. Educational preparation at this level might be in occupational health nursing, in community health nursing, or as a nurse practitioner.

🌀THINK ABOUT IT

Who should supervise the work of occupational health nurses? Why?

Nurses in other settings may also be involved in providing care for health conditions related to work. This fact suggests that nurse practitioners working in ambulatory care settings where occupational conditions may be seen should have a basic grounding in the principles of occupational health.

Standards and Competencies for Occupational Health Nursing

Like other nursing specialties, occupational health nursing should be practiced in accordance with established standards. The AAOHN (1999) has established 11 standards for competent occupational health nursing practice. These standards are summarized below.

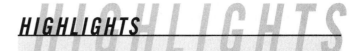

HIGHLIGHTS

Standards of Occupational and Environmental Health Nursing

Assessment: The occupational and environmental health nurse systematically assesses the health status of the individual client or population and the environment.

Diagnosis: The occupational and environmental health nurse analyzes assessment data to formulate diagnoses.

Outcome identification: The occupational and environmental health nurse identifies outcomes specific to the client.

Planning: The occupational and environmental health nurse develops a goal-directed plan that is comprehen-
(continued)

sive and formulates interventions to attain expected outcomes.

Implementation: The occupational and environmental health nurse implements interventions to attain desired outcomes identified in the plan.

Evaluation: The occupational and environmental health nurse systematically and continuously evaluates responses to interventions and progress toward the achievement of desired outcomes.

Resource management: The occupational and environmental health nurse secures and manages the resources that support an occupational health and safety program.

Professional development: The occupational and environmental health nurse assumes accountability for professional development to enhance professional growth and maintain competency.

Collaboration: The occupational and environmental health nurse collaborates with employees, management, other health care providers, professionals, and community representatives.

Research: The occupational and environmental health nurse uses research findings in practice and contributes to the scientific base in occupational and environmental health nursing to improve practice and advance the profession.

Ethics: The occupational and environmental health nurse uses an ethical framework as a guide for decision making in practice.

Source: American Association of Occupational Health Nurses. (1999). *Standards of occupational and environmental health nursing.* Atlanta: Author. Reprinted by permission of American Association of Occupational Health Nurses.

In addition, AAOHN has developed criteria for three levels of competency in practice: competent, proficient, and expert. The competent nurse recognizes a wide range of problems and is comfortable functioning as a clinician, service coordinator, and case manager. The competent nurse tends to rely on company procedures, assessment checklists, and clinical protocols to direct practice. The proficient nurse deftly obtains accurate assessment data and identifies critical aspects of a problem. He or she usually possesses advanced clinical or management skills. The expert provides leadership in the development of occupational health policy and is involved in upper-level administrative practice, consultation, or research. Criteria for each of these three levels of competence have been established for nine aspects of occupation health nursing practice: clinical and primary care; case management; resolution of workforce, workplace, and environmental issues; knowledge of regulatory and legislative issues; management of occupational health services; health promotion and disease prevention; health and safety education; research; and professionalism, which includes maintenance of knowledge by the nurse and mentoring of others (White, Cox, & Williamson, 1999). Criteria for each

level of competence in each of these areas may be reviewed in the article discussed on the companion Web site for this book.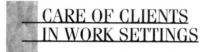

CARE OF CLIENTS IN WORK SETTINGS

Nursing care in work settings is based on the use of the nursing process and includes assessment of the health of the population; development of nursing diagnoses; and planning, implementation, and evaluation of interventions to promote, protect, and restore health.

ASSESSING HEALTH IN WORK SETTINGS

Assessment of employee health status and health needs is undertaken from the perspective of biophysical, psychological, physical environmental, sociocultural, behavioral, and health system factors that influence health and illness in the working population.

Biophysical Considerations

Human biological factors to be addressed in assessing employee health status include those related to maturation and aging, genetic inheritance, and physiologic function.

Maturation and Aging

The age composition of a company's workforce affects its health status. If employees are primarily young adults or adolescents, health conditions that may be noted with some frequency include sexually transmitted diseases, hepatitis, and pregnancy. Younger employees may also be at increased risk of injury due to limited job training and skills. In 1998, there were 7 million persons 16 to 19 years of age in the workforce (U.S. Census Bureau, 1999). Employees aged 14 to 17 years had an injury rate of 4.9 per 100 full-time equivalent employees compared to a rate of 2.9 per 100 for all workers (Division of Safety Research, 2001b).

The health needs of older employees should also be considered. Because of prohibitions on forced retirement at specific ages, many employees are continuing in the workforce beyond the time when they would have retired. Economic need and a desire for continued productivity are two factors that may influence this trend. In 1998, 16.5% of U.S. men and 8.6% of women over 65 years of age were employed (U.S. Census Bureau, 1999). Musculoskeletal capacity diminishes and sensory impairments increase with age, placing older employees at higher risk for occupational injury (Zwerling et al., 1998). Although younger workers experience a higher rate of injury, older workers are at greater risk for occupational death. The occupational death rate for persons over 65 years of age is more than twice that of employees in other age groups (Division of Safety Research, 2001a). The majority of these deaths are due to operation of machinery (Herbert & Landrigan, 2000). In addition to the risk for injury and death, older workers planning to retire in the near future may need assistance with retirement planning and in dealing with retirement issues (see Chapter 19 for a discussion of these issues).

Genetic Inheritance

Genetic inheritance factors likely to be of greatest importance in the workforce are those related to race and gender. For example, in a largely African American labor force, hypertension may be prevalent. In an Asian population, particularly if large numbers are refugees, communicable diseases such as tuberculosis and parasitic diseases may be common.

In 1998, 46% of the total U.S. workforce was women (U.S. Census Bureau, 1999). The gender composition of the employee population also affects the types of health conditions seen. For example, if large numbers of employees are women of childbearing age, there may be a need to provide prenatal or contraceptive services. There would also be a need to monitor more closely environmental conditions that may cause genetic changes or damage to an embryo. Occupational reproductive effects to be monitored include infertility, spontaneous abortion, low birth weight, pre- and postmaturity, birth defects, chromosomal abnormalities, preeclampsia, and an increased incidence of childhood cancers.

⑥THINK ABOUT IT

Should women of childbearing age be prohibited from working in jobs that pose potential health risks for unborn children? Why or why not?

Physiologic Function

An estimated 10 million occupational illnesses and injuries occur in the United States each year (Division of Safety Research, 2000b). Community health nurses in occupational settings must be prepared to recognize and deal with the multitude of illnesses and injuries likely to be encountered in the workplace. Although these vary with the occupational setting, certain conditions are seen commonly in many occupational settings. These include lung diseases, injuries, occupational cancers, cardiovascular disease, and infectious diseases (Herbert & Landrigan, 2000).

Community health nurses working in any occupational setting should be aware of the prevalence of these conditions and of the factors that influence the development of these problems. These contributing factors may be related to the work environment itself or to the personal behaviors of employees within and outside the workplace.

Work-related asthma is a growing concern in occupational settings. Anywhere from 2% to 26% of adult asthma may be work related. Among adults with work-related asthma in one study, 19% experienced exacerbation of prior asthma due to work conditions, and 81% were new onset cases. Industries most often associated with work-related asthma include manufacturing (41.5% of cases), services (31%, with 14% occurring in health service occupations and 9% in education), and public administration (11%, with more than 4% of cases occurring in justice, public order, and safety occupations) (Jajosky et al., 1999). Work-related asthma has been associated with more than 200 asthmogens in various work settings (Herbert & Landrigan, 2000). One particular cause of work-related asthma is latex-induced occupational asthma believed to cause disease in 2.5% to 6% of health care workers. Latex allergy also results in dermatologic sensitivity in 8% to 17% of employees in health care settings (Phillips, Goodrich, & Sullivan, 1999).

Musculoskeletal injuries are the leading cause of lost workdays among U.S. employees (Myers et al., 1999) and include injuries due to the cumulative trauma of repetitive activities as well as acute trauma. Approximately 1.8 million U.S. workers each year experience musculoskeletal injuries such as carpal tunnel syndrome and back injuries, and these injuries lead to 600,000 work absences (*The Nation's Health,* 2001). The annual cost of musculoskeletal workplace injuries is $9.1 billion (*The Nation's Health,* 2000–2001). The causes of carpal tunnel syndrome and other cumulative trauma disorders (CTDs) include repetitive motions, high-force actions, mechanical pressure, awkward posture, and vibration.

Back injury is another significant occupational health problem and accounts for 24% of all work-related injuries. Compensation costs due to back injury amounted to $36 billion in 1992 and accounted for 31% of all compensation costs. In 1990, the average cost of a single back injury was more than $24,000 (Myers et al., 1999). Risks for occupational back pain include overexertion, vibration, and increased body mass index. An increased **work movement index,** or extent of bending, stooping, twisting, and extended reach involved in a job, is also associated with increased risk of back injury (Division of Surveillance, Hazard Evaluations, and Field Studies, 1999; Myers et al., 1999).

A large proportion of cancer deaths each year in the United States are attributable to workplace exposures. These include lung cancer deaths, bladder cancers, and mesotheliomas (USDHHS, 2000a). Other cancers that may result from occupational exposures include those of the blood, bone, larynx, liver, nasal cavity and sinuses, peritoneum, pharynx, pleura, and skin (including scrotal malignancies).

Serious traumatic injuries are those in which multiple injuries occur as a result of trauma, where musculoskeletal injuries are usually confined to localized areas. Approximately 1.1 million occupational deaths occur worldwide each year, with more deaths occurring in developing countries than in developed nations. In 1995, for example, the U.S. occupational fatality rate was 5.5 per 100,000 workers compared to 13.5 per 100,000 in Latin America and the Caribbean and 34 per 100,000 in Korea (Herbert & Landrigan, 2000). From 1980 to 1997, an average of 16 civilian work-related deaths occurred each day in the United States, but fatality rates declined 45% during that period (Division of Safety Research, 2001a). In 1998, the U.S. occupational fatality rate was 4.5 per 100,000 workers for a total of more than 6,000 deaths. Occupations with the highest occupational injury fatality rates are mining (23.6 deaths per 100,000 workers), agriculture (23.3 per 100,000), and construction (14.5 per 100,000) (USDHHS, 2000a).

Injury rates, on the other hand, are highest for manufacturing and transportation, communication, and public utilities employees (4.2 per 100,000 workers), followed by construction (4.0 per 100,000); agriculture, fishing, and forestry (3.8 per 100,000); wholesale trade (3.2 per 100,000); mining (2.7 per 100,000); retail trade (2.6 per 100,000) and service occupations (2.3 per 100,000 workers). In 1998, occupational injuries resulted in lost work time for nearly 3 of every 100 full-time equivalent workers in the United States (USDHHS, 2000a).

For the most part, cardiovascular diseases are influenced by personal risk factors of employees; however, evidence suggests that occupational factors may also contribute to the incidence of cardiovascular diseases. Some of these factors include exposure to metals, dust, and chemical inhalants, noise exposure, and psychological stress. Exposures to carbon disulfide, ethylene compounds, halogenated hydrocarbons, nitroglycerin, and nitrates have also been associated with cardiovascular disease. The extent of one's control over one's job has also been shown to influence cardiovascular mortality. People with greater control tend to have lower mortality rates (Bosma, Peter, Siegrist, & Marmot, 1998; Theorell et al., 1998).

With greater numbers of women working today, there is growing concern for the reproductive and social effects of working conditions. Thus far, 1,000 occupational chemicals have been associated with reproductive effects in animals, but their human effects have not been assessed. Other working conditions, such as heat and radiation, also have reproductive effects. Although the primary concern is the impact on the female reproductive system, evidence indicates that exposure to some of these conditions (e.g., heat) can also affect the reproductive capabilities of men.

Neurotoxic conditions are another concern in occupational health. Some of the conditions encountered include heavy metal poisonings, behavior changes related to chemical exposures, and difficulty concentrating and performing one's job. Specific neurodegenerative disorders, such as presenile dementia, Alzheimer's disease, Parkinson's disease, and motor neuron disease, have also been associated with occupational factors. High prevalence of each of these conditions has been found among teachers, medical personnel, machinists and machine

operators, scientists, writers, entertainers, and clerical workers. Selected conditions are also noted with some frequency among workers exposed to pesticides, solvents, and electromagnetic fields.

Noise-induced hearing loss and infectious diseases are other biophysical considerations in occupational settings. For example, first responders (firefighters, emergency medical technicians) and health care personnel are at increased risk of bloodborne diseases (National Center for Infectious Diseases, 2000), whereas employees in manufacturing, construction, and other high-noise occupations are at greater risk for hearing loss.

With respect to dermatologic conditions arising from occupational factors, occupational health nurses are again in a position to assess the health status of employees. As with other types of health problems, the nurse should be aware of outbreaks of dermatologic conditions that indicate the presence of hazards in the environment and a need for control measures. Conditions encountered include a variety of rashes, pruritus, chemical burns, and desquamation.

The occupational health problems discussed here are only a few of the many physical health problems likely to be encountered by community health nurses working in occupational settings. Each occupational setting contains factors unique to that setting that influence the health of employees. The nurse should be cognizant of the factors operating in any given place, their effects, and the appropriate measures of control.

CRITICAL THINKING IN RESEARCH

The National Institute for Occupational Safety and Health (Rosenstock, Olenec, & Wagner, 1998) developed a set of research priorities for occupational health care. Areas in which a need for further research is needed were grouped into three categories: (a) disease and injury, (b) work environment and workforce, and (c) research tools and approaches. Priority needs for research included the following:

Disease and Injury

- Allergic and irritant dermatitis
- Asthma and chronic obstructive pulmonary disease
- Fertility and pregnancy abnormalities
- Hearing loss
- Infectious diseases
- Low back disorders
- Musculoskeletal disorders of the upper extremities
- Traumatic injuries

Work Environment and Workforce

- Emerging technologies
- Indoor environment

- Mixed exposures
- Organization of work
- Special populations at work

Research Tools and Approaches

- Cancer research methods
- Control technology and personal protective equipment
- Exposure assessment methods
- Health services research
- Intervention effectiveness research
- Risk assessment methods
- Social and economic consequences of workplace illness and injury
- Surveillance research methods

- Which of these areas would be appropriate for nursing research? What special knowledge or expertise might nurses bring to multidisciplinary research in these areas?
- Are there other areas for research that you think might be needed from an occupational health nursing perspective?
- Select two or three of the priority research areas and identify research questions related to each that would be of interest to community health nurses working in occupational health settings.
- What variables would you study if you designed a study to answer one of the research questions you have identified?
- In what type of work setting would you conduct a study of the research question selected? Will the type of setting chosen influence potential findings? In what way?

Immunization is the final physiologic consideration in assessing health needs in the workplace. The nurse assesses the immunization status of employees, with special emphasis on groups of employees who may be at increased risk for certain diseases preventable by immunization. For example, employees who may be at risk for dirty injuries should be assessed for immunity to tetanus, whereas women of childbearing age should be assessed for immunity to rubella. Health care workers, on the other hand, should be particularly assessed for immunity to hepatitis B.

Psychological Considerations

In assessing psychological dimension factors influencing the health of clients in work settings, community health nurses identify psychological health problems prevalent in the population and assess factors contributing to psychological problems. It is estimated that as many as 20% of employees experience some form of psychological problem that reduces their safety and/or job perfor-

mance. Psychological health problems may manifest in substance abuse, violence, psychiatric disorders such as psychoses and neuroses, somatic complaints such as ulcers or fatigue, or a general inability to cope. The nurse can assess individual clients for some of the indicators of psychological health problems presented below.

HIGHLIGHTS

Potential Indicators of Psychological Problems

- Increased absenteeism (especially on Mondays, Fridays, and the day after being paid)
- Mood changes or changes in relationships with others (especially with health care providers)
- Increased incidence of minor accidents on and off the job
- Complaints of fatigue, weakness, or a general decrease in energy
- Sudden weight loss or gain
- Increased blood pressure
- Frequent stress-related illnesses
- Bloodshot or bleary eyes
- Facial petechiae (especially over the nose)

Job strain has also been shown to be associated with higher mortality. *Job strain* has been operationally defined as high job demands coupled with low ability to control demands (Curtis, James, Raghunathan, & Alcser, 1997). In one study, employees with high levels of job strain had higher rates of back injury (Myers et al., 1999). Similarly, job decision latitude (the ability to make decisions on how and when one accomplishes one's work role) has been associated with a variety of health risks. For example, an increase in job decision latitude was found to decrease smoking behaviors in one study (Landsbergis et al., 1998), while choice of work pattern (e.g., shift) has been shown to mitigate the effects of shift work (Fitzpatrick, While, & Roberts, 1999). Low decision latitude (limited ability to make decisions affecting one's work), on the other hand, has been linked to increased risk of coronary heart disease and myocardial infarction (Bosma et al., 1999; Theorell et al., 1998).

Occupational health nurses also need to be able to identify sources of stress in and outside of work settings that may contribute to the development of psychological health problems. Workplace stress has been associated with increased absenteeism, decreased productivity, and increased health care consumption (van der Klink, Blonk, Schene, & van Dijk, 2001). Employees particularly prone to work-related psychological stress include health care and other service personnel, blue-collar workers, and those who work nights or who rotate shifts. Nurses who work with these groups should be particularly aware of the potential for stress-related illnesses.

Other sources of stress in the work setting include work overload, the organizational structure of the company, job insecurity, and interpersonal relationships with co-workers or supervisors. Stress may also be created by sexist or racist attitudes of others in the workplace. Downsizing creates occupational stress, not only for those whose positions are eliminated, but for those who remain as well. In many instances, companies have been accused of going beyond "paring the fat" to becoming virtually "anorexic" (Williams & Cooper, 1999). Remaining employees are left to do more with fewer resources, adding to their stress. Technological advances may also contribute to occupational stress. For example, a person can go almost nowhere without the potential for being interrupted by a business call on a cellular phone or pager.

Perceptions of the source of occupational stress may differ greatly between employees and employers. Sources of stress most frequently identified by workers include lack of control over the content, process, and pace of one's work; unrealistic demands and lack of understanding by supervisors; lack of predictability and security regarding one's job future; and the cumulative effects of occupational and family stressors. Employers, on the other hand, most often perceive employees' lifestyles and health habits as the primary contributors to stress.

Physical Environmental Considerations

Physical environmental factors contribute to a variety of health problems encountered in work settings. Categories of health hazards in the physical environment include chemical hazards, physical hazards (radiation, noise, vibration, and exposure to heat and cold), electrical and magnetic field hazards, fire, heavy lifting and uncomfortable working positions, and potential for falls. Additional hazards that may be present in the workplace include exposure to metallic compounds and allergens and molds (Friis & Sellers, 1999).

Poor lighting or high noise levels may adversely affect vision and hearing, respectively. Heavy objects that must be moved may cause musculoskeletal injuries. In addition, there is the potential for falls or exposure to excessive heat or cold in many workplaces.

The use of toxic substances in work performance is another source of possible health problems related to the physical environment. Toxic substances may be encountered as solids, liquids, gases, vapors, dust, fumes, fibers, or mists. As noted earlier, a great number of toxic substances are present in the work environment that may result in respiratory, dermatologic, and other health problems. Of particular concern in this area is exposure to

A variety of injuries occur as a result of heavy equipment operation.

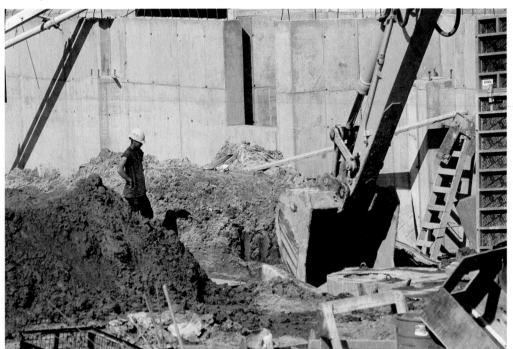

heavy metals (Table 24–1 ■). The adverse effects of occupational exposure to lead, for example, have been known for more than 2,000 years. Despite this knowledge and efforts to minimize occupational exposure to lead and other heavy metals, significant numbers of workers in the United States have the potential for work-related lead exposure, and in many industries no mechanism is in place for biological monitoring of lead levels in employees with potential for exposure. Other metals of concern include mercury, arsenic, and cadmium. Exposure to lead and other metals occurs in a variety of occupations, including those listed in Table 24–1. Areas to be assessed relative to the potential for toxic exposures in the workplace include substances used in the setting and their level of demonstrated toxicity, portals of entry into the human body, established legal exposure limits, extent of exposure, potential for interactive exposures, and the presence of existing employee health conditions that put the individuals affected at greater risk for exposure-related illnesses. The nurse and other personnel would also assess the extent and adequacy of controls to prevent or limit exposures and the availability of and compliance with recommended screening and surveillance procedures.

Equipment may also constitute an occupational health hazard. The use of heavy equipment or sharp tools can result in injury. There is also the potential for hand–arm vibration syndrome in the use of tools that vibrate or visual disturbance related to the use of computer display terminals. Another relatively recent physical hazard generated by widespread computer use is the potential for tendonitis and other similar conditions stemming from the use of word processors. Extreme or awkward postures have been associated with low back problems and repetitive or high-force movements with carpal tunnel syndrome. The nurse in the occupational setting identifies the presence of any hazards in the physical environment that contribute to health problems. In addition, the nurse monitors the status of known hazards and their effects on the health of employees. Some potential questions for evaluating hazardous conditions in work settings are presented below.

HIGHLIGHTS

Evaluating Occupational Hazard Potential

Substances/Conditions Present

- What substances or conditions are associated with production processes (e.g., toxic chemicals, heat)?
- What substances or conditions are associated with clerical processes (e.g., repetitive movements)? With other office processes (e.g., cleaning products, pesticides)?
- What is the typical extent and duration of exposure to hazardous substances or conditions?
- What are the designated exposure limits for substances and conditions in the work setting?

Health Effects

- What research evidence is there for adverse human health effects (e.g., toxicity, teratogenicity, potential for injury) associated with substances used or conditions existing in the work setting?

(continued)

■ **TABLE 24–1** Occupational Sources and Health Effects of Heavy Metal Exposures

METAL	OCCUPATIONAL SOURCES	HEALTH EFFECTS
Antimony	Iron works, red dye manufacture	Irritation, cardiovascular and lung effects
Arsenic	Photographic equipment and supplies	Lung and lymphatic cancer, dermatitis
Cadmium	Soldering, battery manufacture, fuses, paint manufacture and painting, nuclear reactors	Lung cancer, prostatic cancer, renal system effects
Chromium	Steel manufacture, chrome plating, dye and paint manufacture, leather tanning	Lung cancer, skin ulcers, lung irradiation
Lead	Soldering, dispensing leaded gas, cable cutting and splicing; painting, casting, or melting lead; radiator repair, welding, grinding, or sanding lead-painted surfaces; battery manufacture; construction; paper hanging; foundries; plumbing	Kidney, blood, and nervous system effects
Mercury	Metal foil and leaf application, industrial measurement instruments, gold and silver refining	Central nervous system and mental effects
Nickel	Nickel plating, steel manufacture, heating coils, hydrogenation processes	Lung and nasal cancer, skin effects
Tungsten	Steel manufacture, x-ray tubes	Lung and skin effects
Zinc oxide	White paint manufacture	Metal fume fever

- Do low levels of exposure have a cumulative effect?
- What is the usual portal of entry or mechanism of exposure for a specific toxic agent or condition?
- What organ systems are typically affected by specific toxic agents or hazardous conditions?
- What are the usual signs and symptoms of toxicity/ health effects?
- Are there synergistic effects among substances or between substances and other conditions (e.g., heat)?

Employee Considerations

- Do employees have preexisting health conditions that put them at greater risk for toxic effects?
- Do employees engage in other behaviors (e.g., smoking) that increase their risk of toxic effects?
- Do employees use safety equipment and procedures to minimize potential for exposure?

Environmental Considerations

- What are the recommended control practices to prevent or minimize potential for exposure?
- Are the recommended practices in place in a given occupational setting (e.g., ventilation, other engineering controls)?
- Are employees provided with education to prevent or minimize exposure potential?
- Are employees provided with appropriate personal protective devices (e.g., respirators, ear protection)? Do they use protective devices correctly?
- What are the recommended surveillance practices for monitoring environmental conditions and hazardous exposures?
- Are there surveillance systems in place for monitoring the presence or extent of hazardous conditions in the environment?

Health System Considerations

- Are there surveillance systems in place for monitoring employees for evidence of exposure or exposure effects?
- Are surveillance procedures implemented in a systematic way to periodically assess all employees at risk for exposure?
- Are there processes in place for diagnosing and treating health conditions that arise from employee exposures to hazardous conditions?

Sociocultural Considerations

The social environment of the work setting can influence employee health status either positively or negatively. The quality of social interactions among employees, attitudes toward work and health, and presence or absence of racial or other tensions can all affect health status as well as employee productivity.

CULTURAL CONSIDERATIONS

You work in a health agency that employs a number of recent Asian female immigrants in nonprofessional roles (e.g., clerical staff, interpreters, outreach workers). You are responsible for supervising their work. Recently, you have had some difficulties with two or three staff members who either arrive late for work or telephone to indicate that they will not be in because of family responsibilities. At other times, these women have not been able to come to work because their husbands have taken the family's only car and they have no other source of transportation. You know that in their culture, women fulfill traditional gender roles in terms of care of family members and that family responsibilities will always be given priority over work responsibilities. Women also are subservient to their husbands, and if the husband has need of the car, the wife will be expected to do without. Otherwise, these women are good workers, and the interpreters, particularly, provide a much needed function in the agency. How will you handle this situation?

Four spheres of influence in the workplace social environment may affect the health status of individual employees, and the effects of each sphere on health should be assessed by the community health nurse in the occupational health setting. The first sphere of influence involves the health-related behaviors of employees themselves and is addressed in the discussion of behavioral factors affecting health. The other three spheres are more directly related to the social environment of work settings.

The second sphere of influence on health in the workplace occurs among groups of co-workers, and the community health nurse should assess the influence of co-worker groups on the health of individual employees and on the group as a whole. For example, a group of co-workers may decide that they do not wish to be exposed to smoke in their work area. This decision can lead to formal or informal bans on smoking in certain areas. Formal bans may occur when groups of employees request no-smoking policies from company management. When this is not the case, work groups may enforce the decision informally by exerting peer pressure on the smokers in the group. In other words, they can make life unpleasant for those who wish to smoke by ostracizing them or using other social sanctions. Another example of this sphere of social influence lies in the influence that more experienced employees have on the use of safety precautions by younger, less experienced workers who may imitate their behaviors. If older workers effectively use safety practices, younger workers are likely to do so as well; if they do not, younger workers are likely to imitate this behavior and increase their risk of injury.

The third sphere of influence is the management sphere. The nurse assesses management's attitudes toward health and health-related policies and the effects of these policies (or lack of them) on employee health. For example, management may decide on and enforce a no-smoking policy throughout the company, whether or not employees favor such a policy. In fact, smoke-free workplace policies are credited with decreasing annual cigarette consumption by 602 million cigarettes in Australia and 9.7 billion cigarettes in the United States. It is estimated that if all U.S. workplaces were smoke free, there would be 20.9 billion fewer cigarettes smoked each year (Chapman et al., 1999).

Management also makes other kinds of policy decisions that affect employee health. For example, the type of health care coverage provided to employees is a management decision. A policy that provides "well leave" or extra vacation for those who have not taken sick leave may prompt employee efforts to promote health and prevent illness.

For employees to value wellness and health promotive efforts, they must perceive them to be valued by employers. This means that wellness programs and other aspects of occupational health must receive the same degree of emphasis as other areas of business. It has been suggested that companies develop *company wellness policies,* statements of administrative commitment to employee health, and expectations of employees related to health promotion and maintenance, to convey the importance given to health issues. These companies must be seen to abide by, as well as create, such policies.

The last sphere of influence involves legal, social, and political action that influences the health of employees. A prime example of this is the regulation of conditions in work settings by agencies such as the Occupational Safety and Health Administration (OSHA). Through legislation, society can mandate that business and industry create specific conditions that enhance the health of employees. For example, in communities with strong workplace smoking ordinances, an estimated 26% of smokers quit smoking compared to only 19% in communities without such ordinances (Moskowitz, Lin, & Hudes, 2000).

Regulatory agencies have some impact on worksite conditions that influence health. It has been suggested, however, that enforcement of regulations promulgated by federal and state OSHAs should be expanded. It is estimated that, given current resources, the federal program is able to routinely inspect all workplaces only once every 144 years, and state agencies have the capability of inspecting each facility only once every 55 years. Lack of regular inspection and minimal fines (the average fine for a serious violation in 1995 was $763) limit the effectiveness of OSHA regulations. Inspections, on the other hand, have demonstrated their effectiveness in terms of lower injury rates (particularly in the first year after a citation) and changes in areas others than those cited (McQuiston, Zakocs, & Loomis, 1998). Community health nurses in occupational settings may need to report unsafe conditions to promote inspection and corrective action.

On occasion, legislative action may negatively influence employee health. For example, in 2001, the U.S.

Congress overturned an ergnomic standard developed by OSHA claiming that many organizations have already taken action related to the provisions of the standard. OSHA data, however, indicated that as many as 60% of employers have not addressed ergonomic risks to health (*The Nation's Health*, 2001).

Labor unions may also be a social force that influences health for employees. For example, a study in Australia indicated that trade unionism was associated with healthier food services, better sun protection programs, and worksite health programs (Holman, Corti, Donovan, & Jalleh, 1998). The study authors suggested that activity by trade unions might be a means of improving working conditions that influence health.

Additional sociocultural factors that may affect health in the work setting include languages spoken and cultural beliefs and behaviors. For example, employers may provide the traditional Western or Christian holidays, but give no provision for important occasions in other cultural groups. Ethnic and cultural factors may also be the basis for discrimination in the work setting.

One final sociocultural dimension factor within the work setting that is drawing increasing attention is workplace violence. Since 1990, homicide has been the second most common cause of occupational death in the United States, and results in 14% of occupational fatalities each year (Division of Safety Research, 2001a). Contrary to popular belief, few of these crimes are perpetrated by fellow employees; most are robbery related. The risk of exposure to violence in the workplace is increased in jobs in which employees interact with the public, where money is exchanged, or in the delivery of goods or services. Working early in the morning or late at night, working alone, guarding valuables or property, and working with violent people or in volatile situations also increases one's risk of violence. Nonfatal workplace violence also occurs at a rate of 14.8 incidents per 1,000 workers for a total of more than 2 million incidents per year in the United States (U.S. Census Bureau, 1999). Personal safety issues are an important area for occupational health nurses to assess in working with employees.

Social factors outside of the work setting may also influence employees and their relationship to work. For example, family issues affect employee health and productivity. Areas that should be considered by employers in the design of work include dual-career families, single parenthood, changes in gender roles for both men and women, social isolation due to the loss of extended family support, and elder care issues. Each of these factors may impinge on employees' performance and should be considered in the development of worksite policies related to job design (Williams & Cooper, 1999).

Behavioral Considerations

As noted above, behavioral factors exemplified in individual decisions about health-related actions constitute the first sphere of social influence on employee health. Lifestyle factors to be considered here include the type of work performed, consumption patterns, patterns of rest and exercise, and use of safety devices.

Type of Work Performed

The type of work performed by an individual within a company can significantly influence the employee's health. The type of work performed determines the risk of exposure to various physical hazards and level of stress experienced. For example, factory workers in industries using lead may run the risk of lead poisoning, whereas executives in the same companies may be exposed to more stress.

The type of work done also influences the extent of exercise that employees obtain. Construction workers, for example, have ample opportunities for physical activity but also risk serious injury in the use of heavy equipment. Bank tellers, on the other hand, are at risk for cardiovascular and other diseases related to a sedentary lifestyle.

The community health nurse in an occupational setting should be conversant with the variety of jobs performed in that setting. The nurse should also be aware of the health hazards posed by each type of work performed and be alert to signs of health problems deriving from the work itself.

Another aspect of the type of work performed is that of *ergonomics*, the degree of fit between the employee and the job performed. The nurse should assess the degree to which employees are qualified to perform their particular job function and their interest in that job. Employees who work at jobs that do not interest them, that are beyond their capabilities, or that do not provide sufficient challenge may be at greater risk for both emotional and physical health problems than those who are better suited to their jobs. Ergonomics also reflects the design of workstations and their effects on health. For example, the height of a computer keyboard may influence the development of neck and shoulder problems. As noted earlier, the ergonomics standards established by OSHA were overturned by the U.S. Congress, leaving millions of employees at risk for fatigue and injury.

Consumption Patterns

Consumption patterns of interest to the occupational health nurse include those related to food and nutrition, smoking, and drug and alcohol use. The influence of nutrition on health is well established, and the occupational health nurse assesses the nutritional patterns of employees with whom he or she works. In addition, the nurse assesses how the work environment affects eating habits. For example, sufficient opportunity may not be provided for employees to eat despite OSHA regulations regarding time and place for breaks and meals.

The nurse also determines whether food service is available to employees. If there is an employee cafeteria, the nurse may need to assess the nutritional quality of the food provided. If no food services are available in the workplace, the nurse would determine whether they are available nearby, or whether adequate storage facilities exist for employees who bring meals from home.

Smoking is another consumption pattern of concern to the occupational health nurse. Smoking is harmful to health in and of itself. In addition, smoking may increase the adverse effects of other environmental hazards in the work setting, particularly those that affect respiration. Many employers have recently begun to prohibit smoking except in carefully controlled areas in the workplace and have been active in promoting programs to help employees quit smoking. In addition to the health implications, such efforts cut employer expenses. For example, Dupont has estimated that each smoking employee costs $960 more per year than a nonsmoking employee. Similarly, alcohol abuse costs $389 per year per employee affected, and high cholesterol levels cost $370 per employee (Reardon, 1998). The nurse assesses the extent of smoking in the employee population as well as the specific implications of smoking in that particular environment.

⑥THINK ABOUT IT

Should high-risk health behaviors be used as a reason not to employ someone who is otherwise qualified for a particular job? Why or why not?

As noted earlier, employees may have problems with substance abuse. The prevalence of these problems should be monitored and the nurse should be alert to signs and symptoms of substance abuse in the employee population. Overindulgence in other substances, such as caffeine, may also pose a health hazard to employees. Worksite interventions have been shown to be successful in decreasing smoking and other drug use and in reducing fat intake and increasing consumption of fruits, vegetables, and fiber (Bachman, Freedman-Doan, O'Malley, Johnston, & Segal, 1999; Sorensen et al., 1998).

Rest and Exercise

Work places many physical and psychological demands on people. Sometimes these demands result in inadequate rest and recreation, as with the executive who works constantly or the blue-collar worker who holds two jobs in an attempt to make ends meet. Conversely, work may also lead to too much sitting and too little exercise. The majority (56%) of employed persons in the United States, in fact, do not engage in hard physical activity during the workday, and only one quarter of them perform such activities for five or more hours a day. Approximately 23% of employed adults engage in no leisure time physical activity either (National Center for Chronic Disease Prevention and Health Promotion, 2000).

The nurse in the work setting assesses the amount of activity engaged in by employees and the balance between rest and exercise. He or she also obtains information on the types of recreation used by employees and any potential health hazards posed by recreational choices.

Many companies are recognizing the benefits of exercise in terms of both the physical and psychological health of employees. These companies are promoting physical exercise and may even provide facilities for exercise and recreation in the workplace. If this is the case, the nurse should be alert to potential health hazards and the potential for too much exercise. For example, if there is a company pool, the epileptic employee who swims to relieve tension should be cautioned against swimming alone. Similarly, the overweight executive should engage in physical activity cautiously to lessen the risk of heart attack or injury.

Another consideration with respect to rest and exercise is the influence of rotating shifts on employee health and safety. More than 15 million workers in the United States (17%) engage in shift work, and 2.6 million of these people rotate shifts (Erwin, 1998). Shift work has been found to reduce performance and contribute to social isolation, particularly for afternoon shift workers. Other effects of rotating shifts include greater job stress, increased incidence of sleep disorders, decreased mental health, decreased job satisfaction, and lower organizational commitment. Shift rotation also contributes to increased absenteeism and turnover and decreased punctuality (Fitzpatrick et al., 1999).

Use of Safety Devices

A last behavioral factor that is particularly relevant to health in the occupational setting is the use or nonuse of safety devices. Hazards present in the workplace frequently can be mitigated by the use of appropriate safety devices; however, this can occur only if employees use these devices consistently and appropriately.

The community health nurse identifies the need for safety devices and also monitors the extent to which they are used. For example, do individuals working in high-noise areas wear earplugs? Are those earplugs correctly fitted? Do people involved in heavy lifting wear weight belts, or do they ignore the potential for injury? Are heavy shoes or gloves worn in areas with dangerous equipment? Again, the attitude of management toward health promotion and illness prevention strongly influences employee behaviors. When administrators, for example, fail to use hearing protection in high-noise areas, they convey an attitude of disinterest in health, which frequently filters down to employees.

Health System Considerations

Health system factors influencing employee health relate to both external and internal health care systems. The external system reflects the availability and accessibility of health care services outside the workplace, whereas the internal system consists of those services offered within the workplace.

The External System

In assessing employee health status, the community health nurse in the occupational setting gathers information about the use of health services in the community at large. The nurse examines the type of services used and the reasons for and appropriateness of their use. The nurse also assesses the availability of services needed by company employees in the external health care system.

One of the work-related factors influencing use of outside health services is the availability of insurance coverage. Health insurance is an employment benefit for many, but large segments of the working population do not have health insurance coverage. Many of these uninsured workers do not have sufficient income to afford health insurance themselves or out-of-pocket health care expenses. For example, in 1997, 53% of U.S. employees were covered by an employer- or union-provided group health insurance plan. Among workers 15 to 20 years of age, only 22% had employer-provided insurance coverage (U.S. Census Bureau, 1999). Some of those not covered by employer-provided policies had health insurance from other sources (e.g., private or spousal coverage), but others had no insurance at all.

Even for insured employees, medical benefits have steadily declined due to high insurance costs. Co-payments and deductibles have increased at the same time, further limiting access to care for some employees and their families (Bertera, 2000). The occupational health nurse should become familiar with the insurance status of employees in his or her company and with the kinds of benefits covered under group policies where they exist.

The Internal System

The internal health care system consists of those health services and programs provided to employees in the work setting. Three general types of occupational health programs can be found in business and industry: programs aimed at controlling exposure to hazardous conditions; those emphasizing health promotion in the workplace; and comprehensive programs that attempt to meet a variety of employee health needs (Polanyi, Frank, Shannon, Sullivan, & Lavis, 2000).

PROGRAMS TO CONTROL TOXIC EXPOSURES Programs to control or eliminate toxic substances and other hazardous conditions in the workplace usually occur in response to OSHA regulations. Control programs may involve engineering controls, controlled work practices, use of safety equipment or devices, or elimination of toxic substances from the work environment. In industries with this type of program, the community health nurse should assess the efficacy of these control measures and the extent to which they are adhered to in the setting.

HEALTH PROMOTION The second type of program involves both development of organizational policies

of employees, or the total population in the work setting, interventions may be planned at primary, secondary, and tertiary levels of prevention.

Primary Prevention

Primary prevention in the occupational setting is directed toward minimizing the risks for injury and illness and promoting health and well-being.

Health Promotion

Community health nurses in occupational settings educate employees to lead healthier lives. The 1994 National Survey of Worksite Health Promotion Activities indicated that 80% of worksites offered at least one health promotion activity for employees (Reardon, 1998). Generally, these activities fall into one of five categories: programs to promote awareness, motivation programs, behavior change programs, maintenance programs, and culture change programs (Bellingham & Pelletier, 1995).

Awareness programs are designed to make employees aware of the ill effects of unhealthy behaviors and encourage behavior change. General education efforts by the nurse fall into this category. Motivation programs are also geared toward moving employees to take action on their own to change unhealthy behaviors. For example, employees may be rewarded with additional vacation days for maintaining their health. Behavior change interventions are programs designed to assist employees to make changes in their health-related behavior. Work-based smoking cessation programs and exercise programs are examples of this type of health promotion activity. Maintenance programs provide assistance to employees to continue with healthier behaviors and may include such interventions as co-worker support groups as well as increased environmental support for healthy behavior. For example, a nonsmoker support group may be coupled with employer policies prohibiting smoking. Both interventions are designed to help employees who smoke to develop a no-smoking habit. Finally, culture change programs are intended to alter the organizational culture of the work setting to reinforce the importance of health. Actions in these types of programs are directed at both the individual and the organization. For instance, the organization may strive to find effective ways to reduce stress in the work environment while incorporating a health behavior review as part of regular performance appraisals for employees.

⑥THINK ABOUT IT

Should employee participation in health promotion activities be voluntary or mandatory? Why?

Health promotion programs in the occupational setting have been highly successful. Specifically, worksite health promotion programs have been shown to result in better blood pressure control, increased physical activity, decreased weight, smoking cessation, better emotional health, improved productivity and morale, and reduced absenteeism (Allegrante, 1998). Employee assistance, stress management, and other similar programs have also been shown to increase productivity and psychological health among employees as well as to promote more healthful behaviors (Landsbergis et al., 1998; van der Klink et al., 2001). Further research is needed to document the long-term effects and costs of health promotion programs.

Another avenue for health promotion is providing prenatal care to pregnant workers. This could involve referral for prenatal care if this service is not provided by the company health facility. The nurse might also monitor the employee for signs and symptoms of complications of pregnancy. The nurse may find it necessary to function as an advocate for the employee who needs to be relieved of some of her duties as the pregnancy progresses. For example, it may be necessary to move the employee to another position that does not require heavy lifting. The nurse may also be involved in childbirth education for pregnant employees or male employees and their spouses.

Illness Prevention

Preventing illness is the second aspect of primary prevention in the workplace. Illness prevention can involve either employee education or prevention of specific illness through immunization. For example, some industries routinely offer employees influenza immunization to cut down on illness-related absenteeism.

Another aspect of illness prevention involves modifying risk factors. *Risk factors* are personal or group characteristics that predispose one to develop a specific health problem. For example, it is well known that smoking increases one's risk of developing heart disease and lung cancer, so smoking is a risk factor for both of these problems.

Some risk factors can be modified or eliminated, thus decreasing one's chances of developing specific health problems. Again, using smoking as an example, people who quit smoking lower their risk of developing lung cancer. Occupational health nurses can be instrumental in assisting employees to modify risk factors, helping them to prevent health problems. Some risk factors that receive particular attention in the occupational setting are smoking, elevated blood pressure, sedentary lifestyle, stress, and overweight.

Occupational health nurses can work on risk factor modification with individuals or groups of employees. They can also engage in risk factor modification efforts at the company level. One example of this would be efforts to convince company policy makers that a no-smoking policy should be instituted and enforced within the workplace. Nurses can also develop weight standards for job categories in which being overweight is particularly hazardous, or the nurse can recommend the use of safer products in place of toxic substances whenever possible. In health care settings, nurses might work to convince employers that the cost of using nonlatex gloves is outweighed by the savings realized in preventing disability due to latex allergy and latex-induced asthma (Phillips et al., 1999).

At the individual level, the nurse can counsel employees regarding the hazards of smoking, particularly in conjunction with occupational exposure to respiratory irritants. They can also provide assistance to individuals who wish to quit smoking.

Restructuring the work environment can help in minimizing occupational stress as a risk factor for health problems. Efforts in this direction include developing flexible schedules to minimize conflicts with employees' outside responsibilities. The nurse can also facilitate employee input into work-related decisions and strive to minimize role overload and role ambiguity. The nurse can also promote opportunity for social interaction, job security, and career development.

As is obvious, most of these efforts must be undertaken by management, but the nurse can provide management with evidence of related research and can provide the impetus for change in these areas. At the individual level, the occupational health nurse can be aware of the stressors experienced by employees in various jobs in the work setting. The nurse is also in a position to monitor the effects of stress on the individual employee and to counsel employees in stress management.

Injury Prevention

Injury prevention may again entail employee education in a variety of areas. Employees need to be acquainted with safety procedures to prevent accidents. There may also be a need to educate employees in the correct use of safety equipment. For example, individuals working in some areas should wear protective clothing or use breathing apparatus. The nurse should explain the need for safety equipment and be responsible for monitoring its use. This may entail planning periodic visits to certain areas of the workplace to determine whether employees are indeed using safety equipment as directed.

Employees may also be in need of education in other areas related to injury prevention. Handling of hazardous substances, proper use of machinery, need for fluid replacement in high-heat areas, and good body mechanics are all educational topics that may be appropriate in certain industrial settings. Nurses may also provide education on first aid and cardiopulmonary resuscitation.

One aspect of injury prevention in which the nurse may be involved is monitoring hazardous conditions in the workplace. The nurse should be aware of potential hazards and their appropriate management. In the absence of an industrial hygienist, the nurse may plan and conduct environmental testing to detect hazardous levels of chemicals, heat, or noise.

The nurse may need to acquaint management with the occurrence of injuries due to hazardous conditions and advocate changes designed to protect employees from injuries. Recommendations for dealing with the problem of noise-induced hearing loss, for example, include engineering efforts to minimize noise production, use of properly fitted hearing protection devices, education of employees and managers in the use of protective devices and their importance, and periodic audiometric screening. The occupational health nurse may be actively

Injury prevention is an important aspect of primary prevention in work settings.

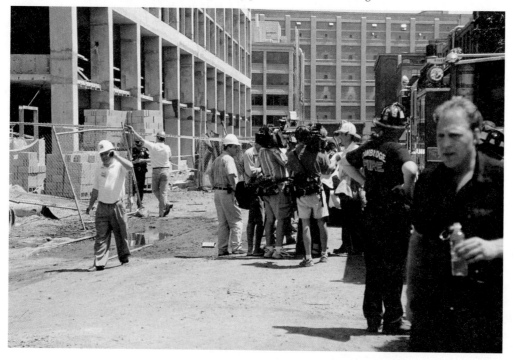

involved in planning and executing the majority of these recommended activities, particularly in screening for hearing loss, fitting protective devices, and educating employees and supervisors. Control of noise-related hearing loss requires commitment on the part of employees and management to the proper use of protective devices. Motivating employees to use these devices and monitoring their use are crucial functions of the occupational health nurse. Emphases in injury prevention, as well as other aspects of primary prevention in work settings, are summarized below.

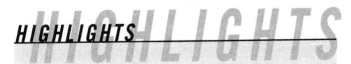

Primary Prevention in Work Settings

Health Promotion
- Awareness
- Motivation
- Behavior change
- Maintenance
- Culture change

Illness Prevention
- Immunization
- Modification or elimination of risk factors
- Stress reduction and management

Injury Prevention
- Safety education
- Use of safety devices
- Safe handling of hazardous substances
- Elimination of safety hazards
- Good body mechanics

Secondary Prevention

Secondary prevention in work settings is aimed at recognizing and resolving existing health problems. General areas of involvement for occupational health nurses include screening, treatment for existing conditions, and emergency care.

Screening and Surveillance

Screening activities can take any of three directions. Screening efforts begin with preemployment assessment of potential employees. Screening may also be conducted at periodic intervals to monitor employee health status. Finally, the work environment may be screened periodically for the presence or absence of hazardous conditions. The community health nurse would be involved in planning and implementing screening efforts at all three of these levels. In fact, in a recent study of occupational

health nurses, 71% of the nurses indicated that they have overall responsibility for screening and surveillance services in their facilities. *Screening* involves testing individual employees for indicators of disease or for risk factors that increase the potential for disease. *Surveillance,* on the other hand, is the analysis of group data to identify trends and problems in the work setting rather than in individual employees (Rogers & Livsey, 2000).

PREEMPLOYMENT SCREENING For many employees, their first interaction with an occupational health nurse is the preemployment screening examination. The purpose of this initial screening is to facilitate employee selection and placement. Hiring an employee for a particular job is in part dependent on his or her physical, mental, and emotional capabilities for performing that job. A similar process may be needed when considering an employee for a change of job. These capabilities can be determined in an initial screening examination. At this time, the nurse usually obtains a complete health history from the employee and conducts a battery of routine screening tests. Nurse practitioners in the occupational setting may also conduct the physical examination.

Based on the information derived from the screening, the nurse may make determinations regarding the person's employability in a particular capacity. To make such determinations, the nurse must be familiar with the types of activities involved and stressors encountered in a particular job. The preemployment screening also provides baseline data for determining the effects of working conditions on the health of employees. Some questions designed to help determine an employee's fitness for a specific job are presented below.

Evaluating fitness for work

Physical Health Considerations
- Does the employee have the physical stamina required?
- Does the employee have any mobility limitations that would interfere with performance?
- Does the employee have sufficient joint mobility to do the job?
- Does the employee have any postural limitations that would interfere with performance?
- Does the employee have the required strength for the job?
- Does the employee have the level of coordination required?
- Does the employee have problems with balance that would interfere with performance?
- Does the employee have any cardiorespiratory limitations?

- Is there a possibility for unconsciousness that would create a safety hazard?
- Does the employee have the required level of visual and auditory acuity?
- Does the employee have communication and speech capabilities required by the job?

Mental and Emotional Health Considerations

- Does the employee have the requisite level of cognitive function (e.g., memory, critical thinking)?
- Will the employee's mental or emotional state (e.g., depression) interfere with performance?
- Does the employee have the required motivational level?
- Does the employee have a substance abuse problem that would interfere with performance?
- Does the employee have effective stress management skills?
- Is there any possibility that the employee might endanger self or others?

Health Care Considerations

- Are there treatment effects that will interfere with performance (e.g., drowsiness from medications)?
- Will subsequent treatment plans interfere with performance (e.g., nausea due to future chemotherapy)?
- What is the employee's prognosis? Will existing conditions improve or deteriorate further?
- Does the employee have any special health needs to be met in the work setting (e.g., diabetic diet)?
- Are any assistive aids or appliances required? Will work processes or setting need to be adapted to accommodate these aids (e.g., space for a wheelchair)?

Task/Setting Considerations

- Are there risk factors in the work setting that would adversely affect the employee?
- What is the level of stress involved in the job?
- Will the employee be working with others or alone? What health effects might this have?
- What are the temporal aspects of the job and how will they affect health (e.g., shift work, early morning or late evening work, length of shift)?
- Is there travel involved in the job? How will this affect employee health?

Source: Cox, R. A. F., & Edwards, F. C. (1995). Introduction. In R. A. F. Cox, F. C. Edwards, & R. I. McCallum (Eds.), *Fitness for work: The medical aspects* (2nd ed.) (pp. 1–24). Oxford: Oxford University Press.

PERIODIC SCREENING The nurse in the occupational setting also plans periodic screening activities to monitor employees' continuing health status. This is particularly true of employees working under hazardous conditions. For example, monitoring devices are used by personnel working with radiation and are periodically checked for exposure limits. Likewise, blood chemistries may be done at periodic intervals to test for exposure to toxic substances. Periodic blood pressure screenings and pulmonary function tests may also be warranted. In some occupational groups such as the armed forces, employees are routinely screened for overweight and for physical capacity.

The types of screening done depend on the type of job performed, the risks involved, and the capabilities required. Some screenings are routinely performed on all employees in a particular setting. For example, employees may receive a routine physical examination at periodic intervals. Other screening tests are performed only on specific employees. For example, lead screening may be done routinely on individuals who work in the company plant, but not on clerical personnel.

Nurses may also be actively involved in providing or promoting routine health screenings that are not related to employees' jobs. For example, the nurse may educate older male employees regarding the need for screening for prostate cancer, or teach men of all ages how to perform testicular self-examination. Similarly, nurses may encourage women to obtain regular Papanicolaou tests and mammography. In one study, for example, an occupational intervention consisting of education, group discussion, and outreach was successful in increasing the extent of cervical cancer screening among women employees. No effect was noted, however, in the rate of breast cancer screening between experimental and control groups (Allen, Stoddard, Mays, & Sorensen, 2001).

Occupational health nurses are frequently responsible for conducting these and other screening tests on employees. They may also interpret test results, explain them to employees, and take action when warranted by positive test results.

ENVIRONMENTAL SCREENING Periodic screening of the environment may also be warranted, and, in the absence of industrial hygienists or safety engineers, the nurse may be responsible for planning and conducting environmental screenings. For example, the nurse may measure noise levels in various work areas at specific intervals to determine areas in which hearing protection is required. Similarly, measurements of volatile chemicals or radiation might be done in high-risk areas.

Treatment of Existing Conditions

The second aspect of secondary prevention is the diagnosis and treatment of existing health problems. Community health nurses are actively involved in planning health interventions for individual employees and should also participate in planning health programs to meet the needs of groups of clients.

Many industries go beyond treating only job-related illnesses and conditions to treating a variety of major and minor conditions. The rationale for the extension of services to non–job-related conditions is that any health problem, physical or emotional, can serve to impair the employee's performance. Also, treatment of these conditions within the work setting itself limits time lost in pursuing outside treatment, saving the company money in the long run.

Depending on the capabilities of the occupational health unit, employees with existing health problems may be referred to the external health care system for problem resolution, or treatment may be provided within the workplace itself. Those occupational health nurses who are nurse practitioners may treat illness in the work setting. Even those nurses who are not nurse practitioners may treat minor conditions on the basis of protocols established in conjunction with medical consultation.

Occupational health nurses also need to plan to monitor the effectiveness of therapy, whether or not that therapy is provided by the occupational health unit. For example, an employee with hypertension might be followed by his or her primary care provider, but the occupational health nurse will monitor medication compliance and effects on the employee's blood pressure. In addition, the nurse will educate the employee regarding the condition and its treatment.

In the case of employees with problems related to substance abuse or stress, the community health nurse usually plans a referral to an appropriate source of assistance. The nurse may also need to function as an advocate for impaired employees, encouraging employers to provide coverage for treatment for psychological as well as physical illness. Nurses may also find it necessary to report substance abuse to supervisory personnel when either the health or the safety of other employees is threatened.

Community health nurses in occupational settings may also be involved in planning and implementing employee assistance programs for employees with psychological problems. An *employee assistance program (EAP)* is a program within the occupational setting designed to counsel employees with psychological problems and assist them in dealing with those problems (Breckon, 1998). EAP programs usually focus on motivating individuals to seek help and on referring the person for needed services.

The nurse can plan to motivate the employee to get help through seven feedback steps performed in sequence until the employee (client) is willing to seek assistance (Csiernik, 1990). First, the nurse discusses with the client (employee) his or her observations of the client's behavior or appearance that indicate the existence of a problem. For example, the nurse might comment on the frequency with which the employee has called in "sick" on Mondays. Second, the nurse comments on several instances of the client's behavior that suggest a psychological problem, making connections between discrete behavioral events to show the employee a definite pattern in his or her behavior. At this point, the nurse might discuss the decline in performance noted for the last few months. Third, the nurse asks the employee to explain the causes for the observed signs and symptoms. Interpreting possible causes for behavior is the fourth feedback step in motivating employees with psychological problems to take action. For instance, the nurse might suggest that one reason commonly associated with frequent Monday absences is weekend binge drinking. The fifth step is to provide suggestions for change that would eliminate or modify factors contributing to the problem. The nurse might suggest a referral to an alcohol treatment center. Sixth, if the employee has not decided to take action by this point, the nurse may need to provide a warning on the progressive nature of most psychological problems and on the possible consequences if no action is taken. For example, the nurse might discuss the potential for accidental injury while under the influence of alcohol or the effects of the client's behavior on his or her family. Finally, the nurse may strongly recommend action to correct the problem. The choice of whether or not to take action, however, remains with the employee (client).

Once the individual is motivated to seek help for the problem, the nurse can make a referral to counselors within or outside the organization. In addition to planning the referral, the nurse should plan activities to support and encourage the employee and to monitor his or her progress in resolving problems. Finally, the community health nurse should plan interventions that help reintegrate the employee into the work setting if an extended absence has been necessary.

Emergency Response

Another aspect of secondary prevention in work settings is response to emergency situations. Nurses may find themselves dealing with both physical and psychological emergencies and should have a basic plan for dealing with various types of emergencies that may arise. Physical emergencies may result from serious accidents or from physical conditions such as heart attack, stroke, seizure disorder, and insulin reaction. Treatment for these emergencies is usually based on established protocols.

With respect to emergencies due to illness, it is helpful if the nurse has prior information related to the employee's condition. For example, if the nurse has prior knowledge that the client is diabetic, the diagnosis of hypoglycemic reaction will be reached and treatment initiated more rapidly than would otherwise be the case. For this reason, occupational health nurses should be well acquainted with employees' health histories.

Psychological emergencies may result in homicide, suicide, or both. Although businesses may have generalized protocols for dealing with such emergencies as threatened homicide or suicide, the nurse faced with such situations will probably need to exercise a great deal of creativity in planning to address a psychological emergency. General considerations include remaining calm and removing others from the immediate vicinity. The nurse *should not* plan any heroic measures that may endanger him- or herself, the employee, or others. Additional interventions are dictated by the situation.

Again, prior identification of employees under excessive stress may help to prevent psychiatric emergencies.

Another psychological emergency with which occupational health nurses may need to deal is sexual assault. Most victims of sexual assault in the workplace are women, and most assaults occur at night when women are working in isolation from co-workers or the public. The nurse who encounters a female employee who has been sexually assaulted should address immediate physical and psychological needs, assess the client for suicidal tendencies, and refer her for counseling. The nurse may also need to act as an advocate with the legal and criminal justice systems and to provide emotional support.

One further type of emergency that requires an occupational health nursing response is the emergency that affects large numbers of people. Examples of mass emergencies are fires or explosions, radiation exposure, and hazardous substance leaks. In addition to providing treatment for those injured in such emergencies, the nurse may be responsible for assisting in evaluating affected areas and in organizing to provide needed care. Occupational health nurses should be involved in planning the overall company response to such situations as well as planning health care in such an eventuality. The role of the nurse in disaster preparedness is discussed in greater detail in Chapter 27. Major emphases in secondary prevention in work settings are summarized below.

ring in the first place, can also be used as tertiary prevention to prevent its recurrence. For example, engineering measures may be used to prevent leakage of a toxic chemical or to prevent subsequent leaks if one has already occurred.

Generally speaking, tertiary prevention is geared toward preventing the spread of communicable diseases, preventing recurrence of other acute conditions, and preventing complications of chronic conditions. Sick-leave policies and employee immunization are examples of tertiary preventive measures that might be taken to stop the spread of influenza in the employee population. By encouraging employees to take advantage of sick-leave benefits when they or family members are ill, the nurse can minimize exposure of others in the occupational setting to communicable diseases and can control the spread of disease. Safety education might prevent a recurrence of accidental injuries due to hazardous equipment, and use of hearing protection might prevent further deterioration of an employee's hearing after noise exposure has already caused some damage. Similarly, treatment of an employee's hypertension can prevent further health problems.

Another aspect of tertiary prevention may be assessing an employee's fitness to return to work after an illness or injury. Assessment considerations in this case would be similar to those in preemployment assessment. Tertiary prevention emphases in occupational settings are summarized below.

HIGHLIGHTS

Secondary Prevention in Work Settings

Screening

- Preemployment screening
- Periodic screening of employees at risk for health problems
- Environmental screening

Treatment of Existing Conditions

Emergency Response

- Physical emergencies
- Psychological emergencies
- Occupational disasters

HIGHLIGHTS

Tertiary Prevention in Work Settings

- Preventing the spread of communicable disease through immunization and sick leave for ill employees
- Preventing the recurrence of other acute conditions
- Preventing complications of chronic conditions
- Assessing fitness to return to work

IMPLEMENTING HEALTH CARE IN WORK SETTINGS

Implementing nursing interventions in work settings frequently involves collaboration with others. Most often, collaboration occurs between the nurse and the employee. In other instances, the nurse may collaborate with health care providers and others within or outside of the occupational setting. For example, the nurse might collaborate with a pregnant employee's primary health care provider to monitor her progress throughout the pregnancy. Implementing the plan of care for an employee with carpal tunnel syndrome might involve collaboration with the primary care provider and with a

Tertiary Prevention

Tertiary prevention in work settings is directed toward preventing a recurrence of health problems and limiting their consequences. The types of tertiary intervention measures employed depend on the problems to be prevented. In many instances, primary prevention measures, which would be used to prevent a problem from occur-

supervisor to facilitate movement to a job that does not necessitate repetitive wrist movements.

When health problems affect groups of employees, implementing the plan of care might involve collaboration with other health care providers and with company management and other personnel. For example, the nurse who has documented an increased incidence of respiratory conditions due to aerosol exposures will advocate plans to resolve the problem. These plans need to be approved by management and implemented by engineering personnel, if engineering controls are required, or by company purchasing agents, if special respiratory protective devices are needed. In the latter instance, the nurse may be involved in determining the types of protective devices needed and recommending their purchase to management.

EVALUATING HEALTH CARE IN WORK SETTINGS

As in all other settings for nursing practice, the effectiveness of health care in work settings must be evaluated. Evaluation can focus on the outcomes of care either for the individual employee or for the total employee population. Evaluation is conducted on the basis of principles discussed in Chapter 15 and focuses on the achievement of expected outcomes and the processes used to achieve those outcomes. For example, the occupational health nurse may evaluate the effectiveness of body mechanics education in decreasing the incidence of back injuries. At the individual level, evaluation might focus on the impact of no-smoking education on an individual employee's smoking behavior. Achievement of objectives related to occupational health can be used to evaluate efforts at the national level. The status of selected national objectives is presented below.

Occupational settings contribute to a wide variety of health problems in individuals and in population groups, yet they also provide an ideal setting for influencing health-related behaviors of employees. Community health nurses employed in occupational settings can do much to promote the health of individual employees and of the general public.

HEALTHY PEOPLE 2010

GOALS FOR THE POPULATION

	Objective	Base	Target
7-5	Increase the proportion of worksites that offer a comprehensive employee health promotion program	95–99%	100%
7-6	Increase the proportion of employees who participate in employer-sponsored health promotion activities	28%	50%
14-3	g. Reduce hepatitis B among occupationally exposed workers (per 100,000)	249	62
14-28	c. Increase hepatitis B vaccine coverage among occupationally exposed workers	71%	98%
20-1	Reduce deaths from work-related injuries (per 100,000 workers)	4.5	3.2
20-2	Reduce work-related injuries resulting in medical treatment, lost work time, or restricted work activity (per 100 full-time workers)	6.6	4.6
20-3	Reduce the rate of injury and illness due to over-exertion or repetitive motion (per 100,000 workers)	675	338
20-5	Reduce deaths from work-related homicides (per 100,000 workers)	0.5	0.4
20-6	Reduce work-related assault (per 100 workers)	0.85	0.60
20-7	Reduce the number of persons who have elevated blood lead levels from work exposures (per million)	93	0
20-8	Reduce occupational skin diseases (new cases per 100,000 workers)	67	47
20-9	Increase the proportion of worksites that provide programs to prevent or reduce stress	37%	50%
20-10	Reduce occupational needlestick injuries among health care workers	600,000	420,000
27-12	Increase the proportion of worksites with formal smoking policies	79%	100%

Source: U.S. Department of Health and Human Services. (2000). *Healthy people 2010* (Conference edition, in two volumes). Washington, DC: Author.

APPLYING YOUR KNOWLEDGE IN PRACTICE

❧ CASE STUDY
Nursing in the Work Setting

You are a community health nurse employed by a large manufacturing plant. On Wednesday you see several employees complaining of abdominal cramping and diarrhea. They all state that their symptoms started at home during the night. You get word from one of the plant supervisors that several of her employees called in sick this morning because of similar symptoms. In checking with other departments, you find that there are a number of absences throughout the plant. Two of the older employees and one whom you know has AIDS have been hospitalized with severe dehydration. All of the people with cramps and diarrhea eat regularly in the cafeteria.

- What are the biophysical, psychological, physical environmental, sociocultural, behavioral, and health system factors operating in this situation?

- What are your nursing diagnoses?
- What outcome objectives do you hope to achieve through intervention?
- What secondary prevention measures will you employ in relation to your diagnoses? Why? What primary preventive measures might have prevented the occurrence of these problems? What tertiary prevention measures are warranted to prevent the recurrence of problems or complications?
- How will you evaluate the effectiveness of your interventions?

❧ TESTING YOUR UNDERSTANDING

- What are some of the advantages of providing health care in work settings? (p. 562)
- What types of health and safety hazards are encountered in work settings? Describe at least one potential control measure for each type of hazard. (pp. 565–570)
- What are some of the biophysical, psychological, physical environmental, sociocultural, behavioral, and health system factors that influence health in work settings? (pp. 565–574)
- What are the spheres of social influence on the health of employees? (pp. 570–571)
- What types of health care programs may be found in work settings? What is the community health nurse's focus in each? (pp. 573–574)

- What are the main areas of emphasis in primary prevention in work settings? Give an example of a community health nursing intervention related to each area. (pp. 576–578)
- Describe the major considerations in secondary prevention in work settings. What activities might a community health nurse be involved in with respect to each? (pp. 578–581)
- What are the areas of emphasis in tertiary prevention in work settings? Describe at least one community health nursing responsibility related to each area of emphasis. (p. 581)

REFERENCES

Allegrante, J. (1998). School-site health promotion for faculty and staff: A key component of the coordinated school health program. *Journal of School Health, 68*, 190–195.

Allen, J. D., Stoddard, A. M., Mays, J., & Sorensen, G. (2001). Promoting breast and cervical cancer screening at the workplace: Results from the Woman to Woman study. *American Journal of Public Health, 91*, 584–590.

American Association of Occupational Health Nurses. (1999). *Standards of occupational and environmental health nursing.* Atlanta: Author.

Anglin, L. T. (1990). *The roles of nurses: A history, 1900 to 1988.* Unpublished doctoral dissertation, Illinois State University.

Bachman, J. G., Freedman-Doan, P., O'Malley, P. M., Johnston, L. D., & Segal, D. R. (1999). Changing patterns of drug use among US

Throughout the world people live in different kinds of environments from crowded and deteriorating inner cities to planned suburban communities to isolated rural areas. Factors in each of these settings influence health in different ways, some positively and others negatively. Prior to the twentieth century, people living in rural areas had generally better health and longer life expectancies than those in cities due to the crowding and poor sanitation that were characteristic of urban life. More recently, however, people in urban areas in developed countries have had access to better health care services and better knowledge of health promotion and illness prevention than those in rural settings (World Health Organization, 2000). Changes in rural and urban environments have resulted in changes in factors that influence health in those settings. In this chapter, we explore some of those factors and their implications for community health nursing as practiced in urban and rural settings.

WHAT IS URBAN? WHAT IS RURAL?

Although 80% of the North American population are described as *urbanized,* and half of the world's population is said to live in urban areas (Hancock, 2000), there is no clear definition of what *urban* means. Nor is there an accepted definition of *rurality.* In fact, the U.S. federal government has changed the definitions of urban and rural frequently, and different definitions are used by different agencies within the federal government, making comparisons between rural and urban areas over time and with respect to different aspects difficult (Wright, Rubin, & Devine, 1998).

Two commonly used sets of definitions of rural and urban come from the U.S. Census Bureau and the Office of Management and Budget (OMB). For the 1990 census, the Census Bureau defined the terms on the basis of population size and density, and an urbanized area was comprised of "one or more places and the adjacent densely settled surrounding territory that together have a minimum population of 50,000 persons" (U.S. Census Bureau, 1999, p. 4). All territory that falls outside of the definition of urbanization is considered "rural." These definitions changed somewhat for 2000 (U.S. Census Bureau, 2000), but since rural/urban delineation data from the 2000 census will not be available until the second quarter of 2002, many statistics reported in this chapter are based on the 1990 definitions.

The OMB system classifies territory in terms of the presence of a city or suburbs and the degree of integration of that territory with city or suburb (Ricketts, Johnson-Webb, & Randolph, 1999).

A set of 10 rural–urban continuum codes used by the U.S. Department of Agriculture differentiates between metropolitan and nonmetropolitan counties based on the degree of urbanization and nearness to central metropoli-

tan areas (National Center for Chronic Disease Prevention and Health Promotion, 1998). These codes are based on the OMB categories and are summarized below.

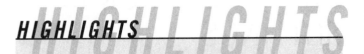

HIGHLIGHTS

Rural–Urban Continuum Codes

Metropolitan Counties

0—Central counties of metropolitan areas with populations of 1 million or more people

1—Metropolitan counties on the fringe of central counties that have populations of 1 million or more people

2—Metropolitan counties with populations of 250,000 to 1 million people

3—Counties in metropolitan areas with populations less than 250,000 people

Nonmetropolitan Counties

4—Urban populations of 20,000 or more people adjacent to a metropolitan area

5—Urban populations of 20,000 or more people, not adjacent to a metropolitan area

6—Urban populations of 2,500 to 19,999 people adjacent to a metropolitan area

7—Urban populations of 2,500 to 19,999, people not adjacent to a metropolitan area

8—Completely rural areas or areas with urban populations of less than 2,500 people (e.g., small towns) adjacent to a metropolitan area

9—Completely rural areas or areas with urban populations of less than 2,500 people, not adjacent to a metropolitan area

Source: Wysong, J. A., Bliss, M. K., Osborne, J. W., Graham, R. P., & Pikuzinski, D. A. (1999). Managed care in rural markets: Availability and enrollment. *Journal of Health Care for the Poor and Underserved, 10*(1), 72–84.

The Montana State University (MSU) rurality index is another approach to defining rurality. Rather than being county based, this index is person based and categorizes individual residents on the basis of their degree of rurality. The advantage of a resident-based index is that it allows comparisons of people within a county who differ from other people in the same county in terms of their rurality. This index allows comparisons between rural and urban populations within the same county. The index for a given individual is derived by creating a weighted score based on the population density of the county and the distance to the nearest emergency services. In the case of persons in a single county, the index is based on distance to emergency services alone (Weinert & Boik, 1998).

One final term that is used in discussion of rural populations is that of *frontier*. A *frontier* area or county is one that has a population density of less than 7 people per square mile (Felt-Lisk, Silberman, Hoag, & Slifkin, 1999). For the most part, in this chapter, we will be using the term *rural* to describe groups with very low population densities (less than 2,500 people), which includes people in small rural communities, and *urban*, or metropolitan, as indicating central metropolitan areas.

URBAN AND RURAL POPULATIONS

In 1996, nearly 80% of the U.S. population resided in metropolitan areas and 20% in nonmetropolitan areas as defined by the OMB. From 1990 to 1996, the urban population increased by nearly 7%, whereas the nonmetropolitan population increased by nearly 6%. The percentage of the population living in rural areas varied considerably by state from 72% in Vermont to just over 3% in California (U.S. Census Bureau, 1999). In 1997, the rural population in the United States included 54 million people (*The Nation's Health*, 1999), and the urban population included more than 213 million (U.S. Census Bureau, 1999).

The rural population can be further categorized as farm and nonfarm populations. In 1990, only 2% of the U.S. population lived on farms, only half of whom depended on agriculture for their income (Wright et al., 1999). The farm population also includes approximately 2.5 million farm laborers, 1.6 million of whom are seasonal workers, and 42% of whom are migrant workers (National Ag Safety Database, 1996).

Rural and urban populations differ considerably in their composition, with rural populations including more young children and elderly individuals (Chase-Ziolek & Striepe, 1999). In fact, approximately one third of the U.S. population over age 65 lives in rural areas (Johnson, 1998), and in 21 states the majority of elderly persons are rural residents (Elnitsky & Alexy, 1998). Approximately 12% of the population in large urban centers are over 65 years of age compared to 17% of rural populations. The difference in age distribution between rural and urban areas is even more striking for persons over 85 years of age who constitute only 1.3% of urban populations and 2.1% of the rural population (Coburn & Bolda, 1999).

The rural elderly are less likely than their urban counterparts to report good to excellent health and more likely to report fair or poor health. Among persons 65 to 69 years of age, one third of rural residents reported fair or poor health compared to only 23% of urban residents. The differences in self-reported health status are even more apparent in older age groups. For example, among persons over 75 years of age, 44.5% of rural residents reported fair or poor health compared to 31% of the urban elderly population (Coburn & Bolda, 1999).

In 1991, 1.2 million children lived on U.S. farms and ranches (Division of Safety Research, 1999). The total number of other children living in rural areas is not available. Farm children, in particular, are at risk for injury, and the National Ag Safety Database (1996) indicates that 150,000 to 200,000 injuries to children occur on farms and ranches every year. This is primarily due to employment of children on family farms. From 1992 to 1996, 300,000 youth aged 15 to 19 years were employed in agricultural production and service sectors. Children in these settings may perform tasks inappropriate to their ages and physical development that are prohibited in other industries. Youth also lack work experience and attention to detail that may place them at increased risk for injury. Finally, youngsters may be hampered by decreased visibility in tractor cabs designed for adults or by control layouts on machinery that was not designed for shorter reach capabilities (Division of Safety Research, 1999).

URBAN AND RURAL COMMUNITY HEALTH NURSING

Rural nursing has been defined as "the provision of health care by professional nurses to persons living in sparsely populated areas" (Long & Weinert, 1998, p. 4). Rural community health nursing originated in 1896 when Ellen M. Wood established an initial rural nursing service in Westchester County, New York. In 1911, Lydia Holman established an independent nursing service in Appalachia, and in 1912, the American Red Cross founded the Rural Nursing Service, which later became the Town and Country Nursing Service (Griffin, 1999). This organization was credited with decreasing infant and overall mortality and improving sanitation, hygiene, and nutrition in rural populations (Anderson & Yuhos, 1993). The Town and Country Nursing Service continued until 1947, when it was disbanded due to the rise of official nursing agencies in state and local health departments. Other rural nursing services were provided by organizations such as the Frontier Nursing Service established by Mary Breckenridge in 1925 (Bigbee, 1993). More recent developments in rural nursing include the Migrant Health Act of 1962, which established the Migrant Health Program (Hibbeln, 1996) and the passage of the Rural Health Clinic Service Act in 1977 (Baer & Smith, 1999). Both of these pieces of legislation provided funding for health care services in rural areas that have addressed some of the health needs of the rural population and increased the use of nurse practitioners as providers of care.

As noted in Chapter 2, urban community health nursing in the United States began primarily with the efforts of Lillian Wald and others in the late 19th century. Occupational health nursing, which was primarily focused on urban manufacturing, also began about this time. Although occupational health risks related to agriculture were recognized as early as 1555 when the effects of breathing grain dust on the lungs of threshers were noted, little attention has been given to occupational health in rural areas until relatively recently. Similarly, Thackrah's report on *The Effects of Arts, Trades, and Professions* in 1832 addressed the effects of poor occupational postures on health, but there was no mention of agricultural occupations—in which bending, twisting, and heavy lifting are common occurrences—as contributing factors (Schenker, 1995).

⑥THINK ABOUT IT

Should rural health care be provided by nurse generalists or specialists? Why? Would your answer be different in relation to nurses in urban settings? Why or why not?

Recent concerns about health influences in rural areas have led to the development of beginning theory related to rural nursing. Key concepts of rural nursing theory include work beliefs and health beliefs, isolation and distance, self-reliance, lack of anonymity, insider/outsider, and old-timer/newcomer (Long & Weinert, 1998). These key concepts and their relationships are summarized below and discussed where relevant throughout the remainder of this chapter. No comparable theory of urban nursing has been noted in the literature.

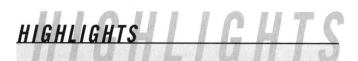

Key Concepts and Relationships in a Theory of Rural Nursing

- *Work beliefs and health beliefs:* Work and health are related. Work is of primary importance, and health is assessed in relation to the ability to work. Health needs are often secondary to work needs.
- *Isolation and distance:* Rural residents often live great distances from health care and other services. Despite these differences, however, they do not generally see themselves as isolated.
- *Self-reliance:* Rural residents are characterized by a strong desire to do and care for themselves. This may result in reluctance to seek help from others, reliance on informal support networks when care is sought, and resistance to seeking care from "outsiders."
- *Lack of anonymity:* Rural communities are close-knit and rural residents may feel a lack of privacy. For rural nurses, this means multiple different relationships with clients that are interrelated. For example, the nurse's credibility as a professional may be linked to perceptions of her performance as a wife and mother as well as to evidence of professional competence. The role diffusion caused by multiple roles within the community may lead to a broader diversity of tasks expected of rural nurses, including expansion into the practice realm of other disciplines.
- *Insider/outsider:* Rural residents prefer to receive services from people well known to them. Rural nurses must become actively involved within their communities in other than professional roles. This may be uncomfortable for nurses who try to maintain a clear separation between their personal and professional lives.
- *Old-timer/newcomer:* Rural residents may continue to perceive people who have lived in the area for several years as "newcomers," and rural nurses new to the area should expect a long period of being considered a newcomer before they are completely accepted by the population.

Source: Long, K. A., & Weinert, C. (1998). Rural nursing: Developing the theory base. In H. J. Lee (Ed.), *Conceptual basis for rural nursing* (pp. 3–18). New York: Springer.

Rural nurses tend to be generalists who may be required to deal with any type of health problem that arises (Tone, 1999). Rural nurses are expected to be competent in multiple areas, and expert in a few. Areas that have been shown in recent research to be most important among rural nurses in hospital settings include the emergency department, obstetrics, intensive coronary care, and general medical surgical nursing (Scharff, 1998). Rural community health nurses should have generalized expertise related to childbearing, child health, injury prevention, health education, and so on. Urban nurses, on the other hand, may have more opportunity for specialization because of the array of other providers available to fulfill other needs in urban areas.

Rural and urban nursing may also differ in the scope of practice. Because of the dearth of health professionals in many rural areas, rural community health nurses may be the only source of health care for many clients. Again, this demands a generalist perspective, but may also mean that the boundaries between nursing and medicine are less distinct that in urban settings. Rural nurses may often be required to engage in what would elsewhere be considered medical practice until a physician arrives, particularly in emergency situations. Even when physicians are present, "newcomer" physicians have been observed consulting with experienced rural nurses regarding treatment options best suited to a given client's situation. Blurring of practice boundaries may also occur between nursing and such disciplines as pharmacy and dietetics in rural hospital settings (Scharff, 1998).

⑥THINK ABOUT IT

How might nursing education institutions help to meet rural community health nurses' needs for an expanded knowledge base? What strategies might work for providing continuing education opportunities for rural nurses? Would the same strategies work for urban nurses? Why or why not?

Care of population groups in both urban and rural settings relies on the nursing process as an organizational framework. However, the factors assessed as influencing health, the health problems identified, and intervention approaches may often differ.

ASSESSING FACTORS INFLUENCING HEALTH IN URBAN AND RURAL SETTINGS

Factors that arise in the biophysical, psychological, physical environmental, sociocultural, behavioral, and health system dimensions influence the health of both rural and urban populations. The types of factors present in each dimension, however, may differ considerably.

Biophysical Considerations

Biophysical considerations related to maturation and aging and their differences in urban and rural settings have already been addressed. Here, we will focus on similarities and differences related to mortality, morbidity related to illness and injury, and levels of immunization. The community health nurse assessing the health of a particular urban or rural population would determine the prevalence of specific biophysical factors in the population and their effects on health status.

Differences between mortality rates in urban and rural areas are controversial. In one study, for example, overall mortality among urban residents was 1.6 times higher than that for rural residents, with even greater differences noted in mortality for urban and rural men. Suburban mortality was also found to be higher than rural mortality except for suburban African American men. Urban residents were found to have 12 times the mortality rate for infections of rural residents, and 2.65 times the mortality of rural dwellers for tumors. These differences persisted even after adjusting for variables such as age, race, sex, education, income, and marital and health status (House et al., 2000). Other authors, however, note no significant differences in overall mortality for rural and urban populations (Ricketts, Johnson-Webb, & Randolph, 1999).

For specific causes of death, though, there are distinct differences between rural and urban populations. For example, mortality related to HIV/AIDS is known to be higher in urban than rural areas, whereas rural residents have higher rates of diabetes mortality and infant and maternal mortality (Chase-Ziolek & Striepe, 1999; Slifkin, Goldsmith, & Ricketts, 2000). Again, these findings vary somewhat among subpopulations, with African American rates for infant mortality lower for rural than urban residents, but much higher for rural American Indian/Alaskan Natives than those in urban areas (23.1 deaths per 1,000 live births in rural areas compared to 14.7 deaths per 1,000 births in urban areas). Similarly, overall mortality for cardiovascular diseases is lower in rural than urban populations, but among Native Americans, mortality is higher for rural residents (Slifkin et al., 2000).

With respect to illness morbidity, more disease seems to be noted in rural than urban populations. Rural areas have been reported as having higher prevalences of hypertension, coronary heart disease, emphysema (Henly, Tyree, Lindsey, Lambeth, & Burd, 1998), diabetes, and HIV infection. Although HIV infection rates remain lower overall in rural than urban areas, recently they have been rising at a faster rate, particularly among rural women, adolescents, and migrant and seasonal workers (Slifkin et al., 2000). In addition, growing numbers of HIV/AIDS cases in rural areas place enormous strain on existing rural health care systems (Anderko & Uscian, 2000).

Disease rates are increasing among many rural minority populations. For example, rural African Americans have higher rates for asthma prevalence than urban dwellers. Conversely, African Americans in urban areas have higher prostate cancer mortality rates than their rural counterparts. High rates of dental caries have been particularly noticeable among rural and Hispanic children (Mueller, Ortega, Parker, Patil, & Askenazi, 1999).

Significant rates of parasitic diseases have been found in rural populations, ranging from 11% to 20% of migrant workers and their families. These high rates are due to lack of access to sanitation facilities, poor housing, and limited education, and seem to be more common among foreign-born workers (Bechtel, 1998).

As noted earlier, rural elderly have poorer self-reported health than older persons living in urban areas. Similarly, rural residents tend to have more functional impairments (Denham, Quinn, & Gamble, 1998; Johnson, 1998). In one study, almost half of rural elderly reported no social support and most had no one to depend on for assistance with functional abilities. These factors, coupled with loss of one's driver's license, increase social isolation among rural elderly people and increase the potential for disabling effects of health impairments.

Injury is a source of both morbidity and mortality in rural and urban populations. Rural injury mortality is 40% higher than in urban areas (U.S. Department of Health and Human Services [USDHHS], 2001). Many of these injuries occur in the context of agricultural occupations. Over the last 50 years, considerable reductions have been made in what are considered urban occupational fatalities related to mining and construction, but little progress has been made in reducing agricultural injuries or fatalities (Schenker, 1995). From 1995 to 1997, more than 117,000 agriculture-related injuries were treated in U.S. emergency departments, with a rate of injury of 1.6 per 100 full-time equivalent employees (Division of Safety Research, 1998). Similarly, the rate of back injury with lost work days was 75.1 per 10,000 full-time agricultural workers (Division of Surveillance, Hazard Evaluations, and Field Studies, 1999a).

Unintentional occupational injuries and fatalities in the urban setting tend to occur in the areas of manufacturing, construction, and transportation and public utilities. Workplace violence also occurs more commonly among members of primarily urban occupations such as taxi drivers and law enforcement (U.S. Census Bureau, 1999).

The final area of assessment of rural and urban health related to the biophysical dimension is that of immunization levels within the population. Oddly enough, there is no consistent difference between settings. Rural residents tend to have slightly higher rates of childhood immunizations than urban dwellers, but older urban residents are more likely than their rural counterparts to be immunized for influenza or pneumonia, particularly among minority groups (Slifkin et al., 2000).

Psychological Considerations

In assessing an urban or rural population, the community health nurse will examine factors in the psychological dimension that influence population health. Actual rural and urban prevalences of mental health problems are probably similar, although rural residents may have slightly lower prevalences of affective disorders (Hartley, Bird, & Demosey, 1999), particularly within minority groups (Mueller et al., 1999). Residents in both areas are subjected to considerable levels of stress. For example, the rural farm population is faced with financial uncertainty, intense time pressures at certain seasons, uncertain weather, and intergenerational conflict that may lead to problems in interpersonal relationships, substance abuse, family violence, and suicide, although the prevalences of these outcomes are no higher than those seen in urban settings (Schenker, 1995). Conversely, it is hypothesized that stressful conditions in urban areas, such as increased noise levels, sensory stimulation and overload, interpersonal conflict, and the vigilance needed regarding crime victimization and accidents, may also contribute to mental health problems (House et al., 2000).

Areas in which differences do exist include the adequacy of mental health services and suicide rates. Rural mental health services are far less adequate than those available in urban areas (Elnitsky & Alexy, 1998). For example, 96% of metropolitan counties have available mental health services compared to only 80% of nonmetropolitan counties. Similarly, nonmetropolitan areas have lower rates of inpatient psychiatric beds (36 per 100,000 population compared to 49 per 100,000 in urban

areas) and psychiatrists (3.9 per 100,000 people versus 14.6 in urban areas) (Hartley et al., 1999).

Finally, rural areas have higher suicide mortality rates than urban settings. In 1995, for example, the nonmetropolitan suicide rate was 17.94 per 100,000 adults compared to 14.91 per 100,000 in urban areas. Similarly, adolescent suicide rates were higher in rural than metropolitan populations (7.45 per 100,000 and 5.6 per 100,000 adolescents, respectively) (Hartley et al., 1999).

Physical Environmental Considerations

Both the built and natural environments affect health status. The *built environment* consists of buildings, spaces, and products created or modified significantly from their natural state by people (Hancock, 2000). The *natural environment* involves natural features of the area, including plant and animal life, terrain, and so on. The community health nurse assessing the health status of a particular rural or urban population would consider the effects of both the built and natural environments and interactions between them on the health of the population.

Differences between the built and natural environments are perhaps the most obvious differences between rural and urban settings. Elements of the built environment are probably more significant influences on health than those of the natural environment in urban settings. Health risks in the urban environment include noise exposures, crowding, and increased potential for environmental pollutants such as air pollution and heavy metals. For example, low-income inner-city children have seven times the risk for elevated blood lead levels as children in other areas (Fitzpatrick, 2000). Central urban areas, however, have the advantage of being more energy efficient than rural or suburban areas. In fact, "suburban sprawl" has been described as being both wasteful of space needed for agricultural purposes and of energy in terms of the need to commute between widely separated residential, commercial, and industrial centers. Carbon monoxide emission levels increase threefold with movement from center city to suburban fringe areas due to motor vehicle use. Urban areas, on the other hand, have been touted as safer in terms of accidents since the accident fatality rate involved for public transit is one twentieth the rate associated with personal automobile use. In addition, urban centers encourage exercise when destinations are within walking distance and contribute to less social isolation than more sparsely settled areas (Hancock, 2000).

In rural settings, the natural environment contributes to a variety of health risks with fewer risks from the built environment. The presence of plants and wild and domesticated animals in the rural environment contribute to the potential for zoonoses (diseases transmitted from animals to people), and plant and animal allergens (National Center for Infectious Diseases, 2001). Dust and extreme weather conditions are other significant aspects of the natural environment in the rural setting that have health consequences. In addition, hilly or steep terrain

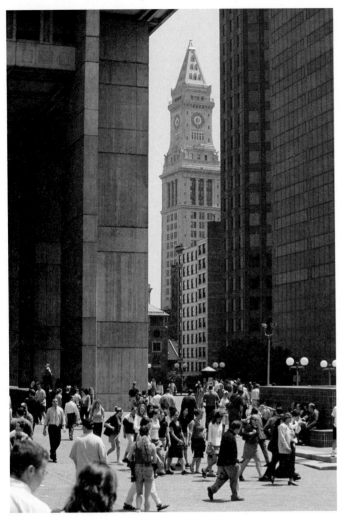

Crowding in urban areas can increase stress, leading to a variety of health effects.

and sinkholes in agricultural areas increase the potential for tractor rollovers, the most common cause of agricultural fatalities (Browning, Westneat, Truszczynska, Reed, & McKnight, 1999). These elements of the natural environment are compounded by features of the built environment when tractors are not equipped with rollover protection and other safety devices. Terrain and its effects on the design of highways combined with great distances to emergency services also contribute to the high incidence of motor vehicle accident fatalities in rural areas.

As noted in Chapter 20, deteriorated housing and lack of affordable housing may affect the health of urban residents, contributing to high levels of homelessness. In rural areas, this component is more apt to reflect the effects of substandard housing that is in poor repair, particularly among the elderly (Griffin, 1999).

The built environment also contributes to health risks in the rural area in the use of pesticides and other chemicals used in agriculture. Improper use of such chemicals and failure to follow safety instructions have resulted in human exposures to toxic and carcinogenic substances (Division of Surveillance, Hazard Evaluations, and Field

Studies, 1999b). Exposure to high noise levels also occurs as a result of some aspects of the built rural environment. In one study, for example, 75% of cabless tractors were found to produce noise levels above the threshold for hearing impairment (Schenker, 1995).

Finally, the built and natural elements combine to create sources of water pollution in rural areas. As noted in Chapter 7, agricultural runoff contaminated with chemical pesticides and heavy metals pollutes drinking water sources as well as local lakes and rivers. According to the Environmental Protection Agency, 91% of drinking water violations involve small water systems serving 25 to 3,300 people, many of which exist in rural areas (USDHHS, 2001).

Sociocultural Considerations

Differences in sociocultural dimension factors between rural and urban settings, while not as immediately obvious as physical environmental factors, are nevertheless quite influential in their effects on population health status. Areas to be considered in assessing rural and urban populations include social values and conditions, economic issues, cultural factors, occupational factors, and factors related to health knowledge and values.

Rural cultures have been described as high-context cultures in which people experience sustained interactions with others. Urban cultures, on the other hand, are low-context cultures in which individuals are more socially isolated and experience greater mobility and frequent changes in relationships (Chase-Ziolek & Striepe, 1999). Urban and rural areas also differ in terms of the potential number of social ties, which are likely to be more numerous in urban areas due to population density (Fitzpatrick, 2000).

Despite the enduring nature of interpersonal relationships in rural settings, long distances and lack of public transportation may lead to social isolation, particularly among the elderly. In addition, the consolidation of many rural schools increases the distance traveled by children to attend and decreases both family time and community involvement (Griffin, 1999).

Rural residents are more likely than urban dwellers to be married and tend to adhere to traditional gender roles. People in urban and rural settings also differ in terms of the likelihood of exposure to strangers and exposure to unconventional norms, including gender norms. Urban areas are more heterogeneous in their population and residents are more likely to be exposed to attitudes and values different from their own (Fitzpatrick, 2000). Depending on the context of these encounters, they may lead to greater tolerance of differences or exhibitions of prejudice and discrimination.

Sustained interpersonal relationships in rural settings lead to the development of trust and informal support networks. These relationships may also result in the lack of anonymity and privacy discussed earlier and lead to less help seeking for problems one does not want known by one's neighbors (Bull, 1998). Urban society, on the

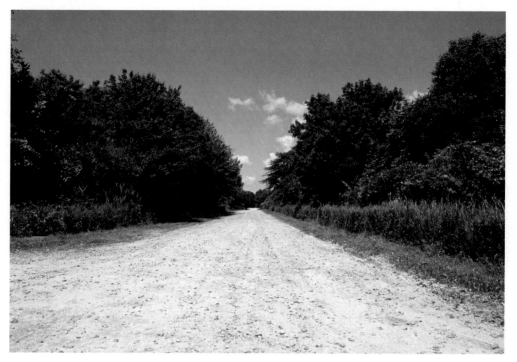

Great distances on poor roads may prevent rural residents from obtaining optimal health care.

other hand, may be characterized by stimulus overload and increasing complexity of interpersonal interactions that may result in a sense of "diffused responsibility" or failure to respond in the face of another's obvious need. Urban residents are twice as likely as rural dwellers to be victims of violence, and murder rates are three times higher in inner city areas than in areas of less population density (Fitzpatrick, 2000). Urban residents generally have less support available from extended family members due to high population mobility (Chase-Ziolek & Striepe, 1999).

Poverty affects health in both urban and rural settings, but those in rural areas are more likely to be poor than their urban counterparts. Rural minorities are three times as likely to be poor as Caucasians (Slifkin et al., 2000). Suburbanites, in particular, are more likely to be better

Threats to personal safety and crime victimization are common problems in many inner city areas.

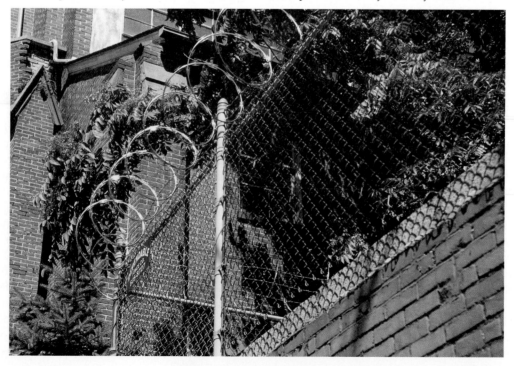

educated and have higher incomes than either rural or inner-city residents (House et al., 2000).

Overall, 16% of rural residents are poor, and the rural population accounts for 27% of the poor in the United States. Half of the 9.1 million nonmetropolitan poor are children and older people. Annual income in rural areas decreases with age, and 28% of rural people over 85 years of age have incomes below poverty level, compared to 24% of those aged 80 to 84 years and 12% of those 60 to 64 (Bull, 1998). In 1990, 11% of the farm population had incomes below poverty level, and 36% of farm children and 11% of elderly were poor. African Americans are disproportionately represented among the farm poor, constituting one third of farm families at poverty level even though they comprise only 6% of the farm population (Wright et al., 1998). Migrant and seasonal farm workers are even worse off, with half of this group below the poverty level. The median family income for seasonal and migrant workers ranges from $7,500 to $10,000 compared to incomes of more than $50,000 for 50% of farm operators and over $100,000 for 25% of this group (Schenker, 1995). Recent changes in immigration laws have made many farm workers ineligible for social services such as Medicaid, WIC, and food stamps, which are available to other poor populations (Ricketts et al., 1999).

The economic situation of migrant workers is further complicated by political inequities. Despite the fact that 80% of migrant workers are U.S. citizens, they are not covered by the National Labor Relations Act, which governs minimum wages. They are also excluded from workers' compensation and unemployment insurance programs in many states (Hibbeln, 1996). Inequities also occur for other segments of the rural population. For example, rural elders have been shown to receive Social Security benefits 10% lower than those residing in urban areas, and some rural elders are not covered at all, having retired from occupations that are not covered by Social Security.

As described in Chapter 20, significant poverty also exists in urban settings, and urban poor families are more likely to be headed by single females than those in rural areas. Rates of homelessness due to poverty and other factors are higher in urban than in rural areas, but the number of homeless people in rural settings is increasing. Rural homeless are apt to be less visible because of the lack of social services and shelters where they might congregate. The rural homeless are also more likely than their urban counterparts to double or triple up in housing with family or friends, increasing their virtual invisibility. Homeless people in rural areas are more likely to be married and to be homeless due to poverty than to mental illness or substance abuse than the urban homeless population (Wright et al., 1998).

Urban settings are more culturally diverse than rural settings, which can be both an advantage and a disadvantage depending on the character of relationships among population groups. Foreign-born persons are more likely to reside in urban than rural settings, and 11% of the

urban population in the United States is foreign-born compared to only 2% of rural residents. Despite traditional resettlement of immigrants and refugees in urban areas, a significant proportion of this population is now migrating to rural areas (Ricketts et al., 1999). Because these immigrants tend to have more health-related needs than their U.S.-born counterparts, they are placing considerable strain on rural health care systems that are already overburdened (Slifkin et al., 2000).

Occupational issues in urban settings are similar to those discussed in Chapter 24. Primary occupations in rural areas include agriculture, mining and other extractive industries, and manufacturing. Agricultural occupations are of two types: agricultural production and agricultural services. Agricultural production encompasses general farming and ranching; agricultural services occupations include custom crop and animal care, horticulture, and landscaping (National Ag Safety Database, 1996).

The primary differences between agricultural occupations and other rural and urban occupations is the absence of regulatory efforts. The Occupational Health and Safety Act of 1970 excluded agricultural workplaces, and this exclusion led to great differences in federal spending for health and safety in rural and urban settings. For example, in 1985, the U.S. federal government spent $181 per miner compared to 30 cents for each agricultural worker (Schenker, 1995). Exclusion from OSHA also means that occupational health and safety regulations are unenforceable on 95% of U.S. farms. In addition, children engaged in work on family farms are not covered by the Fair Labor Standards Act of 1938, which leaves them at risk for hazardous working conditions and injury (Division of Safety Research, 1999). Another disparity lies in the fact that workers' compensation programs do not apply to rural workers in many states (Schenker, 1995).

The last sociocultural dimension factor to be considered in assessing factors influencing health in rural and

CULTURAL CONSIDERATIONS

Traditionally, refugee and immigrant families enter the United States through major metropolitan areas, and the large majority of them remain in these or similar urban centers throughout the country. More recently, however, some refugee groups have begun to relocate to more rural areas. For example, many Laotian Hmong families have moved from San Diego to areas of North Carolina.

- What do you think might be some of the reasons for this migration?
- What are the social implications of an in-migration of such a unique cultural group such as the Hmong into the rural culture of the Southeast?
- What are the implications for community health systems in the North Carolina area?

ETHICAL AWARENESS

Research has indicated that operation of heavy farm machinery—particularly tractors—by children is a serious risk factor for fatal injury. In your rural community, you are aware of several farm families whose use of children in this capacity places them at very high risk. This occurs primarily on small family farms where much of the machinery in use is aging and is not equipped with more modern safety devices, such as rollover protection on tractors. Would you become involved in political activity to ban operation of farm machinery by children under 16 years of age? Why or why not? If not, what other action might you take to protect these children?

urban settings, lies in differences in the definitions of health and illness espoused by rural and urban residents (Mueller et al., 1999). Definitions of health and illness differ widely in urban groups due to the greater heterogeneity of the population as well as greater cultural diversity. Rural definitions tend to be more homogeneous, reflecting a perception that health is synonymous with the ability to work (Earle & Burman, 1998). This definition may lead rural residents to give work needs a higher priority than health needs and to put off seeking health care until conditions become severe. The self-reliance characteristic of rural culture, while often a strength, may also lead to rejection of needed health care services (Bull, 1998). Rural residents also tend to get fewer preventive health services than urban residents. For example, rural children get less well-child care than urban children, with the exception of immunizations (Earle & Burman, 1998).

Residents of rural areas may also have less education and health knowledge than their urban counterparts. In one study, for example, employees in small rural companies had less knowledge of cardiovascular risk factors than those in small urban companies and were less likely to have had any previous screening for risk factors. The absence of preventive programs is due to the lack of an economic base for prevention programs, economic barriers, and inaccessible or nonexistent health services (Williams & Wold, 2000).

Behavioral Considerations

Rural and urban populations also differ with respect to elements of the behavioral dimension as they affect health status. Areas for the community health nurse to consider in assessing a specific rural or urban population include diet, use of tobacco, use of alcohol and other drugs, physical activity, sexual activity, and health-related behaviors.

With respect to diet, rural residents are more likely than their urban counterparts to be overweight (19% of rural populations versus 15% of urban populations),

while urban populations have a slightly greater prevalence of underweight (5.4% versus 5%) (House et al., 2000). Rural and urban populations may also differ in terms of meal patterns, particularly in the case of rural farm families who may plan meals in the traditional pattern connected with the workday, with the heaviest meal at noon. Urban families and nonfarm rural families are more likely to eat their largest meal in the evening.

Adequate nutrition may be particularly problematic for migrant farm workers, who may rely on significant amounts of convenience foods while working and who have limited budgets for providing adequate diets. In addition, English language difficulties may force many families to rely on children to read labels and make food choices, with children selecting foods with high sugar content and few vegetables and fruits. The absence of adequate refrigeration and cooking facilities may further hamper efforts to provide adequate family nutrition. Common health problems in migrant workers with nutritional deficits include anemia, diabetes, obesity, and cardiovascular disease (Hibbeln, 1996).

Tobacco use rates tend to be lower in rural populations than in urban settings, particularly for farm workers (House et al., 2000). The extent of cigarette smoking among rural youth, however, is comparable to that found in urban youth, with approximately 63% of twelfth graders in one study reporting cigarette use in both rural and urban areas. Rural youth, on the other hand, are more likely than their urban counterparts to use smokeless tobacco (40% and 32.5%, respectively) (Clark, Savitz, & Randolph, 1999).

Urban populations have higher rates of use of alcohol and most illegal drugs with the exception of crack cocaine among rural youth. Although overall alcohol use among youth is comparable, rural youth report more involvement with heavy drinking than urban youth (Clark et al., 1999). Among young adults 19 to 32 years of age, more urban residents consume alcohol and report use of marijuana, stimulants, and cocaine than those in rural settings. The only exception to the trend of higher use in urban residents in this age group was cigarettes, where rural populations had higher reported use (Hartley et al., 1999).

In assessing the extent of tobacco and other drug use, the community health nurse should also examine the interactions between these consumption patterns and other features of rural and urban settings. For example, use of alcohol combined with poor rural roads increases the risk of motor vehicle fatalities. Similarly, tobacco use may interact with a variety of urban and rural occupational hazards to increase the risk of multiple health problems.

In the 1996 Behavioral Risk Factor Surveillance Survey, urban areas reported the lowest levels of leisure-time physical inactivity, and rural areas reported the highest levels. Differences between physical inactivity in rural and urban areas were greater for men (12%) than for women (6.7%). Overall, approximately one third of rural residents in that study reported no leisure-time physical activity, possibly related to the older age, lower education level, and lower income of those surveyed in rural areas (National Center for Chronic Disease Prevention and Health Promotion, 1998). 1997 data indicated that 43% of rural populations engaged in no leisure-time physical activity compared to only 39% of urban residents (USDHHS, 2000).

Recent research also indicates a high level of risk behaviors for sexually transmitted diseases in rural communities. Rural high school students in one study reported low perceived risk of HIV infection and limited access to prevention information and displayed limited knowledge of risk factors and condom negotiation skills (Anderko & Uscian, 2000). In another study, rural adolescents reported limited access to contraceptives and few concerns about sexually transmitted disease (STD) exposures, although they did express some concerns about becoming pregnant (Puskar, Tusaie-Mumford, Sereika, & Lamb, 1999). The southern United States accounted for 54% of rural AIDS through 1997, although these rates remain lower than those in southern metropolitan areas. High incidence rates in these rural areas are linked to use of crack cocaine and the exchange of sex for drugs (National Center for HIV, STD, and TB Prevention, 1998). Community health nurses should assess the extent of high-risk sexual behaviors as well as the prevalence of unwanted pregnancy and STDs in both urban and rural populations.

Health-related behaviors are the final behavioral consideration in assessing the health of rural or urban populations. As noted earlier, rural residents tend not to receive preventive health care. In part, this is the result of lack of access to convenient services, but also reflects the definition of health as the ability to work. Rural residents have also been shown to be less likely than their urban counterparts to engage in health-promotive behaviors. For example, 81% of rural adolescents in one study reported never engaging in testicular self-examination or breast self-examination (Puskar et al., 1999). Rural residents have also been found to be less likely to engage in safety practices in the work setting (Griffin, 1999). As noted earlier, older persons in rural settings are also less likely to receive influenza and pneumonia immunizations than those in urban areas, and older rural women are less likely than their urban counterparts to receive mammograms or Papanicolaou smears (Slifkin et al., 2000). Younger rural women may also be less likely to obtain prenatal care than those in urban areas (Denham et al., 1998). Lack of attention to preventive services is even more pronounced in the migrant farm worker population. For example, in one study in Michigan, less than 1% of office visits for migrant children one to four years of age were for health promotion services compared to 34% of visits for nonmigrant children of the same age. Farm workers, in general, receive more care for acute diseases and less care for chronic conditions or health promotion (Schenker, 1995).

Health System Considerations

Significant differences in health care systems in rural and urban areas influence the health of populations in these settings. Areas for consideration in assessing this dimension of health include the availability of and access to health care services, barriers to service use, and the influence of health policies and delivery systems on population health.

Health care services for many rural residents are less accessible, more costly to deliver, narrower in range and scope, and fewer in number than those available to their urban counterparts. This is true for most professional services including those of physicians, dentists, nurses, and social workers and is particularly true of services for the elderly in rural areas.

Nearly three fourths (70%) of federally designated medically underserved areas in the United States are rural, and there is a lack of both basic and specialty health care services in these areas (Griffin, 1999). According to the U.S. Health Resources and Services Administration (HRSA), 40% of rural residents, or 20 million people, lack access to care (*The Nation's Health*, 1999). From 1989 to 1994, the number of rural residents living in primary care shortage areas increased by 4 million (Wysong, Bliss, Osborne, Graham, & Pikuzinski, 1999). Access to care is limited by the availability of providers, long distances to services, lack of health insurance and lower economic levels, lack of a local tax base to support services, and inabilities to use economies of scale to decrease the costs of care (Bull, 1998). For example, rural providers or health care agencies cannot entertain bids from multiple vendors for supplies and equipment because there is frequently only one vendor available.

There is a severe shortage of health care providers in many rural areas. Factors contributing to the difficulty of attracting providers to rural areas include poor Medicare reimbursement, differences between general practice and specialty reimbursement rates, professional isolation, and heavy workloads for the few providers in the area (Baldwin et al., 1998). Although 20% of the U.S. population resides in rural areas, only 9% of physicians practice in these areas (Rosenblatt & Hart, 1999). On average, in 1995, rural counties typically had far fewer physicians per 100,000 population in all categories except family practice/general practice than urban areas. The relative rates of physician coverage in rural and urban areas are presented in Table 25–1 ■. As can be seen in the table, with the exception of family/general practice, rural areas have less than half as many physicians in basic practice areas and less than a third of the number of specialists as urban areas. The lack of access to specialty providers is also seen in the fact that 72% of rural visits are to family or general practitioners compared to only 63% of urban residents where specialists are more widely accessible.

Similar disparities between urban and rural settings are noted with respect to the availability of mental health services. For example, in urban areas there are 14.6

■ **TABLE 25–1**   Rates of Physician Coverage per 100,000 Population by Specialty in Urban and Rural Areas, 1995

SPECIALTY	URBAN	RURAL
Family/general practice	26.1	28.1
General internal medicine	35.4	11.8
General pediatrics	17.5	5.2
General obstetrics/gynecology	13.7	5.1
General surgery	14.6	7.6
Other specialties	134.1	40.1

psychiatrists per 100,000 population compared to 3.9 per 100,000 in rural settings. In addition, 96% of metropolitan counties have mental health services available compared to only 80% of nonmetropolitan counties. Rural areas also have a lower inpatient psychiatric bed rate per 100,000 population (36) than urban areas (49 per 100,000) (Hartley, et al., 1999).

In addition to the shortage of physician providers faced by rural residents in general, members of minority populations in rural settings frequently do not have access to providers who understand their cultures and backgrounds. The problems of recruiting Caucasian providers to rural areas are compounded for ethnic minority providers, who may be faced with lack of acceptance and an even greater perception of being "outsiders" (Mueller et al., 1999).

Nursing shortages are also more acute in rural than urban areas. For example, vacancies for staff nursing positions take approximately 60% longer to fill in rural than urban settings. In addition, rural nurses receive lower wages, and many spouses have difficulty finding work in rural areas. Some nurses are also daunted by the breadth of knowledge required for generalist practice in rural areas as well as by the relative lack of access to further education (Tone, 1999). The outlook is somewhat better for advanced practice nurses (APNs) in rural settings, however, and APNs (and physician assistants) have been suggested as a means of increasing the number of primary care providers in rural areas (Shaw, 1997). In 1996, for example, the ratio of nurse practitioners per 100,000 population was nearly 25 in rural areas compared to 20 in urban settings. Similarly, ratios of nurse anesthetists were 11 per 100,000 population in rural areas and 9.7 in urban areas, while there were 2.5 nurse midwives per 100,000 in rural areas and 1.9 in urban areas. Physician assistants, on the other hand, are more evenly distributed with 11.9 per 100,000 population in rural areas and 11.6 in urban areas (Baer & Smith, 1999). APNs also receive better salaries in rural than urban areas, but may have to contend with greater resistance from more traditional physicians than their urban counterparts (Tone, 1999).

Health care in rural areas is also influenced by the relatively great distances to facilities and the lack of specialized facilities to meet particular needs (e.g., facilities for cancer therapy). Furthermore, small rural hospitals are at

CRITICAL THINKING IN RESEARCH

Boerma, Groenewegen, and van der Zee (1998) conducted a study of the practice patterns of primary care physicians (general practitioners) in rural and urban areas in 30 European countries. They found that physicians in rural areas provided more comprehensive services than those in urban areas regardless of the type of health care system in which they functioned.

• How might you go about conducting a study of the practice patterns of rural and urban nurses?

• Would you use a quantitative or qualitative research methodology? Why?

• How would you recruit your study participants? What inclusion and exclusion criteria would you use for identifying potential subjects? Why would you use the particular criteria selected?

• What kinds of differences do you think you might find in the interventions employed by rural and urban nurses? How would you determine if your assumptions are accurate?

risk for low patient census and closure, further reducing availability of services. From 1980 to 1989, for example, 237 rural hospitals closed, and more than two thirds of hospital closures between 1986 and 1989 occurred in rural areas (Wysong et al., 1999). Limited emergency services and long distances to health care facilities contribute to higher accidental injury mortality rates in rural settings.

Even when health facilities and providers are available, people in rural areas may have more difficulty making use of them than those in urban settings. Distance has already been mentioned as a barrier to health care. Other barriers that are relevant to both urban and rural residents, but are often more prevalent in rural areas, include cost and inconvenience (Earle & Burman, 1998). Rural residents are less likely than their urban counterparts to be insured. Approximately 20% of rural populations are uninsured compared to 16% of those in urban areas. People in rural areas are also more likely than those in urban settings to report delaying care because of cost (10% versus 8%) (Schur & Franco, 1999).

Many rural workers, especially those involved in agriculture, do not have "sick days" and may be unable to take time from work to obtain health care during the hours when facilities are typically open. In one study, mothers of young children cited inconvenience of hours as one of five reasons for not obtaining preventive services for children. Lack of child care and lack of transportation were also reported as barriers to obtaining care (Earle & Burman, 1998).

Managed care has been suggested as a means of increasing the availability of health care services in rural areas, but the promise of this potential solution has yet to be realized. The Health Maintenance Organization (HMO) Act of 1993 set aside 20% of HMO grant funds for rural HMOs. During the first five years of the program's operation, however, only 42 rural projects were funded and 22 of those failed primarily because populations were not sufficiently dense to provide a viable income for the organizations (Wysong et al., 1999).

Despite these setbacks, managed care organizations (MCOs) have made some inroads in rural areas. By 1995, 82% of all counties were within the service area of at least one HMO. At that time, only 14 HMOs were headquartered in rural areas and rural residents comprised only 2.4% of all HMO enrollment in the United States (Wysong et al., 1999). Movement to MCO enrollment for Medicare and Medicaid beneficiaries may increase rural MCO involvement. The Balanced Budget Act of 1997 mandated a new payment scale for Medicare managed care enrollees, which has increased considerably Medicare reimbursement for rural areas. Reimbursement rates, however, are not expected to equal those in urban areas, somewhat decreasing the incentive for MCOs to recruit rural participants. Among counties in the lowest quartile for Medicare reimbursement rates, 92% are rural counties and only 8% are urban (Schoenman, 1999).

Eight states collect HMO enrollment data that permits examination of enrollment figures based on urban or rural residence. In 1995, rural enrollment in HMOs was less than 10% for all but two of these states, and in those states less than 20% of the population were enrolled in HMOs. At the national level, only 10.5% of rural Medicaid recipients are enrolled in MCOs compared to 27% of urban recipients, and in 26 states no rural Medicaid enrollees were involved in MCOs (Moscovice, Casey, & Krein, 1998). In 1998, only 2.6% of rural Medicare recipients were enrolled in MCOs. Roughly 92% of the rural elderly had no access to managed care and only 79% of those in areas adjacent to metropolitan areas had access (Casey, 1999). Urban use of managed care plans is reflected in information presented in Chapter 5.

Urban MCO models may not be appropriate to rural areas. For example, a follow-up study of rural Medicaid managed care enrollment in 10 states indicated that in order for rural managed care to be effective certain conditions needed to be created. These conditions are summarized below.

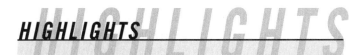

Conditions for Effective Rural Managed Care Systems

- Time to build a provider network that accounts for local use patterns and incorporates local providers already known to the population
- Time to increase rural providers' experience with captitated funding
- Development of effective communication networks with providers
- Accommodation of rural resident's use of mid-level practitioners such as nurse practitioners, rural health clinics, and so on
- Assistance with arrangements for 24-hour coverage for solo providers
- Development of reasonable travel guidelines to obtain services
- Mandates related to maximum distance to specialty care to prevent existing local providers from being excluded

Source: Felt-Lisk, S., Silberman, P., Hoag, S., & Slifkin, R. (1999). Medicaid managed care in rural areas: A ten-state follow-up study. *Health Affairs, 18,* 238–245.

DIAGNOSTIC REASONING AND CARE OF CLIENTS IN URBAN AND RURAL SETTINGS

In rural areas, the etiology of nursing diagnoses is frequently related to a lack of resources and limited access to health care in the community. A nursing diagnosis of "potential for poor infant outcome due to three-hour travel time to nearest maternity delivery service" is common in today's rural health system and requires that the rural nurse providing prenatal care be most astute in assessing this client during her pregnancy. A second nursing diagnosis might be "increased suicide risk due to lack of access to mental health services." Again, this diagnosis is attributable to limited access to health care.

Nursing diagnoses developed for urban populations might also reflect unique factors affecting health in that setting. As an example, the nurse might make a diagnosis of "lack of physical activity due to fear of walking in high crime neighborhoods." Another diagnosis related to urban populations might be "potential for hearing loss among children in schools adjacent to airport."

PLANNING AND IMPLEMENTING CARE IN URBAN AND RURAL SETTINGS

Nursing interventions in rural and urban settings can be directed toward meeting the needs of individual clients, families, or population groups. Community health nurses play pivotal roles in planning intervention strategies for urban and rural populations.

Overall goals for care in urban and rural settings are similar and include:

- Increasing access to health care services and decreasing barriers to their use
- Eliminating or modifying environmental risk factors
- Modifying social conditions that adversely affect health

- Increasing clients' abilities to make informed health decisions
- Developing systems of care that are population appropriate
- Developing equitable health care policies that address the diverse needs of urban and rural populations

Although the goals of care are similar for rural and urban populations, the means by which they are accomplished may be quite different. For example, increasing access to health care in rural settings may revolve primarily around increasing the number and variety of available providers or changing reimbursement rates to attract providers to rural areas. In both urban and rural settings, increasing access may involve dealing with problems of cost, increasing insurance coverage, and developing systems that provide low-cost quality health care to these populations.

Interventions designed to decrease barriers to use of health care services may also differ significantly between urban and rural settings. For example, in urban settings, actions may be needed to increase the ability of providers to communicate with clients from multiple ethnic groups and cultures. With the movement of immigrants to rural areas, some actions along this line will be needed in rural settings as well, but providers are unlikely to be called on to communicate in multiple different languages and with multiple ethnic groups as occurs in urban areas. Decreasing barriers to care in rural settings may involve providing access to transportation services, changing times when services are provided, or finding creative ways to deliver services to great distances in cost-effective ways.

Activities to eliminate or modify environmental risks will also differ greatly between rural and urban settings. For example, skin cancer prevention education should be a high-priority focus among agricultural workers, while interventions to address high urban noise levels or reduce violent crime and gang activity may be more appropriate to urban settings.

In urban settings, action to modify social factors that adversely affect health may involve assisting clients to develop support systems or linking them to available health and social services. Community health nurses may also be involved in activities to promote the availability of affordable housing or to decrease unemployment levels. In rural settings, more focus is needed on providing support and respite for members of informal care networks and changing attitudes to the need for and use of health care services, particularly preventive services.

⑥THINK ABOUT IT

In what ways might health promotion activities for rural populations differ from those designed for urban populations?

Increasing clients' abilities to make informed health decisions usually focuses on the type of decisions to be made and the health problems prevalent in the setting. For example, a rural community health nurse may focus on assisting clients with farm safety issues or use of preventive services. In the urban setting, on the other hand, community assessment data may suggest a need to focus on personal safety and crime prevention.

As noted earlier, the urban model of managed care may not be appropriate to meeting the needs of rural populations, and modified delivery systems may be required. Nurses may be involved in the development and implementation of creative modes of health care delivery in either urban or rural settings. For example, school-based clinics may be an effective mode of providing care in the urban environment. When children travel long distances to consolidated schools, however, the concept of the school as a central community structure that can support health services becomes less meaningful. It may be that parish nursing or some other form of locally based nursing services may be a more appropriate vehicle for delivering nursing services in rural areas.

Finally, community health nurses should be actively involved in developing and promoting national and state health care policies that are equitable and address the diverse needs of both urban and rural populations. For example, nurses may advocate for higher reimbursement rates for providers in rural settings or for other incentives that attract and retain providers in rural communities, or community health nurses might become involved in revisions to policies that prevent both rural and urban immigrants from having access to certain health and social services. Community health nurses working in either rural or urban settings may find a variety of additional sources of information helpful to them. Some of these sources can be accessed through links provided on the companion Web site for this book. ⊕

EVALUATING HEALTH CARE IN URBAN AND RURAL SETTINGS

Nurses providing services in rural and urban settings must evaluate the outcomes of care as well as its cost-effectiveness. One rural nursing clinic's evaluation of services is summarized on the companion Web site for this book. ⊕

Outcomes of care in rural and urban settings may also be evaluated in terms of the accomplishment of the national health objectives. Several of the Healthy People 2010 objectives deal with disparities in health care and health care outcomes between rural and urban populations. These objectives may be viewed on the Healthy People 2010 Web site, which may be accessed through the companion Web site for this book. Data regarding the status of some of these objectives are presented on page 599. ⊕

HEALTHY PEOPLE 2010

GOALS FOR THE POPULATION

Objective		Base	Target
1-1	Increase the proportion of people with health insurance:		
	Metropolitan Statistical Areas (MSAs)	86%	100%
	Non-MSAs	84%	100%
1-5	Increase the proportion of people with a usual primary care provider:		
	MSAs	76%	85%
	Non-MSAs	78%	85%
1-6	Reduce the proportion of families with difficulty in getting care (MSAs and non-MSAs)	12%	7%
7-6	Increase the proportion of employees who participate in employer-sponsored health promotion:		
	MSAs	27%	50%
	Non-MSAs	30%	50%
11-1	Increase the proportion of people with Internet at home:		
	MSAs	28%	80%
	Non-MSAs	22%	80%
20-2d	Reduce injuries in agriculture, forestry, and fishing (per 100 full-time workers over age 16)	7.9	5.5
22-1	Reduce the proportion of people with no leisure-time physical activity:		
	MSAs	39%	20%
	Non-MSAs	43%	20%

Source: U.S. Department of Health and Human Services. (2000). *Healthy people 2010* (Conference edition, in two volumes). Washington, DC: Author.

Community health nursing in urban and rural settings displays some similarities but many differences. Effective community health nurses will be aware of these similarities and differences and will develop health care interventions accordingly. They will recognize that, although a particular intervention has demonstrated effectiveness in one setting, that effectiveness may not translate to other settings.

APPLYING YOUR KNOWLEDGE IN PRACTICE

❧ CASE STUDY
Nursing in a Rural Setting

You are a rural community health nurse assigned to the county health department mobile van visiting a large migrant community at a local farm. Mr. Robert Kelbert is a 64-year-old African American migrant worker who comes into the mobile unit to have his blood pressure medication refilled. He will be in the county for the next 3 to 4 weeks to harvest the soybean crop. He usually attends a rural health clinic in the northern part of the state where he has been receiving his care and medications free.

Today, his blood pressure is 154/98, pulse 88, height 69 inches, and weight 198 pounds. He states he is "worn out" from the heat. He chews tobacco and drinks alcohol "some." He travels and stays with his son and family. His daughter-in-law does the cooking. During your interview, Mr. Kelbert tells you he is worried because two of the migrant workers have been given medicine for lung congestion and one of them has been coughing up blood.

- In what ways is Mr. Kelbert's situation typical of that of rural clients in general? Of migrant farm workers? In what ways is it different?

- What are some of the biophysical, psychological, physical environmental, sociocultural, behavioral, and health system factors operating in this situation?

- List three nursing diagnoses that you would identify for Mr. Kelbert.

- What are your objectives for today's client visit?

- How might your care for Mr. Kelbert differ from that provided to a client you see regularly at the rural health department?

- What primary, secondary, and tertiary prevention measures are appropriate for Mr. Kelbert?

- How will you follow up on this visit?

✿ TESTING YOUR UNDERSTANDING

- Discuss differences in the definitions of *rural* and *urban*. What implications do these definitions have for health care policy? For research? (pp. 586–587)

- What are some of the differences in factors that affect health in rural and urban settings? (pp. 589–597)

- In what two ways do inequities in health policy create barriers to health care in urban and rural settings? (pp. 595–597)

- What are the primary goals for nursing intervention in urban and rural settings? How might accomplishment of these goals differ between settings? (pp. 597–598)

REFERENCES

Anderko, L., & Uscian, M. (2000). The effectiveness of a community-level HIV/STD prevention program in a three-county rural area. *Family & Community Health, 23*(3), 46–58.

Anderson, J., & Yuhos, R. (1993). Health promotion in rural settings. *Nursing Clinics of North America, 28,* 145–155.

Baer, L. D., & Smith, L. M. (1999). Nonphysician professionals and rural America. In T. C. Ricketts III (Ed.), *Rural health in the United States* (pp. 52–60). New York: Oxford University Press.

Baldwin, K. A., Sisk, R. J., Watts, P., McCubbin, J., Brockschmidt, R., & Marion, L. N. (1998). Acceptance of nurse practitioners and physician assistants in meeting the perceived needs of rural communities. *Public Health Nursing, 15,* 389–397.

Bechtel, G. (1998). Parasitic infections among migrant farm families. *Journal of Community Health Nursing, 15,* 1–7.

Bigbee, J. L. (1993). The uniqueness of rural nursing. *Nursing Clinics of North America, 28,* 131–143.

Boerma, W. G. W., Groenewegen, P. P., & van der Zee, J. (1998). General practice in urban and rural Europe: The range of curative services. *Social Science and Medicine, 47,* 445–453.

Browning, S. R., Westneat, S. C., Truszczynska, H., Reed, D., & McKnight, R. (1999). Farm tractor safety in Kentucky, 1995. *Public Health Reports, 114,* 53–59.

Bull, C. N. (1998). Aging in rural communities. *National Forum, 72*(2), 38–41.

Casey, M. M. (1999). Rural managed care. In T. C. Ricketts III (Ed.), *Rural health in the United States* (pp. 113–118). New York: Oxford University Press.

Chase-Ziolek, M., & Striepe, J. (1999). A comparison of urban versus rural experiences of nurses volunteering to promote health in churches. *Public Health Nursing, 14,* 270–279.

Clark, S. J., Savitz, L. A., & Randolph, R. K. (1999). Rural children's health. In T. C. Ricketts III (Ed.), *Rural health in the United States* (pp. 150–158). New York: Oxford University Press.

Coburn, A. F., & Bolda, E. J. (1999). The rural elderly and long-term care. In T. C. Ricketts III (Ed.), *Rural health in the United States* (pp. 179–189). New York: Oxford University Press.

Denham, A., Quinn, S. C., & Gamble, D. (1998). Community organizing for health promotion in the rural South: An exploration of community competence. *Family & Community Health, 21*(1), 1–21.

Division of Safety Research, NIOSH. (1998). Youth agricultural work-related injuries treated in emergency departments—United States, October 1995–September 1997. *Morbidity and Mortality Weekly Report, 47,* 733–737.

Division of Safety Research, NIOSH. (1999). Childhood work-related agricultural fatalities—Minnesota, 1994–1997. *Morbidity and Mortality Weekly Report, 48,* 332–335.

Division of Surveillance, Hazard Evaluations, and Field Studies, NIOSH. (1999a). Back pain among persons working on small or family farms—Eight Colorado counties,

1993–1996. *Morbidity and Mortality Weekly Report, 48,* 301–304.

Division of Surveillance, Hazard Evaluations, and Field Studies, NIOSH. (1999b). Farm worker illness following exposure to carbofuran and other pesticides—Fresno County, California, 1998. *Morbidity and Mortality Weekly Report, 48,* 113–115.

Earle, L. P., & Burman, M. E. (1998). Benefits and barriers to well-child care: Perceptions of mothers in a rural state. *Public Health Nursing, 15,* 180–187.

Elnitsky, C., & Alexy, B. (1998). Identifying health status and health risks of older rural residents. *Journal of Community Health Nursing, 15*(2), 61–75.

Felt-Lisk, S., Silberman, P., Hoag, S., & Slifkin, R. (1999). Medicaid managed care in rural areas: A ten-state follow-up study. *Health Affairs, 18,* 238–245.

Fitzpatrick, K. M. (2000). *Unhealthy places.* New York: Routledge.

Griffin, J. (1999). Parish nursing in rural communities. In P. A. Solari-Twadell & M. A. McDermott (Eds.), *Parish nursing: Promoting whole person health within faith communities* (pp. 75–82). Thousand Oaks, CA: Sage.

Hancock, T. (2000). Healthy communities must also be sustainable communities. *Public Health Reports, 115,* 151–156.

Hartley, D., Bird, D. C., & Demosey, P. (1999). Rural mental health and substance abuse. In T. C. Ricketts III (Ed.), *Rural health in the United States* (pp. 159–178). New York: Oxford University Press.

Henly, S. J., Tyree, E. A., Lindsey, D. L., Lambeth, S. O., & Burd, C. M. (1998). Innovative perspectives on health services for vulnerable rural populations. *Family & Community Health, 21*(1), 22–31.

Hibbeln, J. A. U. (1996). Special populations: Hispanic migrant workers. In S. Torres (Ed.), *Hispanic voices: Hispanic health educators speak out.* New York: National League for Nursing.

House, J. S., Lepkowski, J. M., Williams, D. R., Mero, R. P., et al. (2000). Excess mortality among urban residents: How much, for whom, and why? *American Journal of Public Health, 90,* 1898–1904.

Johnson, J. E. (1998). Stress, social support, and health in frontier elders. *Journal of Gerontological Nursing, 24*(5), 29–35.

Long, K. A., & Weinert, C. (1998). Rural nursing: Developing the theory base. In H. J. Lee (Ed.), *Conceptual basis for rural nursing* (pp. 3–18). New York: Springer.

Moscovice, I., Casey, M., & Krein, S. (1998). Expanding rural managed care: Enrollment and prospects. *Health Affairs, 17,* 172–179.

Mueller, K. J., Ortega, S. T., Parker, K., Patil, K., & Askenazi, A. (1999). Health status and access to care among rural minorities. *Journal of Health Care for the Poor and Underserved, 10,* 230–249.

National Ag Safety Database. (1996). Agricultural Safety. Retrieved April 30, 2001, from the World Wide Web, *http://www.cdc.gov/niosh/nasd.*

National Center for Chronic Disease Prevention and Health Promotion. (1998). Self-reported physical inactivity by degree of urbanization—United States, 1996. *Morbidity and Mortality Weekly Report, 47,* 1097–1100.

National Center for HIV, STD, and TB Prevention. (1998). Risks for HIV infection among persons residing in rural areas and small cities—Selected sites, Southern United States, 1995–1996. *Morbidity and Mortality Weekly Report, 47,* 976–978.

National Center for Infectious Diseases. (2001). Outbreaks of *Escherichia coli* O157:H7 infections among children associated with farm visits—Pennsylvania and Washington, 2000. *Morbidity and Mortality Weekly Report, 50,* 293–297.

The Nation's Health. (1999). Rural hospitals receive means to improve care. *XXIX*(9), 24.

Puskar, K. R., Tusaie-Mumford, K., Sereika, S., & Lamb, J. (1999). Health concerns and risk behaviors of rural adolescents. *Journal of Community Health Nursing, 16,* 109–119.

Ricketts, T. C. III, Johnson-Webb, K., & Randolph, R. K. (1999). Populations and places in rural America. In T. C. Ricketts III (Ed.), *Rural health in the United States* (pp. 7–24). New York: Oxford University Press.

Rosenblatt, R. A., & Hart, L. G. (1999). Physicians and rural America. In T. C. Ricketts III (Ed.), *Rural health in the United States* (pp. 38–51). New York: Oxford University Press.

Scharff, J. E. (1998). The distinctive nature and scope of rural nursing practice: Philosophical bases. In H. J. Lee (Ed.), *Conceptual basis for rural nursing* (pp. 19–38). New York: Springer.

Schenker, M. B. (1995). Preventive medicine and health promotion are overdue in the agricultural workplace. *Wellness Lecture Series.* Davis, CA: University of California.

Schoenman, J. A. (1999). Impact of the BBA on Medicare HMO payments for rural areas. *Health Affairs, 18,* 244–254.

Schur, C. L., & Franco, S. J. (1999). Access to health care. In T. C. Ricketts III (Ed.), *Rural health in the United States* (pp. 25–37). New York: Oxford University Press.

Shaw, J. K. (1997). An assessment of two upstate New York rural counties to determine unmet needs of the Medicaid population. *Journal of the New York State Nurses Association, 28*(1), 12–15.

Slifkin, R. T., Goldsmith, L. J., & Ricketts, T. C. III. (2000). *Race and place: Urban–rural differences in health for racial and ethnic minorities.* Chapel Hill, NC: North Carolina Rural Health Research Program.

Tone, B. (1999). Going rural. *NurseWeek, 12*(6), 1, 8.

U.S. Census Bureau. (1999). *Statistical abstract of the United States, 1999* (119th ed.). Washington, DC: Author.

U.S. Census Bureau. (2000). *Urban and rural classification census 2000: Urban and rural criteria.* Retrieved May 30, 2001, from the World Wide Web, *www.census.gov/www/ua.*

U.S. Department of Health and Human Services. (2000). *Healthy people 2010* (Conference edition, in two volumes). Washington, DC: Author.

U.S. Department of Health and Human Services. (2001). Health equity benefits everyone. *Prevention Report, 15*(2), 1–2.

Weinert, C., & Boik, R. J. (1998). MSU rurality index: Development and evaluation. In H. J. Lee (Ed.), *Conceptual basis for rural nursing* (pp. 449–471). New York: Springer.

Williams, A., & Wold, J. (2000). Nurses, cholesterol, and small work sites: Innovative community intervention comparisons. *Family & Community Health, 23*(3), 59–75.

World Health Organization. (2000). *The world health report 2000: Health systems: Improving performance.* Geneva, Switzerland: Author.

Wright, J. D., Rubin, B. A., & Devine, J. A. (1998). *Beside the golden door: Policy, politics, and the homeless.* New York: Aldine de Gruyter.

Wysong, J. A., Bliss, M. K., Osborne, J. W., Graham, R. P., & Pikuzinski, D. A. (1999). Managed care in rural markets: Availability and enrollment. *Journal of Health Care for the Poor and Underserved, 10*(1), 72–84.

CARE OF CLIENTS IN CORRECTIONAL SETTINGS

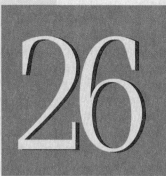

Chapter Objectives

After reading this chapter, you should be able to:

- Discuss the impetus for providing health care in correctional settings.
- Differentiate between basic and advanced nursing practice in correctional settings.
- Describe biophysical, psychological, physical environmental, sociocultural, behavioral, and health system factors that influence health in correctional settings.
- Identify major aspects of primary prevention in correctional settings.
- Describe approaches to secondary prevention in correctional settings.
- Discuss considerations in tertiary prevention in correctional settings.

KEY TERMS

detainees 604
jails 604
juvenile detention facilities 604
lockdown 617
lockup 611
prisons 604
search and seizure 617
TB prophylaxis 616

Media Link

http://www.prenhall.com/clark

Additional interactive resources for this chapter can be found on the companion Web site. Click on Chapter 26 and "Begin" to select the activities for this chapter.

Correctional facilities provide a relatively new practice setting for community health nursing compared to the settings discussed in previous chapters. Correctional nursing, however, is congruent with the primary focus of community health nursing—the health of groups of people—and offers a challenging position for the community health nurse who wishes to expand the frontiers of nursing practice (Hancock, 1999). Corrections nursing frequently involves challenges not encountered in other community health nursing settings. Practice in a correctional setting requires autonomy and excellent assessment skills. Nurses are often responsible for triaging inmates during sick call and identifying those who need to be seen by physicians, nurse practitioners, or other providers. Nurses may also provide routine treatments, including medication, under agency protocols. Nursing in correctional settings operates within the constraints of the security system, which may contribute to increased job stress and frustration. Another source of stress is the fear of litigation by a population that is prone to threats of law suits (Earley, 1999). Although there is some risk to the nurse's physical safety, many correctional nurses feel safer than they would in other settings such as emergency departments.

Another source of stress in the correctional setting is the potential for conflict between nursing values and those of corrections personnel. Some of the potential differences in values are presented below.

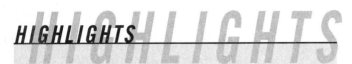

HIGHLIGHTS

Potential Values Differences between Nurses and Corrections Personnel

Nurse	Corrections Personnel
• Individualized care	• Treating all alike
• Health care as priority	• Security as priority
• Basic goodness of client	• Distrust and suspicion of motives
• Display of anger and hostility is normal in response to illness, fear, anxiety	• Display of anger and hostility is unacceptable and warrants a higher level of security
• Trusting relationship	• "Keeper/kept" relationship
• Confidentiality	• Sharing of information necessary for security
• Kindness	• Toughness

Source: Brodie, J. (2000). Caring—The essence of correctional nursing. *Correct Care,* 14(4), 1, 15, 18.

Correctional nursing takes place in three general types of facilities: prisons, jails, and juvenile detention facilities

(American Nurses Association [ANA], 1995). *Prisons* are state and federal facilities that house persons convicted of crimes, usually those sentenced for longer than one year. Municipal or county facilities are usually called *jails* and house both convicted inmates and detainees. Convicted inmates in jails are usually serving sentences under a year in length. *Detainees* are people who have not yet been convicted of a crime. They are being detained pending a trial either because they cannot pay the set bail or because no bail has been set. *Juvenile detention facilities* house children and adolescents convicted of crimes and those who are awaiting trial but who cannot be released in the custody of a responsible adult. Jails and juvenile detention facilities tend to be smaller and house fewer inmates than prisons.

Whatever the size of the facility or the terminology used, nurses working in correctional facilities must be committed to the belief that inmates retain their individual rights as human beings despite incarceration and that they have the same rights to health care as any other individual. Society does not categorically deprive any other group of individuals of access to adequate health care. In fact, there are carefully monitored standards of health care in such institutions as nursing homes, mental health facilities, and orphanages. It has only been as recently as 1979, however, that a program for accrediting health services in prisons was developed by the American Medical Association. Development of accreditation standards occurred at the request of the U.S. Department of Justice following a landmark court decision that depriving inmates of access to health care violated their civil rights (Stringer, 2001). Only since 1985 have published standards for nursing practice in such settings been available (ANA, 1985).

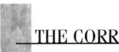

THE CORRECTIONAL POPULATION

In any given year, more than 2 million people are housed in correctional institutions. When those on probation are considered, a total of 6 million people (3% of the U.S. population) are under the jurisdiction of correctional systems (Conklin, Lincoln, & Tuthill, 2000). From 1990 to 2000, the number of people in U.S. prisons and jails increased by 68% (*Correct Care,* 2001b). On average, during most of this time, average growth in this population was 6.5% per year; however, the growth rate slowed to only 3.4% in 1999. In 1999, the rate of incarceration was 476 per 100,000 people. At the end of that year, more than 2 million people were incarcerated in the United States, 65% in federal and state prisons, 30% in local jails, 5% in juvenile facilities, and less than 1% each in territorial prisons, Immigration and Naturalization Service (INS) facilities, and American Indian county jails (*Correct Care,* 2000). According to Department of Justice estimates, 5% of the U.S. population will serve some time in prison within their lifetime (Bureau of Justice Statistics, 2001).

Less than half (47%) of those in state prisons and only 17% of federal prisoners in 1991 had been convicted of violent crimes. Figures indicate a reverse in convictions for drug offenses, which included 21% of those in state prisons but 58% of those in federal institutions (Bureau of Justice Statistics, 2001).

Correctional populations vary greatly in their composition. In 1996, 2.9 million arrestees were juveniles. This constituted 19% of all arrests and 19% of arrests for violent crimes in the United States. These figures were 60% higher than those for 1987, indicating an increase in juvenile crime (Olds et al., 1998). In 1999, 106,000 juvenile offenders were housed in correctional facilities (*Correct Care*, 2000). Youth are often incarcerated for mental health problems when community mental health services are not adequate to meet their needs. Parents may find that they have no alternative for obtaining help for their mentally ill children except to release them to the juvenile justice system. In fact, 23% of parents of juvenile inmates reported being told they would have to release custody of their son or daughter to the courts, and 20% actually had to do so to obtain assistance (Coalition for Juvenile Justice, 2000).

Juvenile inmates tend to have higher prevalences of a variety of physical and mental health conditions than their counterparts in the general population and usually have less access to care prior to incarceration. In one study, for example, 43% of juveniles in detention centers had no previous health care provider and reported high rates of sexual abuse and sexual activity. Asthma was noted in 27% of the population, dental caries in 19%, sexually transmitted diseases in 12%, and scrotal masses were found in 11% of the youth (*Correct Care*, 2001c).

In 2001, women constituted 11% of the total correctional population, but the rate of incarceration for women is growing faster than that for men. Approximately two thirds of women inmates have been convicted of drug offenses (Alemagno, 2001). In 1998, 3.2 million U.S. women were arrested, accounting for 22% of all arrests, and 1% of women in the United States were housed in correctional facilities. Women are perpetrators of 14% of violent crimes (Bureau of Justice Statistics, 2001). Women inmates often have high rates of physical and mental health problems. In one study, for example, 35% of women in correctional settings had syphilis, 27% had chlamydia, and 8% had gonorrhea (National Center for HIV, STD, and TB Prevention, 1998). Women inmates have seroprevalence rates for HIV infection higher than those for men (3.5% versus 2.2%, respectively). These higher prevalence rates are a function of drug use and sale of sex for money or drugs, which is common among incarcerated women. Women in correctional settings also experience more clinical depression (De Groot et al., 1999), and young female offenders are one and a half times as likely to attempt suicide as male juveniles (Coalition for Juvenile Justice, 2000).

Members of ethnic minority groups are disproportionally represented in correctional settings. According to

Department of Justice estimates, 18% of African American men will be incarcerated in federal prisons at some time in their lifetimes compared to 16% of Hispanic men and only 4.4% of Caucasian men. In 1991, 65% of prison inmates and 63% of those in jails were members of ethnic minority groups (Bureau of Justice Statistics, 2001). These and other similar figures have prompted concerns for inequities and prejudice within the justice system. Whether this is indeed the case or not, the fact remains that correctional populations are ethnically diverse, which may result in racial tensions within facilities as well as the need for culturally sensitive health care.

The fastest-growing segment of corrections populations is the elderly, primarily because of extended sentences, with a large proportion of the population growing old in the correctional setting. People over 50 or 55 years of age are considered "old" in correctional systems due to the accelerated aging that occurs in correctional populations (Falter, 1999; Schreiber, 1999). In 1998, people over 50 years of age constituted nearly 12% of the federal inmate population. By 2005, this figure is expected to increase to 16% (Falter, 1999). Both medical and mental health problems increase in older clients. For example, approximately 40% of inmates over age 45 have been found to have medical problems compared to 12% of those under age 24 years. Similarly, the incidence of mental health problems in inmates over 45 years of age was 48% compared to 24% of the younger group (Maruschak & Beck, 2001). In another study, 83% of older inmates had one or more chronic health problems, and 50% had three or more chronic conditions. Conditions reported included hypertension, myocardial infarction, emphysema, diabetes, and functional impairments (Falter, 1999). Correctional facilities are often unprepared to address the health care needs of older inmates, nor are budgets designed to accommodate these needs. For example, it is estimated that health care costs for elderly inmates are approximately three times those of younger age groups and may rise to as much as $60,000 per person (Schreiber, 1999).

THE NEED FOR HEALTH CARE IN CORRECTIONAL SETTINGS

Health care in correctional facilities is an appropriate endeavor for several reasons. First, the right to adequate health care is a constitutionally recognized right arising from the Eighth Amendment, which prohibits "cruel and unusual punishment" of those convicted of crimes. Detainees also have a constitutional right to health care under the Fifth and Fourteenth Amendments, which prohibit punishment of any kind without "due process" (e.g., conviction through the normal legal processes of the nation). In the case of both convicted inmates and detainees, failure to attend to serious illness or injury is interpreted as unusual punishment.

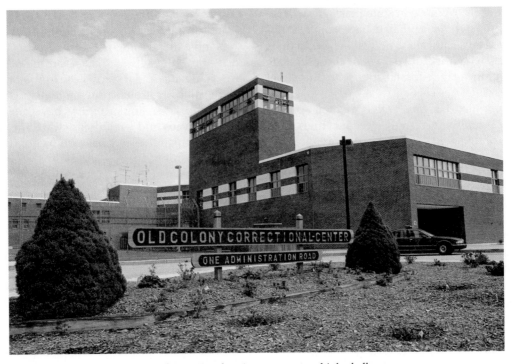

Providing health care to inmates of correctional settings presents multiple challenges.

☺THINK ABOUT IT

If there were no legal mandate to provide health care to inmates in correctional settings, would you choose to spend taxpayers' dollars on care for people convicted of crimes? Would you provide care for some inmates and not for others? If so, for whom and why?

In addition to the constitutional right to health care, correctional care is good common sense for a variety of other reasons. Because of poverty, lower education levels, and unhealthy lifestyles that frequently involve substance abuse, inmates may enter a correctional facility with significant health problems (Leh, 1999). Because many of these individuals cannot afford to pay for care on the outside, the cost of care will be borne by society. Societal costs for this care will be less if interventions occur in a timely fashion, before health problems become severe. Provision of care within the correctional facility also saves taxpayers the cost of personnel and vehicles to transport inmates to other health care facilities. Primary prevention in correctional settings is also cost-effective.

Another possible societal cost of failure to provide adequate health care to inmates lies in the potential for the spread of communicable disease from correctional facilities to the community (Conklin et al., 2000). Environmental conditions and behaviors within correctional facilities lend themselves to the transmission of communicable diseases such as tuberculosis (National Center for HIV, STD, and TB Prevention, 1998). The more than 22 million admissions and releases from U.S. correctional facilities that occur each year put the general public at significant risk for increased incidence of communicable diseases spread from correctional settings (Leh, 1999).

Finally, correctional settings have been described as "inherently unhealthy environments" (Brodie, 2000, p. 15) and may themselves give rise to a variety of health problems. Correctional environments limit inmate autonomy; promote social isolation and communicable diseases; limit exercise; and foster boredom, stress, hostility, and depression. Services are needed to deal with these effects of incarceration as well as the myriad health problems inmates bring with them to correctional settings.

STANDARDS FOR NURSING PRACTICE IN CORRECTIONAL SETTINGS

As noted earlier, the first standards for nursing practice in correctional settings were promulgated by the ANA in 1985. These standards were revised in 1995 and address the scope of nursing practice in correctional settings as well as standards of care and standards of professional performance. Nursing standards for correctional settings are summarized on page 607. The designated standards of care reflect the expected level of care to be provided to individual clients in the correctional setting. The standards of professional performance, on the other hand, are more reflective of the aggregate focus of community health nursing as practiced in correctional settings.

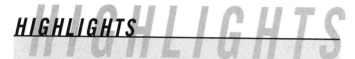

HIGHLIGHTS

Standards for Nursing Practice in Correctional Settings

Standards of Care

Assessment: The nurse collects client health data.

Diagnosis: The nurse analyzes assessment data in determining diagnoses.

Outcomes identification: The nurse identifies expected outcomes individualized to the client.

Planning: The nurse develops a care plan that prescribes interventions to attain expected outcomes.

Implementation: The nurse implements the interventions identified in the care plan.

Evaluation: The nurse evaluates the client's progress toward attainment of outcomes.

Standards of Professional Performance

Quality of care: The nurse systematically evaluates the quality and effectiveness of nursing practice.

Performance appraisal: The nurse evaluates his or her own nursing practice in relation to professional practice standards and relevant statutes and regulations.

Education: The nurse acquires and maintains current knowledge in nursing practice.

Collegiality: The nurse contributes to the professional development of peers, colleagues, and others.

Ethics: The nurse's decisions and actions on behalf of the client are determined in an ethical manner.

Collaboration: The nurse collaborates with the client, significant others, other criminal justice system personnel, and health care providers in providing client care.

Research: The nurse uses research findings in practice.

Resource utilization: The nurse considers factors related to safety, effectiveness, and cost in planning and delivering client care.

Reprinted with permission from: American Nurses Association, *Scope and Standards of Nursing Practice in Correctional Facilities,* © 1995 American Nurses Publishing, American Nurses Foundation/American Nurses Association, Washington, DC.

Some of the standards differentiate between basic and advanced nursing practice in correctional settings. Basic nursing primarily involves provision of care to individuals and families. The advanced practice nurse, on the other hand, can execute all of the responsibilities of the basic nurse, but is also engaged in formulation of policy and in the development, implementation, and evaluation of programs of care for client groups, again incorporating more of the practice of community health nursing. The responsibilities of basic nursing practice include disease prevention and health promotion, recognition and treatment of disease and injury, and counseling. Those of the advanced practice nurse involve supervision of the practice of others, ad-

vanced clinical practice (e.g., treatment of minor illness by nurse practitioners), management, and evaluation of the effects of correctional health care programs (ANA, 1995).

In addition to the standards established for nursing practice in correctional settings by the ANA, the National Commission on Correctional Health Care (NCCHC) has developed standards for health care services in adult and juvenile correctional facilities. These standards are the basis for accreditation of correctional health facilities. The accreditation standards for juvenile facilities have recently been revised and include 71 standards (*Correct Care,* 1999). Some of the areas addressed by the standards are presented below. A similar set of standards exists for adult facilities. In addition, NCCHC is in the process of developing standards and guidelines for the treatment of specific conditions in correctional settings. Areas addressed thus far include chronic asthma, diabetes, epilepsy, HIV infection, high blood cholesterol, and high blood pressure (National Commission on Correctional Health Care, 2001).

HIGHLIGHTS

Areas Addressed by NCCHC Standards for Juvenile Correctional Facilities

- Access to care
- Communication and confidentiality
- Continuity of care
- Credentialing and orientation of staff
- Diet
- Emergency plans and procedures
- Employment of juvenile workers
- Environmental health and safety
- Exercise
- Grievances
- Hygiene
- Infection control
- Informed consent
- Kitchen sanitation
- Pharmaceuticals and medication administration
- Policies and procedures
- Research
- Reporting and notification
- Services (assessment, screening, diagnosis, treatment, oral health, mental health, health education and promotion, family planning, emergency, special needs)
- Staffing levels
- Sexual assault
- Substance abuse
- Suicide prevention
- Therapeutic restraint

Source: Correct Care. (1999). A summary guide to revisions in the 1999 *Standards for Health Services in Juvenile Detention and Confinement Facilities, 13*(2), 18–19.

ETHICAL CONCERNS IN CORRECTIONAL NURSING

There are several ethical considerations that are particularly relevant to nursing in a correctional facility. The right to health care is an ethical as well as legal issue that has already been addressed. Other ethical issues include confidentiality and appropriate use of health care personnel, refusal of care, abuse of prisoners, and advocacy. Confidentiality issues may be a source of conflict in correctional settings when health care providers have access to information that may be of use in criminal proceedings against inmates. Health professionals in correctional institutions may be pressured to divulge client information or to assist with procedures designed to provide evidence for criminal proceedings (e.g., body cavity searches, blood alcohol levels). When these procedures need to be performed by trained personnel (e.g., venipuncture), they should be the task of personnel hired specifically for these types of responsibilities to prevent conflict of interest for health care providers and to avoid jeopardizing a relationship of trust between provider and client. Similarly, health care professionals should not be called upon to engage in security measures or to participate in disciplinary decisions or in execution by lethal injection (ANA, 1995). Assuring appropriate use of personnel in the correctional setting may also mean making sure that nonprofessionals (including inmates) are not allowed to perform medical tasks or dispense medications.

Confidentiality, particularly with respect to HIV status, may be more difficult to achieve in a correctional environment (National Center for HIV, STD, and TB Prevention, 1999a). The intensive nature of treatment and need for multiple doses of medication may serve to label inmates as infected, even when official confirmation of disease is not provided. This potential for lack of confidentiality may act as a deterrent to HIV testing and noncompliance with treatment in infected individuals. Another potential conflict related to confidentiality is the question of whether or not security personnel should be alerted to inmates' HIV-infection status to assure their use of universal precautions (Laird, 1999).

In addition to maintaining confidentiality, nurses may be called on to support an inmate's refusal of care, including forcible administration of psychotherapeutic medications. Inmates have the right to refuse care unless they are determined to be legally incompetent to make that decision. Aggressive or potentially suicidal inmates can, however, be subjected to physical restraint if they are deemed a danger to self or to others. This includes the use of medical isolation when clients suspected of infectious diseases refuse screening procedures or treatment. Medical isolation may also be legitimately employed to protect inmates with symptomatic AIDS from opportunistic infection. Although the U.S. Supreme Court has upheld segregation of HIV-infected inmates, many health care professionals suggest that segregation actually increases the potential for the spread of communicable diseases such as tuberculosis (National Center for HIV, STD, and TB Prevention, 2000). For example, segregation may foster the belief that all others in the institution are uninfected and may lead to high-risk activities (Leh, 1999). In addition, segregation breaches confidentiality and denies segregated inmates access to programs, such as work release and other programs, available to other inmates (Laird, 1999).

Because of the imbalance of power inherent in a correctional setting, there is always the potential for abuse of inmates in the name of punishment. For example, pepper spray is occasionally used as a means of forcing compliance among inmates. Punitive use of such chemicals over and above necessary use for subduing violence has been described as constituting torture and falls within the Eighth Amendment proscription of cruel and unusual punishment (Cohen, 1997). Recent findings also indicate that juvenile inmates may be punished for exhibiting symptoms of mental illness (Coalition for Juvenile Justice, 2000). Preventing this and other forms of abuse of inmates (e.g., denial of health care services) is another ethical aspect of nursing in correctional settings. Finally, nurse advocacy may be needed in the correctional setting. Advocacy may be required at the level of the individual client to ensure that rights are upheld and that appropriate health care services are received or at the aggregate level to assure adequate health care delivery systems in correctional institutions.

ETHICAL AWARENESS

There is considerable controversy regarding the right of corrections personnel to know of the HIV status of inmates, particularly those who are aggressive and might conceivably infect personnel through wounds incurred in fights. To date, no strictly occupational transmission of HIV infection has been documented in correctional settings. Which value do you think should have priority—the inmate's right to privacy or the staff member's right to knowledge that might influence his or her health? Why?

ASSESSING HEALTH IN CORRECTIONAL SETTINGS

Factors in each of the six dimensions of health influence the health status of clients and staff in correctional settings. The nurse assesses factors related to the biophysical, psychological, physical environmental, sociocultural, behavioral, and health system dimensions to identify health problems and to direct interventions to resolve those problems.

Biophysical Considerations

The nurse in the correctional setting needs to assess individual clients for existing physical health problems. He or she also needs to identify problems that have a high incidence and prevalence in the overall institutional population. Particular areas to be considered include communicable diseases, chronic diseases, injury, and pregnancy.

As noted earlier, environmental conditions and behavioral patterns in correctional settings foster the spread of communicable diseases. Although many communicable diseases are found in this population, four of particular concern in correctional populations are tuberculosis, HIV infection and AIDS, hepatitis B, and other sexually transmitted diseases (STDs). Overcrowding and generally poor health status are two of the factors that promote the spread of tuberculosis (TB) in inmate populations. Moreover, co-infection with both TB and HIV is occurring in large segments of some correctional populations (National Center for HIV, STD, and TB Prevention, 2000). A further complicating factor in the problem of tuberculosis in correctional facilities is the prevalence of multidrug-resistant tuberculosis. In 1997, 130,000 U.S. inmates tested positive for latent tuberculosis infection (*Correct Care*, 2001d). The community health nurse working in correctional settings should assess inmates for signs of tuberculosis as well as provide routine screenings for TB according to agency policy. Tuberculin skin test screening in jails may be inappropriate for many inmates who stay only one or two days, so the nurse should ask about TB symptomatology and history of exposure during the intake assessment in order to isolate potentially infectious inmates.

HIV infection and confirmed cases of AIDS are another growing problem in correctional facilities. Many inmates are at increased risk of infection because of injection drug use, and the potential for exposure during incarceration via continued drug use and homosexual activity is high. Between 1991 and 1997, the number of diagnosed cases of AIDS in correctional settings increased by 24% per year. Overall, rates for confirmed cases of AIDS are five times higher in correctional populations than in the general public. In 1997, 2.1% of all state and federal prisoners were infected with HIV (Vitucci, 2000). Inmate deaths due to AIDS, on the other hand, have declined. In 1997, for example, the death rate for AIDS in correctional institutions was 48 per 100,000 inmates, down from 100 deaths per 100,000 inmates in 1995. From 1991 to 1996, AIDS accounted for one third of all deaths in state prisons, but AIDS was responsible for only one fifth of deaths in 1997 (Vitucci, 2000). Rates of HIV infection and AIDS diagnoses vary from one area of the country to another, and nurses should be aware of the overall prevalence of infection in their jurisdictions. Corrections nurses should assess all inmates for history of HIV infection, high-risk behavior, and history or symptoms of possible opportunistic infections.

Drug use behaviors contribute to the increased incidence of tuberculosis and HIV infection in inmates. Such behaviors also place inmates at risk for other STDs and hepatitis B (HBV) and C (HVC). In addition to drug use,

sexual activity and tattooing are other risk factors for HBV and HCV common in correctional populations (Chavez, 1999). In assessing individual inmates for health problems, the nurse should ask about history of STDs and hepatitis B and C and should be alert to the presence of physical signs and symptoms of these diseases.

Chronic illnesses of particular concern in correctional settings include diabetes, hypertension, heart disease, and chronic lung conditions. Seizure disorders are also common, and inmates may also exhibit seizure activity during withdrawal from drugs and alcohol. Diabetes may be particularly difficult to control given the rigid structure of the correctional routine and the need to time hypoglycemic medications, meals, and exercise periods appropriately. The availability of vending machines and the use of commissary privileges as a reward may also complicate dietary control for inmates with diabetes. Many inmates with chronic conditions, particularly those with substance abuse problems, enter the correctional facility after prolonged periods without medications or may not know what medications they have been taking. In many instances, the nurse has to exert considerable ingenuity to obtain an accurate health history from clients, family members, and health care providers in the community. Because of poor overall health status, inmates may also be especially susceptible to exacerbations of chronic conditions. The nurse should assess individual inmates for existing chronic conditions and should also identify problems with high incidence and prevalence in the correctional population with whom he or she works.

In 1997, 11% of state and federal prisoners reported physical health problems, and roughly one fifth of inmates reported developing physical health problems during incarceration. The incidence of medical problems reported increased with the length of time in the correctional setting, with 30% of those incarcerated longer than 72 months reporting problems compared to only 16% of those incarcerated for 12 months or less. Official reports of diagnosed illness among federal prisoners include asthma, diabetes, heart disease, hypertension, and HIV/AIDS. Self-reports by both federal and state prisoners revealed additional problems such as cancer and neurological and musculoskeletal problems. Chronic conditions, particularly when untreated, contribute to functional impairment, and in 1997, 21% of state prisoners and 18% of federal inmates reported a physical or mental impairment that limited their ability to work. A single impairment was reported by 15% to 19% of inmates, but 5% to 7% reported three or more impairments (Maruschak & Beck, 2001).

Injury is another area of physiologic function that should be assessed by the nurse. Injury may result from activities preceding arrest, from actions taken by arresting officers, or from accidents or assaults occurring during incarceration. The nurse should be aware of the potential for internal as well as visible injuries and should assess inmates for signs of trauma. Slightly more than one fourth of state and federal inmates reported injuries that occurred during their incarceration. Approximately two thirds of injuries were due to accidents and the balance were related to fighting (Maruschak & Beck, 2001).

Pregnancy is the final biophysical consideration in assessing the health of correctional populations. As noted earlier, the number of female inmates increases annually. Because of prior drug use and poor health care, pregnant women in correctional settings may be at higher risk for poor pregnancy outcomes than women in the general population. Conversely, incarceration may improve pregnancy outcomes because it interrupts drug use and provides access to prenatal care that the women might not otherwise have (Earley, 1999). Care of pregnant women in correctional settings, however, is often hampered by lack of special diets to support pregnancy, lack of exercise, and inappropriate work assignments. Fetal health may also be compromised by problems encountered in drug and alcohol withdrawal in the correctional setting. Finally, timely transfer of women in labor to obstetrical facilities is often hampered by the security constraints of the correctional facility (Fulco, 2001).

In assessing female inmates, the nurse should ask about the last menstrual period and solicit any symptoms of possible pregnancy. Because drug use can interfere with menses, menstrual history is not always reliable for indicating pregnancy or for suggesting length of gestation

Women in correctional settings may have special needs, including care during pregnancy.

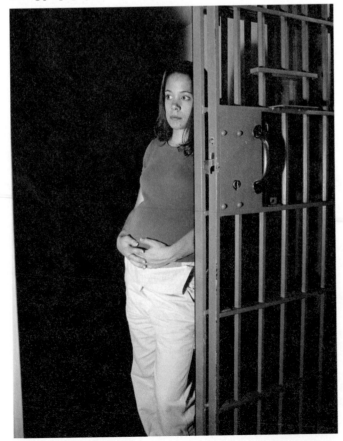

when pregnancy is confirmed. The nurse should also ask about high-risk behavior that may affect the fetus such as smoking, drug and alcohol use, and so on. The pregnant inmate's nutritional status should also be assessed. Other physical problems common in this population that may affect pregnancy outcomes include urinary tract infections and STDs, and the nurse should assess for symptoms of these conditions. Depression and anxiety are also common phenomena among these women.

Psychological Considerations

Assessment in the psychological dimension is particularly important in the correctional setting for a number of reasons. First, many inmates have previously existing mental illness that may have led to their incarceration. In fact, it is not uncommon, since deinstitutionalization, for the mentally ill to be held in jails for lack of any other safe place for them. By law, inmates are entitled to mental health services as well as medical treatment. Mental health services, however, may be lacking in some correctional systems, or the need for these services may go unrecognized. This is particularly true among women inmates and youth.

Correctional institutions have been described by some psychiatrists as "the nation's new mental health hospitals" (cited in Vitucci, 1999a, p. 1). For example, it is estimated that correctional facilities house more than 283,000 mentally ill persons compared to 70,000 persons in public psychiatric hospitals (30% of whom are forensic clients). About 7% of federal prisoners and 16% of state prison inmates reported existing mental health conditions or previous treatment for mental illness. These rates are higher in women with up to 29% of women prisoners in state institutions reporting mental health problems. Inmates with mental health problems frequently have a dual diagnosis of substance abuse. For example, approximately one third of state prisoners and one fourth of federal inmates abuse alcohol. Mental illness contributes to one fifth of violent offenses; inmates with mental health problems are more likely than others to be involved in fights within the correctional setting (Vitucci, 1999c).

The incidence of mental health problems is even higher in incarcerated youth, and 50% to 75% of those in juvenile detention facilities have diagnosable mental disorders. It is estimated that 9% to 13% of young offenders have serious disturbances. Again, the prevalence of dual disorders involving substance abuse is high (50%), probably in attempts to self-medicate distressing symptoms. As noted earlier, juvenile offenders are often punished for symptoms of their disorders leading to withdrawal, depression, and suicidal ideation. Each year, approximately 11,000 boys and 17,000 girls in correctional settings attempt suicide (Coalition for Juvenile Justice, 2000).

Incarceration itself is stressful and can lead to psychological effects including depression and suicide. Correctional nurses should be alert to signs of depression and other mental or emotional distress in inmates, and assessment of suicide potential is a critical part of every intake interview. Suicide is the leading cause of death in jails and "lockups," and is the cause of nearly 100% of deaths among incarcerated juveniles. A *lockup* is a temporary holding facility in which inmates are placed prior to transportation to a jail or other facility. Suicide rates in prisons, on the other hand, are more or less comparable to those in the general population.

Research has indicated that most suicides occur during certain high-risk periods, including within 48 hours of incarceration, after court hearings, after return to the facility from court, after receiving bad news from family members, and after suffering humiliation or rejection. Findings also suggest that suicidal ideation at these times is short-lived. Suicide prevention activities in short-stay units (lockups and jails), then, should focus on reducing the opportunity for suicide at these times. Suicide prevention in long-term facilities, on the other hand, can include psychotherapy and interventions designed to address psychological factors influencing suicidal behaviors (Tartaro, 1999).

Isolation in "safety cells" and physical restraint are some of the interventions that have been employed for inmates who indicate suicidal ideation. Mental health professionals in correctional settings, however, maintain that isolation may increase depression as well as providing greater opportunity for suicide. Close observation is thought to be more effective in suicide prevention, and redesign of correctional units into modular pods to permit routine observation of inmates has been suggested and even implemented in some facilities. Another intervention is the use of a buddy system for surveillance, employing trusted inmates to stay with suicidal peers and report suspicious behavior to personnel (Tartaro, 1999).

Intake screening for suicide is essential; however, nearly half of jails and lockups do not have suicide prevention programs in place. Inmates should be asked on admission about thoughts of suicide as well as observed for signs of drug or alcohol intoxication, which might decrease normal inhibitions for suicidal behavior or increase depression. Inmates can also be inspected for scars from previous suicide attempts. Authorities caution, however, that suicide screening should not be a one-time occurrence, nor should negative screening breed complacence regarding an inmate's potential for suicide (Tartaro, 1999).

The correctional environment may also contribute to sexual assault with its attendant psychological consequences. In addition, many women inmates arrested for prostitution and drug use have histories of sexual abuse (*Correct Care*, 2001c). For men, rape while incarcerated is fairly common. While much sexual activity among male inmates is consensual, the nature of correctional systems places some men at risk for forcible assault. In some correctional systems, homosexual or effeminate males are segregated from the rest of the population for their protection, but forced isolation may also have psychological

consequences or lead to discrimination and assault by other inmates. In assessing clients, particularly those with symptoms of STDs, corrections nurses should be alert to signs of assault and should question clients about this issue. If sexual assault has occurred, the nurse will also need to take action to protect the client from further injury.

Finally, state and federal prison systems may house a number of inmates who have been sentenced to death, creating a need for emotional and psychological support. Corrections nurses working in systems with "death-row" inmates should assess them for evidence of psychological problems and refer them for counseling as appropriate.

Because of the increasing age of corrections populations, nurses may also encounter clients with terminal conditions in the correctional setting. These clients have the same end-of-life care needs as people in the general population. End-of-life care for terminally ill inmates is discussed in more detail later in this chapter.

Physical Environmental Considerations

The physical environment of the correctional setting is constrained by the need for security. Inmates may be relegated to specific spaces at specific times of the day. Because of the tremendous growth in the incarcerated population, jails and prisons are extremely overcrowded and few jurisdictions are not in violation of space standards for inmates. For example, in 1997, state prison inmate censuses were 15% to 24% above capacity; whereas the census in federal institutions was 19% above maximum capacity (Leh, 1999). Other physical environmental problems common in correctional settings include poor ventilation, lack of temperature control, and unsanitary conditions. Lack of funds for maintenance may lead to buildings in poor repair, creating safety hazards for both inmates and staff. Other areas that should be assessed by the nurse include the safety of recreational areas, fire protection, lighting, plumbing, solid waste disposal, and safety of the water supply. Additional considerations include vermin control, noise control, and the presence of high levels of radiation. Because correctional facilities are often situated in areas away from the general population, they may be located in sites with disaster potential such as flooding, earthquake, and so on. The nurse should assess the potential for such disasters as well as the adequacy of the facility's disaster response plan (Paris, 2000; Vitucci, 1999d). Disaster potential may also arise from prison industries. Inmate occupations may also give rise to other physical hazards for individual clients that need to be assessed.

Sociocultural Considerations

Particular elements of the sociocultural dimension that should be assessed in correctional settings include the attitudes of correctional and health personnel toward inmates, the extent of social support available to inmates, the effects of education level and language on the health status of inmates, the potential for violence in the setting, transience, and employment. Security concerns may also hamper provision of health care. The nurse should be alert to the use of excessive force or punitive conditions to which inmates may be subjected. Correctional nurses will also assess the extent of social support available to inmates. Social support may arise from interactions and programs available within the correctional system or from continued interactions with persons or agencies outside the system (e.g., family). Development of social support systems may be particularly important for clients about to be released from the facility.

Concerns for children can be a source of stress for many inmates. Approximately 64% of women inmates with children lived with their children prior to incarceration compared to 44% of fathers, and 31% of the women were single parents (versus 4% of fathers). Four fifths of inmates with children reported that children were currently living with the other parent, 20% with relatives, and 2% had children in foster care. Women inmates were more likely than men to have children placed in foster care (10% versus 2%). Inmates with children, particularly women, are more likely to be convicted on charges related to drugs and alcohol or experience mental health problems than other inmates (Mumola, 2000), suggesting that their children have had long exposure to dysfunctional family settings. Both parent and child may be in need of therapy and the correctional nurse may need to establish close ties with community agencies to address the needs of the children of incarcerated parents.

Problems caused by separation of children from their mothers has led some correctional facilities to allow young children, particularly newborns, to remain with their mothers in custody. Areas for concern in these types of programs that need to be addressed by correctional nurses and other correctional personnel include the security of children and liability issues, costs and mechanisms for providing health care and other services for children, the effects of incarceration on child development, charges of discrimination if pregnant and recently delivered inmates receive special consideration, and lack of interest in parenting by some incarcerated women (Fulco, 2001).

Because members of ethnic minority groups are disproportionately represented among inmate populations, language may prove a significant barrier to providing effective health care for some inmates. Racial and ethnic differences, as well as other factors, may also lead to violence among inmates, and the nurse may need to assess the potential for violence within the population and alert security personnel. Nurses may also need to assess the extent of individual injuries to staff or inmates stemming from inmate violence.

Low socioeconomic level, poverty, and low education levels are all associated with incarceration. All of these factors may adversely affect health status prior to admission to a correctional facility, and education level may influence clients' knowledge of healthful behaviors or understanding of prescribed regimens for existing health problems. Inmate transience is another sociocultural

CULTURAL CONSIDERATIONS

Culturally, Native Americans, as well as some other cultural groups, believe it is inappropriate to look others in the eye while speaking to them. You see a corrections officer grab an inmate by the collar and jerk his head up, saying "Look at me when I talk to you. I want to know when you're lying." You know the inmate is of Native American descent. How would you handle this situation?

dimension factor that may affect health status. Inmates are frequently moved from one facility to another, making completion of treatment for some conditions, contact follow-up for communicable diseases, and continuity of other health services difficult to maintain (National Center for HIV, STD, and TB Prevention, 1999a). Release back into the general population is another factor that may impede continuity of care, particularly in the case of communicable diseases like tuberculosis and HIV/AIDS (*HIV Inside*, 1999).

Some correctional facilities have assets that promote rehabilitation and permit inmates to earn some money. In some states, there are even provisions for inmates to work to repay victims of their crimes. Such opportunities are less readily available to women inmates than men and are rarely adequate to meet the rehabilitation needs of all inmates. The presence of occupational opportunities, however, may contribute to a variety of occupational risks to health that should be assessed by nurses in correctional facilities. Occupational hazards for correctional facility staff, as well as those for inmates, should be considered.

Security concerns within the correctional setting are another sociocultural dimension factor that may influence health by hampering efforts to provide health care services. In some institutions, nurses do not have immediate access to inmates unless security personnel are present. In other instances, transportation of inmates for outside services may be postponed if there are insufficient security personnel available to accompany them. There is also the potential for violence against health care providers and their use as hostages.

Behavioral Considerations

Behavioral dimension factors that influence the health of inmates and staff in correctional settings include diet, substance abuse, smoking, opportunities for exercise and recreation, and sexual activity. Inmates are more likely than the general public to engage in tobacco use and alcohol and drug use and abuse. In 1998, for example, 70% of inmates in local jails were arrested for drug offenses, and half of jail inmates and 57% of state prison inmates reported drug use in the month prior to arrest. Similarly, one fifth of jail inmates and one third of those in state prisons reported prior involvement in substance abuse programs, and 30% of those in jails had prior convictions for drug offenses (Wilson, 2000). Alcohol and tobacco use are also common. With little to occupy their time, inmates may find themselves smoking more after incarceration than before. Smoking, coupled with overcrowding, lack of exercise, and inadequate diet may increase inmates' risk of both communicable and chronic diseases.

The correctional nurse should assess substance use and abuse in individual clients as well as in the inmate population as a whole. The nurse should also assess inmates' nutritional status and particular dietary needs for individual inmates (e.g., those with diabetes). Other behavioral dimension factors that should be assessed include opportunities for and participation in exercise and recreational activities. Potential safety hazards posed by exercise and recreation activities should also be assessed. Sexual activity in correctional settings has already been touched on, but the nurse should assess the extent to which condoms are available and their use within correctional systems. This is particularly important given the high incidence of STDs and HIV infection among inmates.

Health System Considerations

The correctional nurse also assesses the adequacy of the health care system in meeting the needs of the correctional facility population. Depending on several factors, including size and financial capabilities, correctional facilities may take one of two approaches to the provision of health care services for inmates. Services may be provided in-house by staff employed by the facility or the agency may contract with other provider agencies for needed services. In many institutions, a combination of both approaches is used. Some authors report cooperative partnerships between correctional institutions and nonprofit Medicaid managed care organizations (MCOs) in which the corrections department provides primary care services, and the MCO assists with external specialty care, special diagnostic needs, and inpatient care (Mayes, Schilling, & Long, 1998).

Whatever the approach used, the corrections nurse should assess the adequacy of health services for inmates. Minimum services should include both primary and secondary care services. Primary health care services begin with an initial health screening on admission to the facility. This initial screening is a brief immediate evaluation of whether or not it is safe to admit the inmate to the facility given his or her current health status. The initial screening also facilitates correct placement of the inmate within the facility, initiates planning to meet identified health needs, and provides aggregate data for use in overall program planning. Minimal areas to be addressed in this screening include evidence of infectious disease, existing health problems, current medications, evidence of disability or activity limitation, suicide risk, and other special needs (e.g., dietary restrictions, pregnancy, need for dialysis).

The correctional health care system should also make adequate provision for diagnostic and treatment services

with access assured to health personnel evaluation in a timely fashion. In some situations, this may mean curtailing the discretion of corrections personnel in determining whether or not an inmate should be brought to the attention of health care providers. If needed diagnostic and treatment services are not available within the facility, arrangements should be in place for securing these services elsewhere. The need for diagnostic and treatment services extends to dental health and mental health needs as well as care for physical health problems. The nurse should assess the adequacy of in-house services as well as the effectiveness of procedures designed to accomplish outside referrals.

⑥THINK ABOUT IT

In one study conducted with corrections personnel, correctional nurses had less favorable attitudes toward inmates than corrections officers, defense attorneys, students, and members of the general public. Why do you think the nurses' attitudes were so unfavorable? Why might these nurses continue to work in correctional settings with such unfavorable attitudes?

The extent of emergency response capabilities (including suicide prevention programs) and health promotion activities should also be assessed. Recommended health promotion and education emphases for correctional settings include mental health issues, substance abuse, smoking cessation, sexuality issues, nutrition, disease prevention, women's health, hygiene, safety and first aid, cardiovascular health, dental health, and immunization.

The health care system within a correctional setting should also make adequate provision for efforts to control communicable diseases. This means screening programs, provision for isolation of infectious inmates, and follow up on contacts both within and outside the correctional system.

In order for health care services to be adequate to meet clients' needs, health care personnel must be available in adequate numbers and with adequate preparation for practice in correctional settings.

Another assessment consideration related to the health care dimension is inmates' use of health care services prior to their incarceration. For example, the nurse might ask the female inmate when she had her last Pap smear or mammogram. The nurse would also want to explore prior interactions with health care providers related to existing health problems. For example, was the client being seen for hypertension or other health problems? Or has the client not been taking antihypertensive medications because he or she did not have the prescription renewed?

One other feature of the correctional health care system that may affect inmates' health status is the growing tendency to require co-payments for visits to internal health care providers. Through U.S. congressional legislation, the Federal Prisoner Health Care Copayment Act of 1999 allows federal prisons to charge a minimum fee of $2 for inmate-initiated health care visits (Vitucci, 1999b). The intent of this practice is to decrease service utilization rates and generate funds. The point has been made, however, that co-payments may deter inmates from obtaining needed health care and contribute to the spread of communicable diseases as well as increased costs for care of chronic conditions allowed to deteriorate. Correctional nurses may need to be actively involved in evaluating the effect of co-payment systems on the health of inmates and the implications for the health of the general public if legitimate needs for services are not being addressed.

⑥THINK ABOUT IT

What do you think are some of the possible outcomes of requiring co-payment for health care services provided in correctional settings? Do you think co-payment is a good idea? Why or why not?

Features of the correctional setting that influence health are assessed by the community health nurse and used to derive nursing diagnoses. A comprehensive tool for assessing the health status of correctional populations is provided on the companion Web site for this book. Assessment tips for use with correctional populations are provided on page 615. ⬥

DIAGNOSTIC REASONING AND CARE OF CLIENTS IN CORRECTIONAL SETTINGS

Based on information obtained in assessing the dimensions of health, the nurse in the correctional setting "uses independent judgment and available data to formulate diagnoses" (ANA, 1995, p. 7). Diagnoses should be validated with the client, significant others, or other health care providers when possible. Community health nurses working in correctional settings determine nursing diagnoses relevant to individual clients as well as diagnoses related to the health needs of the total population of inmates and staff. For example, an individual diagnosis might be "uncontrolled diabetes mellitus due to substance abuse." A diagnosis related to the population group might be "increased potential for violence due to racial tensions and unrest." This second diagnosis would affect facility personnel as well as inmates since all might be involved in any violence that occurs.

PLANNING AND IMPLEMENTING HEALTH CARE IN CORRECTIONAL SETTINGS

Planning to meet identified health problems in correctional settings may be accomplished by the nurse him or herself or in conjunction with other personnel within and outside the institution. Interventions may take place at the primary, secondary, or tertiary level of prevention.

Primary Prevention

Primary prevention in correctional settings involves both health promotion and illness prevention. Health promotion emphases include adequate nutrition, rest and exercise, health education, prenatal care, and contraceptive services. Preventive efforts center around prevention of communicable diseases, suicide prevention, and violence prevention.

Health Promotion

Health promotion in correctional settings differs from that in other settings in a number of ways. First, the general purpose of health promotion in correctional settings is protection of the health of others rather than to enhance the health of the particular inmate. Second, group health promotion efforts may be hampered by the compulsory nature of one's presence in the institution. For example, inmates may be resistant to health education because they perceive themselves as a "captive audience" with little option regarding participation. Third, the great majority of offenders are men who tend not to be as highly motivated with respect to health promotion as women. Health promotion in correctional settings often needs to focus less on information transmission than on attitude development or change, and behavioral change may not be as easy within the constraints of the correctional setting as in the outside world. In addition, the correctional emphasis on punishment for crimes may result in political interference with health promotion efforts. Finally, given the extensive health problems encountered in this population, there may be little time or resources available for health promotion efforts, which may receive lower priority than curative activities (Burgess, 1999).

However, some correctional health promotion efforts have been shown to be effective. These efforts are characterized by structured, but open and nonthreatening milieu; by the provision of factual information relevant to client motivations; and by attention to the belief systems of participants. For example, programs to promote HIV screening among minority inmates may need to first address perceptions that HIV seroprevalence studies are a means of spreading HIV infection to targeted groups (De Groot et al., 1999). Effective programs also enhance participants' analytic skills and foster their ability to self-evaluate behavior. In addition, they provide practical coping skills relevant to the learners, address the link between behavior and the offense (e.g., between anger management and violent crime, or substance abuse and

assessment tips assessment tips assessment tips

ASSESSING HEALTH IN CORRECTIONAL SETTINGS

Biophysical Considerations

- What is the age, gender, and ethnic composition of the correctional population (inmates and staff)?
- What communicable and chronic health problems are prevalent among inmates? Among staff?
- What is the prevalence of pregnancy among inmates?
- What are the immunization levels in the population?

Psychological Considerations

- What procedures are in place for dealing with suicidal ideation or attempts? Are these procedures followed?
- What is the psychological effect of incarceration? Does the individual inmate exhibit signs of depression? Does the inmate express thoughts of suicide?
- What is the extent of sexual assault among inmates? What are the psychological effects of assault?
- Are there inmates in the setting under sentence of death? If so, what psychological effects does this have? Are there terminally ill inmates in the population?
- What is the prevalence of mental illness among inmates?

Physical Environmental Considerations

- Are there health or safety hazards present in the correctional facility?
- Is there potential for disaster in the area? Is there a disaster plan?

Sociocultural Considerations

- What are the attitudes of health and correctional personnel toward inmates?
- What is the attitude of the surrounding community to the correctional facility and to the inmates?
- What family concerns influence the health of inmates?
- Are there intergroup conflicts within the population? Do these conflicts result in violence?

- What is the extent of mobility in the population?
- Are inmates employed in the correctional setting? Are they employed outside? What health hazards, if any, are posed by the type of work done?
- How do security concerns affect the ability of health care personnel to provide services?

Behavioral Considerations

- Are there inmates with special nutritional needs? How well are they being met? What is the nutritional quality of food served in the correctional setting?
- What are the health-related behaviors of the correctional population? How do they affect health?
- How are medications dispensed in the correctional setting? Are there procedures in place to prevent inmates from selling medications or accumulating them for use in a suicide attempt?
- What is the extent of sexual activity in the correctional setting? To what extent do inmates engage in unsafe sexual practices? What is the availability of condoms in the correctional setting?

Health System Considerations

- What health services are offered in the correctional setting? Are they adequate to meet needs?
- Are there isolation procedures in place for inmates with communicable diseases? Are these procedures followed?
- How are health care services funded? Is funding adequate to meet health needs? Are inmates charged a fee for health care services?
- What is the quality of interaction between internal and external health care services?
- What is the extent of emergency response capability of the correctional facility (e.g., to myocardial infarction, stab wound)?
- What provisions are made for continuity of care after release from the correctional facility?

robbery), and reflect the effects of behavior on others (Burgess, 1999).

Nutritional intake in correctional settings may be far from adequate. The nurse in this setting may need to monitor the diet of inmates and may need to influence administrative decisions regarding the nutritive value of meals served. There may also be a need to suggest changes in food served to facility personnel if meals are provided for them as well. In addition, the nurse may need to make arrangements to meet the special dietary needs of specific inmates based on their health status. Examples include a diabetic diet or a liquid diet for an inmate recuperating from a broken jaw.

Attention should also be given to provisions for adequate rest and exercise by inmates. Nurses may need to advocate for adequate space and facilities for sleeping in inmate housing units. In addition, the nurse should work to assure that time and facilities are provided for inmates to obtain exercise. In some instances, this may mean curtailing certain activities that place inmates at risk because of existing health problems. Nurses can also educate both inmates and staff on the benefits of exercise and suggest forms of exercise congruent with health status and available opportunities.

Both inmates and facility staff may be in need of a variety of health education efforts. Areas of importance include the elimination of risk factors for disease. Education programs that may be planned and implemented by nurses may include smoking cessation campaigns or stress management classes. Education regarding problem solving and positive coping strategies may also benefit both staff and inmates.

Prenatal care is a significant health promotion activity for pregnant female inmates. Areas to be addressed include adequate nutrition, the effects of smoking and other substances on the fetus, parenting skills, discomforts of pregnancy, and planning for child care if the child is delivered while the client is still in custody. Contraceptive education may benefit both pregnant and nonpregnant inmates.

Illness and Injury Prevention

Preventing the spread of communicable diseases in correctional settings is an important primary prevention activity. Possible approaches include the use of universal precautions in the handling of blood and body fluids (see Chapter 28 for a discussion of universal precautions), isolation of infected persons when appropriate, immunization, TB prophylaxis, and education on condom use during sexual encounters. Isolation is appropriate for diseases spread by airborne transmission such as measles and influenza. Isolation of HIV-infected individuals is not generally recommended. Immunization is particularly recommended for HBV, but other immunizing agents may be needed as well depending on the incidence of specific diseases in the general community. For example, measles immunizations may be warranted for all inmates and staff during a measles outbreak in the community. Corrections staff, particularly health care personnel, should definitely receive HBV immunization.

TB prophylaxis is treatment of persons with reactive tuberculin skin tests, but without evidence of active tuberculosis, to prevent their development of disease. Prophylactic treatment is also recommended for persons with HIV infection even in the absence of evidence of tuberculosis. HIV-infected persons with undocumented treatment for tuberculosis should be given directly observed therapy for nine months with isoniazid or two months with rifamycin and pyrazinamide (National Center for HIV, STD, and TB Prevention, 1999b; 2000). Corrections personnel with positive skin tests should also receive prophylaxis. In addition, all inmates and personnel should be educated on infection control procedures and universal precautions (De Groot et al., 1999; National Commission on Correctional Health Care, 1998).

Other avenues for illness and injury prevention include suicide prevention and prevention of violence. The primary mode of suicide prevention is identification of inmates at risk for suicide. Those at risk for suicide should be closely monitored and receive timely referrals for psychiatric services.

Violence prevention activities may need to be directed to both inmates and corrections staff. The purpose of such activities is to teach alternative behavioral responses to violence. Recommended components of violence prevention programs in correctional settings include incorporation of violence assessment (including prior exposure to violence) in intake screening, referral of inmates with a history of personal violence or violence exposures for counseling, education on alternative responses to potentially violent situations for both inmates and corrections staff, and referral of inmates for continued counseling on release. Primary prevention emphases in correctional health care are summarized below.

HIGHLIGHTS

Primary Prevention Activities in Correctional Settings

Health Promotion
- Provision of adequate nutrition
- Provision of opportunities for adequate rest and exercise
- Health education for self-care, risk factor elimination, stress reduction, etc.
- Prenatal care for pregnant inmates
- Contraceptive education

Illness Prevention
- Control of communicable diseases
- Immunization
- Isolation of persons with infectious diseases
- Use of universal precautions for blood and body fluids
- TB prophylaxis
- Education for safe sex
- Suicide prevention
- Violence prevention

Secondary Prevention

Secondary prevention activities in correctional health settings focus on screening and diagnostic and treatment activities.

Screening

Screening activities center around communicable diseases and suicide risk. As noted earlier, assessment for suicide risk should be an integral part of every intake interview. Screening for certain communicable diseases may also be warranted based on client health status and the incidence and prevalence of specific conditions in the surrounding community. Screening for tuberculosis has been identified by the National Commission on Correctional Health Care (1998) as a need for all employees and new inmates. Inmates who will be in custody long enough for the test to be read (48 to 72 hours) should be given a Mantoux skin test (see Chapter 28 for information on tuberculin skin tests), while a chest x-ray is recommended for those in short-stay units. Because of the tendency for HIV-infected individuals to have negative TB skin tests even with active disease, it has been suggested that chest x-ray, anergy testing, and sputum collections may be more appropriate in persons known to be HIV-positive and for those whose HIV status is unknown in areas with high prevalence rates of multidrug-resistant tuberculosis infection (National Center for HIV, STD, and TB Prevention, 2000; National Commission on Correc-tional Health Care, 1998).

Screening for HIV infection is also recommended. Voluntary screening programs have not been very effective due to the multiple barriers to screening encountered in correctional settings. These include fear of disclosure and discrimination if HIV status becomes known, isolation, inability to access programs and services available to noninfected inmates, prohibition of conjugal visits, and so on (Altice et al., 1998). Peer counselor programs have been shown to be effective in promoting HIV screening among inmates. Again, care must be taken to avoid compromising the confidentiality of peer counselors (Flores, 1998). Evidence of HIV infection may also be found during sick call if health care providers are alert to the symptoms of possible opportunistic infections (De Groot et al., 1999).

Rapid screening for syphilis, gonorrhea, and chlamydia has also been suggested for all admissions to correctional facilities, particularly among women. In one study, for example, less than half of jails offered routine STD testing for women, and in those with a routine screening policy, less than half of inmates were screened on admission. Another 52% to 77% of facilities provided screening to women with symptoms or on request. Routine screening promotes early and effective treatment and reduces the cost of follow-up and treatment after release (National Center for HIV, STD, and TB Prevention, 1998). Pregnancy screening for female inmates may also be warranted given the erratic nature of menses in the face of abuse of some drugs, particularly narcotics. Nurses in correctional settings will most likely be responsible for conducting these screenings.

Diagnosis and Treatment

Correctional nurses may also be actively involved in the diagnosis and treatment of existing medical conditions. Many minor illnesses are handled exclusively by nurses working under medical protocols. In other instances, nurses are responsible for implementing medical treatment plans initiated by physicians or nurse practitioners. This may involve giving medications or carrying out treatment procedures. Treatment procedures would be handled in much the same way as in any health care facility. Dispensing medications in a correctional setting, however, requires that the nurse directly observe the client taking the medication, and often only a single dose is dispensed at a time rather than giving the client several doses of medication to be taken at prescribed times. This precaution is necessary because of the potential for inmates to sell medications to other inmates or to stockpile certain medications for use in a suicide attempt. The U.S. courts have upheld the practice of dispensing of medications by corrections personnel, but significant safeguards must be in place to assure that corrections personnel dispense medications correctly and accurately document dispensing (*Correct Care*, 2001a).

Treatment for tuberculosis and HIV infection in correctional settings are complicated by the long-term nature of the therapies. Although not recommended for HIV-infected inmates, those with tuberculosis should be placed in respiratory isolation in negative-pressure rooms until they are no longer communicable. If negative-pressure rooms are not available in the correctional facility, arrangements should be made to transport the inmate to a local hospital with such facilities. Respiratory isolation should also be instituted for all inmates with respiratory symptoms suspicious of TB. Tuberculosis treatment should involve a multidrug regimen, particularly when exposure to multidrug-resistant infection is suspected. Drug susceptibility testing should be carried out on all inmates with active TB, and therapy should rely on directly observed therapy (DOT) (National Commission on Correctional Health Care, 1998).

HIV/AIDS therapy is also difficult in correctional settings because of the number of factors that promote noncompliance. As noted earlier, having to receive multiple doses of medication each day may "tag" inmates as infected and leave them open to discrimination and assault. Security practices such as lockdowns and search and seizure may interfere with dispensing of medications or attendance at support group or education programs. A *lockdown* occurs when inmates are locked in their cells at times when they would ordinarily have greater freedom to come and go throughout the facility, usually in response to a security incident or to permit a search for contraband items (drugs, alcohol, weapons) or a *search and seizure* procedure. During search and seizure, all medications are taken away, so clients in some facilities where self-medication is permitted may have their medications removed and be unable to take doses as directed (Altice et al., 1998). Research has shown that compliance with HIV/AIDS treatment regimens must be at 95% or better to prevent development of resistant viral strains (De Groot et al., 1999).

Strategies that can increase compliance with HIV/AIDS treatment regimens include simplifying the regimen to include fewer doses or combining medications into a single pill, protecting confidentiality, using medications with fewer side effects, and dealing with those side effects that occur. Treatment is also more effective if provided by providers who have expertise with HIV/AIDS.

CRITICAL THINKING IN RESEARCH

In an effort to prevent coercion of inmates to participate in clinical research studies, the federal government promulgated regulations that prohibit the use of inmates as research subjects. Inmates, however, entered a successful class action suit to gain the ability to participate in clinical trials, particularly those pertaining to HIV/AIDS treatment. In response, the Belmont report recommended that inmates not be denied access to participation in clinical trials. Four types of studies were deemed permissible for inclusion of inmates: (1) studies of factors that lead to incarceration, (2) studies on correctional facilities as institutions and their effects on people, (3) conditions that affect inmates as a group (e.g., HIV infection or TB), and (4) studies that offer the potential for specific benefit (e.g., clinical trials of AIDS drugs) (De Groot et al., 1999). In addition, the National Commission on Correctional Health Care developed guidelines for inmate participation in research. These included the need for a compelling reason for the inclusion of inmates in the study, equitable participation by other groups, and research conducted in correctional institutions characterized by openness and absence of the potential for coerced participation (De Groot, 1998).

- How would you design a study that would meet these two sets of conditions for the inclusion of inmates as subjects?
- What would you study?
- How would you recruit inmates as subjects in such a way that you were sure their participation was voluntary?

In larger systems, inmates with HIV infection may be moved to facilities with this expertise or where this expertise is available in the community. Directly observed therapy, while recommended for tuberculosis treatment, may result in noncompliance on release since the client will have no stimulus to take his or her medications. A "buddy system" has been recommended as a substitute for DOT in HIV/AIDS treatment in correctional settings. In a buddy system, inmates on similar drug regimens are paired and observe each other taking medications (De Groot et al., 1999).

Treatment should also be available for substance abuse and mental health problems. Research has indicated that treatment of substance abuse while in prison reduces the likelihood of rearrest by 57% and reduces the return to previous drug use patterns by 37% (National Institute of Drug Abuse, 1998). Similarly, youth who receive structured, meaningful, and sensitive treatment for mental illness exhibit 24% less recidivism than those who are not treated (Coalition for Juvenile Justice, 2000).

Nurses will also be involved in emergency response to life-threatening situations. Emergency situations likely to be encountered include seizures, cardiac arrest, diabetic coma or insulin reaction, attempted suicide, and traumatic injury due to inmate violence. The nurse would respond to these situations with actions designed to relieve the threat to life and stabilize the client's condition prior to transportation to a hospital facility either within or outside the correctional system. Correctional nurses may also find themselves involved in emergency care of large numbers of persons injured in man-made or natural disasters involving the correctional facility. Major foci in secondary prevention in correctional settings are summarized below.

HIGHLIGHTS

Secondary Prevention Activities in Correctional Settings

Screening
- Screening for communicable diseases
  - Tuberculosis
  - HIV infection
  - Hepatitis B
  - Sexually transmitted diseases
- Screening for suicide risk
- Screening for pregnancy

Diagnosis and treatment
- Treatment of existing acute and chronic conditions
- Emergency care for accidental and intentional injuries
- Emergency care in the event of a disaster

Tertiary Prevention

Tertiary prevention in correctional settings focuses on preventing complications of existing conditions, preventing recurrence of problems, rehabilitation, discharge planning, and end-of-life care. Tertiary prevention directed toward preventing complications of existing health problems depends on the conditions experienced by inmates. For example, tertiary prevention for the inmate with diabetes will be directed toward preventing circulatory changes, diabetic ketoacidosis, and hypoglycemia. For the client with arthritis, tertiary prevention will focus on pain management and prevention of mobility limitations.

Tertiary preventive activities may also be directed toward preventing the recurrence of problems once they have been resolved. For example, the nurse may educate an inmate who has been treated for gonorrhea on the use of condoms to prevent reinfection. Rehabilitation activities, on the other hand, may be required for clients who have already suffered consequences of acute health problems. Rehabilitation may be physical, as in the case of an inmate whose arm was fractured in a fight with other inmates, or psychological, as exemplified in care for substance abusers.

Discharge planning is another tertiary prevention activity for inmates who are about to be released back into the general population. The nurse may need to make arrangements for continuing care or arrange for housing or other survival needs. Nurses may also assist clients to anticipate and deal with some of the difficulties that are likely to arise with reintegration into families or communities after prolonged absences.

Discharge planning activities are particularly important for inmates with tuberculosis, AIDS, or substance abuse and mental health problems. Many clients started on tuberculosis treatment will be released prior to treatment completion, and discharge planning for continuity of care is particularly important to assure completion of therapy. In one study, for example, 61% of inmates with positive TB skin tests who were put on medication were released before completing therapy. Only 3% of these inmates were seen at the local TB clinic after release (Tulsky et al., 1998). Continuity of tuberculosis care will require extensive coordination between correctional health staff and local health departments.

Similar efforts must be made to assure continuity of care for inmates with HIV/AIDS. In fact, discharge planning should be begun at entry, particularly in short-stay facilities such as jails. Whenever possible, discharge planning should include probation officers, family members, and local agencies to which the client will be referred (De Groot et al., 1999). In some instances, case managers have joint positions in correctional facilities and community agencies, providing the inmate with a familiar contact on release. Attention should be given not only to continued therapy, but to other health and social service needs that may hold higher priority for the inmate. These may include assistance with housing, drug treatment, education, employment assistance, legal assistance, mental health treatment, and financial help (*HIV Inside*, 1999). Similar types of assistance may also be needed by substance abusers to prevent them from returning to prior drug habits (Alemagno, 2001).

The last aspect of tertiary prevention, end-of-life care, is a growing responsibility in correctional settings. As noted earlier, the number of older people in correctional settings as well as the prevalence of AIDS in this population has increased the number of people who will die while in jail. The problem is compounded by stiffer sentencing and parole laws. The National Prison Hospice Association has been assisting correctional facilities to develop hospice services for terminally ill inmates, and as of 1998, 15 facilities had some form of hospice care in place (Seidlitz, 1998).

End-of-life care in correctional settings involves two major aspects: practical aspects of caring for dying clients and a change in staff values and attitudes. Areas that need to be addressed include protocols for palliative care, particularly pain management irrespective of the client's prior history of drug abuse, and adequate access to pain medication. Other considerations for dying inmates

include increased access by family members, access to chaplains and other spiritual advisors as desired, and family member involvement in care and decision making as appropriate. Memorial rituals to commemorate the deceased are also recommended to provide closure for staff and other inmates (Dubler & Heyman, 1998).

In some jurisdictions, terminally ill inmates may petition for compassionate release, and nurses may need to advocate for such policies. If inmates are released from custody pending death, there is a need to provide for continuity of care so they and their families are not abandoned (Dubler & Heyman, 1998). For example, the correctional nurse may make a referral to a community hospice agency. Tertiary prevention emphases in correctional health care, including end-of-life care, are summarized below.

Nurses working in correctional settings will find themselves in need of additional information on a variety of topics. The companion Web site for this book provides links to some useful sources of information on correctional health nursing as well as health problems that nurses may encounter in that setting.

HIGHLIGHTS

Tertiary Prevention Activities in Correctional Settings

Preventing consequences of acute and chronic health problems

Preventing recurrence of health problems

Rehabilitation
- Physical rehabilitation: restoration of normal function after physical illness or injury
- Psychological rehabilitation: restoration or creation of abilities to cope with the stress of life
- Social rehabilitation: assistance with resumption of life outside of the correctional facility following release

Discharge planning

End-of-life care
- Palliative care
- Spiritual care
- Involvement of family
- Compassionate release and follow-up

EVALUATING HEALTH CARE IN CORRECTIONAL SETTINGS

The principles that guide the evaluation of health care in correctional settings are the same as those applied in other settings. The nurse evaluates the outcomes of care for individual clients in light of identified goals. Correctional nurses may also be involved in evaluating health outcomes for groups of inmates or for the entire facility population, including staff. In addition, the nurse examines processes of care and makes recommendations for improvements in terms of quality, efficiency, and cost-effectiveness.

Correctional facilities present a useful setting in which community health nurses can engage in health-promotive and illness-preventive activities with clients who may have little knowledge of these activities. Clients in correctional settings may be less motivated than those in other settings, but can realize substantial health benefits through the efforts of community health nurses during incarceration and in promoting follow-up on release. Community health nursing efforts in correctional settings also help to prevent the flow of health problems back into the larger population, thereby benefiting society as a whole.

APPLYING YOUR KNOWLEDGE IN PRACTICE

🗶 CASE STUDY
Nursing in the Correctional Setting

You are the only nurse on the night shift in a county jail housing 150 male inmates. A new inmate is admitted to the jail for driving under the influence of alcohol. During your initial history and physical, the inmate tells you that he is on kidney dialysis and missed his last dialysis appointment, which was yesterday. It is Sunday night and your facility does not have dialysis capabilities. The dialysis unit at the local hospital does not function on Sundays except in the case of emergencies. The inmate appears to be in no immediate distress and has normal vital signs and no evidence of edema. He is appropriately alert and oriented despite the odor of obvious alcohol consumption. The watch commander tells you he has no one to spare to transport the inmate to the hospital, and if he goes it will have to be by private ambulance. Your back-up physician is out of town for the weekend and the on-call physician is tied up with an emergency.

- What are the biophysical, psychological, physical environmental, sociocultural, behavioral, and health system factors operating in this situation?
- What are your nursing diagnoses? How would you prioritize those diagnoses?
- What action would you take in this situation? Why?

🗶 TESTING YOUR UNDERSTANDING

- What are the implications, for inmates and for the general public, of providing health care in correctional settings? (pp. 605–606)
- Describe some of the ethical considerations facing nurses in correctional settings. What values are in conflict in each of these areas? (p. 608)
- How do basic and advanced nursing practice in correctional settings differ? (p. 607)
- What are some of the biophysical, psychological, physical environmental, sociocultural, behavioral, and health system factors that influence health in correctional settings? How might these factors differ for inmates and correctional staff? (pp. 608–614)
- What are the major aspects of primary prevention in correctional settings? What activities might nurses perform in relation to each? (pp. 614–616)
- What are the main aspects of secondary prevention in correctional settings? How might community health nurses be involved in each? (pp. 616–618)
- Discuss considerations in tertiary prevention in correctional settings. (pp. 618–619)

REFERENCES

Alemagno, S. A. (2001). Women in jail: Is substance abuse treatment enough? *American Journal of Public Health, 91*, 798–800.

Altice, F., Bellin, E., Bick, J., De Groot, A. S., et al. (1998). *Management of the HIV-positive prisoner.* New York: World Health CME.

American Nurses Association. (1985). *Standards of nursing practice in correctional facilities.* Kansas City, MO: Author.

American Nurses Association. (1995). *Scope and standards of nursing practice in correctional settings.* Washington, DC: Author.

Brodie, J. (2000). Caring—The essence of correctional nursing. *Correct Care, 14*(4), 1, 15, 18.

Bureau of Justice Statistics. (2001). *Criminal offender statistics.* Retrieved June 2, 2001, from the World Wide Web, *http://www.ojp. usdoj.gov/bjs.*

Burgess, R. (1999). Health promotion with offenders. In E. R. Perkins, I. Simnett, & L. Wright (Eds.), *Evidence-based health promotion* (pp. 226–237). New York: John Wiley & Sons.

Chavez, R. S. (1999). Health experts outline epidemiology and treatment of hepatitis C. *Correct Care, 13*(3), 7.

Coalition for Juvenile Justice. (2000). *Handle with care: Serving the mental health needs of young offenders.* Retrieved June 2, 2001, from the World Wide Web, *http://www.juvjustice.org.*

Cohen, M. D. (1997). The human health effects of pepperspray—A review of the literature and commentary. *Journal of Correctional Health Care, 4*, 73–88.

Conklin, T. J., Lincoln, T., & Tuthill, R. W. (2000). Self-reported health and prior health behaviors of newly admitted correctional inmates. *American Journal of Public Health, 90*, 1939–1941.

Correct Care. (1999). A summary guide to revisions in the 1999 *Standards for Health Services in Juvenile Detention and Confinement Facilities. 13*(2), 18–19.

Correct Care. (2000). Nation's prison population growth rate slows. *14*(4), 22.

Correct Care. (2001a). COs passing meds passes court—but wise wardens will mandate controls. *15*(2), 6.

Correct Care. (2001b). Population stats. *15*(2), 21.

Correct Care. (2001c). Study released on health needs of detained youth. *15*(1), 19.

Correct Care. (2001d). Tuberculosis comes roaring back—and the nation responds. *15*(2), 18.

De Groot, A. S. (1998). *HIV Frontline, 34*, 1–2.

De Groot, A. S., DeHovitz, J. A., Fletcher, C., Lancaster, J. L., et al. (1999). *Optimal management of HIV in correctional systems.* New York: World Health CME.

Dubler, N. N., & Heyman, B. (1998). End-of-life care in prisons and jails. In M. Puisis (Ed.), *Clinical practice in correctional medicine.* St. Louis: Mosby.

Earley, J. (1999, spring/summer). Nursing behind bars. *Minority Nurse*, 22–26.

Falter, R. G. (1999). Selected predictors of health services needs of inmates over age 50. *Journal of Correctional Health Care, 6*, 149–175.

Flores, M. (1998). Peer groups offered as way to slow prison AIDS. *Correct Care, 12*(1), 8.

Fulco, S. D. (2001). Babies behind bars: The rights and liabilities of babies and mothers. *Correct Care, 15*(1), 6.

Hancock, P. J. (1999). CCHP employs philosophy of community health nursing. *Correct Care, 13*(2), 4.

HIV Inside. (1999). Ensuring continuity of care for the HIV-positive inmate. *1*(4), 1–5, 8, 11–12.

Laird, L. H. (1999). Myths of HIV in prison settings: Implications for policy and intervention. *Journal of Correctional Health Care, 6*, 177–196.

Leh, S. K. (1999). HIV infection in U.S. correctional systems: Its effect on the community. *Journal of Community Health Nursing, 16*(1), 53–63.

Maruschak, L. M., & Beck, A. J. (2001). *Medical problems of inmates.* Retrieved June 2, 2001, from the World Wide Web, *http://www.ojp. usdoj.gov/bjs.*

Mayes, M. S., Schilling, C., & Long, B. (1998). An alternative approach to managed care. *Correct Care, 12*(1), 9, 11.

Mumola, C. J. (2000). *Incarcerated parents and their children.* Retrieved June 2, 2001, from the World Wide Web, *http://www.ojp.usdoj. gov/bjs.*

National Center for HIV, STD, and TB Prevention. (1998). *Morbidity and Mortality Weekly Report, 47*, 429–431.

National Center for HIV, STD, and TB Prevention. (1999a). Decrease in AIDS-related mortality in a state correctional system—New York, 1995–1998. *Morbidity and Mortality Weekly Report, 47*, 1115–1117.

National Center for HIV, STD, and TB Prevention. (1999b). Tuberculosis outbreaks in prison housing units for HIV-infected inmates—California, 1995–1996. *Morbidity and Mortality Weekly Report, 48*, 79–82.

National Center for HIV, STD, and TB Prevention. (2000). Drug-susceptible tuberculosis outbreak in a state correctional facility—South Carolina, 1999–2000. *Morbidity and Mortality Weekly Report, 49*, 1041–1044.

National Commission on Correctional Health Care. (1998). *Position statement on the management of tuberculosis in correctional facilities.* Chicago: Author.

National Commission on Correctional Health Care. (2001). *Draft recommended correctional clinical guidelines.* Retrieved June 2, 2001, from the World Wide Web, *http://www.ncchc.org.*

National Institute of Drug Abuse. (1998). Later criminal behavior and drug use dramatically reduced by drug treatment beginning in prison. *Correct Care, 12*(1), 1, 15.

Olds, D., Henderson, C. R., Cole, R. Eckenrode, J., et al. (1998). Long-term effects of nurse home visitation on children's criminal and antisocial behavior. *Journal of the American Medical Association, 280*, 1238–1244.

Paris, J. (2000). Georgia inmates and staff coped with natural disaster—Lessons learned from Hurricane Floyd. *Correct Care, 14*(1), 8, 21.

Schreiber, C. (1999). Behind bars: Aging prison population challenges correctional health systems. *NurseWeek, 12*(15), 10.

Seidlitz, A. (1998). National Prison Hospice Association helps facilities deal with inmate deaths. *Correct Care, 12*(1), 10.

Stringer, H. (2001). Prison break. *NurseWeek, 14*(6), 13–14.

Tartaro, C. (1999). Reduction of suicides in jails and lockups through situational crime prevention: Addressing the needs of a transient population. *Journal of Correctional Health Care, 6*, 235–263.

Tulsky, J. P., White, M. C., Dawson, C., Hoynes, T. M., Goldenson, J., & Schecter, G. (1998). Screening for tuberculosis in jail and clinic follow-up after release. *American Journal of Public Health, 88*, 223–226.

Vitucci, N. (1999a). Corrections challenged with treating mentally ill. *Correct Care, 13*(3), 1, 14, 18.

Vitucci, N. (1999b). FOP to implement fee-for-services. *Correct Care, 13*(4), 1, 6.

Vitucci, N. (1999c). More than one quarter million prison and jail inmates identified as mentally ill. *Correct Care, 13*(4), 18.

Vitucci, N. (1999d). Team work and preparation help Louisiana correctional facilities during hurricane Georges. *Correct Care, 13*(1), 1, 9.

Vitucci, N. (2000). Inmate rates of HIV infection and AIDS-related deaths drop. *Correct Care, 14*(1), 7.

Wilson, D. J. (2000). *Drug use, testing, and treatment in jails.* Retrieved June 2, 2001, from the World Wide Web, *http://www.ojp. usdoj.gov/bjs.*

CARE OF CLIENTS IN DISASTER SETTINGS

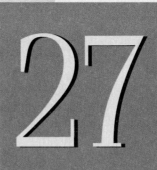

27

Chapter Objectives

After reading this chapter, you should be able to:

- Describe ways in which disaster events may vary.
- Describe the elements of a disaster.
- Identify potential benefits of disaster preparedness.
- Identify biophysical, psychological, physical environmental, sociocultural, behavioral, and health system considerations to be assessed in relation to a disaster.
- Discuss the principles of community disaster preparedness.
- Describe the characteristics of an effective disaster plan.
- Identify the component elements of an effective disaster plan.
- Describe the role of community health nurses in primary, secondary, and tertiary prevention related to disaster situations.

KEY TERMS

community resource maps 632
community risk maps 631
direct victims 633
displaced persons 633
early warning systems 637
emergency consensus 634
indirect victims 633
logistical coordination 638
mitigation 627
preimpact mobilization 628
protein-energy malnutrition (PEM) 645
reconstitution 629
refugees 633
rescue chains 637
restoration 629
triage 638
twinning 635
vulnerability assessment 637

Media Link

http://www.prenhall.com/clark

Additional interactive resources for this chapter can be found on the companion Web site. Click on Chapter 27 and "Begin" to select the activities for this chapter.

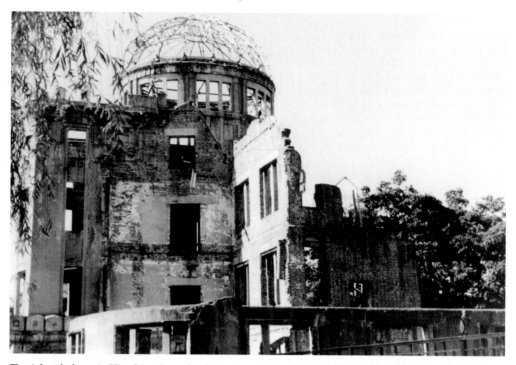

The A-bomb dome in Hiroshima Japan has become an international symbol of the devastation of war.

Throughout history, people have been subjected to unexpected events that cause massive destruction, death, and injury. From 1980 to 1991, the number of people killed, injured, or displaced by disasters more than tripled, from 100 million to 311 million people. Preparation for disasters and effective response when a disaster occurs can help minimize the long-term effects of these events. The United Nations declared the 1990s the Decade for National Disaster Reduction in an effort to combat the sense of fatalism often attached to disasters (Noji, 1997b). This chapter explores the role of the community health nurse in proactive efforts before, during, and after disaster events.

Disasters are events that require extraordinary efforts beyond those needed to respond to everyday emergencies (Noji, 1997c). Emergencies, on the other hand, are serious events that fall within the coping abilities of the individual or community. Disasters test the adaptive responses of communities or individuals beyond their capabilities and lead to at least a temporary disruption of function. Similar to the experience of crisis by individuals or families, what constitutes a disaster for one community may not be perceived as such by another. From 1989 to 2000, the U.S. government spent an average of $10 million a year on disaster relief (Lichterman, 2000). This figure does not include the extent of private spending (e.g., by insurance companies) to remedy the effects of disaster, nor does it convey the extent of death, injury, disease, and grief that result from disasters. Expenditures arising from the September 11, 2001, terrorist attacks on the World Trade Center and the Pentagon as well as subsequent anthrax contamination are likely to be considerably higher. Information about the effects of selected disasters

is summarized below to convey a picture of the multiple effects of these catastrophic events.

Disasters are of even greater concern today than in the past for several reasons. The frequency of disaster events has increased, due in part to increasing technology and the concomitant increase in the potential for technological disasters. Human populations are also more densely populated, increasing the potential for exposure to disaster events as they occur. In addition, because of increasing population sizes, people are more likely to build, live, or work in areas with high disaster potential (Comerio, 1998). Finally, recent events have demonstrated the willingness of some radical groups to engineer massive disasters to achieve their political goals.

HIGHLIGHTS

Selected Effects of Recent Disasters

1991–1994	Economic sanctions against Haiti increased child mortality from 56 deaths per 1,000 children to 61 deaths per 1,000 and increased maternal mortality by 29% (Gibbons & Garfield, 1999).
1995	A bioterrorist attack using sarin nerve gas in Tokyo caused 11 deaths (Wetter, Daniell, & Treser, 2001).
1998	A series of storms in Texas caused 31 deaths and $900 million in damages (National Center for Environmental Health, 2000b).

A cholera epidemic in Rwandan refugee camps caused 1,521 deaths in 30 days (National Center for Environmental Health, 1998).

Hurricane Georges caused 300 deaths in the Dominican Republic and 8 in Puerto Rico. In the Dominican Republic, 170,000 people were still in need of food relief two months after the storm. In Puerto Rico, 28,000 people were housed in government shelters, 700,000 people were without water, and 1 million were without electricity (Epidemiology Program Office, 1998; National Center for Environmental Health, 1999).

1994–1999	International economic sanctions against Iraq more than doubled the mortality rate among children 1 to 4 years of age (*The Nation's Health*, 1999).
1999	An earthquake in Turkey killed 17,000 people and caused 24,000 injuries (Epidemiology Program Office, 1999).
	Hurricane Floyd caused 52 deaths (Epidemiology Program Office, 2000).
2000	Famine in Ethiopia placed 10 million people at risk for starvation (National Center for Environmental Health, 2001).
2001	Terrorist attacks on the World Trade Center in New York and the Pentagon in Washington, DC, resulted in an as yet undetermined number of deaths (estimated at more than 4,000, including more than 300 deaths among rescue workers).
	Mailed dissemination of anthrax spores resulted in an as yet undetermined number of cases and deaths.

TYPES OF DISASTERS

Disasters have traditionally been categorized as natural or man-made (Noji, 1997c). Natural disasters are those produced by epidemics, famine, and forces of nature such as storms, floods, and earthquakes. Man-made, or human-generated, disasters may be either accidental or intentional (Comerio, 1998), and can be further differentiated as complex emergencies, technological disasters, deforestation, material shortages, and other disasters not caused by natural hazards (Noji, 1997c). Complex emergencies are events related to political conflicts such as war and civil strife. Technological disasters occur as a result of technology gone awry, as in the case of an airplane crash or train derailment. Bioterrorism is another type of technological disaster—an intentional one. As noted in Chapter 7, deforestation leads to a variety of effects, including increased potential for natural disasters.

Civil conflicts trigger mass migration and a host of health effects in the migrant population as well as for their host countries. In 1995, it was estimated that one of every 200 people in the world was a refugee or internally displaced. In 1999, approximately 50 military conflicts were going on around the world (Neugebauer, 1999), adding to what has been termed "a demographic epidemic of unprecedented proportions—an epidemic of forced migrations that has had grave public health consequences" (Toole, 1999, p. 13). Overall, an estimated 100 million people are involved in global migration due to adverse conditions in their own regions (McGuire, 1998), including more than 10,000 Afghan refugees who have sought asylum in Pakistan before and after the start of the U.S. war against the Taliban in Afghanistan.

Another category of disaster combines human and natural causes. For example, toxic substances released in a transportation disaster may be widely dispersed by a windstorm. These combined disasters are sometimes referred to as "NA-TECH" disasters (Noji, 1997c). Whether natural or man-made, disasters vary considerably in terms of their frequency, predictability, preventability, imminence, and destructive potential.

Some disasters occur relatively frequently in certain parts of the world. Consequently, people in those areas have some knowledge of what to expect and what can be done to minimize the effects of the event. For example, earthquakes occur periodically in California, and residents in earthquake-prone areas are encouraged to be prepared in the event of a large quake. Similarly, hurricanes and other severe storms are frequently experienced during certain seasons in other parts of the country.

Some disaster events are predictable. The probability of destructive tornadoes increases from April through June in the United States in general, but in North Dakota, most tornadoes occur from June to August (Lillibridge, 1997c). Similarly, many rivers are known to flood periodically with heavy spring rains. Other events, such as a plane crash, a fire in a chemical plant, or a terrorist attack are not predictable.

Some types of disasters are more easily prevented than others. For example, periodic flooding can be prevented by rerouting waterways or by building dams. Others, such as earthquakes, cannot be controlled or prevented. Increased security measures are one attempt to prevent disasters resulting from terrorist activities, but their effectiveness remains to be seen.

Disasters also vary with respect to their imminence in terms of their speed of onset, extent of forewarning, and duration. Some disasters provide evidence of their imminent occurrence and allow time for forewarning and preparation prior to impact. For example, hurricanes can be tracked and their probable path determined. People along that path usually have sufficient warning to take preventive actions that minimize the potential for death and destruction. Other disasters such as fires and explosions occur instantaneously, with no prior warning. In some cases, the disaster event itself is of short duration,

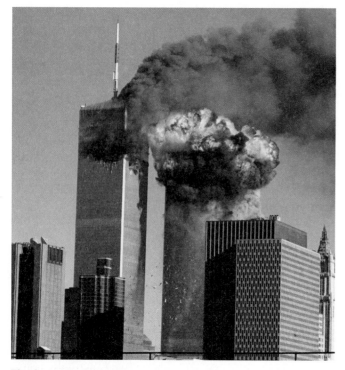

The destruction of the World Trade Center in 2001 was a man-made disaster caused by international terrorists. (Photo courtesy of Corbis/SABA Press Photos, Inc.)

tively small number of people. For example, the effects of a mine cave-in are generally restricted to the area where the mine is located. The effects of war or famine, on the other hand, may be more far-reaching. Many experts distinguish between primary and secondary effects of disasters. Primary disaster effects are the immediate effects of the disaster event itself, such as the extent of death, injury, and destruction of property. Rapid-onset natural disasters, such as earthquakes, often have severe primary effects. Secondary disaster effects are those that occur indirectly as a result of the disaster. Examples include malnutrition due to disruption of food supplies, psychological problems such as posttraumatic stress disorder, or disruption of the U.S. economy following the World Trade Center attack. Disasters also vary in terms of the severity of their effects. Some disasters cause moderate loss of life or property and result in only temporary inability to function, whereas others are devastating. The destructive potential of a nuclear explosion, for example, is far greater than that of a single plane crash.

PUBLIC HEALTH EFFECTS OF DISASTERS

As demonstrated by the figures provided above, disasters have a variety of physical, psychological, social, and economic effects. Many of these effects have consequences for the health of the public. The most obvious effects with public health consequences are, of course, the extent of death and injury that occur in a disaster. Disasters may also increase the potential for communicable diseases and

as in the case of an earthquake or a transportation disaster. At other times, the disaster event lasts some time. Examples of prolonged disasters are epidemics, famine, and war.

Finally, disasters vary in terms of their impact and their destructive potential. Some disasters are fairly limited in scope, affecting a small geographic area or a rela-

Earthquakes leave an aftermath of destruction. (Photo courtesy of AP/Wide World Photos)

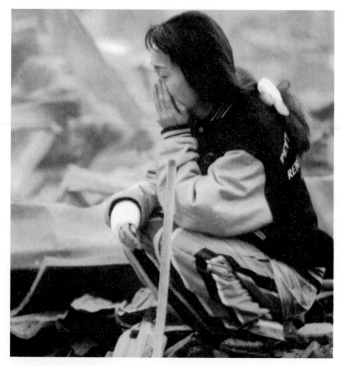

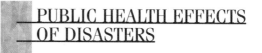

(Photo courtesy of Shinya Inui/Friday/Corbis/Sygma)

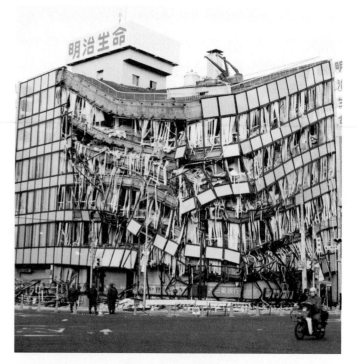

environmental hazards. Floods, for example, may contribute to breeding areas for communicable disease vectors such as mosquitoes and other insects as well as the nuisance and discomfort caused by insect bites and stings (Malilay, 1997b). The crowding that may occur in shelters also contributes to the spread of disease, while migration of large population groups may expose them to new pathogens or lead to exposure of host country residents (Toole, 1997). Explosions and volcanic eruptions may cause emission of toxic gases or radiation in addition to the physical damage that may be caused to structures (Baxter, 1997).

Disasters such as drought and famine, as well as war and civil conflict, may lead to food shortages and malnutrition among the populations affected. Displacement may also contribute to assault and rape, particularly among female refugees (Diaz, 1999). Any number of different types of disasters, including the application of economic sanctions against a nation, may lead to the destruction of the health care infrastructure or disruption of routine health care services (Noji, 1997c; Sidel, 1999). In addition to drought, wind, and flood damage, severe weather conditions may contribute to problems of hypothermia or hyperthermia, particularly among economically disadvantaged segments of the population (Kilbourne, 1997a, 1997b). Finally, all kinds of disasters have the potential for creating transient or long-lasting psychological effects.

ELEMENTS OF A DISASTER

To plan with other members of the community for an effective response to a disaster, community health nurses need to understand the three elements of a disaster: the temporal, spatial, and role elements.

The Temporal Element: Stages of Disaster Response

Disaster experts characterize disasters as cyclic phenomena unfolding in five stages: the nondisaster or interdisaster stage, the predisaster stage, the impact stage, the emergency stage, and the reconstruction or rehabilitation stage (Noji, 1997c).

THE NONDISASTER STAGE
The nondisaster stage, also referred to as the interdisaster phase, is the period of time before the threat of a disaster materializes. This period should be a time of planning and preparation. During this stage, communities should engage in such activities as identifying potential disaster risks and mapping their locations in the community. Vulnerability analysis and capability inventory are other features of this stage in which the community assesses the potential consequences of disasters likely to occur within the community and its ability to cope with these

consequences. Determination of adaptive capacity involves an inventory of resources that are likely to be needed in the event of specific types of disasters.

During the nondisaster stage, the community should also engage in prevention, preparedness, and mitigation activities. *Mitigation* is action taken to prevent or reduce the harmful effects of a disaster on human health or property (Malilay, 1997a). Mitigation is sometimes referred to as "hard" or "soft." Hard mitigation involves construction of the built environment to withstand the force of natural hazards (Lichterman, 2000). Retrofitting or reinforcing major highway overpasses is an example of hard mitigation being used in California to prevent the collapse of highways and bridges in the event of an earthquake. Soft mitigation is intended to minimize the adverse effects of disasters that cannot be prevented, for example, developing communication strategies that enhance the capability of multiunit response to major brush fires.

The final area of activity in the nondisaster planning period is education of both professionals and the public regarding disaster prevention and preparation. Unfortunately, many communities deny the need for disaster planning when they are not faced with the direct threat of a disaster. Even when disaster planning occurs, if the plan is not widely disseminated, disaster response can be impeded. For example, effective response to extensive flooding in Missouri was hampered by failure of the Missouri Department of Health to engage local health departments and regional offices in the development of their disaster plan and to communicate the plan to them once it was developed (Gautam, 1998).

THE PREDISASTER STAGE
The predisaster stage occurs when a disaster event is imminent but has not yet occurred. This stage may also be referred to as the warning (Noji, 1997c) or threat stage. Major activities during this stage are warning, preimpact mobilization, and, in some cases, evacuation. Warning involves apprising members of the community of the imminence of a disaster event and of the actions that should be taken to minimize its consequences. For example, storm warnings are broadcast in many areas when there is potential for a severe storm, but people do not immediately go to a storm cellar or leave the area, because the possibility remains that the storm will bypass the area.

Just as communities may accept or deny the need for disaster planning, members of the community may respond positively or negatively to warnings of possible disasters. Several factors can influence a person's response to warnings of imminent disaster. These factors include the source, content, and mechanism for warning, and individual perceptions and beliefs. Warning messages that are clear, practical, and relevant or that originate from credible sources are more likely to be acted on than vague or impractical warnings. Warnings need to specify the exact nature of the threat and provide specific recommendations for action (World Health Organization, 1989). For example, vague warnings of the potential for additional terrorist activities following the September 11, 2001, attacks provided little direction for action. Specific guidelines on how to handle potentially contaminated mail, on the other hand, were more effective in promoting action. Warnings should also contain sufficient information to allow people to decide on an appropriate course of action. It is sometimes erroneously believed that detailed information about a disaster will cause panic. In effect, failure to provide information usually leads to failure to act on warnings; providing information does not seem to contribute to panic among individual citizens.

Response to a warning is also affected by each individual's perceptions about the possibility of disaster. These perceptions arise from past experiences with disaster, psychological traits, and sociocultural factors. For example, if people have previously been only on the fringes of a hurricane path, they may not perceive a hurricane as a very frightening event, and they may ignore storm warnings. Similarly, if the individual has a fatalistic attitude that one's own actions will not make much difference in the outcome of an event, he or she might not act in response to warnings. Such an attitude may be the result of an individual personality trait or a sociocultural norm in the group.

Warning confirmation also influences the way people respond. Warnings tend to be believed if the source of the warning is official, if the probability of the event is increasing, and if one is in close geographic proximity to the area where the disaster is likely to occur. For example, people who live on a recognized geological fault line are more likely to take warnings about potential earthquakes seriously than those who do not live on a fault.

Finally, belief influences action with respect to warnings. Again, belief in the potential for disaster is enhanced if the source of the warning is an official agency and if that agency has credibility. For example, if there have been numerous false alarms in the past, people are less likely to pay attention to warnings. Belief is also enhanced if the medium of the warning is personal rather than impersonal. People are more likely to evacuate their homes if someone comes to their door to warn them than if they hear a warning on the radio. Previous experience also influences the likelihood of belief. If one has experienced the full force of a hurricane before, one is more likely to believe and act on a hurricane warning than would otherwise be the case.

The frequency with which the warning is received also influences belief, as do observable changes in the situation. For example, if people see evidence of flames on a nearby hill, they are more likely to believe in the imminence of danger posed by a brush fire. Perceived behavior of others can influence belief either positively or negatively. When others act in response to the warning, belief is enhanced. If others appear to be ignoring the warning, however, belief is less likely. Factors influencing responses to disaster warnings are summarized at right.

Preimpact mobilization is action aimed at averting the disaster or minimizing its effects. Categories of activity involved in this stage might include efforts to prevent the disaster or its effects, seeking shelter from the effects of the disaster, evacuating people from areas threatened by the disaster, and implementing plans to deal with the effects of a disaster. For example, in the threat of a flood, people may sandbag river banks to divert floodwaters from a town, or board up windows and tie down equipment when a hurricane is forecast. People may seek shelter from tornadoes or other storms by moving to a basement, a storm cellar, or an interior room of a house. Preimpact mobilization might also involve evacuating people from an area threatened by fire, radiation, or chemical leakage. Finally, the initial phases of a disaster response plan may be implemented. For example, off-duty health care personnel may be called to health facilities in preparation for treating anticipated casualties.

THE IMPACT STAGE

In the impact stage of a disaster, the disaster event has occurred and its immediate effects are experienced by the community. The effects of the disaster impact will vary with the type of disaster, the density of population in the area affected, the predisaster status of the community, and the extent to which mitigating actions have been taken and the community is prepared to deal with the consequences of the specific disaster event that has occurred (Noji, 1997c). One major activity in this stage is the assessment of the impact of the disaster with an inventory of the immediate needs of the community. Inventory is a rapid assessment of the damage to buildings and the type and extent of injuries suffered. This information is used to determine actions needed in carrying out the efforts of the emergency stage.

THE EMERGENCY STAGE

The emergency stage involves the immediate response to the effects of the disaster and can be divided into two phases: an early isolation phase and a later relief phase (Noji, 1997c). In the isolation phase, the response to community needs arises from community members themselves because there has not been time for assistance to arrive from outside sources. If the community is geographically isolated or access to the community is impeded by the disaster, this isolation period will be prolonged. In the relief phase, assistance is provided from sources outside of the area affected by the disaster. The activities performed are essentially the same, although performed by different agents in the two phases, and include search and rescue operations, first aid, emergency medical assistance, establishment or restoration of modes of communication and transportation, surveillance for public health effects of the disaster (e.g., infectious diseases, mental health problems), and, in some cases, evacuation of community members from affected areas.

Some areas experience regular flooding causing loss of life and property. (Photo courtesy of Dennis MacDonald/PhotoEdit)

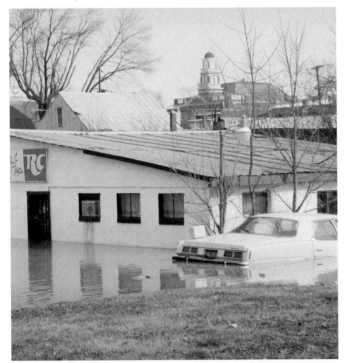

THE RECONSTRUCTION STAGE

In the reconstruction or recovery stage, the focus is on returning the community to equilibrium. This stage can be divided into substages of restoration, reconstitution, and mitigation.

Restoration is the reestablishment of a basic way of life and occurs within the first six months of a disaster. Activities of this stage include returning to or rebuilding homes, replacing lost or damaged property, and continuing life without those who were killed in the catastrophe. At the community level, restoration involves reestablishing community services that may have been disrupted by the disaster. After a flood, for example, people may return to their homes, clean up the mud, and replace water-damaged furniture. Schools reopen, and residents return to work. If a prominent community official was killed in the flood, someone is appointed to fill that post until an election can be held.

Reconstitution occurs when the life of the community has returned, as far as possible, to normal. This return to normal may take from several months to several years, depending on the degree of damage sustained in the disaster. It may take several years after a flood, for example, to restore the landscape of the community to its former state or to replenish the city treasury after disaster costs have depleted it. It may also take some time for individuals to adjust to the loss of loved ones or for the community government to be reconstituted. In extreme disasters, full reconstitution may never occur. For example, many people believe that life in the United States was completely changed by the terrorist attacks on September 11, 2001, and the full effects of that disaster are not yet known.

The final stage of recovery after a disaster is mitigation, which involves future-oriented activities to prevent subsequent disasters or to minimize their effects. For example, a community that has experienced a flood may take engineering action to prevent the likelihood of subsequent floods, or a community that was unprepared for disaster may develop a disaster response plan. Increased security measures and irridiating mail are other examples of efforts aimed at preventing subsequent terrorist activities and their effects. These activities cycle the community back into the nondisaster stage. Stages in the development of and response to a disaster are summarized below.

HIGHLIGHTS

Stages of Community Disaster Response

Nondisaster Stage

- Identification of potential disaster risks
- Vulnerability analysis
- Capability inventory
- Prevention and mitigation
- Public and professional education

(continued)

Predisaster Stage

- Warning
- Preimpact mobilization
- Evacuation

Impact Stage

- Damage inventory
- Injury assessment

Emergency Stage

- Search and rescue
- First aid
- Emergency medical assistance
- Restoration of communication and transportation
- Public health surveillance
- Evacuation

Reconstruction Stage

- Restoration
- Reconstitution
- Mitigation

The Spatial Element

The spatial elements of a disaster refer to the extent of its effects on specific geographic regions. These regions include the area of total impact, the area of partial impact, and outside areas (Figure 27–1 ■).

The area of total impact is the zone where the most severe effects of the disaster are found. In an earthquake, for example, this would include the area where the greatest damage to buildings has occurred and where the greatest number of injuries was sustained.

In the area of partial impact, evidence of the disaster can be seen but the effects are not of the magnitude of those in the total impact area. Using the earthquake example, windows may be broken or objects shaken from shelves in the partial impact area, but buildings are intact. Injuries, if any, are infrequent and relatively minor, or only telephone and electrical services might be disrupted in the partial impact area.

The outside area is not directly affected but may be a source of assistance in response to the disaster. Areas immediately adjacent to the disaster area are called on first to provide assistance, with further outlying areas being involved later as needed.

FIGURE 27–1 ■ *Areas of disaster impact*

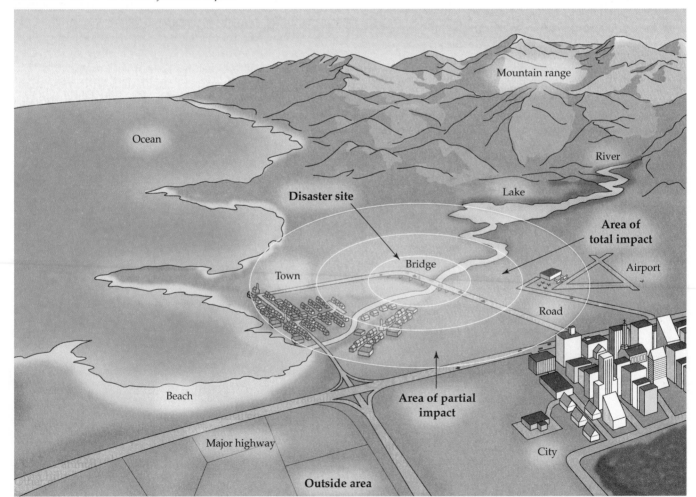

Spatial elements of a disaster vary greatly from event to event. For example, the total and partial impact areas affected by a nuclear accident would be far larger than those affected by a fire at an industrial chemicals plant. The area from which assistance might be requested would also be larger given the greater magnitude of the problem, the number of victims involved, and the damage sustained.

Spatial elements of a potential disaster can also be explored prior to a disaster event. The World Health Organization (1989) recommends the use of community risk maps and community resource maps to help delineate spatial dimensions in disaster planning. *Community risk maps* pinpoint the locations of disaster risks within the community. Risk maps also delineate probable areas

of effect for different types of disasters. Figure 27–2 ■ is an example of a community risk map. Two primary disaster risks are identified in the community risk map in Figure 27–2: a dam and reservoir that could result in flooding and a chemical manufacturing plant on the south side of the river. In addition, this community is in an area that experiences periodic tornadoes. The community risk map delineates the areas of the community likely to be affected by a flood (along the river) and a fire or explosion at the chemical plant. The area affected by a tornado would depend on where the tornado touched down. The map also indicates several pockets of particularly vulnerable populations in areas likely to be affected by disasters. These include residents of a nursing home, prison inmates, and schoolchildren in the vicinity of the

FIGURE 27–2 ■ *Sample community risk map*

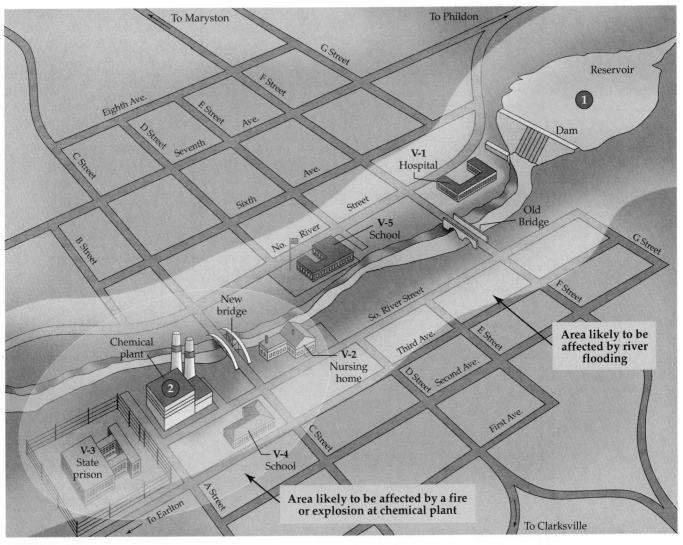

Legend:

● **Disaster risk**
1. Dam and reservoir: potential for flooding
2. Chemical plant: potential for explosion/fire

V **Vulnerable populations**
1. Hospitalized patients
2. Nursing home residents
3. State prison inmates
4. School children
5. School children

chemical plant. These same groups, along with patients at the hospital at F and North River streets and children in the school just north of the river, would be at risk in the event of a flood on the river.

Community resource maps indicate the locations of resources likely to be needed in the event of each of the types of disasters for which the community is at risk. Notations on a community resource map include, for example, potential shelter locations, designated command headquarters (and alternates if advisable), storage places for supplies, areas where heavy equipment is available, health care facilities, and proposed emergency morgue areas for the dead. Resource maps also indicate primary and alternate evacuation and transportation routes. Figure 27–3 ■ is a sample resource map related to the community risks identified in Figure 27–2. Looking at Figure 27–3, we see that city hall is adjacent to the river

and likely to be affected by a flood. Therefore, the command headquarters has been situated at the television station in the northern part of town. It was believed that placement at the station would facilitate communication because of the equipment available there. A southern command post has also been established in the event that both bridges are impassable and response operations on the two sides of the river cannot be coordinated. Because of the potential for splitting the community and lack of access across the river, potential shelter sites have been established and supplies have been stored on both sides of the river. Health services are also available on both sides even if the hospital at F and North River streets has to be evacuated due to flooding. Rescue operations for people stranded along the river would have to be handled from the north side of the river because that is where the boat docks are located. Personnel and supplies can be

FIGURE 27–3 ■ *Sample community resource map*

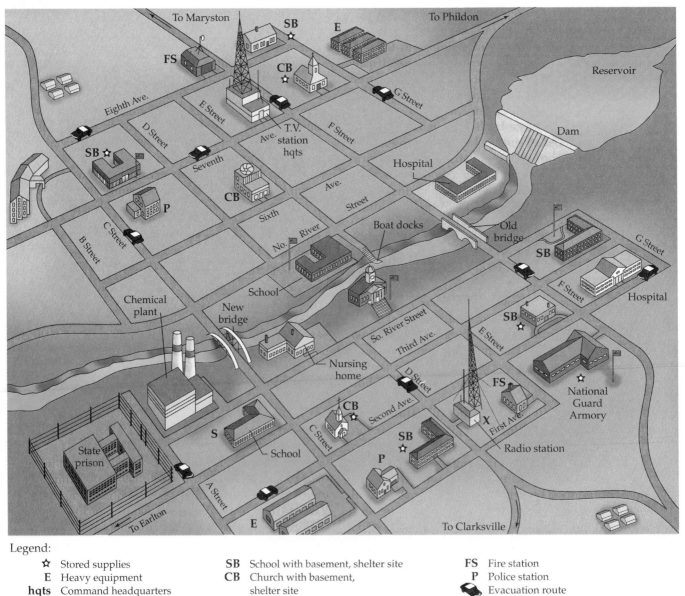

Legend:

☆	Stored supplies	**SB**	School with basement, shelter site	**FS**	Fire station
E	Heavy equipment	**CB**	Church with basement,	**P**	Police station
hqts	Command headquarters		shelter site		Evacuation route
X	Southern command post		Tent shelter site		

brought in from other towns in several different directions and could be brought directly to tent shelter sites if necessary. Only the road from Phildon is likely to be impassable if flooding reaches that far from the reservoir. Both the community risk and resource maps allow disaster planners to visualize what is likely to occur in a disaster event and to plan the most effective response to a disaster.

The Role Element

The final element of a disaster is its role element. Two basic roles for people involved in a disaster are *victim* and *helper roles.*

People may be direct or indirect victims of a disaster. *Direct victims* are those who experience maximum exposure to and effects of the event. *Indirect victims* are friends and family of direct victims. Direct victims may require medical or psychological assistance or help with basic survival necessities. Indirect victims need reassurance and may require help in locating family members affected by the disaster.

Refugees and displaced persons are special categories of direct victims of disasters. *Displaced persons* are those who are forced by the disaster to leave their homes. Displacement may occur for a variety of reasons, including destruction of one's home, temporary hazardous conditions, and war, and may persist for varying periods. *Refugees* are a subgroup of displaced persons defined by the United Nations Convention and the Organization of African Unity as those who have fled their own country for fear of war, civil disturbance, or other forms of violence. Another group of people are *economic refugees,* those who have fled due to poverty, famine, or natural disaster rather than war or persecution. Economic refugees are not recognized by the United Nations and are often not eligible for the kinds of assistance provided to designated refugee populations (McGuire, 1998). In 1999, there were an estimated 22 million refugees and 20 million displaced persons throughout the world (Toole, 1999). These disaster victims constitute populations at high risk for multiple health problems, including malnutrition, trauma, communicable diseases, and psychological problems.

ETHICAL AWARENESS

Arnold (1999) reported that some critics of nongovernment organizations providing disaster relief in war-torn countries suggest that they only prolong the fighting ability of combatants by preventing them from having to negotiate peace to meet the needs of the population. Do you think this is a valid assessment? Why or why not? Should humanitarian organizations refrain from providing aid until one or the other party in a conflict has been soundly defeated in order to prevent further loss of life by prolonging the conflict?

Helpers include designated rescue and recovery personnel as well as community members who help provide care or who assist in the provision of necessities such as food, shelter, and clothing. It is important to remember that victim and helper roles may overlap and that rescue and recovery personnel or other community helpers may themselves have suffered injury or loss as a result of the disaster. For example, significant loss of life in the World Trade Center attacks in 2001 occurred among rescue personnel.

Both victims and helpers are under stress as a result of the disaster. Stressors for victims may be quite obvious and include injury and the loss of loved ones or property. Additional stressors for helpers during the rescue and recovery periods include encounters with multiple deaths that are frequently of a shocking nature, experiencing the suffering of others, and role stress. Frequently, the overwhelming nature of role demands or needs for assistance by victims lead to feelings of helplessness and depression. Other sources of role stress include communication difficulties, inadequacies in terms of resources or staff, lack of access to people needing assistance or resources to help them, bureaucratic difficulties, exhaustion, uncertainties regarding role or authority, and intragroup or intergroup conflicts. Stress may also arise from conflicts between demands of the helper's family members and the needs of victims, and between demands of one's regular job and disaster role.

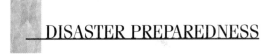

DISASTER PREPAREDNESS

As noted earlier, it is to be hoped that the earlier stages of a community's response to a disaster involve planning for a disaster event. For this to occur, community health nurses and others in the community must have an understanding of the concepts and principles of disaster preparedness.

Benefits of Disaster Preparedness

The need for disaster preparation and plans for disaster response is greater today than at any time in history. Increased population density throughout the world has heightened the potential for widespread effects of disasters. Technologies such as nuclear reactors and dams to provide water and electricity have also contributed to increased potential for disastrous events, as have terrorism and the increased capacity to wage destructive warfare.

The costs of all types of disasters are staggering in terms of death and human suffering as well as dollars. With adequate preparation and timely response, the monetary costs of disaster could be greatly reduced. The savings in human lives that could result is another strong motivation for concerted community efforts in disaster planning.

The need for disaster planning is reinforced by observations that there is less confusion regarding responsibilities and communications when specific agencies have been assigned specific functions in keeping with an overall disaster response plan. In addition, the development of interagency linkages that take place in disaster planning increases the smoothness of response in an actual disaster situation (Paris, 2000). A final reason for concerted disaster planning is that well-developed existing plans can be used in the event of other unforeseen events.

Disaster planning can also increase the adaptive capacity of the community. Planning for a disaster event heightens the community's ability to respond effectively to the aftermath of the disaster. For example, if there is a plan for emergency food and shelter that can be put into operation in the event of a disaster, the number of lives that are disrupted can be minimized. Similarly, if contingency plans exist for different situations, performance of critical functions will be less disrupted than would otherwise be the case. For example, plans may call for casualties to be brought to a certain hospital during a disaster. If that hospital is affected by the disaster and no alternative is planned, the community will be less able to adapt to the situation, care of victims will suffer, and more lives may be lost.

Purposes of Disaster Preparedness

Disaster planning has two major purposes. The first is to reduce the community's vulnerability to the disaster and to prevent it, if possible. For example, when the threat of flood is imminent, work crews may sandbag river banks in an attempt to prevent flooding of homes and businesses. In an area where flooding occurs periodically, a dam might be built to control water flow and prevent flooding. A community's vulnerability to the effects of flooding may also be reduced by locating vital community services on high ground to prevent their disruption by floodwaters.

The second purpose of disaster planning is to ensure that resources are available for effective response in the event of a disaster. This aspect of planning involves determining procedures that will be employed in response to a disaster event and obtaining material and personnel that will be required to implement the disaster plan.

Principles of Disaster Preparedness

Disaster planning should be based on several general principles. First, measures used for everyday emergencies typically are not useful for major disasters. Disasters and everyday emergencies differ in their degree of uncertainty, urgency, and emergency consensus. They also differ in terms of the role played by private citizens. Disasters typically present a greater degree of uncertainty than do everyday emergencies in that the latter tend to be more predictable. For example, the types of activities needed to respond to the usual residential fire are well known and predictable. The precise needs in a disaster situation are largely dependent on the type and extent of the disaster; although some of this can be predicted, the exact extent of needs is uncertain until the event occurs.

Disasters are also attended by a greater degree of urgency than everyday emergencies. Traffic accidents, for example, occur frequently and pose a need for action. People may be trapped in damaged vehicles, and there is a need to get them out. In a large-scale plane crash or train wreck, however, there is less knowledge of what the status of those trapped may be than if an individual were trapped in a single vehicle. There would be an even greater urgency if the train were carrying hazardous materials that might cause further damage.

In a disaster there is also less of an *emergency consensus* or agreement on what must be done and how to do it than is usually true of an everyday emergency. In addition, private citizens may have a very active role in rescue and response activities in a disaster situation, but little or no role in responding to everyday emergencies. In the case of a residential fire, for example, once fire department personnel have arrived, private citizens are expected to stay out of the way rather than assist in fighting the blaze. When a lengthy section of a major highway collapsed during an earthquake in San Francisco, however, residents in the area began immediately to help rescue people trapped in their cars and continued to help with rescue operations after emergency personnel arrived.

A second principle in disaster planning is that plans need to be adjusted to people's needs and not vice versa. If a large portion of the population is non–English-speaking, for example, it is unreasonable to issue disaster warnings only in English in the hope that someone will be available to translate the message. Third, disaster planning does not stop at the development of a written plan. Rather, disaster planning is a continuing process that changes as community circumstances change.

The greater the incorporation of disaster "myths" into the plan, the less effective the plan will be. For example, some individuals believe that disasters inevitably trigger widespread looting and theft when this is not usually the case (Noji, 1997c). If disaster planning focuses on such myths, supplies and personnel will be diverted from necessary activities and directed instead toward preventing events that are unlikely to occur.

A fifth principle is that people in the community affected must be informed. All too frequently, some planners believe that providing the public with detailed information about the disaster and its effects will lead to panic. For this reason, vital information may be withheld, actually leading to a lack of response or to an inappropriate response on the part of the public.

Sixth, in the event of a disaster, people are likely to respond without direction in the absence of a specific disaster plan. The typical response of most community members will be to do what seems best in the circumstances, sometimes even with heroic action. Although such efforts are commendable, they may result in duplication of effort, inefficient use of resources, and confusion.

Seventh, the disaster plan should enlist the support and coordinate the efforts of the entire community. To achieve this end, major components of the community that would be involved in a disaster response should be involved in developing the response plan. Some of those that might be involved include police and fire departments, local governing bodies, major health care facilities, and large corporations. Predisaster incorporation of these various segments of the community limits confusion with respect to authority and direction for disaster-related activities and enhances the smooth operation of a disaster effort.

Eighth, there is a need to link the disaster plan for one area with those of surrounding areas to allow coordination of efforts in the face of widespread catastrophe. Conversely, when help is needed from surrounding areas, that help will better complement local efforts if plans are coordinated. The World Health Organization (1989) referred to this kind of mutual disaster planning between adjacent communities as *twinning.*

There is a need for a general plan that addresses all potential types of disasters in the community. When separate plans exist for different types of disasters, there is potential for confusion regarding roles and responsibilities in any particular situation. If, for example, fire personnel are supposed to have primary authority in disasters involving fires and military personnel in disasters related to destruction of property (e.g., an earthquake), there may be confusion about authority in any disaster involving both. Conversely, in an unanticipated disaster, neither group may take responsibility for decision making, and the response will be hampered by lack of leadership.

In addition, disaster plans should be based as much as possible on everyday working methods and procedures. If one approach to communication is used in dealing with everyday emergencies, the same approach should be used in the event of a major disaster. This eliminates the need for personnel to learn new procedures and prevents confusion about which procedure is applicable in a given situation.

A disaster plan should be flexible enough to fit the specific situation. If the disaster event has eliminated usual means of communication, there should be a contingency plan to adapt to that circumstance. Similarly, if injured victims were to be taken to a specific hospital for treatment after stabilization and that hospital is damaged in an earthquake, there is a need to change the plan to adapt to this situation.

Finally, the plan should not specify responsible persons by name but by position or title. This prevents a need to revise the plan when one person leaves and another takes over the position. For example, the plan may specify that the chief of police be notified of the emergency situation and put the disaster plan into effect. Then, whoever happens to be chief of police will know that it is his or her responsibility to mobilize personnel in the event of a disaster. The principles of disaster planning at the community level are summarized at right.

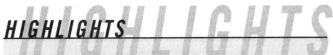

HIGHLIGHTS

General Principles of Disaster Planning

- Measures used for everyday emergencies are not sufficient for major disasters.
- Disaster plans should be adjusted to people's needs and not vice versa.
- Disaster planning does not stop with the development of a written plan, but is a continuous process changing with community circumstances.
- The greater the incorporation of disaster myths, the less effective the disaster plan will be.
- Lack of information, rather than too much information, causes inappropriate response by community members.
- People respond to a disaster situation with or without direction.
- The disaster plan should coordinate the efforts of the entire community so large segments of the citizenry should be involved in its development.
- The community's disaster plan should be linked to those of surrounding areas.
- Plans should be general enough to cover all potential disaster events.
- As much as possible, plans should be based on everyday work methods and procedures.
- Plans should be flexible enough to be used in a variety of situations.
- Plans should specify persons responsible for implementing segments of the plan by position or title rather than by name.

Participants in Disaster Preparedness

Planning community response in the event of a disaster should involve a broad cross-section of the community. Categories of people who should be involved in developing a disaster response plan are those discussed in Chapter 15 and include individuals who have the authority to sanction the plan, those who will implement the plan, beneficiaries of the plan, experts in the area, and those who are likely to resist the plan.

In disaster planning, the people who have authority to sanction a disaster plan are usually local government officials, so local governing bodies should be represented in the planning group. Representatives of those who will implement the plan might include health care professionals (including community health nurses) and personnel from local health care facilities; fire department and police department spokespersons; personnel from major industries in the area; and others who have special capabilities that might be needed in a disaster (e.g., representatives of local radio and TV stations). Beneficiaries of the disaster plan are community residents, so members of

CRITICAL THINKING IN RESEARCH

Community health nurses have the knowledge of the community and the expertise in program planning to make significant contributions to community disaster preparedness. In many instances, however, the only involvement that community health nurses have is in practicing and executing the emergency health care services components of a local disaster plan.

- To what extent do you think community health nurses are involved in disaster planning in your local community? How would you go about discovering if your perceptions of their involvement are correct?
- What barriers might prevent community health nurses from participating in disaster planning? How might you design a study to answer this question?
- How often do community health nurses educate members of the general public regarding disaster preparedness? How might you determine what approaches to community disaster education are most effective?

concerned citizens' groups might be asked to participate in developing a disaster response plan. Consultants in disaster planning may also be invited to participate and to share their expertise. Finally, those who might object to the plan could include people who are concerned with the cost of mounting disaster planning efforts. They should be included in the planning group because they might be able to envision less expensive ways of achieving the goals of disaster planning.

THINK ABOUT IT

Who is involved in disaster planning in your community? What role do community health nurses have in disaster planning? Should that role be expanded? If so, how?

Characteristics of Effective Disaster Plans

Disaster plans can be more or less effective. An effective plan is characterized by several qualities. An effective plan is based on realistic expectations of the effects and needs a disaster will generate. A sound disaster plan is also brief and concise. A lengthy or complicated plan is unlikely to be properly understood or implemented. An effective plan unfolds by stages, designates activities that must be carried out first, and establishes priorities

and timelines appropriate to the situation. In addition, a good disaster plan possesses an official stamp of authority. When a plan is officially sanctioned by all of the participating agencies and governing bodies, those agencies are more likely to cooperate in implementing the plan.

Other characteristics of effective disaster plans include two-way communication and local participation in their development rather than being imposed from above. Effective plans also respond to the direct needs of disaster victims. Finally, effective plans address realistic expectations for data collection that centralize data collection to enable integration of reports, avoid duplication of data collection efforts, distinguish between rapid assessment data and epidemiologic and policy-related information that can be collected later, and address available resources as well as needs (Gautam, 1998). The characteristics of effective disaster plans are summarized below.

HIGHLIGHTS

Characteristics of Effective Disaster Plans

- The plan is based on realistic expectations of effects and needs.
- The plan is brief and concise.
- The plan unfolds and expands by stages.
- The plan possesses an official stamp of authority.
- The plan is developed with local input.
- The plan responds to the direct needs of disaster victims.
- The plan addresses data collection mechanisms that are centralized, avoid duplication of effort, integrate data, distinguish between rapid needs assessment and epidemiologic and policy-related data, and address resource availability as well as needs.

General Considerations in Disaster Preparedness

General considerations in planning the response to a disaster event include designating authority, developing communication mechanisms, providing transportation, and developing a record-keeping system.

AUTHORITY

An effective disaster response plan designates a central authority and delineates the responsibilities that are delegated to specific persons and organizations. For example, if it is clear that evacuation decisions are made by the mayor and implemented by members of a local military installation, while police have the responsibility for keeping roads open, there will be less confusion, and evacuation efforts will be carried out more smoothly. Central authority may be assigned to several people in a hierarchical order so that in the absence of the first person designated, the second person has authority to implement the plan. In this individual's absence, a third person would assume that authority, and so on.

COMMUNICATION

Communication is critical to the effective implementation of a disaster response plan. Modes of communication should be established, and disaster personnel and the general public should be familiarized with them. Specific considerations in this area include how warnings of an imminent disaster will be communicated, how communication between various emergency teams and facilities will be handled, and how communication with the outside world will be facilitated. It is important to remember that normal means of communication may be disrupted during an emergency. There should also be some consideration given to facilitating communication among members of the community. For example, there may be a central bulletin board where messages can be left or a specific agency that is responsible for handling personal communications that permit family members separated by a disaster to locate each other.

TRANSPORTATION

General plans for the provision of necessary transportation must also be considered. There will be a need to transport personnel and equipment to the disaster site as well as to transport victims away from the site. There will also be a need to move personnel to areas where they are most needed. Another consideration with respect to transportation is keeping access roads open so that emergency vehicles can pass. There is a need to provide alternate transportation routes, especially for evacuating people from a high-risk area, in case first-choice routes are blocked.

RECORDS

Records are needed prior to a disaster regarding the availability of supplies and equipment and areas where they are stored. This information should be updated on a regular basis, and a systematic process for its updating should be established. Local institutions such as schools and businesses should be encouraged to keep records of all those present at any given time to allow everyone to be accounted for and to permit the identification of those missing as early as possible.

During the disaster itself, there is a need for a variety of other types of records. Victims need to be identified and their condition and treatment documented. Deaths should also be recorded. Records are also needed of the use of supplies and equipment so that additional materials can be obtained if required. Records of the deployment of rescue personnel are needed to ensure the most effective use of personnel. It would be difficult to develop systematic record-keeping systems during an actual disaster, so it is important that such systems be in place before a disaster occurs.

Critical Health Considerations in Disaster Preparedness

Four critical considerations related to the health aspects of disaster planning have been suggested by the World Health Organization. They are closely related to other elements of a community disaster plan and include early warning systems, vulnerability assessment, rescue chains, and disaster-resistant facilities. *Early warning systems* are planned surveillance systems designed to alert health care personnel of potential large-scale health problems resulting from a disaster. For example, an effective early warning system would identify early cases of communicable disease in a refugee camp, permitting immunization or other control measures to prevent an epidemic. Local surveillance for cases of anthrax or smallpox is another example of an early warning system. *Vulnerability assessment* involves predisaster identification of groups within the population who would be particularly vulnerable to the adverse effects of a disaster. Elderly persons are an example of a highly vulnerable population. The extent and location of vulnerable populations should be determined and plans made for meeting their unique needs in the event of a disaster.

Rescue chains are the logistical component of emergency health care services and reflect plans for moving injured persons to appropriate care facilities. Plans should be made for distribution and transport of persons with specific types of health problems to specific facilities. Rescue chain planning also involves training in mass casualty management for health personnel in designated facilities.

Finally, there is a need for disaster-resistant health care facilities. Disaster-resistant facilities are buildings that can be expected to withstand the effects of most types of disasters without major damage. For this reason, health care and other facilities essential to disaster response should be located above potential flood levels, built to stringent earthquake-resistant building codes, and so on.

Elements of a Typical Disaster Plan

A thorough disaster plan should address notification, warning, control, coordination, evacuation, and rescue. Additional elements of the plan should specify protocols for immediate care, supportive care, recovery, and evaluation.

NOTIFICATION

A disaster plan specifies in a systematic fashion the means of notifying the person or persons who can set the plan in motion. Persons who might be in a position to have advance warning of a disaster (e.g., local weather service personnel) should have a clear understanding of who should be apprised of the potential for disaster. There must also be specific plans for notifying personnel and organizations involved in the disaster response. Notification should always include the fact of occurrence of a disaster, the type of disaster involved, and the extent of damage as far as it is known at the time. Notification should also convey any other relevant information that is known about the situation.

WARNING

The disaster plan should also spell out the procedures for disseminating disaster warnings to the general public. Procedures should specify the content of warnings, who will issue the warnings, and the manner in which warnings will be communicated. For example, the plan might specify that warnings include the type of disaster involved, the area affected, and specific directions on actions to be taken by community members. Warnings may be issued by local radio and TV stations and by police vehicles with loudspeakers, or sirens may be used to alert people if they have been informed beforehand of the meaning of the siren and where to turn for more information. If warnings are to be communicated by media personnel, the plan should specify contact persons at radio and TV stations.

CONTROL

A disaster plan also specifies how the effects of a disaster are to be controlled. Different control efforts are required for different types of disasters, and a community should be prepared to implement a variety of control activities. In the case of an earthquake, for example, control measures are directed at preventing and extinguishing fires before further damage is caused. Again, the procedures, materials, and personnel needed to carry out control measures must be specified in the plan.

LOGISTICAL COORDINATION

Another element of a community disaster plan deals with logistical coordination. *Logistical coordination* is the coordination of attempts to procure, maintain, and transport needed materials. The disaster plan specifies where and how supplies and equipment will be obtained, where these will be stored, and how they will be transported to the disaster site.

Traffic control is another aspect of logistical coordination. The disaster plan should specify personnel and procedures for controlling access to the disaster site. Traffic control procedures should also specify means by which access to the disaster site is ensured for rescue vehicles and vehicles carrying personnel, supplies, and equipment.

EVACUATION

A disaster plan also specifies evacuation procedures. The plan should indicate how those to be evacuated will be notified, what they can take with them, and how the evacuation will be accomplished. The plan may need to specify several contingency evacuation procedures, depending on the type of disaster.

The disaster response plan also provides for the logistics of evacuation, including the personnel needed to carry out the evacuation, how they are to be recruited

and assigned, and how they will be notified. The plan also specifies the forms of transportation to be used during evacuation, where appropriate vehicles can be obtained, and how they will be refueled.

RESCUE

The response plan should specify the process to be used to assess rescue needs and who is responsible for carrying out the assessment. Once the assessment is made, there should be procedures in place for obtaining the appropriate personnel and equipment. For example, in the event of an earthquake, heavy construction equipment and operators are needed, whereas fire department personnel are needed in a fire-related disaster.

The rescue operation should focus on removing victims from hazardous conditions and providing first aid as needed. Rescue personnel should refrain from providing other forms of care as much as possible. This care can be provided by others, thus freeing rescue personnel to carry out the rescue operation.

IMMEDIATE CARE

Provision of immediate care is another consideration detailed in a disaster response plan. *Immediate care* is care required on the spot to ensure a disaster victim's survival or a disaster worker's continued ability to function. Plans for providing immediate care in four areas in the vicinity of the disaster site (Figure 27–4 ■) should be detailed in the disaster response plan. Immediate care begins at the actual site of the disaster, with a rapid initial assessment of all victims by the first health care provider on the scene. This phase of immediate care is geared to correcting any life-threatening problems.

The second area of immediate care is the triage area. *Triage* is the process of sorting casualties on the basis of urgency and their potential for survival to determine priorities for treatment, evacuation, and transportation. Triage decisions are intended to maximize the number of survivors of a disaster event. When victims are easily accessible, triage can take place at the site of the disaster. Victims are then removed to treatment areas based on their triage priority. In a disaster occurring in an enclosed environment (e.g., in a mine or in a building), victims may not be easily accessible and will probably need to be removed to a more distant triage area as they are found.

The triage process usually involves placing color-coded tags on victims. Typically, black tags are attached to victims who are already dead. Red tags indicate top priority and are attached to victims who have life-threatening injuries but who can be stabilized and who have a high probability of survival. Priority is automatically given to injured rescue workers, their family members, hysterical persons, and children. Yellow tags, indicating second priority, are assigned to victims with injuries with systemic complications that are not yet life threatening and who are able to withstand a wait of 45 to 60 minutes for medical attention. Yellow tags are also assigned to victims with severe injuries who have a poor

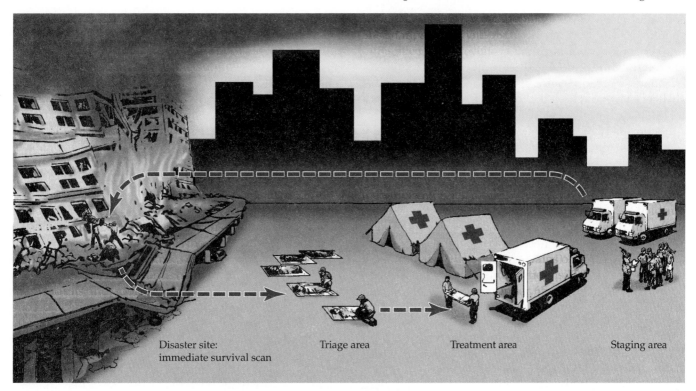

Disaster site:
immediate survival scan

Triage area

Treatment area

Staging area

FIGURE 27-4 ■ *Areas of operation in the rescue phase of disaster response*

chance of survival. Green tags indicate victims with local injuries without immediate systemic complications who can wait several hours for treatment.

The third area of immediate care at the disaster site is the treatment area to which victims are removed after triage. In this area, medical stabilization, temporary care, and emergency surgical stabilization are provided as needed. There may also be a need for psychological first aid at this point. The final area at the site of the disaster is the staging area. It is here that immediate care operations are coordinated and vehicles and personnel are directed to areas of greatest need. The disaster plan should specify the procedures for setting up and operating each of the four areas of immediate care. The plan should also address the supplies, equipment, and personnel needed in each area, how they will be obtained, and how they will be transported to the area.

Another aspect of immediate care that should be addressed in the disaster plan is care of the dead. Plans should be included for procedures to identify bodies and transport them to a morgue of some sort. Records of deaths should be kept, and procedures for rapid disposal of bodies should be specified should contagion be a problem. Plans should also include where and how body bags and identification tags will be obtained.

SUPPORTIVE CARE

Supportive care must also be addressed in an effective disaster response plan. Supportive care includes providing food, water, and shelter for victims and disaster relief workers. Other considerations in this area are sanitation and

waste disposal, providing medications and routine health care, and reuniting families separated by the disaster.

Shelter is required for those who are evacuated from their homes or whose homes are damaged in the disaster. The disaster response plan should specify which community buildings can be used to shelter victims and how victims are to be transported to shelters. There may also be a need to use the homes of private citizens to shelter victims if public shelters are insufficient. When such is the case, the plan should specify how to notify concerned citizens of the need to place victims in their homes and how placement is to be handled. It is helpful to have a list of people willing to provide shelter to others should a disaster occur. In the case of large groups of displaced persons, refugee camps may be set up. Potential camp sites should be carefully selected in relation to possible physical hazards or water runoff.

Within the shelter, there is a need for supplies to sustain daily living. Shelters should have adequate sanitation and sleeping facilities. There should be plans for heating shelters and cooking food if area gas and electrical power systems are disrupted. Mechanisms should also be specified for governance and security within the shelter, particularly if the shelter will be in use for some time. Shelter leaders can be appointed or elected, and persons within the shelter should have a means of providing input into governance in long-term shelter situations.

Food supplies should be planned and obtained prior to a disaster. There should also be a mechanism for obtaining more food and other supplies from outside the community in the event of damage to stores and stockpiled supplies. A source of clean water is needed, and the disaster plan should identify how and where water will be supplied. Equipment for water purification should be stored in case of need (Lillibridge, 1997b). There is also a need to plan for adequate sanitation, waste disposal, and vector control at shelters and throughout the community following a disaster (Malilay, 1997b).

Victims may have other health care needs unrelated to the disaster that need to be met, so plans for providing basic health care in shelters should also be specified. These plans should include stores of medications most likely to be needed by the general public and critical to survival. For example, diabetics will continue to need insulin or oral hypoglycemics, whereas individuals with heart conditions may need a variety of medications. Priority should be given to medications required for serious illnesses rather than for minor conditions. Because communicable diseases spread more rapidly in a debilitated population following a disaster, antibiotics and vaccines should be stored in case of need.

Supportive care also includes psychological counseling for those who are not coping adequately with the situation. Counseling may be required by both victims and disaster workers, and plans should be made to provide crisis intervention services during the response stage of the disaster (Gerrity & Flynn, 1997). For example, following the World Trade Center and Pentagon terrorist attacks, an online self-assessment was established for identifying persons with severe depression related to the attacks (National Mental Health Association, 2001). Psychological support can be provided by comforting and consoling those in distress and by protecting them from the ongoing disaster threat. The disaster plan should include mechanisms for identifying those in need of counseling and providing them with the services required.

Disaster victims may require goal orientation and guidance, and they can be directed to perform specific tasks that help them achieve a sense of control. Support is needed for those who must identify loved ones among the dead. Expression of feelings should be fostered, and victims should be encouraged to make use of available support networks. Immediate referral to mental health personnel may be required in some instances. Structuring the environment and regularizing schedules, particularly in shelters, can also help to reestablish a sense of security.

Some relief from psychological stress can frequently be obtained if victims can be assured that family members are safe. Disaster plans should therefore include mechanisms for locating people and reuniting families. Names of persons admitted to shelters or health care facilities should be recorded and communicated to a central location where others can check for word of loved ones. Deaths should also be reported if the dead can be identified, and information should be kept on the assignment of disaster workers to specific areas. It is helpful if institutions, such as schools and businesses, compile the names of those who were present prior to a disaster so that they can be accounted for afterward.

RECOVERY

Another component of the disaster plan is mechanisms for supporting community rehabilitation. There may be a need to rebuild or repair damaged structures, and plans should be made for obtaining financial and material assistance in these endeavors. Mechanisms should be developed that help victims to process insurance claims as rapidly as possible. There may also be a need for outside assistance in rebuilding, and plans should be made for obtaining that assistance.

Psychological counseling is needed in the aftermath of a disaster, and mechanisms should be developed for identifying and referring those in need of counseling. Postdisaster counseling may be delegated to specific mental health agencies that would plan how postevent counseling will be handled, who will be eligible for care, and procedures for obtaining care. Particular attention should be given to the counseling needs of both disaster workers and victims, because research has indicated the potential for psychological trauma to both as a result of a disaster experience.

Because of today's graphic media coverage of disasters, people who view the disaster and its effects may also develop psychological problems. For example, after the terrorist attacks on the World Trade Center and the Pentagon in 2001, nearly 80% of women and 62% of men surveyed reported experiencing depression. Some people also become obsessed with coverage of the event (The Pew Research Center for the People and the Press, 2001).

EVALUATION

Plans should also be made prior to the disaster for evaluating the effectiveness of the disaster plan and its implementation. Again, consideration should be given to procedures, personnel, and materials needed to carry out the evaluation. Records are needed that permit evaluation of the efficiency and effectiveness of the plan, and procedures should be developed for obtaining and storing data. Plans should also be made for follow-up meetings with disaster workers to provide input into the evaluation process. The focus of these meetings would be on what worked and what did not work and what could be done to improve the plan and its implementation in subsequent disasters. Elements of a typical disaster plan are summarized below.

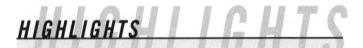

HIGHLIGHTS

Elements of a Typical Disaster Plan

- Mechanisms exist for notifying individuals responsible for authorizing disaster plan implementation.
- Mechanisms exist for warning individuals likely to be affected by the disaster.
- Mechanisms exist for controlling damage due to disaster.

- Procedures are specified for logistical coordination in traffic control and transportation of equipment, supplies, and personnel to the disaster site.
- Procedures are specified for evacuating individuals in the potential disaster area.
- Plans are in place for rescue operations to remove victims from hazardous situations.
- Plans and procedures have been designed to meet immediate care needs of disaster victims related to triage, first aid, transportation to other facilities, and care of the dead.
- Plans and procedures have been designed to provide supportive care to meet ongoing needs of disaster victims and relief workers related to emergency shelter, food and water, sanitation and waste disposal, health care and medications, and reuniting families.
- Mechanisms are in place to provide assistance to victims during the recovery period.
- Mechanisms exist for evaluating the adequacy of the disaster plan in meeting the community's needs.

NURSING RESPONSIBILITIES IN DISASTER PREPAREDNESS

Community health nurses are well suited to assist in the actual development of a disaster plan. Because of their background in program planning and group dynamics, they can help ensure that planning is a systematic rather than a haphazard process. Community health nurses also have knowledge of what the health-related needs of the population would be in a disaster and can provide input regarding needs and vulnerable populations, as well as potential resources for meeting needs.

Another role for community health nurses in disaster preparation is to train rescue workers in triage techniques and basic first aid. Nurses might also help educate personnel who will staff shelters regarding the needs of disaster victims and considerations related to group interactions that will make shelter operations run more smoothly. A final responsibility of community health nurses in the disaster planning stage is educating the public regarding the disaster plan and the need for personal preparation for a disaster.

CARE OF CLIENTS IN DISASTER SETTINGS

Community health nursing care related to disasters involves participation in assessment of disaster situations and planning, implementation, and evaluation of disaster-related services.

ASSESSING THE HEALTH-RELATED DIMENSIONS OF A DISASTER

Assessment in providing disaster care has three aspects: assessing the extent of disaster preparedness, assessing the potential for disaster, and assessing possible effects of a disaster. The first task of community health nurses and others involved in disaster planning is to examine the current level of disaster preparedness in the community. How prepared is the community to respond to a disaster, and how effective is that response likely to be? The World Health Organization has developed a preparedness checklist intended for use in assessing national levels of disaster preparation. This checklist has been adapted for use at the community level as presented below. Answers to the questions posed in the checklist provide direction for comprehensive community disaster planning.

HIGHLIGHTS

Community Disaster Preparedness Assessment

- Is there a community disaster plan? Is the plan being implemented?
- Is there a person in charge of promoting, developing, and coordinating emergency preparation?
- Are emergency preparedness activities coordinated among relevant community agencies?
- What joint emergency preparedness and response activities are undertaken by community agencies?
- Are there operational plans for health response to a disaster?
- Have mass casualty plans been developed?
- What surveillance measures are in place for early detection and response to health emergencies?
- What steps have been taken by environmental health services to prepare for disaster response?
- Have facilities and safe areas been designated as shelter sites in the event of a disaster? What health care provisions have been made?
- What disaster preparedness training has been undertaken with health care personnel?
- What resources are available for rapid health response to disaster (e.g., communications, financing, transport, supplies)?
- Is there a system for updating information on supplies and personnel?
- What opportunities exist to test the effectiveness of the disaster plan?

Identifying the potential for disaster in a particular community involves forecasting the types of disasters possible and the likelihood of their occurrence. The possible types of disasters, of course, vary from community to community. Disaster potential and the probable effects can be systematically assessed by examining factors related to each of the six dimensions of health. The dimensions of health perspective can also be used to assess the effects of an actual disaster.

Biophysical Considerations

One determinant in forecasting potential disasters is that of human biology. Certain groups of people are more likely than others to be affected by a disaster. For example, if the anticipated disaster is an epidemic of influenza, those most likely to be severely affected are the very young and the elderly; however, there also will be illness among the health care workforce that may impede efforts to halt the spread of disease. On the other hand, if there is potential for an explosion in a local chemical plant, those affected are likely to be company employees and persons in surrounding buildings. Again, this might include children if there is a school nearby. In disasters requiring evacuation, the elderly are at particular risk because of potential mobility limitations.

Human biology is also a factor in predicting the types of effects expected as a result of the disaster. In the case of an influenza epidemic, illness potentially accompanied by dehydration and electrolyte imbalance may be expected. In an explosion, expected injuries may consist of burns and trauma (Lillibridge, 1997a), whereas a flood results primarily in drownings (Malilay, 1997a). Terrorist dissemination of anthrax spores, on the other hand, may result in cutaneous, inhalation, or intestinal forms of disease with related symptoms and complications (Centers for Disease Control and Prevention [CDC], 2001).

The overall health status of the community also influences disaster planning requirements. For example, if hypertension is prevalent in the community, provisions need to be made in a disaster plan for ongoing treatment of hypertension or other prevalent diseases. Possible biophysical effects of several types of disasters are presented in Table 27–1 ■.

In the event of disaster, the community health nurse assesses the physiologic effects of the event on human biology. The nurse appraises the extent of injuries incurred by victims and relief workers and may also assess other needs for health care. For example, the nurse might need to assess the health status of a disaster relief worker with diabetes or of a child with a fever. The nurse assists in assessing the health status of groups of people. For example, among refugees from Bhutan housed in refugee camps in Nepal, chronic malnutrition led to a sixfold increase in vitamin A deficiency among adolescents and a high risk of iron deficiency in adolescent females (National Center for Environmental Health, 2000a).

Psychological Considerations

Components of the psychological dimension can also influence the effects of a disaster on health. As noted earlier, a number of psychological factors can affect the way people respond to a warning of disaster. Similarly, psychological factors can influence responses once a disaster has occurred. For example, familiarity with earthquakes may limit panic in some people, whereas those new to the area, who have never before experienced an earthquake, may panic and respond inappropriately. Communities and persons with good coping skills usually respond more effectively in a disaster situation than those who have poor coping skills.

The community health nurse should assess the attitudes of community members toward disaster preparedness. To what extent are individuals and families in the area prepared for potential disasters? Have families in an earthquake-prone region, for example, gathered supplies that will be needed in the event of an earthquake and placed them in an accessible location? Have emergency escape routes from homes, schools, and other buildings been identified? Have families discussed an emergency contact person who can relay messages for and about family members separated in a disaster? Or are these types of preparation largely ignored?

In the event of an actual disaster, the community health nurse assesses the psychological effects of the disaster event. As noted earlier, both victims and relief workers may experience stress related to a disaster, and the nurse should be alert to signs of emotional distress in both groups. Generally, four types of psychological response are seen in disaster victims and rescue workers: psychophysiological responses, behavioral responses, emotional responses, and cognitive responses. Psychophysiological responses include such symptoms as fatigue, tremors, dizziness, and gastrointestinal upset. Behavioral responses may manifest as sleep disturbances, substance abuse, hypervigilance, and so on. Emotional responses include fear and anxiety as well as depression, grief, and other emotional reactions. Finally, difficulties making decisions, confusion, and impaired concentration are examples of cognitive responses (Gerrity & Flynn, 1997). Widespread depression as well as insomnia and difficulty concentrating were experienced by people who viewed the 2001 terrorist attacks on television as well as among direct and indirect victims and rescue workers (The Pew Research Center for the People and the Press, 2001).

Types of immediate psychological responses to disasters range along a continuum from calm, collected action to confusion and hysteria. Plans should be made for services to address each level of response. Health care providers should also keep in mind that psychological responses may change with time and with the progression of the disaster event. The sequence of psychological responses to a disaster parallel the stages of the disaster

■ TABLE 27-1 Biophysical Effects of Selected Disasters

TYPE OF DISASTER	CONSIDERATIONS RELATED TO HUMAN BIOLOGY
All disasters	Greater loss of life and injury among the elderly, young children, and chronically ill and disabled persons
Avalanches	May result in asphyxiation May result in frostbite and other effects of exposure to cold May result in fractures or other forms of trauma
Bioterrorism	May result in widespread communicable disease, death, and disability
Chemical spills or chemical terrorism	May result in chemical burns of the skin May result in respiratory irritation and illness May result in poisoning with a variety of symptoms depending on the chemical involved May result in eye irritation
Earthquakes	May result in crushing injuries and fractures from falling bricks, masonry, and other objects May result in burns suffered in fires and explosions due to ruptured natural gas mains May result in waterborne diseases because of ruptured water mains and lack of safe drinking water May result in electrocutions from fallen power lines
Epidemics	May result in communicable diseases with a variety of symptoms depending on the disease involved
Explosions	May result in burns due to associated fires May result in fractures or crushing injuries due to explosion impact or falling masonry, bricks, and other debris
Famine	May result in developmental delay in young children May result in failure to thrive in nursing infants because of inadequate lactation by mothers May result in protein-energy malnutrition and other nutritional deficiencies
Fire	May result in minor to severe burns May result in respiratory problems due to inhalation of smoke and hazardous fumes from burning objects
Floods	May result in drownings May result in waterborne and insect-borne diseases from contaminated water supplies and insect breeding grounds
Nuclear attacks or radiation leakage	May result in radiation burns or radiation sickness May result in later cancer May result in later infertility, spontaneous abortion, or fetal defects
Storms	May result in crushing injuries due to windblown objects and debris May result in minor to severe lacerations due to flying glass from broken windows
Transportation disasters	May result in crushing injuries and other trauma May result in burns with associated vehicle fires May result in drownings or asphyxiation if disasters occur over water or in tunnels May result in exposure to the elements if disaster occurs in a remote area
Volcanic eruptions	May result in toxic gas or radiation exposures, respiratory or eye irritations

itself (Gerrity & Flynn, 1997). For example, the typical response in the warning stage of a disaster is fight or flight, either of which may be appropriate or inappropriate in a given situation. In the alarm stage, the most likely response is one of anxiety, whereas a feeling of being stunned is typical of the impact stage. During the rescue stage, many people may exhibit mood and attitude extremes. Ambivalence is common in the recovery stage as the reality of loss is acknowledged. Finally, psychological responses in the reconstruction stage may be quite varied. These responses are basically normal unless they are extreme in nature. Even normal response, however, can place one at risk for harm. For example, the feeling of being stunned during the impact stage may lead one to disregard personal safety and to fail to avoid environmental hazards like unsafe masonry in an earthquake area. Psychological recovery occurs for most people within 6 to 12 months of the disaster, but a small segment of the population may exhibit ongoing problems and require therapy.

Physical Environmental Considerations

Many disasters arise out of features of the physical environment. For example, the presence of a river near the community and the likelihood of heavy rainfall both contribute to the potential for flooding, as does the construction of homes and businesses on floodplains. A geological fault, a nuclear reactor, and a chemical plant are other examples of factors in the physical environment that may increase the potential for a disaster.

Elements of the physical dimension can either help or hinder efforts to control the effects of a disaster. For example, limited traffic access to the part of town where an explosives plant is located could hinder movement of emergency vehicles in the event of a fire or explosion. Similarly, the physical isolation of a mountain community may impede rescue efforts in the event of a forest fire or flood. On the other hand, such isolation might spare the community from the effects of an epidemic in the surrounding area.

In conducting a community assessment, the community health nurse identifies physical environmental factors that might contribute to the occurrence of a disaster. The nurse also determines whether the community is prepared for potential disasters. When the community is not prepared, the nurse would advocate the planning activities described earlier in this chapter.

⑥THINK ABOUT IT

What factors in your community contribute to the potential for a disaster event? What interventions could be taken to prevent a disaster? What actions could mitigate the effects of a disaster if one occurs?

The nurse also identifies factors that might impede the community's response in the event of a disaster. The nurse can then share these observations with others involved in disaster planning, and interventions to modify or circumvent these factors can be incorporated into the community's disaster response plan.

Sociocultural Considerations

Sociocultural dimension factors can also influence the way people respond to a disaster and may even give rise to one. For example, the presence of racial tensions could trigger outbreaks of violence in some communities. War is another disaster arising out of social environmental conditions. In assessing a community, the nurse identifies social factors that might contribute to disasters and to the way people respond to them.

Elements of the sociocultural dimension also may increase or limit the effects of a disaster on a community. For example, the economic status of community members and of the community at large may limit the ability of people to prepare for potential disasters or to recover after a disaster event. Language barriers may hamper evacuation or rescue efforts. Strong social networks in the community that can be tied into disaster planning aid in effective disaster response, whereas intragroup friction hampers response effectiveness. The nurse identifies social and cultural factors present within the community that may decrease the effectiveness of the community's response to a disaster and participates in planning efforts to modify these factors. The nurse also identifies social factors that enhance the community's ability to respond effectively in the event of a disaster. Planning groups could then capitalize on these factors in designing an effective disaster plan. For example, well-established cooperative relationships between groups and agencies in the community are an asset in designing and implementing a disaster plan, whereas the presence of relatively isolated cultural groups may impede planning and response efforts.

Another aspect of the social environment that should be assessed is community attitudes toward and participation in disaster planning. Are local government agencies supportive of planning efforts? Do community members exhibit concern for disaster planning and do they follow through on recommendations for disaster preparedness?

Occupational factors are another element of the sociocultural dimension that contribute to the potential for disaster in a community and should be assessed by the nurse. Occupational disasters are events related to a particular business or industry in which more than five deaths occur. In the early part of the twentieth century, occupational disasters, particularly explosions, accounted for 84% of all disaster-related deaths in the United States. Safer equipment and working conditions have reduced these rates considerably (CDC, 1999).

The community health nurse should be aware of industries in the area that pose hazards related to fire or explosion. The potential for radiation exposure or leakage of toxic chemicals in the community should also be determined. The nurse may also want to appraise the extent to which local industries adhere to safety regulations related

CULTURAL CONSIDERATIONS

You live and work in a highly ethnically diverse community in which residents come from multiple different cultural backgrounds and where 38 different languages are spoken. Major sources of disaster potential in the area include the possibility of earthquakes and brush fires. How would you design community notification systems related to evacuation in the event of a major fire accounting for the language barriers to communication and the fatalistic attitudes of some cultural groups in the area?

to hazardous conditions. Community health nurses working in industrial settings would be particularly likely to have access to this type of information. Other community health nurses may need to advocate regular inspection of industrial conditions by the appropriate authorities.

The community health nurse also identifies occupational factors that may enhance a community's abilities to respond effectively in the event of a disaster. The nurse and others involved in disaster planning would explore the adequacy of rescue services and personnel for dealing with potential disasters. Is the number of firefighters in the community, for example, adequate to deal with an explosion and fire in a local chemical plant? Do firefighting units possess the equipment needed to deal with such an event? Planners also assess the existence of other occupational groups that may assist with disaster response. For example, are there construction companies in the community that could supply heavy equipment that might be needed for rescue operations?

In the event of an actual disaster, the nurse might also assess sociocultural factors influencing the community's disaster response. For example, the nurse might identify growing intergroup tensions in shelters for disaster victims or disorganization in efforts to reunite families separated by the disaster. Other areas for consideration include the degree of cooperation among groups providing disaster relief and, following the disaster, the availability of recovery assistance to individuals and families.

Another social response to disasters, particularly those caused by terrorist activities, may include anger and hostility toward groups deemed responsible for the disaster. These emotions may be demonstrated in prejudice, discrimination, and attacks on innocent parties believed to be related to the perpetrators. In a study conducted after the 2001 terrorist attacks in Washington, D.C. and New York, 29% of respondents favored establishing internment camps for legal immigrants from hostile nations (The Pew Research Center for the People and the Press, 2001). News media also reported a variety of unprovoked attacks against Muslims and other ethnic minority groups. Community health nurses may need to be involved in advocacy to prevent discrimination and violence against such groups.

Behavioral Considerations

Behavioral factors related to consumption patterns and even leisure pursuits can also influence the occurrence of disasters and their effects on the health of community members. Consumption patterns such as smoking, drinking, and drug use can contribute to disasters. Smoking, for example, is often the cause of residential fires and forest and brush fires that result in loss of life as well as extensive property damage. Drinking and drug abuse have both been known to contribute to transportation disasters, and they may also contribute to industrial disasters when the abuser is working in a setting with disaster potential. For example, if a person responsible for monitoring the safety of a nuclear reactor is drunk, he or she is unlikely to recognize or respond appropriately to signs of danger. The community health nurse assesses the extent of smoking and substance abuse in the community in relation to the potential for disaster. The nurse may also want to assess (or encourage others to assess) the effectiveness of substance abuse policies in transportation services and industries where there is potential for disaster. Another area for assessment is the extent of safety education in regard to smoking (e.g., not smoking in bed) that occurs in the community.

Consumption patterns may also intensify the effects of a disaster on the health of a population. A community whose members are poorly nourished, for example, is at greater risk for consequences of disaster such as communicable diseases. Substance abuse may limit one's potential for appropriate behavior in an emergency and lead to injury and even death due to failure to respond appropriately. For example, intoxication may prevent someone from fleeing a burning building.

Consumption patterns and their effects are particularly relevant in disasters involving famine and large displaced or refugee populations. Famine is a population-wide condition involving substantial mortality from malnutrition. Common nutritional effects of famine among refugee populations include *protein-energy malnutrition (PEM)*, a severe state of undernutrition that may be either acute or chronic, and deficiencies of specific micronutrients such as vitamin A, iron, vitamin C, niacin, and thiamine.

Lack of exercise in the population can limit their ability to engage in strenuous labor that might be demanded in a disaster situation. Unaccustomed activity may result in exhaustion or heart attack. The nurse assesses the levels of exercise engaged in by the general population. Community health nurses in occupational settings may also be responsible for determining the physical fitness of personnel who would be involved in rescue operations in the event of a disaster (e.g., firefighters).

The leisure pursuits of community members may, on occasion, contribute to the occurrence of a disaster event. Careless campers, for example, could ignite a forest fire, or skiers might trigger an avalanche. Fires can be started by sparks from recreational vehicles. The community health nurse and others involved in disaster planning assess the extent of such leisure pursuits in the community, the existence of safety regulations related to these pursuits, and the degree of adherence to safety regulations. Do campers, for example, refrain from lighting fires in fire-prone areas, or do skiers avoid restricted areas where avalanches are possible?

Leisure pursuits can also enhance the community's response to a disaster event, and the nurse assesses the presence of leisure pursuits that may have this effect. For example, the existence of a group with an interest in wilderness survival may be an advantage in the event of an avalanche or a plane crash in a remote area, or people with citizens-band radios may assist with communications in the event of an emergency.

Health System Considerations

The adequacy of the health care system's response capability in the event of a disaster influences the extent to which a disaster affects a community and the health of its members. Assessing the ability of the health care system to respond to a disaster includes examining facilities and personnel as well as the organizational framework in which they operate. A community that has a variety of health care facilities joined in a cooperative network can respond more effectively to the health care demands of a disaster situation than can a community with limited facilities or where there is no existing system for coordinating joint efforts.

The nurse and other disaster response planners identify the types of health care facilities available in the community and the number and type of health care personnel that could be called on in the event of a disaster. Planners might also determine the existence and adequacy of disaster plans developed by health care facilities. For example, has a local hospital developed a plan for evacuating patients if the hospital is involved in the disaster? Is there a plan for handling mass casualties of various types in the event of a disaster? In one study, for example, only 20% of hospitals surveyed had the capability of responding to biological or chemical weapons incidents (Wetter et al., 2001). Local communities need to assess the likelihood of such incidents in the area and prepare accordingly. As several authors have concluded, however, preventive measures for bioterrorist activities should be placed in priority with other existing public health needs and resources allocated based on those priorities (Geiger, 2001; Sidel, Cohen, & Gould, 2001). This prevents needless expenditure of resources that could be better used to address other, more pressing public health issues.

In 2000, CDC published guidelines for preparedness for and response to biological and chemical terrorism. Acts of chemical terrorism are likely to be overt because their effects tend to be immediate and obvious. Some chemical agents are capable of covert dissemination in food and water, however. Biological terrorism tends to be covert in that its effects are more insidious and occur over sometimes extended incubation periods.

The two main facets of state and local public health preparedness to be assessed by community health nurses and other disaster response planners are the existence of surveillance systems capable of identifying unusual disease patterns and the availability of expertise and resources needed to respond to chemical or biological terrorist attacks. Specific preparation for biological attacks includes:

- Enhancing surveillance and response capabilities
- Providing for diagnostic services
- Establishing effective communication systems
- Educating health care providers on recognition and treatment of diseases caused by bioterrorism
- Educating the general public
- Obtaining and storing needed drugs and vaccines
- Supporting development of diagnostic tests, vaccines, and appropriate treatments (CDC, 2000)

These guidelines were expanded by the National Center for Infectious Diseases (2001) to encompass the specific roles of health care providers in the recognition, reporting, and treatment of high-priority biological agents. Laboratory personnel are also advised to test findings on cultures that would normally be discarded as contaminants when they occur in suspicious circumstances (e.g., febrile illness in a previously healthy person) and to be alert to unusual clusters of laboratory results. Laboratory precautions for handling suspected contaminants are also addressed, and unusual specimens should be sent to specialty laboratories as appropriate.

State health departments are charged with reeducating health care providers to recognize unusual diseases. For example, many U.S. providers will never have seen a case of smallpox and will need to be reminded of typical signs and symptoms of this disease. State health departments also need to remind providers of reporting requirements and procedures, improve capacities for immediate response to suspected bioterrorism, investigate unusual illness clusters, develop and implement plans for collecting and transporting specimens to appropriate laboratory facilities, and reporting suspected release of biological agents to CDC.

Guidelines for public health agency preparation for chemical attacks have also been provided by CDC (2000). Public health responsibilities in this area include developing capabilities for detecting and responding to chemical attacks, educating first responders and health care personnel regarding chemical terrorism, and obtaining and storing supplies of chemical antidotes. Additional responsibilities include developing diagnostic processes for chemical injuries and educating the public about potential effects and actions to be taken in the case of chemical attacks. Educational information for the general public regarding biological and chemical attacks were addressed in Chapter 3. Community health nurses and others assessing disaster preparedness should determine the extent to which state and large local public health agencies (e.g., those in large metropolitan areas) are capable of carrying out these responsibilities.

Assessment of potential avenues for obtaining health care personnel is also important. For example, local professional organizations might serve as a means of contacting and organizing health care providers, or area educational programs for health care professionals may provide a source of manpower.

In the event of an actual disaster there is also a need to assess the effects of the disaster on the health care system and its ability to respond effectively. For example, are facilities badly damaged or unusable for other reasons? In some instances, health care facilities have collapsed in earthquakes or become inaccessible due to flood waters or highway damage.

Assessment tips for assessing disaster potential and the health-related aspects of a disaster are summarized on page 647. A complete assessment tool to guide assessment in disaster situations is available on the companion Web site for this book. 🌐

assessment tips assessment tips assessment tips

ASSESSING HEALTH IN DISASTER SETTINGS

Biophysical Considerations

- What is the age, gender, and ethnic composition of the population involved in the disaster? Are the effects of the disaster likely to be worse for some subgroups than others?
- What is the extent of injury or disease resulting from the disaster?
- What existing health problems are prevalent among those involved in the disaster?
- Are there pregnant women involved in the disaster?

Psychological Considerations

- How does the population respond to disaster warnings?
- What is the extent of community/individual ability to cope with the disaster?
- What is the extent of existing mental illness among those involved in the disaster?
- What is the extent of damage or loss of life involved in the disaster?
- Does the disaster present the potential for continuing damage or loss of life?
- What is the effect of the disaster on rescue workers? On victims? What are the long-term psychological effects of the disaster on the community?

Physical Environmental Considerations

- What physical features of the community create the potential for disaster? What types of disasters are likely to occur?
- What structures are likely to be threatened by a disaster? To what extent are vital structures likely to withstand a disaster?
- What structures could be used as emergency shelters?
- Will weather conditions influence the effects of the disaster?
- Are there elements of the physical environmental dimension that will hinder response to the disaster (e.g., blockage of roads)?
- Have buildings been structurally damaged? Is there potential for additional structural damage? Does structural damage pose further risk to victims? To rescuers?
- Is there a need for sources of shelter for persons displaced by the disaster?
- Is there a safe water source available to victims of the disaster?
- To what extent are animals involved in the disaster? What health effects might this have?

Sociocultural Considerations

- Do relationships in the community have the potential to create a disaster (e.g., civil strife, war)?
- How cohesive is the community? Are community members able to work together for disaster planning? What is the attitude of community members to disaster planning?
- What provisions have been made for reuniting families separated by disaster?
- What is the extent of social support available to disaster victims?
- What is the extent of collaborative interaction among relief agencies involved in the disaster?
- Has the community disaster plan been communicated to residents? How are disaster warnings communicated to residents? Are there language barriers that impede communication in the disaster setting? What is the effect of disaster on normal channels of communication?
- What community groups are responsible for disaster planning? Who is available to provide leadership in responding to the disaster? What is the level of credibility of leaders among those affected by the disaster?
- What community industries pose disaster hazards? What type of hazards are present? To what extent do local industries adhere to safety procedures that would prevent a disaster? Is adherence monitored by regulatory bodies?
- What occupational groups in the community are available to respond to the disaster?
- What is the extent of property damage and loss resulting from the disaster?
- What is the economic status of those affected by disaster? Do they have economic resources available to them? What is the effect of the disaster on the local economy?
- What is the effect of the disaster on transportation?
- What is the effect of the disaster on community services? What community services are available to assist with recovery?
- Is equipment needed to deal with the disaster available and in good repair?

Behavioral Considerations

- To what extent do consumption patterns (e.g., drugs or alcohol) create the potential for disaster in the community?
- Do community members engage in leisure pursuits that pose a disaster hazard? To what extent do community members engage in recreational safety practices that can prevent disasters? What leisure pursuits

(continued)

by community members could enhance the community's disaster response?

- What is the availability of food and water to disaster victims? To rescuers? Are there special dietary needs among those affected by the disaster? What provisions have been made to meet these needs?

Health System Considerations

- How well prepared are health service agencies to respond to a disaster?
- What health care facilities are available to care for disaster victims? What are their capabilities? What

health care personnel are available to meet health needs in a disaster? How can they best be mobilized?

- What is the extent of basic first aid and other health-related knowledge in the community?
- What is the effect of a disaster on health care facilities? Health care services?
- What health care services are needed as a result of disaster? Are available services adequate to meet the need?

DIAGNOSTIC REASONING AND CARE OF CLIENTS IN DISASTER SETTINGS

Based on the assessment of biophysical, psychological, physical environmental, sociocultural, behavioral, and health system factors, the nurse derives nursing diagnoses related to disaster care. These diagnoses may reflect the potential for disaster occurrence, the adequacy of disaster preparation, or the extent of effects in an actual disaster. A diagnosis related to forecasting is "potential for major earthquake damage and injury due to community location on a geological fault." A diagnosis of "inadequate disaster planning due to fragmentation of planning efforts among community agencies" is a possible nursing diagnosis related to disaster preparedness. A diagnosis derived from information about the effects of an actual disaster is "need for additional shelter sites due to destruction of planned shelters by fire."

In the event of an actual disaster, nursing diagnoses might relate to individual clients as well as to the status of the overall community. For example, individual diagnoses include "grief due to loss of husband" and "pain due to leg fracture suffered in the collapse of a wall." Nurses may derive diagnoses related to both helpers and victims, such as "role overload due to need to rescue disaster victims and care for own family" and "stress related to constant exposure to death."

PLANNING HEALTH CARE IN A DISASTER

Activities related to disaster care take place in several areas. Two of these areas, prevention and education, involve primary prevention. The third area of activity, the actual emergency response, reflects secondary prevention, whereas recovery, the fourth area of activity, involves tertiary prevention.

Primary Prevention

Primary prevention is geared toward preventing the occurrence of a disaster or limiting consequences when

the event itself cannot be prevented. Activities to prevent or minimize the effects of a disaster take place during the nondisaster and predisaster stages of disaster response. Community health nurses may be involved in eliminating factors that may contribute to disasters to the extent that they identify these factors and report their existence to the appropriate authorities. For example, the community health nurse working in an occupational setting may note that an employee who is responsible for monitoring pressure levels in a boiler may be drinking heavily. This employee's drinking problem may lead to lack of attention to rising pressures and an explosion and fire in the plant. In such a case, the nurse would call the employee's drinking behavior to the attention of a supervisor.

Community health nurses may also become politically active to ensure that risk factors for potential disasters present in the community are eliminated or modified. For example, the nurse might campaign for stricter safety regulations for nuclear power plants or stricter building safety codes (Noji, 1997a) or serve as a mediator in an attempt to defuse social unrest in the community. Similarly, community health nurses may advocate for "smart sanctions" at the international level when nations impose sanctions on countries that violate basic human rights. Smart sanctions are targeted toward the policy makers or the elite of the nation subject to the sanctions and do not unduly burden the rest of the population, preventing some of the effects of international sanctions discussed earlier (Marks, 1999). Another possibility for action at the societal level is advocating for tax incentives or reduced insurance premiums for citizens who engage in disaster mitigation efforts for their own property (Comerio, 1998).

Community health nurses can also assist in the development of community-as-resource strategies for disaster response. These strategies consist of a series of training programs for disaster preparedness at the individual, neighborhood, and advanced level. Individual-level programs focus on basic family preparedness, reduction of household hazards, preparation of family emergency kits and plans, and developing family notification systems. The second level involves training and development of neighborhood response teams trained to carry out immediate response activities. Advanced training prepares local residents to augment the efforts of public response personnel such as police and firefighters (Lichterman, 2000).

Community health nurses are often involved in educating the public about how to prevent disasters and minimize their consequences. This may involve planning education for individuals, families, or groups of clients on home safety practices to prevent fires and explosions, how to prepare for a possible community disaster, and what to do in the event of a disaster situation.

The nurse would plan to acquaint clients with whom he or she works with the types of disasters possible in their community and about actions they can take to minimize the consequences should an emergency arise. The nurse can also guide clients to resources that help them prepare for the possibility of a disaster. A variety of government agencies publish literature containing guidelines for emergency preparation by individual citizens. One such publication, *In Time of Emergency: A Citizen's Handbook,* is published by the Federal Emergency Management Agency. The American Red Cross publishes the *Family Disaster Plan and Personal Survival Guide.* These and similar publications offer general guidelines for emergency preparation as well as more specific recommendations for certain common types of disasters. Potential topics for family disaster education are presented below.

HIGHLIGHTS

Areas for Client Education Related to Disaster Preparedness

- Install and maintain smoke detectors in homes.
- Bolt bookcases and cabinets to walls in areas with earthquake potential.
- Seek shelter in a reinforced area (e.g., a doorway) during an earthquake and face away from windows. Stay indoors.
- Seek shelter from hurricanes or tornadoes in basements or inner rooms without windows.
- Seek high ground in the event of a flood.
- Drop to the ground and roll about to extinguish flaming clothing, or smother flames with a rug.
- Close doors and windows to prevent the spread of a fire, and place wadded fabric beneath doors to prevent smoke inhalation.
- Determine avenues of escape from the home or other buildings.
- Install fire escape ladders as needed at upper windows.
- Keep stairways and doors free of obstacles to permit an easy way out.
- Identify a place for family members to meet after escape from the home.
- Designate a person living outside the area as a family contact if family members are separated during a disaster.
- Learn community disaster warning signals and their meaning.
- Keep a battery-operated radio and extra batteries available (replace batteries periodically).
- Collect and store, in an accessible location, sufficient emergency supplies for one week, including:
  - Nonperishable foods (including pet foods)
  - Drinking water
  - Warm clothing
  - Bedding (blankets or sleeping bags)
  - Tent or other type of shelter
  - Source of light (flashlights or lanterns)
  - Chlorine bleach for treating suspect water supplies to prevent infection
  - First-aid supplies and first-aid manual
  - Medications needed by family members
- Replace stored food, water, and medications periodically.
- Know where natural gas and water valves are located and how to turn them off. Attach a wrench close to valves.
- Determine what valuables are to be taken if evacuation is required.
- Assign activities related to evacuation (e.g., designate the person responsible for taking the baby or family pets).
- Know the general plan and designated routes for evacuating the community.
- Know where proposed shelters will be located.
- Know what actions should be taken when warning is given.
- Know where to seek additional information.

⑥THINK ABOUT IT

How prepared are you and your family in the event of a disaster? Why doesn't everyone engage in personal disaster preparation?

Secondary Prevention

Secondary prevention involves the response to a disaster occurrence. Implementing the community's disaster plan is a secondary preventive measure. Secondary prevention is geared toward halting the disaster and resolving problems caused by it. Secondary prevention may take place at the community level or at the level of individual victims. For example, efforts to provide food and shelter are secondary preventive measures taken at the group level, whereas treatment of burns and other injuries is secondary prevention related to specific individuals.

Community health nurses are actively involved in the response to an actual disaster event. Areas for involvement include triage, treatment of injuries and other health conditions, and shelter supervision. Community health nurses may be some of several health care providers who perform triage activities described earlier and who determine priorities for treatment, evacuation, and transportation of disaster victims. In planning for triage responsibilities, community health nurses would familiarize themselves with criteria for assigning priority.

Community health nurses may also be involved in treating injuries or other health conditions. This may occur in definitive care sites (hospitals or other health care facilities removed from the disaster site itself) or in shelters. Nurses involved in first aid for victims should plan to update their skills in basic first aid on a periodic basis. Community health nurses, particularly those working in shelters, need to plan to deal not only with existing health conditions, such as hypertension and diabetes, but also with acute conditions. For example, the nurse may encounter a child with a middle ear infection that requires treatment or a woman in labor. In planning for these and similar activities, the nurse should be familiar with procedures included in the disaster plan for care of minor illnesses and dispensing medications for clients with chronic diseases. The nurse needs to know to whom to refer those in need of services and how to arrange for transportation or other needs. The disaster plan may call for nurses to treat minor illnesses on the basis of protocols developed in conjunction with medical personnel. If such is the case, the nurse should become familiar with those treatment protocols. Finally, the nurse needs to plan for activities to monitor clients' health status. For example, the nurse might schedule periodic blood pressure measurements for a disaster relief worker with hypertension.

Community health nurses may also be responsible for supervising and coordinating shelter activities. Responsibilities might include supervising the meeting of health care and other needs by other disaster relief workers; supervising record keeping related to people brought to and released from the shelter; assisting people housed in shelters on a long-term basis to develop some form of governance; and using interpersonal skills to keep the shelter running smoothly.

Community health nurses may also be involved in crisis counseling for both victims and rescue workers, or, since people often turn to family, friends, or community leaders for assistance with emotional needs, nurses may assist in training local resource personnel to help with initial crisis intervention. General principles for such interventions include recognizing that most people are not mentally ill but are experiencing crisis, and that the intent is to provide immediate support and stabilize their emotional status, not to provide therapy. Nurses and others should also keep in mind that distress is a universal response to events like disasters. Finally, resource people should refer those who need professional help to experienced mental health workers (North & Hong, 2000).

A final consideration with respect to secondary prevention is the extent of preparation needed to respond to potential bioterrorism. The greater the likelihood of such events occurring, the greater the need for preparation. The Centers for Disease Control and Prevention Strategic Planning Workgroup (2000) has recommended that state and local jurisdictions be prepared to (1) detect unusual disease patterns or injuries, (2) respond to reports of clusters of unusual events, and (3) conduct epidemiologic investigations, treatment and prophylaxis, or disease prevention and environmental decontamination procedures as needed. These recommendations are based on the usual response to any new or unusual condition encountered in the population and should work equally well for instances of bioterrorism. Secondary preventive activities by community health nurses in a disaster setting are summarized in Table 27–2 ■.

Tertiary Prevention

Tertiary prevention with respect to a disaster has two major goals. The first is recovery of the community and its members from the effects of the disaster and return to normal. The second aspect of tertiary prevention is preventing a recurrence of the disaster.

Community health nurses have responsibilities in both of these areas after the disaster is over. Community health nurses may be called on to provide sustained care to both victims and disaster workers following the disaster. They may also be involved in identifying health and psychosocial problems that require further assistance. Community health nurses should plan to provide counseling or referral for persons with psychological problems stemming from their experiences during the disaster. There may also be a need to refer disaster victims to continuing sources of medical care. Community health nurses may also need to plan referrals for clients in need of social and financial assistance. For example, disaster victims may require help in finding housing or in getting financial aid to rebuild homes or businesses.

Community health nurses may also provide input into interventions designed to prevent future disasters or to minimize their effects. For example, if the disaster involved rioting by members of oppressed groups, the community health nurse might advocate measures to meet the needs of minority group members to prevent further rioting; or community health nurses might campaign for stronger building codes to prevent the collapse of buildings in subsequent earthquakes. Community health nurses can also help to educate the public on disaster preparedness to minimize the effects of subsequent disasters. Tertiary prevention foci in disaster settings and related community health nursing activities are summarized in Table 27–3 ■. Resources to assist nurses with

■ TABLE 27–2   Secondary Preventive Activities by Community Health Nurses in Disaster Settings

SECONDARY PREVENTION FOCUS	RELATED NURSING ACTIVITIES
Triage	Assess disaster victims for extent of injuries. Determine priority for treatment, evacuation, and transportation. Place appropriate colored tag on victim depending on priority.
Treatment of injuries	Render first aid for injuries. Provide additional treatment as needed in definitive care areas.
Treatment of other conditions	Determine health needs other than injury. Refer for medical treatment as required. Provide treatment for other conditions based on medically approved protocols.
Shelter supervision	Coordinate activities of shelter workers. Oversee records of those admitted and discharged from the shelter. Promote effective interpersonal and group interactions among those housed in the shelter. Promote independence and involvement of those housed in the shelter.

primary, secondary, and tertiary prevention aspects of disaster care are available through links provided on the companion Web site for this book.

IMPLEMENTING DISASTER CARE

Prior to the occurrence of a disaster, the community health nurse may be involved in activities preliminary to implementing a disaster plan, particularly in disseminating the plan to others. Dissemination needs to occur among persons and agencies who will have designated responsibilities during a disaster. The community health nurse participating in disaster planning is responsible for communicating elements of the plan to members of the nurse's employing agency. They may also ensure that the plan is disseminated to nursing organizations in the area (e.g., to members of a district nurses' association). The nurse who assumes this responsibility should be sure that the general plan, as well as the specific part to be played by members of the agency or organization, is understood.

The essential features of the community's disaster response plan should also be communicated to the general public so residents will be prepared to follow the plan in the event of a disaster. The community health nurse may be involved in helping to communicate the plan to the public by apprising clients with whom he or she works of relevant aspects of the plan. The public should be alerted to mechanisms that will be used to inform them of a disaster and where to go for additional information. Community members should also know the general procedures to be followed in terms of caring for disaster victims and setting up shelters. They should also be informed of the locations of proposed shelters. Finally, community members should be told of specific disaster preparations that should be undertaken by individuals and families.

■ TABLE 27–3   Tertiary Preventive Activities by Community Health Nurses in Disaster Settings

TERTIARY PREVENTION FOCUS	RELATED NURSING ACTIVITIES
Follow-up care for injuries	Provide continued care for people injured as a result of the disaster or during rescue operations. Monitor response to treatment.
Follow-up care for psychological problems resulting from the disaster	Provide counseling for those with psychological problems resulting from the disaster. Refer clients for counseling as needed. Monitor progress in resolving psychological problems.
Recovery assistance	Refer clients for financial assistance. Provide assistance in finding housing.
Prevention of future disasters and their consequences	Advocate measures to prevent future disasters. Educate the public about disaster preparation to minimize the effects of subsequent disasters.

EVALUATING DISASTER CARE

The final responsibility of community health nurses with respect to disaster care is evaluating that care. Nurses and others involved in the disaster participate in evaluative activities outlined in the disaster plan. Evaluation focuses on the adequacy of the plan for curtailing the disaster and meeting the needs of those involved in it.

In this effort it may be helpful to examine the disaster response in light of the six dimensions of health. Did the plan adequately provide for the needs of the people affected and the kinds of health problems that resulted? Did physical environmental, psychological, or sociocultural dimension factors impede implementation of the plan or limit its effectiveness? What influence did behavioral factors have on plan implementation, if any? Were

health care services adequate to meet the health needs posed by the disaster itself as well as those encountered in the period after the disaster? Data obtained in the evaluative process are used to assess the adequacy of the community disaster plan and to guide revisions of the plan to better deal with future disasters.

The effectiveness of care provided to individual disaster victims should also be assessed. Evaluation in this area focuses on the degree to which individual needs were met and the extent to which problems resulting from the disaster were resolved.

Although disasters occur infrequently in community health practice, community health nurses should be prepared to respond effectively when they do occur. They should also be instrumental in assuring that individual clients and families, as well as communities, are prepared to respond effectively in the event of a disaster.

APPLYING YOUR KNOWLEDGE IN PRACTICE

❧ CASE STUDY
Nursing in the Disaster Setting

Two commuter trains have collided in a tunnel at rush hour. Both trains derailed and one of them struck the side of the tunnel, causing it to collapse on two of the derailed cars. Approximately 300 people were passengers on the two trains, with 50 or more people trapped in the two buried cars. The accident occurred approximately one-quarter mile from the west end of the tunnel and two miles from the east end. Most of both trains lie on the west side of the collapsed portion of the tunnel.

One of the passengers is a community health nurse. The nurse was not injured in the accident and was able

to get out of the wreckage to the west end of the tunnel, where most of the survivors are gathered.

- What are the biophysical, psychological, physical environmental, sociocultural, behavioral, and health system factors that may be influencing this disaster situation?
- What role functions might the community health nurse carry out in this situation?
- What primary, secondary, and tertiary preventive activities might be appropriate in this situation? Why?

❧ TESTING YOUR UNDERSTANDING

- In what ways do disaster events vary? What are the implications of these variations for disaster preparedness? (pp. 625–626)
- What are the three elements of a disaster? How does each influence disaster response? (pp. 627–633)
- What are some of the potential benefits of disaster preparedness? (pp. 633–634)
- How might biophysical, psychological, physical environmental, sociocultural, behavioral, and health system considerations influence a disaster or a community's response to a disaster? (pp. 641–648)

- What are the principles of community disaster preparedness? (pp. 634–635)
- Describe the characteristics of an effective disaster plan. (p. 636)
- What are the elements of an effective disaster plan? (pp. 637–641)
- What is the role of the community health nurse in primary, secondary, and tertiary prevention related to disaster situations? (pp. 648–651)

REFERENCES

Arnold, D. (1999). War & relief: Critics say refugee camps delay necessary defeat. *World View, 14*(4), 9–10.

Baxter, P. J. (1997). Volcanoes. In E. K. Noji (Ed.), *The public health consequences of disasters* (pp. 179–204). New York: Oxford University Press.

Centers for Disease Control and Prevention. (1999). Improvements in workplace safety—United States, 1900–1999. *Morbidity and Mortality Weekly Report, 48,* 461–469.

Centers for Disease Control and Prevention Strategic Planning Workgroup. (2000). Biological and chemical terrorism: Strategic plan for preparedness and response. *Morbidity and Mortality Weekly Report, 49*(RR-4), 1–14.

Centers for Disease Control and Prevention. (2001). Facts about anthrax. Retrieved October 25, 2001, from the World Wide Web, *http://www.bt.cdc.gov.*

Comerio, M. (1998). *Disaster hits home: New policy for urban housing recovery.* Berkley, CA: University of California Press.

Diaz, M. F. (1999). Refugee women: Overcoming the odds. In K. M. Kahill (Ed.), *A framework for survival: Health and humanitarian assistance in conflicts and disasters* (pp. 49–59). New York: Routledge.

Epidemiology Program Office. (1998). Deaths associated with Hurricane Georges—Puerto Rico, September, 1998. *Morbidity and Mortality Weekly Report, 47,* 897–898.

Epidemiology Program Office. (1999). Community needs assessment and morbidity surveillance following an earthquake—Turkey, August, 1999. *Morbidity and Mortality Weekly Report, 48,* 1147–1150.

Epidemiology Program Office. (2000). Morbidity and mortality associated with Hurricane Floyd—North Carolina, September–October, 1999. *Morbidity and Mortality Weekly Report, 49,* 369–372.

Gautam, K. (1998). Organizational problems faced by the Missouri DOH in providing disaster relief during the 1993 floods. *Journal of Public Health Management Practice, 4*(4), 79–86.

Geiger, H. J. (2001). Terrorism, biological weapons, and bonanzas: Assessing the real threat to public health. *American Journal of Public Health, 91,* 708–709.

Gerrity, E. T., & Flynn, B. W. (1997). Mental health consequences of disasters. In E. K. Noji (Ed.), *The public health consequences of disasters* (pp. 101–121). New York: Oxford University Press.

Gibbons, E., & Garfield, R. (1999). The impact of economic sanctions on health and human rights in Haiti, 1991–1994. *American Journal of Public Health, 89,* 1499–1504.

Kilbourne, E. M. (1997a). Cold environments. In E. K. Noji (Ed.), *The public health conse-*

quences of disasters (pp. 270–286). New York: Oxford University Press.

Kilbourne, E. M. (1997b). Heat waves and hot environments. In E. K. Noji (Ed.), *The public health consequences of disasters* (pp. 245–269). New York: Oxford University Press.

Lichterman, J. D. (2000). A "community as resource" strategy for disaster response. *Public Health Reports, 115,* 262–265.

Lillibridge, S. R. (1997a). Industrial disasters. In E. K. Noji (Ed.), *The public health consequences of disasters* (pp. 354–372). New York: Oxford University Press.

Lillibridge, S. R. (1997b). Managing the environmental health aspects of disasters: Water, human excreta, and shelter. In E. K. Noji (Ed.), *The public health consequences of disasters* (pp. 65–78). New York: Oxford University Press.

Lillibridge, S. R. (1997c). Tornadoes. In E. K. Noji (Ed.), *The public health consequences of disasters* (pp. 228–244). New York: Oxford University Press.

Malilay, J. (1997a). Floods. In E. K. Noji (Ed.), *The public health consequences of disasters* (pp. 287–301). New York: Oxford University Press.

Malilay, J. (1997b). Tropical cyclones. In E. K. Noji (Ed.), *The public health consequences of disasters* (pp. 207–227). New York: Oxford University Press.

Marks, S. P. (1999). Economic sanctions as human rights violations: Reconciling political and public health imperatives. *American Journal of Public Health, 89,* 1509–1513.

McGuire, S. Sr. (1998). Global migration and health: Ecofeminist perspectives. *Advanced Nursing Science, 21*(2), 1–16.

National Center for Environmental Health. (1998). Cholera outbreak among Rwandan refugees—Democratic Republic of Congo, April, 1997. *Morbidity and Mortality Weekly Report, 47,* 389–391.

National Center for Environmental Health. (1999). Needs assessment following Hurricane Georges—Dominican Republic, 1998. *Morbidity and Mortality Weekly Report, 48,* 93–95.

National Center for Environmental Health. (2000a). Nutritional assessment of adolescent refugees—Nepal, 1999. *Morbidity and Mortality Weekly Report, 49,* 864–867.

National Center for Environmental Health. (2000b). Storm-related mortality—Central Texas, October 17–31, 1998. *Morbidity and Mortality Weekly Report, 498,* 133–135.

National Center for Environmental Health. (2001). Mortality during a famine—Gode District, Ethiopia, July 2000. *Morbidity and Mortality Weekly Report, 50,* 285–288.

National Center for Infectious Diseases (2001). Recognition of illness associated with the intentional release of biologic agents.

Morbidity and Mortality Weekly Report, 50, 893–897.

National Mental Health Association. (2001). Depression screening. Retrieved September 24, 2001, from the World Wide Web, *http://www.depression–screening.org.*

The Nation's Health. (1999, October). Iraqi children suffer under sanctions. P. 11.

Neugebauer, R. (1999). Mind matters: The importance of mental disorders in public health's 21st century mission. *American Journal of Public Health, 89,* 1309–1311.

Noji, E. K. (1997a). Earthquakes. In E. K. Noji (Ed.), *The public health consequences of disasters* (pp. 135–178). New York: Oxford University Press.

Noji, E. K. (1997b). Introduction. In E. K. Noji (Ed.), *The public health consequences of disasters* (pp. xiii–xvii). New York: Oxford University Press.

Noji, E. K. (1997c). The nature of disaster: General characteristics and public health effects. In E. K. Noji (Ed.), *The public health consequences of disasters* (pp. 3–20). New York: Oxford University Press.

North, C. S., & Hong, B. A. (2000). Project CREST: A new model for mental health intervention after a community disaster. *American Journal of Public Health, 90,* 1057–1058.

Paris, J. (2000). Georgia inmates and staff coped with natural disaster—Lessons learned from Hurricane Floyd. *Correct Care, 14*(1), 8, 21.

The Pew Research Center for the People and the Press. (2001). Overwhelming support for Bush, military response, but American psyche reeling from terror attacks? Retrieved September 24, 2001, from the World Wide Web, *http://www.people–press.org.*

Sidel, V. W. (1999). Can sanctions be sanctioned? *American Journal of Public Health, 89,* 1497–1498.

Sidel, V. W., Cohen, H. W., & Gould, R. M. (2001). Good intentions and the road to bioterrorism preparedness. *American Journal of Public Health, 91,* 716–718.

Toole, M. J. (1997). Communicable diseases and disease control. In E. K. Noji (Ed.), *The public health consequences of disasters* (pp. 79–100). New York: Oxford University Press.

Toole, M. J. (1999). The public health consequences of inaction. In K. M. Kahill (Ed.), *A framework for survival: Health and humanitarian assistance in conflicts and disasters* (pp. 13–25). New York: Routledge.

Wetter, D. C., Daniell, W. E., & Treser, C. D. (2001). Hospital preparedness for victims of chemical or biological terrorism. *American Journal of Public Health, 91,* 710–716.

World Health Organization. (1989). *Coping with natural disasters: The role of local health personnel and the community.* Geneva: World Health Organization.

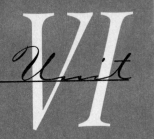

COMMON HEALTH PROBLEMS OF POPULATIONS

ON HEARING THE NEWS OF A PATIENT'S DEATH

Morning light glances off the chrome
of a stripped down car in the alley
slices through window panes
along the edges of drawn shades
opens fire on sheets pulled up
to shield the eyes of sleepers.

This summer sun won't light your eyes.
Not even the cries of the baby reach you.
It's too late, for you went early
just as we thought you might
but not like this
manacled to a bed
in the maternity ward
of D.C. General Hospital.

Hearing the news, I call up your face
a wide-open face with a slow shy smile
as if the shock of life had somehow dazed you.
You took each day
each man
each child
each welfare check
each jail cell
as it came.

It just wasn't in you to ask why or why not
to look ahead or behind.
Since when does someone like you get to choose?
Since when do poor ignorant women take charge
of their lives?

The world for you was
your mother's house, teeming with kin
the street
the welfare office
hospital and
jail.
A heroin high was the only place you ever had
to call your own
and a fix was the only way you knew
to get there.

The judge decided to keep you in jail
those last few months of your pregnancy—
the best he could do for your unborn child.
Why bring another addict into the world?

Oh, it isn't that you never tried to kick.
You'd come to us in pain
with abscesses from dirty needles.
You'd come when the drug supply dried up.
You'd come when there was no money to buy.
You'd come when you felt too tired to sell.

I can do it alone, you said
I can kick.
Just give me a few Valiums.
A little help is all I need.

I suppose we'll never know just how you died.
It was after the baby was born
after they'd taken you back to the ward.
Some people said they heard calls for help.
When they found you, you were hanging
over the side of the bed
dangling by the foot
they'd shackled to the bedframe.

Your family set up a wail that went on for days
alleged foul play
hinted at revenge.
There was gunfire at the wake, they say
and eight motherless children destined for
your mother's house
the street
the welfare office
hospital and
jail.

The last light you saw in the blank night
of your life
was your newborn girl.
Is that why you named her Star?

Reprinted with permission from V. Masson (1999),
Rehab at the Florida Avenue Grill. *Washington, DC:*
Sage Femme Press.

he poem above reflects the multiple tragedies of substance abuse, one of the population health problems addressed by community health nurses.

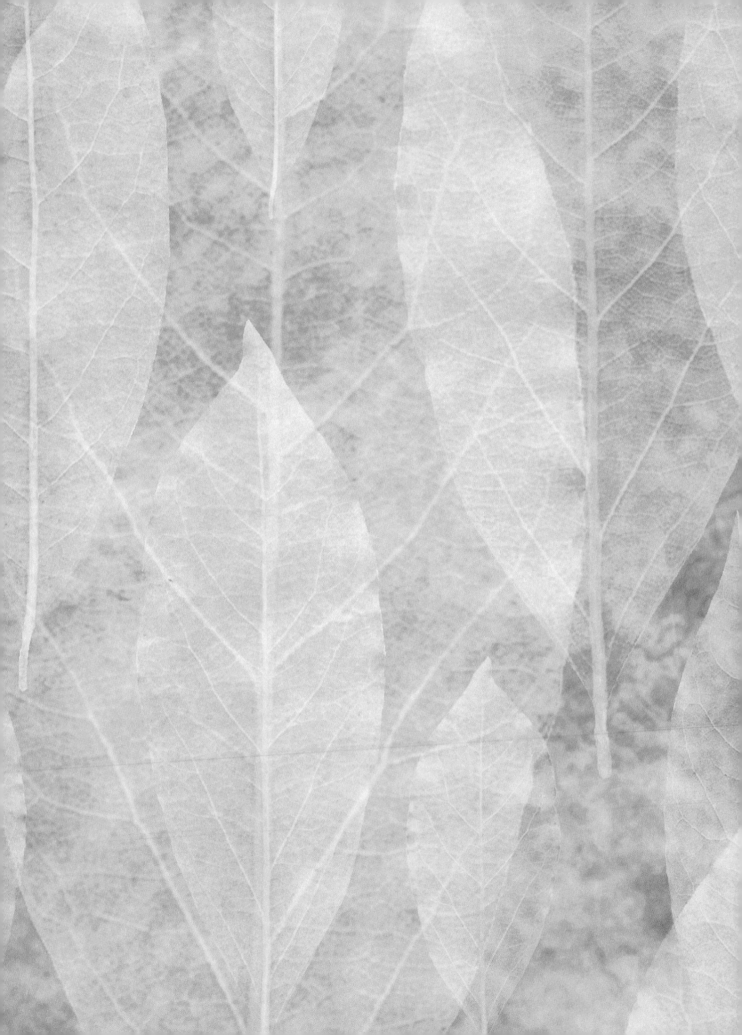

COMMUNICABLE DISEASES

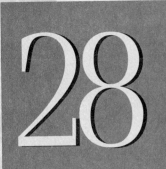

28

Chapter Objectives

After reading this chapter, you should be able to:

■ Describe major trends in the incidence of communicable diseases.
■ Identify the modes of transmission for communicable diseases.
■ Discuss the role of community health nurses in controlling communicable diseases.
■ Describe the influence of biophysical, psychological, physical environmental, sociocultural, behavioral, and health system factors on communicable diseases.
■ Discuss approaches to primary prevention of communicable diseases.
■ Describe major considerations in secondary prevention for communicable diseases.
■ Discuss tertiary prevention of communicable diseases.

KEY TERMS

anergy 667
case fatality rate 664
chain of infection 661
chemoprophylaxis 672
co-infection 660
communicable diseases 658
contact notification 672
directly observed therapy (DOT) 675
elimination 658
eradication 658
incubation period 662
mass screening 674
mode of transmission 661
opportunistic infections (OIs) 664
prodromal period 662
selective screening 674
superinfection 660

Media Link

http://www.prenhall.com/clark

Additional interactive resources for this chapter can be found on the companion Web site. Click on Chapter 28 and "Begin" to select the activities for this chapter.

Communicable diseases are those diseases spread by direct contact with an infectious agent. Communicable diseases affecting humans arise from both human and animal sources. At the beginning of the twentieth century, four communicable diseases—pneumonia, tuberculosis, diarrheal diseases, and diphtheria—accounted for 40% of all deaths in the United States. By 1997, only 4.5% of U.S. deaths were due to the three major communicable disease killers—pneumonia, influenza, and HIV/AIDS (Centers for Disease Control and Prevention [CDC], 1999a). In both the United States and Britain, mortality due to childhood diseases declined 200-fold from 1961 to 1996 (DiLiberti & Jackson, 1999). In spite of the remarkable decline in mortality due to communicable diseases in the United States and other developed nations, these conditions continue to exact a toll in worldwide suffering, death, and economic costs.

TRENDS IN COMMUNICABLE DISEASE INCIDENCE

As noted above, overall mortality from communicable diseases has declined significantly in some parts of the world. These trends are not, however, universal. Because

of the potential for rapid spread of disease throughout the world, community health nurses need to be aware of trends in communicable disease incidence, prevalence, and mortality in their local areas as well as nationally and internationally. Communicable disease incidence also varies among geographic areas in the United States and among ethnic groups. Figure 28–1 ■ presents the distribution of reported pediatric AIDS cases in 1999 by state. Similar maps depicting the distribution of disease by state are provided on the companion Web site for this book. Generally speaking, most communicable diseases have higher incidence rates among ethnic minority groups than among Caucasians, due to a number of social conditions such as poverty and lack of access to care.

One disease, smallpox, has been completely eradicated from the world, although there is potential for its reintroduction through bioterrorism. The goal of the World Health Organization (WHO) is the elimination of several diseases, with their eventual eradication throughout the world. *Eradication* involves eliminating the causative organism of a disease from nature. *Elimination*, on the other hand, is more circumscribed and may involve eliminating a disease from a single country or region or controlling manifestations of the disease so it is

FIGURE 28–1 ■ *Distribution of Pediatric AIDS Cases, by State, 1999*

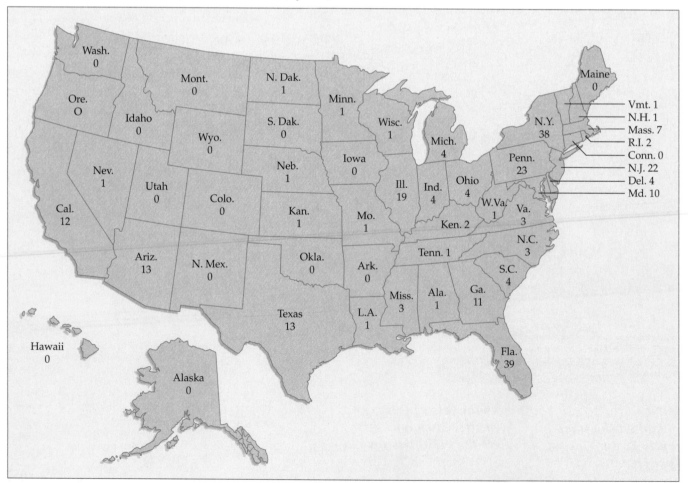

no longer a public health problem. Poliomyelitis has been targeted for eradication and has been eliminated in several areas, and measles has been targeted for elimination in major segments of the world. Currently, three WHO regions have eliminated or are close to eliminating wild poliovirus infection. Most of the world's remaining polio cases occur in only 50 countries (Vaccine Preventable Disease Eradication Division, 1999).

The incidence of vaccine-preventable childhood diseases is diminishing in areas where vaccination coverage is high. For example, prior to the availability of measles vaccine, more than 400,000 cases of measles occurred each year in the United States. With the advent of widespread vaccine use, measles incidence has declined by 99% (Watson, Hadler, Dykewicz, Reef, & Phillips, 1998). In 1999, provisional data indicated that only 100 confirmed cases of measles occurred in the United States, for an incidence rate of 0.04 per 100,000 population, with no measles-related deaths (CDC, 2001a). In contrast to the early 1900s, most of these cases occurred among people over 20 years of age rather than in young children (National Immunization Program, 2000a).

Worldwide, on the other hand, more than 700,000 cases of measles occurred in 1997 (Vaccine Preventable Disease Eradication Division, 1998). Although this figure represents a 48% decrease in incidence since 1990, measles still contributed to over 1 million deaths and $1.5 billion in treatment costs (Orenstein et al., 2000). Table 28–1 ■ presents recent incidence and trend information for vaccine preventable childhood diseases.

Somewhat less favorable trends are noted for other communicable diseases. In 1999, the rate of new cases of AIDS was 16.66 per 100,000 population in the United States (CDC, 2001a). Worldwide, more than 5.3 million new cases of HIV infection occurred, including more than 600,000 children. At the end of 2000, an estimated 36.1 million people in the world were living with HIV infection, and 3 million deaths occurred in that year alone, for a total of 21.8 million deaths since the beginning of the epidemic in 1981. Prevalence rates are significantly higher in some parts of the world than in North America. For example, in 2000, 25.3 million people in sub-Saharan Africa and 5.8 million in Southeast Asia were infected with HIV compared to only 920,000 people in North

■ **TABLE 28–1**   Vaccine Availability, 1999 Incidence per 100,000 U.S. Population, Deaths, and Trends in Childhood Diseases

DISEASE	VACCINE AVAILABLE	1999 INCIDENCE	TRENDS
Diphtheria	1923	0.00	Slight resurgence in incidence in 1960s, peaking in the 1970s; 100% decline in U.S. incidence with vaccine; none of the 41 cases that occurred from 1980 to 1995 had been immunized
Haemophilus influenzae type b (HiB)	1985	0.48	99.7% decline in cases with vaccine, 11 U.S. deaths in 1999
Measles	1963	0.04	Worldwide 48% decline in incidence from 1990 to 1997; 1 million deaths; $1.5 billion costs; 82% global vaccine coverage
Mumps	1967	0.14	99% decrease in U.S. cases from 1968 to 1995; 1 death reported in 1999
Pertussis	1926	2.67	96% decline in U.S. incidence with vaccine
Poliomyelitis	1955	0.00	100% decline in U.S. cases with vaccine; Western Hemisphere declared free of wild poliovirus in 1994, two other WHO regions close to elimination
Rubella	1969	0.10	97% decline in U.S. cases with vaccine; 10% of U.S. young adults susceptible, 4 to 68% in other countries; U.S. incidence of congenital rubella syndrome declined 69% from 1970 to 1996
Tetanus	1927	0.01	47 U.S. cases reported in 1997; 31 cases of neonatal tetanus reported from 1972 to 1978
Varicella	1995	44.56	81 U.S. deaths in 1999

Sources: Bisgard, K. M., Hardy, I. R. B. Popovic, T., Strebel, P. T., et al. (1998). Respiratory diphtheria in the United States, 1980 through 1995. *American Journal of Public Health, 88*, 787–791; California Department of Health Services. (1998). Tetanus among injection drug users—California, 1997. *Morbidity and Mortality Weekly Report, 47*, 149–151; Centers for Disease Control and Prevention. (2001). Summary of notifiable diseases, United States, 1999. *Morbidity and Mortality Weekly Report, 48*(53), 1–101; National Center for Infectious Diseases. (1998). Rubella among crew members of commercial cruise ships—Florida, 1997. *Morbidity and Mortality Weekly Report, 46*, 1247–1250; National Immunization Program. (1998). Neonatal tetanus—Montana, 1998. *Morbidity and Mortality Weekly Report, 47*, 928–930; National Immunization Program. (1999). Impact of vaccines recommended for children—United States, 1990–1998. *Morbidity and Mortality Weekly Report, 48*, 243–248; Prevots, D. R., Burr, R. K., Sutter, R. W., & Murphy, T. V. (2000). Poliomyelitis prevention in the United States: Updated recommendations of the Advisory Committee on Immunization Practices. *Morbidity and Mortality Weekly Report, 49*(RR-5), 1–22; Vaccine Preventable Disease Eradication Division. (1998). Progress toward global measles control and regional elimination, 1990–1997. *Morbidity and Mortality Weekly Report, 47*, 1049–1054; Vaccine Preventable Disease Eradication Division. (1999). Progress toward global poliomyelitis eradication, 1997–1998. *Morbidity and Mortality Weekly Report, 48*, 416–421; and Watson, J. C., Hadler, S. C., Dykewicz, C. A., Reef, S., & Phillips, L. (1998). Measles, mumps, and rubella—Vaccine use and strategies for elimination of measles, rubella, and congenital rubella syndrome and control of mumps: Recommendations of the Advisory Committee on Immunization Practices (ACIP). *Morbidity and Mortality Weekly Report, 47*(RR-8), 1–57.

America. AIDS-related deaths show similar differences with 2.4 million deaths in sub-Saharan Africa and 470,000 in Southeast Asia in 2000 compared to 20,000 deaths in North America (UNAIDS, 2000).

Deaths due to AIDS in the United States have declined somewhat from the peak of the epidemic due primarily to advances in treatment options. In 1997, HIV/AIDS dropped from the eighth to the fourteenth leading cause of death in all age groups (National Center for Health Statistics, 1999). In 1998, the age-adjusted death rate for AIDS was 4.6 per 100,000 population, less than one third of the 1995 rate (15.6 per 100,000) (U.S. Department of Health and Human Services [USDHHS], 2000a).

Generally speaking, incidence rates for sexually transmitted diseases (STDs) have declined in the United States. For example, in 1999, the incidence rate for primary and secondary syphilis was 2.5 per 100,000 persons, an 88% decrease from 1990 (CDC, 2001a). The incidence of congenital syphilis (syphilis passed from infected mother to unborn infant) declined 78% from 1992 to 1998 (Division of Sexually Transmitted Diseases Prevention, 1999a), and in 1998, 80% of U.S. counties reported no cases of primary or secondary syphilis (Gunn, Harper, Brontrager, Gonzales, & St. Louis, 2000). In 1999, the CDC launched a campaign to eliminate syphilis from the United States. Elimination in this instance means a lack of sustained transmission, or transmission to other people, within 90 days of the report of an imported case of syphilis (Division of Sexually Transmitted Diseases Prevention, 2001).

Like the rates for syphilis, the overall 1999 incidence rate of 133.2 per 100,000 people for gonorrhea was less than half of the 1989 rate (297.36 per 100,000) (CDC, 2001a). Gonorrhea incidence, however, was somewhat less evenly distributed over the United States, with 21 states showing more than a 10% increase in incidence from 1997 to 1998 and another 1.2% increase in the following year (Fox et al., 2001). Incidence rates for *Chlamydia trachomatis* show the greatest increase among STDs, rising from 126.6 per 100,000 population in 1995 to 254.1 per 100,000 in 1999 (CDC, 2001a).

Incidence rates for cases of hepatitis vary with the causative agent. In 1999, for example, the incidence rate for hepatitis A virus (HAV) infection was 6.25 per 100,000 people, down from 14.43 per 100,000 in 1989. Similarly, 1999 hepatitis B (HBV) incidence (2.82 per 100,000) was less than one third the incidence of 1989, and hepatitis C (HCV) incidence (1.14 per 100,000) was less than half of the 1989 rate. Despite the decreasing incidence of these three diseases, they continue to cause mortality. In 1999, for example, HAV contributed to 114 deaths and HBV to 1,052 deaths. HCV, however, is the biggest contributor to hepatitis-related deaths, causing more than 3,600 deaths in 1999 (CDC, 2001a).

Hepatitis also contributes to significant health care costs, with hepatitis A costing approximately $200 million per year in medical care and lost work time, hepatitis B accounting for $700 million per year, and hepatitis C for $600 million in annual costs (National Center for Infectious Diseases, 2000a, 2000b, 2000c).

Hepatitis D (HDV) and E (HEV) virus infections occur far less frequently than hepatitis A, B, or C. Hepatitis D occurs only in conjunction with hepatitis B as a co-infection or as a superinfection (National Center for Infectious Diseases, 2000d). *Co-infection* means that the two diseases occur simultaneously, in the case of hepatitis B and D, usually as a result of injection drug use (IDU). *Superinfection* exists when infection with hepatitis D occurs in a person with existing chronic hepatitis B virus infection. Hepatitis E occurs primarily in areas of poor sanitation and, in the United States, is usually diagnosed in travelers returning from endemic areas such as Mexico, Southeast Asia, and northern and eastern areas in Africa (National Center for Infectious Diseases, 2000e).

Two other communicable diseases of interest to community health nurses are tuberculosis (TB) and influenza. A resurgence of tuberculosis was noted with the influx of refugee populations from endemic areas of the world after several years of declining incidence. Approximately one third of the world's population is infected with tuberculosis, and TB contributes to more than 2 million deaths per year (CDC, 2001b), killing more adults worldwide than any other communicable disease (O'Brien, 1998). In 1997, 39% of tuberculosis cases in the United States occurred in foreign-born persons, who had incidence rates 4 to 5 times those of the native-born population (Division of Tuberculosis Elimination, 1998). The 1999 incidence rate for TB was 6.43 per 100,000 people (CDC, 2001a), and TB incidence declined 7% from 1999 to 2000 (CDC, 2001b).

In 1918, an influenza epidemic resulted in 20 million deaths worldwide and 500,000 deaths in the United States (CDC, 1999a). Since then, influenza has caused an average of 114,000 hospitalizations and 20,000 deaths per year (Brammer et al., 2000). Although rates of infection are highest in the young, the elderly are at particular risk for complications (Bridges, Fukuda, Cox, & Singleton, 2001), and influenza is the fifth leading cause of death in people over 65 years of age (National Center for Chronic Disease Prevention and Health Promotion, 1998).

The diseases discussed here are not the only communicable diseases to affect the health of populations. Each year, new emerging and reemerging diseases occur due to a variety of circumstances. For example, diseases once thought controlled are becoming more frequent and harder to treat due to development of antimicrobial-resistant strains of microorganisms. Changes in food preparation and distribution processes are spreading foodborne diseases in much wider geographic areas than in the past. Similarly, environmental changes are increasing human exposures to new pathogens (e.g., hantavirus), and infectious agents have been identified for several chronic conditions (e.g., heart disease, some cancers, and peptic ulcer disease (Binder, Levitt, & the National Center for Infectious Diseases Plan Steering Committee, 1998). In addition, modern ventilation systems have spawned and spread diseases such as Legionnaires' disease. Medical advances, such as transfusions, have increased transmission of bloodborne diseases like hepatitis C, while medical treatments for some conditions (e.g., steroids) produce immunosuppression and susceptibility to communicable diseases. There is also the potential for epidemics of communicable diseases due to bioterrorism. In spite of the advances made in controlling communicable diseases to date, there remains considerable work to be done.

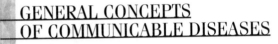

GENERAL CONCEPTS OF COMMUNICABLE DISEASES

Several communicable disease concepts must be understood before control efforts can be undertaken. These include concepts related to the "chain of infection," such as modes of transmission and portals of entry and exit, and the concepts of incubation and prodromal periods.

Chain of Infection

In communicable diseases, epidemiologic factors related to the biophysical, psychological, physical environmental, sociocultural, behavioral, and health system dimensions create what may be termed a chain of infection. A *chain of infection* is a series of events or conditions that lead to the development of a particular communicable disease. The "links" in the chain are the infected person or source of the infectious agent, the reservoir, the agent itself, the mode of transmission of the disease, the agent's portals of entry and exit, and a susceptible new host. The concepts of reservoir, agent, and host were introduced in Chapter 10. This discussion focuses on the remaining links in the chain: modes of transmission and portals of entry and exit.

Modes of Transmission

The *mode of transmission* of a particular disease is the means by which the infectious agent that causes the disease is transferred from an infected person to an uninfected one. Communicable diseases may be spread by any of several modes of transmission: airborne transmission, fecal–oral (gastrointestinal) transmission, direct contact, sexual contact, direct inoculation, insect or animal bite, or via inanimate objects or soil.

AIRBORNE TRANSMISSION

Airborne transmission occurs when the infectious organism is present in the air and is inspired (inhaled) by a susceptible host during respiration. Diseases transmitted by the airborne route include the exanthems (diseases characterized by a rash, such as measles and chickenpox), infections of the mouth and throat (such as streptococcal infections), and infections of the upper and lower respiratory system (such as tuberculosis, pneumonia, influenza, and the common cold). Certain systemic infections are

also products of airborne transmission. Examples of these are meningococcal meningitis and pneumococcal pneumonias, hantavirus pulmonary infections, coccidioidomycosis, anthrax, and smallpox. In the case of anthrax and smallpox, disease may also be transmitted by aerosolized dissemination of microorganisms.

FECAL–ORAL TRANSMISSION

Fecal–oral transmission of an infectious agent may be either direct or indirect. Direct transmission occurs when the hands or other objects (fomites) are contaminated with organisms from human feces and then put into the mouth. Indirect transmission occurs via contaminated food or water. For example, a person with hepatitis A may defecate, fail to wash his or her hands properly, and then prepare a sandwich for someone else. The second person would ingest the virus with the sandwich and, if susceptible, might develop hepatitis A. Additional examples include *Salmonella*- or *Shigella*-caused diarrheas. Botulism is another disease in which the causative organism is ingested with contaminated food or water. Contamination usually occurs by accident through inadequate canning and preserving processes, but could potentially occur as a result of bioterrorist activity. Ingestion anthrax may also result from intentional introduction of spores into food supplies.

DIRECT CONTACT

Direct contact transmission involves skin-to-skin contact or direct contact with mucous membrane discharges between the infected person and another person. Diseases typically spread by this route include infectious mononucleosis, impetigo, scabies, and lice. Smallpox may also be transmitted by contact with the lesions of infected persons. Scabies, lice, and other parasitic diseases also may be transmitted through contact with clothing and other items containing the eggs of the parasites. Similarly, the cutaneous form of anthrax is transmitted by handling contaminated objects (CDC, 2001).

SEXUAL TRANSMISSION

Transmission of diseases via sexual contact is a special instance of direct contact transmission. Diseases spread by this mode of transmission are usually referred to as sexually transmitted diseases (STDs). Diseases spread during sexual intercourse include (but are not limited to) AIDS, gonorrhea, syphilis, genital herpes, and hepatitis B, C, and D. These diseases may also be spread by other modes of transmission. For example, hepatitis B, C, and D and AIDS may be spread by direct inoculation.

TRANSMISSION BY DIRECT INOCULATION

Direct inoculation occurs when the infectious agent (a bloodborne pathogen) is introduced directly into the bloodstream of the new host. Direct inoculation can occur transplacentally from an infected mother to a fetus, via transfusion with infected blood or blood products, through the use of contaminated hypodermic equipment, or through a splash of contaminated body fluid to mucous membrane or nonintact skin. With the advent of several screening tests for blood donors, transmission via transfusion has been significantly decreased (National Center for Infectious Diseases, 2000c). Health care workers are particularly at risk for several communicable diseases caused by bloodborne pathogens. Diseases commonly spread by direct inoculation include AIDS and hepatitis B, C, and D.

TRANSMISSION BY INSECT OR ANIMAL BITE

Insect and animal bites can also transmit infectious agents. For example, the bite of the *Anopheles* mosquito is the mode of transmission for malaria. Similarly, rabies frequently is transmitted via a bite from infected, warm-blooded animals such as dogs, skunks, and raccoons. Lyme disease is transmitted by the bite of an infected tick, and plague can be transmitted by fleas on infected rodents.

TRANSMISSION BY OTHER MEANS

Some communicable diseases are transmitted through contact with spores present in the soil or with inanimate objects. For example, exposure to the bacillus that causes tetanus frequently occurs through a dirty puncture wound. Modes of transmission and typical diseases most often transmitted by each mode are summarized in Table 28–2 ■.

Portals of Entry and Exit

Communicable diseases also differ in terms of the portals through which the infectious agent causing the disease enters and leaves an infected host. Portals of entry include the respiratory system, the gastrointestinal tract, and the skin and mucous membranes.

Portals of exit also differ among communicable diseases. Infectious agents may leave an infected host through the respiratory system or through feces passed from the gastrointestinal tract. Blood and other body flu-

ids such as semen, vaginal secretions, and saliva are the portals of exit for infectious agents causing diseases such as AIDS, gonorrhea, and hepatitis B. The skin acts as a portal of exit as well as a portal of entry for conditions such as impetigo, cutaneous anthrax, and syphilis. Portals of entry and exit and related modes of disease transmission are summarized in Table 28–3 ■.

Incubation and Prodromal Periods

The *incubation period* of a communicable disease is the interval from exposure to an infectious organism to development of the symptoms of the disease (Friis & Sellers, 1999). The length of the incubation period for a particular disease may influence the success of efforts to halt the spread of the disease. Some diseases, such as influenza and scarlet fever, have incubation periods of less than a week. Others typically require incubation periods of one to two weeks (gonorrhea, measles, pertussis, and polio), two to three weeks (rubella, chickenpox, and mumps), or months (viral hepatitis, syphilis). In some diseases, such as AIDS, the incubation period can be years.

The *prodromal period* of a communicable disease is the period between the first symptoms and the appearance of the symptoms that typify the disease. For example, prior to appearance of the jaundice that is characteristic of viral hepatitis, the client may experience prodromal symptoms of nausea, fatigue, and malaise. Similarly, a cough, runny nose, and watery eyes are prodromal symptoms for measles. In many diseases, the prodromal period is the time of greatest ability to infect others.

⊚THINK ABOUT IT

What effect does the length of the incubation period have on efforts to control a specific communicable disease?

■ TABLE 28–2   Modes of Disease Transmission and Typical Diseases

MODE OF TRANSMISSION	DISEASES TRANSMITTED
Airborne	Measles, mumps, rubella, poliomyelitis, *Haemophilus influenzae* type B (HiB) infection, tuberculosis, influenza, scarlet fever, diphtheria, pertussis, hantavirus, respiratory anthrax, coccidioidomycosis, smallpox, plague (pneumonic form)
Fecal–oral/ingestion	Hepatitis A and E, salmonellosis, shigellosis, typhoid, polio (in poor sanitary conditions), botulism, ingestion anthrax
Direct contact	Impetigo, scabies, lice, smallpox, cutaneous anthrax
Sexual contact	Chlamydia, gonorrhea, hepatitis B, C, and D, HIV infection, herpes simplex virus (HSV) infection, syphilis
Direct inoculation	Syphilis, hepatitis A, B, C, and D, HIV infection
Insect or animal bite	Malaria, rabies, Lyme disease, plague (bubonic form)
Other means of transmission	Tetanus, hookworm

■ **TABLE 28–3** **Portals of Entry and Exit for Each Mode of Disease Transmission**

MODE OF TRANSMISSION	PORTAL OF ENTRY	PORTAL OF EXIT
Airborne	Respiratory system	Respiratory system
Fecal–oral/ingestion	Mouth	Feces
Direct contact	Skin, mucous membrane	Skin, mucous membrane
Sexual contact	Skin, mouth, urethra, rectum	Skin lesions, vaginal or urethral secretions
Direct inoculation	Across placenta, bloodstream	Blood
Animal or insect bite	Wound in skin	Blood, saliva
Other means of transmission	Wound in skin, intact skin	Animal feces, soil

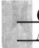

COMMUNITY HEALTH NURSING AND COMMUNICABLE DISEASES

Community health nurses play a variety of roles in controlling communicable diseases in individual clients and in population groups. These roles are incorporated into the nursing process and include assessing factors contributing to communicable diseases as well as the presence and extent of communicable disease in the individual or population, planning and implementing control strategies for communicable diseases, and evaluating the effectiveness of communicable disease interventions.

ASSESSING CONTRIBUTING FACTORS IN COMMUNICABLE DISEASES

Factors in each of the six dimension of health influence the development of communicable diseases in individuals and in population groups, and the community health nurse assesses factors related to each dimension. These factors are discussed in relation to several communicable diseases that are widespread in the U.S. population and that pose pervasive public health problems. A number of other communicable diseases (e.g., hantavirus, Ebola virus, Creutzfeldt–Jakob syndrome, plague, anthrax, and others) occur as sporadic outbreaks in certain populations or particular areas of the country or have potential for use in bioterrorist attacks. Information on factors contributing to these diseases is summarized in Appendix B.

Biophysical Considerations

Biophysical considerations such as age and physiologic health status influence the development of many communicable diseases. In the case of some diseases, age may influence susceptibility to a disease or its effects. As noted earlier, although children more often develop influenza, the elderly are more likely to develop fatal complications. Similarly, children usually have mild or asymptomatic hepatitis A (Bell, Wasley, Shapiro, & Margolis, 1999), while adults are usually sicker. Adults often have more complications with mumps and varicella as well (National Immunization Program, 2000c).

Tuberculosis, on the other hand, seems to occur most often in the very young and the very old.

The elderly are also most at risk for tetanus in the United States because they are the least likely to have been immunized. In addition, older persons seem to develop more severe cases of tetanus with more acute respiratory failure (Khajehdehi & Rezaian, 1997), and mortality rates are slightly higher for persons over 60 years of age (18%) than for younger adults (16% aged 40 to 59 years) (Bardenheier, Prevots, Khetsuriani, & Wharton, 1998). In developing countries with unsafe delivery conditions, neonates are at high risk for tetanus fatality. Neonates are also at risk for diseases that can be passed from mother to child perinatally. Such diseases include HIV infection, syphilis, and hepatitis B and C. For example, an estimated 500,000 neonates were infected with HIV in 1999 (Rosenfield, 2001). The risk of vertical transmission (from mother to child) is approximately 5% in babies born to mothers with HCV infection (National Institute of Diabetes and Digestive and Kidney Diseases, 1999), and when mothers are infected with both HIV and HCV, vertical transmission occurs in 14% to 17% of newborns (Alter et al., 1998). Overall estimated perinatal transmission of HIV seems to be about 25% in untreated mothers, rising to 45% when HIV-infected mothers breast-feed their infants (Rosenfield, 2001). In parts of the world where HIV infection is endemic, such as Africa, the rate of vertical transmission is much higher. Syphilis and rubella during pregnancy cause stillbirths and a variety of congenital anomalies (Fonck et al., 2001). Approximately 90% of untreated infants born to HBV-infected mothers can be expected to become chronic carriers (Corrarino, 1998), and these children are more likely to develop chronic infection (Yusuf et al., 1999).

Age also influences one's chance exposure to some communicable diseases. For example, STDs and hepatitis B, C, and D occur more frequently in younger than older people because of their propensity to engage in high-risk sexual behaviors and injection drug use. An estimated 3 million U.S. adolescents, for instance, are exposed to STDs each year, and HIV/AIDS is the sixth leading cause of death among 15 to 24 year olds in the United States (Division of Sexually Transmitted Diseases Prevention, 1998).

The presence of other physical health conditions may also influence one's propensity to develop certain communicable diseases. For example, HIV infection increases one's risk of a variety of opportunistic infections. *Opportunistic infections (OIs)* are diseases caused by organisms that either do not usually cause illness in humans or that usually cause only mild disease. For example, HIV infection increases the incidence of tuberculosis as well as the rate of progression to active disease (Weis, Foresman, Cook, & Matty, 1999), and influenza mortality is 10 times higher in HIV-infected individuals than in the general population (Bridges et al., 2001). Diabetes also increases influenza mortality approximately fourfold in people 25 to 64 years of age (Valdez, Narayan, Geiss, & Englegau, 1999).

Conversely, the presence of other STDs increases the potential for HIV infection. This is particularly true for STDs that cause lesions such as secondary syphilis and herpes simplex virus (HSV) infection, but also occurs with inflammatory STDs such as gonorrhea, chlamydia, and trichomonas infections (Fox et al., 2001; St. Louis et al., 1998). The presence of several of these diseases also increases one's risk of hepatitis B, particularly among men who have sex with men (MSM) (Remis et al., 2000).

Another biophysical consideration with respect to communicable diseases relates to the effects of the diseases themselves. Most childhood diseases are relatively mild and self-limiting. On occasion, diseases such as varicella, HiB, and mumps result in death as indicated in Table 28–1. The overall case fatality rate for untreated tetanus in unimmunized individuals, however, is 25%. The *case fatality rate* is the number of persons who have a disease who will die as a result of it. Hepatitis B, C, and D often result in chronic liver disease with 20% to 30% of HCV infections resulting in cirrhosis or liver cancer within two to three decades (Lorvick, Kral, Seal, Gee, & Edlin, 2001). HCV is responsible for 30% of liver transplants (Wong, McQuillan, McHutchinson, & Poynard, 2000). Persons with hepatitis B are also at high risk of cirrhosis and liver cancer (Yusuf et al., 1999), and in those with HDV super-infection, 70% to 80% will develop chronic liver disease compared to only 15% to 30% for those with HBV alone (National Center for Infectious Diseases, 2000d).

Psychological Considerations

Psychological considerations may play a part in the development of some communicable diseases. For example, stress has been shown to contribute to the development of active tuberculosis in persons with prior infection. Similarly, psychological factors may lead to risk-taking behaviors such as unprotected sexual activity or injection drug use that increase the risk of STDs, HIV infection, and hepatitis B, C, and D. For example, HIV infection was found to be eight times more prevalent among subjects with severe mental illness than in the general population. Prevalence rates for HBV infection were five times those of the general population, and HCV prevalence was 11 times higher. These results were prob-

ably a function of a high incidence of substance abuse comorbidity in the mentally ill population (Rosenberg et al., 2001).

Communicable diseases may also have psychological consequences for those infected. This is particularly true for conditions that have long-term consequences (e.g., HSV infection, HIV infection, or chronic hepatitis C) or require changes in lifestyle and behavior. In addition, clients with HIV/AIDS may develop dementia that alters behaviors and makes them difficult to care for. Depression may also be a significant consequence of stigmatizing diseases such as HIV infection or tuberculosis in some cultural groups.

Physical Environmental Considerations

Physical environmental factors play a part in the development of diseases spread by airborne transmission and those transmitted by fecal–oral means. Overcrowding contributes to the incidence of such diseases as measles, mumps, rubella, polio, HiB, diphtheria, pertussis, and varicella. Crowded living conditions also enhance the spread of tuberculosis and influenza. Wind factors are an element of the physical environment that would influence the spread of aerosolized pathogens in the event of a terrorist attack.

Sanitation and disposal of both human and animal feces are other factors in the physical environmental dimension that affect the development of communicable diseases, particularly hepatitis A, tetanus, and polio. The organism causing tetanus is found on a variety of surfaces and is more common in areas where there is animal excrement. In addition, home delivery and poor hygiene on the part of untrained midwives in developing countries and some parts of the United States contribute to the development of tetanus in neonates and, occasionally, in postpartum women.

In developing countries, poor environmental sanitation contributes to the incidence of diseases such as hepatitis A and E and poliomyelitis. Sanitation is a less likely factor in the development of these diseases in the United States; however, contaminated food and water supplies have been implicated in several disease outbreaks related to *Escherichia coli*, hepatitis A, botulism, and other enteric pathogens.

Sociocultural Considerations

A variety of social and cultural factors influence the development and course of communicable diseases. For example, congregating with large groups of people indoors during the winter facilitates the spread of airborne diseases, while poverty and poor nutrition increase susceptibility to a variety of diseases, particularly tuberculosis. Congregate living in institutional settings also contributes to the spread of disease. For example, TB outbreaks frequently occur in correctional settings, particularly among HIV-infected inmates (Division of Tuberculosis Elimination, 2000a). College campuses and military installations experience frequent outbreaks of measles among young adults in close quarters who are not immunized or whose immunity levels have declined over time.

Poverty and unemployment, with consequent loss of health insurance, are social factors that may limit the ability of parents to have their children immunized or to provide prompt medical care when illness does occur, resulting in more serious consequences of disease. Pregnant women with low incomes might not receive prenatal care, thus denying them the opportunity to obtain screening and counseling for congenital rubella syndrome, syphilis, HIV infection, and other diseases transmitted from mother to baby.

Language barriers and lower education levels among some ethnic and socioeconomic groups may impede awareness of the need for immunization or other preventive measures for communicable diseases. In addition, the beliefs of some religious sects prohibit immunizations, thus increasing the size of the susceptible population among members of these sects and the community at large. Because of reduced herd immunity (see Chapter 10 for a discussion of herd immunity), the presence of these unimmunized individuals increases the potential for the spread of disease throughout the community.

Occupational factors are another part of the sociocultural dimension that contribute to communicable diseases. Health care workers and "first responders" (e.g., emergency personnel) are at increased risk for blood-borne diseases, and health care workers are frequently exposed to a variety of other communicable diseases. Hepatitis B, for example, causes 100 to 200 deaths in health care personnel each year, and the risk of infection after percutaneous exposure to hepatitis C in health care workers is 1% to 2% (Scharbaugh, 1999), more than three times the risk of HIV in this group (0.3%) (Chiarello et al., 1998). Both employees and children are at risk for hepatitis A when outbreaks occur in child care settings, but risk for hepatitis A infection in health care workers is minimal (Bell et al., 1999). Certain occupations may contribute to the spread of disease as well as increased potential for exposure. For example, food service personnel may spread hepatitis A, and health care workers may expose clients to a number of communicable diseases.

Culture is another aspect of the sociocultural dimension that influences exposure to communicable diseases and attitudes to people who have them. For example, TB has social meaning and significant stigma in many cultures, and people may be reluctant to notify contacts of their exposure to disease for fear of being stigmatized (Poss, 1998). HIV infection and risk behaviors for infection also carry social stigma. For example, nearly one fifth of people in one U.S. survey believed that people who became infected through sexual intercourse or drug use "deserved what they got" (Division of HIV/AIDS Prevention—Intervention, Research, and Support, 2000). Such attitudes have often led to discrimination and victimization of people with stigmatizing diseases. For instance, 20.5% of women, 11.5% of men who have sex with men, and 7.5% of heterosexual men with HIV infec-

tion report being assaulted at least once by an intimate partner, with half the assaults because of their diagnosis (Zierler et al., 2000). Similarly, less tolerant attitudes toward certain sexual behaviors (e.g., homosexuality) in the United States has hampered the development of policies designed to prevent the spread of disease (Michael et al., 1998). Lack of status for women in some cultural groups and dependence on marriage or prostitution for one's livelihood has also made it difficult for women to negotiate condom use or insist on safe sexual activity (Susser & Stein, 2000; UNAIDS, 2000).

Social norms that contribute to high-risk behaviors also foster the spread of some communicable diseases. For example, relaxed sexual mores have led to greater sexual promiscuity and increased risk of exposure to HIV infection, STDs, and some forms of hepatitis. Similarly, a social environment in which it is relatively easy to obtain drugs for injection drug use promotes infection with HIV, syphilis, and hepatitis B, C, and D.

Other social factors that can increase the incidence of childhood diseases include homelessness and other forms of social upheaval and media communications. The fatigue, malnutrition, exposure to cold and crowding, and general debilitation associated with homelessness have contributed to increased pertussis, influenza, and other communicable diseases in homeless populations.

Immigration is another social factor that influences communicable diseases. From 1994 to 1998, 4.9 million immigrants entered the United States legally; another 2.7 million undocumented immigrants arrived as well, primarily from Latin America. Immigrants, especially refugees fleeing their home country, are often infected with a variety of communicable diseases. For example, in 1999, 43% of U.S. cases of TB occurred among foreign-born persons (Lobato, Cegielski, & the Tuberculosis Along the U.S.–Mexico Border Work Group, 2001). Because of the potential for rapid international spread of communicable

CRITICAL THINKING IN RESEARCH

Lobato et al. (2001) have noted the need for international cross-border research between the United States and Mexico to reduce the spread of tuberculosis across the border.

- What potential research questions might be appropriate?
- How would you design a study to answer one or more of the questions you have generated? What type of research methodology would be appropriate to the study? Why?
- How would you select your sample?
- What data would you collect? How would you go about collecting it?

diseases, there is a need to develop cooperative international control programs, particularly between countries that share borders such as Mexico and the United States.

Large population movements may result in sanitation problems or tax the capabilities of local health services to provide immunizations or diagnostic and treatment services. This is particularly true of large influxes of refugee populations in times of war or civil strife. Similarly, breakdown of the social order, as occurred with the disintegration of the former Soviet Union, may disrupt provision of health care services or abilities to procure vaccines. Finally, media reports of adverse reactions to immunization have led some parents to put off immunizing their children, while media attention to the effectiveness of HIV therapy has reduced adherence to safe sexual practices in some segments of the population. Media presentations of sexual activity as desirable behavior have also contributed to the incidence of STDs. Portrayals of popular heroes and heroines as "sexy" and sexually active have fostered imitative behavior, particularly among adolescents.

Political unrest that leads to bioterrorism is another possible factor in the development of communicable diseases. As indicated in Chapter 3, CDC has designated three categories of biological agents with differing degrees of potential use in biological terrorist activities. Category A organisms are those that would most easily lend themselves to intentional dissemination and include anthrax, smallpox, plague, botulism, tularemia, Ebola and Marburg hemorrhagic fevers, and diseases caused by arenaviruses (e.g., Lassa fever). Category B organisms would be slightly less easily disseminated, and category C pathogens have potential for development as biological weapons. (See Chapter 3 and Appendix B for more information about these diseases.)

In addition to social factors that contribute to disease, communicable diseases may have social effects. For example, congenital rubella syndrome and congenital syphilis lead to long-term consequences in newborns that have extensive costs for society. Similarly, treatment of persons with chronic hepatitis or HIV infection pose a costly burden for society, and care of children orphaned by HIV disease in their parents poses another social dilemma (Rosenfield, 2001). On the other hand, social conditions may have positive effects on the incidence and prevalence of communicable diseases. For instance, higher taxes on alcohol and increasing age for legal use of alcohol have been associated with lower incidence of gonorrhea. Alcohol lowers inhibitions to risky sexual behaviors, so control of alcohol use can minimize such behaviors (Division of Sexually Transmitted Diseases Prevention, 2000).

Behavioral Considerations

The major behavioral dimension factors that influence the development of communicable disease are related to diet, sexual activity, and drug use. Malnutrition makes people more susceptible to a number of diseases, particu-

larly TB and childhood diseases in unimmunized populations. Malnutrition may also contribute to more severe disease and a greater chance of complications.

Sexual activity obviously increases the risk of STDs, but hepatitis B and D are also spread by sexual activity (McQuillan et al., 1999). The role of sexual intercourse in the transmission of hepatitis C is not yet clear (National Institute of Diabetes and Digestive and Kidney Diseases, 1999), although increased prevalence is associated with sex for money to support drug use (Diaz et al., 2001).

Certain sexual behaviors increase one's risk of disease over and above just engaging in sexual intercourse. For instance, multiple sexual partners and unprotected intercourse increase exposure to disease (UNAIDS, 2000). In the 1997 Behavioral Risk Factor Surveillance Survey (BRFSS), the median prevalence of multiple sexual partners in participating states was 11%, and a median of 65% of those reporting multiple partners failed to use a condom during their last sexual encounter (Division of HIV/AIDS Prevention—Surveillance and Epidemiology, 2001). Fortunately, sexual activity among adolescents has decreased somewhat in the last few years. For example, from 1991 to 1997, the mean prevalence of sexual activity among high school seniors declined by 7% to 14% in several major U.S. cities (Division of HIV/AIDS Prevention—Intervention, Research, and Support, 1999), and condom use by sexually active adolescents increased by 23% (Division of Sexually Transmitted Diseases Prevention, 1998).

Men who have sex with men (MSM) frequently engage in either receptive or insertive anal sex without the use of a condom, increasing their potential for HIV infection and infection with HBV, HCV, and HDV. Early in the HIV epidemic, many MSM adopted safer sexual practices, but more recent data indicate a return to unprotected anal intercourse (Wolitski, Valdiserri, Denning, & Levine, 2001). Research with male-to-female (MTF) transgender persons also indicates a high incidence of multiple risk behaviors (Clements-Nolle, Marx, Guzman, & Katz, 2001). Some of the reasons for this return to high-risk behaviors include optimism regarding available treatment for HIV, the potential for postexposure treatment, and the possibility of a vaccine to prevent HIV infection (Wolitski et al., 2001). In addition, many MSM are experiencing what has been termed "fatigue" with messages about safe sexual practices to the point where they are often ignored (Fox et al., 2001). Because of the resulting changes in sexual behavior, there is an increasing incidence of gonorrhea and syphilis among MSM (Williams et al., 1999; Wolitski et al., 2001).

Drug use is another behavioral factor that influences the incidence of several communicable diseases. Several STDs are common among crack cocaine and multidrug users. For instance, in one study, 43% of multidrug users were found to be infected with trichomonas, 6% with syphilis, 2.3% with chlamydia, and 1.6% with gonorrhea (Bachmann et al., 2000). HCV prevalence is as high as 90% among injection drug users in some cities (Diaz et al., 2001), and HCV infection has been associated with the sharing of drug apparatus (e.g., cookers and filters) as well as with needle sharing (Hagan et al., 2001). Drug use also increases one's risk of hepatitis B, and both injection and noninjection drug use have been implicated in transmission of hepatitis A (Bell et al., 1999). Nearly one fifth of injection drug users (IDUs) and crack cocaine users in one study had evidence of tuberculosis infection (Malotte, Rhodes, & Mais, 1998). Finally, the incidence of tetanus is increasing among IDUs. From 1995 to 1997, for example, the rate of tetanus infection in this group increased threefold over that in 1991–1994 (Bardenheier et al., 1998). Injection of Mexican black tar heroin has also been associated with an increased risk of wound botulism (California Department of Health Services, 1998). Drug abuse, particularly opiate use, may also result in anergy, reducing the validity of tuberculin tests as a screening tool in this high-risk population. *Anergy* is an inability to react to antigens commonly used in tuberculosis skin testing due to suppression of cellular immunity. Anergy also occurs in the presence of HIV infection, making it more difficult to diagnose TB in HIV-infected individuals.

Smoking, as a behavioral risk factor, also plays a small part in the development of communicable diseases. For example, unimmunized children who live with smokers are more likely to develop *Haemophilus influenzae* type b infection than are other children (Jafari et al., 1999).

assessment tips assessment tips assessment tips

ASSESSING RISK FOR COMMUNICABLE DISEASES

Biophysical Considerations

- What age groups are most likely to develop the disease? Are there differences in disease effects among age groups?
- Are there racial or gender differences in disease incidence?
- What physiologic conditions, if any, increase the risk of disease?
- What are the signs and symptoms of the disease?
- What are the physiologic effects of the disease? What is the effect of the disease in pregnancy?
- What is the mode of disease transmission? What are the physiologic portals of entry and exit?

Psychological Considerations

- Does exposure to stress increase risk of the disease?
- Do psychological factors play a part in the risk of exposure to disease?
- Does the disease have potential psychological consequences (e.g., suicide risk)?

Physical Environmental Considerations

- What effect, if any, do crowded living conditions have on the incidence of the disease?
- Can the disease be transmitted to humans by animals or insects?
- Is the disease spread by contaminated food or water?

Sociocultural Considerations

- Does society condone behaviors that increase the risk of disease (e.g., sexual activity)?
- Does social interaction increase the risk of the spread of disease?
- What are societal attitudes to the disease? Do they hamper control efforts? Is there social stigma attached to having the disease?

- Do occupational factors influence the incidence of the disease?
- Does socioeconomic status affect risk for the disease? Consequences of the disease?
- What effect, if any, do cultural beliefs and behaviors have on incidence of the disease?
- Does the disease have potential as a biological weapon?

Behavioral Considerations

- Does diet play a part in the incidence of the disease (e.g., malnutrition as a risk factor for TB)? Does nutritional status influence the consequences of the disease?
- Does alcohol or drug use contribute to the incidence of the disease?
- Does sexual activity increase the risk of the disease? Do specific sexual behaviors increase the risk of the disease?

Health System Considerations

- What primary preventive measures are available for the disease? Are they widely used?
- To what extent do health care providers educate the public on primary prevention of the disease?
- Is there a vaccine available for the disease?
- Is there a screening test for the disease? If so, are persons at risk for the disease screened?
- How is the disease diagnosed?
- Is there an effective treatment for the disease? Are diagnostic and treatment services for the disease available and accessible to infected persons?
- What are the attitudes of health care providers to persons with the disease?

Health System Considerations

Factors related to the health care system may also influence the development and course of communicable diseases. For example, failure of many providers to give varicella vaccine to children increases the risk of disease and promotes the spread of varicella epidemics. In one study, for instance, only 42% of physicians routinely offered varicella vaccine to susceptible clients in spite of the fact that routine immunization has been recommended by the American Academy of Pediatrics and the American Academy of Family Physicians (Ehresmann, Mills, Loewenson, & Moore, 2000). Charging fees for immunizations may also limit the ability of people in lower socioeconomic groups to become adequately immunized. Similarly, missed opportunities for immunizations and failure to give immunizations because of mythical contraindications also increase the risk of communicable diseases.

Health care providers may also fail to provide screening or health education related to communicable diseases. For example, in a study of Canadian general practitioners and obstetricians, only half routinely asked sexually active clients about condom use or number of sexual partners (Haley, Maheux, Rivard, & Gervais, 1999). Similarly, pregnant women with private insurance were less likely than those with public insurance to be tested for HIV infection, perhaps in the belief that they were less likely to be at risk due to higher economic status (Royce et al., 2001).

When health care providers do educate clients, however, their efforts appear to be effective. For example, in one study of voluntary HIV screening, 28% of men and 18% of women reported being tested on the recommendation of their health care provider or a friend. Similarly, 90% of people with a recent diagnosis of HIV infection reported a change in their sexual behaviors, presumably based on counseling by providers (Division of HIV/AIDS Prevention—Surveillance and Epidemiology, 2000).

Health care providers may also fail to recognize atypical forms of childhood illnesses and treat them effectively. For example, because of its relative infrequency in modern society, providers may lack clinical experience with pertussis or fail to consider it as a possible diagnosis. Similarly, they may fail to consider a diagnosis of HIV in a client with no known risk factors.

Health system factors may also contribute more actively to communicable diseases and their effects. For example, nosocomial infection in hospitals and physicians' offices is a significant factor in the spread of varicella. Contaminated equipment has also been implicated in the spread of bloodborne infections, and transfusion was a source of HIV infection and infection with hepatitis B, C, and D prior to screening of blood donors. Similarly, medical treatment for conditions such as asthma and autoimmune diseases that require immunosuppressive therapy place individuals at greater risk for complications of influenza. In addition, inappropriate prescription of antimicrobials by health care providers has led to the development of antibiotic-resistant strains of several microorganisms.

Provider attitudes to persons with stigmatizing diseases may also influence care. For example, 19% of Canadian dentists in one study were unwilling to treat persons infected with HIV. The reasons given for refusing care were lack of a belief in an ethical responsibility to provide care and fear of cross infection to other clients (McCarthy, Koval, & MacDonald, 1999). Potential questions for exploring health system factors and the influence of factors in the other dimensions of health in the development of communicable diseases are presented on page 667. A communicable disease risk inventory for assessing the risk of communicable diseases in population groups is available on the companion Web site for this book.   ⊛

DIAGNOSTIC REASONING AND CONTROL OF COMMUNICABLE DISEASES

The community health nurse may derive a variety of nursing diagnoses related to communicable diseases. These diagnoses may reflect the health needs of individuals, families, or population groups. Diagnoses may also reflect potential for infection or the presence of active disease. For example, the nurse working with a family may diagnose "inadequate immunization status due to poor knowledge of children's immunization needs." A nursing diagnosis related to an individual client is "potential for infection with tetanus due to increased risk of occupational injury," or "failure to obtain routine immunizations due to lack of transportation." A diagnosis related to the presence of active disease might be "probable tuberculosis as evidenced by cough, weight loss, and night sweats and recent travel to an endemic area."

Nursing diagnoses related to communicable diseases may also be derived for population groups. Diagnoses at the community level may reflect the current incidence of disease or the potential for spread of infection. Examples of such diagnoses are "increased incidence of HCV due to injection drug use" and "potential for increased transmission of HIV infection due to widespread use of unsafe sexual practices among MSM."

Nursing diagnoses may also reflect the presence of risk factors that affect the development of communicable diseases in individuals or population groups. For example, the nurse may diagnose an "increased risk of hepatitis A due to shellfish contamination in local waters" or "increased risk of tuberculosis transmission from refugees from endemic areas."

PLANNING AND IMPLEMENTING CARE RELATED TO COMMUNICABLE DISEASES

Community health nursing interventions related to communicable diseases may reflect primary, secondary, or tertiary levels of prevention.

Primary Prevention

Primary prevention of communicable diseases is directed toward preventing the occurrence of disease. Major emphases in preventing communicable diseases include immunization, chemoprophylaxis, and other preventive measures specific to particular communicable diseases.

Immunization

Immunization is the most effective method of preventing the occurrence of communicable diseases. The concept of immunization originated with William Jenner, and the first smallpox vaccine was developed in 1796, but its use did not become widespread for more than 100 years. Similarly, four other vaccines (rabies, cholera, typhoid, and plague) were developed between 1885 and 1897 but were not widely used. Since 1900, vaccines for 21 other diseases have been developed or licensed for use in the United States (National Immunization Program, 1999).

Widespread use of vaccines is a twentieth century phenomenon, but barriers still exist to the use of immunization services. Some of these barriers include lack of access to services (e.g., due to cost), lack of knowledge regarding the need for immunization, parental concerns regarding the discomfort associated with administration of some vaccines (e.g., localized swelling with DTaP), and

Immunization is one approach to preventing some communicable diseases.

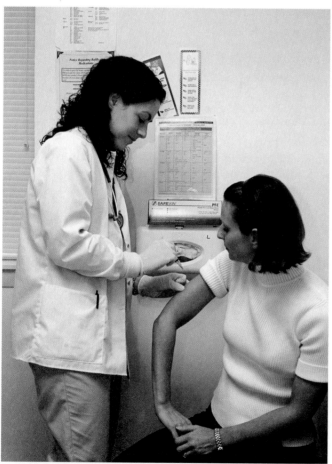

health system limitations such as differences in school entry requirements across jurisdictions, poor enforcement of immunization requirements, and poor data management (Horner & Murphy, 1999). Other system barriers are the failure of providers to encourage immunizations other than those required for school entry and missed opportunities for immunization in the course of providing other services.

Several of the 2010 national health objectives are related to increasing immunization coverage for a variety of communicable diseases (USDHHS, 2000b). Some of these objectives with baseline data and 2010 targets are summarized on page 670. Additional objectives may be viewed on the Healthy People 2010 Web site, which can be accessed through a link provided on the companion Web site for this book. The problem of data management has also been addressed in the objectives with the recommendation to develop population-based immunization registries to consolidate records and generate reminders of subsequent immunization needs. As of 2000, however, only half of jurisdictions that were awarded federal grants for registry development had registries in place, and only 21% of U.S. children under 6 years of age were included in a population-based registry (National Immunization Program, 2001), a decline from the 1998 baseline figure of 32% and far short of the 95% target for 2010.

The extent of vaccination coverage varies among specific communicable diseases. In 1998 and 1999, universally recommended vaccine coverage for children 19 to 35 months of age ranged from 90% for varicella and poliomyelitis to 91.5% for measles, mumps, and rubella to 93.5% for *Haemophilus influenzae* to 95.9% for diphtheria, tetanus, and pertussis (CDC, 1998b; National Immuniza-tion Program, 2000b). Recent changes were made to recommendations for poliomyelitis immunization due to the incidence of vaccine-related disease with oral polio vaccine (OPV). Starting in 2000, all four doses of polio vaccine for U.S. children were to be given with inactivated polio vaccine (IPV), with OPV used only for mass

CULTURAL CONSIDERATIONS

You are an international community health nurse who has been hired to develop and implement a national immunization campaign in India. You know from your study of other cultures that many Hindus, a primary cultural group in India, believe that immunization will anger the goddess Devi, who is responsible for bringing illness and may actually bring about disease rather than preventing it. You are also aware that many parents have discontinued vaccine series because of local inflammation at the injection site. How will you design your immunization campaign to account for these factors?

HEALTHY PEOPLE 2010

GOALS FOR THE POPULATION

Objective		Base	Target
13-1	Reduce new AIDS cases among adolescents and adults (per 100,000 population over age 13)	19.5	1
13-6	Increase the proportion of sexually active persons who use condoms	23%	50%
13-11	Increase the proportion of adults with TB tested for HIV	55%	85%
13-13c	Increase the proportion of HIV-infected persons who receive HAART	54%	95%
13-14	Reduce HIV deaths (per 100,000 population)	4.9	0.8
14-1	Reduce cases of vaccine preventable diseases		
	a. congenital rubella syndrome	7	0
	b. diphtheria	1	0
	c. *Haemophilus influenzae* type b	253	0
	d. hepatitis B	945	9
	e. measles	74	0
	f. mumps	666	0
	g. pertussis (children under 7 years of age)	3,417	2,000
	h. wild virus poliomyelitis	0	0
	i. rubella	364	0
	j. tetanus (persons under 35 years of age)	14	0
	k. varicella	4 mil	400,000
14-6	Reduce new cases of hepatitis A (per 100,000 population)	11.3	4.5
14-8	Reduce new cases of hepatitis C (per 100,000 population)	2.4	1
14-11	Reduce new cases of tuberculosis (per 100,000 population)	6.8	1
14-12	Increase the proportion of people with TB who complete treatment within 12 months	74%	90%
14-13	Increase the proportion of TB contacts and high-risk persons with TB infection who complete prophylactic treatment	62.2%	85%
14-22	Increase the proportion of vaccination coverage among children 19 to 35 months of age for universally recommended vaccines	43%–93%	90%
14-26	Increase the proportion of children in population-based immunization registries	32%	95%
14-28	Increase hepatitis B vaccine coverage in		
	a. hemodialysis patients	35%	90%
	b. men who have sex with men	9%	60%
	c. occupationally exposed workers	71%	98%
14-29	Increase the proportion of adults over 65 years of age vaccinated against		
	a. influenza (annually)	63%	90%
	b. pneumococcal disease (in life time)	43%	90%

Source: U.S. Department of Health and Human Services. (2000b). *Healthy people 2010* (Conference edition, in two volumes). Washington, DC: Author.

immunization campaigns in response to disease outbreaks, children traveling to polio-endemic areas within four weeks of immunization, and children whose parents refuse the recommended number of doses of injectable IPV (but only for the third and fourth doses) (CDC, 1999b). OPV will also continue to be used in endemic areas of the world. IPV is recommended for adults traveling to endemic areas, laboratory workers handling specimens potentially containing poliovirus, those providing care to persons with polio, and unvaccinated adults whose children receive OPV (Prevots, Burr, Sutter, & Murphy, 2000).

Persons younger than 29 years of age in the United States are unlikely to have been immunized against smallpox because vaccination was discontinued in 1972. In the event of a terrorist attack using variola virus, which causes smallpox, this age group would receive priority for use of limited vaccine supplies. It is likely that previously immunized persons, while probably not completely safe, would still have significant levels of immunity. In fact, in one smallpox outbreak in 1902–1903, 93% of people vaccinated as long as 50 years earlier were protected (Cohen, 2001).

Adult vaccine coverage for many of these diseases, however, lags behind child coverage. For example, many adults have not had recent tetanus and diphtheria boosters, and many older adults have never been immunized for tetanus and are at high risk for disease. Unimmunized women of childbearing age or those with waning tetanus immunity increase the risk of congenital rubella syndrome or neonatal tetanus in their infants. Similarly, many adults and adolescents are at risk for varicella and should be immunized.

Vaccines are also available for hepatitis A and B, tuberculosis, and influenza, although many people at risk for these diseases are not adequately immunized. Hepatitis A vaccine is recommended for all children in areas with incidence rates twice the national rate (California Department of Health Services, 1999), for travelers to endemic areas, those with clotting factor disorders or chronic liver disease, and those who encounter occupational risk for infection (e.g., handlers of primates) (Bell et al., 1999). HAV vaccine is also recommended for men who have sex with men. Immunization has been found to be highly effective, and intensive campaigns among persons at risk have been shown to decrease HAV incidence by 16% within 5 months (Division of Viral and Rickettsial Diseases, 1998).

Hepatitis B immunization is recommended for all infants and persons at risk (National Center for Infectious Diseases, 2000b). Research has indicated that infants who receive the first dose of HBV vaccine at birth are more likely to complete the series than those who receive their first dose at 1 to 2 months of age (Yusuf, Daniels, Smith, Coronado, & Rodewald, 2000), and vaccine coverage is higher in states that require HBV immunization for school entry (Yusuf et al., 1999). In 1999, 88% of U.S. children aged 19 to 35 months had received the three-dose series of HBV vaccine (National Immunization Program, 2000b). Unimmunized adolescents, who are at high risk for HBV infection from both sexual and drug use behaviors, should receive two doses of vaccine (CDC, 2000a). HBV vaccine is also recommended for MSM, but a study of vaccine coverage in seven U.S. cities indicated that only about 9% of persons in this group had been immunized (McKellar et al., 2001).

Hepatitis vaccine has been shown to be effective in preventing disease and cost-effective as well. For example, one campaign to immunize sixth graders in British Columbia estimated a net savings of $75 per child immunized. Immunization campaigns were not, however, found to be cost-effective in areas with disease incidence less than 3 cases per 100,000 population (Krahn, Guasparini, Sherman, & Detsky, 1998).

Bacille Calmette–Guerin (BCG) vaccine is used for TB prevention in some parts of the world, but has not been found to be particularly effective. In fact, a recent study of vaccine effectiveness found no overall effect in decreasing TB incidence (O'Brien, 1998). In addition, use of BCG vaccine causes tuberculin skin tests to become reactive and invalidates skin tests as a screening measure for tuberculosis. New vaccines for TB are being developed, and several are currently being tested in animals, so a more effective vaccine may be available in the future.

Influenza vaccine has been shown to be highly effective in preventing disease or mitigating its severity when the vaccine is developed for strains of virus prevalent in a given year. In fact, immunization is 70% to 90% effective among healthy people under 65 years of age. Influenza vaccine is also cost-effective, with an estimated average savings of $13.66 per year per person immunized. Influenza vaccine must be received annually and is recommended for all persons over 65 years of age, people at increased risk for complications due to chronic illness, pregnant women who will be in the second or third trimester of pregnancy during influenza season, people in institutional settings, and people who are at high risk of transmitting the disease to persons in high-risk groups (e.g., health care workers, home care personnel, institutional employees, etc.) (Bridges et al., 2001). Research has indicated that persons with diabetes should be particularly targeted for both influenza and pneumonia vaccines (Valdez et al., 1999).

At present, there are no vaccines for most STDs; for hepatitis C, D, or E; or for HIV infection. Because hepatitis D can only occur in the presence of HBV infection, HBV immunization is an effective prevention measure. There is also some potential for development of a vaccine for HIV infection, although development is complicated by the ease with which the virus mutates and the fact that it is not inherently containable by the human immune system as other vaccine-preventable diseases are. There has been some progress made, however, on vaccines that attack immature HIV cells (Baltimore, 1999). Like HIV, development of a vaccine for HCV infection is hampered by rapid mutation of the virus (Des Jarlais & Schuchat, 2001).

Community health nurses educate the public regarding the need for immunizations. They are also frequently involved in planning, implementing, and evaluating immunization campaigns and in giving immunizations to susceptible individuals. Community health nurses may also advocate for access to immunization services for all segments of the population and may be involved in the enactment and enforcement of immunization policies designed to protect the general public. For example, community health nurses might advocate requirements that college entrants provide evidence of measles immunity or that varicella immunization be required for preschool or elementary school entry.

Chemoprophylaxis and Contact Notification

Another primary preventive measure for communicable diseases is chemoprophylaxis. *Chemoprophylaxis* is the use of medications to prevent the onset of disease in exposed individuals. When individuals are prevented from developing symptomatic disease, they are usually also prevented from spreading the disease to others.

Chemoprophylaxis usually occurs in the context of contact notification. *Contact notification* is the process of identifying persons who have been exposed to a communicable disease, informing them of exposure, testing them for the particular disease, and offering chemoprophylatic treatment to prevent them from becoming symptomatic and exposing others. Contact notification can be carried out in one of two ways: client referral and provider referral. In client referral, individuals who are known to have a communicable disease notify their contacts themselves and refer them for testing and possible treatment. In provider referral, designated health care personnel solicit names of contacts from infected persons and notify the contacts of potential exposure. When given the option, many people with communicable diseases select provider referral as the preferred mechanism of contact notification. In other instances, they may prefer to notify their contacts themselves.

Community health nurses are frequently involved in the provider referral approach to contact notification. The process used is systematic and begins with an interview of the client with a communicable disease. In this interview, the community health nurse explains the need for notification, testing, and possible treatment of contacts, and then elicits names, addresses, and other information that will allow contacts to be located and informed of their exposure. Depending on how the notification system is organized, this same nurse may follow up on contacts whose names were elicited or communicate this information to another health care provider (frequently another community health nurse) who will get in touch with the individuals named. The identity of the client with the communicable disease from whom the names were elicited is not included in the information communicated.

Nurses involved in contact follow-up may make home visits or approach contacts at work or any other place where they can be located. When they approach contacts, nurses should speak to them in a setting that ensures privacy and inform them that they have been exposed to a communicable disease. Nurses frequently need to exercise creativity to prevent others from knowing why the person is being contacted by a nurse.

The nurse who approaches the contact never divulges information about the source of the exposure, but explains that the person has potentially been exposed to a communicable disease. In addition to notifying the contact regarding the exposure, the nurse educates the client about the potential for developing the disease and for spreading it to others and refers the client for testing and treatment for the condition as needed.

☾ THINK ABOUT IT

How would you respond if you were notified that you had been exposed to someone with TB? HIV? Would your response differ depending on how the contact occurred? If so, why? If you had been exposed through sexual contact, would you prefer to be notified by the person who exposed you or by health care personnel? Why?

The purpose of contact notification is to identify persons who may be infected or in need of chemoprophylaxis. Chemoprophylaxis is available for tuberculosis, gonorrhea, syphilis, hepatitis A and B, measles, *Haemophilus influenzae* type B (HiB) infection, diphtheria, and tetanus. Approaches to chemoprophylaxis for communicable diseases include booster vaccination or immediate immunization for unimmunized contacts, immune globulins, antibiotics or antiviral medications, and provision of antitoxins.

Immediate postexposure immunization should be given to people exposed to pertussis, and may be given after exposure to polio, mumps, or rubella, although its efficacy in these three diseases is unknown. Booster immunizations should be given to previously immunized persons exposed to diphtheria, tetanus, and pertussis, and in the case of smallpox exposure.

Immune globulin (IG) is an effective chemoprophylactic measure in measles, tetanus, and varicella, and following exposure to HAV or HBV infection. Hepatitis B IG may also be effective in preventing hepatitis D (National Center for Infectious Diseases, 2000d). Hepatitis A IG may be given prophylactically either prior to exposure (e.g., prior to travel to endemic areas) or postexposure (National Center for Infectious Diseases, 2000a). IG administration does not appear to affect development of diseases such as rubella, mumps (Chin, 2000), HCV infection (Alter et al., 1998), or HEV infection (National Center for Infectious Diseases, 2000e).

Antibiotics and antivirals are used to prevent disease after exposure to diphtheria, pertussis, HiB, TB, many STDs (e.g., gonorrhea, syphilis, and chlamydia), anthrax, and influenza. Contact notification and chemoprophylaxis can prevent the spread of TB as well (Kellner, 1999). TB prophylaxis should be given to all close contacts of persons with TB as well as persons with reactive tuberculin skin tests without evidence of active disease. Prophylaxis for TB is also recommended for persons with HIV infection (Division of Tuberculosis Elimination, 2000b).

Chemoprophylaxis with highly active antiretroviral agents has been shown to be effective in preventing vertical transmission of HIV infection from mother to infant

(Msellati et al., 1999) and in preventing some of the opportunistic infections that occur in people with AIDS (Jones et al., 1999), and may be effective in preventing HIV infection after exposure to a confirmed case (Chiarello et al., 1998). The CDC has developed specific guidelines for the prevention of common opportunistic infections in HIV-infected individuals (Kaplan, Masur, & Holmes, 1999).

Antiviral agents, such as amantadine, rimantadine, or oseltamivir, may be used in conjunction with influenza vaccine for prophylaxis. Use of these agents is recommended for persons immunized after the influenza season has started, for caretakers of persons at high risk for complications due to influenza, and in persons with diminished immune function (Bridges et al., 2001). Finally, tetanus antitoxin may be given as chemoprophylaxis for tetanus (see Chin, 2000, for information on agents used for chemoprophylaxis of specific diseases). Community health nurses are often involved in referring clients for chemoprophylaxis and may provide chemoprophylaxis themselves under protocols. For example, many community health nurses employed in official public health agencies administer IG to persons exposed to hepatitis A and B.

Other Primary Prevention Measures

Other primary prevention measures for communicable diseases may be directed toward the mode of transmission of specific diseases. Primary prevention for tetanus due to puncture wounds, for example, involves educating clients on the use of protective clothing to prevent injuries and the need for adequate cleansing of wounds with soap and water when injuries do occur. For STDs, refraining from sexual activity is the most effective means of preventing diseases. For those who are sexually active, however, use of condoms and refraining from unsafe sexual practices may limit exposure to disease. Use of spermicides may also provide some protection against STDs,

Condoms may help to prevent both sexually transmitted diseases and pregnancy. (Photo courtesy of Church & Dwight Co. Inc. 2001. Trojan-ENZ is a registered trademark of ARMKEL, LLC.)

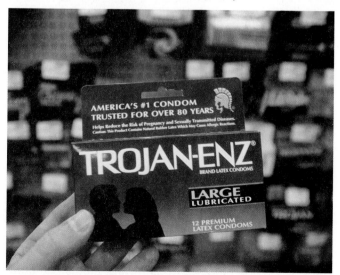

including HIV infection, although the full effect of spermicide use is not yet known (Wittkowski, Susser, & Dietz, 1998). Community health nurses can also educate clients who engage in oral–genital intercourse as a mode of contraception that they continue to be at risk for STD transmission.

Primary prevention for bloodborne diseases such as HIV/AIDS and hepatitis B, C, and D involves prevention of drug use or promotion of harm-reduction strategies such as needle exchanges and education on safer drug use procedures (Division of HIV/AIDS Prevention—Intervention, Research, and Support, 1998). Employment of such harm-reduction strategies in England and Wales, for example, appears to be decreasing the incidence of HCV infection (Hope et al., 2001). Infection among persons with potential for occupational exposure to bloodborne diseases can be prevented by means of universal precautions for the handling of blood and other bodily secretions and excretions. Unfortunately, many such persons fail to use universal precautions, increasing their risk of disease. For example, even though 73% of health care workers in one study reported using universal precautions at all times, only 58% always used gloves when handling blood or bloody equipment, and only 85% used them for cleaning up urine or feces (Knight & Bodsworth, 1998). Screening of blood and tissue donors for HIV and for hepatitis B, C, and D has virtually eliminated transmission of these diseases by means of transfusion (National Center for Infectious Diseases, 2000c). One additional strategy for preventing vertical transmission of HIV infection is delivery by cesarean section prior to rupture of membranes. In some studies, for example, delivery by cesarean section was found to decrease vertical transmission irrespective of whether or not the mother had been treated for HIV infection (Regional Perinatal Programs of California, 1999). In the case of anogenital herpes simplex, cesarean section is recommended for pregnant women who have active lesions present at the time of delivery to prevent transmission of HSV infection to the newborn (Chin, 2000).

For hepatitis A and E, control measures are aimed at improving sanitation, protecting food and water from contamination, and promoting adequate handwashing. Washing fruits and vegetables before eating, boiling contaminated water, and discouraging use of human waste as fertilizer may also serve to prevent both diseases in developing countries.

Prevention of crowding and promotion of adequate nutrition are control measures for conditions such as TB and influenza. Other primary prevention measures include the use of adequate ventilation and ultraviolet light in areas that increase the risk of TB transmission. For example, areas in which aerosol sputum specimens are collected provide an environment conducive to the spread of disease that can be modified using these measures. Providing appropriate facilities for isolating infectious clients in hospitals and other institutions also minimizes the risk of transmission to health care personnel.

Other measures that aid in the control of communicable diseases include legislation requiring screening for specific diseases in high-risk groups, mandatory reporting of cases of communicable disease with contact notification and follow-up, and regulation of potential vehicles of transmission such as insects. Community health nursing involvement in other control measures for communicable diseases generally lies in educating the public and individual clients regarding prevention and in identifying and helping to eliminate risk factors for exposure and disease. Primary prevention strategies for communicable diseases are summarized below.

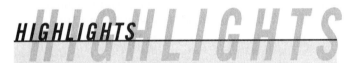

HIGHLIGHTS

Primary Prevention for Communicable Diseases

Immunization

Contact notification

- Client referral
- Provider referral

Chemoprophylaxis

- Immediate immunization or booster dose
- Immune globulins
- Antimicrobial medications
- Antitoxins

Other

- Adequate nutrition, rest, etc.
- Wound care
- Safe sexual practices
- Prevention of drug abuse or promotion of harm-reduction strategies
- Universal precautions
- Sanitation and hygiene (e.g., handwashing)
- Prevention of food and water contamination
- Prevention of crowding
- Ventilation and ultraviolet light
- Legislation
- Advocacy for preventive education and services

Secondary Prevention

Secondary prevention activities in relation to communicable diseases include screening, diagnosis, and treatment. These activities frequently rely on case finding activities by community health nurses. Because they serve large segments of the population who may not receive care from other health care providers, community health nurses are in a unique position to identify possible cases of communicable diseases. Once a person with a potential communicable disease has been identified, the community health nurse may make a referral for further diagnosis and treatment. In some cases, the nurse may be involved in diagnosing and treating communicable diseases on the basis of medically approved protocols.

Screening

Screening is presumptive identification of asymptomatic persons with disease. Screening may involve either selective or mass screening. *Selective screening* is directed toward persons exhibiting risk factors for a particular disease. *Mass screening* involves screening an entire population regardless of the level of risk among individuals (Friis & Sellers, 1999).

Screening is not generally done for communicable diseases that have a short incubation period such as measles, rubella, influenza, and so on. Screening tests are available, however, for diseases such as HIV/AIDS, hepatitis A and B, TB, and STDs such as gonorrhea, syphilis, chlamydia, and HSV infection.

Screening for HIV infection is recommended for all pregnant women and for other persons at risk for infection including injection drug users, men who have sex with men, and those with multiple sexual partners. Because of the close relationship between TB and HIV infection, persons with TB and their close contacts may also benefit from HIV screening (Division of Tuberculosis Elimination, 2000b). From 1987 to 1995, the proportion of the U.S. population screened for HIV infection increased from 16% to 40%, with higher rates of screening in high-risk populations (Anderson, Carey, & Taveras, 2000). Two concerns with respect to HIV screening are confidentiality and the length of time before results are known. MSM are particularly concerned about confidentiality issues because of the twofold potential for stigmatization related to homosexual behavior and to HIV infection (Division of HIV/AIDS Prevention—Surveillance and Epidemiology, 1999). Confidentiality concerns may deter people from being tested or encourage them to use anonymous testing. Anonymous testing, however, makes it impossible to notify persons with positive tests who do not return for their results. For this reason, screening tests that provide same-day results are preferred (UNAIDS, 2000).

Pregnant women and persons at risk should also be screened for STDs and HBV (CDC, 1998b; Corrarino, 1998). Emergency departments and correctional settings have been recommended as sites for STD screening because of the high incidence of STDs in these settings (Division of Sexually Transmitted Diseases Prevention, 1999b; Todd, Haase, & Stoner, 2001). Screening for TB should also be a routine procedure in correctional settings (Tulsky et al., 1998) and among injection drug users (Malotte et al., 1998). TB screening is cost-effective in high-risk groups, but not among those with low risk for infection (CDC, 2000b).

Drug users should be screened for HIV infection as well as hepatitis B and C. Routine screening for HCV is not warranted for health care personnel or first responders unless other risk factors are present. Screening should occur with exposure to HCV-infected blood, however (Division of Viral and Rickettsial Diseases, 2000). Another population that should be screened for HCV are recipients of transfusions prior to 1992 when blood donors began to be tested for HCV. Although attempts have been made to contact blood recipients who received blood from donors known to be infected with HCV, many people have not been located and may be unaware of their risk for disease (Buffington, Rowell, Hinman, Sharp, & Choi, 2001). (See Appendix B for information on screening for selected communicable diseases.)

Community health nurses may refer individuals at risk for disease to appropriate screening resources. Many community health nurses may also be involved in conducting screening examinations and tests and in counseling clients regarding test results and their implications.

⑥THINK ABOUT IT

Should mandatory HIV screening be required for all hospital admissions? For prisoners? Why or why not?

Diagnosis

Diagnosis of many communicable diseases relies on serologic evidence of disease markers or the actual presence of causative organisms. For example, diagnostic tests for syphilis and hepatitis A, B, C, and D rely on the presence of specific antibodies in the blood of infected persons. More sophisticated tests for syphilis, on the other hand, are based on demonstration of the presence of the actual causative organism in the bloodstream and are used when antibody-based tests are inconclusive. Similarly, tests for gonorrhea involve culture of urine or urethral, vaginal, anal, or pharyngeal specimens for growth of *Neisseria gonorrhoeae*, while diagnostic tests for chlamydial infection include culture of specimens for *Chlamydia trachomatis*. Diagnosis of many childhood diseases is based on physical signs and symptoms, with laboratory confirmation for some diseases (e.g., pertussis, diphtheria, tetanus, etc.). Information on specific diagnostic tests for selected communicable diseases is presented in Appendix B.

Community health nurses may refer suspected cases of communicable diseases for diagnostic confirmation. In addition, nurses may educate clients regarding the types of diagnostic procedures likely to be used. Community health nurses may also be involved in conducting some diagnostic tests for communicable diseases. For example, community health nurses in some agencies routinely draw blood for diagnostic tests for syphilis or collect urine samples for gonorrhea testing on the basis of medical protocols.

Treatment

Many communicable diseases are treated with antibiotics or antiviral medications, but some diseases such as varicella and uncomplicated measles are treated symptomatically. Treatment for selected communicable diseases commonly encountered by community health nurses is presented in Appendix B. Other sources of information include the *Report of the NIH Panel to Define Principles of Therapy of HIV Infection* (Feinberg & Kaplan, 1998) and the CDC's *Guidelines for Treatment of Sexually Transmitted Diseases* (CDC, 1998a).

Community health nurses may provide supportive care for clients with self-limiting diseases that have no specific treatment. Supportive care may include educating clients and families about measures to reduce fever or enhance comfort until the disease has run its course. For example, parents should be informed of the dangers in giving aspirin for fever in children. Other supportive measures may include encouraging a low-fat diet in hepatitis A to deal with nausea.

TB treatment, and to a lesser extent HIV therapy, rely on a process called directly observed therapy (DOT). In *directly observed therapy*, a nurse or other health care provider actually watches the client take the medication. DOT has been shown to increase treatment completion rates, particularly in areas with historically low rates of compliance with therapy (Bayer et al., 1998). A modified approach to DOT in which clients take a daily dose of TB medications on their own for four to eight weeks followed by twice weekly DOT has demonstrated 85% completion rates at a 40% reduction in costs (Desvarieux, Hyppolite, Johnson, & Pape, 2001).

Treatment of communicable diseases is complicated by noncompliance and by the development of drug-resistant microorganisms, which is fostered by noncompliance. Gonococcal organisms, for example, exhibit ongoing development of resistance to multiple antibiotics (Division of AIDS, STD, and TB Laboratory Research, 2000), and treatments such as alpha interferon for chronic HCV infection prove effective in only 10% to 40% of cases (National Center for Infectious Diseases, 2000c). HCV treatment also appears to be less effective in the presence of HIV infection (National Institute of Diabetes and Digestive and Kidney Diseases, 1999).

Community health nurses may provide treatment for some communicable disease under medical protocols, but are more likely to be involved in educating clients

ETHICAL AWARENESS

Current recommendations are to treat injection drug users with hepatitis C only after they have ceased using drugs for at least six months (Des Jarlais & Schuchat, 2001). Do you think this is appropriate? Why or why not?

about treatment and promoting compliance. The role of community health nurses in treating communicable diseases may also involve political activity and advocacy. For example, the nurse might be actively engaged in efforts to ensure access to health care for persons with AIDS or to change policies for providing treatment to drug users with chronic HCV infection. Emphases in secondary prevention of communicable diseases are summarized below.

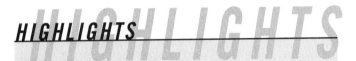

HIGHLIGHTS

Secondary Prevention for Communicable Diseases

Screening
- Case finding and referral of potential cases
- Provision of selective screening
- Provision of mass screening

Diagnosis
- Referral for diagnostic services
- Provision of diagnostic services
- Interpretation of diagnostic results

Treatment
- Provision of antimicrobial medications
- Education regarding treatment
- Promotion of compliance with treatment regimens
- Education for supportive care
  - Fever control
  - Comfort measures
  - Diet
  - Rest
- Advocacy for accessible diagnostic and treatment services

Tertiary Prevention

Tertiary prevention of communicable diseases may occur with individual clients or with population groups. At the individual level, emphasis is on preventing complications and long-term sequelae, monitoring treatment compliance and effects, monitoring treatment side effects and assisting clients to deal with them, and providing assistance in dealing with long-term consequences of some communicable diseases.

Community health nurses can educate clients to prevent complications of communicable diseases with their attendant long-term sequelae. For example, clients with influenza can be encouraged to rest and to refrain from resuming normal activities until they are recovered.

Similarly, parents can discourage scratching in children with varicella to prevent secondary infection in lesions and encourage clients with hepatitis to refrain from alcohol use to prevent further liver damage.

Community health nurses should also monitor clients with HIV infection for signs and symptoms of opportunistic infections and refer them for treatment when OIs are suspected. Nurses may also be involved in assisting clients with prophylactic regimens to prevent opportunistic infections. Clients with HIV infection may also experience a number of nutritional difficulties that may require nursing intervention. For example, weight loss and wasting may occur as a result of reduced food or calorie intake due to anorexia, nausea and vomiting, changes in taste or smell, fatigue, or painful oral or esophageal lesions. Weight loss, loss of muscle mass, and vitamin deficiencies may also result from malabsorption due to lactose or fat intolerance, gastrointestinal infection, malignancies, and so on. Finally, HIV-infected clients may experience metabolic alterations due to HIV, medications, and other circumstances (Keithley, Swanson, Murphy, & Levin, 2000). Community health nurses engaged in tertiary prevention would assist clients to overcome these nutritional deficiencies through nutritional counseling, promoting food and water safety, dealing with medication side effects, and suggesting complementary and alternative nutritional therapies such as the use of nutritional supplements.

Community health nurses also monitor communicable disease treatment compliance and treatment effects, particularly in diseases such as tuberculosis and HIV infection that require long-term therapy. Treatment of chronic hepatitis B, C, or D may also involve prolonged use of medications. In addition, community health nurses monitor the occurrence of adverse effects of treatment. For example, antituberculin drugs may result in hepatitis or visual disturbances, and the nurse should be alert to signs and symptoms of adverse effects.

Similarly, long-term highly active antiretroviral therapy (HAART) has a variety of complications that are only now beginning to manifest in many HIV-infected clients. For example, HAART has been associated with lipodystrophy (redistribution of body fat), hypercholesterolemia, hypertriglyceridemia, insulin resistance and diabetes, and mitochondrial toxicity that may lead to cardiomyopathy, peripheral neuropathy, pancreatitis, and lactic acidosis (*HIV Inside*, 2000). Many of these complications may have life-threatening consequences, and the nurse should closely observe clients receiving HAART for their occurrence.

Treatment for chronic HCV infection may also have multiple side effects such as fatigue, muscle aches, headache, nausea and vomiting, irritability, depression, reversible hair loss, skin rashes and itching, and nasal stuffiness. More serious adverse effects of therapy include bone marrow depression, thyroid disease, bacterial infection, seizures, blood dyscrasias, retinopathy, tinnitus and hearing loss, and suicidal ideation (National Institute of Diabetes and Digestive and Kidney Diseases, 1999).

Promoting treatment adherence in the face of multiple side effects can be difficult. Some strategies that may be effective in promoting compliance include reducing side effects where possible, simplifying the regimen to include fewer doses and fewer pills, establishing client trust in the efficacy of treatment, and tailoring therapy to fit the client's lifestyle whenever possible. Additional approaches may include clarifying treatment instructions and making sure that clients understand them, simplifying distribution systems (e.g., providing easy access to medication refills), and providing frequent follow-up (*HIV Inside*, 1999).

Rehabilitation may be required following some communicable diseases. For example, rehabilitation may be needed to strengthen affected muscles or to promote individual and family adjustment to permanent disabilities from paralytic poliomyelitis. Active and passive range of motion may help restore muscle strength and prevent contractures. Maintaining skin integrity for clients with braces or those confined to bed or wheelchair is also important. Observation for recurrent disease (even many years later) is also needed. Families may also require assistance in financing rehabilitative care and procuring needed equipment and appliances.

Community health nurses may also need to help clients deal with the long-term consequences of communicable diseases. For example, children with anomalies or mental retardation due to congenital rubella syndrome or congenital syphilis will need ongoing care, and their families will need emotional support and assistance in finding resources needed to deal with their children's disabilities. Support may also be needed for long-term behavior changes required to prevent infecting others with HIV or hepatitis. Community health nurses may also need to function as advocates to prevent stigmatization and discrimination and to foster clients' integration into the community to the extent permitted by their health status. For example, nurses may need to educate those who interact with HIV-infected clients about how HIV infection is and is not transmitted. Similarly, when working with children with AIDS, advocacy by the community health nurse may necessitate planning activities that foster normal growth and development in each child.

Assistance may also be needed in dealing with the financial impact of HIV infection and other diseases that have long-term treatment needs. The community health nurse can help in this respect by referring clients and their families to sources of financial assistance. Advocacy by community health nurses may be required to ensure client eligibility for financial assistance programs.

For a few communicable diseases, tertiary prevention with individual clients entails preventing reinfection. This does not apply to the majority of the diseases dis-

cussed in this chapter because they result in immunity. For example, hepatitis A confers immunity against reinfection with hepatitis A, but does not provide immunity to other forms of hepatitis. Similarly, varicella, measles, and mumps usually confer immunity, and clients do not become reinfected. Some diseases, however, do not produce immunity, and reinfection is possible and even likely if clients do not change risk behaviors. For example, clients may be reinfected with gonorrhea or chlamydia with continued unprotected sexual activity. Similarly, reinfection with syphilis is possible unless the disease has progressed to the point of immunity, by which time the risk for long-term complications is quite high. Community health nurses need to educate clients about the potential for reinfection and the need for behavior changes to reduce the risk of reinfection. For example, nurses might educate clients about the need for condoms during sexual intercourse or educate IDUs on harm-reduction strategies such as not sharing needles or other drug paraphernalia.

Tertiary prevention at the community level is directed toward preventing the spread of disease and providing access to long-term care services. Measures to prevent the spread of disease in the population include many primary prevention measures for individuals such as immunization and identification, notification, and prophylactic treatment of contacts. Isolation of infected persons may also prevent further spread of some communicable diseases within the community. Changes in risk behaviors among persons who are chronic carriers of infection can also serve to prevent dissemination of disease.

Health systems must also be in place to meet the tertiary prevention needs of clients with communicable diseases. At the level of public policy, community health nurses may need to plan political activity to ensure necessary funding for assistance programs for clients experiencing long-term needs related to the effects of communicable diseases. Strategies for tertiary prevention of communicable diseases are summarized below.

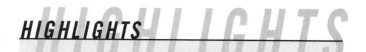

HIGHLIGHTS

Tertiary Prevention for Communicable Diseases

Monitoring treatment compliance

Monitoring treatment
- Monitoring effectiveness
- Identifying and dealing with side effects
- Identifying and referring for adverse effects

• Dealing with complications
- Preventing complications
- Rehabilitation

(continued)

• Promoting adjustment to long-term consequences
• Advocacy for long-term care services as needed

Preventing reinfection
• Education for safe sexual practices
• Referral for drug abuse treatment
• Promotion of harm-reduction strategies

Preventing the spread of disease
• Mass immunization
• Contact notification
• Screening of blood and tissue donors
• Screening and treatment of infected pregnant women
• Isolation of infected persons
• Promotion of behavior change

Effective community health nursing care for communicable diseases may necessitate obtaining information not addressed in this chapter. Some sources of relevant information are provided on the companion Web site for this book.

⑥THINK ABOUT IT

Does the role of the community health nurse in controlling communicable diseases differ with the disease to be controlled? If so, how does it differ?

EVALUATING CARE RELATED TO COMMUNICABLE DISEASES

Evaluating primary prevention related to communicable diseases with individual clients is based on the prevention of occurrence of disease. If drug users educated for harm reduction do not develop HBV or HIV infection, intervention has been successful. At the community level, the effectiveness of primary prevention of communicable diseases is reflected in declining incidence and prevalence rates.

The effectiveness of secondary prevention is reflected in communicable disease mortality and continued morbidity. For example, HAART for HIV infection has decreased HIV/AIDS-related mortality and prolonged survival time for infected persons. Similarly, the effectiveness of TB therapy is reflected in the number of clients whose TB has been cured.

Evaluation of tertiary preventive measures focuses on the extent to which complications of communicable diseases have been prevented, the extent to which reinfection occurs for those diseases where reinfection is a possibility, and the extent of disability and adverse consequences resulting from communicable diseases. Evaluation of each of the three levels of prevention is also reflected in the national objectives related to communicable diseases presented earlier in this chapter.

Although remarkable progress has been made in controlling communicable diseases, they remain significant contributors to morbidity and mortality in the United States and throughout the world. Community health nurses can be actively involved in preventing communicable diseases and in identifying and treating them when they do occur.

APPLYING YOUR KNOWLEDGE IN PRACTICE

✺ CASE STUDY
A Communicable Disease

Jane is an 18-year-old college student. She lives in the dorm with her roommate Sally. Shortly after Jane returned from Christmas vacation, she developed a fever and a rash. She didn't feel too badly, but Sally persuaded her to see a doctor. Because it was Saturday, Jane went to the emergency department (ED) of the local hospital. The physician there made a diagnosis of rubella. Later that night, he and the nurses in the ED became very busy with victims of a multicar accident. As a result, no one completed the health department form reporting Jane's rubella until two days later.

By the time a community health nurse contacted Jane to complete a rubella case report, Sally and several other girls in Jane's dorm also developed rubella. Sally gave it to her boyfriend, who exposed those in his classes. One of the women in his English class is pregnant.

- What primary preventive measures could have been employed to prevent this situation? What primary prevention measures are appropriate at this point?

- What secondary and tertiary measures by the community health nurse are appropriate at this time?

- What roles will the community health nurse perform in dealing with this situation?

✿ TESTING YOUR UNDERSTANDING

- What are some of the major trends in communicable disease incidence in the United States? How do these trends differ from those worldwide? What factors are influencing those trends? (pp. 658–661)

- What are the major modes of transmission of communicable diseases? What effect has technology had on disease transmission? (pp. 661–662)

- What roles do community health nurses play in the control of communicable diseases? (pp. 663–678)

- How do biophysical, psychological, physical environmental, sociocultural, behavioral, and health system factors influence the incidence and control of communicable diseases? (pp. 663–668)

- What are the major approaches to primary prevention of communicable diseases? (pp. 669–674)

- What are the major considerations in secondary prevention of communicable diseases? (pp. 674–676)

- What are the foci of tertiary prevention in the control of communicable diseases? (pp. 676–678)

REFERENCES

Alter, M. J., Margolis, H. S., Bell, B. P., Bice, S. D., et al. (1998). Recommendations for prevention and control of hepatitis C virus (HCV) infection and HCV-related chronic disease. *Morbidity and Mortality Weekly Report, 47*(RR-19), 1–39.

Anderson, J. E., Carey, J. W., & Taveras, S. (2000). HIV testing among the general US population and persons at increased risk: Information from national surveys, 1987–1996. *American Journal of Public Health, 90*, 1089–1095.

Bachmann, L. H., Lewis, I., Allen, R., Schwebke, J. R., et al. (2000). Risk and prevalence of treatable sexually transmitted diseases at a Birmingham substance abuse facility. *American Journal of Public Health, 90*, 1615–1618.

Baltimore, D. (1999). Can we make an AIDS vaccine? *National Forum, 79*(3), 35–37.

Bardenheier, B., Prevots, D. R., Khetsuriani, N., & Wharton, M. (1998). Tetanus surveillance—United States, 1995–1997. *Morbidity and Mortality Weekly Report, 47*(SS-2), 1–13.

Bayer, R., Stayton, C., Desvarieux, M., Healton, C., Landesman, S., & Tsai, W. (1998). Directly observed therapy and treatment completion for tuberculosis in the United States: Is universal supervised therapy necessary? *American Journal of Public Health, 88*, 1052–1058.

Bell, B. P., Wasley, A., Shapiro, C. N., & Margolis, H. S. (1999). Prevention of hepatitis A through active or passive immunization: Recommendations of the Advisory Committee in Immunization Practices (ACIP). *Morbidity and Mortality Weekly Report, 48*(RR-12), 1–37.

Binder, S., Levitt, A. M., & the National Center for Infectious Diseases Plan Steering Committee. (1998). Preventing emerging infectious diseases: A strategy for the 21st century. *Morbidity and Mortality Weekly Report, 47*(RR-15), 1–14.

Brammer, T. L., Izurieta, H. S., Fukuda, K., Schmeltz, L. M., et al. (2000). Surveillance for influenza—United States, 1994–95, 1995–96, and 1996–97 seasons. *Morbidity and Mortality Weekly Report, 49*(SS-3), 13–28.

Bridges, C. B., Fukuda, K., Cox, N. J., & Singleton, J. A. (2001). Prevention and control of influenza: Recommendations of the Advisory Committee on Immunization Practices. *Morbidity and Mortality Weekly Report, 50*(RR-4), 1–44.

Buffington, J., Rowell, R., Hinman, J. M., Sharp, K., & Choi, S. (2001). Lack of awareness of hepatitis C risk among persons who received blood transfusions before 1990. *American Journal of Public Health, 91*, 47–48.

California Department of Health Services. (1998). Tetanus among injection drug users—California, 1997. *Morbidity and Mortality Weekly Report, 47*, 149–151.

California Department of Health Services. (1999, April 2). The ACIP recommends universal pediatric hepatitis A immunization for California. *Miniupdate*, 1–2.

Centers for Disease Control and Prevention. (1998a). 1998 guidelines for treatment of sexually transmitted diseases. *Morbidity and Mortality Weekly Report, 47*(RR-1), 1–116.

Centers for Disease Control and Prevention. (1998b). National vaccination coverage levels among children aged 19–35 months—United States, 1998. *Morbidity and Mortality Weekly Report, 47*, 829–830.

Centers for Disease Control and Prevention. (1999a). Control of infectious diseases. *Morbidity and Mortality Weekly Report, 48*, 621–629.

Centers for Disease Control and Prevention. (1999b). Recommendations of the Advisory Committee on Immunization Practices: Revised recommendations for routine poliomyelitis vaccination. *Morbidity and Mortality Weekly Report, 48*, 590.

Centers for Disease Control and Prevention. (2000a). Alternate two-dose hepatitis B vaccination schedule for adolescents aged 11–15 years. *Morbidity and Mortality Weekly Report, 50*, 261.

Centers for Disease Control and Prevention. (2000b). Targeted tuberculin testing and treatment of latent tuberculosis infection. *Morbidity and Mortality Weekly Report, 50*, 261.

Centers for Disease Control and Prevention. (2001a). Facts about anthrax. Retrieved October 25, 2001, from the World Wide Web, *http://www.bt.cdc.gov.*

Centers for Disease Control and Prevention. (2001b). Summary of notifiable diseases, United States, 1999. *Morbidity and Mortality Weekly Report, 48*(53), 1–101.

Centers for Disease Control and Prevention. (2001c). World TB Day—March 24, 2001. *Morbidity and Mortality Weekly Report, 50*, 201.

Centers for Disease Control and Prevention Strategic Planning Workgroup. (2000). Biological and chemical terrorism: Strategic plan for preparedness and response. *Morbidity and Mortality Weekly Report, 49*(RR-4), 1–14.

Chiarello, L. A., Cardo, D. M., Panlilio, A. L., Bell, D. M., et al. (1998). Public Health Service guidelines for the management of health care worker exposures to HIV and recommendations for postexposure prophylaxis. *Morbidity and Mortality Weekly Report, 48*(RR-7), 1–33.

Chin, J. (Ed.) (2000). *Control of communicable diseases manual* (17th ed.). Washington, DC: American Public Health Association.

Clements-Nolle, K., Marx, R., Guzman, R., & Katz, M. (2001). HIV prevalence, risk behaviors, health care use, and mental health status of transgender persons: Implications for public health intervention. *American Journal of Public Health, 91,* 915–921.

Cohen, J. (2001). And now the good news about smallpox. Retrieved October 30, 2001, from the World Wide Web, *http://www. content.health.msn.com.*

Corrarino, J. E. (1998). Perinatal hepatitis B: Update and recommendations. *MCN, 23,* 246–253.

Des Jarlais, D. C., & Schuchat, A. (2001). Hepatitis C among drug users: Deja vu all over again? *American Journal of Public Health, 91,* 21–22.

Desvarieux, M., Hyppolite, P., Johnson, W. D., & Pape, J. W. (2001). A novel approach to directly observed therapy for tuberculosis in an HIV-endemic area. *American Journal of Public Health, 91,* 138–141.

Diaz, T., Des Jarlais, D. C., Vlahov, D., Perliss, T. E., et al. (2001). Factors associated with prevalent hepatitis C: Differences among young adult injection drug users in lower and upper Manhattan, New York City. *American Journal of Public Health, 91,* 23–30.

DiLiberti, J. H., & Jackson, C. R. (1999). Long-term trends in childhood infectious disease mortality rates. *American Journal of Public Health, 89,* 1883–1885.

Division of AIDS, STD, and TB Laboratory Research. (2000). Fluoroquinolone-resistance in *Neisseria gonorrhoeae,* Hawaii, 1999, and decreased susceptibility to azithromycin in *N. gonorrhoeae,* Missouri, 1999. *Morbidity and Mortality Weekly Report, 49,* 833–837.

Division of HIV/AIDS Prevention—Intervention, Research, and Support. (1998). Update: Syringe exchange programs—United States, 1997. *Morbidity and Mortality Weekly Report, 47,* 652–655.

Division of HIV/AIDS Prevention—Inter-vention, Research, and Support. (1999). Trends in HIV-related sexual risk behaviors among high school students—Selected U.S. cities, 1991–1997. *Morbidity and Mortality Weekly Report, 48,* 440–443.

Division of HIV/AIDS Prevention—Intervention, Research, and Support. (2000). HIV-related knowledge and stigma—United States, 2000. *Morbidity and Mortality Weekly Report, 49,* 1062–1064.

Division of HIV/AIDS Prevention—Surveillance and Epidemiology. (1999). Anonymous or confidential HIV counseling and voluntary testing. *Morbidity and Mortality Weekly Report, 48,* 509–513.

Division of HIV/AIDS Prevention—Surveillance and Epidemiology. (2000). Adoption of protective behaviors among persons with recent HIV infection and diagnosis—Alabama, New Jersey, and Tennessee, 1997–1998. *Morbidity and Mortality Weekly Report, 49,* 512–515.

Division of HIV/AIDS Prevention—Surveillance and Epidemiology. (2001). Preva-lence of risk behaviors for HIV infection among adults—United States, 1997. *Morbiity and Mortality Weekly Report, 50,* 262–265.

Division of Sexually Transmitted Diseases Prevention. (1998). Trends in sexual risk behaviors among high school students—United States, 1991–1997. *Morbidity and Mortality Weekly Report, 47,* 749–752.

Division of Sexually Transmitted Diseases Prevention. (1999a). Congenital syphilis—United States, 1998. *Morbidity and Mortality Weekly Report, 48,* 757–761.

Division of Sexually Transmitted Diseases Prevention. (1999b). High prevalence of chlamydial and gonococcal infection in women entering jails and juvenile detention centers—Chicago, Birmingham, and San Francisco, 1998. *Morbidity and Mortality Weekly Report, 48,* 793–796.

Division of Sexually Transmitted Diseases Prevention. (2000). Alcohol policy and sexually transmitted disease rates—United States, 1981–1995. *Morbidity and Mortality Weekly Report, 49,* 346–348.

Division of Sexually Transmitted Diseases Prevention. (2001). Primary and secondary syphilis—United States, 1999. *Morbidity and Mortality Weekly Report, 50,* 113–117.

Division of Tuberculosis Elimination. (1998). Tuberculosis morbidity—United States, 1997. *Morbidity and Mortality Weekly Report, 47,* 253–257.

Division of Tuberculosis Elimination. (2000a). Drug-susceptible tuberculosis outbreak in a state correctional facility housing HIV-infected inmates—South Carolina, 1999–2000. *Morbidity and Mortality Weekly Report, 49,* 1041–1044.

Division of Tuberculosis Elimination. (2000b). Missed opportunities for prevention of tuberculosis among persons with HIV infection—United States, 1996–1997. *Morbidity and Mortality Weekly Report, 49,* 685–687.

Division of Viral and Rickettsial Diseases. (1998). Hepatitis A vaccination of men who have sex with men—Atlanta, Georgia, 1996–1997. *Morbidity and Mortality Weekly Report, 47,* 708–711.

Division of Viral and Rickettsial Diseases. (2000). Hepatitis C virus infection among firefighters, emergency medical technicians, and paramedics—Selected locations, United States, 1991–2000. *Morbidity and Mortality Weekly Report, 49,* 660–665.

Ehresmann, K. R., Mills, W. A., Loewenson, P. R., & Moore, K. A. (2000). Attitudes and practices regarding varicella vaccination among physicians in Minnesota: Implications for public health and provider education. *American Journal of Public Health, 90,* 1917–1920.

Feinberg, M. B., & Kaplan, J. E. (1998). Report of the NIH Panel to Define Principles of Therapy of HIB Infection. *Morbidity and Mortality Weekly Report, 47*(RR-5), 1–82.

Fonck, K., Claeys, P., Bashir, F., Bwayo, J., Fransen, L., & Temmerman, M. (2001). Syphilis control during pregnancy: Effectiveness and sustainability of a decentralized program. *American Journal of Public Health, 91,* 705–707.

Fox, K. K., del Rio, C., Holmes, K. K., Hook, E. W., et al. (2001). Gonorrhea in the HIV era:
A reversal in trends among men who have sex with men. *American Journal of Public Health, 91,* 959–964.

Friis, R. H., & Sellers, T. A. (1999). *Epidemiology for public health practice* (2nd ed.). Gaithersburg, MD: Aspen.

Gunn, R. A., Harper, S. L., Brontrager, D. E., Gonzales, P. E., & St. Louis, M. E. (2000). Implementing a syphilis elimination and importation control strategy in a low-incidence urban area: San Diego County, California, 1997–1998. *American Journal of Public Health, 90,* 1540–1544.

Hagan, H., Thiede, H., Weiss, N. S., Hopkins, S. G., Duchin, J. S., & Alexander, E. R. (2001). Sharing of drug preparation equipment as a risk factor for hepatitis C. *American Journal of Public Health, 91,* 42–46.

Haley, N., Maheux, B., Rivard, M., & Gervais, A. (1999). Sexual health risk assessment and counseling in primary care: How involved are general practitioners and obstetrician–gynecologists? *American Journal of Public Health, 89,* 899–902.

HIV Inside. (1999). Ensuring continuity of care for the HIV-positive inmate. *1*(4), 1–5, 8, 11.

HIV Inside. (2000). Complications associated with long-term antiretroviral therapy. *2*(1), 1, 3–4, 7–8.

Hope, V. D., Judd, A., Hickman, M., Lamagni, T., et al. (2001). Prevalence of hepatitis C among injection drug users in England and Wales: Is harm reduction working? *American Journal of Public Health, 91,* 38–42.

Horner, S. D., & Murphy, L. (1999). Creating alternative immunization clinics to maintain and improve community immunization rates. *Journal of Community Health Nursing, 16,* 121–132.

Jafari, H., Adams, W. G., Robinson, K. A., Plikaytis, B. D., Wenger, J. D., and the *Haemophilus influenzae* study group. (1999). Efficacy of *Haemophilus influenzae* type b conjugate vaccines and persistence of disease in disadvantaged populations. *American Journal of Public Health, 89,* 364–368.

Jones, J. L., Hanson, D. L., Dworkin, M. S., Alderton, D. L., et al. (1999). Surveillance for AIDS-defining opportunistic illnesses, 1992–1997. *Morbidity and Mortality Weekly Report, 48*(SS-2), 1–22.

Kaplan, J. E., Masur, H., & Holmes, K. K. (1999). The USPHS/IDSA guidelines for the prevention of opportunistic infections in persons infected with human immunodeficiency virus. *Morbidity and Mortality Weekly Report, 49*(RR-10), 1–66.

Keithley, J. K., Swanson, B., Murphy, M., & Levin, D. G. (2000). HIV/AIDS and nutrition: Implications for disease management. *Case Management, 5*(2), 1–9.

Kellner, P. (1999). A century of tuberculosis nursing: Changing challenges. *Journal of the New York State Nurses Association, 30*(1), 9–15.

Khajehdehi, P., & Rezaian, G. (1997). Tetanus in the elderly: Is it different from that in younger age groups? *Gerontology, 44,* 172–175.

Knight, V. M., & Bodsworth, N. J. (1998). Perceptions and practice of universal blood and body fluid precautions by registered nurses at a major Sydney teaching hospital. *Journal of Advanced Nursing, 27,* 746–751.

Krahn, M., Guasparini, R., Sherman, M., & Detsky, A. S. (1998). Costs and cost-effectiveness of a universal, school-based hepatitis B vaccination program. *American Journal of Public Health, 88,* 1638–1644.

Lobato, M. N., Cegielski, J. P. & the Tuberculosis Along the U.S.–Mexico Border Work Group. (2001). Preventing and controlling tuberculosis along the U.S.–Mexico border. *Morbidity and Mortality Weekly Report, 50*(RR-1), 1–27.

Lorvick, K., Kral, A. H., Seal, K., Gee, L., & Edlin, B. R. (2001). Prevalence and duration of hepatitis C among injection drug users in San Francisco, Calif. *American Journal of Public Health, 91,* 46–47.

Malotte, C. K., Rhodes, F., & Mais, K. E. (1998). Tuberculosis screening and compliance with return for skin testing reading among active drug users. *American Journal of Public Health, 88,* 792–796.

McCarthy, G. M., Koval, J. J., & MacDonald, J. K. (1999). Factors associated with refusal to treat HIV-infected patients: The results of a national survey of dentists in Canada. *American Journal of Public Health, 89,* 541–545.

McKellar, D. A., Valleroy, L. A., Secura, G. M., McFarland, W., et al. (2001). Two decades after vaccine license: Hepatitis B immunization and infection among young men who have sex with men. *American Journal of Public Health, 91,* 965–971.

McQuillan, G. M., Coleman, P. J., Kruszon-Moran, D., Moyer, L. A., Lambert, S. B., & Margolis, H. S. (1999). Prevalence of hepatitis B virus infection in the United States: The National Health and Nutrition Examination Surveys, 1976 through 1994. *American Journal of Public Health, 89,* 14–18.

Michael, R. T., Wadsworth, J., Feinlieb, J., Johnson, A. M., Laumann, E. O., & Wellings, K. (1998). Private sexual behavior, public opinion, and public health policy related to sexually transmitted diseases: A US–British comparison. *American Journal of Public Health, 88,* 749–754.

Msellati, P., Meda, N., Welffens-Ekra, C., Leroy, V., et al. (1999). Zidovudine and reduction in vertical transmission of HIV in Africa. *American Journal of Public Health, 89,* 947–948.

National Center for Chronic Disease Prevention and Health Promotion. (1998). Influenza and pneumococcal vaccination levels among adults aged > 65 years—United States, 1997. *Morbidity and Mortality Weekly Report, 47,* 797–802.

National Center for Health Statistics. (1999). Mortality patterns—United States, 1997. *Morbidity and Mortality Weekly Report, 48,* 664–668.

National Center for Infectious Diseases. (2000a). *Viral hepatitis A—Fact sheet.* Retrieved June 13, 2000, from the World Wide Web, *http://www.cdc.gov/ncidod/diseases/hepatitis/a/fact.*

National Center for Infectious Diseases. (2000b). *Viral hepatitis B—Fact sheet.* Retrieved June 13, 2000, from the World Wide Web, *http://www.cdc.gov/ncidod/diseases/hepatitis/b/fact.*

National Center for Infectious Diseases. (2000c). *Viral hepatitis C—Fact sheet.* Retrieved June 13, 2000, from the World Wide Web, *http://www.cdc.gov/ncidod/diseases/hepatitis/c/fact.*

National Center for Infectious Diseases. (2000d). *Hepatitis D virus.* Retrieved June 13, 2000, from the World Wide Web, *http://www.cdc.gov/ncidod/diseases/hepatitis/d.*

National Center for Infectious Diseases. (2000e). *Hepatitis E virus.* Retrieved June 13, 2000, from the World Wide Web, *http://www.cdc.gov/ncidod/diseases/hepatitis/e.*

National Immunization Program. (1999). Impact of vaccines universally recommended for children—United States, 1990–1998. *Morbidity and Mortality Weekly Report, 48,* 243–248.

National Immunization Program. (2000a). Measles—United States, 1999. *Morbidity and Mortality Weekly Report, 49,* 557–560.

National Immunization Program. (2000b). National, state, and urban area vaccination coverage levels among children aged 19–35 months—United States, 1999. *Morbidity and Mortality Weekly Report, 49,* 585–589.

National Immunization Program. (2000c). Varicella outbreaks among Mexican adults—Alabama, 2000. *Morbidity and Mortality Weekly Report, 49,* 735–736.

National Immunization Program. (2001). Progress in development of immunization registries—United States, 2000. *Morbidity and Mortality Weekly Report, 50,* 3–7.

National Institute of Diabetes and Digestive and Kidney Diseases. (1999). *Chronic hepatitis C: Current disease management.* Washington, DC: Author.

O'Brien, R. J. (1998). Development of new vaccines for tuberculosis: Recommendations of the Advisory Council on Immunization Practices (ACIP). *Morbidity and Mortality Weekly Report, 47*(RR-13), 1–6.

Orenstein, W. A., Strebel, P. M., Papania, M., Sutter, R. W., Bellini, W. J., & Cochi, S. L. (2000). Measles eradication: Is it in our future? *American Journal of Public Health, 90,* 1521–1525.

Poss, J. E. (1998). The meanings of tuberculosis for Mexican migrant farmworkers in the United States. *Social Science & Medicine, 47,* 195–202.

Prevots, D. R., Burr, R. K., Sutter, R. W., & Murphy, T. V. (2000). Poliomyelitis prevention in the United States: Updated recommendations of the Advisory Committee on Immunization Practices. *Morbidity and Mortality Weekly Report, 49*(RR-5), 1–22.

Regional Perinatal Care Programs of California. (1999, spring). HIV transmission: Mode of delivery and risk of vertical transmission. *Perinatal Care Matters,* 2–3.

Remis, R. S., Dufour, A., Alary, M., Vincelette, J., et al. (2000). Association of hepatitis B virus infection with other sexually transmitted diseases in homosexual men. *American Journal of Public Health, 90,* 1570–1574.

Rosenberg, S. D., Goodman, L. A., Osher, F. C., Schwartz, M. S., et al. (2001). Prevalence of HIV, hepatitis B, and hepatitis C in people with severe mental illness. *American Journal of Public Health, 91,* 31–37.

Rosenfield, A. (2001). Where is the M in MTCT? The broader issues in mother-to-child transmission of HIV. *American Journal of Public Health, 91,* 703–704.

Royce, R. A., Walter, E. B., Fernandez, M. I., Wilson, T. E., et al. (2001). Barriers to universal prenatal HIV testing in 4 US locations in 1997. *American Journal of Public Health, 91,* 727–733.

Scharbaugh, R. J. (1999). The risk of occupational exposure and infection with infectious disease. *Nursing Clinics of North America, 34,* 493–508.

St. Louis, M. E., Levine, W. C., Wasserheit, J. N., DeCock, K. M., et al. (1998). HIV prevention through early detection and treatment of other sexually transmitted diseases—United States. *Morbidity and Mortality Weekly Report, 47*(RR-12), 1–24.

Susser, I., & Stein, Z. (2000). Culture, sexuality, and women's agency in the prevention of HIV/AIDS in Southern Africa. *American Journal of Public Health, 90,* 1042–1048.

Todd, C. S., Haase, C., & Stoner, B. P. (2001). Emergency department screening for asymptomatic sexually transmitted diseases. *American Journal of Public Health, 91,* 461–464.

Tulsky, J. P., White, M. C., Dawson, C., Hoynes, T. M., Goldenson, J., & Schecter, G. (1998). Screening for tuberculosis in jail and clinic follow-up after release. *American Journal of Public Health, 88,* 223–226.

UNAIDS. (2000). *AIDS epidemic update: 2000.* Retrieved January 4, 2001, from the World Wide Web, *http://unaids.org.*

U.S. Department of Health and Human Services. (2000a). *Health, United States, 2000.* Washington, DC: Author.

U.S. Department of Health and Human Services. (2000b). *Healthy people 2010* (Conference edition, in two volumes). Washington, DC: Author.

Vaccine Preventable Disease Eradication Division. (1998). Progress toward global measles control and regional elimination, 1990–1997. *Morbidity and Mortality Weekly Report, 47,* 1049–1054.

Vaccine Preventable Disease Eradication Division. (1999). Progress toward global poliomyelitis eradication, 1997–1998. *Morbidity and Mortality Weekly Report, 48,* 416–421.

Valdez, R., Narayan, V., Geiss, L. S., & Englegau, M. M. (1999). Impact of diabetes mellitus on mortality associated with pneumonia and influenza among non-Hispanic black and white US adults. *American Journal of Public Health, 89,* 1715–1721.

Watson, J. C., Hadler, S. C., Dykewicz, C. A., Reef, S., & Phillips, L. (1998). Measles, mumps, and rubella—Vaccine use and strategies for elimination of measles, rubella, and congenital rubella syndrome and control of mumps: Recommendations of the Advisory Committee on Immunization Practices (ACIP). *Morbidity and Mortality Weekly Report, 47*(RR-8), 1–57.

Weis, S. E., Foresman, B., Cook, P. E., & Matty, K. J. (1999). Universal HIV screening at a major metropolitan TB clinic: HIV prevalence and high-risk behaviors among TB patients. *American Journal of Public Health, 89,* 73–75.

Williams, L. A., Klausner, J. D., Whittington, W. L. H., Handsfield, H. H., Celum, C., & Holmes, K. K. (1999). Elimination and reintroduction of primary and secondary

Because of the effectiveness of control measures developed for many previously fatal communicable diseases, chronic health problems have largely replaced communicable diseases as the leading causes of death and disability in the United States. Each year, millions of people experience the suffering and the economic costs associated with chronic problems, and many die as a result. Diabetes, for example, kills one American every three minutes and costs $98 million per year in health care expenditures (Juvenile Diabetes Foundation International, 1998).

Chronic health problems are those that are present for extended periods and that are characterized by one or more distinctive features. These features may include nonreversible pathological changes, a need for lifestyle adjustment, or a prolonged period of supervision and care by health professionals. Chronic conditions include disease entities, injuries with lasting consequences, and other enduring abnormalities.

Chronic health problems may be either physical or emotional, and both types of chronic conditions are addressed in the national health objectives developed for the year 2010 (U.S. Department of Health and Human Services [USDHHS], 2000b). These objectives may be viewed at the Healthy People 2010 Web site through the link provided on the companion Web site for this book. In this chapter, we address chronic physical health problems. Chronic emotional conditions are addressed in Chapter 30.   ◈

EFFECTS OF CHRONIC HEALTH PROBLEMS

Chronic health problems can arise from a variety of sources. For example, a person might develop a chronic disability as a result of a serious accident or because of arthritis. Other chronic conditions arise out of other disease processes such as cardiovascular disease, chronic respiratory diseases, and cancer. Some chronic conditions, such as some cancers, may result in death. Others, although not fatal, cause persistent pain and disability.

The effects of chronic health conditions are not only experienced by individuals. Population groups and society at large are also affected by the consequences of chronic health problems.

Personal Effects

The advent of a chronic condition has many personal effects for individual clients. The consequences of disease and injury include impairment, disability, and handicap. A fourth consequence is personal economic burden. According to the World Health Organization, *impairment* refers to the "loss of psychological, physiological, or anatomical, structure or function." *Disability,* on the other hand, is a limitation in functional ability resulting from impairment (Larson, 1998, pp. 529–530). In 1998,

approximately 13% of the U.S. population experienced some form of activity limitation due to a chronic condition (USDHHS, 2000a).

⑥THINK ABOUT IT

What chronic physical condition would be most devastating for you personally? Why? What effects do you think this condition would have on your life?

Activity restrictions often require a change in lifestyle. Individuals with arthritis, for example, may need to adjust to their inability to do some things that they have done in the past or may need to learn to use special implements to accomplish everyday tasks like closing a zipper or buttoning a shirt. Similarly, clients with chronic respiratory conditions may find that they are less able to engage in vigorous activity than in the past and may require more frequent rest periods, and the client seriously injured in an automobile accident may need to adjust to using a wheelchair. Frequently, such physical limitations make it necessary to rely on others to perform routine tasks of daily living. This enforced dependence on others may, in turn, adversely affect an individual's self-image.

Even when activities are not restricted, the presence of a chronic health problem usually requires lifestyle adjustments. For the person with diabetes or a heart condition, for example, changes in diet are required. The person with diabetes may also need to make changes in eating

CRITICAL THINKING IN RESEARCH

Much of the research on the effect of disabilities is based on secondary analysis of data from multiple studies in which *disability* is defined in multiple ways. Some authors argue that a standard definition of disability should be developed to facilitate comparison of the findings of different studies. Others suggest that since disability is often defined on the basis of the perceptions of the person experiencing it, continued research using multiple different definitions of the term would provide more meaningful information for those interested in disability and its affects on health and life (Joslyn, 1999).

- What are the advantages and disadvantages of each position?
- Which position would you adopt? Why?
- If you were planning to conduct a study related to disability, how would you define this variable?

ETHICAL AWARENESS

Many chronic conditions involve considerable pain that is frequently only lessened, but never eliminated. Other conditions result in significant disabilities that severely diminish clients' quality of life. How would you respond to a client who tells you he is considering assisted suicide because he can no longer live with the consequences of his condition? Would your response be different if he were considering euthanasia for a family member in intractable pain, rather than for himself? Why or why not?

patterns. This might mean not skipping meals or not eating on the run.

Pain also accompanies a number of chronic conditions and is often unremitting. The client with arthritis or cancer, for example, may have to endure a long period of pain despite the continued use of analgesics. The constant battle with chronic pain can be disheartening and can lead to depression and possible suicide.

The third consequence of chronic conditions is *handicap*, which is the disadvantage resulting from impairment or disability that impedes role fulfillment in one's usual roles (Larson, 1998). The pain, lifestyle changes, decreased activity levels, and impaired mobility associated with chronic conditions can contribute to social isolation. The chronically ill individual may be less able to interact with others in familiar patterns or be unable to engage in activities that friends and family enjoy. Consequently, this person may feel left out unless concerted efforts are made to incorporate him or her into family and community life. Only approximately 70% of disabled individuals socialize with family and friends, for example, compared to 85% of the nondisabled (National Organization on Disability, 2000).

Finally, chronic health problems often entail considerable financial burden. Most chronic conditions require the individual to take prescribed medications for the rest of his or her life and the cost can escalate rapidly. Add to this the cost of frequent visits to health care providers to monitor the condition and the effects of therapy. Moreover, many individuals with chronic conditions require expensive special equipment or services. Disabled individuals have been found to be more than twice as likely as those who are not disabled to put off needed health care because of costs and are four times more likely to have health needs that are not covered by health insurance (National Organization on Disability, 2000). Dis-abled individuals are also more likely to live in poverty and rates of disability are three times higher among the poor than the nonpoor (USDHHS, 2000a).

Chronic conditions may have at least one positive personal effect, however. Research has indicated that persons with one or more chronic conditions exhibit greater readiness to change unhealthful behaviors than those

without chronic illness (Boyle, O'Connor, Pronk, & Tan, 1998). Such changes may lead to better overall health in the long term.

Population Effects

Chronic conditions also affect the general population. These effects are reflected in financial costs, mortality, and morbidity.

SOCIETAL COSTS

Chronic health problems cost society millions of dollars each year. Societal costs of chronic health conditions include the direct monetary costs of health care as well as the indirect costs of lost productivity and use of limited resources. In 1992, for instance, asthma resulted in expenditures of $65 million and accounted for nearly 5% of all ambulatory care visits (Health Care and Aging Studies Bureau, 1999). Similarly, cardiovascular disease accounts for more than 6 million hospitalizations each year and has a total financial burden of $108 billion (Suminski et al., 1999). Direct and indirect costs for diabetes amounted to $98 million in 1997 (Valdmanis, Smith, & Page, 2001), and the lifetime costs of diabetes for someone diagnosed at age 3 is more than $600,000 (Juvenile Diabetes Foundation International, 1998). Accidental injuries also contribute a major portion of societal costs related to chronic conditions, and long-term management costs for heart failure are estimated to be $10 billion per year (Blaha, Robinson, Pugh, Bryan, & Havens, 2000). It would seem clear from these cost figures alone that the United States can no longer bear the burden of chronic disease and must take steps to control these and other chronic conditions.

MORBIDITY

Societal costs of chronic health conditions are measured not only in dollars but also in terms of the extent of morbidity resulting from these conditions. Although some progress has been made in preventing mortality due to chronic conditions, their prevalence has been increasing over the years. Because the reporting of chronic health conditions is not mandatory, however, prevalence figures probably grossly underrepresent the extent of these conditions in the population.

For example, hypertension affects approximately 50 million people in the United States. Approximately one third of people with hypertension are unaware of their disease; 15% remain untreated; 26% receive treatment, but their hypertension remains uncontrolled. Only 27% of those with hypertension have achieved good control of their disease (Goldsmith, 2000).

Although overall cancer incidence rates declined by 0.7% from 1990 to 1995 (Wingo, Ries, Rosenberg, Miller, & Edwards, 1998), cancer remains a serious concern in the United States and worldwide. Each year, approximately 182,000 women develop breast cancer, and in 2000 more than 41,000 deaths due to breast cancer were anticipated.

Similarly, 12,800 new cases and 4,600 deaths due to cervical cancer were expected (Lawson, Henson, Bobo, & Kaeser, 2000). In that same year, 47,700 new diagnoses of malignant melanoma and 180,400 cases of prostate cancer were expected to be diagnosed (Centers for Disease Control and Prevention [CDC], 2000; National Center for Chronic Disease Prevention and Health Promotion, 2000).

Various forms of heart disease affect major segments of the U.S. population as well. Cardiovascular disease is the leading cause of work-related disability in U.S. men and has a prevalence rate of 192 per 100,000 population (Suminski et al., 1999). Congestive heart failure is also prevalent, with 4.8 million people affected in the United States (Cardiovascular Health Bureau, 1998a). At the global level, by 2020 it is anticipated that ischemic heart disease and cerebrovascular disease together will account for 10% of the global burden of disease (Ustun, 1999).

Approximately 16 million individuals in the United States have diabetes mellitus, a third of whom are not aware of their diagnosis. Each year, roughly 798,000 new diagnoses of diabetes are made, with 1,700 diagnoses made daily (National Diabetes Information Clearinghouse, 2000, 2001). From 1935 to 1993, the prevalence of diabetes in the U.S. population increased 80% (Hunt, Pugh, & Valenzuela, 1998) and tripled in the last 30 years to affect an estimated 6% of the U.S. population (Elder & Muench, 2000). The rate of increase in diabetes prevalence is higher in blacks than in whites. For example, from 1980 to 1996, diabetes prevalence increased 18% for the population as a whole, but increased 50% for black men compared to only 10% in white women. In 1996, the overall age-adjusted incidence for diabetes in the United States was 2.79 per 100,000 population (National Center for Chronic Disease Prevention and Health Promotion, 1999). Selected subgroups in the United States affected by diabetes include 10.9% of Puerto Ricans, 9.6% of African Americans and Mexican Americans, 9.1% of Cuban Americans, and 6.2% of white Americans. Diabetes prevalence among Native Americans varies from 5% to as much as 50% in some tribal groups (National Diabetes Information Clearinghouse, 2000).

Asthma affects about 17 million Americans, and its prevalence increased 75% from 1980 to 1994 (National Center for Environmental Health, 1998). These figures include a 160% increase among children under 4 years of age and a 74% increase for children aged 5 to 14 years (Mannino et al., 1998). As noted in Chapter 16, asthma accounts for more school absences than any other condition. Asthma is also a significant problem in the workplace, where hypersensitive individuals may be exposed to small but significant amounts of respiratory irritants (Jajosky et al., 1999).

Arthritis is another chronic condition with significant health effects experienced by 43 million people in the United States. By 2020, arthritis may affect 60 million people. Arthritic conditions include osteoarthritis, rheumatoid arthritis, gout, ankylosing spondylitis, and

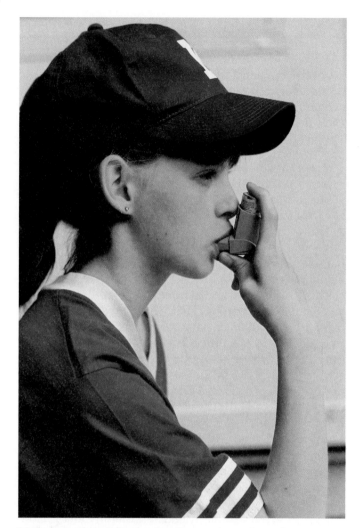

Morbidity and mortality due to asthma are increasing each year.

juvenile rheumatoid arthritis. From 1990 to 1997, the prevalence of arthritis increased by 750,000 cases per year, and in 1997, the self-reported prevalence of arthritis was 16.1 per 100 population. People with arthritis are three times more likely to report fair or poor health and experience an average of 4.2 more days of poor physical health, 1.6 more days of poor mental health, and 2.3 more days of activity limitation than those without the disease. In 1997, activity limitation occurred in nearly three of every 100 people with arthritis (Health Care and Aging Studies Bureau, 1999, 2000, 2001).

Some of the increase in incidence and prevalence figures for chronic health problems is attributable to better diagnosis as well as to the ability to prevent deaths due to these conditions. These and similar figures for other chronic conditions, however, indicate that Americans are making little progress in the primary prevention of chronic health problems.

MORTALITY

Many chronic health conditions contribute to increased mortality and loss of productive years of life among the population. As with morbidity figures, mortality figures also provide only a partial picture of the extent of chronic health problems within the population; however, they can provide information on patterns and trends in chronic conditions over time.

Despite a marked decline in mortality, cardiovascular disease has been the leading cause of death in the United States since 1921, and stroke has been the third leading cause of death since 1938. Together, these two conditions account for 40% of all U.S. deaths. In 1995, ischemic heart disease caused 21% of U.S. deaths and 65% of heart-related deaths. From 1950 to 1999, overall cardiovascular disease mortality declined 60%, with a 58% decline for ischemic heart disease. Similarly, the mortality rate due to stroke decreased 70% from 1950 to 1996. Unfortunately, some subpopulations have shown less decline than others. For example, black Americans have three to four times the risk of cardiovascular death as white Americans at specific ages; Native Americans have 1.3 to 2 times the risk; and Hispanics have 1.3 times the risk of death. Differences in mortality risk tend to diminish in older adults. These differences may be the result of higher prevalence of risk factors in minority populations, poorer access to health care services, or less use of services due to fear, lack of trust, transportation problems, and so on (Cardiovascular Health Bureau, 1998a, 1998b, 1999, 2000a, 2000b).

In 1998, cardiovascular disease contributed to 460,000 deaths, 44% of which were caused by myocardial infarction (CDC, 2001). The overall age-adjusted death rate for heart disease in 1998 was 126.6 per 100,000 population (USDHHS, 2000a).

After several years of increasing cancer mortality, cancer deaths decreased by 0.5% from 1990 to 1995 (Wingo et al., 1998). The U.S. age-adjusted mortality rate for all forms of cancer was 123.6 per 100,000 population in 1998. Some forms of cancer are greater contributors to mortality than others. The 1998 mortality due to lung cancer (37 per 100,000 population), for example, was nearly twice that for breast cancer (18.8 per 100,000).

Cancer mortality, like that for cardiovascular disease, is higher in some groups than in others. For example, in 1998 the overall mortality rate for cancers was 208.1 per 100,000 people for black men, 146.2 per 100,000 for white men, 95.7 per 100,000 for Native American men, 92.6 per 100,000 for Hispanic men, and 91.1 per 100,000 for Asian men. Similar differences were noted between groups for women (USDHHS, 2000a). Breast cancer survival rates also display marked subgroup differences. Although overall five-year survival rates increased to 85% from 1989 to 1995, rates increased only 71% for black women (Phillips, Cohen, & Tarzian, 2001). In 2000, malignant melanoma was expected to result in 47,700 new cases and 9,600 deaths (CDC, 2000).

Other chronic conditions also contribute to mortality figures for the nation. Diabetes mellitus, for example, accounted for 13.6 deaths per 100,000 population in 1998. This figure somewhat underrepresents the extent of the problem, as diabetes may contribute to death without being reported on death certificates. Again, the rate of diabetes mortality for black Americans and Native Americans is more than twice that of white Americans, while that for Hispanic Americans is more than 50% higher (USDHHS, 2000a). Overall, adults with diabetes have 2.6 times the risk of death as those without diabetes (Tierney et al., 2001), and diabetes decreases life expectancy by approximately 15 years (Juvenile Diabetes Foundation International, 1998).

Mortality due to chronic obstructive pulmonary disease (COPD) and allied conditions increased fivefold from 1950 to 1998 and constituted the fourth leading cause of death in the United States in 1998. The 1998 mortality rate for COPD was 21.3 per 100,000 population (USDHHS, 2000a). Asthma mortality increased by more than a third from 1960 to 1977 then more than doubled by 1995 to 17.9 deaths per million population. Although most asthma morbidity occurs in children, adults over 35 years of age account for 85% of asthma-related mortality (Mannino et al., 1998). Finally, chronic liver disease and cirrhosis caused 7.2 deaths per 100,000 people in 1998, and constituted the eighth leading cause of death. Accidents were the fourth leading cause of death at 30.1 deaths per 100,000 population (USDHHS, 2000a).

⓺THINK ABOUT IT

Given the limited resources available for health care services, do you think U.S. priority should be given to dealing with problems of communicable diseases or chronic diseases? Would priorities be different elsewhere in the world?

COMMUNITY HEALTH NURSING AND CONTROL OF CHRONIC PHYSICAL HEALTH PROBLEMS

Community health nurses are actively involved in efforts to control chronic physical health problems and their effects for individuals and populations. These efforts involve assessment, planning and implementation of control programs, and evaluation of their effectiveness.

ASSESSING FACTORS INFLUENCING CHRONIC PHYSICAL HEALTH PROBLEMS

Community health nurses use their assessment skills to assess for risk factors that contribute to chronic health problems and for existing chronic conditions and their effects. Factors related to the biophysical, psychological, physical environmental, sociocultural, behavioral, and health system dimensions can increase the risk of the individual or a population group with respect to a particular chronic condition. Conversely, the presence of a chronic health problem might affect factors in each of these areas.

Biophysical Considerations

Human biological factors related to age, sex, race and ethnicity, specific genetic inheritance, and physiologic function can increase one's risk of developing several chronic health problems. Ethnic and racial differences in incidence, prevalence, and mortality have already been discussed, but the concepts of race and ethnicity as risk markers for chronic disease will be addressed here.

Maturation and Aging

Many people think of chronic health problems as occurring primarily among the elderly, despite the fact that 6.5% of U.S. children experience some form of disability related to a variety of chronic conditions (Newacheck & Halfon, 1998), many of which were discussed in Chapter 16. Both the young and the elderly, for example, are at higher risk for accidental injuries and resulting disabilities. In part, this increased risk is due to maturational events of childhood and aging. The inability of a young infant to roll over or support his or her head contributes to suffocation as the leading cause of accidental death and disability in this age group. Similarly, normal toddler development involves a great deal of experimentation that may lead to accidental injury and disability if close supervision and safety precautions are not employed. The risk taking and feelings of invulnerability characteristic of preadolescent and adolescent development place young people at risk for motor vehicle and firearms accidents. Among the elderly, death and disabilities due to fires and falls are of the greatest concern. Typical causes of accidental injury and disability for selected age groups are presented in Table 29–1 ■.

Some chronic conditions and their effects are more prevalent in adults. For example, despite the popular belief that people with arthritis are elderly, most cases of

arthritis have their onset in the fourth decade of life. For women over age 45, for example, arthritis is the major cause of activity limitation. Older persons do, however, tend to experience greater disability as a result of this condition. The prevalence of COPD tends to increase dramatically in the fifth through the seventh decades of life. The incidence of malignant neoplasms, in general, also increases with advancing age, and 85% of prostate cancer occurs in men over 65 years of age (National Center for Chronic Disease Prevention and Health Promotion, 2000). Diabetes prevalence is also higher in the elderly (18%) than in children (0.16%) (National Diabetes Information Clearinghouse, 2001). Mortality due to chronic disease also, unsurprisingly, increases with age. For example, cardiovascular disease mortality among people over 85 years of age is almost 20 times higher than for those aged 65 to 74 years (Cardiovascular Health Bureau, 1998a). As noted earlier, asthma mortality is also higher for adults than for children.

Gender

One's gender can also influence the risk of developing a variety of chronic health conditions. Women, for example, have lower incidence rates for hypertension, and those who do have hypertension are more likely than men to have their blood pressure under control. Men are more than twice as likely as women to die of chronic liver disease and unintentional injuries, and about one and one-half times more likely to die of heart disease or malignant neoplasms than women. Similarly, men have higher risks for death from stroke, COPD, and diabetes (USDHHS, 2000a); however, arthritis prevalence for women exceeds that for men at all ages (U.S. Census Bureau, 1999).

Race and Ethnicity

For many chronic conditions, ethnic or racial factors function as risk markers rather than risk factors. *Risk markers* are factors that help to identify persons who may have an elevated risk of developing a specific condition but that do not themselves contribute to its development. For many chronic diseases, race and ethnicity are probably markers for differences in health behaviors, access to health care, and other factors that contribute to the development of disease. For example, when socioeconomic status is controlled, there is very little difference in mortality rates for cardiovascular disease between black Americans and their white counterparts. Socioeconomic status and access to health care are also believed to contribute to differences in asthma mortality between blacks and whites (Mannino et al., 1998) but do not completely explain these differences, suggesting that there may be some other underlying factors operating (Grant, Lyttle, & Weiss, 2000).

Genetic Inheritance

Some chronic diseases seem to be associated with genetic predisposition. Thus, community health nurses should

■ **TABLE 29–1** **Typical Causes of Injury and Disability**

AGE GROUP	TYPICAL CAUSES OF INJURY AND DISABILITY
Infants (birth–1 year)	Suffocation, aspiration of food and other objects, fire, drowning
1–9 years	Motor vehicle accidents, drowning, poisoning, fires
10–14 years	Motor vehicle accidents, drowning, firearms, fires
15–64 years	Motor vehicle accidents, occupational injury, falls, fires
Over 65 years	Falls, fires

obtain a family history of chronic diseases to help determine the individual client's risk for these conditions. Genetic inheritance is thought to be a major contributing factor for some cancers, for diabetes, and for cardiovascular disease.

In assessing the potential for chronic health problems in individual clients, the nurse obtains a family history and constructs a genogram as described in Chapter 14. Positive findings related to chronic conditions with a genetic component direct the assessment to possible signs and symptoms of existing chronic health problems.

Physiologic Function

Assessment of physiologic factors related to chronic conditions focuses on three areas: presence of physiologic risk factors, physiologic evidence of existing chronic health problems, and evidence of physiologic consequences of chronic conditions.

Certain physiologic conditions may predispose one to develop some chronic health problems. Activity limitations and impaired balance and mobility, for example, may contribute to injuries with long-term consequences, particularly in elderly individuals, whereas hypertension, elevated serum cholesterol, and diabetes are all physiologic factors in the development of cardiovascular disease. Diabetes also tends to increase the risk of stroke.

Obesity is a physiologic factor that can contribute to diabetes, and co-existent hypertension may increase the risk of diabetic complications such as blindness. Obesity also places greater strain on joints and may exacerbate the effects of arthritis on affected joints.

Past infection may also be implicated in the development of some chronic conditions. For example, viral infection is suspected as a contributing factor in both cancer and diabetes. A history of recurrent respiratory infections, particularly a history of severe viral pneumonias early in life, has been found to be associated with COPD. Respiratory allergy and asthma may also be predisposing physiologic factors in COPD, whereas viral infection may be a predisposing factor in childhood asthma. There is also some evidence to suggest that chronic *Chlamydia pneumoniae* infection may be a risk factor for coronary heart disease (Nieto, 1999). Other physiologic conditions may be complicated by the existence of chronic illnesses. For example, diabetes places both the pregnant woman and her child at increased risk of adverse outcomes (National Diabetes Information Clearinghouse, 2000). Conversely, pregnancy complicates diabetes control.

In addition to assessing individual clients for the presence of physiologic risk factors for chronic health problems, the community health nurse examines the incidence and prevalence of these risk factors in the general population to determine the potential for chronic health problems in the community. The nurse also assesses individual clients and groups of people for indications of existing chronic health problems. Finally, the nurse assesses clients with existing chronic conditions for evidence of related physical effects. Assessment considera-

tions related to physiologic risk factors, signs and symptoms of existing chronic conditions, and evidence of physical problems related to selected conditions are summarized in Table 29–2 ■.

Psychological Considerations

The major psychological factor contributing to chronic health problems is stress. Stress can result in carelessness and contribute to accidents that lead to chronic disability. Similarly, stress has been implicated as a contributing factor in the development of cancer and cardiovascular disease. Stress may also lead to poor compliance with control measures in persons with diabetes, resulting in diabetic complications. Depression and anxiety have also been associated with the onset of cardiovascular disease and with coronary heart disease survival. Conversely, myocardial infarction increases one's risk for major depressive disorder (Neugebauer, 1999). Similarly, bereavement due to the loss of a child has been linked to the development of some cancers and with increased cancer mortality when diagnosis occurs before the loss, but not afterwards (Levav et al., 2000).

In addition to assessing individual clients for levels and sources of stress and the adequacy of their coping mechanisms, the community health nurse assesses the psychological effects of chronic health problems on persons experiencing them. Psychological effects of chronic and debilitating conditions occur in response to perceived loss. Aspects of loss and considerations in dealing with them are addressed in the discussion of tertiary prevention of chronic physical health problems.

Physical Environmental Considerations

Physical environmental factors contribute to chronic health problems such as long-term sequelae of accidents, cancer, and COPD. Road conditions, weather, dangerous conditions for swimming, and other physical safety hazards can contribute to accidents that result in permanent physical disability, and the nurse assesses the existence of these types of hazardous conditions in the community.

The community health nurse also assesses the environment for pollutants that may be carcinogenic. Air pollution, in particular, contributes to COPD and asthma. Other environmental factors that may influence chronic respiratory conditions, particularly those with an allergic basis, include house dust, mites, molds, tobacco smoke, and occupational exposures to respiratory irritants. Increases in particulate matter and sulfur dioxide have been associated with increases in systolic blood pressure (Ibald-Mulli, Stieber, Wichman, Koenig, & Peters, 2001). Low-level exposures to lead have also been linked to increased hypertension in women (Korrick, Hunter, Rotnitzky, Hu, & Speizer, 1999). The effects of environmental pollution on health were addressed in more detail in Chapter 7.

Community health nurses should also be concerned with the concept of environmental justice. Many environmental hazards are located in low-income neighborhoods,

■ **TABLE 29–2   Assessment Considerations Related to Selected Chronic Physical Health Problems**

CONDITION	PHYSIOLOGIC RISK FACTORS	SIGNS AND SYMPTOMS	POTENTIAL EFFECTS
Arthritis	Previous injury, obesity	Painful, swollen joints, limited range of motion	Contractures, mobility limitations, inability to perform activities of daily living (ADLs)
Cancer	Cervical dysplasia, viral infection	Weight loss, change in bowel or bladder habits, changes in voice quality, pain, skin changes, palpable lumps or growths, persistent cough, rectal bleeding or blood in stool	Debility, pain, death
Cardiovascular disease	Hypertension, hypercholesterolemia, diabetes, atherosclerosis, obesity, infection	Chest pain, shortness of breath on exertion, fatigue, arrhythmias, elevated blood pressure, cardiac enlargement, edema	Debility, myocardial infarction, death
Cerebrovascular disease	Hypertension, atherosclerosis, congenital anomaly, heart disease, diabetes, polycythemia	Headaches, confusion, vertigo, parasthesia of extremities, transient ischemic attacks, slurred speech, weakness	Paralysis, aphasia, incontinence, death
Chronic obstructive pulmonary disease	Asthma, respiratory allergy, frequent respiratory infections	Shortness of breath on exertion, cough, weakness, weight loss, diminished libido	Debility, inability to perform ADLs, heart failure
Diabetes mellitus	Obesity, viral infection	Polyuria, polydipsia, polyphagia, weight loss, frequent infections (especially monilia)	Ketoacidosis with nausea, anorexia, vomiting, air hunger, and coma; diabetic retinopathy, poor wound healing and infection, sensory loss, postural hypotension, male impotence, nocturnal diarrhea, death
Hypertension	Atherosclerosis	Headache, blurred vision, dizziness, flushed face, fatigue, epistaxis, elevated blood pressure	Heart disease, stroke, death

further increasing the effects of poverty and other social factors on health (American Lung Association, 1999). Advocacy is required to prevent the location of hazardous industries in low-income residential areas and to promote elimination of existing hazards.

The other aspect of the physical environment related to chronic health problems is its effect on the functional abilities of persons with existing chronic conditions. From this perspective, the nurse assesses the need to adapt the environment to accommodate the needs of the client with a chronic condition. For example, does the home have a shower to make personal hygiene easier for the person with arthritis who may have difficulty getting in and out of a bathtub? Or does the home of the person with cardiovascular disease or COPD have numerous stairs that cause the individual to become short of breath? Similarly, the nurse assesses for potential barriers that limit access to community services for persons with chronic disabilities. Long distances to health care facilities that are encountered in rural environments also place clients with chronic health problems at risk for deterioration of their conditions (Davis & Magilvy, 2000).

Sociocultural Considerations

The sociocultural dimension contributes to the development of chronic health problems primarily in terms of social support for unhealthful behaviors and factors that enhance or impede access to health care. Social norms that condone or promote behaviors such as smoking, drinking alcohol, and a sedentary lifestyle contribute to the development of a variety of chronic health problems.

Social factors also include role modeling of healthful behaviors. Sociocultural dimension factors may also promote health and healthy behaviors and impede the development of chronic health problems. For example, social pressures to quit smoking may motivate many smokers to abandon their habit. Similarly, no-smoking policies in work settings have led to an overall decrease in smoking in many instances. Much of California's decrease in lung cancer deaths has been attributed to tobacco control initiatives and prohibition of smoking in all public venues (Office on Smoking and Health, 2000). The existence of strong social support networks has also been shown to reduce the risk of cardiovascular disease.

Culture may play a role in the extent of support for healthy or unhealthy behaviors that influence the development of chronic health conditions. For example, in many cultures, use of alcohol is discouraged, so the risk of chronic liver disease due to alcohol intake is reduced. Conversely, nondrinkers would not benefit from the potential positive effects of moderate alcohol intake on cardiovascular disease risk (Wannamethee & Shaper, 1999). Cultural factors may also influence compliance with treatment regimens for chronic conditions. For example, in some cultural groups, health care providers are expected to provide remedies that resolve a problem immediately and group members have difficulty conceiving of conditions that require life-long use of medications. Similarly, as discussed in Chapter 6, many cultural remedies may counteract or potentiate the effects of medications prescribed for chronic health conditions.

Social environmental factors such as low income, low education levels, and unemployment may prevent access to health care for persons who have existing chronic conditions. Lack of care leads to the development of complications that might be averted if adequate treatment and monitoring are available. These types of socioeconomic factors explain some of the differences in survival rates for members of different ethnic groups who have cancer, and particularly explain the poor survival rates of African Americans with cancer. Income may also affect health behaviors. For example, sedentary lifestyle has

been shown to be inversely related to income levels, with those at lower levels engaging in less physical activity.

Occupational factors are another element of the sociocultural dimension that can contribute to the development of chronic health problems. As noted in Chapter 24, safety hazards in the work environment can result in accidents that lead to chronic disability. Clients' occupations may also increase their potential for exposure to various carcinogens found in the workplace. Repetitive movements involved in some jobs can lead to joint injuries and subsequent arthritis. Occupations involving exposure to organic and inorganic dusts or noxious gases increase the probability of COPD, with employment in plastics factories and cotton mills particularly associated with increased incidence of COPD.

Work-related stress has also been shown to increase the risk of some chronic health problems. For example, low job control and an imbalance between effort expended and rewards achieved have been associated with coronary heart disease (Bosma, Peter, Siegrist, & Marmot, 1998).

The community health nurse assesses the jobs performed by individual clients and identifies any risk factors for chronic health problems posed by the work environment or the work performed. The nurse also assesses the community for potential occupational risk factors related to chronic health problems by determining the major employers and occupations present in the community and the types of products, services, and processes involved.

The community health nurse also assesses the social effects of chronic health problems on those clients experiencing them. For example, the nurse might note that the physical effects of arthritis or COPD may prevent clients from engaging in activities that provided them with opportunities for social interaction in the past, thus resulting in social isolation.

Legislative factors can also influence health behaviors and consequent chronic health problems. For example, smoking has been shown to decrease when cigarette prices or taxes increase. Similarly, bicycle helmet use increases when use legislation is enforced.

In addition, the nurse should assess the adequacy of the client's social support network for dealing with the problems posed by chronic health problems. Areas to be considered include those who make up a client's social support network, the assistance provided by each, the adequacy of the network for meeting the client's needs, and the extent to which the network is appropriately used. For example, the nurse might note that the client's support network is not sufficiently broad to meet his or her needs or that the client is not using the existing network as fully as possible.

CULTURAL CONSIDERATIONS

The concept of chronic diseases is difficult for members of many cultural groups to understand. It is particularly difficult for people to grasp the concept of needing to take medication for the rest of one's life as is the case in many chronic diseases. Select a cultural group in your own area whose members believe that with treatment a condition should be cured. How would you convey to them, in culturally congruent terms, the need for life-long therapy?

Behavioral Considerations

Behavioral factors are the major contributors to the development of most chronic health problems. Behavioral considerations to be assessed by the nurse include consumption patterns, exercise, and other behaviors.

Consumption Patterns

Consumption patterns that play a role in the development and course of chronic health problems include diet and the use of tobacco and alcohol. Poor dietary patterns contribute to chronic diseases such as diabetes and cardiovascular disease and to obesity, which is a risk factor for both of these conditions. According to figures from the 1999 Behavioral Risk Factor Surveillance System (BRFSS), the median prevalence of overweight in the United States was 54% (Holtzman, Powell-Griner, Bolen, & Rhodes, 2000).

Cholesterol consumption patterns are well-known correlates of cardiovascular disease, and excess blood cholesterol is a prevalent problem throughout the United States. A large percentage of the fat consumed by Americans comes from animal sources known to be high in cholesterol. In 1997, a median of 29% of people in states participating in the BRFSS reported being told that they had elevated blood cholesterol levels (Holtzman et al., 2000). In addition, as the percentage of calories derived from fat increases, intake of more healthful foods such as fruits, vegetables, and dietary sources of vitamins A and C, folates, and fiber decreases. As a result, not only does increased fat intake contribute to obesity and thereby to chronic disease, it may also contribute to a variety of dietary deficiencies.

Diet has also been implicated in the development of some forms of cancer. Baseline data for the national health objectives for 2010 indicate that only 28% of the U.S. population eats two or more servings of fruit a day, and only 36% consume less than 10% of their calories as saturated fat. Similarly, only 46% of the population meet daily dietary recommendations for calcium intake, a preventive measure for osteoporosis (USDHHS, 2000b). Other nutrients may also have protective effects. For example, consuming whole-grain products rather than refined grains may decrease the risk for diabetes (Liu et al., 2000).

Use of tobacco is another consumption pattern highly correlated with the development of a variety of chronic health problems. Worldwide, tobacco use contributed to more than 4 million deaths in 1999, and this figure is expected to increase to 10 million by 2030 (Sussman, 2000).

Tobacco use remains one of the primary behavioral factors contributing to cancer of the lungs, bladder, mouth, pharynx, larynx, and esophagus. Smoking, for example, is credited with causing 80% of deaths due to cancers of the lungs and bronchi (Office on Smoking and Health, 2000). Smoking has also been found to influence the incidence of cardiovascular disease and complications of diabetes and COPD. The association between smoking and cardiovascular disease is supported by findings that people who quit smoking reduce their risk of coronary heart disease by about half after a year of abstinence from tobacco. Smoking cessation also markedly reduces the risk of premature death in persons with existing car-

ETHICAL AWARENESS

Many chronic physical health problems are the result of personal behaviors such as smoking or not using seat belts. Others are primarily the result of conditions over which the individual has little control (e.g., pollution or an occupational exposure). Do you think that people whose conditions are the result of external factors, rather than personal behaviors, should receive priority for treatment if health care resources are not sufficient to provide care for all? Why or why not?

diovascular disease. Smoking has been found to interact with diabetes to result in greater risk of complications. Smoking is also the primary contributing factor in the development of COPD. In addition to being the single most significant factor in the development of this disease, smoking interacts with all other contributing factors to increase the potential for COPD. In the 1997 BRFSS, 23% of the U.S. population reported current smoking (Holtzman et al., 2000), and one third of more than 15,000 adolescents responding to the 1999 Youth Risk Behavior Survey (YRBS) reported current tobacco use (Kann et al., 2000).

Alcohol use also contributes to the development of certain chronic health problems and their consequences. For example, alcohol is implicated in motor vehicle accidents, bicycling accidents, fires, falls, and boating accidents, many of which result in chronic disability. Alcohol abuse also contributes to mortality due to chronic liver disease, but moderate alcohol use appears to have a protective effect for coronary heart disease regardless of the type of alcoholic beverage consumed (Wannamethee & Shaper, 1999).

In assessing the influence of consumption patterns on chronic health problems, the community health nurse identifies consumption patterns that place individuals at risk for chronic conditions. The nurse also determines the prevalence of high-risk consumption patterns in the community. In addition, the nurse explores unhealthful consumption patterns with clients who have existing chronic diseases and determines their effects on the course of the condition. For example, the nurse would determine whether a client with diabetes is adhering to a diabetic diet. The nurse also assesses for factors related to food preferences and modes of preparation that may impede adherence to special diets.

THINK ABOUT IT

Should healthful behavior be legislated (e.g., helmet-use laws, smoking prohibitions)? Why or why not?

Exercise and Leisure Activity

Exercise, or the lack of it, can influence the development and course of some chronic conditions. Exercise may enhance the control of diabetes or contribute to hypoglycemic reactions. The community health nurse should assess the extent of the diabetic client's exercise in relation to his or her dietary intake and the amount of insulin used to determine the potential for hypoglycemic reaction related to exercise.

Physical activity has also been shown to be directly related to the incidence of heart disease. Several studies have documented that adults with active lifestyles have significantly lower risk of developing heart disease than their less active contemporaries. A sedentary lifestyle, on the other hand, is closely associated with obesity, a risk factor for cardiovascular disease. In the 1997 BRFSS, more than one fourth of the U.S. adult population continued to report no leisure-time physical activity (Holtzman et al., 2000). The association of lack of exercise, obesity, and cardiovascular risk holds true for children as well as for adults.

Television viewing is frequently a component of a sedentary lifestyle and has been shown to be associated with obesity. Watching television is the third most time-consuming activity in the United States, and the typical adult watches TV an average of four hours each day. As viewing time increases, physical fitness declines. The nurse assessing an individual client or a community for risk factors related to exercise or its lack would determine the extent of regular exercise obtained by the individual or the proportion of sedentary individuals who make up the population.

Other Behaviors

Other lifestyle behaviors that might influence the development and course of chronic diseases include the practice of self-assessment behaviors for breast and testicular cancers and the use of safety devices and precautions.

Despite the advantages of early detection of breast cancer through breast self-examination, few women engage in this practice on a regular basis, and even fewer men engage in regular testicular examinations. In assessing this aspect of lifestyle and its effects on chronic health problems, the nurse would ascertain how often individual clients engage in breast or testicular self-examination. The nurse would also assess the extent to which these practices are employed within the community to determine the community's potential for increased mortality due to breast and testicular cancer.

The use of safety devices and safety precautions can prevent accidents that may result in chronic disability, and the nurse should determine the extent to which individual clients and their families practice safety measures. Are there smoke detectors in the home? Are hazardous items, such as sharp objects and poisons, stored appropriately? Is there potential for falls owing to multiple obstacles in the homes of elderly persons? Do family members consistently use seat belts? Seat belt use is an important behavioral factor in preventing motor vehicle fatalities. In the 1997 BRFSS, roughly two thirds of respondents reported consistent seat belt use (Holtzman et al., 2000). Other safety factors to be considered include the use of bicycle or motorcycle helmets, occupational safety equipment, and so on. Community health nurses would also explore the presence or absence of legislation mandating their use and the extent to which such legislation is enforced.

The community health nurse also appraises the extent to which these and similar safety conditions and practices are found in the general population or in the work setting. Are smoke detectors and sprinkler systems present in public buildings or in businesses and industries? Is seat belt use mandatory in the jurisdiction and, if so, is it enforced? Are appropriate safety equipment and safety precautions employed in work settings?

Other behaviors can contribute to or prevent skin cancer. For example, reducing direct exposure to sunlight (particularly from 10 A.M. to 4 P.M.), using sunscreen protection, and wearing a broad-brimmed hat can minimize the risk of malignant melanoma. According to the Centers for Disease Control and Prevention (2000), 70% of U.S. adults do not routinely engage in these behaviors, but 75% of children do.

Health Care System Considerations

Health care system factors may contribute to the development of chronic health problems or influence their course and consequences. The failure of health care professionals to educate their clients and the general public on the effects of diet, exercise, smoking, alcohol, and other factors in the development of chronic health problems contributes to the increased incidence of these conditions. In one study, for example, only 19% of general medical or gynecological visits included counseling related to physical activity; 23% included counseling on diet; 10% on weight reduction; and only 41% addressed smoking cessation for clients who smoked (Division of Adolescent and Community Health, 1998).

The extent of screening services for existing chronic conditions may influence their course and effects. It is estimated that diabetic screening programs, for example, detect only about half of the population affected by this disease (National Diabetes Information Clearinghouse, 2000).

The extent to which low-cost screening procedures for various forms of cancer are available varies considerably throughout the country. Although screening services may often be obtained from private health care providers, they are often costly and many low-income people are prevented from taking advantage of them.

Even in those states where screening services are provided, they may not be used effectively. In 1997, for example, a median of 77% of adult women included in the BRFSS reported having had a clinical breast examination by a health care professional in the last two years, and 75% reported having had a mammogram (Holtzman et al., 2000). Research has repeatedly shown provider recommendations regarding screening procedures is linked to seeking screening. In addition, referral to a primary care provider for clients without a regular source of health care has also increased the proportion of women who received screening for cervical cancer (Gill & McClellan, 2001).

Health care system factors influence the availability and quality of treatment obtainable for persons with chronic conditions. The aggressiveness of treatment received also affects the outcome of chronic health conditions. Some studies, for example, suggest that poorer cancer survival rates among low-income populations may be related to reduced access to care. The quality of treatment received for diabetes may also vary widely and affect the consequences of this disease. Medical technology, on the other hand, has greatly reduced mortality from cardiovascular and cerebrovascular diseases. This is largely due to a concerted effort to control hypertension, smoking, and diet.

⑥THINK ABOUT IT

What are some of the reasons for the increased prevalence of chronic physical health problems in the United States? Could the same be said of developing countries in the world?

In assessing individual and community risk for chronic health problems, the community health nurse determines the extent of preventive, diagnostic, and treatment services offered to community residents as well as their cost and accessibility. The nurse also assesses the extent to which available services are used and possible reasons for nonuse if indicated.

Risk factors related to the biophysical, psychological, physical environmental, sociocultural, behavioral, and health system dimensions all influence the development and outcomes of chronic physical health problems. Risk factors for selected chronic conditions are summarized in Appendix C, Factors in the Epidemiology of Selected Chronic Physical Health Problems. Tips for assessing risk for chronic physical health problems are presented on page 695. A Chronic Disease Risk Factor Inventory tool is also available on the companion Web site for this book.

■ DIAGNOSTIC REASONING AND CARE OF CLIENTS WITH CHRONIC PHYSICAL HEALTH PROBLEMS

Nursing diagnoses are derived from information collected relative to the incidence and prevalence of chronic health problems in the population and the factors contributing to these conditions. These diagnoses may relate to individual clients or to the general population. Examples of nursing diagnoses related to an individual client are "potential for cardiovascular disease due to smoking and sedentary lifestyle" and "uncontrolled diabetes due to inability to adhere to diabetic diet." At the group level, the nurse might derive diagnoses such as "increased prevalence of lung cancer due to smoking and occupational exposure to carcinogens." In each case, the nursing diagnosis contains a statement of the probable cause or etiology of the problem that directs interventions designed to resolve it.

■ PLANNING AND IMPLEMENTING CARE IN THE CONTROL OF CHRONIC PHYSICAL HEALTH PROBLEMS

Planning interventions related to chronic health problems for individual clients is based on the understanding of contributing factors derived from the assessment. It is particularly important to involve the client and his or her family in planning solutions to chronic health problems because the client or a significant other will probably be responsible for implementing the plan. By involving the client and members of the client's family, the nurse can tailor the plan of care to the client's circumstances. It is important to remember that the presence of a chronic health problem affects many facets of life for the client and his or her family. Effective planning accounts for these effects and minimizes the consequences of chronic illness for client and family alike.

When chronic health problems exist at the community or group level, the nurse collaborates with other members of the community to plan health programs that address the problems identified. For example, if the prevalence of cardiovascular disease is particularly high in the community, programs to prevent and control cardiovascular disease might be developed. In planning these programs, the nurse and other health planners employ the general principles of health programming discussed in Chapter 15.

Control of chronic diseases requires "complete disease management" which involves prevention, optimal self-management, and optimal professional care (Fries, Koop, Sokolov, Beadle, & Wright, 1998). Prevention, the first aspect of disease management reflects the primary prevention level of intervention. Self-management and professional care each reflect both secondary and tertiary levels of prevention.

Primary Prevention

Nursing strategies for primary prevention of chronic conditions focus on two major areas: health promotion and risk factor modification. Both aspects of primary prevention can be applied to individual clients or to population groups.

Health Promotion

General health promotion is aimed at making people healthier and reducing their chances of developing a

assessment tips assessment tips assessment tips

ASSESSING RISK FOR CHRONIC HEALTH PROBLEMS

Biophysical Considerations

- What age groups are most likely to develop the problem? What age groups will be most seriously affected?
- Are there racial or gender differences in disease incidence?
- Is there a genetic predisposition to the problem?
- Are there other physiologic conditions that increase the risk of developing the problem?
- What are the signs and symptoms of the problem?
- What are the physiologic effects of the problem? Does the problem limit functional abilities?

Psychological Considerations

- Does exposure to stress increase risk of the problem?
- What are the psychological effects of the problem?
- What is the extent of adaptation to the problem?

Physical Environmental Considerations

- Do environmental pollutants contribute to the problem?
- What effect, if any, do weather conditions have on the problem?
- Does the problem necessitate environmental changes (e.g., installation of ramps for a wheelchair)?

Sociocultural Considerations

- Do social norms support behaviors that increase the risk of developing the problem (e.g., smoking)?
- What are societal attitudes to the problem? Do they hamper control efforts? Is there social stigma attached to having the problem? What social support systems are available to people with the problem?
- Do occupational factors influence the incidence of the problem?
- Does socioeconomic status influence the effects of the problem?

- What effect, if any, do cultural beliefs and behaviors have on incidence of the problem? On treatment of the problem?
- What effect, if any, does legislation have on risk factors for the problem?

Behavioral Considerations

- Do dietary factors influence the incidence of the problem? Does having the problem necessitate dietary changes?
- Does alcohol or drug use contribute to the incidence of the problem? What effect does alcohol or drug use have on the course of the problem?
- What effect does physical activity have on the incidence of the problem?
- Does smoking contribute to the incidence of the problem?
- What effects do self-care behaviors (e.g., breast self-examination) have on the course of the problem?

Health System Considerations

- Do health system factors contribute to the development of the problem?
- What primary preventive measures are available for the problem? Are they widely used? To what extent do health care providers educate the public on primary prevention of the problem?
- Is there a screening test for the problem? If so, are persons at risk for the problem adequately screened?
- How is the problem diagnosed? Are diagnostic and treatment services for the problem available and accessible to those who need them?
- Can the problem be controlled with conventional medical therapy? Are there alternative therapies that may contribute to the control of the problem? Do alternative therapies pose health risks themselves?
- What is the attitude of health care providers to persons with the problem?

variety of health problems including chronic conditions. Health promotion at both the individual and group levels involves education for a healthier lifestyle, political activity to create conditions that promote health, and immunization for selected conditions.

EDUCATION　Health education efforts in primary prevention of chronic health problems focus on diet, exercise, and coping skills. The nurse employs the principles of health education discussed in Chapter 11 to educate both individual clients and the general public on basic nutrition and specific nutritional requirements based on age and activity level. For example, to prevent obesity the nurse would teach parents about the nutritional needs of infants and young children and encourage a well-balanced diet with minimal amounts of junk food. Similarly, the nurse would teach a pregnant woman, a nursing mother, or a physically active person about their specific nutritional needs. The nurse would also try to inform the general public about proper nutrition.

Exercise is another area in which health education may be required, and nurses would plan to inform both individual clients and the general public about the need for regular exercise. The nurse might also assist clients to plan ways to incorporate exercise into their daily routine or develop plans for exercise programs in the community or for employees of local businesses.

Teaching general coping skills is another way for community health nurses to promote health and prevent chronic health problems that are influenced by stress. In this respect, the nurse might assist a harried mother of several small children to develop ways of coping with stress, or the nurse might assist school personnel to develop a program to teach basic coping skills as part of elementary and secondary school curricula. Another approach might be to plan a program to foster adequate coping among employees of local businesses.

POLITICAL ACTIVITY Political activity related to primary prevention focuses on measures to promote access to preventive health services and to create a healthful environment. Nursing involvement in efforts at this level include planning strategies to influence health policy making discussed in Chapter 4. For example, community health nurses might campaign for better access to prenatal care for pregnant women or legislation to prevent or reduce pollution so as to prevent its contribution to chronic respiratory conditions and other chronic health problems.

Political activity by community health nurses might also be required to establish and enforce policies and legislation that foster healthful behaviors. For example, failure to enforce laws related to sale of tobacco products to minors has enabled youngsters to purchase tobacco. Conversely, enforcement of seat belt legislation has reduced motor vehicle accident fatalities by approximately 10,000 deaths per year (USDHHS, 1999).

IMMUNIZATION Although immunization is generally considered a primary preventive measure for communicable diseases, it can also serve to prevent some chronic conditions and their effects. For example, immunization of persons at risk for hepatitis B can serve to eliminate this risk factor for chronic liver disease and cirrhosis. Those clients with existing liver disease should receive pneumococcal vaccine and annual immunizations for influenza as should persons with diabetes and COPD.

Risk Factor Modification

Activities designed to eliminate or modify risk factors include quitting smoking, reducing weight, controlling hypertension, using safety and protective devices, and creating environments free of safety hazards. Additional problem-specific risk factor modification strategies include the use of aspirin to prevent myocardial infarction, hormone replacement therapy to prevent both osteoporosis and cardiovascular disease, and use of antioxidants (Nieto, 1999). Again, educational efforts by community health nurses are an important aspect of risk

factor modification, and nurses would plan to educate both individual clients and the general public about the elimination or modification of identified risk factors for chronic health problems.

SMOKING Some progress has been made in eliminating smoking as a risk factor for chronic health problems. Two general approaches have been used in this area: personal efforts and public activity. Personal efforts are designed to keep people from ever starting to smoke and encouraging smokers to quit. Among adults, these efforts have been relatively successful, and as of 1997, less than 23% of the adult population in the United States were smokers (Holtzman et al., 2000). Unfortunately, the prevalence of tobacco use among adolescents is somewhat higher, at nearly 33% in 1999 (Kann et al., 2000). Some ethnic minority groups also have higher rates of tobacco use. For example, approximately 31% of Native Americans smoke (Behavioral Surveillance Bureau, 2000).

Community health nurses can educate smokers regarding the hazards of smoking and direct them to sources of assistance to quit smoking. In addition, the community health nurse can provide support and encourage family members to support the smoker's efforts to quit. Nurses can also educate young people regarding the hazards of smoking and develop programs that discourage them from initiating the habit. Finally, nurses can educate individual clients and groups of people to eliminate other forms of tobacco use such as snuff and chewing tobacco.

Community health nurses may also be involved in political activity to limit smoking. Legislative and regulatory activities to control smoking can be of two types: legislation controlling smoking in public places and taxation of tobacco sales. In Great Britain, for example, prohibitively high taxes on cigarettes and other forms of tobacco have greatly reduced tobacco use. Legislation has also been effective in controlling smoking behavior by limiting smoking in public places (Office on Smoking and Health, 2000). Another area of public effort to reduce smoking lies in workplace restrictions, and community health nurses can be active in promoting no-smoking policies in business and industry.

OBESITY Control efforts for obesity have been less extensive than those for smoking. Health education related to caloric intake and fat consumption, particularly saturated fats, is required, and community health nurses should educate individual clients about the need to consume fewer calories and to reduce fat consumption. Dietary recommendations related to the year 2010 health objectives include reducing fat intake to less than 30% and saturated fat to less than 10% of total caloric intake (USDHHS, 2000b). Community health nurses can educate clients about reading package labels to determine the fat and caloric content of various foods. They can also inform clients about foods that are low in saturated fats and about food preparation methods that minimize fat consumption.

Development of modified food products also assists in controlling fat intake. Community health nurses can encourage the food industry to pursue research on food modification. They can also campaign for legislation to require accurate labeling of food packages and disclosure of food contents.

Regular exercise can also be emphasized as a control strategy for obesity, as well as a means of counteracting the effects of a sedentary lifestyle, itself a risk factor in many chronic conditions. Community health nurses can encourage overweight or sedentary clients to incorporate more exercise into their daily routine. Nurses may also be involved in planning exercise programs for groups of overweight or sedentary clients in the community or in work settings.

Prevention of obesity and diet modification can also help to prevent the onset of other chronic health problems. For example, decreased fat consumption and lower blood cholesterol are two of several factors contributing to the tremendous declines in cardiovascular disease mortality since 1950 (Cardiovascular Health Bureau, 1999). Prevention of obesity, weight loss, and supervised exercise programs may also help to decrease the incidence and disabling effects of arthritis (Health Care and Aging Studies Bureau, 2001).

HYPERTENSION   In addition to being a chronic condition itself, hypertension is a risk factor for several other chronic health problems and their complications. For this reason, efforts to control hypertension constitute primary prevention for cardiovascular and cerebrovascular diseases as well as for complications of diabetes. In fact, up to 50% of the decrease in stroke mortality from 1980 to 1990 is attributed to the combined effects of hypertension control and smoking cessation (Zhan, Cloutterbuck, Keshian, & Lombardi, 1998). Reductions of diastolic blood pressure by 5 to 6 mm Hg has been found to reduce stroke incidence by 35% and occurrence of myocardial infarction by 16% (Goldsmith, 2000). Hypertension control is particularly important in some segments of the population with continuing high rates of mortality from cardiovascular diseases. For example, it is estimated that control of systolic blood pressure below 140 mm Hg would decrease the incidence of coronary heart disease by 34% in African American men and 19% in women (Gillum, Mussolino, & Madans, 1998).

Community health nurses should educate individual clients and the general public regarding the effects and signs and symptoms of hypertension. They can also identify people with hypertension and be involved in planning hypertension screening programs or in referring clients with elevated blood pressures for further evaluation and treatment.

The second aspect of hypertension control is encouraging behaviors that promote control of existing hypertension. Community health nurses can educate hyperten-

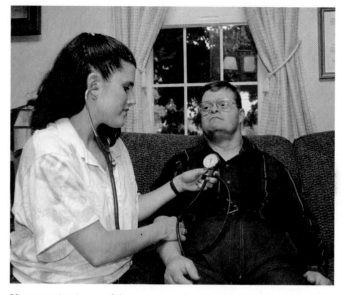

Hypertension is one of the most prevalent chronic health conditions.

sive clients on the appropriate use of antihypertensive medications and potential side effects. In addition, nurses should convey to clients the need to continue with therapy and to report any adverse effects of treatment to their primary care providers.

SAFETY PRECAUTIONS   The use of safety devices and other safety precautions can modify risk factors for accidents that may lead to chronic disability. Community health nurses can encourage clients to install smoke detectors in residences, provide adequate supervision for small children, store hazardous items appropriately, and remove hazards that promote falls for the elderly. They can also promote the use of seat belts in vehicles and campaign for legislation that makes seat belt use mandatory in all vehicles. Community health nurses can promote use of safety devices and safety precautions in the work setting to prevent accidental injury. Programs to prevent sports and occupational injuries will also help to prevent arthritis (Health Care and Aging Studies Bureau, 2001). Finally, community health nurses can motivate clients to use sunscreen and protective clothing to prevent melanoma. Primary prevention goals in the control of chronic physical health problems and related community health nursing activities are summarized in Table 29–3 ■.

⑥THINK ABOUT IT

If you could choose only one target population, what would be the "ideal" group for interventions designed to prevent chronic conditions? Why?

■ **TABLE 29-3** Goals for Primary Prevention and Related Community Health Nursing Interventions in the Control of Chronic Physical Health Problems

PRIMARY PREVENTION GOAL	NURSING INTERVENTIONS
1. Health promotion	1. Promote client health.
a. Provide prenatal care.	a. Educate clients and public about the need for prenatal care. Refer to or provide prenatal care.
b. Maintain appropriate body weight through adequate nutrition.	b. Educate clients and public about adequate nutrition.
i. Breast-feed infants.	i. Obtain diet history and identify poor food habits.
ii. Delay introduction of solid foods.	ii. Assist with breastfeeding.
iii. Avoid use of food as pacifier or reward.	iii. Assist with menu planning and budgeting.
iv. Establish healthy food habits from childhood.	iv. Refer for food-supplement plans as needed.
	v. Encourage use of nonfood reward systems.
c. Engage in graduated program of exercise.	c. Educate public about need for exercise. Assist clients to plan appropriate exercise programs.
d. Develop coping skills.	d. Teach coping skills.
2. Risk factor modification	2. Screen for risk factors. Educate public regarding risk factors.
a. Quit smoking and prevent initiation of smoking.	a. Foster self-help groups for smokers and overeaters.
	i. Educate nonsmokers about the hazards of smoking.
	ii. Promote no-smoking policies in public places and in the workplace.
b. Decrease dietary intake of saturated fats, cholesterol, sodium, and alcohol.	b. Educate and help clients plan adequate nutritional intake.
c. Identify and treat existing health problems that are risk factors for chronic illness (hypertension, obesity).	c. Screen for and refer clients with existing conditions.
	i. Educate clients regarding therapy for existing disease.
	ii. Adjust therapy to client's situation when possible.
	iii. Monitor for compliance, therapeutic effects, and side effects.
d. Eliminate environmental pollutants contributing to chronic conditions.	d. Educate public about pollution. Become politically active on environmental legislation.
e. Decrease exposure to sources of radiation (x-ray, sunlight).	e. Educate public about risks of radiation.
	i. Discourage sunbathing.
	ii. Encourage use of sunscreen and protective clothing.
f. Eliminate occupational exposure to hazardous substances.	f. Monitor occupational safety conditions.
g. Prevent occupational and sports injuries.	g. Promote occupational safety and use of protective sports equipment.
h. Eliminate or modify effects of emotional stress. Avoid stressful situations when possible.	h. Assist clients to identify stressful situations. Explore with clients ways of decreasing stress.
i. Engage in other behaviors to modify risk factors.	i. Promote other risk modification behaviors.
	i. Promote use of hormone replacement therapy.
	ii. Promote use of aspirin and antioxidants.

Secondary Prevention

Secondary prevention activities in the control of chronic illness are aimed at dealing with chronic health problems once they have occurred. The three major foci at this level of prevention are screening for existing chronic conditions, early diagnosis, and prompt treatment of these conditions.

Screening

Although the prevalence of many chronic conditions in the population has been increasing, there is less evidence of both upper and lower body limitations that may lead to disability. In all likelihood, this improvement in health status despite increased incidence of disease is due to earlier diagnosis and more effective disease management (Freedman & Martin, 2000). Screening is the first step in early diagnosis of many chronic health problems.

Screening tests are available for several chronic health problems. Pap smears, for example, are used to screen women for cervical cancer, and breast self-examination and mammography assist in early detection of breast cancer. Testicular self-examination is an equally important screening procedure for men. Early detection of colorectal cancers is assisted with annual fecal occult blood tests and digital rectal examinations. Additional screening tests that have been recommended for colorectal cancer include flexible sigmoidoscopy every five years or colonoscopy every 10 years (National Colorectal Cancer Action Campaign, 2000). Similarly, screening for prostate cancer has been recommended annually for men over 50 years of age either on a routine basis or based on provider determination of need (Steele, Miller, Maylahn, Uhler, & Baker, 2000). Dermatologic screening for skin cancers and hypertension and diabetes screenings are readily available and easily accessible in most areas.

Community health nurses play an important role in screening for chronic illness. They are conversant with the prevalence of various risk factors in the community and can plan screening programs needed to detect conditions related to the most prevalent risk factors. They may also plan to motivate client participation in screening by educating the public regarding the need for screening. Research has indicated that knowledge of risk factors alone does not motivate the general public to seek screening opportunities (Suminski et al., 1999), so motivational activities must go beyond educational campaigns. For example, community health nurses may be actively involved in referring clients for screening services and linking disease prevention to other goals valued by clients (e.g., the ability to continue working).

Interpretation of test results and referrals for further diagnosis and treatment of suspected conditions are also functions of community health nurses in secondary prevention of chronic health problems. (See Chapters 17 and 18 for recommendations for routine screening tests for men and women.) In addition to routine screening recommendations, persons with specific risk factors for chronic conditions should be screened as needed.

At the population level, community health nurses may need to advocate for available and accessible screening services for underserved segments of the population. For example, lack of health insurance and presence of fee-for-service insurance (as opposed to managed care enrollment) has been associated with lack of cancer screening in women under 65 years of age. Conversely, the combination of Medicare and supplemental insurance has been linked to cancer screening in older women (Hsia et al., 2000). Community health nurses may also need to educate and motivate providers to recommend screening procedures to their clients since provider recommendation has been shown to be a strong predictor of prostate screening in men and cervical cancer screening in women (Epidemiology Program Office, 2000; Gill & McClellan, 2001).

Early Diagnosis

The effects of many chronic health conditions can be minimized when they are diagnosed and treated early in the course of the disease. As noted earlier, positive screening test results are always an indication of a need for further diagnostic testing. Persons with obvious symptoms associated with chronic diseases should also be referred for diagnostic evaluation.

Community health nurses frequently engage in case finding with respect to chronic diseases, identifying community members with possible symptoms of disease and referring them for diagnosis and treatment as appropriate. Community health nurses are also active in educating clients and the general public regarding signs and symptoms of chronic diseases and the need for medical intervention. Community health nurses who are nurse practitioners may also be involved in making medical diagnoses of chronic illnesses.

Prompt Treatment

The third aspect of secondary prevention in the control of chronic health problems is the treatment of existing conditions. Treatment considerations in chronic conditions include stabilizing the client's condition as rapidly as possible, establishing a medical treatment regimen, promoting self-management, and preventing progression of the disease by monitoring treatment effectiveness.

STABILIZING THE CLIENT'S CONDITION   Community health nurses may need to provide emergency care to stabilize clients who are experiencing some chronic conditions. For example, the client having a heart attack may need cardiopulmonary resuscitation (CPR); emergency care is also required for the client in diabetic coma. Community health nurses may actually provide emergency care in situations of this type or may educate clients and the public in emergency care procedures. Once the client has been stabilized, the nurse would refer the client to an appropriate source of medical care.

ESTABLISHING A TREATMENT REGIMEN   The medical treatment regimen for a chronic health problem may involve medication, radiation, chemotherapy, surgery, or other types of therapy. Although nurse practitioners may be involved in providing some of these forms of care, most community health nurses are not. They are, however, involved in preparing clients for treatments both physically and psychologically, and they provide supportive measures as needed during therapy. For example, the nurse may administer intravenous pain medication to clients in the terminal stages of cancer or help clients deal with the side effects of radiation or chemotherapy.

Nurses also educate clients about their treatment and motivate them to comply with treatment recommendations. For example, community health nurses can educate clients with hypertension about antihypertensive medications and their effects and side effects as well as about diet, weight loss, and the need for continued medical supervision.

At the community level, community health nurses may be politically involved in efforts to ensure the presence and accessibility of prompt treatment for chronic conditions. They may also be involved in planning health care programs for the treatment of a variety of chronic health problems using the principles of health program planning discussed in Chapter 15.

MOTIVATING COMPLIANCE Many persons with chronic conditions are noncompliant in following prescribed recommendations. Reasons for noncompliance include inability to understand recommendations, inconvenience of required actions, disruption of lifestyle, financial or situational constraints, and lack of belief in the severity of the problem or the efficacy of treatment.

Monitoring client compliance with therapy for chronic conditions is an important community health nursing function. Identifying and eliminating factors in a client situation that promote noncompliance may foster compliance instead. Clients may be physically or mentally unable to comply with recommendations. Clients who cannot remove the childproof cap, cannot get into the tub for a sitz bath, or cannot remember to take their medication will not be compliant because of sheer inability. These are some of the considerations the nurse must make when planning to enhance client compliance with the recommended treatment plan. This is also further reason for incorporating the client and/or family members in the design of the treatment plan.

Other clients may be noncompliant because treatment requires too great an alteration in lifestyle. In this case the nurse can plan adjustments in the treatment plan to more closely fit the client's lifestyle. For example, the nurse can assist the client who has diabetes to incorporate culturally preferred foods into a diabetic diet. Research has indicated that clients themselves modify treatment regimens to better fit their lives. To do so safely and effectively, they need knowledge about areas that can reasonably be modified and areas where modifications are hazardous (Hunt et al., 1998). Examples of modifications that diabetic clients have made on their own include substitution of herbal remedies, eating less of regularly prepared foods, or eating more fruits and vegetables when they cannot afford their diabetic medications (Eid & Kraemer, 1998). People with chronic diseases may also tend to rely on medication for disease control, ignoring recommendations for behavior change intended to accompany medication use. In addition, many people may engage in both medication use and behavior change when they experience physical symptoms of disease and ignore them when they do not (Hunt et al., 1998). Clients may also alter medication regimens without consulting their health care providers or be quite irregular in their use of medications (Kyngas & Lahdenpera, 1999).

Situational constraints can also lead to noncompliance. Clients who cannot afford to purchase their medication will not take it. Lack of running water may make warm soaks difficult for the arthritic client. The effort of bringing water from a well and heating it on the stove may be more detrimental to inflamed joints than doing nothing. The nurse plans measures to eliminate situational barriers to clients' compliance with treatment plans. For example, the nurse may plan a referral to assist a client to obtain Medicaid coverage to help pay for medical expenses, or help the client plan for other ways to provide moist heat to arthritic joints.

Noncompliance may also result when the client has a vested interest in being ill. Clients who use illness to get attention or qualify for disability benefits are unlikely to comply fully with a treatment program. In such cases, community health nurses must identify the goal of the client's noncompliance. They may then be able to help the client plan other means of achieving that goal and motivate greater compliance.

Finally, lack of motivation can contribute to noncompliance. Clients may lack motivation owing to a poor self-concept or because of discouragement. The nurse, family members, and friends can help improve the client's self-concept by encouraging independence, helping the client accomplish short-term goals, and positively reinforcing accomplishments. Above all, the client must be accepted by family and friends as a unique individual worthy of respect.

Discouragement can be abated through realistic goal setting and achievement of short-term goals. Emotional support by the nurse, provided through opportunities for the client to express feelings of fear and frustration, as well as positive reinforcement of accomplishments, can help to alleviate discouragement and foster compliance. Another way to deal with this type of noncompliance is referral to an appropriate self-help group.

PROMOTING SELF-MANAGEMENT *Self-management* of chronic health problems involves handling the day-to-day treatment of the disease and its effects. Self-management involves adherence to the treatment regimen with modifications as warranted by the situation. The classical example of client self-management is the alteration of insulin dosage based on blood glucose levels, presence of illness, and so on. Clients with diabetes also engage in self-management when they increase caloric intake to cover periods of intense physical activity. Clients with other chronic conditions may also engage in self-management. For example, clients with cardiovascular disease and COPD may regulate periods of rest and physical activity on the basis of symptoms of fatigue or overexertion. Similarly, clients and/or family members may regulate use of pain medication based on need in cases of terminal illness due to cancer. Clients with arthritis or other conditions causing chronic pain may also engage in self-management of pain relief.

It is estimated that effective self-management of chronic disease can decrease health care costs by 7% to 17%. Even greater reductions in expenditures are possible when self-management or family management takes place in terminal illness. An estimated 18% of health care expenditures, for example, occur in the last year of life and involve intensive services that do not affect prognosis or comfort in terminally ill clients (Fries et al., 1998). Self-management of arthritis using the self-help course designed by the Arthritis Foundation has also been found to decrease pain and minimize the number of visits to health care providers (Health Care and Aging Studies Bureau, 2001).

Effective self-management requires knowledge and confidence on the part of clients that they can deal with most of their care themselves. Clients also need to be able to determine when self-care is not appropriate and professional care is needed. Community health nurses can educate clients regarding self-management of disease and determination of the need for professional care. Nurses may also need to motivate clients to engage in self-management as appropriate. For example, although self-monitoring of blood glucose is a standard feature of diabetes management, only 30% to 65% of clients in various surveys actually engaged in regular glucose monitoring (Division of Diabetes Translation, 2000). A description of a model for chronic illness care based on self-management is provided on the companion Web site for this book. 🌐

MONITORING TREATMENT EFFECTS The nurse involved in secondary prevention for chronic health problems also monitors clients for the presence of side effects related to treatment. For example, the nurse may note that a client is experiencing postural hypotension due to antihypertensives and will then educate the client about the need to change position gradually and will continue to monitor blood pressure levels to be sure that they do not drop too low.

At the same time, the nurse monitors the therapeutic effects of treatment. For instance, the nurse may obtain periodic blood pressure measurements for the client with hypertension. In the event the nurse determines that anti-hypertensive therapy has not noticeably affected the client's blood pressure, the nurse would make sure that the client is taking the medication appropriately and refer the client to his or her primary provider for further follow-up.

The goal of monitoring therapeutic effectiveness of interventions may also require community health nurses to advocate for routine treatment-monitoring services. For example, although effective diabetes management includes annual dilated eye examinations, foot examinations, and glycosylated hemoglobin determinations, clients with diabetes may not receive these services. In fact, in one national study, the percentage of diabetic clients who received these services ranged from a low of 17% for glycosylated hemoglobin in some areas to 81% for a dilated eye examination in others (Division of Diabetes Translation, 2000). Goals for secondary prevention of chronic physical health problems and related community health nursing interventions are summarized in Table 29–4 ■.

■ **T A B L E   2 9 – 4   Goals for Secondary Prevention and Related Community Health Nursing Interventions in the Control of Chronic Physical Health Problems**

SECONDARY PREVENTION GOAL	NURSING INTERVENTIONS
1. Screening	1. Screen for existing chronic diseases.
a. Perform periodic health examinations.	a. Educate public about need for health examinations. Provide periodic examinations.
b. Periodically screen for chronic disease.	b. Educate public about need for periodic screening. Plan and implement screening programs for high-risk groups.
2. Early diagnosis	2. Educate public about warning signs and symptoms of chronic disease.
	a. Engage in case finding and refer for diagnosis as appropriate.
	b. Prepare client for diagnostic procedures (physically and emotionally).
	c. Conduct diagnostic tests as appropriate.
3. Prompt treatment	3. Assist with management of chronic disease.
a. Stabilize condition as soon as possible.	a. Provide emergency care as needed.
	i. Educate public to provide emergency care (CPR).
	ii. Refer for further treatment.
b. Establish treatment regimen.	b. Prepare client for treatment procedures (physically and emotionally).
i. Medication	i. Carry out treatment regimen.
ii. Radiation	ii. Provide supportive measures during treatment (relief of pain).
iii. Chemotherapy	iii. Educate clients about medications: dosage, side effects, etc.
iv. Surgery	iv. Encourage client compliance with treatment.
c. Promote self-management.	c. Educate and motivate clients for self-management.
d. Prevent disease progression.	d. Monitor therapeutic effects of treatment.
	i. Monitor side effects.
	ii. Refer for follow-up as needed.

Tertiary Prevention

In tertiary prevention the aim is to promote the client's optimal level of function despite the presence of a chronic health problem. This entails preventing further loss of function in affected and unaffected systems, restoring function, monitoring health status, assisting the client to adjust to the presence of a chronic condition, and providing end-of-life care as needed.

Preventing Loss of Function in Affected Systems

Chronic health problems frequently result in some loss of function in organ systems affected by the condition, and tertiary prevention activities should be planned to prevent further loss of function in these systems. Activities may be planned to minimize losses or to eliminate risk factors that might lead to adverse consequences of the condition. Such activities on the part of the community health nurse might include motivating client compliance with treatment recommendations and assisting clients to identify and change risk factors that may lead to further loss of function. For example, the client with arthritis may be assisted to identify safety factors in the home that might contribute to falls, leading to further mobility limitation, or the client who has had a myocardial infarction may be assisted to plan a regimen of diet and exercise that will prevent future infarcts.

Preventing Loss of Function in Unaffected Systems

Chronic health problems may also result in loss of function in other physical and nonphysical systems not directly affected by the condition. For example, the client with arthritis may develop skin lesions due to limited mobility, or the client with COPD may become malnourished because meal preparation is too exhausting.

Nursing interventions will be directed toward preventing both physical and social disability. Physical complications of chronic conditions may be prevented by activities such as teaching breathing exercises to clients with COPD, providing good skin care for the client with arthritis, and teaching foot care for clients with diabetes. Clients may also need help in managing fatigue, a frequent effect of chronic health problems, particularly COPD and asthma (Small & Lamb, 1999). Prevention of additional physical effects may also entail immunization. Clients with diabetes, for example, are in particular need of influenza and pneumonia immunizations (Division of Diabetes Translation, 1999).

Nurses can also help prevent social disability by encouraging clients to interact with others, assisting clients to maintain their independence as much as possible, assisting with necessary role changes within the family, and referring the client to appropriate self-help groups. At the group level, community health nurses can work to prevent social isolation of those with chronic illnesses by advocacy and political activities to ensure access to services. They can also work to educate the public and to develop positive attitudes to persons with chronic or disabling conditions.

Restoring Function

The restoration aspect of tertiary prevention focuses on regaining as much lost function as is possible given the client's situation. Particular areas of function to be considered include bed activities, positioning, range of motion, transfer abilities, dressing, bowel and bladder control, hygiene, locomotion, and eating. Other functional considerations include vision, hearing, speech, mental ability, and capacity for social interaction. The nurse, together with the client and his or her significant others, can foster renewed abilities to perform these functions. For example, the nurse may develop a plan and teach the client and family how to reestablish bowel control following a stroke, or the nurse might assist the client with passive and active range-of-motion exercises to restore function after a broken arm has healed.

Other interventions may necessitate referral to other health care providers. For example, clients may need physical therapy to regain lost function after a stroke. Clients may also need rehabilitation services following myocardial infarction or to minimize the effects of arthritis. Community health nurses may assist individual clients to obtain these services or advocate for their availability and accessibility in the community.

Monitoring Health Status

Another aspect of tertiary prevention in the control of chronic health problems is monitoring clients' health status. The nurse would be actively involved in periodic reassessment, being particularly alert to changes in circumstances that may affect health. For example, the nurse may note that termination of unemployment benefits will limit the client's capacity to pay for health care. In this case, a referral might be made for additional financial assistance.

The nurse monitors the client's overall health status as well as the status of the chronic condition. When warranted, the nurse refers the client for medical follow-up. For example, the nurse may note that a client disabled by a serious accident is developing pressure sores due to long periods in a wheelchair. In this case, the nurse would suggest interventions to heal the pressure sores and prevent their recurrence or refer the client for medical assistance for severe lesions.

Promoting Adjustment

Clients may display one of two perspectives in their adjustment to the presence of a chronic physical health condition or may shift between them at different points in the disease experience (Paterson, 2001). In the "illness in the foreground" perspective, the client focuses on the illness and the attendant loss, suffering, and burden that accompany the illness. This perspective may be beneficial when it assists the client to conserve energy and other resources, but is self-absorbing and may interfere with interpersonal interactions. The "wellness in the foreground" perspective permits the client to focus on the positive aspects of life and state of health, but may lead to ignoring symptoms of deterioration and the need to seek professional care.

Adjustments to the presence of a chronic disease occur in both functional and psychological realms. Functional adjustments reflect changes in lifestyle necessitated by the illness. Such changes may involve diet, activity patterns, restrictions (e.g., limiting alcohol use or caloric intake), and the need to take medications. Some diseases necessitate learning special skills. For example, insulin-dependent diabetic clients need to learn to give themselves insulin injections, and hypertensive clients may need to learn how to take their blood pressure. In other chronic conditions, such as arthritis, there may be a need for special apparatus to assist in performing routine activities. The need for medication may also necessitate budgetary changes that the client must adjust to.

Psychological adjustments are also necessary. Psychological adjustment to a chronic condition may be required in a number of areas. Self-esteem is one of these areas. A chronic disease may make a client more dependent on others and less able to engage in activities that promote a positive self-image. For example, the client may need to stop working or begin to rely on others for assistance with basic functions such as eating and toileting. This dependence may be demeaning to one who has been self-reliant. The nurse should encourage the client to maintain as many functions as possible and help families to see the client's need for independence.

Loss of independence also necessitates adjustments in one's sense of control. Clients may feel they are not in control of events when the food they eat or the activities they perform are dictated in part by the chronic health problem. For some clients, noncompliance with recommendations might be an attempt to regain control over their own lives. Nurses can help prevent noncompliance by providing the client with other avenues for exercising control. Ways of doing this include involving the client in planning interventions and providing, whenever possible, choices in which the client can exercise control over actions and outcomes.

Guilt may also require adjustments in the way clients think about themselves. Because behavioral factors are widely known to make a significant contribution to the majority of chronic conditions, clients may feel guilty about behaviors that may have contributed to their current health problems. The nurse can help clients explore their feelings and assist them to turn from an irredeemable past to present behaviors that minimize the effects of health problems.

Another area that may require adjustment for clients with chronic conditions is that of intimacy. Among men, for example, some chronic conditions or their treatments may result in impotence. In other cases, pain or changes in self-image may limit a client's ability to maintain intimate relationships with others. Another potential problem may be the withdrawal of significant others. Clients and their families can be encouraged to discuss intimacy issues openly, and significant others can be assisted to find ways of fulfilling intimacy needs that are congruent with the presence of a chronic health problem.

Stigma is another psychological issue in adjustment to a chronic health problem. Many chronic health conditions are stigmatized by the general population. *Stigmatization* is a social process of attaching meaning to behavior and individuals on the basis of certain traits or characteristics. Stigmatization tends to occur in response to three types of attributes: physical deformities, character blemishes, and tribal stigma based on race or religion (Joachim & Acorn, 2000). Some chronic health conditions create visible physical evidence, such as the malformed joints often seen in arthritis or the need to use a wheelchair or other assistive devices. Knowledge of others, such as seizure disorder or mental retardation, may be perceived as evidence of inferiority.

Clients with visible evidence of disease may attempt to deal with stigma by minimizing the perceived consequences of the disease or covering them up as much as possible while still acknowledging their existence. Those whose condition is invisible are faced with decisions of whether to disclose their chronic illness, how much to disclose, and to whom. Clients who fear rejection on the basis of stigma attached to the disease may attempt to pass themselves off as healthy, but then endure the stress of possible discovery and loss of credibility as well as rejection (Joachim & Acorn, 2000). Community health nurses can assist clients to deal with perceptions of stigma and to make decisions regarding disclosure. For clients suffering from the psychological effects of stigmatization, referrals for counseling services may be warranted. Nurses may also engage in public education campaigns to diminish the stigma attached to certain chronic conditions.

In caring for clients who have chronic illnesses, the nurse must plan to assist them to return to a normal level of functioning as far as this is possible. In addition to the assistance of the nurse, it may be appropriate to refer the client to a relevant self-help group. Self-help groups can be particularly helpful in dealing with the psychosocial adjustments required by a chronic condition. Clients may be able to relate better to persons experiencing similar problems than to the authority figures represented by health care professionals.

Referral to self-help groups and other assistance may also be needed for family members who experience caregiver burden. *Caregiver burden* is the effect of the stress of caring for a family member with a physical or mental illness on those providing the care (Faison, Faria, & Frank, 1999). Caregiver burden can stem from the extent of care required or from behaviors exhibited by the family member receiving care. For example, caregivers in one study experienced significant depression, particularly when the person to whom care was given exhibited behavioral disturbances. In this study it was unclear whether the depression stemmed from the difficulty of dealing with the behavior disturbance or behavior disturbance occurred because depression prevented the caretaker from providing adequate care (Washio & Arai, 1999). In either event, the caretakers were, themselves, in need of assistance. For an insightful description of caregiver burden, see the summary of an article provided on the companion Web site for this book. 🌐

Community health nurses can refer clients and caregivers to self-help groups or other community agencies that provide assistance in dealing with problems arising from chronic health conditions. Community health nurses should determine the availability of such agencies within their own communities and identify the services provided and eligibility requirements for each type of service so as to make appropriate referrals. Links to some of the resources nurses might use in assisting clients with chronic diseases are provided on the companion Web site for this book. 🌐

End-of-Life Care

A few chronic physical health problems are terminal in nature, and community health nurses may be involved in providing care to clients who are facing death and to their families. Recent literature contends that nurses are often ill-prepared to provide end-of-life care and that certain core competencies are required for effective care of dying clients and their families (White, Coyne, & Patel, 2001). These competencies are summarized below.

HIGHLIGHTS

Core Competencies for End-of-Life Care

- Ability to talk with clients and their families about dying
- Effective pain control
- Comfort care
- Palliative care
- Ability to recognize impending death
- Ability to deal with one's own feelings
- Ability to deal with anger expressed by clients and families
- Knowledge of legal and ethical issues in palliative care
- Knowledge about advance directives and their support
- Ability to incorporate religious and cultural beliefs and values
- Knowledge of hospice services

Source: White, K. R., Coyne, P. J., & Patel, U. B. (2001). Are nurses adequately prepared for end-of-life care? *Journal of Nursing Scholarship, 33,* 147–151.

Tertiary prevention related to individuals with chronic health problems focuses on assisting clients to adjust to their condition and on preventing additional problems. Tertiary prevention at the community level might involve planning and implementing programs to assist with client adjustment or political activity to ensure the availability of tertiary prevention programs. Tertiary prevention goals and related nursing interventions are summarized in Table 29–5 ■.

EVALUATING CARE OF CLIENTS WITH CHRONIC PHYSICAL HEALTH PROBLEMS

Evaluating care related to chronic health problems is done in terms of care outcomes. Care may be evaluated in relation to the individual client or to a population group. In the case of the individual client, the nurse evaluates the status of the chronic condition as well as the client's adjustment to having a chronic health problem. If interventions, both medical and nursing, have been effective, the condition will be controlled or may even be improving. Failing improvement, the condition will provide the least disruption possible to the life of the client and his or her significant others. Evaluative criteria reflect both the client's physiologic status and his or her quality of life.

When the recipient of care is a community or population group, evidence of success in controlling chronic health problems lies primarily in changes in morbidity and mortality figures. Are there fewer cases of hypertension or cardiovascular disease in the population now than before the initiation of control efforts? Are there fewer disabilities due to accidental injuries? Do those individuals with diabetes live longer or have fewer hospitalizations for diabetic complications? Based on the evaluative data, decisions can be made regarding the need to attempt other control strategies or to continue with current measures.

Evaluation of population-based control strategies may focus on the status of national objectives for 2010 for selected chronic diseases. Baseline and target information for several of these objectives is presented on page 706.

Chronic physical health problems have largely replaced communicable diseases as the major contributors to death and disability in developed countries. Significant morbidity and mortality due to chronic physical conditions is also seen throughout the world. Community health nurses are actively involved in efforts to educate the public to prevent these diseases as well as in the design and implementation of programs to provide diagnostic, treatment, and support services for persons with existing disease.

■ **T A B L E   29–5**   **Goals for Tertiary Prevention and Related Community Health Nursing Interventions in the Control of Chronic Physical Health Problems**

TERTIARY PREVENTION GOAL	NURSING INTERVENTIONS
1. Preventing further loss of function in affected systems Decrease risk factors for recurrence, exacerbation, or development of crises.	1. Motivate client to comply with treatment regimen. Assist client to identify risk factors amenable to change. Assist client to identify ways of decreasing risk factors.
2. Preventing loss of function in unaffected systems a. Prevent physical disability.	2. Assist client to maintain function in unaffected systems. a. Prevent physical complications of illness through: i. Breathing exercises ii. Skin care iii. Range-of-motion exercises iv. Adequate nutrition and fluids Provide physical care as required. Refer for assistance with physical care as needed
b. Prevent social disability.	b. Accept client as a unique person. Encourage interaction with others. Assist significant others to deal with feelings about client's illness. Assist client to maintain independence as much as possible. Assist with identification of need for changes in family roles. Work to change public attitudes toward the disabled. Promote legislation to aid chronically ill to maintain their independence.
3. Restoring function	3. Assist with planning and implementation of programs to regain function (bowel training, physical therapy). Teach client and others to carry out program and evaluate effects.
4. Monitoring health status	4. Monitor client health status. Identify changes in client situation that affect health. Refer for follow-up as appropriate.
5. Promoting adjustment a. Deal with feelings about disease.	5. Assist client to adjust to presence of chronic disease. a. Accept client at his or her level of development and acceptance of disease. Encourage client to discuss fears and apprehensions. Refer to self-help groups as appropriate.
b. Adjust lifestyle to accommodate chronic disease and its effects. c. Adjust environment to meet changed needs.	b. Assist client to identify needed changes in lifestyle. Assist client to plan and carry out lifestyle changes. c. Identify need for self-help devices and help client obtain them. Identify environmental changes needed to foster independence. Assist client to make necessary environmental changes.
d. Adjust self-image.	d. Assist client to adjust to change in self-image. Refer for counseling as needed.
e. Adjust to expense of chronic care. f. Deal with stigma.	e. Refer for financial aid as needed. f. Assist with decisions regarding disclosure. Assist client to cope with effects of stigma. Educate public to minimize stigma.
6. Adjusting to death	6. Provide end-of-life care. a. Pain management b. Comfort care c. Palliative care d. Encouraging advance directives e. Referral to hospice services as needed

HEALTHY PEOPLE 2010

GOALS FOR THE POPULATION

Objective	Base	Target
2-2 Reduce the proportion of adults with chronic joint symptoms with limitation in activity	27%	21%
2-9 Reduce the overall number of cases of osteoporosis in adults	10%	8%
4-4 Reduce the rate of new cases of end-stage renal disease (per million population)	289	217
4-7 Reduce kidney failure due to diabetes (per million population)	113	78
5-2 Prevent diabetes (new cases per 1,000 population)	3.1	2.5
5-5 Reduce the diabetes death rate (per 100,000 population)	75	45
5-7 Reduce deaths from cardiovascular disease in persons with diabetes (per 100,000 persons with diabetes)	343	309
6-4 Increase the proportion of adults with disabilities who participate in social activities	95.4%	100%
6-6 Increase the proportion of adults with disabilities reporting satisfaction with life	87%	96%
12-1 Reduce coronary heart disease deaths (per 100,000 population)	205	166
12-7 Reduce stroke deaths (per 100,000 population)	60	48
12-9 Reduce the proportion of adults with high blood pressure	28%	16%
12-10 Increase the proportion of adults with high blood pressure whose blood pressure is under control	18%	50%
12-14 Reduce the proportion of adults with high total blood cholesterol levels	21%	17%
19-1 Increase the proportion of adults who are at a healthy weight	42%	60%
22-1 Reduce the proportion of adults who engage in no leisure time physical activity	40%	20%
24-1 Reduce activity limitations among persons with asthma	19.5%	10%
24-9 Reduce the proportion of adults with activity limitations due to chronic lung and breathing problems	2.2%	1.5%
27-1a Reduce cigarette smoking by adults	24%	12%
27-2b Reduce cigarette smoking by adolescents	36%	16%

Source: U.S. Department of Health and Human Services. (2000). *Healthy people 2010* (Conference edition, in two volumes). Washington, DC: Author.

APPLYING YOUR KNOWLEDGE IN PRACTICE

✷ CASE STUDY
A Chronic Physical Health Problem

You have just started working as a community health nurse for the Wachita County Health Department in Mississippi. During your employment interview, the nursing supervisor mentioned that one of your responsibilities would be to participate in developing plans for dealing with the high rate of hypertension in the county. The incidence rate for hypertension here is three times that of the state and twice that of the nation. The population of the county is largely African American, with high unemployment rates and little health insurance. Folk health practices are quite common, one of them being drinking pickle brine for a condition called "high blood." Although this condition is not related to high blood pressure, the two terms are frequently confused by lay members of the community and professionals alike. Dietary intake is typical of the rural South, consisting of a variety of fried foods, beans and other boiled vegetables, and corn bread.

Few health services are available in the county itself, although there is a major hospital 50 miles away. There are two general practitioners in the area and one pediatrician. The health department holds well-child, immunization, tuberculosis, and family planning clin-

ics regularly, and all are well attended. Transportation is a problem for many community residents.

- What are the biophysical, psychological, physical environmental, sociocultural, behavioral, and health system factors influencing the incidence and prevalence of hypertension in this county?
- Write two objectives for your efforts to resolve the county's problem with hypertension.
- What primary, secondary, and tertiary prevention activities might be appropriate in dealing with the problem of hypertension? Which of these activities might you carry out yourself? Which would require collaboration with other community members? Who might these other people be?
- How would you evaluate the outcome of your interventions?

❧ TESTING YOUR UNDERSTANDING

- What are some of the personal effects and population effects of chronic physical health problems? (pp. 684–687)
- What are some of the biophysical, psychological, physical environmental, sociocultural, behavioral, and health system factors that influence the development of chronic physical health problems? Do these factors differ among chronic diseases? (pp. 688–694)
- What are the major strategies for primary prevention of chronic physical health problems? Give an

example of an activity that a community health nurse might perform in relation to each. (pp. 694–698)

- Identify at least three aspects of the treatment of chronic physical health problems. What is the role of the community health nurse with respect to each? (pp. 698–701)
- What are the major considerations in tertiary prevention of chronic physical health problems? How might a community health nurse be involved in each? (pp. 702–704)

REFERENCES

American Lung Association. (1999, spring/summer). American Lung Association focuses on environmental justice as asthma rates soar in low-income neighborhoods. *Breathe Easy, 1.*

Behavioral Surveillance Bureau. (2000). Prevalence of selected risk factors for chronic disease and injury among American Indians and Alaskan Natives—United States, 1995–1998. *Morbidity and Mortality Weekly Report, 49,* 79–82.

Blaha, C., Robinson, J. M., Pugh, L. C., Bryan, Y., & Havens, D. S. (2000). Longitudinal nursing case management for elderly heart failure patients: Notes from the field. *Nursing Case Management, 5*(1), 32–36.

Bosma, H., Peter, R., Siegrist, J., & Marmot, M. (1998). Two alternative job stress models and the risk of coronary heart disease. *American Journal of Public Health, 88,* 68–74.

Boyle, R. G., O'Connor, J., Pronk, N., & Tan, A. (1998). Stages of change for physical activity, diet, and smoking among HMO members

with chronic conditions. *American Journal of Health Promotion, 12,* 170–175.

Cardiovascular Health Bureau. (1998a). Change in mortality from heart failure—United States, 1980–1995. *Morbidity and Mortality Weekly Report, 47,* 633–637.

Cardiovascular Health Bureau. (1998b). Trends in ischemic heart disease death rates for blacks and whites—United States, 1981–1995. *Morbidity and Mortality Weekly Report, 47,* 945–949.

Cardiovascular Health Bureau. (1999). Declines in deaths from heart disease and stroke—United States, 1900–1999. *Morbidity and Mortality Weekly Report, 48,* 649–656.

Cardiovascular Health Bureau. (2000a). Age-specific excess deaths associated with stroke among racial/ethnic minority populations—United States, 1997. *Morbidity and Mortality Weekly Report, 49,* 94–97.

Cardiovascular Health Bureau. (2000b). Prevalence of selected cardiovascular disease risk factors among American Indians

and Alaska Natives—United States, 1997. *Morbidity and Mortality Weekly Report, 49,* 461–465.

Centers for Disease Control and Prevention. (2000). *Preventing skin cancer: The nation's most common cancer.* Retrieved April 30, 2001, from the World Wide Web, *http://www.cdc.gov/cancer.*

Centers for Disease Control and Prevention. (2001). American Heart Month—February 2001. *Morbidity and Mortality Weekly Report, 50,* 89.

Davis, R., & Magilvy, J. K. (2000). Quiet pride: The experience of chronic illness by rural older adults. *Journal of Nursing Scholarship, 32,* 385–390.

Division of Adolescent and Community Health. (1998). Missed opportunities in preventive counseling for cardiovascular diseases—United States, 1995. *Morbidity and Mortality Weekly Report, 47,* 91–95.

Division of Diabetes Translation. (1999). Diabetes preventive-care practices in managed-care organizations—Rhode Island, 1995–1996. *Morbidity and Mortality Weekly Report, 48,* 958–961.

Division of Diabetes Translation. (2000). Levels of diabetes-related preventive-care practices—United States, 1997–1999. *Morbidity and Mortality Weekly Report, 49,* 954–958.

Eid, J., & Kraemer, H. (1998). Mexican-American experience with diabetes. *Journal of Nursing Scholarship, 30,* 393.

Elder, N. C., & Muench, J. (2000). Diabetes care as public health. *Journal of Family Practice, 49,* 513–514.

Epidemiology Program Office. (2000). Screening with prostate-specific antigen test—Texas, 1997. *Morbidity and Mortality Weekly Report, 49,* 818–820.

Faison, K. J., Faria, S. H., & Frank, D. (1999). Caregivers of chronically ill elderly: Perceived burden. *Journal of Community Health Nursing, 16,* 243–253.

Freedman, V., & Martin, L. G. (2000). Contribution of chronic conditions to aggregate changes in old-age functioning. *American Journal of Public Health, 90,* 1755–1760.

Fries, J. F., Koop, C. E., Sokolov, J., Beadle, C. E., & Wright, D. (1998). Beyond health promotion: Reducing need and demand for medical care. *Health Affairs, 17,* 70–84.

Gill, J. M., & McClellan, S. A. (2001). The impact of a referral to a primary physician on cervical cancer screening. *American Journal of Public Health, 91,* 451–454.

Gillum, R. F., Mussolino, M. E., & Madans, J. H. (1998). Coronary heart disease risk factors and attributable risks in African-American women and men: NHANES I epidemiologic follow-up study. *American Journal of Public Health, 88,* 913–917.

Goldsmith, C. (2000). Hypertension: Still the silent killer. *NurseWeek, 13*(5), 16–17.

Grant, E. N., Lyttle, C. S., & Weiss, K. B. (2000). The relation of socioeconomic factors and racial/ethnic differences in US asthma mortality. *American Journal of Public Health, 90,* 1923–1925.

Health Care and Aging Studies Bureau. (1999). Impact of arthritis and other rheumatic conditions on the health care system—United States, 1997. *Morbidity and Mortality Weekly Report, 48,* 349–353.

Health Care and Aging Studies Bureau. (2000). Health-related quality of life among adults with arthritis—Behavioral Risk Factor Surveillance System, 11 states, 1996–1998. *Morbidity and Mortality Weekly Report, 49,* 366–369.

Health Care and Aging Studies Bureau. (2001). Prevalence of arthritis—United States, 1997. *Morbidity and Mortality Weekly Report, 50,* 334–336.

Holtzman, D., Powell-Griner, E., Bolen, J. C., & Rhodes, L. (2000). State- and sex-specific prevalence of selected characteristics—Behavioral Risk Factor Surveillance System, 1996 and 1997. *Morbidity and Mortality Weekly Report, 49*(SS-6), 1–39.

Hsia, J., Kemper, E., Kiefe, C., Zapka, J., et al. (2000). The importance of health insurance as a determinant of cancer screening: Evidence from the Women's Health Initiative. *Preventive Medicine, 31,* 261–270.

Hunt, L. M., Pugh, J., & Valenzuela, M. (1998). How patients adapt diabetes self-care rec-

ommendations in everyday life. *Journal of Family Practice, 46,* 207–215.

Ibald-Mulli, A., Stieber, J., Wichman, H. E., Koenig, W., & Peters, A. (2001). Effects of air pollution on blood pressure: A population-based approach. *American Journal of Public Health, 91,* 571–577.

Jajosky, R. A. R., Harrison, R., Reinisch, F., Flattery, J., et al. (1999). Surveillance of work-related asthma in selected U.S. states using surveillance guidelines for state health departments—California, Massachusetts, Michigan, and New Jersey. *Morbidity and Mortality Weekly Report, 48*(SS-3), 1–20.

Joachim, G., & Acorn, S. (2000). Stigma of visible and invisible chronic conditions. *Journal of Advanced Nursing, 32,* 243–248.

Joslyn, E. (1999). Disability and health care expenditure data: A wide range of user experience is more important than standard definitions of disability. *Disability and Rehabilitation, 21,* 382–384.

Juvenile Diabetes Foundation International. (1998). *Diabetes facts.* Retrieved April 22, 2001, from the World Wide Web, http://www.jdfcure.org.

Kann, L., Kinchen, S. A., Williams, B. I., Ross, J. G., et al. (2000). Youth risk behavior surveillance—United States, 1999. *Morbidity and Mortality Weekly Report, 49*(SS-5), 1–94.

Korrick, S. A., Hunter, D. J., Rotnitzky, A., Hu, H., & Speizer, F. E. (1999). Lead and hypertension in a sample of middle-aged women. *American Journal of Public Health, 89,* 330–335.

Kyngas, H., & Lahdenpera, T. (1999). Compliance of patients with hypertension and associated factors. *Journal of Advanced Nursing, 29,* 832–839.

Larson, P. D. (1998). Rehabilitation. In I. M. Lubkin & P. D. Larson (Eds.), *Chronic illness: Impact and interventions* (4th ed.) (pp. 528–547). Boston: Jones and Bartlett.

Lawson, H. W., Henson, R., Bobo, J. K., & Kaeser, M. K. (2000). Implementing recommendations for the early detection of breast and cervical cancer among low-income women. *Morbidity and Mortality Weekly Report, 49*(RR-2) 37–55.

Levav, I., Kohn, R., Iscovich, J., Abramson, J. H., Tsai, W. Y., & Vigdorovich. (2000). Cancer incidence and survival following bereavement. *American Journal of Public Health, 90,* 1601–1607.

Liu, S., Manson, J. E., Stampfer, M. J., Hu, F. B., et al. (2000). A prospective study of whole-grain intake and risk of type 2 diabetes mellitus in US women. *American Journal of Public Health, 90,* 1409–1415.

Mannino, D. M., Homa, D. M., Pertowski, C. A., Ashizawa, S., et al. (1998). Surveillance for asthma—United States, 1960–1995. *Morbidity and Mortality Weekly Report, 47*(SS-1) 1–27.

National Center for Chronic Disease Prevention and Health Promotion. (1999). *Statistics: Diabetes surveillance, 1999.* Retrieved April 22, 2001, from the World Wide Web, http://www.cdc.gov/diabetes/statistics/surv1999.

National Center for Chronic Disease Prevention and Health Promotion. (2000). *Prostate cancer: Can we reduce deaths and preserve quality of life?* Retrieved April 30, 2001, from the

World Wide Web, http://www.cdc.gov/cancer/prostate.

National Center for Environmental Health. (1998). Forecasted state-specific estimates of self-reported asthma prevalence—United States, 1998. *Morbidity and Mortality Weekly Report, 47,* 1022–1025.

National Colorectal Cancer Action Campaign. (2000). *Colorectal cancer: Health professionals facts on screening.* Washington, DC: Centers for Disease Control and Prevention.

National Diabetes Information Clearinghouse. (2000). Why November is National Diabetes Month: The disturbing statistics behind diabetes. *Gourmet Connection.* Retrieved April 22, 2001, from the World Wide Web, http://www.gourmetconnection.com.

National Diabetes Information Clearinghouse. (2001). *Diabetes statistics.* Retrieved April 22, 2001, from the World Wide Web, http://niddk.nih.gov/health/diabetes.

National Organization on Disability. (2000). *The 2000 N.O.D./Harris survey of Americans with disabilities.* Retrieved September 19, 2000, from the World Wide Web, http://www.nod.org/hs2000.

Neugebauer, R. (1999). Mind matters: The importance of mental disorders in public health's 21st century mission. *American Journal of Public Health, 89,* 1309–1311.

Newacheck, P. W., & Halfon, N. (1998). Prevalence and impact of disabling chronic conditions in childhood. *American Journal of Public Health, 88,* 610–617.

Nieto, F. J. (1999). Cardiovascular disease and risk factor epidemiology: A look back at the epidemic of the 20th century. *American Journal of Public Health, 89,* 292–293.

Office on Smoking and Health. (2000). Declines in lung cancer rates—California, 1988–1997. *Morbidity and Mortality Weekly Report, 49,* 1066–1069.

Paterson, B. L. (2001). The shifting perspectives model of chronic illness. *Journal of Nursing Scholarship, 33,* 21–26.

Phillips, J. M., Cohen, M. Z., & Tarzian, A. J. (2001). African American women's experiences with breast cancer screening. *Journal of Nursing Scholarship, 33,* 135–140.

Small, S., & Lamb, M. (1999). Fatigue in chronic illness: The experience of individuals with chronic obstructive pulmonary disease and with asthma. *Journal of Advanced Nursing, 30,* 469–478.

Steele, C. B., Miller, D. S., Maylahn, C., Uhler, R. J., & Baker, C. T. (2000). Knowledge, attitudes, and screening practices among older men regarding prostate cancer. *American Journal of Public Health, 90,* 1595–1600.

Suminski, R. R., Anding, J., Smith, D. W., Zhang, J. J., Utter, A. C., & Kang, J. (1999). Risk and reality: The association between cardiovascular disease risk factor knowledge and selected risk-reducing behaviors. *Family and Community Health, 21*(4), 51–62.

Sussman, D. (2000). Going beyond Joe Camel. *NurseWeek, 13*(5), 14.

Tierney, E. F., Geiss, L. S., Engelgau, M., Thompson, T., et al. (2001). Population-based estimates of mortality associated with diabetes: Use of a death certificate check box in North Dakota. *American Journal of Public Health, 91,* 84–92.

U.S. Census Bureau. (1999). *Statistical abstract of the United States, 1999* (119th ed.). Washington, DC: Author.

U.S. Department of Health and Human Services. (1999). Seat belts still save lives. *Prevention Report, 14*(3), 1–2.

U.S. Department of Health and Human Services. (2000a). *Health United States, 2000.* Washington, DC: Author.

U.S. Department of Health and Human Services. (2000b). *Healthy people 2010* (Conference edition in two volumes). Washington, DC: Author.

Ustun, T. B. (1999). The global burden of mental disorders. *American Journal of Public Health, 89,* 1315–1318.

Valdmanis, V., Smith, D. W., & Page, M. R. (2001). Productivity and economic burden associated with diabetes. *American Journal of Public Health, 91,* 129–130.

Wannamethee, S. G., & Shaper, A. G. (1999). Type of alcoholic drink and risk of major coronary heart disease events and all-cause mortality. *American Journal of Public Health, 89,* 685–690.

Washio, M., & Arai, Y. (1999). Depression among caregivers of the disabled elderly in southern Japan. *Psychiatry and Clinical Neurosciences, 53,* 407–412.

White, K. R., Coyne, P. J., & Patel, U. B. (2001). Are nurses adequately prepared for end-of-life care? *Journal of Nursing Scholarship, 33,* 147–151.

Wingo, P. A., Ries, L. A. G., Rosenberg, H. M., Miller, D. S., & Edwards, B. K. (1998). *Cancer incidence and mortality, 1973–1995, A report card for the U.S.* Atlanta, GA: American Cancer Society.

Zhan, L., Cloutterbuck, J., Keshian, J., & Lombardi, L. (1998). Promoting health: Perspectives from ethnic elderly women. *Journal of Community Health Nursing, 15*(1), 31–44.

COMMUNITY MENTAL HEALTH PROBLEMS

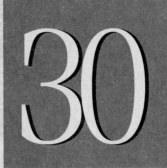

Chapter Objectives

After reading this chapter, you should be able to

■ Discuss the personal and societal impact of mental illness and mental health problems.
■ Describe factors influencing the development of mental health problems.
■ Identify symptoms characteristic of selected mental health problems.
■ Discuss strategies for preventing mental health problems.
■ Discuss approaches to treatment of mental health problems and the community health nurse's role in each.
■ Describe areas of emphasis in maintenance therapy for mental health problems.

KEY TERMS

Media Link

http://www.prenhall.com/clark

Additional interactive resources for this chapter can be found on the companion Web site. Click on Chapter 30 and "Begin" to select the activities for this chapter.

Mental illness is a growing problem throughout the world and community health nurses may often find themselves involved in efforts to promote mental health and prevent mental illness as well as activities required for the treatment of clients with mental illness. *Mental health* is the ability to successfully perform mental functions, to engage in productive activities and meaningful interpersonal relationships, and to adapt to change and cope with adversity. *Mental illness,* on the other hand, encompasses a wide variety of diagnosable mental disorders characterized by changes in thinking, mood, or behavior associated with stress or impaired function. *Mental health problems* involve signs and symptoms of mental distress that are of insufficient duration or intensity to qualify as mental disorders diagnosed on the basis of accepted criteria (U.S. Public Health Service [USPHS], 1999). In this chapter we use the term mental health problems to refer to the composite of conditions that result in impaired function.

THE EFFECTS OF MENTAL HEALTH PROBLEMS

Mental health problems have burdensome effects for individuals and their families as well as for society as a whole. Some of these effects will be presented here.

Personal Effects

Suffering and disability are the two most prominent effects of mental health problems for the individuals they affect. There is no objective measure of the suffering endured, but measures of disability are discouraging. Approximately 20% of the U.S. population is affected by mental illness in any given year, and 44 million people have diagnosable mental disorders. Among these, 19% have a mental disorder alone, 6% have addictive disorders alone, and 3% experience both mental and addictive disorders. Approximately 9% of the population have significant functional impairment due to mental illness, and for 7% of people, this impairment lasts for more than a year (USPHS, 1999).

Schizophrenia, one of the most disabling of mental disorders, affects 1% of the world's population and 2.5 million people in the United States. Schizophrenia accounts for 10% of permanently and totally disabled people and contributes to 20% to 30% of homelessness in the United States (Lehman, 1999). According to the National Comorbidity Study, 17% of the U.S. population had experienced a major depressive disorder at some time in the past, and 10% had experienced one or more major depressive episodes in the previous year (Neugebauer, 1999). Worldwide, the extent of disability due to major depression equals that caused by blindness or paraplegia; the extent of disability due to schizophrenia is similar to that caused by paraplegia and quadriplegia. Overall, depressive disorders outranked all other mental and

physical conditions in the number of years lived with disability (Ustun, 1999).

THINK ABOUT IT

Discuss the possible relationships between homelessness and mental health problems.

In one study, clients with depression enrolled in managed care plans had poorer mental, role, and social function than those with chronic physical health problems. When clients had both chronic medical problems and depression, their level of function was even worse (Wells & Sherbourne, 1999). Mental health problems not only result in mental disability, but they also cause physical and social impairments. In one study, for example, depressed elderly clients were 1.6 times more likely than the nondepressed to experience disability related to performance of activities of daily living (ADLs) and 1.7 times more likely to have mobility limitations (Penninx, Leveille, Ferrucci, van Eijk, & Guralnik, 1999).

Family Effects

Mental health problems also exact a toll on the families of people that experience them. The family costs of mental disorders are both economic and emotional. In Chapter 19, we reviewed the effects of caregiving for family members with Alzheimer's disease. Other chronic mental health problems also have family effects. For example, many caregivers for persons with schizophrenia are aging parents. In one study in the United States, caregivers spent up to 15 hours a week caring for family members with schizophrenia, with average annual expenditures of $3,540 for care. In another study in the United Kingdom, one in 10 families experienced financial difficulties stemming from the care of clients with schizophrenia (Frangou & Murray, 2000). Because health insurance usually provides minimal reimbursement for mental health services, much of the financial burden of care is borne by family members.

Clients with mental illness may have difficulty holding a job because of the impairments resulting from their conditions. Unemployment and underemployment may lead to poverty for the individual and the family (Lehman, 1999). In addition, family caretakers may be forced to take time from work or even stop working, further diminishing family income.

Major mental disorders may prevent family members from carrying out their expected family roles. Mental illness in a family member also increases stress for the entire family and may contribute to family communication problems and perceptions of social stigma for both client and family.

Societal Effects

Mental illness and less severe mental health problems also pose a burden for society in general. Mental disorders are the leading cause of disability in the world (Norquist & Hyman, 1999), and overall accounted for 9.7% of the global disease burden (Ustun, 1999).

According to the World Health Organization (1999), neuropsychiatric conditions (which include substance abuse disorders) account for 10% of the global burden of disease, as measured by disability adjusted life years (DALYs), in low- and middle-income countries and 23% in high-income countries. These figures compare to cardiovascular diseases, which account for 10% and 18% of the burden of disease in low- to middle- and high-income countries, respectively. The burden of disease due to neuropsychiatric conditions is expected to increase to 15% of the total global disease burden by 2020, with unipolar depression alone emerging as the second highest contributor.

In addition to the burden of disability posed by mental disorder, society experiences considerable economic burden as well. As noted earlier, schizophrenia affects 1% of the world's population and accounts for 1.6% of the world's total health care budget (McCann, 2000). In 1996, the direct costs of care for mental illness in the United States was $69 billion, excluding an additional $17.7 billion for Alzheimer's care and $12.6 billion for treatment of substance abuse disorders (USPHS, 1999). In one study in the United Kingdom, the indirect costs of lost productivity resulting from mental illness was approximately four times higher than the direct costs (Frangou & Murray, 2000). In 1997, total U.S. expenditures for mental illness (due to treatment, social services, disability payments, lost productivity, and premature mortality) amounted to more than $150 billion (National Center for Chronic Disease Prevention and Health Promotion, 1998). In general, these figures indicate the magnitude of mental health problems as a community health issue.

The importance of chronic mental health problems in the United States is highlighted by the number of objectives related to these disorders in the national health objectives for the year 2010 (U.S. Department of Health and Human Services [USDHHS], 2000b). Some of these objectives are presented at the end of this chapter. The complete set of objectives for mental health and mental disorders can be viewed on the Healthy People 2010 Web site accessible through a link on the companion Web site for this book.

COMMUNITY HEALTH NURSING AND MENTAL HEALTH PROBLEMS

As noted earlier, community health nurses may play a significant part in the control of mental health problems with individuals and with population groups. Effective control includes assessment of risks for and factors influencing mental health problems, as well as the planning, implementation, and evaluation of health care programs directed toward mental health.

ASSESSING FACTORS INFLUENCING MENTAL HEALTH PROBLEMS

Factors in each of the six dimensions of health influence risk for and the course of mental health problems for individuals and for communities. Community health nurses will be actively involved in assessing for these risks as well as for the presence of mental illness in individual clients and in the population as a whole.

Biophysical Considerations

Biophysical factors influencing mental health problems include genetics, maturation and aging, and physiologic function.

Genetics

Various studies of families, twins, and adopted children provide strong evidence that some people have a genetic predisposition to develop schizophrenia. For example, the lifetime risk of developing schizophrenia for someone with one or more family members with schizophrenia is 10 times greater than for those with no family history of the disease (Frangou & Murray, 2000). Additional evidence of a genetic contribution to disease is seen in the incidence of schizophrenia in 50% of identical twins whose twin is affected, but in only 10% to 15% of nonidentical twins (Lehman, 1999). The fact that concordance is not perfect in identical twins, however, suggests the modifiability of genetic predisposition through environmental factors.

Genetic contributions to vulnerability are implicated in other mental health problems as well, including bipolar depression, early onset depression, autism, attention deficit hyperactivity disorder (ADHD), anorexia nervosa, panic disorder, and so on. It should be noted, however, that heredity plays a role in transmission of vulnerability to disease, not in transmission of disease itself. Furthermore, genetic research has indicated that it is not a single gene that causes most of these diseases, but a complex interaction of multiple genes (USPHS, 1999).

Genetic factors may even have differential effects in the development of a single mental disorder. For example, three basic genetic forms of familial schizophrenia have been identified: dopamine psychosis, neurodegenerative schizophrenia, and schizophrenia caused by genetic failure in neurologic development during the second trimester of pregnancy (Flaskerud, 2000).

Maturation and Aging

Mental health problems may have differential effects on different age groups. For example, depression is a common problem in the elderly, with 3% of community-dwelling elderly persons in the United States affected.

Depression in the elderly is often misdiagnosed or inadequately treated (Davis & Mathew, 1998). Overall, an estimated 20% of people in the United States over the age of 55 have some form of mental disorder, including 11% with anxiety disorders, 4.4% with mood disorders, 6.6% with severe cognitive impairment, and 0.6% with schizophrenia (USPHS, 1999).

☉THINK ABOUT IT

How would you differentiate a mood disorder characterized by depression from other causes of apparent depression in an elderly client?

Schizophrenia is rarely seen in young children and has a typical onset in late adolescence (Lehman, 1999). Other disorders are seen more frequently in children. For example, 21% of U.S. children have mental disorders that result in at least mild functional impairment. An estimated 5% to 9% have "serious emotional disturbances." The relative percentages of children aged 9 to 17 years affected by specific problems is as follows: anxiety disorders—13%, disruptive disorders—10.3%, and mood disorders—6.2% (USPHS, 1999). Prevalences found among adolescents include 10% to 40% for depressed mood, 5% for depressive syndrome, and 0.4% to 8.7% for clinical depression. Co-morbidity of depression and substance abuse is also high among adolescents (Kelder et al., 2001).

Physiologic Function

The interaction between mental health and physiologic factors is complex. The presence of physiologic conditions may increase one's risk for mental health problems. Conversely, mental health problems may pose risks for physiologic effects. Finally, the presence of either mental or physical conditions may complicate control of problems in the other realm.

There is considerable evidence that mental health problems have a physiologic basis in brain chemistry and that neurophysiologic deficits are a major contributor to mental illness. Similarly, the presence of chronic physical illness, infection, malnutrition, and the effects of hormones and physical trauma have all been shown to play a part in the development of mental health problems. Infectious agents such as human immunodeficiency virus (HIV) and syphilis, for example, are implicated in the development of some forms of dementia, and one form of sudden onset obsessive–compulsive disorder in children has been linked to streptococcal pharyngitis (USPHS, 1999).

Physiologic differences also account for differential effects of psychotropic drugs in different racial and ethnic groups. There is also some indication that biological markers for mental illness differ among racial ethnic groups. For example, African Americans have lower monoamine oxidase activity in schizophrenia than do Caucasians (Flaskerud, 2000).

Mental health problems may also increase one's risk for physical illness. For example, anxiety and depression have been shown to increase the risk for the onset of coronary heart disease (CHD) and to affect survival in persons with existing CHD. Conversely, people recovering from myocardial infarction are at increased risk for major depressive disorders (Neugebauer, 1999).

Complications of birth and pregnancy and exposure to influenza in the second trimester of pregnancy have been linked to the incidence of schizophrenia in adult children of affected women. Pregnancy does not seem to result in greater risk for rehospitalization among women with schizophrenia (as depression does), but schizophrenic women may have delusions regarding the pregnancy that are associated with high risk of complications due to noncompliance with prenatal care recommendations (Frangou & Murray, 2000). Mental health problems of all kinds may also interfere with treatment compliance for physical health conditions.

Psychological Considerations

Psychological considerations to be addressed in assessing factors influencing mental health problems include psychological risk factors, psychiatric co-morbidity, coping skills, suicide potential, and characteristic manifestations of mental health problems for which the nurse would assess individual clients.

Psychological Risk Factors for Mental Health Problems

Personality traits, difficult temperament, experience of stressful life events, and below-average intelligence are some of the psychological factors that have been associated with the development of mental health problems.

Some people's personalities appear to place them at increased risk for mental health problems. For example, people who are excessively critical or who have difficult temperaments may alienate others, giving them less social support for dealing with everyday sources of stress that we all encounter.

Psychological stress appears to play an important part in development of mental disorders. Stress and an emotionally charged environment are implicated in symptomatic relapses in clients with schizophrenia. Conversely, decreasing stress and increasing personal and interpersonal competencies appears to contribute to mental health and to control of existing mental health problems. Stressful life events may contribute to situational depression or exacerbate major depressive disorders.

Psychiatric Co-morbidity

Clients with one mental disorder may concurrently experience other disorders. This co-occurrence of two mental disorders is referred to as *dual diagnosis*, a term commonly used to indicate the presence of a substance abuse disorder with one or more other psychiatric diagnoses. Although dual diagnosis most often incorporates a substance abuse disorder with some other mental health problem, other forms of co-morbidity may occur. For example, 25% of people with schizophrenia experience depression at any one time, and 80% of schizophrenics will experience depression prior to their first psychotic episode (Frangou & Murray, 2000).

Research has indicated that people with dual diagnoses are more likely to be noncompliant with therapy, engage in violence, attempt suicide, and have a higher risk for homelessness than those with a single diagnosis. They also tend to engage in high-risk sexual behaviors that increase their risk for HIV and other sexually transmitted diseases (STDs). Finally, persons with dual diagnoses use significantly more health services than those with only one psychiatric diagnosis (Gafoor & Rassool, 1998).

Coping Skills

The extent of an individual's coping abilities mediates the effect of stress on both physical and mental health. Coping strategies are culturally determined, and different cultural groups may display different approaches to coping with life's stress. For example, Asian clients would tend to avoid dwelling on unpleasant circumstances. African Americans, on the other hand, might be more likely to attempt to overcome adversity by increased striving, at the same time minimizing the significance of the stress (USPHS, 1999).

Some clients with mental health problems may turn to substance use or abuse as a coping strategy, which may contribute to the potential for dual diagnosis. Other clients may engage in other, more or less adaptive coping strategies for dealing with stress or with symptoms. Research has indicated, for example, that clients with schizophrenia have fairly well developed coping skills used to control their symptoms. Some of these coping strategies are healthier than others and can be encouraged by community health nurses working with clients with schizophrenia and their families. One category of coping skill displayed by schizophrenic clients dealt with behavior control by means of passive or active distraction (e.g., listening to music or reading versus playing an instrument or writing poetry), rest or physical activity (e.g., running), or indulgence (e.g., eating, drinking, or smoking). Other coping strategies included socializing with and talking to others, avoiding thinking about or ignoring misperceptions, shifting one's attention to other thoughts, engaging in future planning or problem solving, seeking medical care, prayer, and acceptance of symptoms. One final strategy, symptomatic behavior (e.g., telling voices to "shut up" or doing as told by voices) is a less healthy approach to dealing with symptoms of schizophrenia (Kingdon & Turkington, 1994).

Suicide Potential

Both the stress that contributes to the development of mental disorders and the hopelessness often associated with having a mental disorder place clients at increased risk for suicide, and community health nurses must be particularly alert to evidence of suicidal ideation in clients with mental health problems. Depression, in particular, whether due to major depressive, unipolar, or bipolar disorder, or to situational factors, increases the potential for suicide. The nurse should explore with the client any suicidal tendencies or thoughts of suicide. Suicide tends to occur most frequently when clients are recovering from an episode of depression; this is because the severely depressed client probably does not have the energy to commit suicide. Suicide is addressed in more depth in Chapter 32.

Characteristic Manifestations of Selected Mental Health Problems

In their work with individual and family clients in the community, community health nurses are in a position to identify those with signs and symptoms suggestive of mental health problems. In order to effectively identify those individuals with problems, community health nurses need to be conversant with signs and symptoms typical of the most commonly encountered mental disorders.

The fourth edition (text revised) of the *Diagnostic and Statistical Manual of Mental Disorders (DSM-IV-TR)* of the American Psychiatric Association (2000) addresses several classes of psychiatric diagnoses that are summarized below. It is beyond the scope of this book to describe each of these disorders or even each of the major categories of illness, and the reader is referred to the *DSM-IV-TR* or to a general psychiatric nursing textbook for greater depth of coverage. However, characteristic signs and symptoms of three types of conditions will be addressed here: psychoses (of which schizophrenia is the most common), mood disorders, and anxiety disorders. Substance abuse disorders are addressed in Chapter 31.

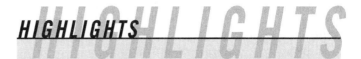

DSM-IV-TR Classes of Mental Disorders

- Disorders most often diagnosed in infancy, childhood, or adolescence (e.g., autism, ADHD)
- Cognitive disorders (e.g., dementia, Alzheimer's disease)
- Mental disorders due to general medical conditions
- Substance-related disorders (e.g., alcohol dependence)
- Schizophrenia and other psychotic disorders
- Mood disorders (e.g., major depressive disorder, unipolar and bipolar disorders)
- Anxiety disorders (e.g., panic disorder, phobia, obsessive–compulsive disorder, posttraumatic stress disorder)

(continued)

- Somatoform disorders (disorders manifesting as physical symptoms without an underlying physiological cause
- Factitious disorders (simulation of physical or mental illness for the purpose of obtaining medical treatment, e.g., Munchhausen syndrome)
- Dissociative disorders (e.g., dual personality)
- Sexual and gender identity disorders
- Eating disorders (e.g., anorexia nervosa, bulimia nervosa)
- Sleep disorders
- Impulse control disorders (e.g., kleptomania)
- Adjustment disorders
- Personality disorders (e.g., antisocial personality disorder)

Source: U.S. Public Health Service. (1999). *Mental health: A report of the surgeon general.* Washington, DC: Author.

Psychoses are characterized by both positive and negative symptoms. Positive symptoms involve the experience of something that should not be there and include hallucinations, delusions, and other symptoms. Negative symptoms, on the other hand, involve the absence of thoughts or behaviors that should be present (USPHS, 1999). Negative symptoms are more disabling than positive symptoms because of their greater impact on one's ability to function effectively in society (Lehman, 1999). Both positive and negative symptoms of psychoses are presented below.

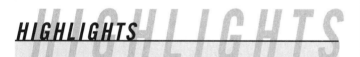

HIGHLIGHTS

Positive and Negative Symptoms of Psychoses

Positive Symptoms

- *Hallucinations:* Sensory experiences that occur without any sensory input (may occur in any sensory modality)
- *Delusions:* Distortions of inferential thinking that lead to misperceptions of experiences and erroneous beliefs
- *Disorganized, loose, or illogical thoughts:*
  - *Loose associations:* Wandering from one topic to another
  - *Tangentiality:* Oblique relationships between topics
  - *Incoherence:* Words strung together without producing any coherent meaning
- *Disorganized behavior:* Unusual modes of dress, inappropriate sexual behavior, unpredictable agitation

Negative Symptoms

- *Flattened or blunt affect:* Lack of emotional response, facial inexpressiveness, diminished body language

- *Concrete thinking:* Inability to abstract from concrete examples
- *Anhedonia:* Inability to experience pleasure
- *Poor motivation, lack of spontaneity and initiative*

A mood disorder is a disturbance in mood that manifests mainly as depression but can also involve elation or mania. In the *DSM-IV-TR,* mood disorders include major depressive disorder, unipolar and bipolar disorder, as well as other forms of depression such as dysthymic disorder. Symptoms characteristic of the two mood extremes in mood disorders, depression and mania, are summarized below.

HIGHLIGHTS

Characteristic Signs of Depression and Mania

Depression

- Persistent sadness or despair
- Disturbances in sleep patterns
  - Difficulty falling asleep
  - Early morning awakening
  - Difficulty waking up
- Alterations in eating habits
  - Significant weight gain
  - Significant weight loss
- Diminished energy level
- Decreased interest in sex
- Difficulty concentrating
- Social withdrawal

(The presence of one or more of these symptoms can indicate that a client is experiencing depression.)

Mania

- Persistent euphoria
- Grandiosity (inappropriately high self-esteem)
- Psychomotor agitation
- Decreased sleep
- Racing thoughts and distractibility
- Poor judgment and impaired impulse control
- Rapid or pressured speech

Anxiety disorders include such conditions as panic attacks, phobias, generalized anxiety disorder, obsessive–compulsive disorder, and posttraumatic stress disorder. Symptoms are those engendered by any sensation of fear and are summarized on page 717.

HIGHLIGHTS

Symptoms of Anxiety Disorders

- Feelings of fear/dread
- Trembling, restlessness
- Muscle tension
- Rapid heart rate
- Dizziness, lightheadedness
- Increased perspiration
- Cold hands and feet
- Shortness of breath

Source: U.S. Public Health Service. (1999). *Mental health: A report of the surgeon general.* Washington, DC: Author.

Physical Environmental Considerations

Physical environmental factors influence the development and course of some mental health problems. For example, chronic exposure to lead and other toxins may cause mental retardation and other forms of mental illness (USPHS, 1999). There is also evidence that schizophrenia may be triggered by neurotropic virus infections, anoxia, and radiation exposures in the environment (Flaskerud, 2000). Similarly, rehospitalization for serious mental illness has been associated with increased population density. Possible explanations for this association might be greater familiarity with the client and earlier identification of behavior changes preceding relapse by family and friends in areas of low population density or the increased stress that accompanies increased population density (Husted & Jorgens, 2000).

Seasonal changes may also contribute to mental health problems as in the case of seasonal affective disorder. *Seasonal affective disorder (SAD)* is a form of depression that varies with the seasons resulting in depression in the fall and winter when exposure to natural light is diminished and euthymia (positive mood) in spring and summer when natural light is more abundant. There is some evidence, however, that the occurrence of SAD is mediated by cultural factors. In northern Norway, for example, which has extreme seasonal changes, SAD is uncommon. Possible explanations include cultural perceptions that the changes in season are important, seasonal celebrations that promote connectedness with others, and rituals that assist one in coping with seasonal changes (Stuhlmiller, 1998).

Sociocultural Considerations

A number of sociocultural dimension factors influence risk for and treatment of mental health problems. These factors include societal disorganization, social and economic factors, family relationships, social support, culture, and societal attitudes to mental illness. As noted in

Chapter 27, social upheaval such as war and disaster increase the incidence of mental health problems in the populations affected, particularly when the effects are long-lasting. Immigration, which may result from social upheaval, has also been linked with a high incidence of mental disorders (Frangou & Murray, 2000).

Mental health problems are also influenced by more contained social events. For example, the risk of depression increases with recent divorce or separation, unemployment, and bereavement (Armstrong, 1999). Inability to work and stresses associated with low income have also been associated with mental illness, as have overcrowding and living in an area with a high rate of disorganization (USPHS, 1999).

Family interactions may also influence the development and course of mental health problems. For example, severe marital discord, large family size, paternal criminality, maternal mental disorder, and placement in foster care have all been associated with increased risk of mental illness (USPHS, 1999). Research has linked schizophrenia with hereditary communication difficulties with one's parents, compounding the disorientation experienced by the client with schizophrenia (Wuerker, 2000). High parental levels of expressed emotion conveying criticism, hostility, or stifling overinvolvement have been shown to be linked to relapse in clients with schizophrenia. High levels of negative emotional expression have also been associated with anorexia nervosa and depression. Conversely, warmth and positive family relationships may have a protective effect against mental health problems or assist family members to cope more effectively when they do occur (Frangou & Murray, 2000).

⑥THINK ABOUT IT

What effect does dysfunctional family communication have on schizophrenia?

Social support may assist clients to cope with the stresses of life and prevent mental health problems. Lack of social support, on the other hand, may increase the risk of mental illness, contributing to feelings of isolation and poor social skills common among people with mental health problems. Some interventions to increase social interaction and social support networks have been beneficial for clients with mental illness. In one study, for example, befriending by trained volunteers was thought to be beneficial by all clients involved, and 67% reported improved social skills as a result of the program (Bradshaw & Haddock, 1998). Other research has indicated, however, that increasing clients' social support networks might not have a positive effect until sufficient symptom control has been achieved for clients to perceive social support positively (Clinton, Lunney, Edwards, Weir, & Barr, 1998).

The effects of culture on mental health are many and pervasive. Culture defines what constitutes mental illness for members of a group, and that definition may not always conform to the diagnostic criteria established in the *DSM-IV-TR*. What may be seen as abnormal behavior or feelings in one culture may be perfectly normal in another. Similarly, culture mediates one's experience of distress and how one expresses that distress. Culture, for example, creates what are known as "idioms of distress" or typical ways of expressing mental discomfort. In many cultural groups, for example, mental distress is expressed in terms of somatization. *Somatization* is the expression of mental or emotional distress in terms of physical symptoms. Diagnostic criteria contained in the *DSM-IV-TR* are based on Western Anglo experience, and it is unclear how applicable diagnostic criteria are with members of other cultural groups (USPHS, 1999). Some cultures also have recognized culture-bound syndromes generally reflecting concepts of mental illness that are culture specific and fall outside Western psychiatric practice. Culture-bound syndromes were discussed in Chapter 6.

Cultural differences in diagnostic criteria, expressions of distress, and meanings and value attributed to different symptoms may result in misdiagnosis in cross-cultural encounters. Language barriers between provider and client also increase the potential for misdiagnosis, as do diagnostic measurements that are not linguistically or culturally sensitive (Flaskerud, 2000).

Culture also influences expectations regarding treatment that may enhance or impede compliance with therapy. Members of many cultural groups engage in the use of herbal remedies. For this reason, they may expect psychotropic medications to act rapidly as most herbals do. The need to build effective blood levels of medications may be difficult for clients in these cultural groups to understand. Inability to see immediate results may lead to discontinuation of pharmacotherapy. Herbal therapies may also interact with prescription medications to impede or enhance their effects, contributing to therapeutic ineffectiveness or adverse reactions to medications (Flaskerud, 2000).

Culture also contributes to the way people view mental illness and to the degree of stigmatization encountered by those who experience mental illness. Stigmatization is characterized by bias, distrust, stereotyping, fear, embarrassment, anger, and avoidance. Stigmatization has the effect of reducing willingness to seek help and thereby reduces access to needed care. For example, it is estimated that stigmatization prevents approximately two thirds of people with mental illness from seeking care (USPHS, 1999). This response to perceived stigma is also mediated by culture, however. For example, in one study, African American subjects indicated greater willingness to seek care for a hypothesized mental health problem and less embarrassment than Caucasian subjects (Diala et al., 2001).

Stigmatization of the mentally ill may also decrease their access to needed resources and opportunities such as those related to employment or housing. For the individual, stigma leads to low self-esteem, hopelessness, and social isolation. Clients with mental illness are faced with the same kinds of decisions regarding disclosure that were discussed in the context of chronic physical health problems in Chapter 29. At the population level, stigmatization influences public willingness to pay for services for the mentally ill (USPHS, 1999).

Studies of the U.S. population have indicated continuing unfavorable attitudes toward the mentally ill. In one study, for example, public perceptions of mental illness were strongly linked to fears of potential violence and a desire for limited interaction with the mentally ill. These effects were stronger for some forms of mental disorder than others. Subjects were most likely to perceive cocaine addicts as potentially violent (87%), followed by alcohol abusers (71%), people with schizophrenia (61%), depressed persons (33%), and "troubled persons" (17%). The extent of desire to maintain social distance from people affected by these conditions occurred in a similar rank order and ranged from 90% of people who did not want to interact with cocaine addicts to 29% of people who would avoid a troubled person (Link, Phelan, Bresnahan, Stueve, & Pescosolido, 1999). In another report of the same study (Pescosolido, Monahan, Link, Stueve, & Kikuzawa, 1999), study subjects perceived alcohol and drug abusers and schizophrenics as unable to manage money and likely to be violent, and a significant percentage of subjects were willing to coerce individuals into involuntary treatment, believing it was justified based on the perceived risk of injury to self or others.

Other evidence of societal attitudes toward mental illness lies in the number of the mentally ill who are incarcerated in correctional facilities. Jails and prisons have been described as the "provider of last resort" for the mentally ill (Hagar, 1999). Approximately 210,000 severely mentally ill persons are housed in U.S. jails and prisons

CULTURAL CONSIDERATIONS

You are seeing Su-Chen, a 20-year-old single Asian woman who lives with her parents. Su-Chen is being treated for schizophrenia at the local mental health clinic after a referral from the student health center at the community college where she is enrolled. You have been asked to visit her because she has not been keeping appointments at the clinic. When you arrive at the home, Su-Chen tells you that her father will not allow her to continue to be seen at the clinic because he is afraid that their neighbors will find out that she is mentally ill. She is doing well and is free of symptoms at present, but she is almost out of her medications. The clinic will not authorize a refill unless she is seen by the provider.

- What cultural factors are operating in this situation?
- How will you address Su-Chen's needs?

ETHICAL AWARENESS

Hagar (1999) has noted that current legislation requiring that seriously mentally ill persons be a clear danger to themselves or others before involuntary commitment is considered, prevents them from receiving necessary services when they are too seriously ill to be able to make informed decisions regarding refusal of care. He argued that legislation should be changed to allow more effective involuntary intervention for the seriously mentally ill who refuse treatment. He noted that changes in the law will not eliminate requirements for due process prior to involuntary treatment and that such changes were being considered in California. What do you think about the proposal to broaden the potential for involuntary treatment of the mentally ill? Can it be justified on ethical grounds?

compared to only 70,000 in public mental hospitals, 30% of whom are forensic detainees (Vitucci, 1999). As noted in Chapter 26, correctional institutions are mandated to provide treatment for mental illness (unless refused by the client); however, there are few follow-up programs that ensure continuity of care on release and no legal way to maintain treatment compliance in this population (Hagar, 1999).

Behavioral Considerations

Personal behaviors also influence the development and course of mental health problems, but it is often difficult to determine the direction of influence. In some studies, for example, depression and anxiety in adolescents predicted experimental smoking that was linked with eventual daily smoking (Patton et al., 1998). Depressed mood has also been found to predict initiation of marijuana use (Kelder et al., 2001). In other studies, smoking was associated with an increased risk of depression among adolescents, but depression was not associated with smoking initiation (Wu & Anthony, 1999). In still other studies, depression has been linked to substance abuse and smoking. Major depressive disorders were three to four times more common among drug abusers than among nonabusers, and the extent of substance abuse and major depressive disorder co-morbidity has been shown to be 20% to 30%, with depression antedating substance abuse by an average of 4.5 years (Kelder et al., 2001).

⑥THINK ABOUT IT

What is your personal risk of developing a depressive disorder? What factors are contributing to that risk? What could you do about them?

Physical activity and sexual activity are two other behavioral considerations in an assessment of mental health problems. For example, depressed elderly clients have been shown to be less physically active than nondepressed elderly, leading to greater disability in performance of ADLs and greater mobility limitations (Penninx et al., 1999). Sexual activity is an area that is often ignored in the care of clients with mental illness, and there is a need for attention to the meeting of sexual needs as well as for the assessment of high-risk sexual behaviors that may be exhibited by some mentally ill individuals. Sexuality issues are complicated by possible links with childhood sexual abuse, the sexual content of positive symptoms in clients with schizophrenia, sexual disinhibition in some conditions, and medication side effects such as diminished libido and disabling extrapyramidal effects that promote distancing and social isolation by other people. Use of safe sexual practices and contraception are other sexual behaviors that should be assessed (McCann, 2000).

Health System Considerations

The mental health system consists of four aspects: the general medical or primary care sector, the specialty mental health care sector, the social services sector, and the volunteer support network sector, all of which appear to be inadequate to meet the need for care. Less than one third of adults and fewer children in need of mental health services receive them. An estimated 15% of the U.S. adult population uses mental health services in a given year, 11% from general or special care sectors, 5% from the social service sector, and 3% from the voluntary sector. Just over half of those served (8%) have diagnosable mental illnesses, and the remaining 7% experience mental health problems. An additional 21% of children receive some type of mental health services in a year (USPHS, 1999).

Both psychotherapy and pharmacologic therapy for mental illness have proved to be effective when provided in primary care settings. Few such settings are equipped to provide this care, however, given the need for an organized treatment program, regular follow-up and compliance monitoring, and access to mental health specialists for consultation or treatment of more severe disease (Schulberg, Katon, Simon, & Rush, 1998). Neither primary care nor specialty mental health services are well equipped to address the mental health needs of minority group members, and cultural biases on the part of providers may lead to under- or overdiagnosis as well as inappropriate treatment (USPHS, 1999).

Health system bias against those with mental illness is also seen in the relative level of expenditures for mental health care as compared to physical health care. In 1994, per capita expenditures for mental health services in the United States amounted to $128 (USDHHS, 2000a), far less than that spent on physical health care. Insurance spending for mental health services averages $3 to $8 per person per month, compared to $150 per person per month for medical care (Simon, 1999).

In 1997, total Medicaid costs were $23.1 billion for general hospitalization compared to only $2 billion for mental hospital costs (U.S. Census Bureau, 1999). Alcohol, drug, and mental health care costs borne by employers fell from 9% in 1989 to 4% in 1995 in spite of increased need and documented inadequacy of treatment to meet that need. Similarly, the average length of stay for inpatient mental health care declined from 12.6 days in 1988 to 8.6 days in 1995 without a concomitant increase in outpatient mental health services. It is estimated that every day of reduced hospital stay increases the risk of rehospitalization for mental illness by 3%. There is also evidence of a widening gap between employer coverage for mental health care and coverage of physical care as well as higher co-payments and increasing lifetime limits on care for mental illness (Mechanic & McAlpine, 1999). Some authors argue that higher co-payments for mental health services are based on a perception that mental health care is "discretionary" rather than necessary, and there appears to be a systematic trend in managed care organizations to cut

assessment tips assessment tips assessment tips

ASSESSING RISK FOR MENTAL HEALTH PROBLEMS

Biophysical Considerations

- Is there a family history of mental health problems?
- Is there any existing physical health condition that may contribute to mental health problems? What effects do personal physical health conditions or those of family members have on mental health? Do physical health problems or their treatment cause signs and symptoms suggestive of the mental health problems?
- Does the presence of a mental health problem complicate treatment of physical health conditions?

Psychological Considerations

- What life stresses is the client experiencing? Does stress contribute to or exacerbate mental health problems? How does the client cope with stress?
- What signs and symptoms does the client exhibit that suggest the presence of mental health problems?
- What is the extent of adaptation to the mental health problem? How does the client cope with the problem?
- Is there existing psychiatric co-morbidity? If so, what form does it take?
- Is the client at risk for suicide as a result of the mental health problem?

Physical Environmental Considerations

- What effect, if any, do weather conditions have on the client's mental health?
- Do environmental pollutants contribute to the incidence of mental health problems?

Sociocultural Considerations

- What are the effects of mental health problems on social interactions (with family and others)?
- What are societal attitudes to the problem? Do they hamper control efforts?
- Is there social stigma attached to having the problem? What effect does stigma have on clients' willingness to seek care?

- What effect, if any, do cultural beliefs and behaviors have on mental health problems?
- Does the mental health problem contribute to the risk of homelessness for the client?
- What social support systems are available to the client?
- How do social factors (e.g., unemployment) influence the problem?
- How does the mental health problem affect the client's ability to work?

Behavioral Considerations

- Does alcohol or drug use influence the problem or its effects? Are alcohol or drugs used in an effort to self-manage symptoms?
- What effect, if any, does exercise have on the problem?
- Does smoking influence the problem?
- What effect does the problem have on self-care behaviors?

Health System Considerations

- What is the attitude of health care providers to persons with mental health problems?
- Are health care providers alert to signs and symptoms of mental health problems?
- What treatment facilities are available to persons with mental health problems? How adequate are they? What types of therapy are available? How effective are they?
- Are diagnostic and treatment services available and accessible to persons with mental health problems?
- Does the client exhibit treatment side effects or adverse effects?
- Does treatment for other health problems cause or exacerbate the mental health problem?

costs in the area of mental health care to offset increasing costs in other areas (Simon, 1999). Tips for assessing health system factors, as well as other types of factors, influencing risk for mental health problems are presented on page 720.

DIAGNOSTIC REASONING AND CARE OF CLIENTS WITH MENTAL HEALTH PROBLEMS

Community health nurses may make a variety of nursing diagnoses related to mental health problems. These diagnoses can reflect the health needs of an individual client, the client's family, or a population group. For example, the nurse might diagnose "impaired reality orientation due to schizophrenic episode" in an individual client or an "exacerbation of depression due to family stress." Another nursing diagnosis at this level might reflect "disruption of family function due to exhibition of symptoms of schizophrenia" on the part of one member.

Nursing diagnoses may also be made that reflect mental health problems affecting population groups. For example, the community health nurse might diagnose an "increased incidence of schizophrenia in the homeless population" or "inadequate treatment facilities for persons with chronic mental health problems due to reduced program funds."

PLANNING AND IMPLEMENTING CARE FOR CLIENTS WITH MENTAL HEALTH PROBLEMS

The surgeon general's report on mental health (USPHS, 1999) made several recommendations with respect to mental health care in the United States. These recommendations included the need to reduce the stigma attached to mental illness, improve public awareness of the availability of effective treatment for most mental health problems, ensure the supply of providers and services for those in need, and ensure the use of state-of-the-art treatments. Additional recommendations addressed the need to tailor treatment to the age, gender, race, and culture of those affected; to facilitate early entry into treatment; and to reduce financial barriers to treatment (USPHS, 1999). Community health nurses can be actively involved in efforts to address these recommendations.

Many people in the mental health field believe that the public health concepts of primary, secondary, and tertiary prevention are not helpful in dealing with mental health problems. These difficulties arise in the application of the secondary prevention element of diagnosis due to the difficulty of diagnosing mental disorders in the absence of objectively verifiable signs of disease and the need to rely on subjective information from clients. In addition, the definitions of psychiatric disorders change over time, making diagnosis even more difficult. Also, there are no

screening procedures for most mental disorders, another element of secondary prevention. For this reason, these concepts have been recast as prevention, treatment, and maintenance. In this conceptualization, *prevention* is similar to primary prevention and involves preventing the occurrence of mental health problems. *Treatment* encompasses the identification and standard treatment of persons with mental illness or mental health problems, including prevention of co-occurring disorders. *Maintenance* incorporates some elements of secondary and tertiary prevention such as ongoing treatment and monitoring treatment effects (USPHS, 1999). Each of these three levels of care will be discussed here.

Prevention

Prevention of mental health problems and mental disorders involves both promotion of protective factors and risk factor reduction. Promotion of coping abilities and resilience can help prevent the development of mental health problems. *Resilience* is the ability to withstand chronic stress or to recover from traumatic and stressful events. Community health nurses can assist individual clients to develop coping skills that will increase their resilience in the face of adversity. In addition, nurses can be instrumental in developing programs that promote coping in school, work, or other settings.

Community health nurses are also actively involved in risk-reduction efforts. The support provided to clients with mental distress and efforts to ameliorate or eliminate sources of stress may prevent the occurrence of mental health problems (Armstrong, 1999). For example, referral for financial assistance may alleviate economic stresses that can contribute to depression. The nurse may also refer clients experiencing situational stressors such as divorce or care of a chronically ill family member to support groups to help them deal with stress. Assisting clients and families to expand social support networks may also prevent mental health problems.

Treatment

Early entry into treatment for mental disorders requires identification of those in need of treatment. Community health nurses should be knowledgeable about and alert to signs and symptoms of mental illness. They also need to be conversant with the kinds of services available to the individual client and within the population. When appropriate services are not available, community health nursing intervention may focus on advocacy and assurance of access to needed services.

Effective referral for services for clients in need of them requires that community health nurses have an understanding of the process of help seeking in mental illness. This process begins with a recognition of a problem and the determination that the problem is serious enough to seek care. The determination is then made as to the possible origin of the problem as either physical or mental in nature. At this point, the person needs to

CRITICAL THINKING IN RESEARCH

Carney et al. (1998) conducted a study using guided focus groups to determine how physicians in primary care went about making a diagnosis of depression. They found that physicians used three approaches to the diagnosis of depression: exclusion of all biomedical causes first, focus on psychosocial factors first, or a combination of the two. If you conducted a similar study of community health nurses and their recognition of the need for referral for depression, do you think the findings would be similar? Would findings differ for different groups of clients? If so, how? How would you go about conducting your study?

decide whether or not to seek help and, if so, where help should be sought. The decision to seek care is then followed by activities to obtain care. Once care has been obtained, there is the further decision of whether or not to continue with care or to adhere to care recommendations (USPHS, 1999). Community health nurses may assist clients in making decisions throughout the process as indicated in Table 30–1 ■.

The surgeon general's report on mental illness in the United States stresses the availability of effective treatment for the majority of mental health problems and notes that, in many cases, clients have multiple options for treatment (USPHS, 1999). In general, treatment for mental health problems is more cost-effective than non-

■ **TABLE 30–1** **Stages of the Help-Seeking Process and Related Community Health Nursing Interventions**

STAGE	POSSIBLE INTERVENTIONS
Problem recognition	Informing of problems observed by the nurse Education regarding normal and abnormal findings
Determination of seriousness	Review of the effects of the problem on client's life, family interactions, etc.
Determination of nature of problem as physical or mental	Exploration of meaning of symptoms from client's perspective Exploration of alternative explanations of problem
Choice of seeking care or not seeking care	Review of possible consequences of either decision
Choice to continue or not continue care	Review of consequences of continuing or not continuing care

treatment. For example, the estimated cost of treating depression (including medication, visits to providers, etc.) amounts to $50 to $75 per month compared to the cost savings of excess service use by clients with depression of $100 to $150 per month. There is an additional cost savings for treatment of $300 per month in preventing lost work productivity (Simon, 1999). Cost-effectiveness can also be viewed in terms of DALYs averted (Ustun, 1999).

Several general approaches may be implemented for the treatment of mental illness. These approaches include pharmacotherapy, individual or group psychotherapy, family intervention, and use of self-help groups. Multimodal therapy involves a combination of approaches. It is beyond the scope of this book to discuss these therapeutic approaches in detail, but each will be addressed briefly. The reader can find additional information in a general psychiatric nursing textbook or from some of the resources available through links on the companion Web site for this book.

Pharmacotherapy relies on the use of medications alone or in conjunction with other treatment approaches to mental illness. Most pharmacologic agents used in the treatment of mental disorders alter the action of neurotransmitters in the brain, either increasing or decreasing their activity. Major categories of pharmacotherapeutic agents include antipsychotics (neuroleptics), antidepressants, stimulants (used for ADHD), antimanic medications, anxiolytics, and cholinesterase inhibitors (used for Alzheimer's disease) (USPHS, 1999). The role of community health nurses with respect to pharmacotherapy for mental disorders lies primarily in monitoring and motivating medication compliance, monitoring therapeutic effects, assisting with side effects, and identifying adverse effects.

Community health nurses, as well as other providers who deal with clients with mental health problems, need an awareness of ethnopsychopharmacology. *Ethnopsychopharmacology* is the study of ethnic and cultural alterations in response to medication. These alterations reflect genetic differences in drug metabolism as well as cultural practices related to medication adherence, placebo effect, diet and its effects on medication absorption and effect, and the concomitant use of traditional therapies. Members of many ethnic groups have slowed drug metabolism compared to Caucasians, which may result in higher blood levels with typical dosages, leading to adverse effects (USPHS, 1999).

Monitoring clients on psychotropic medications for side effects is an important role for community health nurses. Any of several different classes of antipsychotic drugs may be used in the initial treatment of clients with schizophrenia. Some clients will not respond to initial drug therapy or may experience adverse effects or annoying side effects that may limit compliance with the therapeutic regimen. In such cases, alternative drugs may be tried until the desired effect is achieved.

Antidepressant medications are effective in all forms of depressive disorders and may be used alone or in conjunction with other therapies. Because depression and anxiety often go hand in hand, both symptoms can be treated pharmacologically. Several categories of antidepressant and antianxiety agents are commonly prescribed. Two classes of antidepressants have been prescribed since 1960, tricyclics like amitriptyline (Elavil) and imipramine hydrochloride (Tofranil), and monoamine oxidase (MAO) inhibitors like phenelzine sulfate (Nardil) and tranylcypromine sulfate (Parnate).

Although the reason for their effectiveness is not known, both types of antidepressants share one property: the ability to boost the action of serotonin and norepinephrine. While the tricyclics block reabsorption of these neurotransmitters, MAO inhibitors interfere with enzymes that break them down. When a client is started on a traditional tricyclic, he or she spends several weeks taking progressively larger doses. The health care provider uses blood tests to determine the effective serum concentration, which is different for each individual. Because an overdose of tricyclics can be extremely toxic, resulting in low blood pressure, heart disturbances, blurred vision, constipation, dizziness, sluggishness, and weight gain, many providers often prescribe too little. Because the therapeutic range is so narrow, too little medication is often ineffective. The MAO inhibitors can cause a hypertensive response to foods containing retsin (e.g., chocolate, cheese, wines). Many people choose depression over these side effects.

The community health nurse caring for clients on antidepressant medications educates them about the medication and its therapeutic and toxic effects as well as potential side effects. Fluoxetine (Prozac) is one of the most commonly prescribed antidepressants in the United States. Prozac works like a tricyclic that focuses on serotonin. Although Prozac takes three weeks to become effective, there is no blood monitoring, because a dose of 20 to 40 mg is usually effective. There is less risk of overdose, and the most common side effects are nuisance effects such as headaches, nausea, insomnia, nervousness, weight loss, decreased sexual interest and loss or delay of orgasm, and a slight risk of seizures. In rare cases, suicidal thoughts and overtly violent behavior have been traced to Prozac. A small number of clients develop a "caffeine syndrome" in which they become restless and sometimes experience tremors.

Antianxiety agents, sedatives, and hypnotics are often prescribed when symptoms of anxiety are related to depression. These classes of drugs share similar pharmacologic properties, and they can be effective in small doses to relieve anxiety and in larger doses to induce sleep. The benzodiazepines are the most commonly used antianxiety agents. These include chlordiazepoxide hydrochloride (Librium) and diazepam (Valium), both of which are widely prescribed and widely abused. Other drugs in the benzodiazepine family include lorazepam (Ativan), alprazolam (Xanax), clonazepam (Klonopin), and triflupromazine (Vesprin). Drugs in the benzodiazepine family offer rapid, effective, and safe treatment for anxiety states. They have a low addiction potential

and do not affect the metabolism of medications taken concurrently, although caffeine interferes with their effectiveness. The major side effect of the benzodiazepines is drowsiness, and community health nurses should warn clients not to drive when they feel drowsy.

The barbiturates (secobarbital [Seconol]) are a group of sedative–hypnotic drugs. These are often contraindicated in treating anxiety states because they are very addictive, used in suicide attempts, depress the central nervous and respiratory systems, and depress rapid eye movement (REM) sleep, possibly resulting in the insomnia these drugs are intended to control.

Lithium, one of the commonly used drugs in the control of mania, has a very narrow gap between therapeutic levels and toxic levels. For this reason, blood levels must be monitored frequently. When lithium is first prescribed, daily blood tests may be necessary, decreasing to weekly and, finally, to monthly checks during maintenance. Significant side effects are correlated with blood levels above 1.5 mEq/L.

Community health nurses educate clients who are on lithium about the need to drink eight glasses of water a day, eat foods high in potassium (lithium can deplete potassium levels), and watch for early signs of toxicity. The nurse also monitors the client closely for signs of lithium toxicity, which are summarized below. The nurse refers the client back to the psychiatrist if signs of toxicity are evident. The nurse also reinforces the need for periodic checks of blood levels of lithium to ensure early identification of toxic levels.

HIGHLIGHTS

Signs of Lithium Toxicity

Confusion	Seizures
Dizziness	Slurred speech
Hyperactive reflexes	Somnolence
Incontinence	Stupor
Nausea	Thirst
Polyuria	Tremor
Restlessness	Vertigo

Psychotherapy may be used with individual clients or with groups of people. The intent of psychotherapy is to develop an understanding of one's problems and ways of dealing with them. Several different approaches to psychotherapy are used, including psychodynamic therapy, behavior therapy, and humanistic therapy. Psychotherapy may not be effective with clients from some cultural groups because it is incongruent with cultural norms of not dwelling on or thinking about problems. Family intervention is directed toward alleviation of inappropriate family dynamics that promote stress and result in mental distress. The community health nurse's primary role with respect to psychotherapy and family interventions is referral of clients for services.

Self-help groups are designed to promote mutual support, education, and personal growth among people who share similar kinds of mental health problems. Many self-help groups focus on the concept of recovery. *Recovery* involves restoration of a meaningful life rather than symptom relief, which is the emphasis in the medical model of care. In many cases, recovery does not imply a return to full function or the ability to discontinue medication use in chronic mental illnesses (USPHS, 1999). Self-help groups will be discussed in more detail in the context of substance abuse disorders in Chapter 31.

Maintenance

Several authors have noted a need to focus on disease management rather than crisis-oriented care for chronic mental health problems (Lehman, 1999; Ustun, 1999). Maintenance involves long-term management of chronic mental illness and focuses on rehabilitating the client and preventing relapse. The goal of maintenance in chronic mental illness is to maintain the client's level of function and to prevent *recidivism* or frequent rehospitalization. Maintenance may include medications and a variety of other interventions. Community health nurses may be asked to follow clients with diagnoses of chronic mental illness to provide support, encourage compliance, and monitor the effects of treatment. Community health nurses can assist clients to plan regular lifestyles and to minimize sources of stress in their lives. Clients should also be cautioned about potential interactions of medication and alcohol use. The nurse can also help clients and their families to identify symptoms that signal a symptomatic relapse and to seek professional assistance when these symptoms are noted.

In addition, community health nurses can educate clients and their families regarding medication side effects and ways to deal with them as well as educating them about serious adverse effects that should be reported to their health care providers.

Many chronic mental disorders are cyclical, and there are exacerbations and remissions. In the first session with a depressed client, for example, it is useful to the family and helpful to the clinician to draw a timeline that reflects the client's history of mood swings over several years. Trends might begin to appear that alert nurse and family to times with increased potential for symptoms. Nurses must rely heavily on family members' monitoring of the prodromal signs of mania because clients who have bipolar disorder are notoriously poor at identifying these signs in themselves. For this reason, the nurse should make family members thoroughly conversant with prodromal signs of mania. Not sleeping is often the first sign of a person moving toward mania. If the client has difficulty sleeping more than two nights, the nurse and the psychiatrist should be notified.

It is important that community health nurses learn to assess levels of depression and suicide risk and refer clients at risk to a mental health provider immediately if they are not already involved in ongoing therapy. Community health nurses are also using approaches such as diary writing and physical exercise to help individuals deal more effectively with depressive symptoms. Open lines of communication are imperative among nurse, mental health provider, family, and client, particularly at times when the client is deeply depressed or actively suicidal.

Persons with chronic mental illness often have a high incidence of physical health problems and sometimes lack the capacity to seek health care in today's complex delivery systems. The community health nurse may be in the situation of following a person for a physical health problem who suddenly begins to show signs of mental illness. The nurse's role in this case is to refer the client for further diagnosis and treatment, as well as to assist in addressing the physical health problem. The community health nurse also refers clients who are exhibiting signs of exacerbation of their disorders.

EVALUATING CONTROL STRATEGIES FOR MENTAL HEALTH PROBLEMS

Evaluation of mental health interventions occurs at the individual and family level as well as the population level. Evidence of effective intervention for the individual client may lie in diminished mental distress or a decrease in symptoms of a specific mental disorder. Similarly, effective family care may result in improved family dynamics or decreased disruption of family life by a mentally ill family member.

At the population level, evidence of effective primary prevention activities would lie in decreased incidence and prevalence of mental disorders as well as decreased reports of mental distress in the population. National health objectives for 2010 may also be used as guidelines for evaluating mental health care, particularly care related to secondary and tertiary prevention. Baseline data and 2010 targets for selected objectives are provided on page 725.

Because of their presence in the community and familiarity with many community members experiencing adverse life situations, community health nurses are in a position to identify clients at risk for mental health problems. Nurses can engage in activities designed to ameliorate these risks and to promote resilience and coping. Community health nurses are also able to recognize clients with symptomatic mental illness and refer them for mental health services. Assisting clients with chronic mental illness to adjust to their conditions and live as normally as possible is another significant role for community health nurses. Finally, community health nurses may be actively involved in advocacy to assure that culturally appropriate preventive, diagnostic, and treatment services are available to those in need of them.

HEALTHY PEOPLE 2010

GOALS FOR THE POPULATION

Objective	Base	Target
18-3 Reduce the proportion of homeless adults who have serious mental illness	25%	19%
18-4 Increase the proportion of people with serious mental illness who are employed	42%	51%
18-9 Increase the proportion of adults with serious mental disorders who receive treatment		
a. Adults 18–54 years of age with serious mental illness	47%	55%
b. Adults over 18 years with depression	23%	50%
c. Adults over 18 years with schizophrenia	60%	75%

Source: U.S. Department of Health and Human Services. (2000). *Healthy people 2010* (Conference edition, in two volumes). Washington, DC: Author.

APPLYING YOUR KNOWLEDGE IN PRACTICE

✂ CASE STUDY
Caring for the Client with a Mental Health Problem

You are the community health nurse assigned to see Donna for a well-baby visit several weeks after she delivered a healthy son. Donna is 39 and has been married to Jack, 48, for a year. Stephen is their first child. When you arrive at Donna's house, you note that she and her family live in a comfortable home in an upper-middle-class neighborhood. Donna answers the door, and you see that her eyes and nose are red as though she has been crying. You explain the purpose of your visit and examine the baby, who is in a freshly painted nursery with a bright mobile over the crib and plenty of stuffed animals and toys around. Stephen is neat, clean, and appears to be well fed, happy, and healthy.

When you finish with the baby, you ask how Donna is doing. Donna bursts into tears. She tells you that she has been feeling desperately unhappy since her pregnancy began. She has been feeling so depressed, she reports, that she is not sure she will be able to get out of bed anymore to take care of her son. You say, "Tell me about this past year." Donna tells you that this is a first marriage for her and for Jack, and neither of them has children from previous relationships. In their discussions prior to marriage, she and Jack had never resolved their differences about having children. Donna was ambivalent about having a child; her husband was sure he did not want one. Because they are

devout Roman Catholics, they used the rhythm method of birth control. When Donna told Jack she was pregnant after two months of marriage, he became very angry and blamed Donna for tricking him into having a baby. Although she had not tricked him, Donna felt guilty and blamed herself for becoming pregnant. Terrified that Jack would leave her if she told him how she felt, she kept all her own feelings of sadness, anger, and depression inside. She did not want to be a single parent. Abortion was never considered because of their religious beliefs.

During the pregnancy, Jack was emotionally withdrawn, depressed, and refused to take part in any activity related to the upcoming birth. Donna's sister attended Lamaze classes with her and coached her during the birth because Jack would not attend. Donna felt jealous of the women whose husbands were so attentive during these classes. Ever since her son's birth, Donna says that she has had "postpartum depression." She has told no one how depressed she feels because she is afraid she will have to be hospitalized as she was several times in her late twenties and early thirties for episodes of clinical depression.

When you do a genogram with her, you discover a family history of depression. Both her grandmother and mother suffered bouts of deep depression, and her grandmother had been hospitalized for a year in a psychiatric institution following menopause. Donna's father is an emotionally withdrawn man whose only sister committed suicide when she was 40. Donna's sister has an eating disorder; she is bulimic.

Now that Donna has been home for three weeks with her son, she sees her sister twice a week. Jack is pleased that they have a son, and he is beginning to spend time after he comes home from work playing with Stephen. Donna cannot understand why it makes her angry instead of happy that Jack is becoming involved with their child. Because Jack has refused to support them in a manner that would allow Donna to stay home with Stephen, Donna must return to work after her six-week maternity leave. She is afraid she will be unable to function at work and has yet to find a day care facility for Stephen. Donna worries about these things and has difficulty both in falling asleep and in getting up during the night to feed her son. She says she cries "at the drop of a hat" and has lost

weight. She weighs less now than before she was pregnant. She has little interest in anything, including her baby, and she says that life does not really seem worth living anymore.

- Does Donna have any typical signs of depression? If so, describe them.
- How would you assess her potential for suicide?
- Do you think Donna's depression is "normal" postpartum depression or clinical depression requiring psychiatric assessment and treatment? Why?
- Based on your assessment, will you follow Donna yourself or refer her to a psychiatrist or mental health worker?
- How will you involve Donna's husband and sister in the plan of care?
- What other interventions might be warranted with this family?

🦋 TESTING YOUR UNDERSTANDING

- What are some of the personal, family, and societal effects of mental health problems? (pp. 712–713)
- What are some of the factors that influence the development and progression of mental health problems? (pp. 713–721)
- Describe symptoms characteristic of schizophrenia. What forms of disorganized speech are commonly associated with schizophrenia? Give an example of each. (p. 716)
- How do symptoms of mood disorders differ from those of anxiety disorders? (pp. 716–717)

- What are the major strategies for preventing mental health problems? (p. 721)
- What are the major approaches to treatment of mental health problems? How might community health nurses be involved in each? (pp. 721–724)
- What are the areas of emphasis in maintenance therapy for mental health problems? Give an example of community health nursing involvement in each. (p. 724)

REFERENCES

American Psychiatric Association. (2000). *Diagnostic and statistical manual of mental disorders* (4th ed., Text Revision). *(DSM-IV-TR).* Washington, DC: Author.

Armstrong, E. (1999). Role of the community nurse in caring for people with depression. *Nursing Standard, 13*(35), 40–43.

Bradshaw, T., & Haddock, G. (1998). Is befriending by trained volunteers of value to people suffering from long-term mental illness? *Journal of Advanced Nursing, 27,* 713–720.

Carney, P. A., Rhodes, L. A., Eliassen, S., Badger, L. W., et al. (1998). Variations in approaching the diagnosis of depression: A guided focus group study. *Journal of Family Practice, 46,* 73–82.

Clinton, M., Lunney, P., Edwards, H., Weir, D., & Barr, J. (1998). Perceived social support and community adaptation in schizo-

phrenia. *Journal of Advanced Nursing, 27,* 955–965.

Davis, K. M., & Mathew, E. (1998). Pharmacologic management of depression in the elderly. *The Nurse Practitioner, 23*(6), 16, 17, 26, 28, 31–32, 41–42, 44–47.

Diala, C. C., Muntaner, C., Walrath, C., Nickerson, K., LaVeist, T., & Leaf, P. (2001). Racial/ethnic differences in attitudes toward seeking professional mental health services. *American Journal of Public Health, 91,* 805–807.

Flaskerud, J. H. (2000). Ethnicity, culture, and neuropsychiatry. *Issues in mental health nursing, 21,* 2–29.

Frangou, S., & Murray, R. M. (2000). *Schizophrenia* (2nd ed.). London: Martin Dunitz.

Gafoor, M., & Rassool, G. H. (1998). The coexistence of psychiatric disorders and substance misuse: Working with dual diagnosis

patients. *Journal of Advanced Nursing, 27,* 497–502.

Hagar, R. (1999). Legislative action. *NAMI California Statement: The state's voice on mental illness, XIX*(6), 1.

Husted, J., & Jorgens, A. (2000). Population density as a factor in the rehospitalization of persons with serious and persistent mental illness. *Psychiatric Services, 51,* 603–605.

Kelder, S. H., Murray, N. G., Orpinas, P., Prokhorov, A., et al. (2001). Depression and substance use in minority middle-school students. *American Journal of Public Health, 91,* 761–766.

Kingdon, D. C., & Turkington, D. (1994). *Cognitive-behavioral therapy of schizophrenia.* New York: Guilford Press.

Lehman, A. F. (1999). Quality of care in mental health: The case of schizophrenia. *Health Affairs, 18,* 52–65.

Link, B. G., Phelan, J. C., Bresnahan, M., Stueve, A., & Pescosolido, B. A. (1999). Public conceptions of mental illness: Labels, causes, dangerousness, and social distance. *American Journal of Public Health, 89,* 1328–1333.

McCann, E. (2000). The expression of sexuality in people with psychoses: Breaking the taboos. *Journal of Advanced Nursing, 32,* 132–138.

Mechanic, D., & McAlpine, D. D. (1999). Mission unfulfilled: Potholes on the road to mental health parity. *Health Affairs, 18,* 7–21.

National Center for Chronic Disease Prevention and Health Promotion. (1998). Self-reported frequent mental distress among adults—United States, 1993–1996. *Morbidity and Mortality Weekly Report, 47,* 325–333.

Neugebauer, R. (1999). Mind matters: The importance of mental disorders in public health's 21st century mission. *American Journal of Public Health, 89,* 1309–1311.

Norquist, G., & Hyman, S. E. (1999). Advances in understanding and treating mental illness: Implications for policy. *Health Affairs, 18,* 32–47.

Patton, G. C., Carlin, J. B., Coffey, C., Wolfe, R., Hibbert, M., & Bowes, G. (1998). Depression, anxiety, and smoking initiation: A prospective study over 3 years. *American Journal of Public Health, 88,* 1518–1522.

Penninx, B. W. J. H., Leveille, S., Ferrucci, L., van Eijk, J. Th. M., & Guralnik, J. M. (1999). Exploring the effects of depression on physical disability: Longitudinal evidence from the established populations for epidemiologic studies of the elderly. *American Journal of Public Health, 89,* 1346–1352.

Pescosolido, B. A., Monahan, J., Link, B. G., Stueve, A., & Kikuzawa, S. (1999). The public's view of the competence, dangerousness, and need for legal coercion of persons with mental health problems. *American Journal of Public Health, 89,* 1339–1345.

Schulberg, H. C., Katon, W., Simon, G., & Rush, J. (1998). Treating major depression in primary care practice. *Archives of General Psychiatry, 55,* 1121–1127.

Simon, G. E. (1999). Economic evidence and policy decisions. In M. Maj & N. Sartorius (Eds.), *Depressive disorders* (pp. 452–455). New York: Wiley.

Stuhlmiller, C. M. (1998). Understanding seasonal affective disorder and experiences in northern Norway. *Image: Journal of Nursing Scholarship, 30,* 151–156.

U.S. Census Bureau. (1999). *Statistical abstract of the United States, 1999* (119th ed.). Washington, DC: Author.

U.S. Department of Health and Human Services. (2000a). *Health, United States, 2000.* Washington, DC: Author.

U.S. Department of Health and Human Services. (2000b). *Healthy people, 2010* (Conference edition, in two volumes). Washington, DC: Author.

U.S. Public Health Service. (1999). *Mental health: A report of the surgeon general.* Washington, DC: Author.

Ustun, T. B. (1999). The global burden of mental disorders. *American Journal of Public Health, 89,* 1315–1318.

Vitucci, N. (1999). Corrections challenged with treating mentally ill inmates. *Correct Care, 13*(3), 1, 14.

Wells, K. B., & Sherbourne, C. D. (1999). Functioning and utility for current health of patients with depression or chronic medical conditions in managed, primary care practices. *Archives of General Psychiatry, 56,* 897–904.

World Health Organization. (1999). *The world health report, 1999: Making a difference.* Geneva, Switzerland: Author.

Wu, L., & Anthony, J. C. (1999). Tobacco smoking and depressed mood in late childhood and early adolescence. *American Journal of Public Health, 89,* 1837–1840.

Wuerker, A. K. (2000). The family and schizophrenia. *Issues in Mental Health Nursing, 21,* 127–141.

SUBSTANCE ABUSE

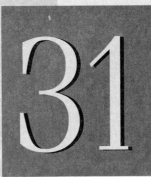

31

Chapter Objectives

After reading this chapter, you should be able to:

- Differentiate among theories of substance abuse.
- Identify criteria for diagnosing psychoactive substance dependence.
- Distinguish between psychoactive substance dependence and abuse.
- Identify substances that lead to dependence and abuse.
- Describe personal, family, and societal effects of substance abuse.
- Discuss aspects of community health nursing assessment in relation to substance abuse.
- Identify major approaches to primary prevention of substance abuse.
- Describe the components of the intervention process in secondary prevention of substance abuse.
- Identify general principles in the treatment of substance abuse.
- Describe treatment modalities in substance abuse control.
- Discuss harm reduction and its role in control of substance abuse.

Media Link

http://www.prenhall.com/clark

Additional interactive resources for this chapter can be found on the companion Web site. Click on Chapter 31 and "Begin" to select the activities for this chapter.

Most drugs are used appropriately for medicinal purposes, but substance abuse is a growing world problem. The illegal drug trade is big business, and the fact that many substances with the potential for abuse also have legitimate use has made control of substance abuse difficult. *Drug use* is the taking of a drug in the correct amount, frequency, and strength for its medically intended purpose. *Drug abuse* or misuse, on the other hand, is the deliberate use of a drug for other than medicinal purposes in a manner that can adversely affect one's health or ability to function.

In the United States, the abuse of alcohol and other drugs and the use of tobacco products are of particular concern. For example, more than 929,000 people in the United States sought substance abuse treatment in 1997 (U.S. Census Bureau, 1999). The magnitude of concern for problems of substance use and abuse is also seen in the development of more than 40 national health promotion and disease prevention objectives for the year 2010 related to tobacco use and the abuse of alcohol and other drugs. These objectives can be reviewed on the Healthy People 2010 Web site accessible through links on the companion Web site for this book. Baseline data and targets for selected objectives are provided at the end of this chapter.

In this chapter, perspectives on causes of abuse and trends in substance use and abuse are examined. Risk factors contributing to all forms of substance abuse, signs and symptoms of specific types of abuse, and community health nursing interventions in the control of substance abuse are addressed. The focus of the chapter is the abuse of psychoactive substances addressed by the *Diagnostic and Statistical Manual of Mental Disorders*, Fourth Edition (Text Revision) *(DSM-IV-TR)* of the American Psychiatric Association (2000).

PSYCHOACTIVE SUBSTANCES: DEPENDENCE AND ABUSE

Substance abuse involves the inappropriate use of psychoactive substances. *Psychoactive substances* are drugs or chemicals that alter ordinary states of consciousness, including mood, cognition, or behavior (Insel & Roth, 1998). The *DSM-IV-TR* recognizes abuse of several substances under umbrella diagnoses of psychoactive substance dependence and psychoactive substance abuse. The *psychoactive substance dependence syndrome* is a cluster of cognitive, behavioral, and physiologic symptoms that indicate impaired control over the use of a psychoactive substance and continued use despite adverse consequences (American Psychiatric Association, 2000). Diagnosis of psychoactive substance dependence is based on the signs and symptoms presented at right.

HIGHLIGHTS

Signs and Symptoms of Psychoactive Substance Dependence

- Increasing amounts of substance used, or use extending over a longer period than intended
- Persistent desire for the substance or one or more unsuccessful attempts to control its use
- Increased time spent in obtaining, using, or recovering from the effects of the substance
- Frequent symptoms of intoxication or withdrawal interfering with obligations
- Elimination or reduction of important occupational, social, or recreational activities as a result of substance use
- Continued use of the substance despite recurrent problems caused
- Increased tolerance to the substance
- Experience of characteristic withdrawal symptoms
- Increased substance use to decrease withdrawal symptoms

Psychoactive substance abuse involves maladaptive patterns of substance use that do not meet the criteria for dependence. Criteria for a diagnosis of abuse include continued use of a substance (or substances) despite persistent or recurrent physical, psychological, or social problems related to its use or recurrent use of the substance in physically dangerous situations (e.g., driving while intoxicated). Because substance abuse is a precursor to dependence, the term *substance abuse* is used throughout this chapter in discussing the role of the community health nurse in its prevention and control.

PERSPECTIVES ON CAUSATION IN SUBSTANCE ABUSE

The trajectory of substance abuse usually includes four phases: experimental or social use, problematic use and abuse, dependence and addiction, and recovery and relapse (Allen, 1998). Not every user, however, progresses from initial experimentation to dependence. What explains progression to abuse and dependence in some people and not in others?

At present, there is no definitive answer to this question. An important trend to be noted, however, is the changing historical perspective on abusive disorders. For many years, society perceived substance abuse, particularly drunkenness, as a character defect and a vice. This view was largely supplanted in the twentieth century by the biomedical concept of substance abuse and dependence as disease (Muller, 1999). This model, however, does not effectively address the current propensity for recreational use of drugs (Lennings, 2000). There is also some evidence that public opinion is drifting back toward a concept of blame for the user based on the perception that use and abuse are personal choices, the consequences of which are to be endured by the user (Muller, 1999). The most recent genre of theories of causation in substance abuse, biopsychosocial theory, suggests that abuse is a product of the interaction of multiple genetic, psychological, and environmental factors (Allen, 1998). These factors will be discussed later in this chapter.

PSYCHOACTIVE SUBSTANCES AND THEIR USE

Psychoactive substances are abused because of their desirable initial effects. Some of these effects and the drugs associated with them are presented in Table 31–1 ■. Unfortunately, many psychoactive drugs with potential for abuse have rebound effects that are usually the opposite of their initial effects and lead to repeated use to eliminate the undesirable symptoms created by the rebound. These adverse effects are discussed later in this chapter. Because of the phenomenon of tolerance, the user requires larger and larger doses of many drugs to combat rebound effects and to achieve the desired pleasurable effect. *Drug tolerance* is an adaptation of the body to a substance such that previous doses do not have the desired effect. Psychoactive substances commonly involved in either dependence or abuse are presented below.

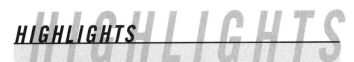

HIGHLIGHTS

Substances Commonly Involved in Substance Abuse or Dependence

- Alcohol
- Sedatives, hypnotics, and anxiolytics
- Opioids
- Cocaine
- Amphetamines
- Hallucinogens
- Cannabis
- Inhalants
- Steroids
- Nicotine

Alcohol

The alcohol contained in alcoholic beverages is ethyl alcohol created by the fermentation of grain mixtures or the juice of fruits and berries. After ingestion, alcohol is rapidly absorbed into the bloodstream through the gastrointestinal tract and functions as a central nervous system (CNS) depressant.

Although moderate alcohol intake has been found to have positive health effects, alcohol abuse remains a serious problem in the United States and elsewhere in the world. In 1998, 16% of the U.S. adult population reported binge drinking (more than five alcoholic drinks on a single occasion), with 8% of those 12 to 17 years of age engaged in this practice (U.S. Department of Health and Human Services [USDHHS], 2000a). Approximately 40% of college students in 1996 exhibited a drinking problem (USDHHS, 1998), and the 1999 Youth Risk Behavior Surveillance (YRBS) indicated that 31.5% of high school students in participating states and cities engaged in periodic heavy drinking (Kann et al., 2000). Nearly 10% of the U.S. population (8 million people) meet diagnostic criteria for alcohol dependence, and 7% qualify as abusers (USDHHS, 2000b).

Sedatives, Hypnotics, and Anxiolytics

A second group of drugs frequently abused are the sedatives, hypnotics, and anxiolytics. Sedatives are used to calm nervousness, irritability, and excitement, whereas hypnotics induce sleep. Many drugs have sedative effects in lower doses and hypnotic effects in higher doses. Anxiolytics (also known as antianxiety agents or minor tranquilizers) are used to reduce anxiety and tension and promote sleep. All three types of drugs are CNS depressants.

These drugs are frequently prescribed for symptoms of nervousness, anxiety, or difficulty sleeping. Unfortunately, their prescription for legitimate use often creates dependence. In low doses, these drugs produce a mild state of euphoria, reduce inhibitions, and create feelings of relaxation and decreased tension. Their major pharmacologic action is CNS depression. Drugs involved in this category of substance abuse include tranquilizers such as chlordiazepoxide hydrochloride (Librium) and diazepam (Valium); barbiturate sedatives; nonbarbiturates such as hydroxyzine hydrochloride (Atarax) and meprobamate (Equanil); and hypnotics such as methaqualone hydrochloride (Quaalude) and diphenhydramine hydrochloride (Nytol, Sleep-eze, Sominex). Because of their widespread use for both legitimate and illegitimate reasons and their easy availability, precise figures on the abuse of these drugs are difficult to obtain. In 1997, however, an estimated 0.4% of the U.S. population over 12 years of age engaged in nonmedical use of tranquilizers (U.S. Census Bureau, 1999).

Opioids

Opioids are also CNS depressants and are derived naturally from the opium poppy or created synthetically. Opioids bind to CNS cell receptors to mimic the action of naturally produced endorphins that relieve pain. In

■ **TABLE 31–1**   **Selected Psychoactive Substances, Street Names, Typical Routes of Administration, and Effects Promoting Abuse**

SUBSTANCE	STREET NAMES	TYPICAL ROUTE OF ADMINISTRATION	EFFECTS PROMOTING ABUSE
Alcohol	Beer, wine, spirits, booze, various brand names	Orally ingested	Relaxation, decreased inhibitions, increased confidence, euphoria
Sedatives, hypnotics, and anxiolytics		Orally ingested, injected	Calming effect, decreased nervousness and anxiety, ability to sleep, relaxation, mild intoxication, loss of inhibition
Barbiturates			
Amytal	Blues, downers		
Nembutal	Yellows, yellow jackets		
Phenobarbital	Phennie, purple hearts		
Seconal	Reds, F-40s, Redbirds		
Tuinal	Rainbows, tooies		
Quaalude	Ludes, 714s, Q's, Quay, Quad, mandrex		
Tranquilizers (minor)	Tranks, downs, downers, goof balls, sleeping pills, candy		
Dalmane			
Equanil/Miltown	Muscle relaxants, sleeping pills		
Librium			
Valium			
Serax			
Opioids			
Codeine	Schoolboy	Orally ingested	Pain relief, euphoria
Demerol	Demies, dolls, dollies, Amidone	Injected	
Dilaudid	Little D, Lords	Injected	
Heroin	Smack, junk, downtown, H, black tar, horse, stuff	Injected, smoked, sniffed	
Methadone	Meth, dollies	Injected	
Morphine	M, Miss Emma, morph, morpho, tab, white stuff, monkey	Injected	
Opium	Blue velvet, black stuff, Dover's powder, paregoric	Orally ingested, smoked, injected	
Percodan	Perkies	Orally ingested	
Cocaine	Coke, snow, uptown, flake, crack, bump, toot, c, candy	Snorted, injected, smoked	Increased alertness, confidence, euphoria, reduced fatigue
Amphetamines		Orally ingested	Increased alertness, confidence, decreased fatigue, euphoria
Benzedrine	Bennies, pep pills, uppers, truck drivers		
Biphetamine	Black beauties		
Desoxyn	Co-pilots		
Dexedrine	Dex, speed, dexies		
Methedrine	Meth, crank, speed, crystal, go fast		
MDMA	Ecstasy		
Hallucinogens		Orally ingested, smoked, injected	Altered perceptions, mystical experience
Phencyclidine	Angel dust, krystal, DOA, hog, PCP, peace pill	Smoked, orally ingested, injected	Dreamlike state producing hallucinations

SUBSTANCE	STREET NAMES	TYPICAL ROUTE OF ADMINISTRATION	EFFECTS PROMOTING ABUSE
Hallucinogens (continued)			
LSD	Acid, microdot, cubes		
MDA	The love drug		
Mescaline	Cactus, mesc		
Peyote	Buttons		
Psilocybin	Magic mushrooms, shrooms, sacred mushrooms		
Cannabis		Smoked, orally ingested	Relaxation, euphoria, altered perceptions
Hashish	Kif, herb, hash		
Hashish oil	Honey, hash oil		
Marijuana	Grass, ganja, weed, dope, reefer, Thai sticks, pot, Acapulco gold, roach, loco weed, Maui wowie, joint, Mary Jane		
Inhalants		Inhaled	Relaxation, euphoria, intoxication
Amyl nitrate	Poppers		
Butyl nitrate	Locker room, rush		
Nitrous oxide	Laughing gas		
Nicotine	Various brand names of tobacco products	Smoked, chewed	Relaxation, mild stimulation

addition to relief of pain, opioids create a psychological euphoria that prompts continued use.

Chronic heroin use occurs in approximately 810,000 people in the United States (Goldsmith, 2000a). In 1997, the prevalence of current heroin use among persons aged 12 years and older was less than 1% (U.S. Census Bureau, 1999), but health care providers in many areas of the country are reporting increased use, particularly among young people. In 1997, 2.4% of high school students reported ever using heroin (Kann et al., 2000), and the mean age for initiation of heroin use decreased from 27.4 years in 1998 to 17.6 years in 1997 (Goldsmith, 2000a).

There is growing concern regarding abuse of the synthetic opioid oxycodone (or oxycontin). Oxycontin is a time-release form of oxycodone intended for extended relief of pain. Street drug users have found, however, that chewing or crushing and inhaling or injecting the tablets invalidates the time-release mechanism, resulting in a rapid and powerful high similar to that achieved with morphine. Several deaths have been reported due to drug overdoses with this drug (About, 2001).

Cocaine

Cocaine is a stimulant derived from the leaves of the coca plant. Its use produces euphoria and a sense of competence. Other desired effects include increased energy and clarity of thought. Unlike many of the other drugs presented here, the pleasurable effects of cocaine are extremely short acting (approximately 30 minutes) and

are followed by an intense letdown and craving for another dose.

Use of cocaine may be accompanied by the practice of "freebasing." Normally, to maintain its stability, cocaine is combined with a hydrochloride base, creating a substance that is usually only about 25% cocaine. *Freebasing* involves the use of heat and ether to free the cocaine from its hydrochloride base, thus creating a purer product that produces a more intense effect. Because of the combination of heat and the highly volatile and explosive ether, freebasing is an extremely dangerous practice. To eliminate the need for freebasing, drug dealers created *crack*, a stable form of cocaine without the hydrochloride base that can be smoked rather than inhaled, for a more rapid and more intense effect.

Next to alcohol, cocaine is the abusive substance of greatest concern because of the rapid escalation in its use and its severe adverse effects. In 1998, 0.8% of persons over 12 years of age in the United States reported using cocaine at least once in the preceding month, and similar figures were noted for those 12 to 17 years of age (USDHHS, 2000a). In the 1999 YRBS, 4% of high school students reported cocaine use in the prior 30 days (Kann et al., 2000).

Amphetamines

Amphetamines are CNS stimulants manufactured chemically. Amphetamines have, on occasion, been prescribed to assist weight loss and relieve fatigue, but they are not recommended for either condition. Amphetamines and similar drugs produce feelings of euphoria, energy, confidence, increased ability to concentrate, and improved physical performance. They are often used by truck drivers and students who wish to stay awake to study or by athletes desiring to improve their performance. In 1997, stimulant use was reported by 0.3% of the U.S. population (U.S. Census Bureau, 1999). Current use of amphetamines was reported by a median of 8.9% of high school students in 1999 YRBS surveys in participating states and cities (Kann et al., 2000).

Amphetamines lend themselves to chemical modifications to create "designer" or "club" drugs. **Designer drugs** are modifications of legal drugs whose use in their original form is restricted. Club drugs are used at group activities known as *raves* or *trances*, and include 3,4-methylene-dionymethamphetamine (MDMA), better known as "ecstasy"; ketamine; gammahydroxybutyrate (GHB); and Rohypnol (a tranquilizer), the so-called "date rape" drug (Vo, 2000). Club drugs may cause brain damage and coma as well as long-term effects on memory and learning abilities, seizures, malignant hyperthermia, paranoia, and hostility. Although exact figures on use of these drugs is not known, one 1999 study found ecstasy use as high as 5.6% of high school seniors and another noted a 10-fold escalation in illegal possession arrests (Sutherland, 2001; Vo, 2000).

Hallucinogens

Phencyclidine (PCP) was originally developed as an anesthetic, but its use was discontinued because of its many adverse side effects. The effects of PCP are variable and may include stimulation or depression of the CNS or hallucinations. Its more desirable effects include heightened sensitivity to stimuli, mood elevation, a sense of omnipotence, and relaxation. Unfortunately, PCP has some serious adverse effects. PCP-induced psychosis constitutes a psychiatric emergency, and PCP use may lead to seizures, coma, and death.

Other hallucinogens or psychedelic drugs, such as *d*-lysergic acid diethylamide (LSD), mescaline, peyote, and psilocybin mushrooms, alter experience to create hallucinations. They also distort the distinction between self and the environment to make the user extremely vulnerable to environmental stimuli. Common effects of these drugs include changes in mood (euphoria or terror and despair), heightened sensation or synesthesia (merging of the senses so colors, for example, are experienced as odors or vice versa), changes in perceptions of time and objects, and changes in relationships leading to depersonalization and feelings of merging with other people and objects.

In 1997, 9.6% of the U.S. population over the age of 12 reported ever having used hallucinogens. Current use of hallucinogens was reported by 0.8% of the population (U.S. Census Bureau, 1999).

Cannabis

Cannabis species of plants are the source of marijuana and hashish. The primary psychoactive substance in these drugs is delta-9-tetrahydrocannabinol (THC). THC may be inhaled by smoking marijuana or hashish or ingested and produces relaxation, euphoria, and occasionally altered perceptions of time and space. Marijuana use may contribute to exacerbation of other mental health problems such as schizophrenia and depression.

Current marijuana use in the general population has declined from 9.7% in 1985 to 5.1% in 1997 (U.S. Census Bureau, 1999), but has shown a sharp increase among adolescents to more than twice the target for the year 2000 objectives (USDHHS, 1998). In 1998, for example, 8% of those 12 to 17 years of age reported current use of marijuana, with the highest use occurring among 16 and 17 year olds (15% and 14%, respectively) (USDHHS, 2000a). Similarly, in the 1999 YRBS survey, a median of 27% of youth reported marijuana use in the last month (Kann et al., 2000).

Inhalants

Inhalants are abused by sniffing products such as airplane model glue, nail polish remover, gasoline, aerosols, and anesthetics such as nitrous oxide. They usually produce a sense of euphoria, loss of inhibition, and excitement. Inhalants are often used by people who do not have the financial resources to support more expensive drug habits. In addition to a variety of adverse physical effects such as kidney and heart damage, there is the potential for suffocation while inhaling these substances from a plastic bag. Because of their volatile nature, explosion is another hazard presented by inhalants.

Inhalant use is particularly common among adolescents. Approximately 15% of adolescents reported ever having used inhalants in the 1999 YRBS, and 4.2% reported inhalant use on one or more occasions in the last 30 days (Kann et al., 2000). Overall use in the United States in 1997 was reported at 0.4% of the population (U.S. Census Bureau, 1999).

Steroids

Most steroid use occurs under medical direction for treatment of a variety of conditions in which immunosuppression is a desired outcome (e.g., severe arthritis and other inflammatory conditions). Steroids are abused by a small segment of the population, however, particularly adolescents. For example, in 1999, 3.7% of high school students reported ever having used steroids for nonmedical reasons (Kann et al., 2000).

Anabolic steroids may be used by adolescents and athletes because of their potential to increase strength and weight and to improve body image and athletic performance. It is estimated that as many as 80% of body builders and 50% of other athletic competitors use these drugs (McHenry & Salerno, 1998).

Prolonged use of anabolic steroids leads to acne, diminished breast size, ovulatory and menstrual difficulties, deepened voice, clitoral enlargement, and male-pattern baldness in women. In men, effects of prolonged use include continuing erections (priapism), difficult urination, gynecomastia, and impotence. Both men and women may experience liver impairment, urinary calculi, anemia, gastrointestinal problems (e.g., anorexia, nausea), and insomnia (McHenry & Salerno, 1998).

Nicotine

Nicotine, the last of the abusive substances included in the *DSM-IV-TR* categories of psychoactive substance dependence and abuse, is the psychoactive substance present in tobacco smoke. Nicotine produces feelings of well-being, increases mental acuity and ability to concentrate, and heightens one's sense of purpose. Nicotine may also exert a calming effect on the smoker. Unfortunately, nicotine also contributes to a host of adverse physical effects, including heart disease, several forms of cancer, and chronic respiratory diseases. Although a great deal of progress has been made in efforts to limit tobacco use in the United States, its use among young people continues to be relatively prevalent.

Because of the highly addictive nature of nicotine and its adverse health effects, all forms of tobacco use should be discouraged. Unlike moderate alcohol use, even moderate smoking produces negative effects on health. Nicotine, unlike many other abused substances, has no medical applications.

Efforts to eliminate smoking in the U.S. population have been somewhat successful. For example, in 1997, 29.6% of people over 18 years of age smoked compared to 39% in 1985 (U.S. Census Bureau, 1999). Results of efforts to eliminate smoking among young people have been less effective. In 1999, for example, 33% of high school students reported current tobacco use (Kann et al., 2000).

EFFECTS OF SUBSTANCE ABUSE

Substance abuse contributes to adverse effects for the abusing individual, for his or her family, and for society at large.

Personal Effects

The effects of substance abuse on the individual are physical, psychological, and social. Physical effects include increased morbidity directly related to the effects of the drug or drugs abused, as well as increased potential for exposure to diseases such as AIDS and hepatitis when abuse involves use of contaminated needles or results in sexual promiscuity as a means of financing a drug habit or because of lowered inhibitions. Other physical effects of substance abuse include physical deterioration due to malnutrition and poor hygiene. Some drugs, such as alcohol, nicotine, and barbiturates, also result in withdrawal symptoms when the drug is removed from the client's system. The *withdrawal syndrome* caused by these and other drugs is a complex of symptoms usually including severe discomfort, pain, nausea, vomiting, and, possibly, convulsions. Some drugs also produce chromosomal changes that cause congenital malformations in children as well as increased potential for spontaneous abortion. Death is the ultimate adverse effect of drug use and may result from a drug overdose, from withdrawal, or from the long-term effects of drug use such as cirrhosis, cancer, and cardiovascular disease. Assessment for both short-term and long-term physical effects of specific substances is discussed later in this chapter.

In addition to the desired effects that promote drug use and abuse, psychological effects of drug abuse can include personality disturbances, anxiety, and depression. Organic mental disorders characterized by hallucinations, delusions, dementia, delirium, and disorders of mood or perception may also be caused by substance abuse. In addition, substance abuse may trigger exacerbations of existing mental disorders.

Preoccupation with the abused substance can lead to a variety of social problems for the substance abuser. Relationships with family and friends may be impaired, or abusers may become incapable of or disinterested in performing their jobs and may be fired. For example, job loss has been found to be twice as likely for problem drinkers as for nondrinkers, particularly in times of economic uncertainty. Substance abuse may also lead to poor educational outcomes, limiting the abuser's employability. For instance, alcohol dependence prior to age 18 has been associated with a 50% decrease in educational attainment (Muller, 1999). Unemployment can lead to difficulties in obtaining housing and can contribute to homelessness. Futhermore, the need to obtain money to support a drug habit or to obtain necessities may lead to criminal activity.

Family Effects

The effects of substance abuse on the family of the abuser can be many and severe. These families are characterized by frequent conflict, anger, ambivalence, fear, guilt, confusion, mistrust, and violence as a mode of conflict resolution. The family frequently becomes socially isolated in efforts to cover up the problem of abuse and so are not able to make use of sources of assistance that might be available to them (Grant, 2000). Substance abuse may also be a factor in poor parental role execution, leading to neglect and abuse of children (Ehrmin, 2001).

The effects of parental alcoholism on children have been widely studied. An estimated 25% of U.S. children under 18 years of age are exposed to alcohol abuse by family members (Grant, 2000). Children exposed to parental alcoholism are predisposed to alcohol abuse themselves. They are also more likely to display conduct disorders and delinquency, anxiety disorders, and impaired physical health. In fact, health care costs have been found to be 100% higher in families with alcoholic members than in other families (Gruenwald, Treno, Taff, & Klitzner, 1997).

Family members may exhibit the phenomenon of co-dependence. A *co-dependent* is a person in a continuing relationship with the substance abuser, whose behavior enables the abuser to continue his or her drug-dependent existence (Insel & Roth, 1998). Co-dependents practice maladaptive behaviors to cope with the problem of abuse. Characteristics of co-dependents are summarized below.

HIGHLIGHTS

Characteristics of Co-dependents

- Assumption of responsibility for others' feelings or behaviors
- Difficulty in identifying and expressing feelings
- Excessive worry over the response of others to one's feelings
- Difficulty in forming or maintaining close relationships
- Fear of rejection
- Unrealistic expectations of self and others
- Difficulty making decisions
- Tendency to minimize or deny personal feelings or needs
- Emotional dependence on others
- Reluctance to ask for help
- Reluctance to share problems with others
- Steadfast, though misplaced, loyalty to others
- Need to be needed
- Perfectionism
- Depression
- A need to control
- Anxiety

Direct exposure of children to psychoactive substances has a variety of adverse physical and psychological effects. Children with perinatal exposure to alcohol, nicotine, or other drugs may be lower in birth weight, be particularly irritable and difficult to comfort, and experience poor school performance later in life. Drug use during pregnancy may also contribute to premature labor. Home exposure to tobacco smoke also affects the health status of children and may contribute to a variety of respiratory conditions as well as childhood cancers. The health effects of drug exposures for children are discussed in more detail later in this chapter.

☺THINK ABOUT IT

Would you be willing to be a foster parent for a drug-exposed infant? Why or why not?

Societal Effects

Societal effects of substance abuse include increased morbidity and mortality, higher economic costs, and increased crime. Physical morbidity related to psychoactive substance abuse was addressed in relation to personal effects of substance abuse. At the societal level, abuse leads to increased incidence and prevalence of these conditions.

MORTALITY

As noted earlier, substance abuse also leads to increased mortality, either directly as a result of drug overdose or withdrawal or indirectly due to other conditions related to abuse. The contribution of smoking to increased mortality was discussed in Chapter 29. An estimated 14,000 lives are lost each year to drug abuse, and 40% of emergency department visits and 90% of drug-related deaths are due to cocaine and heroin use alone (Drucker, 1999). Three fourths of all poisoning deaths in the United States in 1995 were related to drug use. From 1985 to 1995, the rate of drug poisonings in males tripled (Fingerhut & Cox, 1998), and deaths due to opiate use increased by 25% from 1994 to 1998 (National Center for Injury Prevention and Control, 2000).

Drug-related mortality rates increased from 3.8 per 100,000 population in 1987 to 4.7 per 100,000 in 1996. Increased mortality was more pronounced in some groups than in others, increasing 21% for blacks and 40% for Hispanics during the same time period (USDHHS, 1998). Mortality for particular drugs also varies by city. For example, San Francisco General Hospital experiences four nonfatal heroin overdoses and at least one death every day (Goldsmith, 2000a).

Mortality related to alcohol abuse is of particular concern. In spite of decreases in the number of alcohol-related motor vehicle fatalities, 38% of motor vehicle fatalities in 1999 involved alcohol (U.S. Department of Transportation, 1999). Alcohol use is also implicated in other injury fatalities, including falls, drowning, and burns (Gruenwald et al., 1997). In addition to accident fatalities, alcohol is a factor in other deaths, including homicide; suicide; deaths due to cancers of the lip, oral cavity, pharynx, esophagus, stomach, liver, and larynx; cardiovascular deaths; and deaths due to respiratory diseases, digestive diseases, and diabetes mellitus.

COST

Substance abuse also affects society in terms of its economic costs. Together, drug and alcohol abuse cost society $276 billion in preventable health care expenditures (Sutherland, 2001). Federal drug enforcement activities account for 67% of the $16 million drug budget and another $20 billion are spent by state and local governments on enforcement (Drucker, 1999). Societal costs for fetal alcohol syndrome are estimated to range from $75.6 million to $321 million per year (Egeland et al., 1998). Without doubt, drug and alcohol abuse are costly public health problems that the nation can ill afford.

CRIME

One final social effect associated with the abuse of many substances (excluding nicotine) is increased crime. In 1997, there were 1.2 million drug-related arrests in the United States, 14% of them in people under 18 years of age and 34% in the 18- to 24-year age group. The drug arrest rate was 725.9 per 100,000 population. The majority of these arrests (82%) involved illegal possession of drugs, but 18% were related to production and sale of illicit drugs. Drug and alcohol use have also been implicated in other crimes not strictly related to drugs. For example, 52% of those incarcerated in state and federal prisons for murder in 1997 were under the influence of drugs or alcohol. Similarly, drugs and alcohol figured in 56% of negligent manslaughter and robbery convictions in state correctional systems, 52% of assault convictions, and 45% of sexual assaults (U.S. Census Bureau, 1999).

COMMUNITY HEALTH NURSING AND CONTROL OF SUBSTANCE ABUSE

To control problems of substance abuse, community health nurses must identify those persons and groups at risk for substance abuse and its adverse effects, as well as those who are actually experiencing problems of abuse. The nursing process provides a framework for identifying these people and for planning, implementing, and evaluating interventions to assist them in controlling substance abuse.

ASSESSING THE SUBSTANCE ABUSE SITUATION

Several aspects of community health nursing assessment relate to problems of substance abuse. These include assessing for risk factors, for signs of abuse and dependence, for intoxication, for signs of withdrawal, and for long-term physical and psychological effects of substance abuse. Because of the negative connotations associated with substance abuse, the nursing assessment must be conducted with tact and with an accepting and a nonjudgmental, nonthreatening approach. Nurses must first examine their own attitudes toward substance abuse and work through any negative feelings that may interfere with nurse–client interactions. If clients sense a disparaging or judgmental attitude on the part of the nurse, they are less likely to respond truthfully to questions about their use of psychoactive substances.

Assessing for Risk Factors

The epidemiology of substance abuse indicates that there are contributing factors in five of the six dimensions of health. Community health nurses should keep in mind that the interplay of biological, psychological, and sociocultural factors that lead to substance abuse are unique to each individual, and all areas of clients' lives should be assessed in relation to the potential for substance abuse.

Biophysical Considerations

Human biological factors influencing substance abuse and its effects include genetic inheritance, maturation and aging, and physiologic function.

GENETIC INHERITANCE   A growing body of evidence suggests that substance abuse is associated with some form of genetic predisposition. Studies of adopted children, for example, indicate that alcohol abuse by one or both of the biological parents is associated with alcohol abuse by the child, even if the adoptive parents are nonabusers. Further support for a genetic predisposition for alcoholism comes from the increased risk of alcohol abuse in the second twin if the first of monozygotic twins is alcohol dependent when compared with dizygotic twins.

Research indicating similar ways of processing alcohol and other drugs (e.g., opioids) in the brain suggests that there may also be a genetic component in the abuse of drugs other than alcohol. In assessing individuals and families for the level of risk for substance abuse, the community health nurse prepares a detailed genogram that includes information about the family history of substance abuse as well as the presence of physical and emotional illnesses with a genetic component.

Gender, race, and ethnicity are other factors that may influence substance abuse. For example, men were three times more likely than women to engage in binge drinking and seven times more likely to report chronic drinking in the 1997 BRFSS (Holtzman, Powell-Griner, Bolen, & Rhodes, 2000). With respect to racial or ethnic factors, Asians and African Americans are the ethnic groups most likely to abstain from alcohol use altogether. In 1997, for instance, only 7% of Asians and 9% of African Americans reported binge drinking compared to 19% of Native Americans, 16% of Hispanics, and 14% of Caucasians (Bolen, Rhodes, Powell-Griner, Bland, & Holtzman, 2000).

Age influences one's risk of exposure to drugs and alcohol through social factors. For example, young people are more likely to be exposed to peer influence for drug use or smoking than are older people. Adolescents and preadolescents are particularly vulnerable to this type of influence because of their developmental need to conform to peer expectations and to be part of a group. Often, being part of the group depends on engaging in behaviors that place the individual at risk, such as sexual activity, smoking, and drug and alcohol use. Younger age at onset of alcohol, tobacco, and marijuana use has been linked to greater risk of progression to hard drugs (Golub & Johnson, 2001). Risk for dependence also increases with younger age of initiation of use. For instance, the risk of alcohol dependence for those who start using alcohol at 14 years of age or younger is 40% compared to only 10% in those who initiate alcohol use after age 20. In fact, the risk of dependence has been shown to decrease by 14% for every year of delayed initiation (Grant & Dawson, 1997). Fortunately, the majority of young people who experiment with drugs, however, appear to "grow out of" their use (Drucker, 1999). Community health nurses working with young people should assess their level of maturity and their ability to resist pressure to conform. The elderly have relatively low levels of substance abuse.

One's age also influences the effects of drug exposure, and perinatal exposures to drugs and alcohol have a variety of adverse effects on the fetus. Some psychoactive substances, such as alcohol, amphetamines, and cocaine, have teratogenic effects when taken during pregnancy. *Teratogenic substances* are those that cause physical defects in the developing embryo. Other drugs do not affect fetal development per se, but have other adverse health effects for the neonate or long-term effects for the child. For example, fetal alcohol exposure may result in prenatal and postnatal growth deficits, CNS abnormality, and delayed psychomotor development, and both cocaine and tobacco have been associated with spontaneous abortion (Ness et al., 1999). Fetal, neonatal, and developmental effects of selected psychoactive substances are presented in Table 31-2 ■.

It is estimated that 1 in every 10 babies born in the United States has been exposed to tobacco, alcohol, or illicit drugs in utero. During 1996–1997, for example, 13% of pregnant adult women reported smoking during pregnancy, 14% reported alcohol use, 1% reported binge drinking, and 2% reported use of illicit drugs (USDHHS, 2000b). Community health nurses are often involved in assisting either biological or foster parents to care for these children. Fetal alcohol syndrome (FAS) is a condition resulting from maternal alcohol consumption during pregnancy and is characterized by growth retardation, facial malformations, and CNS dysfunctions that may include mental retardation. Overall, estimated incidence rates for FAS in the United States range from 3 to 22 babies per 10,000 live births, contributing to 1,300 to 8,000 babies born with FAS each year (National Center on Birth Defects and Developmental Disabilities, 2001). Long-term effects of FAS include inability to hold down a job, impulsivity, social withdrawal, poor judgment, and mental retardation.

Even those infants exposed to moderate amounts of alcohol during pregnancy may have long-term effects. It is estimated that three to four times as many infants have fetal alcohol effects as have FAS (USDHHS, 2000a). Approximately 1 in 29 pregnant women continues to

■ **TABLE 31–2**   Fetal, Neonatal, and Developmental Effects of Perinatal Psychoactive Substance Exposure

SUBSTANCE	FETAL EFFECTS	NEONATAL EFFECTS	DEVELOPMENTAL EFFECTS
Alcohol	Growth deficiency, microcephaly, stillbirth, low birth weight (LBW), joint and facial anomalies, cardiac and kidney anomalies	Acute withdrawal with sedation, seizures, poor feeding	Developmental delay, low IQ, hyperactivity
Sedatives, hypnotics	Sedation at delivery	Tremors, hypertonicity, poor suck, high-pitched cry	Unknown
Opioids	Intrauterine growth retardation, microcephaly, prematurity, hyperactivity	Withdrawal with tremors, hypertonicity, poor feeding, diarrhea, seizures, irritability	Increased rate of sudden infant death syndrome (SIDS)
Cocaine	Spontaneous abortion	Tremors, hypertonicity, muscle weakness, seizures	Developmental delay, increased rate of SIDS
Amphetamines	Intrauterine growth retardation, biliary atresia, transposition of great vessels	Stillbirth, LBW, cardiac anomalies, withdrawal	Poor school performance
Hallucinogens	Agitation at delivery, microcephaly	Irritability, poor fine-motor coordination, sensory input problems	Unknown
Cannabis	Bleeding problems in delivery	Sedation, tremors, excessive response to light	Unknown
Inhalants	Unknown	Unknown	Unknown
Nicotine	Intrauterine growth retardation, microcephaly	Jitteriness, poor feeding	Poor school performance, increased rate of SIDS

drink throughout pregnancy, increasing the potential for fetal alcohol effects in their offspring (National Center on Birth Defects and Developmental Disabilities, 2001).

In general, the prevalence of drug and alcohol use declines with increasing age. For example, in 1997 only 1.7% of those seeking treatment for substance abuse were over 65 years of age (U.S. Census Bureau, 1999). However, there may be older clients with substance abuse problems who are not diagnosed because health care providers are not alert to signs and symptoms of abuse in this age group. Elderly clients who do abuse drugs and alcohol are at increased risk for adverse effects of abuse because of decreased ability to metabolize them. In addition, aging itself results in cell loss in target organs, thus increasing their sensitivity to the effects of alcohol and other drugs.

In working with newborns and young children, the community health nurse is alert to signs of perinatal drug exposure. He or she also assesses for risk factors that would make the child or older person particularly vulnerable to substance abuse and its effects.

PHYSIOLOGIC FUNCTION   The relationship between substance abuse and physiologic function is bidirectional. Persons with chronic physical health problems or disability may abuse drugs or alcohol as an escape from pain, depression, or stress related to the disability. Substance abuse may stem from a desire for gratification when other avenues are denied or as a method of regaining control over one's choices and actions. In working with disabled clients, community health nurses assess clients' responses to disability and their vulnerability to substance abuse as a means of coping with disability.

Conversely, substance abuse may result in a variety of physiologic health problems. For example, substance abuse disorders increase the risks of death and disability due to cirrhosis, heart disease, and lung cancer (Neugebauer, 1999). Injection drug users also have a high risk of impairment due to drug impurities and infection. As we saw in Chapter 28, injection drug use is associated with high incidence of HIV infection and hepatitis B, C, and D. Tetanus and abscesses at the injection site also occur with injection drug use (California Department of Health Services, 1998). One major metropolitan hospital, for instance, spends more than $18 million per year to treat drug-related abscesses (Goldsmith, 2000a). As noted earlier, substance use and abuse may also contribute to long-term physical consequences related to accidental injury.

Psychological Considerations

Both personality traits and the presence of psychopathology may contribute to problems of substance abuse. There seem to be some commonalities in the personalities of substance abusers regardless of the type of substance abused. Personality traits that may place one at risk for substance abuse include rebelliousness and nonconformity that may lead to substance abuse as an expression of defiance or as an escape from the constraints and expectations of the adult world. Other common traits in abusers are a greater tolerance of deviant behavior, a poor self-concept, and passive surrender to their belief of their own inevitable failure in life. Abusers of psychoactive substances also tend to be impulsive, unable to value themselves, and have poor tolerance for frustration and anxiety. They may also have difficulty in acknowledging their feelings and in developing interests and deriving pleasure from them. In addition, people who abuse psychoactive substances frequently feel alienated from those around them and are socially isolated. They may also feel powerless, and they usually have poor coping skills.

Substance abusers also tend to display a common set of defense mechanisms that include denial, projection, rationalization, and conflict minimization and avoidance. Abusers frequently deny that they have a problem with substance abuse and assert that they can change their behavior. They may exhibit inability to accept responsibility for their own behavior in other areas as well, and they frequently project or transfer the blame for their own behavior onto others. They also rationalize their behavior without developing true insights into the reason for that behavior. They tend to try to avoid conflict, and may turn to substance abuse as a means of escaping from the stress generated by conflict rather than engaging in positive modes of conflict resolution. Their thinking is characterized by an all-or-nothing quality, and they often make decisions that are inflexible and narrow in scope.

The presence of definite psychopathology also places many people at increased risk of substance abuse, and substance abuse is frequently an attempt to relieve or mask the symptoms of underlying psychiatric disorders. As noted in Chapter 30, clients with dual diagnoses are less compliant with therapy and more likely to be violent than those with substance abuse disorder alone (Gafoor & Rassool, 1998).

Psychological factors are also implicated in tobacco use. For example, depression has been linked to smoking as well as to initiation of drug and alcohol use in adolescents (Kelder et al., 2001). Smokers do not tend to display the psychopathology, alienation, or defense mechanisms typical of other substance abusers; however, young people who begin smoking in the face of current social pressures not to smoke may be exhibiting the defiance that is typical of those who abuse other substances.

Substance abuse may have psychological consequences as well. For example, paranoia has been associated with the use of the club drug ketamine as well as with PCP. Guilt associated with substance abuse and its effects on family members, particularly children, may contribute to relapse after drug treatment unless clients are assisted to deal with their feelings of guilt (Ehrmin, 2001).

Sociocultural Considerations

Factors in the sociocultural dimension may also contribute to problems of substance abuse. These factors can exist within the family unit, one's peer group, or society at large. Within the family, research indicates that perceived disapproval of marijuana as well as perceived risks of harm can influence use in adolescents. Reductions in perceived harm and disapproval have been linked to recent increases in use (Bachman, Johnston, & O'Malley, 1998). Similarly, the use of alcohol or drugs by parents or older siblings may influence drug use by children. Families with low cohesion, high levels of conflict, few shared interests and activities, poor coping strategies, and marital dissatisfaction increase the risk of substance abuse in their members. Families encountering multiple stressors and who have inadequate resources are also at risk. Episodes of violence within the family can also lead family members to abuse substances as a means of escape from family tensions. Community health nurses should assess families for conditions that may contribute to substance abuse by family members.

Peer influence is another factor in the social environment that may contribute to substance abuse. In adolescents and preadolescents in particular, pressure from peers to smoke, drink, or use other psychoactive drugs is a powerful motivator for initiating these behaviors. School performance, truancy, and religious commitment are additional sociocultural factors that influence substance use in adolescents (Bachman et al., 1998). In working with young people, in particular, the nurse carefully assesses peer attitudes toward substance use and abuse as well as the degree to which the individual feels a need to conform to peer-dictated norms.

Social factors such as poverty, unemployment, and discrimination may create a sense of hopelessness and powerlessness that leads to substance abuse as an escape or to enhance one's own feelings of competence. These factors might explain the higher prevalence of some forms of substance abuse among members of minority groups and the poor. Societal attitudes to drug use and abuse also influence the extent of substance abuse in the population. For example, attitudes that promote incarceration rather than treatment are not only ineffective but more costly than substance abuse treatment (Drucker, 1999). Societal action to restrict access to drugs, on the other hand, may be more effective. For example, increasing the minimum legal drinking age has decreased both motor vehicle accident fatalities and suicide among adolescents (Birckmayer & Hemenway, 1999). Similarly, enforcement of zero tolerance laws prohibiting blood alcohol at any level in adolescent drivers is credited with halving the alcohol fatality rate in people under 21 years of age since 1982 (*The Nation's Health*, 1998).

⑥THINK ABOUT IT

Should marijuana use be legalized? If so, for whom?

Culture also seems to play a part in the development of alcohol abuse. Cultural attitudes and modes of introducing alcohol use to young people can either contribute to or impede the development of alcohol abuse. Religion is an aspect of culture that may strongly influence drug use. Strong religious affiliation, whatever the denomination, is associated with reduced risk of drug and alcohol abuse. Cultural factors also influence when drug use behaviors are accepted and when they are not. For example, smoking and use of hallucinogenics are part of traditional religious rituals in some Native American groups. Alcohol use also varies among cultural groups in terms of when and where it occurs, who drinks, levels of alcohol use considered acceptable, what is drunk, and how and why people drink. For example, use of alcohol in many cultures is celebratory in nature; in others it is part of normal dietary patterns (e.g., in France and Italy). Similarly, in some cultural groups alcohol is used by only certain segments of the population (e.g., adults), while in others it is consumed by all. Cultures in which alcohol use is generally disapproved may create a mystique that promotes inappropriate use among the young (e.g., among some conservative Protestant groups in the southern United States). When alcohol use is perceived as manly or desirable, it is embraced; when it is perceived as stupid or disgusting, it tends to be avoided (Heath, 2000). For example, in many Latino cultures and among the Irish, drinking is perceived as related to manly adulthood, and youngsters may begin alcohol use to demonstrate adult behaviors.

In assessing individuals, families, and communities for potential for substance abuse, the community health nurse investigates both the influence of cultural norms and sources of stress on the use of psychoactive substances. In addition, the nurse looks for risk factors such as poverty and unemployment that increase stress and prompt substance abuse.

Other societal factors that contribute to substance abuse should also be assessed, including general norms for abusive behaviors and the availability of psychoactive

CULTURAL CONSIDERATIONS

Among some cultural groups, drinking is considered evidence of adulthood. Because of this perception, young people in these cultural groups may engage in alcohol use, thinking it makes them appear older and more sophisticated.

- What cultural groups are you aware of that have this perception?
- How might programs to prevent alcohol use by adolescents be developed to address these perceptions?
- What cultural groups are familiar to you where drinking alcohol is not considered a mark of adulthood? What is the relative incidence of alcohol abuse in these groups?

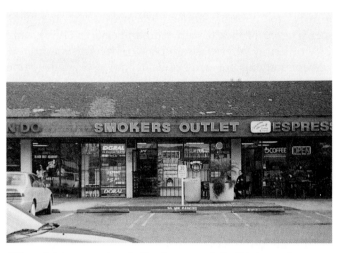

Although tobacco use has declined among adults, it is increasing among young people.

substances. Media portrayals of drinking and smoking as desirable behaviors influence use of these substances. Ready availability of amphetamines in southern California, where methamphetamine labs abound, make this a drug of choice in the area and increase its abuse relative to other psychoactive substances.

Occupation is another sociocultural dimension factor that may contribute to substance abuse. Some occupational groups are at increased risk for substance abuse. People whose work involves drinking or occurs in places where drinking occurs are at higher risk for alcohol abuse than those who do not work in such settings (Muller, 1999). Similarly, there is a relatively high incidence of substance abuse among health care providers because of easy access to controlled drugs. Use of psychoactive substances has been found to vary by nursing specialty area, with emergency department nurses 3.5 times more likely to use cocaine or marijuana than women's health nurses, oncology nurses and nurse administrators more likely to engage in binge drinking, and psychiatric nurses more likely to smoke (Trinkhoff & Storr, 1998). Job dissatisfaction has been shown to contribute to both smoking and drinking behavior in the employed population in general (Muller, 1999).

ETHICAL AWARENESS

You interact socially with one of the nurses who works in the health department with you. She drinks heavily at many of the social events where you encounter her. Recently she has called in sick two or three times on the day after her regular days off. You know that she had been drinking heavily the day before these incidents. You have not noticed alcohol on her breath at work, nor has her work performance been impaired when she is present. Should you inform your supervisor, who seems to accept her stories of illness, that this nurse has an alcohol problem?

Employer attitudes to and sanctions for alcohol, drug, and tobacco use also influence the extent of use among employees. For example, prevalence of drug use declined significantly in military recruits after the initiation of routine screening, and smoking prevalence decreased after smoking was banned during basic training (Bachman, Freedman-Doan, O'Malley, Johnston, & Segal, 1999). As of 1995, 90% of employers with 50 or more employees had adopted alcohol or drug policies (USDHHS, 1998). By 1999, 79% of worksites had formal smoking policies that prohibited smoking or limited it to specifically designated areas (USDHHS, 2000b).

Unemployment and attendant stress and hopelessness may contribute to substance abuse. The effects of unemployment are also seen in the aftermath of substance abuse. Alcohol abusers, for example, are discriminated against in the job market, even when in recovery. Such discrimination leads to increased alcohol abuse. Unemployment is linked to risk of relapse after treatment, but employment is associated with treatment completion (Muller, 1999).

Substance abuse may also lead to other socially stigmatized behaviors. For example, many female drug abusers may engage in prostitution to support their drug habit (Ehrmin, 2001).

Behavioral Considerations

Behavioral factors that influence substance abuse are related to consumption patterns and leisure activities. The community health nurse assesses individual and family consumption patterns related to tobacco, alcohol, and medications. The nurse should ascertain the frequency and amount of substance use as well as the appropriateness of its use. For example, the nurse might determine whether sedatives are in fact being used as prescribed, whether they are kept away from young people in the home, and whether they are ever used in conjunction with alcohol. Nurses should also determine the extent of alcohol use by families. Many people, for example, do not consider taking medications with an alcohol base as drinking, but may be receiving a hefty dose of alcohol through repeated use. Similarly, Mexican American families might return to Mexico to obtain medications such as paregoric (an opioid preparation used for diarrhea) without even knowing about their potential for abuse. The nurse also asks about medicinal uses of alcohol, particularly with children, such as giving alcohol for teething pain or to quiet a fretful child.

Recreational activities can contribute to the use of psychoactive substances in that alcohol and tobacco use are frequent adjuncts to such activities. People tend to drink and smoke when they socialize with others. Friday or Saturday night binges are a relatively common phenomenon, when people can "let go" and drink because they know they will have time to recover before returning to work on Monday. Next to alcohol, marijuana is the most widely used recreational drug, but cocaine is also used recreationally and has the connotation of high status, glamour, and excitement. PCP and the club drugs are also used for recreational purposes.

⑥THINK ABOUT IT

What risk factors for substance abuse are present in your own life? What are you currently doing, or what can you do to eliminate or minimize your risks for substance abuse?

Certain high-risk behaviors associated with substance abuse increase the potential for long-term consequences. The most common form of co-morbidity is polydrug use, which is common among young drug users (Lennings, 2000). Combining alcohol with drug use also increases one's risk of morbidity and mortality, and certain drugs are more likely to be used in combination with alcohol than others. For example, cocaine users have been found to have higher alcohol abuse co-morbidity than opioid users (Preisig & Fenton, 1999).

Sharing of needles and other drug apparatus is a high-risk behavior that increases the risk of infection in injection drug users (IDUs). Research has indicated that some drug users engage in selective sharing only with members of a close-knit group. When local prevalence of infectious diseases such as HIV infection and hepatitis is low, selective sharing can minimize the risk of infection. However, frequent group turnover increases the potential for introduction of disease that, once introduced, progresses rapidly through the group (Valente & Vlahov, 2001). IDUs may also share cigarette filters used to strain drugs prior to injection. Since these filters are not fine enough to eliminate bacteria and viruses, they, too, are a potential source of infection (Caflish, Wang, & Zbinden, 1999).

Health System Considerations

Many of the psychoactive substances with abuse potential originated within the health care system. Opioids were widely used for pain control even during the American Civil War and are still the drug of choice for relief of severe pain. Cocaine and PCP were first used as surgical anesthetics, and marijuana may have some medical use in the treatment of glaucoma and chronic pain. Sedatives and hypnotics are widely used for controlling anxiety, and amphetamines were originally developed as diet aids, although they no longer have any accepted medical use.

Several aspects of the U.S. health care system have contributed to the growing problem of substance abuse. Lack of attention to educating clients and the public about the hazards of substance abuse and failure to identify clients with substance abuse problems have impeded

efforts to control abuse. According to the U.S. Department of Health and Human Services (1998), only 23% of family physicians and 63% of internists routinely screened clients for drug and alcohol use. At the same time, some health care providers have actively fostered drug abuse by prescribing psychoactive drugs inappropriately or by not monitoring the extent of clients' use of these drugs.

The health care system also impedes control of substance abuse by failing to provide adequate treatment for persons affected. For example, health insurance coverage for treatment for substance abuse is minimal at best. Provision of adequate treatment of substance abuse may be further impeded by negative feelings on the part of health care providers toward those who abuse psychoactive substances. Studies have indicated, for example, that despite knowledge of the effectiveness of harm-reduction strategies and the prevalence of periodic relapse during substance abuse treatment, many programs expel clients who revert to drug use during treatment (Lennings, 2000). Many clients in need may not have access to services. For example, many shelters for the homeless refuse abusers despite the fact that a large proportion of homeless individuals abuse alcohol and other drugs. It may also be difficult for pregnant abusers or women with children to find appropriate treatment programs.

⑥THINK ABOUT IT

What factors make control of substance abuse so difficult? How could these factors be modified or eliminated?

The health care system may pose additional barriers to care that are particularly burdensome for some population groups. For instance, most treatment programs are geared toward the needs of younger people and may not recognize the unique needs of the elderly substance abuser. Certainly Medicare, in the implementation of the DRG (diagnosis-related group) system, does not take note of the extended time needed to safely detoxify the elderly substance abuser. In addition, because older people are often considered nonproductive members of society, priority for placement in treatment facilities may be given to younger people. Tips for assessing risk factors for substance abuse in individuals and in the population are presented on page 743. A Substance Abuse Risk Factor Inventory is also provided on the companion Web site for this book. 🌐

Assessing for Signs of Substance Abuse

In addition to assessing individuals, families, and communities for risk factors that may contribute to substance abuse, the nurse should assess individual clients for

assessment tips assessment tips assessment tips

ASSESSING RISK FOR SUBSTANCE ABUSE

Biophysical Considerations

- Are there existing physical health problems contributing to substance abuse? What effects does substance abuse have on efforts to control existing physical health problems (e.g., diabetes)?
- Is there a family history of substance abuse?
- Does the client exhibit signs of intoxication or withdrawal? Does the client exhibit long-term effects of substance use or abuse?
- What influence, if any, does age have on the effects of substance abuse?
- Is the client pregnant? What effects will substance abuse have on the fetus?

Psychological Considerations

- Does the client have a poor self-image?
- What are the client's life goals? Are they realistic?
- Does the client exhibit poor impulse control? What is the client's level of frustration tolerance?
- What life stresses is the client experiencing? What is the extent of the client's coping abilities? What defense mechanisms does the client display?
- Is there underlying psychopathology contributing to substance abuse?

Sociocultural Considerations

- To what extent do social mores contribute to substance abuse?
- What effect does legislative activity have on substance abuse?
- Does the client's peer network support substance use and abuse? Is substance use a regular part of social interaction?
- Does the client's family exhibit characteristics of co-dependence?
- What cultural or religious values or practices influence substance abuse?

- Has the client been a victim or perpetrator of family violence?
- What social factors (e.g., unemployment) contribute to substance abuse?
- How readily available are abused substances?
- What contribution, if any, does occupation make to substance abuse? What is the effect of substance abuse on the client's ability to work?
- What is the contribution of substance abuse to criminal activity? To homelessness?
- What is the extent of substance abuse among homeless individuals?

Behavioral Considerations

- What substances are abused? Is there evidence of multisubstance abuse?
- Are abused substances used recreationally? Is substance use associated with leisure activities?
- To what extent does the client engage in other high-risk behaviors (e.g., driving while intoxicated, high-risk sexual activity)?

Health System Considerations

- What is the attitude of health care providers to clients with substance abuse problems?
- Are health care providers alert to signs and symptoms of substance abuse?
- To what extent do health care providers educate clients about substance abuse?
- What health system factors contribute to substance abuse (e.g., inappropriate prescription of psychoactive drugs)?
- What treatment facilities are available to substance abusers? To special populations of substance abusers (e.g., pregnant women, adolescents)?
- Does the client have financial access to substance abuse treatment?

general indications of existing abuse. Such assessment is particularly needed for clients with psychiatric disorders because of the high rates of dual diagnosis. General indicators that a person has a problem with abuse of a psychoactive substance include frequent intoxication, preoccupation with obtaining and using the substance, binge use, changes in personality or mood, withdrawal, problems with family members related to use of the substance, problems with friends or neighbors, problems on the job (absenteeism, poor performance, interpersonal difficulties), and conflicts with law enforcement officials.

Additional indicators include belligerence, financial problems, inability to discontinue substance use despite attempts, continued use of the substance despite related health conditions and other problems, and increasing tolerance to the substance.

Assessing for Intoxication

Another aspect of the community health nurse's assessment related to substance abuse is assessing individuals for signs of intoxication. *Intoxication* is a state of diminished physical or mental control that occurs as a result of the current use of psychoactive drugs. Intoxication with different drugs may be reflected in differing symptoms. For example, cocaine intoxication is characterized by disinhibition, impaired judgment and impulsivity, grandiosity, and compulsively repeated actions. Other common symptoms include hypersexuality, hypervigilance, and hyperactivity. Nicotine intoxication, on the other hand, is characterized by increased blood pressure, heart rate, and muscle tone. Signs of intoxication with selected psychoactive substances are presented in Table 31–3 ■.

Assessing for Withdrawal

The physiologic dependence engendered by some psychoactive substances leads to withdrawal or abstinence syndrome when the substance is withheld. A withdrawal syndrome is a complex of symptoms that accompany abstinence from a psychoactive substance, usually characterized by severe discomfort, pain, nausea, vomiting, and, possibly, convulsions. The severity of withdrawal may vary with the abusive substance and the degree of dependence experienced by the client. The community health nurse working with clients who may abuse psychoactive substances assesses the client for signs of withdrawal. Typical withdrawal symptoms for selected psychoactive substances are presented in Table 31–4 ■.

Withdrawal can be extremely dangerous and may even be life threatening, especially for vulnerable clients. Withdrawal is a particularly serious event for pregnant women, when both mother and fetus are at risk, and for the elderly. The community health nurse should be alert in assessing these clients for signs of withdrawal. Interventions during the withdrawal phase are addressed later in this chapter.

The physical and psychological discomfort and the deep depression that may occur with withdrawal from psychoactive drug use may lead to suicide. The community health nurse assessing clients for withdrawal symptoms should also carefully assess them for potential suicide. Clients should be monitored carefully and asked about suicidal thoughts.

Assessing for Long-Term Effects of Substance Abuse

In addition to assessing clients for signs and symptoms of intoxication and withdrawal, community health nurses should also assess individual clients for symptoms of long-term effects of substance abuse. These effects can be physical or psychological and vary with the psychoactive substance. For example, long-term effects of alcohol abuse include malnutrition, cirrhosis, and liver cancer, and typical effects of phencyclidine abuse are psychoses and insomnia. Typical long-term effects that should be considered with specific substances are presented in Table 31–5 ■. The community health nurse assessing the health of population groups assesses morbidity and mortality related to these long-term effects of substance abuse in the population.

■ TABLE 31–3   Signs of Intoxication with Selected Psychoactive Substances

SUBSTANCE	TYPICAL INDICATIONS OF INTOXICATION
Alcohol	Decreased alertness, impaired judgment, slurred speech, nausea, double vision, vertigo, staggering, unpredictable emotional changes, stupor, unconsciousness, increased reaction time
Sedatives, hypnotics, anxiolytics	Slurred speech; slow, shallow respiration; cold and clammy skin; nystagmus; weak and rapid pulse; drowsiness, blurred vision, unconsciousness; disorientation; depression; poor judgment; motor impairment
Opioids	Sedation, hypertension, respiratory depression, impaired intellectual function, constipation, pupillary constriction, watery eyes, increased pulse and blood pressure
Cocaine	Irritability, anxiety, slow weak pulse, slow shallow breathing, sweating, dilated pupils, increased blood pressure, insomnia, seizures, dysinhibition, impulsivity, compulsive actions, hypersexuality, hypervigilance, hyperactivity
Amphetamines	Sweating, dilated pupils, increased blood pressure, agitation, fever, irritability, headache, chills, insomnia, agitation, tremors, seizures, wakefulness, hyperactivity, confusion, paranoia
Hallucinogens	Dilated pupils, mood swings, elevated blood pressure, paranoia, bizarre behavior, nausea and vomiting, tremors, panic, flushing, fever, sweating, agitation, aggression, nystagmus (PCP)
Cannabis	Reddened eyes; increased pulse, respirations, and blood pressure; laughter; confusion; panic; drowsiness
Inhalants	Giddiness, drowsiness, increased vital signs, headache, nausea, fainting, stupor, fatigue, slurred speech, disorientation, delirium
Nicotine	Headache; loss of appetite; nausea; increased pulse, blood pressure, and muscle tone

■ TABLE 31–4 Indications of Withdrawal from Selected Psychoactive Substances

SUBSTANCE	INDICATIONS OF WITHDRAWAL
Alcohol	Anxiety, insomnia, tremors, delirium, convulsions
Sedatives, hypnotics, anxiolytics	Anxiety, insomnia, tremors, delirium, convulsions (may occur up to 2 weeks after stopping use of anxiolytics)
Opioids	Restlessness, irritability, tremors, loss of appetite, panic, chills, sweating, cramps, watery eyes, runny nose, nausea, vomiting, muscle spasms, impaired coordination, depressed reflexes, dilated pupils, yawning
Cocaine	*Early crash:* agitation, depression, anorexia, high level of craving, suicidal ideation *Middle crash:* fatigue, depression, no craving, insomnia *Late crash:* exhaustion, hypersomnolence, hyperphagia, no craving *Early withdrawal:* normal sleep and mood, low craving, low anxiety *Middle and late withdrawal:* anhedonia, anxiety, anergy, high level of craving exacerbated by conditioned cues *Extinction:* normal hedonic response and mood, episodic craving triggered by conditioned cues
Amphetamines	Fatigue, hunger, long periods of sleep, disorientation, severe depression
Hallucinogens	Slight irritability, restlessness, insomnia, reduced energy level, depression
Cannabis	Insomnia, hyperactivity, decreased appetite
Inhalants	None reported
Nicotine	Nervousness, increased appetite, sleep disturbances, anxiety, irritability

DIAGNOSTIC REASONING AND CONTROL OF SUBSTANCE ABUSE

Community health nurses make nursing diagnoses related to substance abuse at two levels. The first level is diagnoses related to individuals who have problems of substance abuse and their families. For example, the nurse might make a diagnosis for the individual client of "increased risk of substance abuse due to family history of alcohol abuse" or "abuse of sedatives due to increased life stress and poor coping skills." Nursing diagnoses related to the family of a substance abuser might include

■ TABLE 31–5 Long-Term Effects Associated with Abuse of Selected Psychoactive Substances

SUBSTANCE	LONG-TERM EFFECTS OF ABUSE
Alcohol	Malnutrition; impotence; ulcers; cirrhosis; esophageal, stomach, and liver cancers; organic brain syndrome; deafness
Sedatives, hypnotics, anxiolytics	Potential for death due to overdose from increasing doses due to tolerance, impaired sexual function
Opioids	Lethargy, weight loss, sexual disinterest and dysfunction, increased susceptibility to infection and accidents, constipation
Cocaine	Damage to nasal tissue, high blood pressure, weight loss, muscle twitching, paranoia, hallucinations, disrupted sleeping and eating patterns, irritability, liver damage
Amphetamines	Depression, paranoia, hallucinations, weight loss, impotence
Hallucinogens	Memory loss, inability to concentrate, insomnia, chronic or recurrent psychosis, flashbacks
Cannabis	Chromosome changes, reduced sperm count, impaired concentration, poor memory, reduced alertness, inability to perform complex tasks
Inhalants	Organic brain syndrome, liver and kidney damage, bone marrow damage, anemia, hearing loss, nerve damage
Nicotine	Cardiovascular disease, lung cancer, bladder cancer, chronic disease, diabetic complications

"co-dependency due to family feelings of guilt related to daughter's cocaine abuse" and "school behavior problems due to children's anxiety over mother's alcoholism."

At the second level, the community health nurse might make diagnoses of community problems related to substance abuse. For example, the nurse might diagnose an "increased incidence of motor vehicle fatalities due to driving under the influence of psychoactive drugs," or "increased prevalence of drug abuse among minority group members due to discrimination and feelings of powerlessness." Another community-based diagnosis is "increased prevalence of fetal alcohol syndrome due to alcohol abuse among pregnant women."

PLANNING AND IMPLEMENTING CONTROL STRATEGIES FOR SUBSTANCE ABUSE

Strategies for controlling problems of substance abuse can involve primary, secondary, or tertiary prevention. Resources to assist community health nurses in control efforts for substance abuse are available through links provided on the companion Web site for this book.

Primary Prevention

There are three major goals for primary prevention of substance abuse: (a) to prevent nonusers from initiating use of psychoactive substances, (b) to prevent progression from experimentation to chronic use, and (c) to prevent expansion to the use of other substances. Using smoking as an example, primary prevention may be aimed at preventing the initiation of smoking in the first place, preventing movement from occasional smoking to regular use of tobacco, and preventing movement from tobacco use to the use of other drugs such as marijuana. Primary prevention efforts to control substance abuse usually focus on two approaches: education and risk factor modification.

Education

Education usually focuses on acquainting the public, particularly young people, with the hazards of substance abuse. Both general public education campaigns and school-based education programs have shown moderate success in limiting the use of psychoactive substances; however, they tend to be more effective in moderating the effects of substance abuse such as preventing drug-related motor vehicle fatalities. One of the criticisms of school-based programs is that they may not be reaching groups at greatest risk for substance abuse, those with a family history of abuse or who display characteristics associated with potential abusers. Merely providing information on the consequences of substance use and abuse has been shown to be insufficient to curb use. Instead, education programs should emphasize the development of life skills related to decision making, refusal, and critical analysis that affect substance use

decisions. In addition, education should address interpersonal communication, problem solving, and stress management to provide practical approaches to factors that promote substance use and abuse (Allen, 1998).

Community health nurses may be involved in educating individual clients and families or in providing substance abuse education for groups of people. In either case, the nurse would employ the principles of teaching and learning discussed in Chapter 11.

Risk Factor Modification

Risk factor modification can occur with individuals, families, or society at large. Community health nurses may assist individuals to modify factors that put them at increased risk for substance abuse. For example, the nurse might assist clients experiencing stress to eliminate or modify sources of stress in their lives, or the nurse can assist clients and families to develop more effective coping skills.

In addition, the nurse may make referrals for social services to eliminate financial difficulties and other sources of stress. Or, the nurse might assist a harried single parent to obtain respite care. Nurses can also assist families to plan means of enhancing family communication and cohesion to minimize the risk of substance abuse among children.

At the societal level, community health nurses can engage in political activity to control access to and limit the availability of psychoactive substances as well as to modify societal factors that contribute to abuse. For example, the nurse might advocate enforcement of laws

CRITICAL THINKING IN RESEARCH

Watson (1999) suggested that brief interventions in primary care settings may be effective in preventing the development of health problems in people whose level of alcohol use puts them at risk. She also suggested that nurses without specialist education in treatment of abuse disorders may be able to effectively engage in such brief interventions. Watson notes, however, that there is no evidence that nonspecialist nurses have the knowledge to accurately assess their client's level of alcohol intake or that they have knowledge of the levels at which alcohol use becomes problematic.

- How would you conduct a study to determine if generalist nurses do, in fact, have these capabilities?
- How would you recruit study participants? Who would you invite to participate in the study? Who would you exclude from the study? Why?
- If your study findings indicated that generalist nurses do, indeed, have the requisite knowledge, how would you design an intervention study to test the effectiveness of brief intervention by nurses?

restricting the sale of alcohol and tobacco to minors, or the nurse might work to reduce discrimination against members of minority groups or to ensure a minimal income for all families.

Secondary Prevention

Secondary prevention is employed when there is an existing problem with substance abuse. The goal in secondary prevention is early intervention aimed at those who have not yet developed irreversible pathological changes due to substance abuse. Secondary prevention begins with screening for excessive or inappropriate use of psychoactive substances. Routine screening should be undertaken in multiple settings in which clients are seen. Research has shown that a single screening question related to problem drinking (e.g., "Have you consumed more than five alcoholic drinks on any occasion in the last three months?"), can accurately identify most clients with drinking problems (Taj, Devera-Sales, & Vinson, 1998).

Once screening indicates a substance use problem, planning secondary prevention necessitates mutual goal setting by the nurse and the family of the person experiencing the problem. Goals relate to intervention, treatment for substance abuse, and harm reduction.

Intervention

Intervention, in terms of substance abuse, is the act of confronting the substance abuser with the intent of making a referral for assistance in dealing with the abuse. The goal of the intervention is to elicit an agreement from the individual involved to be evaluated for a possible problem with substance abuse.

Community health nurses may facilitate intervention by families of individual abusers but are not usually the interveners themselves. In this respect, the family, rather than the abuser, is the community health nurse's client.

Many families may not see themselves as clients, and the community health nurse may need to reinforce the idea that substance abuse is a family disorder to motivate family members to engage in intervention. To this end, the first step in preparing for intervention is providing the family or significant others with basic information about substance abuse and the defense mechanisms used by both the abuser and his or her significant others. In this way, family members can be helped to see their role as co-dependents or enablers of the abusive behavior. The nurse also educates family members about the intervention process, their responsibility for that process, and some of the feelings that they may experience during intervention.

In assisting family members to prepare for intervention, the nurse aids them to determine who should be involved. It may be that some members will not be able to follow through with confronting the individual with his or her behavior and should be asked not to participate in the intervention. Individuals who should be involved in the intervention include those who are close to and concerned for the abuser, those who may be able to influence the abuser's behavior in a positive way, and those who are able to engage in the intervention.

Next, the nurse assists those who will be involved in the intervention to identify in writing the causes for their concern and to describe how they felt when significant events related to substance abuse occurred. Areas that the group should plan to address during the intervention are the problem as they perceive it, statements about the individual's behavior that indicate a problem of substance abuse, effects of the abuse problem, and their concern for the individual.

Prior to the intervention, the group should arrange an appointment for an evaluation for substance abuse to take place immediately after the intervention session, as it is wise to follow through on the referral as soon as possible while the individual is motivated to seek help. It is suggested that appointments be made in more than one facility so the individual can exercise some choice in the matter and will feel less coerced.

The group planning the intervention should also consider potential roadblocks to the success of the effort. For example, the individual might be concerned about the cost of care or about the need for child care while he or she is in treatment. If anticipated, these difficulties can be circumvented.

The nurse can also assist family members to plan their response to the individual's possible refusal to comply with a request for evaluation for substance abuse. If the wife plans to threaten divorce if the husband does not seek help, will she be able to carry through this threat in the face of his refusal? The nurse can help the family plan for these contingencies and work through feelings created by the proposed intervention by helping group members practice the intervention (who will say what, when, and so on). Practice should also include who will sit nearest the individual (those with the greatest influence) and between the abuser and the door and who will initiate the intervention.

Once the group is ready for the intervention, the individual should be brought to the place selected and the intervention initiated. Just prior to the intervention, while waiting for the individual to arrive, the nurse may remind family members why they are there and what is planned. The nurse is present to keep the intervention moving, but is not otherwise an active participant.

If the individual agrees to be evaluated, one or more of the group members should accompany him or her to the evaluation appointment to prevent a potential suicide attempt. While this is occurring, the nurse may meet with the other members of the group to discuss their feelings about the process and its outcome. If the intervention has not been successful, the nurse can reassure group members and assist them to plan a subsequent intervention.

Treatment

Treatment for substance abuse is based on several general principles that are discussed below. It also employs several different treatment modalities and should incorporate early treatment where possible, measures for managing withdrawal and cravings, treatment for consequences of abuse, and assistance with building a foundation for recovery.

GENERAL PRINCIPLES OF SUBSTANCE ABUSE TREATMENT

Treatment for problems of substance abuse varies somewhat depending on the type of substance involved. There are, however, some general principles that guide treatment for substance abuse. First, a combination of modalities of treatment is usually more effective than a single mode. Treatment should also be geared to individual problems, responses, and resources. For example, issues of aging related to retirement, physical loss, and loss of significant others leading to social isolation are issues that may need to be addressed with the elderly person but may not be factors in substance abuse by others. Similarly, the effects of physical disability must be dealt with in the handicapped person who abuses psychoactive substances, whereas this is not likely to be an issue with most other clients.

The third principle is that treatment should be administered by both professionals and laypersons. For example, a combination of professional psychotherapy and participation in a self-help group such as Alcoholics Anonymous may be far more effective in dealing with alcohol abuse than either mode by itself. Family members or significant others should also be actively involved in treatment to assist them to refrain from enabling behaviors that allowed the individual to continue his or her substance abuse.

Another major principle is the need for detoxification before any further treatment can be undertaken. In addition, associated psychopathology requires psychiatric treatment, not just the assistance of a self-help group. Feelings of guilt regarding substance abuse and its effects on loved ones may need to be addressed to prevent relapse. Social and vocational rehabilitation may also be needed to reintegrate the person into the family and into society at large. Finally, treatment may also encompass interventions for physical, psychological, and social problems resulting from substance abuse. General principles of substance abuse treatment are summarized below.

- Treatment should be provided by both professionals and laypersons.
- Family members and significant others, as well as the client, should be involved in treatment decisions.
- Detoxification and achievement of sobriety constitute the first step in treatment.
- Associated psychopathology requires psychiatric treatment.
- Guilt related to substance abuse and its effects on others will need to be addressed to prevent relapse.
- Social and vocational rehabilitation may be required to reintegrate the substance-abusing individual into the family and society.
- Treatment may also be required for physical, psychological, and social consequences of substance abuse.

TREATMENT MODALITIES FOR SUBSTANCE ABUSE

Treatment modalities that may be employed include biological methods, psychosocial methods, sociotherapies, and self-help groups. Biological methods use medication or other physiologically based therapies (such as acupuncture) to help the abuser deal with the symptoms of withdrawal or to handle cravings for the substance involved (Allen, 1998). For example, Librium and Valium may be used to help the alcohol abuser relieve the anxiety caused by alcohol withdrawal, while disulfiram (Antabuse) may be given to modify the craving for alcohol. Similarly, methadone may be used to control cravings for heroin. Psychosocial methods of treatment include individual, group, and family therapy; behavior modification; contracting; and aversion or relaxation therapies. Sociotherapy involves participation in therapeutic communities and residential programs where clients learn new lifestyles consistent with sobriety. Finally, self-help groups consist of people who are abusers of the same substance and who provide for each other understanding and support in conquering their substance abuse habit. For example, Alcoholics Anonymous is a self-help group for alcohol abusers, and Potsmokers Anonymous is a self-help group for marijuana abusers. Treatment modalities typically used for specific types of substance abuse are indicated in Table 31–6 ■.

Community health nurses may plan involvement in treatment for substance abuse in a number of ways. First, nurses might identify cases of substance abuse and plan to refer clients and their families to treatment resources in the community. Nurses may also educate the general public on the signs and symptoms of substance abuse as well as the availability of treatment facilities. In addition, community health nurses can monitor the use of medications during withdrawal (if this is done on an outpatient basis) or on a long-term basis.

Community health nurses might also be involved in psychosocial therapies in referring clients to sources of group, individual, or family therapy, or the nurse might

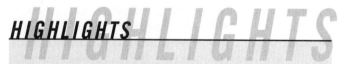

HIGHLIGHTS

General Principles of Treatment for Substance Abuse

- A combination of modalities is usually more effective than a single treatment modality.
- Treatment should be tailored to the problems, responses, and resources of the individual abuser.

■ **TABLE 31–6** Treatment Modalities Typically Used for Selected Forms of Psychoactive Substance Abuse

SUBSTANCE	TYPICAL TREATMENT MODALITIES
Alcohol	Detoxification; psychotherapy; group therapy; family therapy; self-help groups (Alcoholics Anonymous, Al-Anon); pharmacologic therapy (disulfiram, short-term use of tranquilizers or antidepressants); residential programs; referral for vocational rehabilitation and social services as needed
Sedatives, hypnotics, anxiolytics	Detoxification; psychotherapy and group therapy (for underlying psychiatric disorders)
Opioids	Pharmacologic therapy (methadone, opioid antagonists); therapeutic communities (Synanon, Odyssey House, Daytop, Phoenix House); group therapy; assistance with social skills, vocational training and job placement; family therapy; self-help groups (Narcotics Anonymous, Chemical Dependency Anonymous); psychotherapy
Cocaine	Hospitalization; self-help groups; contingency contracting (client agreement to urinary monitoring and acceptance of aversive contingencies for positive results); pharmacologic therapy (tricyclic antidepressants)
Amphetamines	No established treatment guidelines; may be similar to treatment for cocaine abuse
Hallucinogens	Detoxification; psychotherapy (for underlying psychiatric disorders); group therapy; residential programs
Cannabis	Same as for hallucinogens; self-help groups
Inhalants	Psychosocial interventions; psychotherapy (for underlying psychiatric disorder); sociodrama; vocational rehabilitation; family therapy; social support services
Nicotine	Aversive conditioning; desensitization; substitution; hypnotherapy; group therapy; relaxation training; supportive therapy; abrupt abstinence

reinforce contracts made for reducing the use of substances. This is particularly true in measures to help clients stop smoking. In this instance, community health nurses may initiate behavioral contracts with clients to enable them to gradually cut down on tobacco consumption or to quit smoking for gradually lengthened periods.

Community health nurses' involvement with therapeutic communities and self-help groups usually occurs in the form of referrals for these types of services. In some instances, however, community health nurses are actively involved in initiating support groups.

At the community level, nursing efforts to control substance abuse might include political activity to support the development of adequate treatment facilities, especially those geared to the needs of currently underserved population groups such as pregnant women, the homeless, and the elderly. Community health nurses might also be involved in political activity and advocacy to encourage insurance coverage of treatment for substance abuse.

The goals of treatment for substance abuse include intervening early for persons who have not yet become abusers but who use psychoactive substances; managing withdrawal and reducing cravings for the substance involved; and building a foundation for recovery.

EARLY TREATMENT   For some psychoactive substances, such as cocaine, use at any level frequently leads to abuse because of the vicious rebound cycle that occurs. For other substances, like alcohol, sedatives, and tran-

quilizers, moderate use may be acceptable when these substances are used appropriately. Some authors suggest early intervention with people using these substances to allow them to use the substance in moderation. To this end, brief treatment is undertaken to stabilize and to moderate use of the substance in question so that it does not reach the level of abuse. *Brief intervention* involves time-limited, direct strategies to reduce substance use in nondependent users whose consumption rates put them at risk for problems associated with substance use (Watson, 1999). For example, the college student who admits to binge drinking can be reminded of the potential for and consequences of alcohol-related motor vehicle accidents and helped to explore reasons for their drinking behavior as well as safer means of meeting the goals of the behavior. Programs of this type involve teaching clients self-control skills and skills for decision making about responsible behavioral choices.

MANAGING WITHDRAWAL AND CRAVINGS   For clients who have already reached a level of substance abuse that does not admit to moderate use or with substances for which there is no level of moderate use, the goal of treatment is abstinence and long-term sobriety (Goldsmith, 2000b). The first step to abstinence is detoxification, which often involves supporting the client through withdrawal. Community health nurses may be involved in referring clients to detoxification facilities and in supporting them during detoxification.

Persons who are at risk for serious consequences of withdrawal should always go through detoxification under medical supervision. Of particular concern are pregnant women and the elderly. Many of the drugs used to mitigate the adverse symptomatology of withdrawal from psychoactive substances are contraindicated in pregnancy. For example, Valium and Librium, both of which may be used to combat the anxiety and sleeplessness that may accompany withdrawal, may be teratogenic and should not be given to the pregnant substance abuser. Similarly, detoxification procedures may need to be modified for older adults because of their tendency to be overmedicated by relatively small doses of medication.

Community health nurses may monitor medication use during withdrawal or on a long-term basis, and they should be alert to the potential for use of medications for suicide purposes and to the potential for abuse of some of the substances used (e.g., Valium). The nurse should assess clients on medications for suicide potential and should monitor mood changes closely. The nurse should also educate clients and their families as to the adverse effects of combining medications with alcohol or other psychoactive drugs. Because disulfiram (Antabuse), in particular, is contraindicated in both pregnant women and clients with cardiac arrhythmias and pulmonary disease, the nurse should monitor clients for evidence of these conditions.

Other nursing considerations related to withdrawal and craving include maintaining levels of hydration and nutrition. Hydration is particularly important for the client who abuses alcohol because of the diuretic effects of alcohol. Nutrition is important for most drug abusers because substance abuse frequently leads to a disinterest in food in favor of consumption of the abusive substance. Decreased intake of stimulants such as caffeine is also advisable. Treatment can also be enhanced by a regular program of exercise that will improve self-esteem, prevent excessive weight gain, and stimulate the release of endorphins. Community health nurses can educate clients on the need for hydration and nutrition and suggest exercise. Vigorous aerobic exercise should not be undertaken before a thorough medical assessment of cardiovascular status has been conducted. In the interim, however, the nurse can suggest a program of stretching exercises.

DEALING WITH CONSEQUENCES OF ABUSE   Substance abuse may lead to a variety of physical, psychological, and social consequences with which community health nurses need to assist clients. Community health nurses may provide treatment for physical consequences of substance abuse and assist clients to deal with psychological and social consequences. For example, they may treat abscesses due to injection drug use or refer clients for treatment if necessary. Other examples include assisting clients in recovery to deal with the feelings of guilt engendered by their behavior and its effects on loved ones, or helping them to regaining custody of children placed in foster care.

BUILDING A FOUNDATION FOR RECOVERY   Treatment for substance abuse is more than a matter of detoxification and modification of cravings for the drug in question. It is usually a total program of modification that results in changes in modes of thinking and acting. This may be achieved through professional therapy as discussed above, participation in self-help groups, changes in environment and lifestyle, self-image enhancement, and development of new coping skills and new patterns of family interaction.

Self-help groups have been shown to be quite effective in dealing with many health problems. The effectiveness of these groups stems from several assumptions. First, the emotional support of others with similar problems reduces the social isolation experienced by many clients with substance abuse problems. Second, a collective self-identity emerges through group participation, allowing group members to develop new personal self-concepts. Third, group participation permits sharing of experiential knowledge and practical suggestions for coping with problems encountered. Finally, group participation fosters a more active orientation to health, greater reliance on individual and group support systems, and less dependence on health care providers.

Community health nurses may be involved in the initiation of self-help groups or in subsequent support of such groups. Nurses also refer individual clients to groups as appropriate. Nurses should function as facilitators of the group process, not as "leaders" or active participants in the group unless they also experience the condition involved.

Community health nurses can facilitate the work of self-help groups in several ways. These include monitoring and directing active involvement by group members, encouraging the sharing of experiences and solutions to common problems, encouraging provision of mutual aid, and encouraging utilization of professional assistance as needed. Other facilitative measures include emphasizing personal responsibility for and control over events, maintaining positive pressure for behavior change, and emphasizing the need for positive coping strategies. Finally, the nurse should facilitate group interaction by providing the least amount of personal input possible.

Nurses can also assist clients to plan changes in their environment to minimize stresses that may contribute to substance abuse. For example, the nurse can refer a client for help with financial difficulties or for respite from the care of a handicapped child or elderly parent. Socially isolated older persons who abuse substances can be linked to sources of social support, and unemployed persons can be assisted to find employment or to learn skills that enhance their employability.

Community health nurses can also help clients develop stronger self-images by reinforcing their successes and helping them realistically examine their failures and their expectations for themselves. In addition, nurses can help clients who abuse psychoactive substances to develop alternative ways of coping with stress by taking action to modify stressors or changing their perceptions of and responses to stressors.

Treatment efforts are also needed for members of the abuser's family to enable them to recover from co-dependence. Goals in the care of families of substance abusers include stabilizing the family system, making changes in family interactions, and developing mechanisms for maintaining those changes. Family stabilization may be achieved by linking families to needed support services and engaging in the crisis intervention strategies described in Chapter 14. The nurse can also make referrals for marital or family therapy as needed and can assist families to identify their use of defense mechanisms similar to those used by the substance abuser.

The community health nurse might also provide families with anticipatory guidance about the negative effects of life change events and help them deal with these events without resorting to substance abuse. Family members may also need help in working through resentment related to substance abuse and subsequent behaviors by the abuser.

Building positive experiences in the life of the family also fosters cohesion and helps to stabilize the family. The community health nurse can assist the family to plan activities in which all members can participate. It is particularly important to integrate the substance-abusing member into these occasions to prevent further alienation.

The community health nurse can also assist families to develop new patterns of interaction. For example, the nurse might help the family realign members into the more usual husband–wife coalition rather than parent–child coalitions by improving family communication and developing joint problem-solving skills. The nurse can also assist family members to identify and express feelings and learn negotiating strategies.

Harm Reduction

An alternative approach to the control of substance abuse is based on the philosophy of harm reduction. Traditionally, the goal of policy development and implementation related to substance abuse has been a reduction in drug use. It has been suggested that a more appropriate focus would be to reduce the harm to society resulting from drug abuse. *Harm reduction* is an approach to drug use that focuses on moderation of substance use and minimization of its harmful effects (Lennings, 2000). Approaches to harm reduction include provision of methadone to heroin users, needle exchange programs, provision of syringe filters, initiation of outpatient wound clinics for injection abscesses, and wound

care programs at needle exchange sites (Caflish et al., 1999; Goldsmith, 2000a; Langendam, van Brussel, Coutinho, & van Ameijden, 2001). Provision of Narcan, a narcotic antagonist, to opiate addicts has even been suggested as a means of preventing deaths from overdose (Goldsmith, 2000a).

Tertiary Prevention

Tertiary prevention is aimed at preventing a relapse into prior substance-abusing behaviors by the individual or into enabling behaviors by family members and significant others. Approaches to relapse prevention include cognitive/behavioral strategies such as avoiding risk situations and enhancing coping, lifestyle changes such as job change, and other strategies such as cue extinction and pharmacologic management (e.g., methadone use) (Allen, 1998). Community health nurses can contribute to these efforts by providing emotional support to recovering abusers and their families and by linking them with other sources of support. Other tertiary prevention measures might include efforts to eliminate or modify stressors that contribute to relapse. For example, assisting the recovering abuser to find work can alleviate the stress of unemployment and financial worries.

The nurse can also reinforce the individual's motivation to abstain from drug use by commending and highlighting successes and periods of sobriety. Development of positive coping skills may also prevent relapse. Other tertiary prevention needs may involve providing information on resources, providing respite from onerous burdens of care, or helping individuals plan time for themselves. Table 31–7 ■ lists primary, secondary, and tertiary prevention goals and related nursing interventions in the control of substance abuse.

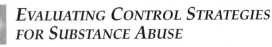 ### EVALUATING CONTROL STRATEGIES FOR SUBSTANCE ABUSE

Evaluating interventions with individual substance abusers and their families focuses on the extent to which problems of substance abuse have been resolved. Has the abuser been able to remain sober for extended periods? Have stresses contributing to substance abuse been modified?

At the level of the community, the nurse could evaluate the effects of intervention programs on the incidence and prevalence of substance abuse as well as indicators of morbidity and mortality related to abuse. The nurse evaluating the effects of programs directed at substance abuse might examine the extent to which national health promotion and disease prevention objectives have been met in the community. Evaluative information on efforts to meet the national objectives for 2010 is presented on page 752.

HEALTHY PEOPLE 2010

GOALS FOR THE POPULATION

Objective		Base	Target
26-1	Reduce deaths and injuries due to alcohol-related motor vehicle crashes:		
	a. Deaths (per 100,000 population)	6.1	4
	b. Injuries	122	65
26-2	Reduce cirrhosis deaths (per 100,000 population)	9.4	3
26-3	Reduce drug-induced deaths (per 100,000 population)	5.1	1
26-4	Reduce drug-related hospital emergency visits	542,544	350,000
26-9	Increase the proportion of adolescents who remain alcohol and drug free		
	c. Alcohol	19%	29%
	d. Illicit drugs	46%	56%
26-11	Reduce the proportion of people engaging in binge drinking in the last month		
	c. Adults	16%	6%
	d. Adolescents	8.3%	3%
26-12	Reduce average annual alcohol consumption (gallons per person)	2.19	2
26-13	Reduce the proportion of adults who exceed guidelines for low-risk drinking		
	a. Females	72%	50%
	b. Males	74%	50%
26-14c	Reduce steroid use by 12th graders	1.7%	0.4%
26-15	Reduce inhalant use by adolescents	4.4%	0.7%
26-17	Increase the proportion of adolescents who perceive great risk associated with substance abuse:		
	a. Alcohol	47%	80%
	b. Marijuana	31%	80%
	c. Cocaine	54%	80%
26-20	Increase the number of admissions to treatment for injection drug use (per year)	167,960	200,000
27-1a	Reduce cigarette smoking by adults	24%	12%
27-2	Reduce tobacco use by adolescents	43%	21%
27-4	Increase the age of first use of tobacco		
	a. By adolescents	12	14
	b. By young adults	15	17
27-5	Increase smoking cessation attempts by adults	43%	75%
27-6	Increase smoking cessation during pregnancy	12%	30%
27-8	Increase insurance coverage for treatment of nicotine dependence in:		
	a. Managed care programs	75%	100%
	b. Medicaid programs	24%	51%
27-10	Reduce the proportion of nonsmokers exposed to environmental tobacco smoke	65%	45%
27-11	Increase tobacco-free environments in schools	37%	100%
27-12	Increase the proportion of worksites with formal smoking policies	79%	100%

Source: U.S. Department of Health and Human Services. (2000). *Healthy people 2010* (Conference edition, in two volumes). Washington, DC: Author.

■ **TABLE 31–7** Primary, Secondary, and Tertiary Prevention Goals and Related Community Health Nursing Interventions in the Control of Substance Abuse

GOAL OF PREVENTION	NURSING INTERVENTIONS
Primary Prevention	
1. Positive coping skills	1. Teach coping skills.
2. Strong self image	2. Foster and reinforce development of strong self-image.
3. Public education on the hazards of substance abuse	3. Educate clients and public.
4. Policies and programs to prevent abuse	4. Engage in political activity and advocacy.
Secondary Prevention	
1. Early detection of persons with substance abuse problems	1. Engage in case finding.
2. Early intervention for persons with problems related to substance abuse	2. Assist families to plan and carry out intervention.
3. Treatment of substance abuse	3. Refer client for treatment. Monitor client during treatment.
4. Treatment for consequences of substance abuse	4. Refer for or provide assistance in dealing with physical, psychological, and social consequences of abuse.
5. Public education on signs of abuse and resources available	5. Educate clients and public.
6. Treatment facilities	6. Engage in political activity to support treatment facilities and programs.
7. Insurance coverage for treatment	7. Engage in political activity and advocacy.
Tertiary Prevention	
1. Support for abusers	1. Provide emotional support and encouragement; refer to support groups.
2. Lifestyle changes that discourage abusive behavior	2. Assist with lifestyle changes.
3. Modification of stressors that contribute to substance abuse	3. Assist with modification of stressors.

APPLYING YOUR KNOWLEDGE IN PRACTICE

✛ CASE STUDY
Caring for the Client with a Substance Abuse Problem

You have been working with the Schumacher family for the last several months. The youngest child, who is 18 months old, has multiple physical handicaps and has been in and out of the hospital numerous times for surgery. He is currently enrolled in physical and occupational therapy programs to promote his development. You have been following this child and working with the family to meet his needs. On your most recent home visit, Mrs. Schumacher voiced concern about her husband's drinking.

Since the birth of the baby, Mr. Schumacher has gone on periodic drinking binges. Initially, these occurred about once a month, but lately he has been getting drunk almost every weekend. This week Mrs. Schumacher had to call her husband's office, where he is employed as a civil engineer, to tell his employer that her husband was ill. Actually, he was too hung over to go to work. She has tried to talk to her husband about his drinking,

but he becomes angry and storms out of the house. When he returns, he is drunk. Each time, after he sobers up, he is repentant and promises not to drink again. Mrs. Schumacher thinks her husband's drinking is the result of his worry about financial problems.

Since Mr. Schumacher's drinking problem has escalated, the older children have been reluctant to bring friends home because they are embarrassed by their father's drunken behavior. They have begun to ask Mrs. Schumacher rather pointed questions about their father, such as "Is daddy an alcoholic?" They know that their grandfather, Mr. Schumacher's father, died of cirrhosis stemming from alcoholism. Mrs. Schumacher says she has told the children their father is not an alcoholic but is just tired and has been under a lot of stress at work.

Mr. Schumacher has always been a successful provider for the family and did not drink much before the baby was born. He did well in school, completing a master's degree in engineering, and was promoted to a new position with his engineering firm about two years ago. His job pays relatively well, but because their health insurance did not cover the baby when he was born, they have had to pay all of the new infant's medical expenses out of pocket. Mrs. Schumacher says they have exhausted their savings and indicates that they are having some difficulty meeting mortgage payments on their house. She would like to work but would have trouble finding someone to care for the baby, who has a tracheostomy and requires periodic suctioning. She has discussed her willingness to work with her husband, but he insists that he is not going to have his wife working when the children need her at home and that he will take care of things.

- What are the biophysical, psychological, sociocultural, behavioral, and health system factors influencing the health of this family?

- What are the health problems evident in this situation? Develop several nursing diagnostic statements related to these problems.
- What evidence of co-dependence is present in this family situation?
- What client care objectives would you set in working with this family?
- What primary, secondary, and tertiary intervention strategies should be employed with this family? Why?
- How would you evaluate the effectiveness of your interventions with the Schumacher family? What evaluative criteria would you use? How would you obtain the evaluative data needed?

✂ TESTING YOUR UNDERSTANDING

- What are the criteria for diagnosing psychoactive substance dependence? Give examples of behaviors that might demonstrate these criteria. (p. 730)
- Distinguish between psychoactive substance dependence and abuse. (p. 730)
- What are the psychoactive substances that most often lead to dependence and abuse? (pp. 731–735)
- Describe some of the personal, family, and societal effects of substance abuse. (pp. 735–737)
- What are the five aspects of community health nursing assessment in relation to substance abuse? (pp. 737–745)
- What are the major approaches to primary prevention of substance abuse? How might community health nurses be involved in each? (pp. 746–747)

- What are the components of the intervention process in secondary prevention of substance abuse? What might be the role of the community health nurse in the intervention process? (p. 747)
- What are the general principles in the treatment of substance abuse? (p. 748)
- What are the major treatment modalities in substance abuse? What is the role of the community health nurse with respect to each? (pp. 748–749)
- What is harm reduction and how does it relate to control of substance abuse? (p. 751)

REFERENCES

About. (2001). Narcotic oxycontin: Savior or killer? Retrieved August 22, 2001, from the World Wide Web, *http://headaches.about*.

Allen, K. (1998). Essential concepts of addiction for general nursing practice. *Nursing Clinics of North America, 33*, 1–13.

American Psychiatric Association. (2000). *Diagnostic and statistical manual of mental disorders* (4th ed., text revision) (DSM-IV-TR). Washington, DC: Author.

Bachman, J. G., Freedman-Doan, P., O'Malley, P. M., Johnston, L., & Segal, D. R. (1999). Changing patterns of drug use among U.S. military recruits before and after enlistment. *American Journal of Public Health, 89*, 672–677.

Bachman, J. G., Johnston, L. D., & O'Malley, P. M. (1998). Explaining recent increases in students' marijuana use: Impacts of perceived risks and disapproval, 1976 through 1996. *American Journal of Public Health, 88*, 887–892.

Birckmayer, J., & Hemenway, D. (1999). Minimum-age drinking laws and youth suicide, 1970–1990. *American Journal of Public Health, 89*, 1365–1368.

Bolen, J. C., Rhodes, L., Powell-Griner, E. E., Bland, S. D., & Holtzman, D. (2000). State-specific prevalence of selected health behaviors, by race and ethnicity—Behavioral Risk Factor Surveillance System, 1997. *Morbidity and Mortality Weekly Report, 49*(SS-2), 1–60.

Caflish, C., Wang, J., & Zbinden, R. (1999). The role of syringe filters in harm reduction among injection drug users. *American Journal of Public Health, 89*, 1252–1254.

California Department of Health Services. (1998). Tetanus among injecting drug users. *Morbidity and Mortality Weekly Report, 47*, 149–151.

Drucker, E. (1999). Drug prohibition and public health: 25 years of evidence. *Public Health Reports, 114*, 14–29.

Egeland, G. M., Perham-Hester, K. A., Gessner, B. D., Ingle, D., Berner, J. E., & Middaugh, J. P. (1998). Fetal alcohol syndrome in Alaska, 1977 through 1992: An administrative prevalence derived from multiple data sources. *American Journal of Public Health, 88,* 781–786.

Ehrmin, J. T. (2001). Unresolved feelings of guilt and shame in the maternal role with substance-dependent African American women. *Journal of Nursing Scholarship, 33,* 47–52.

Fingerhut, L. A., & Cox, C. S. (1998). Poisoning mortality, 1985–1995. *Public Health Reports, 113,* 218–233.

Gafoor, M., & Rassool, G. H. (1998). The coexistence of psychiatric disorders and substance misuse: Working with dual diagnosis patients. *Journal of Advanced Nursing, 27,* 497–502.

Goldsmith, C. (2000a). The new face of heroin: Nurses seeing younger users. *NurseWeek, 13*(13), 13.

Goldsmith, C. (2000b). Tough lessons: Alcohol treatment programs debate abstinence vs. moderation. *NurseWeek, 13*(20), 28–29.

Golub, A., & Johnson, B. D. (2001). Variation in youthful risks of progression from alcohol and tobacco to marijuana and to hard drugs across generations. *American Journal of Public Health, 91,* 225–232.

Grant, B. F. (2000). Estimates of US children exposed to alcohol abuse and dependence in the family. *American Journal of Public Health, 90,* 112–115.

Grant, B. F., & Dawson, D. A. (1997). Age at onset of alcohol use and its association with DSM-IV alcohol abuse and dependence: Results from the National Longitudinal Alcohol Epidemiologic Survey. *Journal of Substance Abuse, 9,* 103–110.

Gruenwald, P. J., Treno, A. J., Taff, G., & Klitzner, M. (1997). *Measuring community indicators: A systems approach to drug and alcohol problems.* Thousand Oaks, CA: Sage.

Heath, D. B. (2000). *Drinking occasions: Comparative perspectives on alcohol and culture.* Philadelphia: Brunner/Mazel.

Holtzman, D., Powell-Griner, E. E., Bolen, J. C., & Rhodes, L. (2000). State- and sex-specific prevalence of selected characteristics—Behavioral Risk Factor Surveillance System, 1996 and 1997. *Morbidity and Mortality Weekly Report, 49*(SS-6), 1–39.

Insel, P., & Roth, W. T. (1998). *Core concepts in health* (8th ed.). Mountain View, CA: Mayfield.

Kann, L., Kinchen, St. A., Williams, B. I., Ross, J. G., et al. (2000). Youth risk behavior surveillance—United States, 1999. *Morbidity and Mortality Weekly Report, 49*(SS-5), 1–94.

Kelder, S. H., Murray, N. G., Orpinas, P., Prokhorov, A., et al. (2001). Depression and substance use in minority middle-school students. *American Journal of Public Health, 91,* 761–766.

Langendam, M. W., van Brussel, G. H. A., Coutinho, R. A., & van Ameijden, E. J. C. (2001). The impact of harm-reduction-based methadone treatment on mortality among heroin users. *American Journal of Public Health, 91,* 774–780.

Lennings, C. J. (2000). Harm minimization or abstinence: An evaluation of current policies and practices in the treatment and control of intravenous drug using groups in Australia. *Disability and Rehabilitation, 22*(1/2), 57–64.

McHenry, L. M., & Salerno, E. (1998). *Mosby's pharmacology in nursing* (20th ed.). St. Louis: Mosby.

Muller, R. (1999). Alcoholism today: The rebirth of ideologies of individual blame. In D. Ladewig (Ed.), *Basic and clinical science of substance related disorders* (pp. 56–63). Basel, Switzerland: Karger.

National Center for Injury Prevention and Control. (2000). Unintentional opiate overdose deaths—King County, Washington, 1990–1999. *Morbidity and Mortality Weekly Report, 49,* 636–640.

National Center on Birth Defects and Developmental Disabilities. (2001). *Fetal alcohol syndrome.* Retrieved April 21, 2001, from the World Wide Web, http://www.cdc.gov/ncbddd.

The Nation's Health. (1998, August). Zero tolerance laws reach all 50 states. P. 7.

Ness, R. B., Grisso, J. A., Hirschinger, N., Markovic, N., et al. (1999). Cocaine and tobacco use and the risk of spontaneous abortion. *New England Journal of Medicine, 340,* 333–339.

Neugebauer, R. (1999). Mind matters: The importance of mental disorders in public health's 21st century mission. *American Journal of Public Health, 89,* 1309–1311.

Preisig, M., & Fenton, B. T. (1999). Comorbidity research in substance abuse disorders. In D. Ladewig (Ed.), *Basic and clinical science of substance related disorders* (pp. 29–39). Basel, Switzerland: Karger.

Sutherland, J. A. (2001). Craving to rave: The agony of ecstasy abuse. *NurseWeek, 14*(8), 19.

Taj, N., Devera-Sales, A., & Vinson, D. C. (1998). Screening for problem drinking: Does a single question work? *Journal of Family Practice, 46,* 328–335.

Trinkhoff, A. M., & Storr, C. L. (1998). Substance use among nurses: Differences between specialties. *American Journal of Public Health, 88,* 581–585.

U.S. Census Bureau. (1999). *Statistical abstract of the United States, 1999* (119th ed.). Washington, DC: Author.

U.S. Department of Health and Human Services. (1998, May 6). *Healthy people 2000 progress review: Substance abuse, alcohol and other drugs.* Washington, DC: Author.

U.S. Department of Health and Human Services. (2000a). *Health, United States, 2000.* Washington, DC: Author.

U.S. Department of Health and Human Services. (2000b). *Healthy people 2010* (Conference edition, in two volumes). Washington, DC: Author.

U.S. Department of Transportation. (1999). *Traffic safety facts 1999.* Retrieved November 17, 2000, from the World Wide Web, http://www.nhtsa.dot.gov/people/ncsa.

Valente, T. W., & Vlahov, D. (2001). Selective risk taking among needle exchange participants: Implications for supplemental interventions. *American Journal of Public Health, 91,* 406-411.

Vo, K. (2000). The party's never over. *NurseWeek, 13*(4), 33.

Watson, H. E. (1999). Minimal interventions for problem drinkers: A review of the literature. *Journal of Advanced Nursing, 30,* 513–519.

SOCIETAL VIOLENCE

Chapter Objectives

After reading this chapter, you should be able to:

- Compare types of societal violence.
- Discuss the influence of biophysical, psychological, sociocultural, behavioral, and health system factors on societal violence.
- Identify major foci in primary prevention of societal violence.
- Describe approaches to the secondary prevention of societal violence.
- Discuss considerations in tertiary prevention of societal violence.
- Discuss the role of community health nurses in controlling societal violence.

KEY TERMS

battering 759
child abuse 758
critical incident stress 766
elder abuse 759
emotional abuse 758
intimate partner violence (IPV) 759
neglect 758
physical abuse 758
psychological battering 759
sexual abuse 758

Media Link

http://www.prenhall.com/clark

Additional interactive resources for this chapter can be found on the companion Web site. Click on Chapter 32 and "Begin" to select the activities for this chapter.

Violence is a pervasive phenomenon in our society. In part, this is a function of the American heritage and the activities required to carve a nation from a wild and uncivilized land. Violence has historically been seen as a mode of resolving conflict and even of ensuring support of law and order. The vigilante approach to justice on the Western frontier is one example of the use of violence to protect society.

In societies in which survival is subjected to physical threats that must be countered by physical force, violent behavior may be more or less of a necessity. Some authorities, however, contend that humankind has failed to adapt to changes in survival needs and has continued to exercise proclivities to violence that are not warranted in today's society. Societal violence has become a global as well as national concern.

Societal violence costs million of dollars in hospital care alone and results in millions of days of lost work productivity. Add to this the personal costs of victimization as well as the mounting cost of police and other protective services and related court costs, and it becomes apparent that the United States cannot afford the current level of violence and must do something to contain it. Evidence of public concern for problems of societal violence are found in a number of objectives related to violence and injury prevention in the national objectives for 2010 (U.S. Department of Health and Human Services [USDHHS], 2000b). These objectives may be viewed by accessing the Healthy People 2010 Web site through links available on the companion Web site for this book.

Family violence, assault and homicide, and suicide are forms of violence that are of particular concern to society and, hence, to community health nurses who are charged with promoting the health of the population. Violence contributes to a variety of physical and psychological health problems that can be prevented by community health nursing efforts to modify factors that contribute to violence against self or others.

TRENDS IN SOCIETAL VIOLENCE

Family Violence

Family violence encompasses child abuse, intimate partner abuse, and elder abuse. In many families, these forms of abuse are intertwined, creating an intergenerational transmission of violence in which children who are subjected to or witness violence in the family internalize violence as a mode of family interaction (McClellan & Killeen, 2000). These children then become abusive or enter abusive relationships in adulthood. These abusive relationships may also carry over into care of aging parents, particularly if the parents were abusive themselves.

CHILD ABUSE

Child abuse involves intentional physical or mental harm to a child by someone responsible for the child's welfare. Several different types of child abuse occur in the context of family–child interactions. These include physical abuse, emotional abuse, sexual abuse, and physical or emotional neglect. *Physical abuse* involves intentional injury of a child by a caretaker that results in harm. *Emotional abuse* consists of either verbal or behavioral actions that have negative emotional consequences for the child. Constant belittling of a child is an example of emotional abuse. *Sexual abuse* is any involvement of a child in an act designed to provide sexual gratification to an adult. Both child pornography and sexual intercourse with a child are examples of sexual abuse. In 1993, an estimated 300,000 U.S. children were subjected to known sexual abuse (Division of Violence Prevention, 2001). *Neglect* is failure to provide for a child's physical, educational, or emotional needs. In physical neglect, caretakers fail to provide the child with the material requirements for healthy growth. Physical neglect may include failure to feed or clothe a child appropriately or failure to provide needed medical attention. Finally, emotional or psychological neglect involves failure to provide a child with the love and affection needed for optimal emotional development (Nester, 1998).

An estimated 1 million children are abused each year in the United States, amounting to 15 of every 1,000 children under 18 years of age (Eckenrode et al., 2000). There has been an increase in substantiated cases of child abuse from 1.4 million cases in 1986 to 3.1 million cases in 1995. Most of this increase, however, is due to increased recognition and reporting of child abuse rather than an actual increase in incidence. More than half of these incidents (54%) involve physical neglect, 25% involve physical abuse, 11% involve sexual abuse, and 3% involve emotional abuse or neglect. Another 6% of children are subjected to multiple forms of abuse (Nester, 1998).

There has also been a 48% increase in the number of fatalities related to child abuse since 1985. It is a serious indictment of the child protective system that 46% of the children who died as a result of abuse had had prior involvement with child protective services (CPS). More than four fifths (82%) of these children were under 5 years of age, and 41% were under 1 year of age. Almost half of the deaths (49%) were the result of physical abuse, 40% were due to neglect, and 11% were due to a combination of both (Nester, 1998).

Perpetrators of child abuse tend to be family members, typically parents, and mothers and fathers are equally involved, accounting for 21% of incidents each. Other perpetrators include mothers' boyfriends (9%), babysitters (8%), and stepfathers (5%) (Nester, 1998). A very small percentage of children are abused by older siblings.

⑥ THINK ABOUT IT

How would you feel about providing services to a woman who abuses her children? Would you be able to work effectively with this type of client? Why or why not?

INTIMATE PARTNER VIOLENCE

It is estimated that one of every six couples in the United States experiences at least one instance of intimate partner violence in a given year (Schafer, Caetano, & Clark, 1998). *Intimate partner violence (IPV)* refers to physical, psychological, or sexual abuse by a current or former intimate partner (Rodriguez, Bauer, McLoughlin, & Grumbach, 1999). Each year 1.5 million women and more than 834,000 men are raped or physically assaulted by an intimate partner, and 25% of women and 8% of men will be subjected to IPV in their lifetimes (Division of Violence Prevention, 2000b; 2000e). Intimate partners include spouses, ex-spouses, boyfriends or girlfriends, or former boyfriends or girlfriends, and risk of severe violence may actually be higher once a relationship has been terminated than during the relationship (Campbell & Soeken, 1999).

Intimate partner violence also includes "battering." *Battering* is chronic and continuing violence of one partner against another that is characterized by vulnerability, entrapment, and loss of control of one's life on the part of the abused partner. *Psychological battering* exists when there is no current physical or sexual abuse being perpetrated, but fear of potential abuse keeps the victim subservient (Coker, Smith, McKeown, & King, 2000). Battering is believed to occur in a predictable cycle that includes a period of growing tension in the batterer that culminates in a specific incident of battering and that is followed by a period of remorse and forgiveness (Walker, 2000). Research on intimate partner violence is difficult because of the potential vulnerability of subjects. For a discussion of the ethical implications of research with this population, please see a summary of a related article provided on the companion Web site for this book. 🌐

Estimated annual costs for care of victims of IPV is $67 million (Schafer et al., 2000). Approximately 85% of victims of IPV are women (Division of Violence Prevention, 2000d). Approximately 20% of emergency department visits are believed to be due to IPV and 25% of homicides involving female victims are extreme instances of intimate partner violence. In one study, more than 23% of women and 16% of men reported experiencing IPV, but women were more likely than men to report injuries as a result (22% and 7.5%, respectively) (Division of Violence Prevention, 2000c). In another study, 63% of women abused in the previous year sought medical care for related injuries (Division of Violence Prevention, 1998a), and approximately 1 million U.S. women seek care for abuse-related injuries each year (Glass & Campbell, 1998).

Intimate partner violence occurs throughout the world in all nations, and in all social, economic, religious, and cultural groups. IPV is often referred to as *gender-based violence* because in many cultures it arises in part from women's subordinate social status (Heise, Ellsberg, & Gottemoeller, 1999). Like child abuse, several different forms of IPV occur including physical and sexual abuse, threats of physical or sexual violence, stalking, and emotional or psychological abuse (Saltzman, Fingerhut, Rand, & Visher, 2000). Other measures by which intimate partners exert coercive control include threats to children, belongings, and pets, and control of financial assets (Campbell & Soeken, 1999).

Intimate partner violence and child abuse tend to co-occur in families. In some studies, 40% to 60% of mothers of abused children are themselves abused compared to only 13% of mothers whose children were not abused. Women who engaged in chronically violent behaviors toward male partners had a 38% probability of also abusing a male child. Men who abused their female partners had a 100% probability of also abusing a male child (National Center for Injury Prevention and Control, 1999). Even when children are not themselves abused, witnessing family violence has profound psychological and social consequences that will be discussed later in this chapter. It is estimated that as many as 10 million children may witness family violence each year (Gomby, 2000).

Intimate partner violence also occurs outside the family constellation. In a series of state studies, 14.5% to 24% of adolescent girls and 3% to 10% of boys reported physical or sexual violence during dating. In another study, 59% of young people overall reported experiencing dating violence in the last year. Girls were more likely to report severe violence than boys. For example, nearly 18% of girls reported forced sexual intercourse compared to less than 1% of boys (Molidor, Tolman, & Kober, 2000). Women in general are five times more likely to experience forced sexual activity than are men (Division of Violence Prevention, 2000a).

ELDER ABUSE

Elder abuse is purposeful physical or psychological harm directed toward elderly persons. Elder abuse can occur within families or in institutional settings such as nursing homes and other residential facilities for the elderly. The

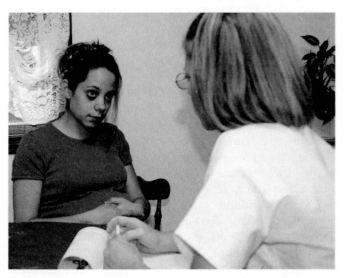

Pregnant women should be routinely asked about family violence.

focus of this chapter, however, is on abuse of older persons by family members.

An estimated 4% to 10% of the U.S. population over 65 years of age experience abuse, and it is estimated that 820,000 to 1.8 million adults are abused each year (Champion, 1998; Hogstel & Curry, 1999). Half of the perpetrators of this abuse are children or grandchildren of the victims, and 40% are elderly spouses (Champion, 1998). As was true of the other categories of family violence discussed here, several forms of elder abuse occur, many of them similar to the types of abuse found among children and couples. Types of abuse that may be encountered by community health nurses working with elderly clients include physical and sexual abuse, neglect, emotional abuse, financial or material exploitation, violation of personal rights, and abandonment. Physical abuse of the elderly may include injury, inappropriate restraint, or overmedication. Neglect may involve failure to meet physical or emotional needs, failure to attend to medical needs, or self-neglect by the older person him- or herself. Emotional abuse may consist of verbal abuse or disrespect or social isolation. Older clients may also be financially exploited when their funds or material goods are appropriated by others rather than used to meet their needs. Older clients' personal rights may be violated if they are not allowed to participate in decisions regarding their lives when they are capable of making such decisions. Finally, older clients may be abandoned or deserted by those responsible for their care. Of these various types of abuse, physical and financial abuse are the most common (Hogstel & Curry, 1999).

Assault and Homicide

Considerable societal violence also occurs outside of the family unit. Multiple forms of physical assault take place each day in the United States with the most extreme form of assault resulting in homicide. Homicide rates have declined significantly in recent years, decreasing 30% from 10 per 100,000 population in 1990 to 7 per 100,000 in 1997. These figures are somewhat misleading in that part of the decline in homicide-related fatalities lies in better medical care for those who have been assaulted. Some authors believe a more accurate indicator of societal violence is the rate of aggravated assault. An aggravated assault is one in which a weapon is used or in which serious injury is inflicted (U.S. Census Bureau, 1999). From 1957 to the mid-1990s the rate of aggravated assault in the United States increased from 60 cases per 100,000 population to 440 per 100,000 (Grossman, 2000). In 1997, the U.S. rate of aggravated assault was 382 per 100,000 persons, indicating a slight decline in incidence. Other forms of assault have also declined but remain sources of societal problems. For example, the rate of forcible rape decreased from 36.8 per 100,000 people in 1980 to 35.9 in 1997 after a peak incidence of 42.8 in 1994.

Although schools are often perceived as safe places for children, violence occurs in schools on a regular basis.

During the 1996–1997 school year, for example, 10% of U.S. public schools reported one or more serious violent crimes, including murder, rape or other sexual assault, suicide, robbery, and fighting with a weapon. The majority of these reports originated in high schools, with 21% of U.S. high schools reporting such crimes; however, reports also arose in 19% of middle schools and 4% of elementary schools (Riner, 1999).

Frequently, societal violence involves the use of weapons, which are readily available among the general public. Evidence of this is seen in the fact that more than 17% of high school students in the 1999 Youth Risk Behavior Surveillance (YRBS) surveys admitted carrying a weapon in the last 30 days and that more than 70 incidents of weapons carrying occurred for every 100 students. Rates of weapons carrying and fighting are even higher for students in alternative high schools, those being most at risk for resorting to violence due to prior aggressive behavior. In a 1998 survey, nearly one third of students in alternative high schools reported carrying a weapon in the last 30 days, and nearly 60% had been involved in a fight, with 11% being treated for injuries sustained in a fight (Grunbaum et al., 1999).

Fear of violence is a significant problem in society. More than 50% of students participating in the 1999 YRBS reported missing school on one or more days due to fear of violence, and nearly 11% of students in alternative high schools missed school because of fear. Another 7.7% of students had experienced threats or actual injury at school (Grunbaum et al., 1999; Kann et al., 2000). Adolescents are not the only ones who experience fear of violence. Although elderly people make up only a small proportion of homicide victims in the United States (5% in 1996), fear of victimization may significantly interfere with the quality of life for older community residents (Stevens et al., 1999).

In 1998, homicide, the most extreme instance of assault, was the third leading cause of death in children 1 to 14 years of age, the second leading cause of death in those aged 15 to 24 years, and the fourth leading cause of death for those 25 to 44 years of age. The overall homicide death rate for that year was 7.3 per 100,000 people, with rates of 8.5 per 100,000 people for children under 1 year of age and 2.6 for those over age 65. The highest homicide rate for any age group was 14.8 among those 15 to 25 years of age (USDHHS, 2000a). Although homicide rates among people over 65 years of age are decreasing, they remain the group with the highest rate during commission of a felony (Bureau of Justice Statistics, 1998). Among the elderly, the highest rates of homicide occur among those 85 years of age or older, or the most vulnerable of the elderly (Stevens et al., 1999).

Disproportionate rates of homicide occur in some groups. For example, in 1998, the homicide rate for black men was 43.1 per 100,000 population compared to only 4.4 for non-Hispanic white men. The rate for Native American men was also high, at 14.9 per 100,000 people (USDHHS, 2000a). Overall, African Americans are six

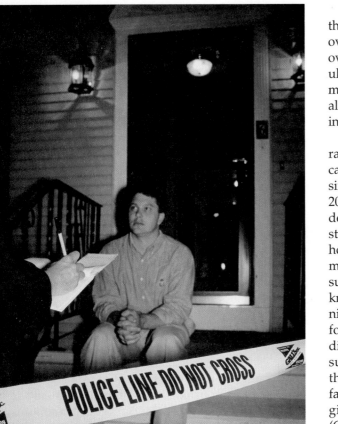

Multiple forms of physical assault occur each day in the United States, with the most extreme resulting in homicide.

times more likely than their white counterparts to be victims of homicide and, based on national figures, seven times more likely to commit homicides. Similarly, men are nine times more likely than women to commit homicides and more likely to be victims (Bureau of Justice Statistics, 1998).

Suicide

Suicide is another serious problem in the United States and worldwide. In 1998, the overall age-adjusted suicide rate in the United States was 10.4 per 100,000 people, down slightly from 10.6 per 100,000 in 1997 (USDHHS, 2000a). Elsewhere in the world, rates are even higher, at 41.2 per 100,000 people in Russia, 30.9 per 100,000 in Hungary, and 26.1 per 100,000 in Finland in 1997 (U.S. Census Bureau, 1999). Like homicide, rates of suicide differ among subpopulations. For example, since 1979, suicide and homicide have alternated as the second and third leading causes of death among young Native Americans, and from 1979 to 1992 the overall suicide rate for this group was 1.5 times that for the general U.S. population (Division of Violence Prevention, 1998c).

The highest suicide rates for any age group occur in those over 85 years of age, at 21 of every 100,000 people over age 85 in 1998 (USDHHS, 2000a). In 1996, people over 65 years of age comprised only 13% of the U.S. population, but accounted for 20% of all suicides. Approximately 82% of suicides in older persons occur among men, although rates declined 15% among elderly men (and 25% in women) from 1990 to 1996 (Stevens et al., 1999).

Older people are not the only ones to experience high rates of suicide. In 1998, suicide was the third leading cause of death in persons 15 to 24 years of age and the sixth leading cause in those age 5 to 14 years (USDHHS, 2000a). In the 1999 YRBS, nearly 20% of high school students had considered suicide and more than 28% had stopped one or more usual activities due to sadness or hopelessness. In this survey, 14.5% of the students had made a plan for suicide and 8.3% had actually attempted suicide (Kann et al., 2000). It is estimated that for every known suicide attempt, 100 to 200 attempts go unrecognized (Thompson, Eggert, Randell, & Pike, 2001). Figures for students in alternative high schools are even more distressing, with 25% of those surveyed contemplating suicide and more than 15% attempting suicide. More than 7% of those surveyed required medical care for failed suicide attempts. Unlike older persons, adolescent girls are more likely to attempt suicide than are boys (Grunbaum et al., 1999).

COMMUNITY HEALTH NURSING AND CONTROL OF SOCIETAL VIOLENCE

ASSESSING FACTORS INFLUENCING SOCIETAL VIOLENCE

Factors in five of the six dimensions of health influence one or more of the forms of societal violence presented in this chapter. Generally speaking, violence results from a combination of factors in several areas. Areas to be addressed include biophysical, psychological, sociocultural, behavioral, and health care system considerations.

Biophysical Considerations

Biophysical considerations include both factors that contribute to violence and those that arise as a consequence of violence. For example, children with special needs are more likely to be abused than normal children. An estimated 13.5% of disabled children are physically abused, as are children born prematurely, those with colic, and those with other chronic health conditions. When physical difficulties in the child are combined with immaturity on the part of the parent (e.g., adolescent parents) the potential for abuse is even greater. As one author expressed it, "Abuse is more likely to occur with high-risk parents who are responsible for a high-risk child" (Nester, 1998, p. 62).

Pregnancy is a biophysical risk factor for abuse of women, and approximately 20% of pregnant women are abused (Parker, McFarlane, Soeken, Silva, & Reel, 1999; Rodriguez et al., 1999). Sexual abuse also increases the risk of pregnancy as well as the risk of sexually transmitted diseases (STDs) (Heise et al., 1999). In one study, for example, pregnant women who were abused were 2.5 times more likely to have STDs than those who were not abused (Martin et al., 1999). Abuse during pregnancy may lead to depression; suicide attempts; and tobacco, drug, and alcohol use and abuse, which increase the potential for complications of pregnancy, low birth weight, and fetal distress (Parker et al., 1999). Approximately one fourth of miscarriages are the result of intimate partner violence (Farella, 2000).

Older clients made vulnerable by poor health and other forms of dependence are also at greater risk of abuse than those who are more independent and in better health (Champion, 1998). Physical abuse at any age may lead to a variety of physical consequences including injury, impairment, poor subjective health, and multiple chronic somatic complaints (Heise et al., 1999). Approximately 10% to 21% of abused women require medical care for injuries received, 70% of which occurs in emergency departments (Division of Violence Prevention, 2000e). Abused women are also more likely than their nonabused counterparts to be hospitalized, with hospitalization for digestive problems nine times more likely, and hospitalizations for injury or poisoning 3.6 times more likely than for other women (Kernic, Wolf, & Holt, 2000).

Physical signs and symptoms may also indicate the presence of current abuse. Physical and other indicators of child abuse are presented in Table 32–1 ■. Indicators of intimate partner violence and elder abuse are presented in Tables 32–2 ■ (page 764) and 32–3 ■ (page 765).

Biophysical factors do not seem to play a contributing role in homicide outside of the differential effects of age and gender discussed above. The one exception is in the small number of combined murder–suicide incidents in which elderly persons with seriously ill spouses may kill their spouse and then kill themselves. Long-term disability and intractable pain, however, may be factors in depression that may result in suicide in all age groups. There is also some indication that obesity is linked to suicide, with women with high body mass index (BMI) more likely to engage in suicidal ideation than nonobese women. In men the association seems to be reversed, with increased thoughts of suicide occurring in men with low BMI (Carpenter, Hasin, Allison, & Faith, 2000).

Psychological Considerations

As was the case with biophysical considerations, psychological factors serve as both contributors to and consequences of violence. For example, caregiver resentment, fatigue, family conflict, and personality traits have been found to contribute to elder abuse (Hogstel & Curry, 1999). Similarly, grief at the loss of a loved one may also

contribute to abuse (Farella, 2000). The presence of psychiatric disorders also increases the potential for all forms of violence. Personality factors such as risk-taking preferences, depression, stress, and excessive temper have also been associated with weapons carrying in adolescents, which may be a precursor to violence (Simon, Richardson, Dent, Chou, & Flay, 1998).

Psychological factors that may contribute to family violence include poor coping skills, the emotional climate in the family, personality traits of the abuser or the victim, and the presence of psychopathology. Families with poor coping skills have difficulty dealing with situational stressors that create tension, resulting in violence. Constant family crises or upheavals indicative of poor coping abilities are frequently characteristic of abusive families.

The emotional climate in the family can also contribute to abuse. Families that exhibit increased emotional tension and anxiety, with little display of visible affection or emotional support, are considered emotionally impoverished and are at risk for violence. Similarly, family communication patterns that are non-nurturing, destructive, or ambiguous may also indicate risk for family violence. Couples that experience intimate partner violence have been found to have poorer communication skills and less satisfying relationships than other couples, and tend to engage in mutual exchange of negative communication (McClellan & Killeen, 2000). These couples are also characterized by poor conflict negotiation skills, poor problem-solving skills, and defensiveness on the part of both members (Lloyd, 2000).

The distribution of power within the family is another element of the emotional climate that may lead to abuse. Abusive families are characterized by autocratic decision making and power struggles between members. Abusers tend to abuse the power they have over other family members when they feel their power is threatened. Various studies of elder abuse, for example, have indicated that some abusers are economically dependent on the victims of abuse, and abuse may be an indication of frustration over their helplessness.

Personality traits of either the abuser or the victim can influence the incidence of family violence. Abusers and victims alike tend to have poor self-esteem. Abusers may also be emotionally immature, hostile, and unable to cope with problems in a healthy manner. They frequently feel personally insecure and inadequate, although they often appear successful to others.

Child abusers tend to have unrealistic expectations of children, particularly as sources of warmth and love. When they are disappointed in these expectations, abuse may occur. For example, children who are irritable, who cry often, or who do not care to be cuddled may be perceived as rejecting the parent. For parents with low self-esteem, this perceived rejection can set the stage for abuse. Some authors suggest that this response becomes stronger over time and occurs in stages. In earlier stages, the parent exhibits poor tolerance for stress and disinhibition of aggression in the face of stress. This stage leads

■ TABLE 32–1   Physical and Psychological Indications of Child Abuse

TYPE OF ABUSE	PHYSICAL INDICATIONS	PSYCHOLOGICAL INDICATIONS
Neglect	Persistent hunger Poor hygiene Inappropriate dress for the weather Constant fatigue Unattended physical health problems Poor growth patterns	Delinquency due to lack of supervision School truancy Begging or stealing food
Physical abuse	Bruises or welts in unusual places or in several stages of healing; distinctive shapes Burns (especially cigarette burns; immersion burns of hands, feet, or buttocks; rope burns; or distinctively shaped burns) Fractures (multiple or in various stages of healing, inconsistent with explanations of injury) Joint swelling or limited mobility Long-bone deformities Lacerations and abrasions to the mouth, lip, gums, eye, genitalia Human bite marks Signs of intracranial trauma Deformed or displaced nasal septum Bleeding or fluid drainage from the ears or ruptured eardrums Broken, loose, or missing teeth Difficulty in respirations, tenderness or crepitus over ribs Abdominal pain or tenderness Recurrent urinary tract infection	Wary of physical contact with adults Behavioral extremes of withdrawal or aggression Apprehensive when other children cry Inappropriate response to pain
Emotional abuse	Nothing specific	Overly compliant, passive, and undemanding Extremely aggressive, demanding, or angry Behavior inappropriate for age (either overly adult or overly infantile) Developmental delay Attempted suicide
Sexual abuse	Torn, stained, or bloody underwear Pain or itching in genital areas Bruises or bleeding from external genitalia, vagina, rectum Sexually transmitted disease Swollen or red cervix, vulva, or perineum Semen around the mouth or genitalia or on clothing Pregnancy	Withdrawn Engages in fantasy behavior or infantile behavior Poor peer relationships Unwilling to participate in physical activities Wears long sleeves and several layers of clothes even in hot weather Delinquency or running away Inappropriate sexual behavior or mannerisms

to poor management of stress, resulting in acute crises and provocation. Later stages are characterized by chronic patterns of anger and abuse in response to provocation by the child (Wolfe, 1999).

Abused women tend to be dependent, passive, and reluctant to make changes. Some authors attribute these characteristics to feelings of learned helplessness in which the woman can no longer predict with any accuracy that any action she may take will have the desired effect, leading to loss of motivation for any action

(Walker, 2000). Grief and guilt are other frequent feelings exhibited by victims of intimate partner violence.

Consistent themes in the psychological origins of youth suicide include the presence of conflict. Conflict may be either interpersonal, in which adolescents disagree strenuously with parents and other significant others, or intrapsychic, in which there are marked discrepancies between self-expectations and perceived performance. These conflicts escalate over time, and suicidal behavior may be an attempt to resolve the conflict motivated by

■ **TABLE 32-2   Physical and Psychological Indications of Intimate Partner Violence**

PHYSICAL INDICATIONS	PSYCHOLOGICAL INDICATIONS
Chronic fatigue	Casual response to a serious injury or excessively emotional response to a relatively minor injury
Vague complaints, aches, and pains	Frequent ambulatory or emergency room visits
Frequent injuries	Nightmares
Recurrent sexually transmitted diseases	Depression
Muscle tension	Anxiety
Facial lacerations	Anorexia or other eating disorder
Injuries to chest, breasts, back, abdomen, or genitalia	Drug or alcohol abuse
Bilateral injuries of arms or legs	Poor self-esteem
Symmetric injuries	Suicide attempts
Obvious patterns of belt buckles, bite marks, fist, or hand marks	
Burns of hands, feet, buttocks, or with distinctive patterns	
Headaches	
Ulcers	

perceptions of death as the only available method of resolution (Aldridge, 1998).

Psychological consequences of abuse are many and varied and may arise both from the experience of being abused and witnessing abuse. For example, childhood sexual abuse has been linked to 14 subsequent mood, anxiety, and substance abuse disorders in women and five disorders in men, with depression and substance abuse particularly prevalent (Molnar, Buka, & Kessler, 2001). Consequences of abuse among women include posttraumatic stress disorder (PTSD), depression, anxiety, phobias, panic disorder, eating disorders, sexual dysfunction, and low self-esteem. The primary psychological response of women to abuse is depression (Campbell & Soeken, 1999), but other effects also occur with alarming frequency. For example, in a review of several studies, the mean prevalence of depression among abused women was found to be 48%, with suicidality occurring in 18% and PTSD in 64%, and dose-response relationships were noted for the extent of abuse and the occurrence of depression and PTSD (Golding, 1999). Abused women are 3.6 times more likely to be hospitalized for psychiatric diagnoses and nearly five times more likely to attempt suicide than nonabused women (Kernic et al., 2000).

Consequences of witnessing abuse among children include emotional and behavioral problems, anxiety, depression, poor school performance, low self-esteem, disobedience, nightmares, physical complaints, and aggression. Similar findings are noted for children who are themselves abused, but the combination of both experiencing and witnessing abuse has been found to have more severe effects on children than either condition alone (Heise et al., 1999). Children's response to witnessing violence has been found to be more severe with poor maternal adjustment to abuse, particularly for girls (Cummings, Pepler, & Moore, 1999).

Sociocultural Considerations

Sociocultural factors play a considerable part in the occurrence of societal violence. Social disorganization theories of homicide, for example, suggest that the inability of communities to realize the common values of their members and maintain social controls on behavior contribute to homicide. In other theoretical perspectives, homicide is an instrumental act designed to obtain money or property denied one because of economic hardship or lack of opportunity. A third perspective posits that homicide arises out of a subculture of violence in which violence is perceived as a legitimate means of conflict resolution (Cubbin, Pickle, & Fingerhut, 2000).

Cultural themes also influence intimate partner violence. In many cultural groups, men are believed to have a right to control women. Norms granting financial and physical control of women lend themselves to multiple forms of abuse. A consistent set of events seems to trigger IPV in cultures in which women are expected to be subservient to men. These events include disobedience, talking back, not having meals ready at the expected time, perceived failures in household or child care, questioning the male about money or girlfriends or expressing suspicion of infidelity, going out without permission, and refusing sex (Heise et al., 1999). Subservience in marriage makes it particularly difficult to refuse sexual intimacy or unsafe sexual practices, particularly when reinforced by abuse or fear of violence. This then places these women at higher risk for sexually transmitted diseases (STDs). In multiple studies worldwide, men who were abusive in the home have been shown to be more likely to have extramarital relationships and higher incidence of STDs than nonabusive men (UNAIDS, 1999).

Other sociocultural factors have been shown to influence violence as well. For example, IPV is five times more

■ **TABLE 32–3   Physical and Psychological Indications of Elder Abuse**

TYPE OF ABUSE	PHYSICAL INDICATIONS	PSYCHOLOGICAL INDICATIONS
Neglect	Constant hunger or malnutrition Poor hygiene Inappropriate dress for the weather Chronic fatigue Unattended medical needs Poor skin integrity or decubiti Contractures Urine burns/excoriation Dehydration Fecal impaction	Listlessness Social isolation
Emotional abuse	Hypochondria	Habit disorder (biting, sucking, rocking) Destructive or antisocial conduct Neurotic traits (sleep or speech disorder, inhibition of play) Hysteria Obsessions or compulsions Phobias
Physical abuse	Bruises and welts Burns Fractures Sprains or dislocations Lacerations or abrasions Evidence of oversedation	Withdrawal Confusion Fear of caretaker or other family members Listlessness
Sexual abuse	Difficulty walking Torn, stained, or bloody underwear Pain or itching in genital area Bruises or bleeding on external genitalia or in vaginal or anal areas Sexually transmitted diseases	Withdrawal
Financial abuse	Inappropriate clothing Unmet medical needs	Failure to meet financial obligations Anxiety over expenses
Denial of rights	Nothing specific	Hesitancy in making decisions Listlessness and apathy

common in households with annual incomes under $15,000 than in those with incomes over $50,000 (Division of Violence Prevention, 2000a). Victims of IPV may also stay in abusive relationships because of limited resource availability and social isolation (Tyson & Fleming, 1999). Lack of social resources, both tangible social support and emotional support provided by friends and family, have also been linked to child abuse (Hall, Sachs, & Rayens, 1998). Economic factors and the cultural factor of ageism contribute to abuse of elderly individuals (Hogstel & Curry, 1999). Strong associations between homicide and urbanization and socioeconomic conditions have also been found (Cubbin et al., 2000). Similarly, lack of employment, lack of educational opportunity, community history of suicide, and loss of traditional spiritual practices and language have been linked to higher inci-

dence of suicide among Native Americans (Division of Violence Prevention, 1998c). Social factors associated with increased suicide potential among adolescents include poor school performance and long absences from school (Thompson et al., 2001), as well as lack of social

CULTURAL CONSIDERATIONS

Women in many cultural groups adhere to cultural norms that permit men to control their lives even when this control is harmful to themselves and to their children. What would you do if you were working with a woman who was being abused but refused to leave her husband because of her cultural beliefs and values?

connectedness and interpersonal conflict (Aldridge, 1998).

The social response to violence also influences its occurrence. Cultural factors, for example, influence the willingness of persons outside the intimate relationship to take action when IPV is suspected. The incidence of abuse tends to be higher in cultures in which family matters are considered "private" (Heise et al., 1999). Legal alternatives open to victims may also influence response to violence. For example, women may be more likely to seek a restraining order or protection order (PO) against an abusive partner than to press criminal charges. POs entail automatic legal responses to their violation without the emotional and financial costs of lengthy court proceedings. POs also help to deter retaliation against the victim for taking action. An estimated 22% of abused women seek POs in the face of physical abuse (Division of Violence Prevention, 2000e). One study of the effectiveness of POs indicated that the incidence of physical abuse declined from 68% to 23%. Other studies have shown declines of 40% to 50%. However, POs have been shown to be less effective in lower socioeconomic groups who may have less to lose by violating them (Carlson, Harris, & Holden, 1999).

Social factors may also have protective effects against societal violence. For example, social connectedness is known to be inversely related to suicide, and social support and regular church attendance have been shown to be protective of abuse among Latino women (Lown & Vega, 2001). Similarly, having social power outside the family and intervention by family members have a protective effect in preventing the abuse of women (Heise et al., 1999).

Another social factor that influences societal violence is media attention. Some authors contend that unbalanced media attention to some types of homicide (e.g., of children or by children) provides the public with an inaccurate view of the problem that hampers their ability to engage in effective problem solving (Sorenson, Manz, & Berk, 1998). Others suggest that exposure to media violence is a causal factor in homicide and suicide. For example, the claim is made that murder rates tend to double with the introduction of television into new areas and that "the data linking violence in the media to violence in society is superior to that linking cancer and tobacco" (Grossman, 2000, p. 12). The media no longer presents extensive coverage of youth suicides, for example, because of the known effect seen in cluster suicides. The contention is made that similar coverage of adolescent homicide creates inappropriate role models for vulnerable teenagers throughout the country. In some counties, in fact, reporting of the names and images of juvenile criminals is prohibited in efforts to prevent "copycat" violence (Grossman, 2000).

The availability of lethal weapons, particularly guns, is another social factor that influences violence. Firearms are used in approximately 70% of homicides and in 60% of suicides. In one study, 12% to 57% of households in the states surveyed have firearms, and in as many as 23% of these households firearms are kept loaded (Powell, Jacklin, Nelson, & Bland, 1998). Counterclaims are made, however, that guns are more often used for defense than in the commission of a crime (2 million incidents per year versus 430,000 respectively) (Lott, 2000).

Occupation is another social factor to be addressed in assessing contributions to societal violence. Nurses, as well as members of other occupational groups, are at increased risk for both suicide and assault. In fact, suicide is the fifth most common cause of death among nurses, as high as six times the rate for the general population in some studies. Nurses are also more likely than the general public to be successful in suicide attempts due to their greater knowledge of the lethality of various methods. Increased suicide rates among nurses have been attributed to high job stress and "critical incident stress." *Critical incident stress* is the stress that accompanies experiencing or witnessing events that cause unusual emotional upset (Bellanger, 2000).

Occupation is also implicated in some homicides. In 1990, homicide became the second leading cause of occupational deaths in the United States, accounting for 13.5% of all occupational deaths from 1980 to 1994 (Division of Safety Research, 1998). While nurses may experience homicide, they are more likely to be subjected to milder forms of assault. In one survey of nurses in Colorado, for instance, 32% of nurses reported being subjected to threats or to assault. It has been hypothesized that the increase in assault suffered by nurses in the work setting is a result of changing norms of acceptable behavior (Morgan, 1999), and "a nursing culture where showing signs of distress is discouraged" (*Legislative Network for Nurses*, 1998, p. 4).

Behavioral Considerations

Behavioral factors also contribute to societal violence. For example, alcohol abuse by a male partner was found to be the strongest correlate of intimate partner violence

⑥THINK ABOUT IT

You encounter a situation in which an Asian refugee mother has inflicted several round lesions on her three-year-old daughter's abdomen in the process of "coining" her to cure a stomachache. One of the lesions has become infected. Would you report the mother to child protective services? Why or why not?

CRITICAL THINKING IN RESEARCH

Dorfman et al. (1997) examined local television news stories related to young people or violence or both to determine whether or not the stories were framed episodically or thematically. Episodically framed stories focused on the events that had occurred without addressing the context in which they occurred. Thematic stories, on the other hand, included material on trends and conditions related to the events covered. They contended that thematically framed stories help to define violence as a public health issue, whereas episodic stories address violence as a criminal justice issue and that the approach taken influences policy makers to assume either a preventive public health approach or a punitive criminal justice approach to the control of societal violence. Their findings included the following:

- Violence dominated news coverage.
- Crime details dominated coverage of violence.
- More than half of the stories about youth related to violence.
- More than two thirds of stories on violence related to youth.
- Most of the coverage reflected an episodic framework rather than a thematic framework.
- What are the implications of the findings of this study for public policy related to violence? Do you think the direction policy making is likely to take is an appropriate one? Why or why not?
- What would the effects be if news coverage related to young people were more positive in nature? Why do you think news coverage focuses on the negative side of youth behavior?
- Do you think news media coverage of youth behaviors has changed over time? How would you find out if your assumption was true or false?
- Do you think a study of print news media would result in similar findings? How would you go about doing such a study? What types of print news media would you examine?

in one study (Coker, Smith, et al., 2000). In many instances, the effects of social factors such as unemployment and lack of opportunity are exacerbated by drug or alcohol use leading to an increased potential for violence (Margolin, John, & Foo, 1998). Behavioral factors such as smoking may also contribute to suicide. For example, nurses who smoke are four times more likely than nonsmokers to commit suicide, while excessive caffeine intake appears to be associated with a decreased risk of suicide (Bellanger, 2000). Some studies have indicated

that the link between smoking and suicide involves a dose response relationship, with former smokers 1.4 times more likely, light smokers 2.5 times more likely, and heavy smokers 4.3 times more likely to commit suicide than nonsmokers (Miller, Hemenway, & Rimm, 2000).

Conversely, violence may lead to high-risk behaviors. For example, sexual abuse may contribute to high-risk sexual behaviors in victims, increasing the potential for unwanted pregnancy or STDs (Heise et al., 1999). The mean prevalence of alcohol abuse among abused women in a review of multiple studies was 18.5%, while the mean prevalence of drug abuse was 9% (Golding, 1999).

Health System Considerations

Health system factors contributing to violence relate primarily to the failure of health care providers to identify clients at risk for or experiencing violence. Providers are generally able to deal with the physical effects of intimate partner violence or attempted suicide or homicide but may be less adept at dealing with underlying causes or addressing safety issues (Sword, Carpio, Deviney, & Schreiber, 1998). According to the Division of Violence Prevention (1998b), only 16% of physicians, 31% of nurse practitioners or physicians assistants, and 21% of nurses reported routinely screening women for intimate partner violence, and 29%, 8%, and 57% of respondents, respectively, reported being unsure how to screen for IPV. Often, screening occurs only in the face of suggested evidence of abuse. For

ETHICAL AWARENESS

Some states have passed legislation mandating reporting of physical abuse of women. Some authors, however, maintain that such laws are paternalistic and assume that abused women are incapable of making their own decisions. These authors also note the biases that occur in current reporting systems for child and elder abuse, whereby black and Latin American families are disproportionately reported as abusive. In addition, mandatory reporting may put women at risk for subsequent abuse, particularly since the criminal justice system has a poor record of acting expeditiously to deal with cases of abuse (Glass & Campbell, 1998).

- Do you think that mandatory reporting should be legislated?
- What are the ethical implications of mandatory reporting of intimate partner violence?
- Do these implications differ for mandatory reporting of abuse of children or elderly persons? Why or why not?

example, 79% of primary care physicians reported screening injured clients for abuse, but only 10% routinely screened new patients, and only 9% included screening in routine checkups. Similarly, only 11% of physicians reported screening prenatal patients for abuse (Rodriguez et al., 1999). In some studies, fewer than 5% of battered women are accurately identified by health care providers (Glass & Campbell, 1998).

Even when abuse is suspected or confirmed, providers may be hesitant to report findings. For instance, 59% of California family physicians reported that they might not comply with mandatory reporting of IPV if the client objected to reporting (Rodriguez, McLoughlin, Bauer, Paredes, & Grumbach, 1999). Barriers to reporting abuse of older clients also exist. For example, some providers report confidentiality issues, fear regarding the response of the abuser, desires to avoid involvement in court proceedings, distrust of the effectiveness of follow-up, and doubt of their own abilities to accurately recognize abuse as reasons for not reporting abuse (Hogstel & Curry, 1999).

Numerous biophysical, psychological, sociocultural, behavioral, and health system factors contribute to the occurrence of violence in individual clients and families and in society at large. Tips for assessing risk for violence are presented below. The companion Web site for this book also provides tools for assessing risk for societal violence, the Family Violence Risk Factor Inventory, and the Suicide Risk Factor Inventory.   ✪

DIAGNOSTIC REASONING AND CONTROL OF SOCIETAL VIOLENCE

Nursing diagnoses may be derived from assessment data related to individual clients and families or population groups. An example of a nursing diagnosis for an individual client might be "potential for child abuse due to increased stress of single parenthood and care of disabled child." A population-based diagnosis might be "increased potential for violence due to prevalence of weapons carrying among high school students."

PLANNING AND IMPLEMENTING CONTROL STRATEGIES FOR SOCIETAL VIOLENCE

Community health nurses are actively involved in planning control strategies for societal violence at primary, secondary, and tertiary levels of prevention. Resources to assist nurses in these efforts are available through links provided on the companion Web site for this book.   ✪

Primary Prevention

Primary prevention of all of the forms of societal violence discussed here focuses on three major approaches, increasing personal aversion to violence as a means of resolving conflict, increasing personal abilities to deal with stress, and eliminating or reducing factors that contribute to stress.

---

assessment tips assessment tips assessment tips

ASSESSING RISK FOR VIOLENCE

Biophysical Considerations
- Are there physical considerations that place clients at risk for IPV or suicide (e.g., disability, pregnancy)?
- Is there physical evidence of abuse?

Psychological Considerations
- What is the level of stress experienced by potential abusers or suicide victims? What coping skills are employed? How effective is coping?
- Is there evidence of psychiatric disorder? Depression?
- Do potential victims or perpetrators of violence exhibit poor self-esteem? Poor impulse control?
- Is there a negative emotional climate in the setting?

Sociocultural Considerations
- Do sociocultural norms support violence?
- Is there intergenerational evidence of violence?
- Are social interactions positive or negative?
- Do societal conditions contribute to stress (e.g., unemployment, homelessness)?

- Do cultural or religious values influence the risk of violence positively or negatively?
- Are there adequate social support networks available to members of society?
- Are there occupational risks for violence?
- What is the societal response to violence? What is the media response to violence?

Behavioral Considerations
- Is there evidence of substance abuse in the situation?
- What is the extent of smoking behavior?
- Is there evidence of high-risk sexual behavior?

Health System Considerations
- Are health care providers alert to risk for or evidence of violence?
- What is the response of health care providers to evidence of violence or potential for violence?

Increasing aversion to violence may be accomplished by teaching alternative methods of conflict resolution and by imposing cultural and social sanctions against violent behavior. For example, in societies in which violence is not perceived as an acceptable approach to interpersonal conflict, less violence occurs. Similarly, strong religious convictions may deter attempted suicide. Community health nurses can be actively involved in teaching positive modes of conflict resolution, anger management, and coping strategies and in activity to change societal attitudes toward the acceptability of violence.

Community health nurses can also assist clients and families at risk to develop effective parent–child and intimate partner relationships by providing anticipatory guidance, assistance with communication, and so on. For instance, the nurse can educate new parents about child behavioral cues and appropriate parental responses as well as provide reinforcement for positive responses. In addition, the nurse can suggest activities that will enhance the bond between parents and child (e.g., reading to or playing with the child), and educate parents regarding appropriate forms of discipline (Nester, 1998).

Community health nurses can also help to remove or reduce factors that contribute to stress and the potential for abuse. For example, the nurse might refer caretakers of an elderly client for respite services, assist an unemployed parent to find employment, or increase social support networks for socially isolated families. Treatment of substance abuse problems in the individual or family may also decrease the potential for violence. Crisis intervention and hotlines may also prevent suicide.

Specific prevention of financial abuse of older clients may involve four options to safeguard their funds and property. These options include a financial representative trust, durable power of attorney, designation of a representative payee, and joint tenancy (Weiler, 1989).

In a *financial representative trust,* the older person transfers to a trustee, selected by him- or herself, responsibility for managing his or her property. In this type of arrangement, the trustee is required to manage the older person's assets in a particular manner for the benefit of the older person or others designated (e.g., grandchildren).

A *durable power of attorney* is a written document in which the older person grants another person the authority to act in his or her stead. The durable power of attorney comes into force only when the older person (the "principal") chooses to relinquish control of his or her affairs to the designated person or when the principal becomes incapacitated.

A *representative payee* is a person or organization that receives payments as a substitute for the beneficiary. For example, an older person may make arrangements for his or her Social Security benefits to be paid to a specific family member who uses that money to meet the beneficiary's financial obligations. This type of arrangement is restricted to payments to veterans, recipients of Social Security and Supplemental Security Income, and retirees

from railroad companies or state agencies. The agreement covers only that one source of the older person's income. The person receiving the money is required by law to use the funds for the care of the beneficiary, and the agency remitting the checks may demand an accounting of expenditures.

In *joint tenancy,* the person is co-owner of the assets covered with one or more designated others. All parties involved have the use of funds or property covered under joint tenancy. In the event of the death of one party, ownership automatically devolves on other members of the joint tenancy agreement. Advantages and disadvantages of these four methods of preventing financial abuse of older people are summarized in Table 32–4 ■. The community health nurse can assist older clients at risk for financial abuse to evaluate these financial management options and select those best suited to their needs. If the older person needs help in implementing the alternative suggested, the nurse could refer the individual to a source of assistance.

⑥THINK ABOUT IT

What recommendations would you have for reducing violence in school settings?

At the societal level, community health nurses may be involved in the development of legislation to regulate media coverage of violence or access to lethal weapons. Another legislative strategy that has had some success in curbing youth suicide is increasing the legal drinking age to 21 (Birckmayer & Hemenway, 1999).

Secondary Prevention

Secondary prevention of family violence involves identification of abuse and treatment for its immediate effects. Identification requires screening for those at risk for abuse. Routine use of a simple screening tool for IPV in prenatal clinics increased the propensity of providers to screen for abuse to 88% and increased detection of abuse from 0.8% of clients to 7% (Wiist & McFarlane, 1999). Routine screening for IPV and child abuse has been suggested in maternal–child health services, reproductive health services, mental health services, and emergency departments (Heise et al., 1999). Routine screening of men as potential abusers during primary care visits has also been suggested, particularly among men who are depressed, report a history of abuse in childhood, or engage in heavy alcohol use (Oriel & Fleming, 1998).

Some authors have suggested the use of administrative sanctions against health care providers who fail to screen for IPV as directed by agency protocols (Larson, Rolniak, Hyman, MacLeod, & Savage, 2000). Others,

■ TABLE 32–4   **Advantages and Disadvantages of Financial Arrangements to Prevent Financial Abuse of the Elderly**

TYPE OF FINANCIAL ARRANGEMENT	ADVANTAGES	DISADVANTAGES
Financial representative trust	Legal accountability for use of funds Ability to specify use of funds and beneficiaries	Cost of establishing and administering trust
Durable power of attorney	Financial needs met if older person becomes incapacitated Ability to designate person to control funds Retention of control of funds by older person until he or she chooses to relinquish it or becomes incapacitated	Limited measures to safeguard older person if designee does not use funds as intended
Representative payee	Limited control of funds by designated payee Legal responsibility to use funds for the benefit of the stated beneficiary Mechanism for demanding accounting of use of funds	Restrictions on types of funds covered
Joint tenancy	Ability of older person to designate recipient of funds Automatic right of survivorship eliminates inheritance taxes	Both parties have access to and use of property, and the joint tenant may use them for his or her own benefit and not that of the older person

however, caution that failure to screen clients for IPV may reflect personal experiences with violence and, in the absence of effective occupational programs to help employees deal with the aftermath of violence, mandatory screening may do more harm than good (Johnson, 2001). Some jurisdictions have found that educating the public, including perpetrators of violence and those who know them, regarding the risk factors for and inappropriateness of violent behaviors has led to self-report of abusive behavior and initiation of treatment prior to filing of a criminal complaint. Similarly, parents have been found to report and seek assistance for teenage children with sexual behavior problems prior to major offenses as a result of public education campaigns (Division of Violence Prevention, 2001).

Once evidence of family violence has been detected, treatment focuses on assessing the client for immediate danger, providing appropriate care for the consequences of violence, documenting the client's condition, developing a safety plan, and making needed referrals to community services (Heise et al., 1999). Intervention may include referring an abused family member to a shelter or removing a dependent victim from the abusive situation. Secondary prevention at this point also includes treatment for the perpetrator of violence and for family members who witness violence.

Secondary prevention also involves mandatory reporting of suspected child abuse and, in some jurisdictions, reporting of intimate partner violence or elder abuse. Reports are generally made initially by telephone to the appropriate agency and are followed, usually within 48 hours, by a written report. (Sample reporting forms are included in Appendix D.) In making a report, the community health nurse should be careful to focus on objective evidence that suggests abuse and to report exactly what he or she has seen or verbatim reports of those involved.

When IPV involves sexual assault or rape, or when such events occur outside intimate relationships, community health nurses should refer victimized clients to a local emergency department for assessment. Most emergency departments have sexual abuse response (SART) teams that have extensive background in assessment and care of persons who have been sexually assaulted. Members of SART teams also have expertise in the collection of forensic evidence that may be used in criminal proceedings against the abuser. Community health nurses should encourage victims of sexual abuse and other intimate partner violence to report the event and to seek help in an emergency department. Clients should be particularly cautioned not to "clean themselves up" following the assault as this destroys physical evidence of the assault.

⑥THINK ABOUT IT

What considerations would lead you to decide to remove a victim of abuse from an abusive situation? Under what circumstances would you recommend leaving the victim in the home?

Several well-designed studies have indicated that treatment of perpetrators of family violence is effective, although there is insufficient data to determine that certain interventions work better than others or work better for certain groups of abusers (Davis & Taylor, 1999). In one study, abused pregnant women provided with empowerment counseling experienced less subsequent abuse than those in a control group (Parker et al., 1999). Couples therapy for abusive husbands has also been shown to be effective even in the face of significant PTSD in the abused women (Schlee, Heyman, & O'Leary, 1998). In other studies, 53% to 85% of abusive men who complete treatment programs remain nonabusive for up to two years. Unfortunately, one third to one half of male abusers do not complete therapy (Heise et al., 1999). Community health nurses can be instrumental in referring abusive clients to treatment programs and in motivating them to continue treatment.

Secondary prevention also involves the early identification of persons who are contemplating suicide or homicide and intervention to prevent the act or limit the consequences. Nurses, teachers, and counselors may recognize the signs of impending suicide or escalating aggression and should take immediate action. Such action might include counseling, referral, or hospitalization if the danger appears imminent. Community health nurses may also be involved in educating individuals who work with young people, the elderly, and others at risk for suicide to recognize indicators of a potential suicide attempt. Indications of suicide risk are summarized below.

HIGHLIGHTS

Indications of Suicide Risk

- Family history of suicide
- History of prior suicide attempt
- Recent serious loss (particularly in the last six months)
- Signs of depression
- Expression of feelings of hopelessness or helplessness
- Display of anxiety, irritability, or panic
- Absence of references to future goals or activities
- Frequent or persistent thoughts of suicide
- Carefully thought-out plan for suicide
- Lethal method selected for suicide with reduced likelihood of rescue
- Suicide planned for near future
- Behavior designed to "put one's house in order" (e.g., making a will, giving away prized possessions)

Tertiary Prevention

Tertiary prevention of societal violence involves dealing with the consequences of violence and preventing its recurrence. Interventions intended for the individual or family level include providing treatment for long-term physical or psychological effects of violence. For example, abused women may need a referral for treatment for PTSD, or children who witness or experience abuse can be referred for counseling. Similarly, the loved ones of suicide or homicide victims may need assistance in dealing with their loss. Another tertiary prevention measure for suicide and homicide is control of media representations that promote copycat events.

Tertiary prevention of family violence also entails changing circumstances that promote violence. For example, the community health nurse may assist abusive parents to understand the needs and behavioral cues of their children or help caregivers of disabled children or elderly family members to find respite. Other potential tertiary strategies for elder abuse include providing alternatives to home care of the elderly and increasing community support services for persons who are caring for older family members. Nurses may also assist family members to improve coping and communication skills as well as to improve self-esteem. This is particularly important for victims of child abuse if the intergenerational cycle of abusive behavior is to be broken. Goals for primary, secondary, and tertiary prevention of societal violence and related community health nursing interventions are summarized in Table 32–5 ■ (on page 772).

EVALUATING CONTROL STRATEGIES FOR SOCIETAL VIOLENCE

The effectiveness of control strategies for societal violence can be evaluated at the level of the individual client or family or at the population level. For example, the nurse might determine whether or not child abuse has been prevented in a family at high risk for abuse, or whether subsequent instances of abuse have been experienced by an older client or pregnant woman. At the population level, the community health nurse might look for changes in suicide or homicide rates or the frequency of reports to child protective services to evaluate the effectiveness of population-based interventions. In assessing such efforts, community health nurses and others might evaluate the extent to which national objectives related to violence and suicide have been achieved. Baseline and target information for selected objectives are presented on page 773.

■ **TABLE 32–5** **Goals for Primary, Secondary, and Tertiary Prevention of Societal Violence and Related Community Health Nursing Interventions**

GOAL OF PREVENTION	NURSING INTERVENTIONS
Primary Prevention	
1. Development of effective coping skills	1. Teach coping skills and stress management skills.
2. Development of self-esteem	2. Foster self-image. Advocate school programs to foster self-esteem in young people.
3. Development of realistic expectations of self and others	3. Educate parents on child development. Educate caregivers on needs of the elderly. Help clients recognize strengths.
4. Develop effective parenting and interpersonal skills	4. Teach parenting skills. Teach and role model effective communication skills.
5. Treatment of psychopathology or substance abuse	5. Refer for treatment.
6. Promotion of nonviolent conflict resolution	6. Teach nonviolent conflict management strategies.
7. Provision of emotional and material support	7. Refer to sources of assistance as needed. Assist in development or expansion of social support networks.
8. Reduction of risk behaviors	8. Encourage clients not to frequent places where homicides occur and not to use drugs and alcohol in circumstances in which interpersonal conflict is likely.
9. Decreased availability of weapons, drugs, and alcohol	9. Engage in political activity to promote control of weapons and limit access to drugs and alcohol.
10. Change in societal attitudes toward violence	10. Teach nonviolent modes of conflict resolution. Teach problem-solving and decision-making skills. Discuss approaches to discipline.
11. Development of policies that discourage violence and protect potential victims	11. Engage in political activity and advocacy. Promote positive attitudes toward the elderly and disabled.
Secondary Prevention	
1. Identification of persons at risk for violence	1. Engage in case finding. Teach teachers and counselors to recognize signs of abuse or potential for violence. Screen for evidence of abuse or potential for violence.
2. Provision of counseling for persons at risk for violence	2. Refer for counseling.
3. Provision of treatment for victims of violence	3. Engage in political activity and advocacy to ensure adequate treatment facilities.
4. Identification of episodes of violence	4. Report instances of violence.
5. Provision of safe environments	5. Remove victims of abuse to safe environments as needed. Plan with victims for achieving a safe environment. Refer to a shelter as needed. Arrange for involuntary commitment if the person is a clear danger to self or others.
6. Provision of treatment for violent persons	6. Refer for treatment. Advocate for availability of treatment services and facilities. Provide emotional support to both victims and perpetrators.
Tertiary Prevention	
1. Prevention of suicide clusters and copycat murders	1. Assist in the development of community response plans. Advocate for control of media exposures to violence.
2. Provision of care to families of homicide and suicide victims	2. Assist family members to work through feelings of grief and guilt. Assist families to find positive ways to cope with loss. Refer for counseling as needed.
3. Treatment of consequences of violence	3. Refer for physical and psychological treatment services as needed. Advocate for available services for victims and perpetrators of violence.
4. Reduction of sources of stress	4. Refer to sources of assistance. Develop or expand social support networks. Provide respite care as needed. Assist with employment and other social needs.

HEALTHY PEOPLE 2010

GOALS FOR THE POPULATION

Objective	Base	Target
15-4 Reduce the proportion of people living in homes with firearms that are loaded and unlocked	19%	16%
15-32 Reduce homicides (per 100,000 population)	6.2	3.2
15-33 Reduce		
a. Maltreatment of children (per 1,000 children)	13.9	11.1
b. Child maltreatment fatalities (per 100,000 children)	1.7	1.5
15-34 Reduce the rate of physical assault by current or former intimate partners (per 1,000 population)	4.5	3.6
15-35 Reduce the annual rate of rape or attempted rape (per 1,000 population)	0.9	0.7
15-36 Reduce sexual assault other than rape (per 1,000 population)	0.6	0.2
15-37 Reduce physical assaults (per 1,000 population)	31.1	25.5
15-39 Reduce weapon carrying by adolescents on school property	8.5%	6%
18-1 Reduce the suicide rate (per 100,000 population)	10.8	6.0
16-2 Reduce the rate of suicide attempts by adolescents (12-month average)	2.6%	1%

Source: U.S. Department of Health and Human Services. (2000). *Healthy people 2010* (Conference edition, in two volumes). Washington, DC: Author.

APPLYING YOUR KNOWLEDGE IN PRACTICE

✽ CASE STUDY
Caring for a Physically Abused Client

On a routine postpartum visit, your client, Mrs. Montanez, mentions that she is very concerned about her next-door neighbor, Mrs. Abood, who is pregnant. Mrs. Montanez tells you that she thinks Mr. Abood beat his wife last night. She heard shouting during the night, and this morning she noticed that Mrs. Abood had a black eye that she said she got when she ran into the bedroom door in the dark. Before leaving the apartment complex, you knock on the Aboods' door, but no one answers. You leave your card asking Mrs. Abood to call you.

When Mrs. Abood phones the next day, you explain that you were responding to the concern of a friend for her safety and ask if she is in need of assistance. Mrs. Abood tells you that there is nothing wrong. When you mention that Mrs. Montanez described some injuries, she denies that her husband is abusive. She states that she is receiving prenatal care from a private

physician, will contact him if she has any problems with the pregnancy, and is not in need of your services. You accept her refusal of help, but you inform her that you are available and can be reached by phone if she needs assistance at some time in the future.

A month later you receive a call from Mrs. Abood, who asks to see you. She indicates that she is afraid to have you come to her home lest her husband return while you are there. She agrees to meet you at the health department when she comes to get a copy of her daughter's immunization record for school entry.

When you see Mrs. Abood, she admits that her husband beat her the previous day. This is the second time he has assaulted her since she became pregnant. She has several bruises on her face and one particularly large bruise on her abdomen where her husband hit her. Mrs. Abood says that her husband is very jealous and does not believe the baby is his. She insists that she has been faithful to her husband and has tried to convince him of this. She says her husband gets angry because she "shows herself off to other men and gives them a come-on." She comments, "I guess he's right. I do wear shorts a lot, because they're comfortable in this hot weather. I really should try to respect his wishes more."

Mrs. Abood has tried to convince her husband that the baby is his. She has stopped going out with female friends and even tries to avoid talking to the mailman and other males who come to the house. She has not even been to see her family because her husband refuses to go with her and accuses her of meeting her lover on these excursions.

Since the beating yesterday, Mrs. Abood says she is afraid for her own safety as well as that of her unborn child. She says that her husband loves their 3-year-old daughter and would not hurt her.

Mrs. Abood has never worked, although she completed nursing school before she got married. She feels as though she should get away from her husband even though she still loves him; however, she has no money to support herself and her daughter. She does not feel

she can go to relatives because her husband would be able to find her there and bring her back home. She is also afraid that if she leaves him, her husband will attempt to get custody of their daughter.

- What are the health problems evident in this situation? What are the biophysical, psychological, sociocultural, behavioral, and health system factors influencing these problems?
- What considerations are important in planning care for Mrs. Abood?
- What secondary prevention measures would be warranted to deal with existing health problems? Describe specific actions that you would take to resolve these problems.
- What could be done in terms of tertiary prevention to prevent further consequences or recurrence of health problems in this situation?
- What primary prevention measures might have prevented the development of the health problems in this situation? How might you, as a community health nurse, be involved in such measures?

✿ TESTING YOUR UNDERSTANDING

- What are the major types of societal violence of concern to community health nurses? (pp. 758–761)
- What biophysical, psychological, sociocultural, behavioral, and health system factors influence societal violence? In what ways are these influences similar among the types of violence described in the chapter? In what ways do they differ? (pp. 761–768)
- What are the major foci in primary prevention of societal violence? What roles do community health nurses play in each? (pp. 768–769)

- What are the major approaches to secondary prevention of societal violence? Give an example of a community health nursing activity related to each approach. (pp. 769–771)
- What are the major considerations in tertiary prevention of societal violence? How might community health nurses be involved in tertiary prevention activities? (p. 771)

REFERENCES

Aldridge, D. (1998). *Suicide: The tragedy of hopelessness.* Philadelphia: Jessica Kingsley.

Bellanger, D. (2000). Nurses and suicide: The risk is real. *RN, 63*(10), 61–64.

Birckmayer, J., & Hemenway, D. (1999). Minimum-age drinking laws and youth suicide, 1970–1990. *American Journal of Public Health, 89,* 1365–1368.

Bureau of Justice Statistics. (1998). *Homicide trends in the United States: 1998 update.* Retrieved June 2, 2001, from the World Wide Web, *http://www.ojp.usdoj.gov/bjs/homicide.*

Campbell, J. C., & Soeken, K. L. (1999). Women's responses to battering: A test of the model. *Research in Nursing and Health, 22,* 49–58.

Carlson, M. J., Harris, S. D., & Holden, G. W. (1999). Protective orders and domestic violence: Risk factors for re-abuse. *Journal of Family Violence, 14,* 205–226.

Carpenter, K. M., Hasin, D. S., Allison, D. B., & Faith, M. S. (2000). Relationships between obesity and DSM-IV major depressive disorder, suicide ideation, and suicide attempts: Results from a general population study. *American Journal of Public Health, 90,* 251–257.

Champion, J. D. (1998). Family violence and mental health. *Nursing Clinics of North America, 33,* 201–215.

Coker, A. L., Smith, P. H., McKeown, R. E., & King, M. J. (2000). Frequency and correlates

of intimate partner violence by type: Physical, sexual, and psychological battering. *American Journal of Public Health, 90,* 553–559.

Cubbin, C., Pickle, L. W., & Fingerhut, L. (2000). Social context and geographic patterns of homicide among US black and white males. *American Journal of Public Health, 90,* 579–587.

Cummings, J. G., Pepler, D. J., & Moore, T. E. (1999). Behavior problems in children exposed to wife abuse: Gender differences. *Journal of Family Violence, 14,* 133–156.

Davis, R. C., & Taylor, B. G. (1999). Does batterer treatment reduce violence? A synthesis of the literature. In L. Feder (Ed.), *Women and domestic violence: An interdisciplinary approach* (pp. 69–93). New York: Haworth Press.

Division of Safety Research. (1998). Fatal occupational injuries—United States, 1980–1994. *Morbidity and Mortality Weekly Report, 47,* 297–302.

Division of Violence Prevention. (1998a). Lifetime and annual incidence of intimate partner violence and resulting injuries—Georgia, 1995. *Morbidity and Mortality Weekly Report, 47,* 849–853.

Division of Violence Prevention. (1998b). Rural health-care providers' attitudes, practices, and training experience regarding intimate partner violence—West Virginia, March 1997. *Morbidity and Mortality Weekly Report, 47,* 670–673.

Division of Violence Prevention. (1998c). Suicide prevention evaluation in a Western Athabaskan American Indian tribe—New Mexico, 1988–1997. *Morbidity and Mortality Weekly Report, 47,* 257–261.

Division of Violence Prevention. (2000a). Intimate partner violence among men and women—South Carolina, 1998. *Morbidity and Mortality Weekly Report, 49,* 691–694.

Division of Violence Prevention. (2000b). *October is domestic violence awareness month.* Retrieved April 21, 2001, from the World Wide Web, *http://www.cdc.gov/ncipc/dvp.*

Division of Violence Prevention. (2000c). Prevalence of intimate partner violence and injuries—Washington, 1998. *Morbidity and Mortality Weekly Report, 49,* 589–592.

Division of Violence Prevention. (2000d). Role of victims' services in improving intimate partner violence screening by trained maternal and child health-care providers—Boston, Massachusetts, 1994–1995. *Morbidity and Mortality Weekly Report, 49,* 114–117.

Division of Violence Prevention. (2000e). Use of medical care, police assistance, and restraining orders by women reporting intimate partner violence—Massachusetts, 1996–1997. *Morbidity and Mortality Weekly Report, 49,* 485–488.

Division of Violence Prevention. (2001). Evaluation of a child sexual abuse prevention program—Vermont, 1995–1997. *Morbidity and Mortality Weekly Report, 50,* 77–78, 87.

Dorfman, L., Woodruff, K., Chavez, V., & Wallack, L. (1997). Youth and violence on local television news in California. *American Journal of Public Health, 87,* 1311–1316.

Eckenrode, J., Ganzel, B., Henderson, C. R., Smith, E., et al. (2000). Preventing child abuse and neglect with a program of nurse home visitation: The limiting effects of domestic violence. *Journal of the American Medical Association, 284,* 1385–1391.

Farella, C. (2000). Love shouldn't hurt: Understanding domestic violence. *Nursing Spectrum, 1*(2), 14–16.

Glass, N., & Campbell, J. C. (1998). Mandatory reporting of intimate partner violence by health care professionals: A policy review. *Nursing Outlook, 46,* 279–283.

Golding, J. M. (1999). Intimate partner violence as a risk factor for mental disorders: A meta-analysis. *Journal of Family Violence, 14,* 99–132.

Gomby, D. S. (2000). Promise and limitations of home visitation. *Journal of the American Medical Association, 284,* 1430–1431.

Grossman, D. (2000). Teaching kids to kill. *National Forum, 80*(4), 10–14.

Grunbaum, J. A., Kann, L., Kinchen, S. A., Ross, J. G., et al. (1999). Youth Risk Behavior Surveillance—National Alternative High School Youth Risk Behavior Survey, United States, 1998. *Morbidity and Mortality Weekly Report, 48*(SS-7), 1–44.

Hall, L. A., Sachs, B., & Rayens, M. K. (1998). Mother's potential for child abuse: The roles of childhood abuse and social resources. *Nursing Research, 47,* 87–95.

Heise, L., Ellsberg, M., & Gottemoeller, M. (1999). Ending violence against women. *Population Reports, Series L*(11), 1–38. Retrieved April 26, 2000, from the World Wide Web, *http://jhuccp.org.*

Hogstel, M. O., & Curry, L. C. (1999). Elder abuse revisited. *Journal of Gerontological Nursing, 25*(7), 10–18.

Johnson, R. M. (2001). Emergency department screening for domestic violence. *American Journal of Public Health, 91,* 651.

Kann, L., Kinchen, S. A., Williams, B. I., Goss, J. G., et al. (2000). Youth Risk Behavior Surveillance—United States, 1999. *Morbidity and Mortality Weekly Report, 49*(SS-5), 1–94.

Kernic, M. A., Wolf, M. E., & Holt, V. L. (2000). Rates and relative risk of hospital admission among women in violent intimate partner relationships. *American Journal of Public Health, 90,* 1416–1420.

Larson, G. L., Rolniak, S., Hyman, K. B., MacLeod, B. A., & Savage, R. (2000). Effect of an administrative intervention on rates of screening for domestic violence in an urban emergency department. *American Journal of Public Health, 90,* 1444–1448.

Legislative Network for Nurses. (1998). ANA conference on worker safety highlights dangers nurses face. *15,* 155–156.

Lloyd, S. A. (2000). Intimate violence: Paradoxes of romance, conflict, and control. *National Forum, 80*(4), 19–22.

Lott, J. R. (2000). When gun control costs lives. *National Forum, 80*(4), 29–32.

Lown, E. A., & Vega, W. A. (2001). Prevalence and predictors of physical partner abuse among Mexican American women. *American Journal of Public Health, 91,* 441–445.

Margolin, G., John, R. S., & Foo, L. (1998). Interactive and unique risk factors for husbands' emotional and physical abuse of their wives. *Journal of Family Violence, 13,* 315–344.

Martin, S. L., Matza, L. S., Kupper, L. L., Thomas, J. C., Daly, M., & Cloutier, S. (1999). Domestic violence and sexually transmitted diseases: The experience of prenatal care patients. *Public Health Reports, 114,* 262–268.

McClellan, A. C., & Killeen, M. R. (2000). Attachment theory and violence toward women by male intimate partners. *Journal of Nursing Scholarship, 32,* 353–360.

Miller, M., Hemenway, D., & Rimm, E. (2000). Cigarettes and suicide: A prospective study of 50,000 men. *American Journal of Public Health, 90,* 768–773.

Molidor, C., Tolman, R. M., & Kober, J. (2000). Gender and contextual factors in adolescent dating violence. *The Prevention Researcher, 7*(1), 1–4.

Molnar, B. E., Buka, S. L., & Kessler, R. C. (2001). Child sexual abuse and subsequent psychopathology: Results from the National Comorbidity Study. *American Journal of Public Health, 91,* 753–760.

Morgan, L. (1999). In harm's way: Nurses face increasing abuse in the workplace. *NurseWeek, 12*(17), 13.

National Center for Injury Prevention and Control. (1999). The co-occurrence of intimate partner violence against mothers and abuse of children. Retrieved April 21, 2001, from the World Wide Web, *http://www.cdc.gov/ncipc/factsheets.*

Nester, C. B. (1998). Prevention of child abuse and neglect in the primary care setting. *Nurse Practitioner, 23*(9), 61–62, 67–68, 73.

Oriel, K. A., & Fleming, M. F. (1998). Screening men for partner violence in a primary care setting. *Journal of Family Practice, 46,* 493–498.

Parker, B., McFarlane, J., Soeken, K., Silva, C., & Reel, S. (1999). Testing an intervention to prevent further abuse to pregnant women. *Research in Nursing & Health, 22,* 59–66.

Powell, K. E., Jacklin, B. C., Nelson, D. E., & Bland, S. (1998). State estimates of household exposure to firearms, loaded firearms, and handguns, 1991 through 1995. *American Journal of Public Health, 88,* 969–972.

Riner, M. A. (1999). Stopping school violence in its tracks. *NurseWeek, 12*(22), 16–17.

Rodriguez, M. A., Bauer, H. M., McLoughlin, E., & Grumbach, K. (1999). Screening and intervention for intimate partner abuse. *Journal of the American Medical Association, 282,* 468–474.

Rodriguez, M. A., McLoughlin, E., Bauer, H. M., Paredes, V., & Grumback, K. (1999). Mandatory reporting of intimate partner violence to police: Views of physicians in California. *American Journal of Public Health, 89,* 575–578.

Saltzman, L. E., Fingerhut, L. A., Rand, M. R., & Visher, C. (2000). Building data systems for monitoring and responding to violence against women: Recommendations from a workshop. *Morbidity and Mortality Weekly Report, 49*(RR-11), 1–16.

Schafer, J., Caetano, R., & Clark, C. L. (1998). Rates of intimate partner violence in the United States. *American Journal of Public Health, 88,* 1702–1704.

Schlee, K. A., Heyman, R. E., & O'Leary, D. (1998). Group treatment for spouse abuse: Are women with PTSD appropriate participants? *Journal of Family Violence, 13,* 1–20.

Simon, T. R., Richardson, J. L., Dent, C. W., Chou, C., & Flay, B. R. (1998). Prospective psychosocial, interpersonal, and behavioral predictors of handgun carrying among adolescents. *American Journal of Public Health, 88,* 960–963.

Sorenson, S. B., Manz, J. G. P., & Berk, R. A. (1998). News media coverage and the epidemiology of homicide. *American Journal of Public Health, 88,* 1510–1514.

Stevens, J. A., Hasbrouck, L. M., Durant, T. M., Dellinger, A. M., et al. (1999). Surveillance for injuries and violence among older adults. *Morbidity and Mortality Weekly Report, 48*(SS-8), 27–50.

Sword, W., Carpio, B., Deviney, L., & Schreiber, H. (1998). Woman abuse: Enabling nursing students to respond. *Journal of Nursing Education, 37*(2), 88–91.

Thompson, E. A., Eggert, L. L., Randell, B. P., & Pike, K. C. (2001). Evaluation of indicated suicide risk prevention approaches for potential high school dropouts. *American Journal of Public Health, 91,* 742–752.

Tyson, S., & Fleming, B. (1999). Conceptualizing battered women as a vulnerable population. *Nursing Clinics of North America, 34,* 301–312.

UNAIDS. (1999). *Global summary of the HIV/AIDS epidemic.* Retrieved August 24, 2000, from the World Wide Web, *http://www. unaids.org/epidemic_update/report.*

U.S. Census Bureau. (1999). *Statistical abstract of the United States, 1999* (119th ed.). Washington: Author.

U.S. Department of Health and Human Services. (2000a). *Health, United States, 2000.* Washington, DC: Author.

U.S. Department of Health and Human Services. (2000b). *Healthy people 2010* (Conference edition, in two volumes). Washington, DC: Author.

Walker, L. E. A. (2000). *The battered woman syndrome* (2nd ed.). New York: Springer.

Weiler, K. (1989). Financial abuse of the elderly: Recognizing and acting on it. *Journal of Gerontological Nursing, 15*(8), 10–15.

Wiist, W. H., & McFarlane, J. (1999). The effectiveness of an abuse assessment protocol in public health prenatal clinics. *American Journal of Public Health, 89,* 1217–1221.

Wolfe, D. A. (1999). *Child abuse: Implications for child development and psychopathology.* Thousand Oaks, CA: Sage.

APPENDIX A

NURSING INTERVENTIONS FOR COMMON HEALTH PROBLEMS IN CHILDREN

The interventions presented here are general guidelines that the community health nurse can use to educate parents for home care of health problems commonly encountered among young children.

■ **TABLE A–1** Nursing Interventions for Common Health Problems in Children

ORGAN SYSTEM	PROBLEM	INTERVENTIONS
Gastrointestinal	Spitting up	Burp baby more frequently.
		Keep infant upright for short time after feeding.
		Check size of nipple hole.
		Change to soy formula.
	Colic	Give small amounts of warm water.
		Exert gentle pressure on abdomen with infant's legs and thighs bent.
	Mild diarrhea or vomiting	Begin oral rehydration to prevent dehydration.
		Do not discontinue feedings.
		Seek medical help if condition continues or worsens.
	Constipation	Increase fluid intake.
		Add bulk to diet.
		Encourage regular toileting habits.
		Discourage postponing defecation.
		Avoid use of laxatives or enemas.
Respiratory	Mild respiratory infection	Increase fluid intake.
		Use a cold mist humidifier to ease breathing.
		Do not use Vicks or other aromatic substances.
		Seek medical help for severe or persistent cough, difficulty breathing, stridor, or nasal flaring.
Integumentary	Diaper rash	Wash diapers with mild soaps and rinse thoroughly.
		Add ¾ cup vinegar to last rinse to remove ammonia.
		If using disposable diapers, use ones that allow air circulation.
		Change diapers frequently, thoroughly cleaning diaper area.
		Do not use powders or lotion in diaper area.
		Leave diaper area exposed when possible.
	Allergic dermatitis	Explore changes in foods or soaps.
		Eliminate possible causative substances.
		Seek medical help for severe rashes or secondary infection.

(continued)

■ **TABLE A–1** **Nursing Interventions for Common Health Problems in Children** *(continued)*

ORGAN SYSTEM	PROBLEM	INTERVENTIONS
Integumentary *(continued)*	Cradle cap	Scrub scalp with soap and soft washcloth during bath.
		Brush scalp with soft brush after bath.
		Do not use oil or lotion on scalp.
	Minor abrasions and lacerations	Wash with soap and water.
		Keep clean.
Urinary	Urinary tract infection	Seek medical assistance.
	Bedwetting	Limit fluid intake after dinner.
		Empty bladder before bed.
		Awaken child to urinate before parents go to bed.
		Do not make an issue of the problem.
		If problem is severe or continues beyond age 6, seek medical attention.
Musculoskeletal	Sprains and fractures	Perform basic first aid and immobilize injured area.
		Seek medical attention.
	Leg cramps	Increase calcium intake.
		If severe or persistent, seek medical attention.
Neurological	Headache	Give nonaspirin analgesic according to child's age and size.
		If severe or recurrent, seek medical attention.
	Hearing problem	Seek medical attention.
	Vision problem	Seek medical attention.
	Delayed speech	Discourage older children and parents from talking for child.
		Encourage child to verbalize needs before meeting them.
		Seek medical attention for prolonged delay.
	Speech defect	Seek medical attention.
Other	Fever	For temperature over 102°F, give nonaspirin antipyretic.
		For high or persistent fever, seek medical attention.
	Suspected abuse	Report to child protective services.
		Refer family to Parents Anonymous or other support groups.
	Night terrors	Use a nightlight or leave bedroom door open.
		Use bedtime rituals of checking for "monsters" if helpful.
		Use a "guardian" stuffed animal to scare away monsters.
		Comfort the child after waking and stay until child returns to sleep.
		Seek assistance for persistent terrors or those related to a real traumatic event.
	Jealousy of new baby	Prepare siblings for birth of another child.
		Have child assist with care of newborn.
		Emphasize positive aspects of being older.
		Accept regressive behavior and do not belittle child.
		Spend time with just the older child.
		Encourage friends and relatives to pay attention to older child as well as new baby.
	Sibling rivalry	Mediate arguments.
		Encourage children to work out their own differences.

TABLE A–1 Nursing Interventions for Common Health Problems in Children *(continued)*

ORGAN SYSTEM	PROBLEM	INTERVENTIONS
Other *(continued)*	Sibling rivalry *(continued)*	Encourage compromise.
		Give reasons for differences in privileges.
		Use role-play with older children to give insight into feelings and behaviors of others.
	Tantrums	Ignore behavior if possible.
		Remove child to bedroom if disturbing others.
		Do not give in to child's demands.
	Bedtime	Complete bedtime rituals and put child in bed.
		Ignore crying for 15 to 20 minutes. If the child does not stop, see what is wrong.
		If child gets up, put him or her back to bed.
		Place several safe toys in bed with child and allow play until the child falls asleep.
	Poor self-esteem	Praise child for accomplishments.
		Correct mistakes without denigrating child.
		Help child identify and strengthen talents.
		Assist child to accept limitations.
		Seek assistance for severe depression or low self-esteem on the part of child.

APPENDIX B

INFORMATION ON SELECTED COMMUNICABLE DISEASES

ANTHRAX (CUTANEOUS FORM)

Agent: Bacillus anthracis

Reservoir: Herbivores (domestic and wild)

Incubation: 1 to 7 days

Communicability: Rare person-to-person transmission; spore-infected articles and soil may spread infection for years to decades

Contributing factors: Infected livestock; importation of hair, wool, and hides contaminated with spores; intentional contamination of articles handled by people; animal husbandry–related occupations; spread of spores from contaminated soil during periods of flooding

Modes of transmission: Handling of contaminated articles, possibly by the bite of insects that have been feeding on contaminated livestock carcasses

Immunization: Not usually used in the general public, reserved for military personnel and those at greatest risk of exposure

Screening: Suggested for those suspected of exposure

Prophylaxis: Antibiotics following exposure

Treatment: Penicillin, doxycycline, fluoroquinolones

Contact notification: None

Reporting: Mandatory in most states

Symptoms: Initial itching followed by papular, then vesicular lesions with skin sloughing

Complications: Rarely fatal

Prevention: Immunization of humans at risk as well as animals at risk (annual); education of animal handlers; handwashing and thorough washing of clothes of persons working in industries with potential for exposure; washing, disinfection, or sterilization of raw animal materials; incineration of infected animal carcasses; engineering controls on effluents and wastes generated by industries that use animal products; treatment of symptomatic animals

Disinfection: Use of hypochlorite, formaldehyde, cobalt irradiation, steam sterilization, autoclaving, or burning

ANTHRAX (INHALATION FORM)

Agent: Bacillus anthracis

Reservoir: Herbivores (domestic and wild)

Incubation: 1 to 7 days

Communicability: Rare person-to-person transmission; spore-infected articles and soil may spread infection for years to decades

Contributing factors: Aerosolized exposure or intentional contamination of articles handled by people

Modes of transmission: Inhalation of aerosolized spores, handling of contaminated articles

Immunization: Not usually used in the general public, reserved for military personnel and those at greatest risk of exposure

Screening: Suggested for those suspected of exposure

Prophylaxis: Antibiotics following exposure

Treatment: Penicillin, doxycycline, fluoroquinolones

Contact notification: None

Reporting: Mandatory in most states

Symptoms: Initial mild upper respiratory symptoms followed by respiratory distress and shock in 3 to 5 days

Complications: Shock and death

Prevention: Immunization of humans at risk as well as animals at risk (annual); education of animal handlers; handwashing and thorough washing of clothes of persons working in industries with potential for exposure; washing, disinfection, or sterilization of raw animal materials; incineration of infected animal carcasses; engineering controls on effluents and wastes generated by industries that use animal products; treatment of symptomatic animals

Disinfection: Use of hypochlorite, formaldehyde, cobalt irradiation, steam sterilization, autoclaving, or burning

ANTHRAX (INTESTINAL FORM)

Agent: Bacillus anthracis

Reservoir: Herbivores (domestic and wild)

Incubation: 1 to 7 days

Communicability: Rare person-to-person transmission, spore-infected articles may spread infection for years to decades

Contributing factors: Use of infected livestock as food, intentional contamination of food supplies

Modes of transmission: Ingestion of spores or contaminated meat

Immunization: Not usually used in the general public, reserved for military personnel and those at greatest risk of exposure

Screening: Suggested for those suspected of exposure

Prophylaxis: Antibiotics following exposure

Treatment: Penicillin, doxycycline, fluoroquinolones

Contact notification: None

Reporting: Mandatory in most states

Symptoms: Initial nausea, anorexia, vomiting, and fever followed by abdominal pain, vomiting blood, and severe diarrhea

Complications: Septicemia and death

Prevention: Immunization of humans at risk as well as animals at risk (annual); education of animal handlers; handwashing and thorough washing of clothes of persons working in industries with potential for exposure; washing, disinfection, or sterilization of raw animal materials; incineration of infected animal carcasses; engineering controls on effluents and wastes generated by industries that use animal products; treatment of symptomatic animals

Disinfection: Use of hypochlorite, formaldehyde, cobalt irradiation, steam sterilization, autoclaving, or burning

BOTULISM

Agent: Clostridium botulinum toxins

Reservoir: Soil, multiple animals

Incubation: 12 to 36 hours

Communicability: No person-to-person transmission

Contributing factors: Contamination of food during canning or preservation, untreated wound infection with anaerobic conditions

Modes of transmission: Ingestion of contaminated food

Immunization: None

Screening: None

Prophylaxis: Use of cathartics, high enemas, and gastric lavage after ingestion of known contaminated foods

Treatment: Administration of botulinum antitoxin

Contact notification: Case finding for others exposed to source

Reporting: Mandatory in most states

Symptoms: Lethargy, blurred or double vision, dysphagia, and dry mouth with possible vomiting and diarrhea followed by cranial nerve impairment and descending paralysis

Complications: Respiratory failure

Prevention: Proper food canning, preservation, and storage techniques, destruction of contaminated foods

CHLAMYDIA (GENITAL INFECTION)

Agent: Chlamydia trachomatis

Reservoir: Humans

Incubation: Probably 7 to 14 days

Communicability: Unknown, relapse possible

Contributing factors: Vaginal or rectal sexual contact, birth to an infected mother

Modes of transmission: Sexual contact, perinatal exposure during passage through the birth canal

Immunization: None

Screening: Routinely recommended for sexually active adolescent girls or women with multiple or new sexual partners

Prophylaxis: Antibiotics following sexual exposure or for infants born to infected mothers

Treatment: Tetracycline, doxycycline, erythromycin, or azithromycin

Contact notification: Sexual contacts

Reporting: Mandatory in most states

Symptoms: Frequently asymptomatic; *males* may have urethritis with burning on urination, urethral itching, penile discharge; *females* may have mucopurulent vaginal discharge, pelvic pain, and dyspareunia

Complications: Epididymitis, infertility, prostatitis, proctitis (in receptive anorectal contact), pelvic inflammatory disease (PID), preterm delivery, neonatal conjunctivitis, otitis media, or pneumonia

Prevention: Monogamy, condom use

COCCIDIOIDOMYCOSIS

Agent: Coccidioides immitis (fungus)

Reservoir: Soil

Incubation: 1 to 4 weeks

Communicability: No person-to-person transmission

Contributing factors: Occupational exposure to dust in endemic areas (road construction, archeology, migrant farm work), reactivation and disseminated disease common in those who are immunocompromised

Modes of transmission: Inhalation of contaminated dust

Immunization: None

Prophylaxis: None

Treatment: Usually self-limiting, amphotericin B for severe infection, fluconazole for meningeal infection, ketoconazole or itraconazole for chronic infection

Contact notification: None

Reporting: In selected endemic areas

Symptoms: Asymptomatic or fever, cough, chills

Complications: Lung fibrosis or cavitation, disseminated disease, meningitis

Prevention: Dust control measures

CREUTZFELDT–JAKOB ("MAD COW") DISEASE

Agent: Unidentified, suspected to be a self-replicating prion

Reservoir: Humans

Incubation: 15 months to 30 years

Communicability: During symptomatic illness

Contributing factors: Use of donor tissue from infected patients, possibly consumption of contaminated animals increases susceptibility

Modes of transmission: Unknown except in the case of infected donor tissue

Immunization: None

Prophylaxis: None

Treatment: No specific treatment

Contact notification: None

Reporting: Individual cases not usually reported

Symptoms: Confusion, progressive dementia, and ataxia

Prevention: Avoid use of infected donor tissue

DIPHTHERIA (PHARYNGOTONSILLAR, LARYNGEAL)

Agent: Corynebacterium diphtheriae

Reservoir: Humans

Incubation: 2 to 5 days

Communicability: Usually 2 weeks or less, reduced by antibiotic therapy

Contributing factors: Lack of immunization or waning immunity, occupational risk among health workers, immunocompromise increases susceptibility

Modes of transmission: Airborne, raw milk, contact with articles soiled with discharge from lesions (rare)

Immunization: Routine use of diphtheria–tetanus–pertussis (DTaP) vaccine (Td for persons over age 7)

Prophylaxis: Penicillin or erythromycin, and booster dose of diphtheria toxoid or full immunization series

Treatment: Diphtheria antitoxin and penicillin or erythromycin

Contact notification: None

Reporting: Mandatory in most states

Symptoms: Sore throat with patchy, grayish membrane over pharynx, tonsils, uvula, and soft palate; cervical lymphadenopathy

Complications: Myocarditis with progressive congestive failure, neuropathies

Prevention: Immunization of susceptible individuals

EBOLA VIRUS HEMORRHAGIC FEVER

Agent: Ebola virus

Reservoir: Unknown

Incubation: 2 to 21 days

Communicability: As long as blood and secretions contain the virus (recorded up to 75 days)

Contributing factors: Living in endemic areas, primate handlers, exposure to contaminated syringes and needles, caring for persons with infection (health workers)

Modes of transmission: Direct contact with infected blood and secretions, organs, or semen

Immunization: None

Prophylaxis: None

Treatment: Supportive only

Contact notification: None

Reporting: Mandatory in most states

Symptoms: Headache, malaise, myalgia, high fever, maculopapular rash, severe diarrhea and vomiting and internal and external hemorrhage

Complications: Liver and kidney dysfunction, dehydration, spontaneous abortion and hemorrhage

Prevention: Isolation of infected individuals

ESCHERICHIA COLI DIARRHEA (HEMORRHAGIC)

Agent: E. coli (shiga toxin producing)

Reservoir: Cattle, humans, some deer in North America

Incubation: 2 to 8 days

Communicability: 1 to 3 weeks (shorter in adults, longer in children)

Contributing factors: Contaminated and inadequately cooked beef, raw milk, fruit and vegetables contaminated with feces, alfalfa sprouts, transmission in child care centers, custodial institutions, swimming in contaminated water

Modes of transmission: Ingestion of contaminated food and, occasionally, water

Immunization: None

Prophylaxis: None

Treatment: Fluid and electrolyte replacement

Contact notification: Exclude from food-handling occupations and care of children until negative stool cultures obtained

Reporting: Mandatory in most states

Symptoms: Mild and nonbloody to bloody diarrhea with abdominal cramping

Complications: Hemolytic uremic syndrome (HUS), thrombotic thrombocytopenic purpura

Prevention: Management of slaughterhouse procedures to minimize contamination, pasteurization of milk, irradiation of beef, thoroughly cook ground beef, chlorinate water supplies and swimming pools, good hygiene, especially handwashing

GONORRHEA

Agent: Neisseria gonorrhoeae

Reservoir: Humans

Incubation: Usually 2 to 7 days

Communicability: Until treated

Contributing factors: Social mores condoning sexual activity, overuse of antibiotics leading to resistant strains, contact with multiple sexual partners, sexual abuse of young children

Modes of transmission: Sexual contact

Immunization: None

Screening: Sexually active individuals with multiple partners, pregnant women

Prophylaxis: Antibiotics after exposure

Treatment: Ceftriaxone and doxycycline

Contact notification: Sexual contacts

Reporting: Mandatory in all states

Symptoms: Vary with site of infection; usually associated with penile discharge and burning on urination in urethritis in heterosexual males and with anal discharge, tenesmus, and pruritus in rectal infection; may be associated with vaginal discharge, foul odor, and bleeding after intercourse in females; sore throat in oral infection

Complications: PID, endometritis, infertility, increased risk of ectopic pregnancy, prostatitis, arthritis, endocarditis, neonatal conjunctivitis

Prevention: Monogamy, use of condoms, avoiding multiple sexual partners

HAEMOPHILUS INFLUENZAE TYPE B (HIB)

Agent: Haemophilus influenzae type b

Reservoir: Humans

Incubation: Typically 3 to 4 days

Communicability: Until organism is no longer present in discharges from nose and mouth

Contributing factors: Lack of immunization, day care for young children

Modes of transmission: Contact with respiratory secretions, droplets

Prophylaxis: Rifampin to household contacts, day care group

Treatment: Penicillin, ampicillin, chloramphenicol

Contact notification: Household and day care contacts

Reporting: Mandatory in most states

Symptoms: Of presenting disease (meningitis, otitis media, etc.)

Complications: Otitis media, meningitis, bacteremia, sepsis

Prevention: Immunization of all young children

HANTAVIRUS (PULMONARY)

Agent: Hantavirus (multiple strains)

Reservoir: Rodents

Incubation: 2 weeks

Communicability: No person-to-person transmission

Contributing factors: Working in dusty areas with infected rodents

Modes of transmission: Inhalation of dust contaminated with urine, feces, saliva of infected rodents

Immunization: None

Prophylaxis: None

Treatment: Symptomatic, ribavirin IV administered early in the disease may be beneficial

Contact notification: None

Reporting: In selected endemic counties

Symptoms: Fever, myalgias, chills, nonproductive cough, headache, nausea, vomiting, diarrhea, malaise

Complications: Hypotensive shock, hemorrhage, severe oliguria, fulminant adult respiratory distress syndrome (ARDS)

Prevention: Rodent control, proper cleaning and disposal of rodent excreta

HEPATITIS A

Agent: Hepatitis A virus (HAV)

Reservoir: Humans, nonhuman primates

Incubation: Average 28 to 30 days

Communicability: Latter half of incubation period to a few days after onset of jaundice

Contributing factors: Contamination of food and water supplies, poor sanitation

Modes of transmission: Fecal–oral, sexual contact (homosexual males), contaminated food or water, direct inoculation (rare)

Immunization: Hepatitis A vaccine

Prophylaxis: Immune globulin (IG)

Treatment: Symptomatic

Contact notification: Household and sexual contacts, day care center classroom contacts

Reporting: Mandatory in all states

Symptoms: Abrupt onset of fever, malaise, anorexia, nausea and vomiting, abdominal discomfort followed by jaundice; adults more likely to be symptomatic than children

Complications: Rare

Prevention: Sanitation, personal hygiene (handwashing), adequate cooking of contaminated foods, immunization of susceptible individuals

HEPATITIS B

Agent: Hepatitis B virus (HBV)

Reservoir: Humans

Incubation: Average 60 to 90 days

Communicability: Several weeks before and after symptom onset; may be lifelong carrier

Contributing factors: Health care occupations, lack of immunization of susceptible individuals, injection drug use, multiple sexual partners

Modes of transmission: Sexual contact, direct inoculation, transplacental transfer

Immunization: Hepatitis B vaccine

Screening: Pregnant women, persons with other sexually transmitted diseases (STDs), blood and tissue donors

Prophylaxis: Hepatitis B immune globulin and/or immunization

Treatment: Symptomatic, alpha interferon or lamivudine for chronic infection

Contact notification: Household or sexual contacts, drug partners

Reporting: Mandatory in all states

Symptoms: Insidious onset of anorexia, abdominal discomfort, nausea and vomiting, followed by jaundice

Complications: Fulminant hepatitis, chronic liver disease, cirrhosis, liver cancer

Prevention: Immunization of infants and persons in high-risk groups; monogamy, condom use, blood donor screening, drug abuse treatment; avoid needle sharing; blood and body fluid precautions

HEPATITIS C

Agent: Hepatitis C virus (HCV)

Reservoir: Humans

Incubation: Average 6 to 9 weeks

Communicability: 1 or more weeks prior to onset of symptoms, may persist indefinitely

Contributing factors: Injection drug use, occasionally multiple sexual partners, tatooing, body piercing

Modes of transmission: Direct inoculation, sexual contact (less often)

Immunization: None

Screening: Blood and tissue donors

Prophylaxis: None

Treatment: Symptomatic, alpha interferon for chronic infection

Contact notification: Drug partners

Reporting: Varies among jurisdictions

Symptoms: Insidious onset of anorexia, vague abdominal discomfort, nausea and vomiting, jaundice

Complications: Cirrhosis, hepatoma, chronic hepatitis

Prevention: Same as for hepatitis B, except immunization

HEPATITIS D (DELTA)

Agent: Hepatitis D virus (HDV)

Reservoir: Humans

Incubation: 2 to 8 weeks

Communicability: Prior to onset, potentially through all phases of active infection and during chronic infection

Contributing factors: Concurrent or chronic HBV infection, injection drug use

Modes of transmission: Direct inoculation, sexual contact

Immunization: Immunization for HBV prevents infection

Prophylaxis: None

Treatment: Symptomatic

Contact notification: None

Symptoms: Abrupt onset of symptoms similar to HBV; always associated with coexistent HBV infection

Complications: Chronic infection, fulminant hepatitis

Prevention: Same as for hepatitis B

HEPATITIS E

Agent: Hepatitis E virus (HEV)

Reservoir: Humans, may include domestic swine

Incubation: 26 to 42 days

Communicability: Unknown

Contributing factors: Poor sanitation, contamination of food and water supplies with fecal material

Modes of transmission: Fecal–oral, contaminated water

Immunization: None

Prophylaxis: None

Treatment: Symptomatic

Contact notification: None

Reporting: Mandatory in most states

Symptoms: Similar to HAV

Complications: 20% fatality in pregnant women

Prevention: Sanitation, hygiene

HIV INFECTION

Agent: Human immunodeficiency virus (HIV)

Reservoir: Humans

Incubation: 2 months to 10 years

Communicability: Unknown, presumed lifelong

Contributing factors: Permissive sexual mores, multiple sexual partners, injection drug use, presence of other STDs (especially those with lesions)

Modes of transmission: Sexual contact, direct inoculation, transplacental transfer, breast-feeding

Immunization: None

Screening: Blood and tissue donors, sexually active persons with multiple or new sexual partners, gay men, injection drug users, pregnant women

Prophylaxis: Antiviral agents

Treatment: Antiviral agents

Contact notification: Sexual partners, drug use partners who share needles, clients of infected health care professionals, recipients of blood or tissue from infected donors

Reporting: Mandatory in all states

Symptoms: Fatigue, malaise, recurrent and sustained opportunistic infections

Complications: Multiple organ damage, dementia, multiple life-threatening opportunistic infections

Prevention: Monogamy, condom use, drug treatment; avoid needle sharing; screen blood and organ donors, use of autologous transfusion when possible

HERPES SIMPLEX VIRUS (HSV) GENITAL INFECTION

Agent: Herpes simplex virus type 2

Reservoir: Humans

Incubation: 2 to 12 days

Communicability: 7 to 12 days, initial lesion; 4 to 7 days, recurrent lesions

Contributing factors: Multiple sexual partners, early onset of sexual activity

Modes of transmission: Sexual contact, passage of neonate through birth canal during periods of active lesions

Immunization: None

Screening: Pregnant women

Prophylaxis: None

Treatment: Symptomatic, antiviral agents

Contact notification: Pregnant women

Reporting: Not ordinarily reportable, but reporting of neonatal cases mandatory in some states

Symptoms: Painful genital lesions

Complications: Meningitis, disseminated neonatal infection with liver involvement, neonatal encephalitis

Prevention: Monogamy, condom use

HUMAN PAPILLOMAVIRUS INFECTION (HPV)

Agent: Human papillomavirus

Reservoir: Humans

Incubation: Usually 2 to 3 months

Communicability: Unknown, probably in the presence of lesions

Contributing factors: Multiple sexual partners, early onset of sexual activity

Modes of transmission: Sexual contact

Immunization: None

Prophylaxis: None

Treatment: Application of liquid nitrogen except in pregnant women

Contact notification: Sexual contacts

Reporting: Not reportable in most cases

Symptoms: Painful genital lesions

Complications: Cervical dysplasia and uterine cervical cancer

Prevention: Monogamy, condom use, cesarean section in the presence of multiple lesions

INFLUENZA

Agent: Influenza viruses A, B, C

Reservoir: Humans (animals for new subtypes)

Incubation: 1 to 3 days

Communicability: 3 to 5 days after onset of symptoms (7 days in children)

Contributing factors: Fatigue, immunosuppression, age, chronic disease (especially cardiac, pulmonary, and renal disease and diabetes), malnutrition, crowding, stress, occupational exposure among health care workers, teachers

Modes of transmission: Airborne

Immunization: Annual use of influenza vaccine for high-risk individuals

Prophylaxis: Amantadine or rimantadine in high-risk persons (type A only)

Treatment: Symptomatic, amantadine or rimantadine within 48 hours of onset

Contact notification: None

Reporting: Outbreaks only

Symptoms: Fever, headache, myalgia, prostration, coryza, sore throat, cough, nausea, vomiting, diarrhea

Complications: Pneumonia, bronchiolitis

Prevention: Immunization of persons at risk; general health promotion

LEGIONELLOSIS (LEGIONNAIRE'S DISEASE)

Agent: Several strains of *legionellae*

Reservoir: Aqueous

Incubation: Typically 5 to 6 days

Communicability: No person-to-person transmission known

Contributing factors: Immunosuppression, poorly maintained air filters on cooling units, water heaters, etc.

Modes of transmission: Airborne

Immunization: None

Prophylaxis: None

Treatment: Erythromycin

Contact notification: Not applicable

Reporting: Reportable in selected areas

Symptoms: Anorexia, malaise, myalgia, headache, fever and chills, nonproductive cough, abdominal pain, diarrhea

Complications: Respiratory failure

Prevention: Regular cleaning of cooling towers and other devices

LYME DISEASE

Agent: Borrelia burgdorferi

Reservoir: Ticks found on deer and wild rodents

Incubation: Usually 7 to 10 days

Communicability: No person-to-person transmission

Modes of transmission: Bite of infected tick

Immunization: Vaccine available, but long-term efficacy unknown

Prophylaxis: None

Treatment: Doxycycline, amoxicillin, tetracycline

Contact notification: Source case finding if outside endemic areas

Reporting: Mandatory in all states

Symptoms: Distinctive skin lesion, followed by malaise, fatigue, fever, headache, stiff neck, myalgias, migratory arthralgia, lymphadenopathy

Complications: Aseptic meningitis, varied neuropathies

Prevention: Use insect repellent, wear long-sleeved light-colored clothes, check for ticks regularly, tick control measures

MEASLES

Agent: Measles virus

Reservoir: Humans

Incubation: Average 10 days

Communicability: Beginning of prodrome to 4 days after onset of rash

Contributing factors: Lack of immunization, malnutrition, crowding, immunosuppression

Modes of transmission: Airborne

Immunization: Routine use of measles–mumps–rubella (MMR) vaccine

Prophylaxis: MMR within 72 hours of exposure; measles immune globulin for children under 1 year within 6 days of exposure

Treatment: Symptomatic

Contact notification: None

Reporting: Mandatory in most states

Symptoms: Prodrome of fever, conjunctivitis, cough, coryza, and Koplik's spots, followed by rash on face and spreading downward

Complications: Otitis media, pneumonia, croup, encephalitis, diarrhea

Prevention: Routine immunization of all susceptible individuals

MUMPS

Agent: Mumps virus

Reservoir: Humans

Incubation: Usually 18 days

Communicability: 6 to 7 days before swelling to 9 days after

Contributing factors: Lack of immunization

Modes of transmission: Airborne

Immunization: Routine use of MMR vaccine

Prophylaxis: None

Treatment: Symptomatic

Contact notification: None

Reporting: Reportable in some areas

Symptoms: Pain and swelling in parotid area accompanied by difficulty swallowing; redness and swelling around Stensen's duct

Complications: Orchitis, encephalitis (rare), hearing loss, pancreatitis

Prevention: Immunization of susceptible individuals

PERTUSSIS

Agent: Bordetella pertussis

Reservoir: Humans

Incubation: 7 to 10 days

Communicability: Early catarrhal stage to 3 weeks after cough begins

Contributing factors: Lack of immunization, crowded living conditions, high mortality with malnutrition and multiple enteric and respiratory infections

Modes of transmission: Airborne, contact with respiratory discharges

Immunization: Routine use of DTaP vaccine

Prophylaxis: DTaP booster and erythromycin

Treatment: Erythromycin may reduce communicability

Contact notification: Nonimmune persons

Reporting: Reportable in selected endemic areas

Symptoms: Initial catarrhal stage followed by paroxysmal whooping cough

Complications: Pneumonia, encephalopathy, severe dehydration

Prevention: Immunization of susceptible individuals

PLAGUE

Agent: Yersinia pestis

Reservoir: Wild rodents

Incubation: 1 to 7 days

Communicability: Person-to-person transmission unusual except with contact with discharge from suppurating buboes in the bubonic form, pneumonic form may be transmitted person to person, infected fleas may be communicable for months

Contributing factors: Uncontrolled rodent populations, overcrowding, hunting, trapping, camping in areas with infected rodents

Modes of transmission: Bite of infected fleas or inhalation of respiratory droplets (pneumonic form)

Immunization: Somewhat effective against bubonic, but not pneumonic, form

Screening: None

Prophylaxis: Disinfestation with insecticide, use of tetracycline or chloramphenicol for close face-to-face contacts

Treatment: Streptomycin, tetracycline, chloramphenicol

Contact notification: In epidemic situations

Reporting: Mandatory throughout the world

Symptoms: Bubonic: fever, chills, myalgia, nausea, sore throat, headache, lymphadenopathy in nodes draining the area of the initial flea bite with swelling, inflammation, tenderness and suppuration; pneumonic: pneumonia with fever, headache, weakness, bloody or watery cough

Complications: Septicemia, shock, disseminated intravascular coagulation, death

Prevention: Surveillance of rodent populations, rodent control, rodent-proofing buildings, sanitation, use of insect repellents in endemic wildlife areas, treating pets in endemic areas with insecticides

POLIOMYELITIS

Agent: Poliovirus, types 1, 2, 3

Reservoir: Humans

Incubation: 7 to 14 days

Communicability: Unknown, possible 36 to 72 hours after exposure to 10 days after symptoms occur

Contributing factors: Crowding, malnutrition, poor sanitation in developing countries, use of oral polio vaccine (OPV) for immunization, lack of immunization

Modes of transmission: Airborne, contaminated milk and food, fecal–oral in areas with poor sanitation

Immunization: Routine use of inactivated polio vaccine (IPV) in developed countries, OPV in developing countries

Prophylaxis: None

Treatment: Symptomatic

Contact notification: Close contacts

Reporting: Mandatory in most countries throughout the world, in all states in the United States

Symptoms: Fever, headache, gastrointestinal disturbance, stiffness of neck and back with or without paralysis

Complications: Respiratory failure, paralysis

Prevention: Immunization of susceptible children and adults; sanitation

ROCKY MOUNTAIN SPOTTED FEVER

Agent: Rickettsia rickettsii

Reservoir: Ticks found on dogs, rodents, and other animals

Incubation: 3 to 14 days

Communicability: No person-to-person transmission

Contributing factors: Work or recreation in tick-infested areas

Modes of transmission: Bite of an infected tick

Immunization: None

Prophylaxis: None

Treatment: Tetracycline or chloramphenicol if tetracycline is contraindicated

Contact notification: None

Reporting: Mandatory in most states

Symptoms: Malaise, deep muscle pain, severe headache, chills, conjunctival injection, maculopapular rash beginning on extremities and spreading to rest of body including palms and soles followed often by a petechial rash

Prevention: Frequent inspection for and removal of ticks, wearing long-sleeved clothing, use of tick repellent, use of tick repellent collars on dogs

RUBELLA

Agent: Rubella virus

Reservoir: Humans

Incubation: 14 to 17 days

Communicability: 1 week before to 4 or more days after onset of rash

Contributing factors: Crowding, lack of immunization, immunosuppression

Modes of transmission: Airborne, transplacental inoculation

Immunization: Routine use of MMR vaccine (contraindicated in pregnancy)

Screening: Women of childbearing age as precursor to immunization

Prophylaxis: IG for pregnant women (value questionable)

Treatment: Symptomatic

Contact notification: Pregnant women

Reporting: Mandatory in all states

Symptoms: Prodrome of mild fever, headache, and malaise, followed by discrete maculopapular rash, occipital node enlargement

Complications: Arthralgia and arthritis, encephalitis, thrombocytopenia, congenital abnormalities and spontaneous abortion

Prevention: Immunization of susceptible individuals, especially women of childbearing age

SALMONELLOSIS

Agent: Salmonella enterica (proposed new nomenclature)

Reservoir: Humans, poultry, swine, cattle, rodents, iguanas, tortoises, turtles, chicks, dogs, cats

Incubation: Typically 12 to 36 hours

Communicability: Throughout infection (may extend to 1 year in some people)

Contributing factors: Poor sanitation, poor handwashing, contamination of food, inadequate cooking, failure to wash fruits and vegetables, care of infants and incontinent adults, immunosuppression

Modes of transmission: Fecal–oral and ingestion of contaminated foods

Immunization: None

Screening: Household contacts who are food handlers or caretakers of children or in institutional settings

Prophylaxis: None

Treatment: Rehydration and electrolyte replacement for most cases, for severe cases or immunocompromised individuals ciprofloxacin, amoxicillin, ampicillin, trimethoprim–sulfamethoxazole or chloramphenicol may be given, but antibiotic resistance develops easily

Contact notification: Household contacts

Reporting: Mandatory in all states

Symptoms: Acute enterocolitis with headache, abdominal pain, diarrhea, nausea, vomiting, fever

Complications: Dehydration, septicemia, septic arthritis, endocarditis, meningitis, pericarditis, pneumonia, pyelonephritis

Prevention: Adquate sanitation and hygiene in the preparation and processing of food; avoidance of raw or undercooked eggs and meat; adequate refrigeration; adequate cleansing of utensils with hot soapy water; exclusion of persons with diarrhea from food handling, child care, institutional care; avoidance of chicks and turtles, etc. as pets; irradiation of food

SMALLPOX

Agent: Variola virus

Reservoir: Currently only in laboratory storage

Incubation: 7 to 19 days

Communicability: From earliest lesions to disappearance of all scabs

Contributing factors: Bioterrorism, secondary spread due to contact with infected persons

Modes of transmission: Inhalation of aerosolized virus, contact with infected lesions of cases

Immunization: Not currently used

Screening: None

Prophylaxis: Vaccinia IG available through the Centers for Disease Control and Prevention (CDC), use of vaccine within 4 days of exposure

Treatment: None at present, supportive therapy and antibiotics for secondary infection of lesions

Contact notification: Close contacts

Reporting: Mandatory throughout the world

Symptoms: Fever, malaise, headache, prostration, back pain, followed in 2 to 4 days with lesions progressing through macular, papular, vesicular, pustular, and crusted stages all at the same stage in a given part of the body

Complications: Severe prostration, hemorrhage, and death

Prevention: Immunization (not generally given at present)

SYPHILIS

Agent: Treponema pallidum

Reservoir: Humans

Incubation: 10 to 90 days (usually 3 weeks)

Communicability: In stages with lesions

Contributing factors: Permissive sexual mores, multiple sexual partners, sex for drugs, injection drug use, maternal infection, concurrent HIV infection increases potential for neurosyphilis

Modes of transmission: Sexual contact, direct inoculation, transplacental transfer

Immunization: None

Screening: Routine screening of sexually active individuals with multiple or new partners, pregnant women

Prophylaxis: Antibiotics after exposure

Treatment: Penicillin

Contact notification: Sexual contacts to primary, secondary, and early latent syphilis; persons sharing needles

Reporting: Mandatory in all states

Symptoms: Vary with stage of disease

Primary: Painless chancre or lesion at site of infection (usually genitalia, lips, etc.); may be accompanied by localized lymphadenopathy in the area of the lesion

Secondary: Coppery, macular rash (may be found in all areas but particularly on palms and soles); may be accompanied by malaise and generalized lymphadenopathy

Latent: Asymptomatic

Late: Depends on organ system affected

Congenital: Hutchinson's teeth and raspberry molars, saddle nose, snuffles, rash if in secondary stage

Complications: Dementia, major organ damage, meningitis, tabes dorsalis, cardiovascular syphilis, congenital infection with multiple anomalies, spontaneous abortion

Prevention: Monogamy, condom use, drug abuse treatment; avoid needle sharing; screening of blood donors

TETANUS

Agent: Clostridium tetani

Reservoir: Humans and animals, soil

Incubation: 3 to 21 days

Communicability: Not directly communicable

Contributing factors: Lack of immunization, work or recreation in areas with potential for dirty injuries (especially in areas where animal excreta is common), injection drug use, poor hygiene during birth

Modes of transmission: Introduction of tetanus spores via wound in skin or unhealed umbilicus

Immunization: Routine use of DTaP vaccine

Prophylaxis: Tetanus–diphtheria (Td) booster for immunized persons; tetanus immune globulin (TIG) or tetanus antitoxin and Td for unimmunized individuals

Treatment: TIG or antitoxin and penicillin

Contact notification: None

Reporting: Mandatory in all states

Symptoms: Painful muscular contractions with progressive rigidity, especially in muscles of neck and shoulders

Complications: Respiratory paralysis and death

Prevention: Immunization of susceptible individuals, prevent injury, cleanse injuries thoroughly, control animal feces; asepsis during deliveries

TUBERCULOSIS

Agent: Mycobacterium tuberculosis

Reservoir: Humans, cattle, other animals

Incubation: 4 to 12 weeks

Communicability: During periods of respiratory expulsion of bacteria

Contributing factors: Malnutrition, fatigue, stress, pregnancy, immunosuppression, concurrent HIV infection, crowding, social disruption (e.g., in war, famine)

Modes of transmission: Airborne, contaminated milk

Immunization: Bacille Calmette–Guérin (BCG) vaccine for selected individuals

Screening: High-risk populations, child care and institutional workers, health care providers

Prophylaxis: Isoniazid for close contacts, persons with positive tuberculin tests and no evidence of active disease

Treatment: Antituberculin agents (multidrug regimen)

Contact notification: Close contacts

Reporting: Mandatory in all states

Symptoms: Cough, hemoptysis, unexplained weight loss, night sweats

Complications: Pulmonary cavitation, disseminated disease, extrapulmonary disease (kidneys, brain, bone, etc.)

Prevention: Improve social conditions, promote general health

FACTORS IN THE EPIDEMIOLOGY OF SELECTED CHRONIC PHYSICAL HEALTH PROBLEMS

Information presented here includes epidemiologic factors associated with the incidence of selected chronic physical health problems. The health problems addressed are arthritis, cancer, cardiovascular and cerebrovascular disease, chronic obstructive pulmonary disease (COPD), diabetes mellitus, obesity, and conditions resulting from accidental trauma. Factors related to each condition are organized in terms of the six dimensions of health.

EPIDEMIOLOGIC FACTORS ASSOCIATED WITH ARTHRITIS

Biophysical Considerations

- There may be a genetic predisposition to arthritis. Asians and Native Americans have low incidence rates for arthritis.
- The onset of arthritis usually begins in the fourth decade of life.
- Older persons usually have greater disability from arthritis.
- Women are more likely than men to develop arthritis.
- Previous injury to bones and joints may predispose one to arthritis.
- Obesity increases stress on joints and may exacerbate arthritis.
- Pregnancy may cause a temporary remission in arthritis symptoms.

Behavioral Considerations

- Occupational or recreational factors that contribute to injury may lead to arthritis in later life.
- Overeating may lead to obesity and increased severity of arthritis.

Health System Considerations

- Many people with arthritis engage in self-care rather than seek medical help.
- Medical treatment for arthritis has limited effects.

EPIDEMIOLOGIC FACTORS ASSOCIATED WITH CANCERS

Biophysical Considerations

- Genetic inheritance may predispose one to cancer.
- Incidence and survival rates for cancer vary among ethnic and racial groups.
- Males have higher mortality rates for most forms of cancer than females have.
- Genital herpes simplex virus (HSV) infection may contribute to cervical cancer.

Physical Environmental Considerations

- Exposure to sunlight increases the risk of skin cancer.
- Cancer incidence is higher in urban than in rural areas.
- Environmental pollutants can contribute to cancer incidence.

Sociocultural Considerations

- Occupational exposures can contribute to cancer.

Behavioral Considerations

- Smoking increases one's risk of several forms of cancer.
- Lack of dietary fiber and increased fat in the diet have been linked to increased risk of colon cancer.
- Alcohol consumption may be associated with increased cancer risk (especially liver cancer).
- Self-screening health practices such as breast self-examination and testicular self-examination increase one's chances of cancer survival.

Health System Considerations

- Lack of emphasis on screening has contributed to cancer mortality.
- Aggressiveness of treatment influences cancer survival rates.

EPIDEMIOLOGIC FACTORS ASSOCIATED WITH CARDIOVASCULAR AND CEREBROVASCULAR DISEASE

Biophysical Considerations

- Genetic inheritance may predispose one to cardiovascular or cerebrovascular disease.
- Cardiovascular disease is more common in young African Americans and older whites.
- Females have lower mortality rates for cardiovascular and cerebrovascular disease than do males.
- Racial differences in incidence of cardiovascular and cerebrovascular disease probably reflect differences in the prevalence of other biological risk factors such as hypertension, increased serum cholesterol, and diabetes.
- Infection with *Chlamydia pneumoniae* may increase the risk of coronary heart disease.

Psychological Considerations

- Stress in the environment can contribute to cardiovascular and cerebrovascular disease.
- Major depressive disorder may increase the risk of heart attack.
- Anger and anxiety contribute to hypertension and heart attack.

Physical Environmental Considerations

- Cumulative lead exposure may contribute to hypertension as a risk factor for coronary heart disease.

Sociocultural Considerations

- High income and educational levels are associated with decreased mortality due to cardiovascular and cerebrovascular disease.

Behavioral Considerations

- Sedentary lifestyle increases the risk of cardiovascular and cerebrovascular disease.
- Smoking increases the risk of cardiovascular and cerebrovascular disease.
- Overeating and increased fat and cholesterol consumption contribute to cardiovascular and cerebrovascular disease.
- Moderate alcohol use may reduce the risk of cardiovascular disease.

Health System Considerations

- Attention to elimination of risk factors has decreased the incidence of cardiovascular and cerebrovascular disease.
- Access to emergency services reduces mortality due to cardiovascular and cerebrovascular disease.

EPIDEMIOLOGIC FACTORS ASSOCIATED WITH COPD

Biophysical Considerations

- Some evidence supports a genetic predisposition to COPD.
- Recurrent respiratory infections early in life can contribute to COPD later in life.
- Respiratory allergies and asthma can increase the risk of COPD.

Physical Environmental Considerations

- Environmental pollution can contribute to or exacerbate COPD.
- COPD is more prevalent in highly industrialized urban areas than in rural areas.
- Exposure of nonsmokers to tobacco smoke exacerbates COPD.

Sociocultural Considerations

- Occupational exposure to dusts or gases increases the risk of COPD.

Behavioral Considerations

- Smoking increases the risk of COPD and interacts with other contributing factors to increase the risk still more.

Health System Considerations

- Lack of emphasis on primary prevention contributes to COPD.
- Treatment of COPD is minimally effective.
- Overuse of β-agonists and underuse of corticosteroids contribute to asthma mortality.

EPIDEMIOLOGIC FACTORS ASSOCIATED WITH DIABETES MELLITUS

Biophysical Considerations

- Genetic predisposition is a contributing factor in diabetes.
- Native Americans and African Americans have higher incidence rates of diabetes than do other racial/ethnic groups.
- The presence of hypertension complicates diabetes.
- Diabetes is a risk factor for heart disease and stroke.
- Viral infection may increase the risk of diabetes.
- Pregnancy complicates diabetes control.

Physical Environmental Considerations

- Diabetes is more prevalent in industrialized countries.

Behavioral Considerations

- Affluence increases incidence rates of diabetes.
- Smoking may be a risk factor in the development of diabetes.

- Smoking interacts with diabetes to increase the risk of heart disease and stroke.
- Overeating and consequent overweight contribute to diabetes.
- Moderate alcohol use may have a protective effect for development of diabetes.
- Alcohol use contributes to diabetes mortality in those with the disease.
- Exercise can contribute to diabetes control.

Health System Considerations

- Lack of emphasis on screening leads to later diagnosis and poor control of diabetes.
- Lack of access to health care influences diabetes control.
- Failure to monitor treatment effects can contribute to increased diabetes mortality.

EPIDEMIOLOGIC FACTORS ASSOCIATED WITH OBESITY

Biophysical Considerations

- There may be a slight genetic predisposition to obesity.
- Obesity occurs in all age groups, both sexes, and all ethnic groups.

Sociocultural Considerations

- Prevalence of junk food contributes to obesity.
- Fast-paced life leads to poor nutrition and obesity.
- Occupations that contribute to a sedentary lifestyle also contribute to obesity.
- Cultural dietary preferences may contribute to or prevent obesity.

Behavioral Considerations

- Consumption of excess calories, especially fats, contributes to obesity.
- Sedentary lifestyle and lack of exercise contribute to obesity.

Health System Considerations

- Lack of emphasis on nutrition education contributes to poor dietary habits and obesity.
- Treatment of obesity is less effective than it might be because of high rates of noncompliance.

EPIDEMIOLOGIC FACTORS ASSOCIATED WITH TRAUMA DUE TO ACCIDENTS

Biophysical Considerations

- Drowning, poisoning, and suffocation are common accidents among young children.

- Firearms injuries are common among preadolescents and adolescents.
- Motor vehicle accidents affect all age groups, but occur most often among adolescents and young adults.
- The elderly are particularly susceptible to the effects of falls and fires.
- The presence of physical disability increases the risk of accidental injury.

Psychological Considerations

- Depression or worry may contribute to lack of attentiveness and subsequent accidents.

Physical Environmental Considerations

- Improper storage of hazardous materials increases accident risk.
- Use of space heaters contributes to fires and burn injuries.
- Absence of smoke detectors in buildings contributes to fire injuries.
- Road conditions and automobile crashworthiness influence motor vehicle accidents and their effects.

Sociocultural Considerations

- Easy access to firearms contributes to accidental injuries.
- Occupations involving heavy labor or motor vehicle operation increase the risk of accidents.

Behavioral Considerations

- Alcohol and drug use and abuse contribute to accidents.
- Recreational activities pose a variety of accident hazards.
- Failure to use safety devices increases the risk of injury.
- Common use and improper storage of medications contribute to poisoning.

Health System Considerations

- Lack of emphasis on safety education has contributed to accidental injuries.
- Access to emergency services influences accident survival rates.
- Long-term consequences of accidents are affected by the availability of rehabilitation services.

APPENDIX D

SUSPECTED ABUSE REPORT FORMS

The forms included here are examples of the type used to report suspected abuse and violence. Generally, cases of suspected or confirmed abuse are reported immediately by telephone and followed with a completed reporting form within 24 to 48 hours. Whenever feasible, specific events leading to suspicion of abuse should be described as fully as possible, including information about specific behavior observed or exact words of those describing events. Community health nurses should become familiar with specific forms used in their local jurisdictions, including special forms for reporting spouse and elder abuse if required.

MEDICAL SERVICES
DOMESTIC VIOLENCE AND VIOLENT
INJURY REPORT

California Penal Code sections 11160 and 11161 require hospitals and physicians to report immediately, both by telephone and in writing, all injuries resulting from the use of a gun or knife or other deadly weapon, or otherwise inflicted in violation of the criminal law, whether by act of the patient or of another person. <u>EXCEPTION:</u> Any physical or psychological condition brought about solely by the voluntary self-administration of any narcotic or restricted dangerous drug is not reportable.

Time of call to police _____   By _____
Print name

REASON FOR REPORT

_____ Gunshot
_____ Knife wound (or from other deadly weapon)
_____ Injury from other criminal law violation

PATIENT'S NAME: _____

PATIENT'S ADDRESS: _____

PATIENT'S WHEREABOUTS: _____
_____

(Facility Name and Address)

_____ Other (specify) _____

NATURE AND EXTENT OF INJURY: _____
_____
_____

_____   _____
Date/Time   Signature of Attending Physician
                                  (or other reporting party)

TELEPHONE REPORT GIVEN TO _____ *of* _____
Name/ID # of officer   Agency

                    _____ *by* _____
                    Date/Time   ED Staff

Original: Law Enforcement Agency
Yellow: Patient's Chart
Pink: District Attorney, Domestic Violence Unit

If officer does not respond, mail yellow and pink copies to the District Attorney, Domestic Violence Unit, 101 W. Broadway, San Diego, California 92101. Mail original to appropriate law enforcement agency with jurisdiction where the battery occurred.

SUSPECTED CHILD ABUSE REPORT
To Be Completed by Reporting Party
Pursuant to Penal Code Section 11166

A. CASE IDENTIFICATION	*TO BE COMPLETED BY INVESTIGATING CPA* VICTIM NAME: _____ REPORT NO./CASE NAME:_____ DATE OF REPORT: _____

B. REPORTING PARTY

NAME/TITLE

ADDRESS

PHONE ( )	DATE OF REPORT	SIGNATURE OF REPORTING PARTY

C. REPORT SENT TO

☐ POLICE DEPARTMENT   ☐ SHERIFF'S OFFICE   ☐ COUNTY WELFARE   ☐ COUNTY PROBATION

AGENCY	ADDRESS	
OFFICIAL CONTACTED	PHONE ( )	DATE/TIME

D. INVOLVED PARTIES

VICTIM

NAME (LAST, FIRST, MIDDLE)	ADDRESS	BIRTHDATE	SEX	RACE
PRESENT LOCATION OF CHILD		PHONE ( )		

SIBLINGS

NAME	BIRTHDATE	SEX	RACE	NAME	BIRTHDATE	SEX	RACE
1.				4.			
2.				5.			
3.				6.			

PARENTS

NAME (LAST, FIRST, MIDDLE)	BIRTHDATE	SEX	RACE	NAME (LAST, FIRST, MIDDLE)	BIRTHDATE	SEX	RACE
ADDRESS				ADDRESS			
HOME PHONE BUSINESS PHONE ( ) ( )				HOME PHONE BUSINESS PHONE ( ) ( )			

E. INCIDENT INFORMATION

IF NECESSARY, ATTACH EXTRA SHEET OR OTHER FORM AND CHECK THIS BOX. ☐

1. DATE/TIME OF INCIDENT	PLACE OF INCIDENT *(CHECK ONE)* ☐ OCCURRED ☐ OBSERVED

IF CHILD WAS IN OUT-OF-HOME CARE AT TIME OF INCIDENT, CHECK TYPE OF CARE:
☐ FAMILY DAY CARE   ☐ CHILD CARE CENTER   ☐ FOSTER FAMILY HOME   ☐ SMALL FAMILY HOME   ☐ GROUP HOME OR INSTITUTION

2. TYPE OF ABUSE: *(CHECK ONE OR MORE)*   ☐ PHYSICAL   ☐ MENTAL   ☐ SEXUAL ASSAULT   ☐ NEGLECT   ☐ OTHER

3. NARRATIVE DESCRIPTION:

4. SUMMARIZE WHAT THE ABUSED CHILD OR PERSON ACCOMPANYING THE CHILD SAID HAPPENED:

5. EXPLAIN KNOWN HISTORY OF SIMILAR INCIDENT(S) FOR THIS CHILD:

SS 8572 (REV.7/87)   *INSTRUCTIONS AND DISTRIBUTION ON REVERSE*

DO NOT submit a copy of this form to the Department of Justice (DOJ). A CPA is required under Penal Code Section 11169 to submit to DOJ a Child Abuse Investigation Report Form SS-8583 if (1) an active investigation has been conducted and (2) the incident is **not** unfounded.

Blue and   Social Services Dept.
Green   P.O. Box 11341
Copies to: San Diego, CA 92111

Police or Sheriff-WHITE Copy; County Welfare or Probation- BLUE Copy; District Attorney-GREEN Copy; Reporting Party-YELLOW Copy

INDEX

Brown Report, 26, 31
Built environment, in urban and rural settings, 590
Bureau of Indian Affairs, 24, 28

C

Caida de mollera, 133
Campaigning, policy development and, 74
Canada
    health care system, 31
        access and coverage, 49, 52
        autonomy, 48, 49, 51–52
        costs, 47, 51
        decision making in, 46, 51
        funding, 47, 51
        outcomes, 49–50
        satisfaction, 50, 52
    health promotion in, 28
    nursing education in, 26
    school nursing in, 23
Canadian National Association of Trained
    Nurses, Public Health Section, 31
Canadian Red Cross Society, 26
Cancer, 791
    as a chronic physical health problem,
        685–86, 687, 688, 689, 690, 693, 694,
        699
    communicable diseases and, 664
    gay, bisexual, and transgender men and,
        424
    international mortality, 55
    lesbian, bisexual, and transgender women
        and, 399
    men and, 415–16, 431, 432, 433
    occupational health and, 565–66
    older clients and, 447
    substance abuse and, 735, 739
    women and, 390
Cannabis, 733, 734
Capitation
    approaches to, 84–85
Cardiovascular disorders/diseases. *See* Heart
        disease
CARE, 53
Care of the dying, home visiting and, 504
Care of the sick, home visiting and, 504
Care map, case management and, 260
Caregiver/caregiving/caretaker/caretaking
    burden and, 703–4
    client-oriented community health nursing
        role as, 178
    men's health and, 420
    mental health problems and, 712
    women's health and, 393
Carpal tunnel syndrome, occupational health
        and, 565
Case-control studies, 217
Case fatality rates, 214, 664
Case finder
    population-oriented community health
        nursing role as, 184
Case finding
    definition, 184
    home visiting and, 503
Case management
    cost-effective care and, 95
    criteria for case selection in, 255–57
    definition, 252

ethical issues in, 254–55
goals of, 254
impetus for, 252–53
legal issues in, 254–55
models for, 253–54
plan, developing, 260–61
process, 266
standards for, 254
Case Management Society of America, 252,
    254
Case manager
    as client-oriented community health nurs-
        ing role, 182
Categorically needy, 92
Catholic Relief Services, 53
Causality/Causation, disease
    criteria for, 211–12
    cultural theories of, 115
    definition, 210
    historical theories of, 210–11
    sufficient-component models of, 210–11
Center for Emergency Preparedness and
        Response, 56
Center for Mental Health Services, 44
Center for Substance Abuse Prevention
        (CSAP), 44
Center for Substance Abuse Treatment
        (CSAT), 44
Centers for Disease Control and Prevention
        (CDC), 43–44
    recommendations for physical activity in
        young people, 552
Centralization/decentralization
    international health system comparisons,
        46–47, 51
    locus of decision making and, 46–47, 51
Cerebrovascular disorders/diseases, 792
    as chronic physical health problem, 690
    men's health and, 430
Chadwick, Edwin, 18, 30
Chain of infection, 661
CHAMPUS/TRICARE. *See* Civilian Health
        and Medical Program of the
        Uniformed Services
Change, 270–76
    activities leading to, 274
    approaches to, 273–74
    conflict resolution in, 284
    decision making in, 283
    driving forces in, 271
    evaluating, 276
    field theory and, 270–71
    goals and objectives for, 273
    implementing, stages in, 275–76
    organizational capacity for, 272
    planning for, 272–75
    process of, 270–76
    resistance to, 275–76
    restraining forces in, 271
    stages of personal, 270, 271
    stage theory of, 271
    theories of, 270–71
Change agent
    as population-oriented community health
        nursing role, 185
    community health nurse as, 276
    definition, 185
Change process, components of, 277
Charms, use of protective, 120
Chemical and gaseous health hazards, 155–58

Chemoprophylaxis, communicable diseases
        and, 672–73
Cheyenne, death practices of, 128
Chickenpox. *See* Varicella
Child care, health effects of, 370–71
Child health
    assessing, 358–73
    behavioral considerations in, 369–71
    biophysical considerations in, 358–62
    child care and, 370–71, 378
    dental care and, 378–79
    evaluating care for, 382–83
    exposure to hazardous substances and, 371
    health system considerations and, 371–73
    immunization and, 362, 378
    implementing care for, 382
    minor illness care and, 380
    nutrition in, 369, 374–76
    parenting support for, 379
    physical environmental considerations in,
        366–68
    planning care for, 373–82
    primary prevention in, 374–79
    promoting growth and development in,
        374
    promoting safety in, 376–78
    psychological considerations in, 362–66
    respite care and, 381
    rest and exercise in, 369–70
    screening and, 380
    secondary prevention in, 380–81
    sociocultural considerations in, 368–69
    tertiary prevention in, 381–82
    treatment regimens and, 380
Child Health Act of 1967, 28, 32
Childrearing
    discipline and, 304
Children
    abuse of, 358
    as aggregate, 353–84
    asthma and, 356
    attention deficit hyperactivity disorder in,
        358
    autism and, 356
    congenital anomalies and, 355
    developmental disorders and, 356
    diabetes and, 356
    fetal alcohol and drug exposure in, 357–58
    fetal alcohol syndrome in, 357
    handicapping and chronic conditions in,
        356–57
    health problems of, 354–58
    HIV/AIDS in, 355
    infant mortality and, 354
    learning disability and, 356
    low birth weight and, 354–55
    nursing interventions for common health
        problems in, 777–79
    physical environmental considerations in,
        366–68
    safety, 366–68
    school performance and, 371
    unintentional injury in, 355–56
Children's Health Insurance Program,
        (CHIP), 93
Chinese population
    culture and, 108, 121, 128, 129, 131
    filial piety and, 108–9
    healers, 132

Guide to Special Features

HIGHLIGHTS

CASE STUDIES